KV-213-024

Orthopaedic
Rehabilitation
Second Edition

14/00
mm 496
35.00

CHICHESTER HEALTH LIBRARIES
DUNHILL LIBRARY
ST RICHARD'S HOSPITAL
CHICHESTER
WEST SUSSEX
PO19 4SE

This book is to be returned on or before
the last date stamped below.

23.	17 FEB 1999	
27. JAN	-7 JAN 2000	
JUL	1 5 OCT 2003	
	- 6 DEC 2004	
	1 7 SEP 2007	
	- 5 JAN 2009	
	3 0 MAR 2009	
30.	1 3 OCT 2010	

Chichester Health Libraries
COPY NUMBER   9601098

Orthopaedic Rehabilitation
Second Edition

Edited by

Vernon L. Nickel, M.D.

Professor Emeritus
Department of Orthopaedic Surgery
University of California, San Diego, School of Medicine
La Jolla, California
Former Director
Department of Rehabilitation
Donald N. Sharp Memorial Community Hospital
San Diego, California
Former Medical Director and Chief
Surgical Services
Rancho Los Amigos Medical Center
Downey, California

Michael J. Botte, M.D.

Assistant Professor
Department of Orthopaedics
University of California, San Diego, School of Medicine
Chief
Section of Hand and Foot Surgery
Department of Orthopaedics
University of California, San Diego, Medical Center
Chief
Rehabilitation Medicine
Veterans Administration Hospital
La Jolla, California

Churchill Livingstone
New York, Edinburgh, London, Melbourne, Tokyo

Library of Congress Cataloging-in-Publication Data

Orthopaedic rehabilitation / edited by Vernon L. Nickel, Michael J.
    Botte. — 2nd ed.
        p. cm.
    Rev. ed. of: Orthopedic rehabilitation. 1982.
    Includes bibliographical references and index.
    ISBN 0-443-08726-1
    1. Physically handicapped—Rehabilitation.   I. Nickel, Vernon L.
II. Botte, Michael J. III. Orthopedic rehabilitation.
    [DNLM: 1. Orthopedics. 2. Rehabilitation.   WE 168 0763]
RD797.077 1992
617.3—dc20
DNLM/DLC
for Library of Congress   91-46101
                                                              CIP

Second Edition © Churchill Livingstone Inc. 1992
First Edition © Churchill Livingstone Inc. 1982

All rights reserved. No part of this publication may be reproduced, stored in a retrieval system,
or transmitted in any form or by any means, electronic, mechanical, photocopying, recording,
or otherwise, without prior permission of the publisher (Churchill Livingstone Inc., 650
Avenue of the Americas, New York, NY 10011).

Distributed in the United Kingdom by Churchill Livingstone, Robert Stevenson House, 1–3
Baxter's Place, Leith Walk, Edinburgh EH1 3AF, and by associated companies, branches, and
representatives throughout the world.

Accurate indications, adverse reactions, and dosage schedules for drugs are provided in this
book, but it is possible that they may change. The reader is urged to review the package information data of the manufacturers of the medications mentioned.

The Publishers have made every effort to trace the copyright holders for borrowed material. If
they have inadvertently overlooked any, they will be pleased to make the necessary arrangements at the first opportunity.

Acquisitions Editor: *Robert Hurley*
Copy Editor: *David Terry*
Production Designer: *Jill Little*
Production Supervisor: *Sharon Tuder*
Production services provided by Bermedica Production, Ltd.
Cover design by Paul Moran

Printed in the United States of America

First published in 1992   7 6 5 4 3 2 1

To Anna,
who married me over fifty years ago.
V.L.N.

To my mother, Verona L. Minning-Botte, M.D.,
and my father, Joseph M. Botte, M.D.,
for all their love and support through all the years.
M.J.B.

We would like to thank
Carlene K. Wright and Susan Gonda
for their high level of professional skill and dedication to this book.

A very special thanks
to our editorial assistant, Catherine F. Fix,
for her diligent review and diplomatic critical assessment
of all the chapters.
Vernon L. Nickel, M.D.
Michael J. Botte, M.D.

Contributors

Jean–Jacques Abitbol, M.D.
Assistant Professor, Department of Orthopaedics, University of California, San Diego, School of Medicine, La Jolla, California

Reid Abrams, M.D.
Assistant Professor, Department of Orthopaedics, University of California, San Diego, School of Medicine, La Jolla, California

Wayne H. Akeson, M.D.
Professor and Chairman, Department of Orthopaedics, University of California, San Diego, School of Medicine, La Jolla, California

I.J. Alexander, M.D.
Assistant Professor, Division of Orthopedic Surgery, Department of Surgery, Northeastern Ohio Universities College of Medicine, Rootstown, Ohio; Active Staff Member, Crystal Clinic, Akron, Ohio

A. Amendola, M.D., F.R.C.S.(C)
Assistant Professor, Division of Orthopaedic Surgery, Department of Surgery, University of Western Ontario Faculty of Medicine, London, Ontario, Canada

David Amiel, Dip. Ing.
Associate Adjunct Professor, Department of Orthopaedics, University of California, San Diego, School of Medicine, La Jolla, California

David F. Apple, Jr., M.D.
Associate Clinical Professor, Division of Orthopaedic Surgery, Department of Orthopaedics, and Clinical Assistant Professor, Department of Rehabilitation Medicine, Emory University School of Medicine, Atlanta, Georgia

Steven Becker, M.D.
Assistant Clinical Professor, Division of Orthopedics, Department of Surgery, University of California, Irvine, College of Medicine, Irvine, California

Matthew Berchuck, M.D.
Assistant Professor, Department of Orthopaedics, University of California, San Diego, School of Medicine, La Jolla, California

Katherine S. Black, M.S., P.T.
Director, Department of Clinical Services, Donald N. Sharp Memorial Community Hospital, San Diego, California

Sue C. Bodine-Fowler, Ph.D.
Assistant Professor, Department of Orthopaedics, University of California, San Diego, School of Medicine, La Jolla, California

Michael J. Botte, M.D.
Assistant Professor, Department of Orthopaedics, University of California, San Diego, School of Medicine; Chief, Section of Hand and Foot Surgery, Department of Orthopaedics, University of California, San Diego, Medical Center; Chief, Rehabilitation Medicine, Veterans Administration Hospital, La Jolla, California

Richard M. Braun, M.D.
Associate Clinical Professor, Department of Orthopaedics, University of California, San Diego, School of Medicine, La Jolla, California; Instructor, Department of Orthopaedic Surgery, University of Southern California School of Medicine, Los Angeles, California; Consultant in Upper Extremity Surgery, Department of Surgery, Rancho Los Amigos Medical Center, Downey, California

Ruth Cox Brunings, M.S.W.
Director of Social Work, Rancho Los Amigos Medical Center, Downey, California

Robert T. Burks, M.D.
Assistant Professor, Division of Orthopedic Surgery, Department of Surgery, and Director, Sports Medicine, University of Utah School of Medicine, Salt Lake City, Utah

Thomas P. Byrne, O.T.C., O.P.A.C.
Senior Orthopaedic Technician, Department of Orthopaedics, University of California, San Diego, Medical Center, La Jolla, California

Douglas Cairns, Ph.D.
Head Clinical Psychologist, Department of Psychology, Rancho Los Amigos Medical Center, Downey, California

Kevin E. Calvo, C.P.
Clinical Prosthetist, Bionics, Orthotics and Prosthetics, Inc., San Diego, California; Consultant, Department of Orthotics and the Prosthetics Clinic, University of California, San Diego, Medical Center, La Jolla, California; Consultant, Department of Rehabilitation Medicine, Veterans Administration Hospital, La Jolla, California; Consultant, Scripps Memorial Hospital, La Jolla, California; Consultant, Children's Hospital and Health Center, San Diego, California

Mary Kay Campbell, P.T.
Private practice, San Diego, California

Daniel A. Capen, M.D.
Associate Clinical Professor, Department of Orthopaedic Surgery, University of Southern California School of Medicine, Los Angeles, California; Chief, Spinal Injury Service, Rancho Los Amigos Medical Center, Downey, California

Mark S. Cohen, M.D.
Resident, Department of Orthopaedics, University of California, San Diego, Medical Center, La Jolla, California

F. Richard Convery, M.D.
Professor, Department of Orthopaedics, University of California, San Diego, School of Medicine, La Jolla, California

Martha Minteer Convery, M.D.
Clinical Professor, Department of Orthopaedics, University of California, San Diego, School of Medicine, La Jolla, California

William P. Cooney III, M.D.
Professor, Division of Hand Surgery, Department of Orthopedic Surgery, Mayo Medical School; Head, Section of Hand Surgery, Mayo Clinic, Rochester, Minnesota

Richard D. Coutts, M.D.
Adjunct Professor, Department of Orthopaedics, University of California, San Diego, School of Medicine, La Jolla, California; Chief, Department of Orthopaedics, Donald N. Sharp Memorial Community Hospital, San Diego, California

Margaret Cullen, O.T.R.
Senior Occupational Therapist, Hand Rehabilitation Center, University of California, San Diego, Medical Center, La Jolla, California

Sylvia Davila, L.P.T., C.H.T.
Clinical Instructor, Department of Physical Therapy, University of Texas Medical School at San Antonio; Director, Hand Rehabilitation Associates of San Antonio, Inc., San Antonio, Texas

Shelli L. Dellinger, O.T.R., C.H.T.
Senior Hand Therapist, Hand Rehabilitation Center, University of California, San Diego, Medical Center, La Jolla, California

Mary Patricia Dimick, O.T.R., C.H.T.
Director, Therapy Programs, University of California, San Diego, Medical Center, La Jolla, California

Cindy Dowdy, O.T.R., C.V.E.
Supervisor, Work Evaluation Center, University of California, San Diego, Medical Center, La Jolla, California

Bruce Foerster, M.D.
Private practitioner in orthopaedic surgery, St. Albans, Vermont

Harold J. Forney, M.D.
Associate Clinical Professor, Department of Orthopaedics, University of California, San Diego, School of Medicine; Chief, Amputation Service, Veterans Administration Hospital, La Jolla, California; Director, Limb Defect Clinic, Children's Hospital and Health Center, San Diego, California

Steven R. Garfin, M.D.
Professor, Department of Orthopaedics, University of California, San Diego, School of Medicine, La Jolla, California

Douglas E. Garland, M.D.
Clinical Professor, Department of Orthopaedics, University of Southern California School of Medicine, Los Angeles, California; Chief, Neurotrauma Service, Department of Surgery, Rancho Los Amigos Medical Center, Downey, California

Richard H. Gelberman, M.D.
Professor, Department of Orthopedic Surgery, Harvard Medical School; Chief, Division of Hand and Upper Extremity Service, Department of Orthopaedic Surgery, Massachusetts General Hospital, Boston, Massachusetts

Harris Gellman, M.D.
Associate Clinical Professor, Department of Orthopaedics, University of Southern California School of Medicine, Los Angeles, California; Director, Spinal Injury/Upper Extremity Clinic, Rancho Los Amigos Medical Center, Downey, California

Irene S. Gilgoff, M.D.
Clinical Associate Professor, Department of Pediatrics, University of Southern California School of Medicine, Los Angeles, California; Attending Pediatrician, Department of Pediatrics, and Co-Director, Muscular Dystrophy Association of America Clinic, Rancho Los Amigos Medical Center, Downey, California

Mary Lou Harris, M.S., C.R.C.
Associate Professor, Part-time Faculty, Department of Administration, Rehabilitation, and Postsecondary Education, School of Education, San Diego State University; President, WorkAble Solutions, Etc., San Diego, California

M. Mark Hoffer, M.D.
Professor and Chief, Division of Orthopedic Surgery, Department of Surgery, University of California, Irvine, College of Medicine, Irvine, California

Peggy Hollingsworth-Fridlund, R.N.
Truma Nurse Coordinator, Division of Trauma, University of California, San Diego, Medical Center, San Diego, California

Robert N. Hotchkiss, M.D.
Assistant Professor, Division of Orthopedics, Department of Surgery, Cornell University Medical College; Chief, Hand Service, The Hospital for Special Surgery, New York, New York

David B. Hoyt, M.D., F.A.C.S.
Associate Professor, Division of Trauma, Department of Surgery, University of California, San Diego, School of Medicine; Chief, Division of Trauma, and Director, Surgical Intensive Care Unit, Department of Surgery, University of California, San Diego, Medical Center, La Jolla, California

John D. Hsu, M.D., C.M., F.A.C.S.
Clinical Professor, Department of Orthopaedics, University of Southern California School of Medicine, Los Angeles, California; Chairman, Department of Surgery, Chief, Department of Orthopaedics, and Co-Director, Muscular Dystrophy Association of America Clinic, Rancho Los Amigos Medical Center, Downey, California

Christopher Jobe, M.D.
Assistant Professor, Department of Orthopedic Surgery, Loma Linda University School of Medicine, Loma Linda, California

Frank W. Jobe, M.D.
Clinical Professor, Department of Orthopaedics, University of Southern California School of Medicine, Los Angeles, California

Christopher Jordan, M.D.
Chief, Stroke Service, Rancho Los Amigos Medical Center, Downey, California

Carol K. Kasper, M.D.
Professor, Division of Hematology, Department of Medicine, University of Southern California School of Medicine; Director, Hemophilia Center, Orthopaedic Hospital, Los Angeles, California

Kenton R. Kaufman, Ph.D.
Director of Orthopedic Research, Motion Analysis Laboratory, Children's Hospital and Health Center, San Diego, California

Mary Ann E. Keenan, M.D.
Professor, Departments of Orthopedic Surgery and Physical Medicine and Rehabilitation, Temple University School of Medicine; Chairman, Department of Orthopaedic Surgery, Albert Einstein Medical Center, Philadelphia, Pennsylvania

Ann Koeneke-Varley, M.S., C.C.C.
Programs Manager, Donald N. Sharp Memorial Community Hospital, San Diego, California

Martin Koffman, M.D.
Assistant Clinical Professor, Department of Orthopaedics, University of Southern California School of Medicine, Los Angeles, California

Kenneth P. Kozole, B.S.M.E., O.T.R.
Lead Rehabilitation Engineer, Rehabilitation Technology Service, Donald N. Sharp Memorial Community Hospital, San Diego, California

Joy N. Langworthy, O.T.R.L., C.H.T.
Certified Hand Therapist, The Wrist and Hand Center of Tampa, Tampa, Florida

Richard L. Lieber, Ph.D.
Associate Professor, Department of Orthopaedics, Biomedical Sciences Graduate Program, University of California, San Diego, School of Medicine, La Jolla, California; Principal Investigator, Skeletal Muscle Physiology Laboratory, Department of Orthopaedics, Veterans Administration Medical Center, La Jolla, California

Charles E. Lowrey, M.D.
Fellow in Joint Reconstruction, Department of Orthopaedics, University of California, San Diego, School of Medicine, La Jolla, California

James V. Luck, Jr., M.D.
Clinical Professor, Department of Orthopaedics, University of Southern California School of Medicine; President and Medical Director, Orthopaedic Hospital, Los Angeles, California

Carol McGough, M.S., O.T.R.L.
Former Director, Department of Occupational Therapy, Braintree Hospital, Braintree, Massachusetts

John W. Michael, M.Ed., C.P.O.
Director and Assistant Clinical Professor, Department of Prosthetics and Orthotics, Duke University School of Medicine, Durham, North Carolina

Vert Mooney, M.D.
Professor, Division of Orthopaedic Surgery, Department of Orthopaedics, University of California, San Diego, School of Medicine, La Jolla, California

Mark S. Myerson, M.D.
Director, Foot and Ankle Services, Union Memorial Hospital; Assistant Professor, Department of Orthopedic Surgery, The Johns Hopkins University School of Medicine, Baltimore, Maryland

Vernon L. Nickel, M.D.
Professor Emeritus, Department of Orthopaedic Surgery, University of California, San Diego, School of Medicine, La Jolla, California; Former Director, Department of Rehabilitation, Donald N. Sharp Memorial Community Hospital, San Diego, California; Former Medical Director and Chief, Surgical Services, Rancho Los Amigos Medical Center, Downey, California

Meenal Patel, M.D.
Voluntary Staff, Department of Anesthesiology, University of Southern California School of Medicine, Los Angeles, California; Physician Specialist Anesthesiologist, Department of Anesthesiology, Rancho Los Amigos Medical Center, Downey, California

Jacquelin Perry, M.D.
Professor, Department of Orthopaedics, University of Southern California School of Medicine, Los Angeles, California; Chief, Pathokinesiology Service, Rancho Los Amigos Medical Center, Downey, California

Marilyn Pink, M.S., P.T.
Director, Department of Biomechanics, Centinela Hospital, Inglewood, California

John M. Rayhack, M.D.
Associate Professor, Department of Orthopedic Surgery, University of South Florida College of Medicine, Tampa, Florida

Steven P. Ringel, M.D.
Professor, Department of Neurology, University of Colorado School of Medicine, Denver, Colorado

Joanne Sandberg-Cook, R.N.C., M.S., C.C.R.N.
Nurse-Practitioner, Department of Rheumatology, Braintree Hospital, Braintree, Massachusetts

Richard F. Santore, M.D.
Associate Clinical Professor, Department of Orthopaedics, University of California, San Diego, School of Medicine, La Jolla, California; Senior Partner and Chief Financial Officer, Orthopedic Medical Group, San Diego, California

Ann H. Schutt, M.D.
Associate Professor, Department of Physical Medicine and Rehabilitation, Mayo Medical School; Consultant, Department of Physical Medicine and Rehabilitation, Mayo Clinic, Rochester, Minnesota

Stephen C. Shoemaker, M.D.
Clinical Instructor, Department of Orthopaedic Surgery, University of California, San Diego, School of Medicine, La Jolla, California; Attending Orthopaedic Surgeon, Department of Surgery, Scripps Institute for Medicine and Science, San Diego, California; Private practitioner, San Dieguito Orthopaedic Medical Group, Encinitas, California

Thomas C. Simmons, P.T., A.T.C.
Director, Scripps Memorial North County Sports Rehabilitation Center, Encinitas, California

David B. Simon, M.D.
Clinical Instructor, Department of Neurosciences, University of California, San Diego, School of Medicine; Chief, Department of Neurology, Sharp Cabrillo Hospital, San Diego, California

Michael J. Skyhar, M.D.
Clinical Instructor, Department of Orthopaedic Surgery, University of California, San Diego, School of Medicine, La Jolla, California; Attending Orthopaedic Surgeon, Department of Surgery, Scripps Institute for Medicine and Science, San Diego, California; Private practitioner, San Dieguito Orthopaedic Medical Group, Encinitas, California

Kim L. Stearns, M.D.
Fellow in Adult Reconstructive Surgery, Orthopedic Medical Group, San Diego, California

Claire M. Stiles, M.D.
Former Chief, Department of Anesthesiology, Rancho Los Amigos Medical Center, Downey, California

David H. Sutherland, M.D.
Professor Emeritus, Department of Orthopaedics, University of California, San Diego, School of Medicine, La Jolla, California; Medical Director, Department of Pediatric Orthopedics, Children's Hospital and Health Center, San Diego, California

Jeffery Sutherland, M.D.
Chief, Department of Orthopedic Surgery, Children's Hospital and Health Center, San Diego, California

Robert M. Szabo, M.D.
Associate Professor, Department of Orthopaedic Surgery, University of California, Davis, School of Medicine, Davis, California; Chief, Hand and Upper Extremity Service, University of California, Davis, Medical Center, Sacramento, California

Sara Wells–Rawson, O.T.R.
Former Supervisor, Department of Occupational Therapy Children's Hospital and Health Center, San Diego, California

Dennis R. Wenger, M.D.
Associate Clinical Professor, Department of Orthopaedics, University of California, San Diego, School of Medicine, La Jolla, California; Director, Department of Pediatric Orthopedics, Children's Hospital and Health Center, San Diego, California

Honora K. Wilson, M.S.W.
Social Work Consultant, Rancho Los Amigos Medical Center, Downey, California

Serena Young, M.D.
Associate Clinical Professor, Division of Orthopedic Surgery, Department of Surgery, University of California, Irvine, College of Medicine; Assistant Orthopedic Chief, Adult Brain Injury Service, Rancho Los Amigos Medical Center, Downey, California; Orthopedic Staff Member, Special Team for Amputations, Mobility and Prosthetics (STAMP Program), Veterans Administration Hospital, Long Beach, California

Jack E. Zigler, M.D.
Clinical Professor, Department of Orthopaedics, University of Southern California School of Medicine, Los Angeles, California; Chief, Spinal Injury Service, Rancho Los Amigos Medical Center, Downey, California

Ephraim M. Zinberg, M.D.
Private practitioner in hand and microvascular surgery, Boca Raton, Florida

Foreword

Rehabilitation is a therapeutic program designed to minimize the consequences of a permanent or protracted disability. It stands in sharp contrast to standard medical care, which concentrates on curing the patient's pathologic process and rests on the assumption that function will be recovered spontaneously. Consequently, failure to cure is considered an unfortunate consequence of an imperfect system, an event to be tabulated as a statistical reminder of improvement needed. The patient is left alone to cope with the residuals.

The basic difference between curative and rehabilitative medicine lies in the direction of effort. The focus of curative medicine is on reversing the primary disease process; every procedure is directed that way. Rehabilitation concentrates on restoring function; emphasis is placed on preventing contractures, developing muscle strength, stimulating latent control, training the patient to use residual function in an effective manner, providing assistive devices, and guiding patient and family in accommodating to an altered way of life.

Rehabilitation is a therapeutic program that works most effectively when integrated with the curative process. Attention to pathology and attention to function are then exercised simultaneously, and the debilitating consequences of uninterrupted bed rest are avoided. The therapeutic continuum gradually shifts from an emphasis on control of pathologic processes to one of restoration of function.

By necessity, rehabilitation is a multidisciplinary program. There must be an appropriate blend of physical therapy, occupational therapy, communication therapy, medical social work, psychology, vocational counseling, prosthetics, orthotics, recreational therapy, rehabilitation-focused nursing, medicine, and reconstructive surgery.

Thus, for a person with a catastrophic disability, normal function is not possible, but effective performance and reentry into active society may often be achieved if all the measures influencing a patient's capacity to function are provided.

Jacquelin Perry, M.D.
Professor
Department of Orthopaedics
University of Southern California
School of Medicine
Los Angeles, California
Chief
Pathokinesiology Service
Rancho Los Amigos Medical Center
Downey, California

Preface

This new edition of *Orthopaedic Rehabilitation* offers comprehensive coverage of the major areas of rehabilitation in chronic neuromuscular skeletal afflictions. The book has been expanded with over twenty new chapters and twelve useful appendices. In addition to coverage of the basic science of rehabilitation, new chapters now provide in-depth discussion of rehabilitation according to specific anatomic region. Our aim is to provide a comprehensive text that is useful as a general reference in most rehabilitation institutes, as well as a primary textbook for orthopaedic residents and general orthopaedic surgeons. The scope of the book will appeal to various members of the rehabilitation team including allied health professionals (nurses, physical therapists, occupational therapists, speech therapists, orthopaedic residents in training, and general orthopaedic surgeons) as well as internists, anesthesiologists, and neurologists. The book serves as a useful reference for any of the other health professionals involved in the rehabilitation process, such as other physicians, primary care specialists, physiatrists, and general surgeons.

The book includes five sections: I. The Rehabilitation Team, covering rehabilitation, nursing, physical therapy, occupational therapy, and other topics; II. Rehabilitation Facilities, with discussion of the general rehabilitation center, the hand rehabilitation center, the spinal cord injury center, motion analysis, and injured worker programs; III. Basic Science Aspects of Rehabilitation, with coverage of neuromuscular physiology including function and plasticity, the biological basis of musculoskeletal rehabilitation, the deleterious effects of mobilization, and muscle spasticity; IV. Generalized Disorders, including cerebral palsy, stroke, traumatic brain injury, spinal cord injury, poliomyelitis, muscular dystrophy, and other subjects; and V. Rehabilitation According to Anatomic Region, with chapters on the hand, wrist, elbow, shoulder, spine, hip, knee, ankle, and foot. In addition, there is a comprehensive series of appendices on assorted topics, including various aspects of musculoskeletal anatomy, the terminology of orthopaedic surgery and rehabilitation including terms of position, direction, and movement, normal ranges of motion, coma scales, and others.

Vernon L. Nickel, M.D.
Michael J. Botte, M.D.

Contents

SECTION III: BASIC SCIENCE ASPECTS OF REHABILITATION

SECTION IV: GENERALIZED DISORDERS

Section I

THE REHABILITATION TEAM

1 General Principles of Orthopaedic Rehabilitation

VERNON L. NICKEL

Two principles are fundamental to the planning of a rehabilitation program. First, the sequelae of the original insult, whether it was trauma or disease, must be minimized as much as possible. Second, all preventable complications should be forestalled, but if they do happen, they should be dealt with aggressively. When these basic rules are strongly enforced, the application of good rehabilitation techniques will most likely obtain the maximal effect in the shortest time at the lowest cost.

A good illustration of the first concept involves the treatment of the patient with spinal cord injury. The spine must be reduced and maintained in a stable position at the earliest possible moment to allow for optimal recovery and forestall additional neurologic loss. Some devastating complications that can and should be prevented are bladder infections, decubitus ulcers, contractural deformities, and muscle atrophy from disuse. These medical problems, combined with the severe psychosocial deficits that many patients will develop under the circumstances, can impede or halt the rehabilitation process.

ORGANIZATION OF THE REHABILITATION SERVICE

The concept of an approach to chronic disease by categories was applied with great success in the treatment of respiratory poliomyelitis.[1,2] It is our firm conviction that this approach is far more effective in the rehabilitation setting than grouping patients together regardless of diagnosis. This trend, which began after World War II, is referred to as comprehensive rehabilitation. Whenever the size of the service and the availability of personnel permit, patients should be grouped according to disease category. Grouping by the physician's medical specialty, which is customary in acute-care hospitals, does not apply to rehabilitation. The organization of this book is based on that belief.

An important component in any rehabilitation service is the need to provide high-quality medical care and discipline. Excellence can and must be the expectation in the chronic as well as the acute-care hospital setting. The centers for respiratory poliomyelitis established in the early 1950s by the National Foundation for Infantile Paralysis,[3] in which the disease was managed as a category and patients were treated by physicians of different specialties, are excellent examples of how standards of excellence were sought and achieved. More recently, many spinal cord injury centers are following their example.[4]

DIRECTION

Confusion over the proper procedure for directing a rehabilitation service is a major impediment to its effective organization. Physicians in the acute-care setting are accustomed to prescribing medications and ordering precise therapeutic programs for their patients. They expect nurses and other health professionals to follow those directions exactly. In the rehabilitation environment, this model of care is not workable. It may, in fact, be a barrier to the development of a good program. The rehabilitation patient has direct contact with the physician and a variety of health professionals, each of whom is expert in dealing with the patient's problems. What these professionals need is general direction and supervision, in many ways like the activities of the coach of a professional football team, who coordinates and acts as a catalyst for the team yet leaves the details of execution to subordinate specialists.

The term *prescription* is a misnomer for the directions given to allied health professionals by physicians, because it is impossible to detail all the procedures to be followed. These are designed by the experienced therapist, who is accustomed to exercise professional judgment in such matters. This may be difficult for some professionals to accept, but a prescription cannot and should not be attempted. Unfortunately, some physicians still write fairly detailed directions (commonly called "prescriptions") in the rehabilitation setting. Allied health professionals usually ignore these directions, chiefly because they may be impractical and often impossible to carry out. It is much more pertinent for the physician to give general directions and leave the details to other trained health professionals.

However, this does not mean that medications need not be ordered with precision. In this respect, the nurse on the rehabilitation service should be encouraged to exercise more independent judgment than is usually the case in the acute medical-surgical ward.

Physicians and administrators who are somewhat doubtful about the idea of extensive delegation of responsibility might be reminded of coronary care units, in which nurses specializing in heart problems have taken over a number of functions previously considered the domain of the physician. If responsibility can be delegated to specifically trained nurses when life itself is at risk, physicians should surely be willing to give authority to competent health professionals in chronic disease situations of less immediate threat to life and limb.

By letting others have a share in making decisions, physicians can then use their time more efficiently and direct the care for a large number of patients.[5] This does not mean that the physician abdicates responsibility. The ability of the rehabilitation team to turn to strong leadership and have prompt, ready access to expert medical guidance is central to the concept of delegation.

TIMING

It is difficult to determine when an active rehabilitation program should begin, but the general rule is the earlier the better. Rehabilitation is not a separate process occurring when an inpatient or outpatient is transferred from an acute-care hospital, a physicians's office, or the home to a rehabilitation center. Astute physicians and their colleagues in the allied health professions understand that, for patients requiring rehabilitation, the conventional progress of healing to an eventual cure is not likely to happen, and that the patient will need a formal, organized program. As soon as this is recognized, planning and treatment should be aimed at lessening the consequences of major and permanent loss of function. The loss will not be only physical; the patient may well sustain mental and emotional problems.

PATIENT SELECTION

The extent and complexity of a rehabilitation program will depend on many factors. For example, one patient may have backache because a large ruptured disc produces severe symptoms and disability. When the disc is removed surgically, the patient recovers and returns to his usual occupation in a relatively short time. In contrast, another patient may exhibit a similar problem but have significant neurologic sequelae. The patient has considerable permanent loss of function, with the added problems of depression and a lack of confidence. The first patient needs little or no rehabilitation, whereas the second would benefit greatly from a well-structured, intensive rehabilitation program staffed by allied health professionals specially instructed in rehabilitating patients with spinal complaints. Without access to such an effective program, the second patient might suffer marked impairment in ambulating (which could have been corrected by proper bracing), chronic renal disability from continued catheterization, and other preventable problems, such as loss of motivation or the breaking up of family relationships.

Another example is the elderly person with Parkinson's disease who falls, fractures a hip, and undergoes total hip replacement. This patient is much more likely to resume ambulation in a rehabilitation setting than in the usual medical-surgical ward. A younger person with a fractured hip and no neurologic problems would not require transfer to a rehabilitation setting under normal conditions. Stroke victims should be considered rehabilitation candidates as soon as their medical condition stabilizes and they have the potential to resume some form of activity. A patient with spinal cord injury and severe neurologic loss will always require an intensive rehabilitation program.

The rehabilitation effort is costly and the process is lengthy, because the problems involved are not straightforward or simple. They require many different kinds of professional personnel to deal with them. The expense is fully justified, however, because every dollar spent in rehabilitating patients with chronic conditions results in manifold dollar savings when these patients eventually return to society.[6]

More awareness of the relatedness of rehabilitation to the spectrum of acute care is needed among orthopaedists, neurologists, and other physicians so that they might recognize more quickly the kind of patient who requires rehabilitation. The physician who has seen the patient from the beginning of the initial injury or illness is the appropriate one to continue treatment when it is clear that a rehabilitation program is needed. This physician has paid careful attention to preserving the patient's life and to immediate physical well-being and has also been alert to the barriers that commonly impede or detract from a rehabilitation program. A doctor who has a positive attitude toward preventing complications and who points out the potential remaining to the patient is making a realistic assessment of both the disability and the potential for rehabilitation. The allied health specialists also contribute to this assessment, and

their involvement is essential in planning the program.

THE SCOPE OF REHABILITATION

The scope of rehabilitation has not been clearly demarcated and is still undergoing rapid change. Previously hospitalization was intrinsic to rehabilitation, but the current emphasis is increasingly on outpatient care. The team effort that has worked so well in hospitals can function equally well in an outpatient setting so long as the organizational structure is suitable.

For many years, too, rehabilitation focused chiefly on children. Orthopaedists devoted themselves to such conditions as poliomyelitis, clubfoot, dislocated hips, and cerebral palsy. In the era when it was customary for these children to spend long periods of time in hospitals, the Shriners' hospitals for disabled children provided excellent care.[7] Today, because of improved surgical procedures, extended periods of hospitalization are seldom indicated. Rehabilitation professionals now try to see that children spend only a short time away from their homes. Modern rehabilitation efforts, of course, extend to adults crippled by a whole range of disorders.

The modern approach to rehabilitation was greatly stimulated by World War II because of the numbers of war-wounded amputees. Rehabilitation was done largely on an outpatient basis, except for surgical procedures; amputation clinics became an example to emulate as a model of the "categories" approach to a disease process. Amputation centers at that time were concentrated in Veterans Administration hospitals.[8] The outstanding level reached during the 1950s is reflected in the fact that the post of clinic chief of the amputation rehabilitation service was considered a high honor and an important professional achievement. It is unfortunate that the interest and the activity on behalf of amputees have dissipated and that the quality of amputee care has deteriorated accordingly.

Poliomyelitis is probably the disease that has been treated with the most success from the rehabilitation standpoint. It is fair to state that for a few years before the development of vaccines, almost every patient with poliomyelitis received adequate care. This changed to some degree with the advent of respiratory poliomyelitis because of the complex nature of the problem, but after the organization of special centers in this area, excellent rehabilitative care was given to these patients.[9]

This is not true for many other disease catergories. Only a small percentage of patients with stroke receive complete care. Similarly, many patients with head injuries are not given the medical treatment they require. Until recently, patients with spinal cord injury were scattered in many different areas of a region, and the cost of care was prohibitive. As centers for spinal care are established across the United States, outcomes are improving and costs are dropping.[10]

GOALS AND LIMITATIONS

Two facets of any treatment plan that must be kept in mind are assistance in making the best return to function or preservation of residual physical abilities, and the greater enhancement of that potential function by proper apparatus, training in substitute skills, and surgical prodedures. Any reasonable means should be used to increase function beyond that which the patient could achieve alone. Operations, strengthening, training, fitting with correct appliances, and auxiliary devices all aid the rehabilitation team in attaining these goals.

The process of defining goals requires a high level of expertise, as well as the combined experience of the entire rehabilitation team. Once the initial effort is made and the goal-setting process is constantly under review, realistic predictions and limitations can be established. Poor goal setting, for example, would be the expectation that an elderly person with an above-knee amputation and marked cardiovascular impairment will ambulate with an above-knee prosthesis. Continuing an extended period of training to reach the goal of ambulation must be avoided. In addition to the economic cost, the patient, family, and staff will suffer inevitable disappointment and frustration in the effort to attain an unachievable goal. Progres-

sively accurate goal setting, with the patient's residual assets kept in mind, is founded on the professional team's level of expertise, the rehabilitation environment, optimal medical care (which includes surgical procedures), and well-designed aids such as prosthetic and orthotic devices.

Goals can gradually be extended with the application of rehabilitation engineering to the severely disabled patient. For instance, high quadriplegics who are unable to propel their own wheelchairs will be able to consider vocational independence as a rational goal once they have properly fitted wheelchairs with adequate seating to control pressure and electrical controls that permit the driving of a van tailored to their needs.

In viewing the totality of the problems of drastically handicapped persons, physicians are subject to many preconceived notions and prejudices. Physicians generally spend most of their time treating conditions in their offices or a hospital for acute care. Reluctance to treat chronically handicapped persons may arise from lack of personal experience in such care and from the disturbing realization that complete recovery is unlikely.[11] The potentially dangerous psychological impediment that must be overcome is that all health professionals have *cure* as their goal. With this mindset, they experience a sense of failure with anything less than a cure. Because many younger orthopaedic surgeons have trained only in acute-care settings, this "cure syndrome" is ever present.

Another psychological hurdle is that our society, including people in the biomedical sciences, considers walking to be the ultimate goal of recovery. Ambulation, however, frequently is overemphasized. Although walking obviously is tremendously important, for many patients with chronic crippling disorders it may not be as essential as having effective use of the hands. It is far more important that the disabled individual be able to take care of personal needs and function socially and vocationally than it is for that person to be able to walk. Patients, relatives, friends, and staff members need to be educated in rational expectations by professionals who themselves have a clear understanding of what constitutes an appreciable functional ability.

TRIAGE

Triage is defined as "the sorting out and classification of casualties of war or other disasters to determine the priority of need and proper place of treatment" (Dorland's Illustrated Medical Dictionary). The term as applied to medical care was reputedly first used at the Battle of Waterloo, when Napoleon's surgeon ordered his medical aides to concentrate their efforts and supplies on the wounded soldiers who would benefit most from them, rather than treating those who were beyond help or others less severely injured and not in immediate need of care.

Triage is vital to a successful rehabilitation program. It must be invoked with firmness when selecting patients with chronic disabling conditions for rehabilitation. Priority of treatment should be weighted toward persons who can make significant gains from the therapy. The steadily increasing numbers of patients who request rehabilitative care make it imperative that leaders of rehabilitation teams exercise some discrimination in selecting candidates for their programs to ensure that the greatest good is accomplished for the greatest number of people.

The total social and medical resources needed to rehabilitate everyone who could conceivably benefit would be enormous. Even if such unlimited resources became available, it would be most inappropriate to devote them to the ongoing care of patients with little potential for functional gains. Costly treatment must be promptly curtailed after it appears that gains are minimal or nonexistent, even when the patients' families apply strong pressure to extend therapy. To preserve a physical system or body part that no longer has any functional menaing is not good medicine, and it is not good rehabilitation. It is, in fact, bad rehabilitation. Just preserving the body is not rehabilitation; life must be worthwhile for the individual.

The decision process of triage is determined by the availability of resources. These consist of the physical plant, the social and economic support for the patient, and the accessibility and expertise of various physicians and allied health professionals. It requires equating the therapeutic potential of maximal effort with the cost, time, and personnel involved in it. Therapeutic potential can be defined as the achieving of a reasonably good functional level on the patient's return to society. This would encompass a person's physical condition, emotional and psychological attitudes, social situation, and vocational possibilities.

Measuring the value of any rehabilitation effort is not simple. One method is based on economics, represented by what disabled persons contribute to society or by the reduction in the cost of care when they gain independence. However, further experience is urgently needed to estimate rehabilitation outcomes more accurately, because many handicapped people with no earning capacity have made important contributions to the arts, sciences, and family management. It is even more difficult to evaluate the joy a happy person can bring to those around him. An unforgettable example is a woman with poliomyelitis who suffered frightful paralysis. She required permanent use of respiratory equipment and had lost the function of her arms and legs. This patient went home to a strongly supportive family and despite her condition assisted her relatives and her community. She had a forceful personality and an active brain. With these assets left to her, she managed her household efficiently.

PREVENTABLE BARRIERS TO SUCCESSFUL REHABILITATION

A patient's rehabilitation is often seriously and sometimes disastrously impeded by complications. Such conditions as decubitus ulcers, bladder infections, contractural deformities, unnecessary muscle atrophy, skeletal deformities, noxious spasticity, psychological regression, and social deterioration will increase the expense and extent of a rehabilitation program. These complications are singularly offensive to knowledgeable rehabilitationists, because they know that with few exceptions such complications could and should be prevented. Prevention is relatively simple and much less costly than treatment. In addition, major complications may not be completely correctable; the residuals that persist add to the patient's already serious loss of function. Typical, avoidable complications are discussed briefly here and in further detail in subsequent chapters.

Decubitus Ulcers

One of the best examples of a preventable condition is decubitus ulcers,[12] which, until recently, were believed to be an inevitable sequel to a condition such as spinal cord injury. Even if a large decubitus ulcer has healed, often with major surgical intervention required, a patient will still be much more susceptible to their recurrence.

Decubitus ulcers are caused by unrelieved pressure, often over an excessive period of time, making the body tissue necrotic. It is not neurologic loss that alters the physiology of the skin and subcutaneous tissue. Factors such as hydration, spasm, protein depletion, rough bedding, moisture, and lack of cleanliness contribute to a patient's propensity for developing these lesions. The optimal solution to the problem is to relieve pressure and avoid as many contributing variables as possible in patients who are at risk.[13]

There are three clinical stages of decubitus ulcer. In the first, the skin is persistently red; this resolves quickly with the relief of pressure. The first stage offers the best opportunity to prevent later stages and their serious consequences. In the second stage, the skin shows bluish discoloration or blistering. These signs mean that some cutaneous necrosis has already occurred. With aggressive treatment the sore may heal, although a longer period of time will be required. In the third and final stage, the skin becomes white (ischemic blanching) or black (actual necrosis), which represents the death of all layers of the skin in varying degrees in the subcutaneous and other underlying tissues. This stage always results in large ulcerations, and when this stage occurs the patient becomes increasingly vulnerable to new sores. Accordingly, it behooves the entire staff—and especially the nurse—to exert great diligence in seeing that no lesion progresses beyond the first stage.

Bladder Infections

The inability to urinate at will is a common problem for patients with a neuromusculoskeletal disorder. The condition of most of these patients has improved with the advent of intermittent catherization. Bladder infection is a grave complication requiring efficient therapy as a preventive or, if neccessary, a curative measure. The consequences of the indiscriminate and unquestioned use of an indwelling catheter for prolonged periods can usually be obviated early in the treatment program.[14]

Contractural Deformities

Research on the development of contractural deformities supports the idea of a vigorous program of prevention.[12] The rehabilitation nurse, working with the physical and occupational therapists on a program of positioning and ranges of motion, can in most instances eliminate this distrubing complication.

The nursing profession is to be commended for pursuing a thorough program of intervention and tracking concerning factors likely to cause contractural deformities. It is well established that daily range-of-motion exercises are a good preventive measure.[1] In addition, the practical step of turning a patient to the prone position at intervals is most effective in discouraging contractures of the hips and knees. In this maneuver, the feet are placed over the edge of the bed against the footboard and the shoulders are elevated.[13] Unfortunately, the correction of contractural deformities remains the most common surgical procedure in most rehabilitation units.

Atrophied Muscles

Patients who have already sustained a loss of functional muscle strength from disease or trauma often suffer additional wasting and weakness as a result of muscle disease. Beginning an active exercise program as early as possible following the acute episode is the best way to maintain maximal muscle strength.[11]

Poor Nutrition

The recovery of patients from major trauma may be considerably hindered by inadequate nourishment. The same deficiency may be true for patients with longstanding chronic diseases. Detailed assessments of a patient's specific dietary requirements and careful supervision by the dietitian are clearly indicated during the rehabilitation program.[15]

Noxious Spasticity

Whenever noxious spasticity interferes with a patient's function, prompt action should be taken to reduce the spasticity. There are few instances in which it cannot be controlled by medication, nerve injection, tenotomy, or tendon transfer. Medication, however, should be used sparingly because of frequent adverse side effects.[11]

Social and Psychological Problems

Skilled professionals who are familiar with the host of social adjustments necessary in cases of severe, chronic disability are as essential to the rehabilitation effort as those who deal with the physical disability itself. The term *social pressure sore*[16] points up dramatically the implication of such problems and the aspects of prevention that must be considered.

Historically, an attitude of helplessness and hopelessness has prevailed in the treatment and rehabilitation of patients with most of the chronic crippling disorders. The psychologist specializing in clinical psychology who has expertise in dealing with various disease entities is of invaluable help to the rehabilitation program. It is vitally important to stress that the patient must focus on the possibilities and abilities remaining — not on what has been lost.[17]

PROGNOSES

It is difficult to assign a prognosis for a patient with a serious multiorgan chronic disorder. Not only are there primary physical deficits being evaluated but these deficits are also compounded by social, psychological, and vocational factors. Physicians who have had minimal contact with rehabilitation services are prone to be more gloomy in their prognoses than is warranted. Unless the prognosis is obvious, or until they gain more experience in the rehabilitation setting, physicians should avoid being specific. The team conference — a group discussion characterized by frequent interchange of ideas among professionals from various backgrounds — is an extremely useful way to arrive at a prognosis. It fosters the establishment of reasonable goals and constantly emphasizes what the patient can still do and can learn to do.

SURGICAL INTERVENTION IN REHABILITATION

Many professionals in rehabilitation settings have had little or no contact with surgeons, and a bias against surgical procedures clearly exists. One reason for this prejudice is that the rehabilitation hospital has been used inappropriately as a dumping ground for patients with failed surgical procedures. This practice obviously is not rehabilitation in the best sense. Furthermore, in many cases, the busy surgeon tends to focus attention on the merits of the surgical procedure and may not be sufficiently interested in or knowledgeable about the patient's total problem or sphere of activities. For instance, a quadriplegic patient who has been operated on for a hand problem may develop decubitus ulcers and bladder infections during the acute-care phases of the hospitalization because these complications were not given proper attention.

Another reason for the bias against surgery is that some physicians who are not successful in pursuing a surgical career may opt for a less demanding area of patient care and enter the rehabilitation field. These persons may nurture and retain a subconscious or open antisurgical bias.

Surgical procedures in the rehabilitation setting should be recognized as having the potential for major complications, just as in acute medicine, and should be performed by physicians who have some specific perspective on the patient and the problems the patient faces as a whole, plus an extensive general understanding of the rehabilitation process. Surgery is advocated when the risk involved is exceeded by reasonable gains in the patient's potential to function. An example of wise surgical decision making is choosing a simple operation to correct a contractural deformity rather than engaging in a costly, time-consuming period of stretching the deformity, which will often yield a poor end result. The same choice — that is, the choice of surgery — is also valid for noxious spasticity, closure of decubitus ulcers, stabilization of joints, and tendon transfers. Because this is a text on orthopaedic rehabilitation, the theme of effective surgical intervention pervades it throughout.

SUMMARY

Initially orthopaedists confined themselves to the practice of treating musculoskeletal disorders, or what is now called orthopaedic rehabilitation. During the last few decades, however, they have treated primarily acute diseases and trauma in acute-care settings. We believe that orthopaedic surgeons must once again devote themselves to caring for patients with chronic crippling conditions and accept responsibility for leadership in this regard.[18]

Several reasons make the return to this original obligation compelling. Acute ailments are better cared for and not neglected. More orthopaedic surgeons are trained and available to rehabilitation. Finally, the rehabilitation population contains an increasing number of elderly men and woman. They will inevitably develop a variety of neuromusculoskeletal complaints, but their mortality rate will not be as high as it would have been decades ago. Accordingly, the number of people who will require rehabilitation is increasing.

When orthopaedic surgeons assume the role of rehabilitation team leader with the same intellectual and professional dedication that they have applied to acute care, the results are extremely promising. They can direct a large program that will consume a comparatively small portion of their total professional time. This would require simply an adjustment in attitude, because the actual techniques used differ very little from those employed in treating acute illnesses. The well-trained orthopaedic surgeon is fully qualified to direct the rehabilitation of patients with chronic crippling conditions. The rewards are as great and the challenges as inspiring as those to be found in any other part of professional life.[19]

REFERENCES

1. Nickel VL: Sir Robert Jones Lecture: Orthopedic rehabilitation—challenges and opportunities. Bull Hosp Jt Dis 29:1, 1968
2. Nickel VL: Orthopedic rehabilitation—challenges and opportunities. Clin Orthop 63:153, 1969
3. Affeldt JE: Concept of patient care in a respiratory and rehabilitation center. p. 618. In ? (ed): Poliomyelitis: Papers and Discussions Presented at the Fourth International Poliomyelitis Conference. JB Lippincott, Philadelphia, 1958
4. Inman VT: Specialization and the physiatrist. Arch Phys Med Rehabil 45:765, 1966
5. Affeldt JE, Nickel VL, Perry J, Kriete BC: Intensive rehabilitation. Recent experience in a chronic disease hospital. Calif Med 91:193, 1959
6. Nickel VL: Rehabilitating the injured worker. p. 29. In: Proceedings of the 1965 Conference on Occupational Health. California Medical Association, ?, 1965
7. Wilson PD: Whither orthopedics? Bull Hosp Jt Dis 24:1, 1963
8. Klopsteg PE, Wilson PD: Human Limbs and Their Substitutes. Hafner Publishing, New York, 1968
9. Affeldt JE, West HF, Landauer KS et al: Functional and vocational recovery in severe poliomyelitis. Clin Orthop 12:16, 1958
10. Pierce DS, Nickel VL (eds): The Total Care of Spinal Cord Injuries. Little, Brown, Boston, 1977
11. Perry J: Orthopedic rehabilitation. p. 1. In Goldsmith HS (ed): Practice of Surgery. Harper & Row, New York, 1972
12. Edberg E: Physical therapy for thoracic and lumbar paraplegia. p. 225. In Pierce DS, Nickel VL (eds): The Total Care of Spinal Cord Injuries. Little, Brown, Boston, 1977
13. Thomas EL: Nursing care of the patient with spinal cord injury. p. 249. In Pierce DS, Nickel VL (eds): The Total Care of Spinal Cord Injuries. Little, Brown, Boston, 1977
14. Guttmann L, Frankel H: The value of intermittent catheterization in the early management of traumatic paraplegia and tetraplegia. Paraplegia 7:38, 1969
15. Mitchell HS: Nutrition in Health and Disease. 16th Ed. JB Lippincott, Philadelphia, 1976
16. Kahn E: Social bracing in rehabilitation. J Am Phys Ther Assoc 47:692, 1967
17. Vash C: The Psychology of Disability. Springer-Verlag, New York, 1981
18. Shands AR: A few remarks on physical medicine, rehabilitation, and orthopedic surgery. South Med J 54:420, 1961
19. Paterson D: Who cares? Bull Am Acad Orthop Surg 29(2):18, 1981

2 The Rationale and Rewards of Team Care

VERNON L. NICKEL

Most physicians, including orthopaedic surgeons, have not concerned themselves as much with the care of chronic disabilities as they could and should have. For many years, the chief reason for this neglect has been the press of work in acute-care hospitals. Now that acute ailments generally are better looked after and enough specialists are available, it is time that these specialists devote themselves to chronic crippling conditions with the same attention. One factor compounding the problem of care for chronic diseases is a fortuitous one — the mortality rate of patients with such conditions is being progressively lowered. More and more patients are surviving their acute episodes, which means there is a growing population of persons requiring rehabilitation.

I believe that at least 25 percent of all patients with chronic neuromusculoskeletal diseases could be aided significantly by the rehabilitation process. Unfortunately for these patients, there is only a limited acceptance of coverage of rehabilitation by third-party payers, such as Blue Cross, Medicare, and Medicaid. Also, in contrast to the excellent example of the crippled children's services in correcting orthopaedic conditions and rehabilitating children, the orthopaedic profession has not assumed that degree of responsibility for rehabilitation of disabled adults. This deficiency was attested to and deplored by the profession's greatest leader, Sir Robert Jones.[1-3]

Because the techniques and skills the physician needs for treating chronic and acute disorders are so similar, a person trained in acute-care orthopaedics also is well qualified to lead a rehabilitation team for chronic neuromusculoskeletal disorders. The rehabilitation team leader should not be chosen on the basis of specialty, but rather on the basis of interest in the particular disease category. For that matter, physicians who are not orthopaedists could be well qualified to direct programs of neuromuscular rehabilitation.[4]

Physical medicine developed largely to fill a void that other expanding specialties created through their neglect. In some areas, the physiatrists are still the only group that concerns itself with the rehabilitation process. The skills of the many disciplines needed in the rehabilitation process cannot be fully encompassed or learned by one person.[5,6]

Occasionally, an allied health professional is chosen to direct the rehabilitation effort. This usually proves unsatisfactory. Although certain aspects of rehabilitation may not require close direction by a physician, because delegation can be extensive, the overall program should be coordinated and led by a physician.

In the sections that follow, the need to discard the myth of the physician as an omnipotent being who can successfully deal with all aspects of the rehabilitation process is emphasized. The skills of each health professional required for a competent rehabilitation service and the improvement in patient care that will result when all members are permitted to work to their full potential are highlighted here. Other chapters describe in more detail the history and contributions of specific allied health professionals in rehabilitation. Delegation of authority and teamwork have been traditional and expected in the operating room and the intensive care unit but they are not as commonplace in rehabilitation. Unfortunately, isolation and bickering among specialties have erected severe hurdles that have hampered progress severely.

NURSING

The nurse is the key person on the rehabilitation team, by virtue of skills and interest in the rehabilitation process. The nursing profession has been one of the first to give status and recognition to its members who have specialized in the field of rehabilitative nursing.

The background and experience of nurses uniquely qualify them to step into roles for which they may not have specific training, to do what needs to be done under the existing circumstances, and then to step back when the specialists arrive to take over. At no time during this process does the nurse lose professional dignity or status.[7,8]

In contrast to the acute-care setting, the nurse's pattern of operation changes somewhat in the rehabilitation environment. Rather than performing every task for patients, the rehabilitation nurse must encourage and direct patients to expend maximum effort in their own care. Nurses must never hover over their patients. Rather, they must instill self-confidence and help the patient in the relearning program. Patients are required to feed and dress themselves even though this is not the easiest path for the patients or the professionals caring for them.

Patients on rehabilitation services have many demands on their time and are kept busy. Their schedules may require that routine nursing care be done early or late in the day or on weekends, or even be omitted. Priority must be given to the tasks that will speed up the patients' return to the outside community.

In a rehabilitation setting, nurses assume responsibility for many activities that are not a part of acute care. At a rehabilitation facility, nurses do positioning, turning, and range of motion exercises, and they constantly work to prevent decubitus ulcers and contractural deformities. They are well aware of how these complications can devastate a patient's rehabilitation.

The nurse recognizes the intense competition for the patient's time among the various rehabilitation services and apportions it among the other professional services. It is not merely a question of freeing the physician from this chore, but rather that the nurse is best suited to supervise the patient's day most effectively. Broad professional interests, skills, and 24-hour-a-day presence with the patient eminently qualify a nurse to assume this responsibility.[9]

Nurses are rapidly assuming charge of arranging and maintaining continuity of care.[9] They are best qualified to plan and extend care into the patient's home environment, and they certainly are most effective in coordinating this effort.

ENGINEERING AND KINESIOLOGY

Rehabilitation engineers bring the scientific and technical knowledge of their profession to the clinical environment of chronic disability. Engineers are recruited from two main sources: the traditional specialties of electrical and mechanical engineering and the newer field of bioengineering. Engineers applying advanced technology to the problems of rehabilitation can well be compared to engineers who participate in space programs. The difficulties a physically disabled person has are similar in concept to those encountered by humans in space. In each case, the engineer must manipulate the environment with the tools of science and technology in order to improve the quality of life for someone at a physical disadvantage. Rehabilitation engineers work to refine diagnostic as well as therapeutic measures. Their contribution to improved diagnostic tests is best represented by spinal cord monitoring; their progress in upgrading therapeutic methods is exemplified by functional electrical stimulation.

An important example of engineering research in the service of the disabled is that of kinesiology. Kinesiology does for persons with motor dysfunction what cardiologic assessment has done for those with heart disease. Kinesiology has made it possible for therapists and surgeons to measure limb function with reproducible precision, with excellent results for amputations, total joint replacement, and gait in cerebral palsy. Surgical decisions regarding muscle transplants in cerebral palsy and stroke have already been markedly improved. It is now possible to evaluate several aspects of phasic muscle activity, including gait velocity, stride length, and force and timing.

The kinesiology laboratory also has provided a rich opportunity for the physician, the therapist, and the engineer to work together in a scientific milieu that encourages pooling of knowledge and wholehearted professional cooperation.

PHYSICAL THERAPY

Traditionally the physical therapist has had a comfortable and rewarding professional relationship with the orthopaedic surgeon; this is even more true in the rehabilitation setting. In orthopaedic rehabilitation, physical therapists help prevent and correct deformities, strengthen and train weakened muscles, and administer a variety of special therapeutic measures to improve function, and they are highly skilled in the employment of special equipment and in training patients in its use. Their duties do not include using such modalities as massage, ultrasound, ultraviolet or infrared radiation, diathermy, diapulse, or whirlpool baths. *These have no place whatsoever in rehabilitation.*

In the early years of this century, physical therapists were instrumental in cooperating with orthopaedic surgeons in developing accurate muscle grading techniques. Their work contributed greatly to the care of thousands of poliomyelitis patients. Today there is a similar need for methods to grade spasticity,[10] and physical therapy is expected to be prominent in solving this problem.

OCCUPATIONAL THERAPY

The profession of occupational therapy has assumed important new dimensions in recent years. Although occupational therapists once were assigned only diversional or recreational activities,[7,11] they now are concentrating their efforts on improving upper extremity function, teaching patients how to carry out activities of daily living, and performing vocational testing. Never again should occupational therapists be wasted on the valuable professional resources of anything less than functional training.

Many orthopaedic surgeons have little or no knowledge of what a professional occupational therapist is and can do. Certainly these trained therapists are ideal partners for the surgeon in pioneering better hand surgery, better upper extremity function, and better neurologic testing and training. They are invaluable assistants to the orthopaedic surgeon and deserve the highest level of support.[12]

ORTHOTICS AND PROSTHETICS

After World War II, the field of prosthetics led the way in medicine for enlisting technology on behalf of serving the disabled. The introduction of plastics, the prefabrication of component parts for prostheses, and the strong emphasis on high standards of education for those wishing to become prosthetists greatly advanced the care given to amputees and improved the status of the field itself. Today, the duties of prosthetists are not confined to fabricating and fitting devices. These professionals also confer with the surgeon about the possibilities for immediate fitting and work with the physician, the occupational and physical therapists, and the social worker in orchestrating the patient's return to a stable life in the community.

The role of the orthotist is changing, much as the prosthetist's function did after World War II. Research, training, and clinical applications of knowledge promise rapid progress in orthotics.[13,14] The orthotist is a vital member of the rehabilitation team, providing the expertise and professional training needed to fit patients with assistive devices. New and better braces and assistive devices make possible many activities that were impossible for patients not so long ago. The orthopaedic surgeon is vitally interested in the progress being made in orthotics, especially as it relates to a rehabilitation program. Cooperation is essential between these two facets of medical care, because their combined efforts often help a dependent person become a productive, independent one.

SOCIAL WORK

Patients with chronic diseases often suffer devastating even crippling social problems in addition to their other disabilities. When a person's diminished wage-earning capacity is added to an impaired capability for self-care, the blow to the patient's self-esteem can easily cause withdrawal and isolation from the surroundings. Constructive social planning is necessary in a good rehabilitation program to prevent such behavior; thus, the social worker is an integral part of the rehabilitation team.[15]

Orthopaedic surgeons should encourage and expand the social workers' activities on the rehabilitation team. The professional contribution of social workers to patients' physical well-being and mental restoration is substantial and demands cooperation from all members of the team.

CLINICAL PSYCHOLOGY

The clinical psychologist not only helps the patient adjust to disability but also helps other members of the professional rehabilitation team to understand the severe psychological problems of patients with chronic crippling disabilities.[16] Clinical psychologists are well trained in experimental designs and the scientific method. They provide leadership for others who might not have as firm a background in validating information. The clinical psychologist has been far more successful in rehabilitation than the psychiatrist, who, except in isolated instances, has not participated effectively on the rehabilitation team. Psychiatrists have had the tendency to consider patients with long-term disability to be mentally ill. Psychologists, however, have seen them as normal people who have been disrupted or disturbed.

VOCATIONAL COUNSELING

Society has long recognized the tremendous financial and social benefits gained by returning a patient with a chronic physical disability to gainful employment.[17,18] Historically, orthopaedics has lead this effort more than any other specialty, as best exemplified by the success in caring for people with residuals of poliomyelitis and returning a large number of them to the work force.[19] From beginning to end, the efforts of the medical and allied health workers are pointed toward developing the disabled person's physical, intellectual, and emotional resources to their maximum potential for functioning as a productive member of society.

Although poliomyelitis is no longer a problem in the United States, rehabilitation professionals need to maintain the aggressive attitude that it spawned and apply that attitude to employable adults with other chronic physical disorders. The vocational counselor — trained to lead patients through the frustrating steps to becoming an independent wage earner — is the person educated to do just that. The total rehabilitation process itself culminates in vocational preparation. All states now have very active and well-funded programs to create conditions conducive to helping many patients with disabilities of varying severity. These programs are led by vocational counselors.

REFERENCES

1. Girdlestone GR: The Robert Jones tradition. J Bone Joint Surg [Br] 30:187, 1948
2. Jones R: The problem of the cripple. Practitioner 112:1, 1924
3. Jones R: An address on the domain of orthopaedic surgery. Br Med J 1:295, 1931
4. Sarmiento A, McCullough NC: The orthopaedist and rehabilitation. Clin Orthop 41:111, 1965
5. Inman VT: Specialization and the physiatrist. Arch Phys Med Rehabil 45:765, 1966
6. Shands AR: A few remarks on physical medicine, rehabilitation, and orthopedic surgery. South Med J 54:420, 1961
7. Goldthwait JE: The backgrounds and foregrounds of orthopaedics. J Bone Joint Surg [Br] 15:279, 1933
8. Knoche FJ, Knoche LS: Orthopedic Nursing. FA Davis, Philadelphia, 1951
9. Stanton J: Rehabilitation nursing related to stroke. Clin Orthop 63:39, 1969
10. Riebel JD, Nashold BS Jr: Electronic method of measuring and recording resistance to passive muscle stretch. J Am Phys Ther Assoc 42:21, 1962
11. Nickel VL: The therapist and the profession, p. 1. In: Proceedings of the American Occupational Therapy Association Conference. American Occupational Therapy Association, Washington, DC, 1960
12. Yerxa EJ: Authentic occupational therapy. Am J Occup Ther 21:1, 1967
13. Jones R: Treatment of fractures of the thigh. Br Med J 1:1086, 1914
14. Snelson R, Conry J: Recent advances in functional arm bracing correlated with orthopedic surgery for the severely paralyzed upper extremity. Orthop Prosthet Appl J 12:41, 1958
15. Kahn E: Social bracing in rehabilitation. J Am Phys Ther Assoc 47:692, 1967
16. Wendland LV: Psychologists at work. Am Psychol Assoc Bull 22:1, 1964
17. Rusk HA: The advantage of disadvantage. Bull Hosp Jt Dis 16:1, 1955
18. Wright BA: Physical Disability: A Psychological Approach. Harper, New York, 1960
19. Nickel VL: Sir Robert Jones Lecture: Orthopedic Rehabilitation — challenges and opportunities. Bull Hosp Jt Dis 29:1, 1968

3 Rehabilitation Nursing

JOANNE SANDBERG-COOK

The Association of Rehabilitation Nurses has defined rehabilitation nursing as "a specialty within the scope of professional nurse practice. [It] is the diagnosis and treatment of human responses of individuals and groups to actual or potential health problems stemming from altered functional ability and altered lifestyle."[1] This definition implies a holistic approach to the "patient" that is not disease centered. (In the field of rehabilitation nursing, use of the term *client* is preferred in order to emphasize this.) Rather, it encompasses the whole person, family, and community and focuses on health and on the interaction of the clients with their environments.

Rehabilitation nurses work with the rehabilitation team to maintain or improve function and prevent complications that can extend or prolong disability. Because of the nurses' holistic focus, they are ideal team coordinators and patient advocates. All other members of the rehabilitation team provide intermittent services. Nurses provides 24-hour care with continuous reinforcement of the services of the other disciplines. Without knowledgeable nursing intervention, the rehabilitation program can fail.

KNOWLEDGE, SKILLS, AND APTITUDES

The professional nurse practicing rehabilitation nursing functions in a variety of institutional and community settings. Basic nursing preparation, specialized education, and experience with disabled clients either as a generalist or within specialty areas such as neurology, rheumatology, or orthopaedics are fundamental requirements. In addition, current rehabilitative technologies and therapies require unique knowledge and skills.[1]

Although all professional nurses are familiar with and practice some basic rehabilitative techniques, nurses working within a rehabilitation setting are emerging as experts in the care of persons with chronic, disabling conditions. They must be grounded in the basic principles of rehabilitation—prevention of further problems, and restoration of function—as well as having an in-depth understanding of anatomy, physiology, and kinesiology, especially concerning musculoskeletal and nervous systems. This knowledge base allows for an understanding of the various pathophysiologic alterations affecting disabled clients.

Nurses must also have a solid understanding of the psychological effects of long-term illness and permanent disability to be able to meet the needs of clients during the various stages of adjustment. They must be familiar with ways of communicating with clients who are having trouble expressing themselves. In addition, nurses must be aware of the ways in which the clients' current physical problems have bearing on their families and community, previous life tasks, and role responsibilities.[2]

Finally, rehabilitation nurses must possess infinite patience. Their actions are more slowly paced than those of their acute-care counterparts. The rehabilitation nurses' role is to encourage clients to do as much for themselves as possible, rewarding every success and even effort with praise and encouragement. Standing aside and allowing clients to "do for themselves" takes more time and patience than doing it for them. Teaching and reinforcing self-care skills requires self-discipline and persistence. Ensuring the safety of newly disabled clients requires an awareness of potential hazards as well as sensitivity to the clients' need for independence. Monitoring the condition of skin, and the functioning of bowel and bladder and preventing the complications of immobility requires well-honed observational skills and a firm knowledge base. Although the data base for each member of the rehabilitation team is similar, it is the nurse who contributes the unique, holistic perspective and approach.

PLANNING NURSING CARE

Nursing care encompasses two broad categories of activity. The dependent function of the nurse includes those activities ordered by the physician and carried out by the nurse. This includes dispensing prescribed medications and treatments that are part of the client's medical regimen. Independent nursing includes those areas of rehabilitation that are uniquely addressed by nurses, which are founded on educational preparation and state practice acts. In the formative years of the profession, leaders focused on skills that were necessary for nursing practice. By 1955 nurses were becoming aware of the need for a broad theoretical base on which to build this practice. Between 1955 and 1965 they were concerned with the specific functions of nursing practice. The term *nursing process* was coined by these nursing leaders, and in 1967 a faculty group at The Catholic University of America in Washington, DC, identified the phases of nursing process as assessing, planning, implementing, and evaluating.[3] Nursing diagnosis (see later discussion) was added to basic nursing process in the early 1970s.

Nursing process is a step-by-step method of problem solving that is a method for assessing, analyzing, prioritizing, correcting, and reevaluating human problems.[4] This scientific approach to the client's problems allows for individualized care regardless of medical diagnosis. It also encourages the identification of problems that are solved by independent nursing action in concert with the other members of the rehabilitation team.

In 1986 the American Nurses' Association, in conjunction with the Association of Rehabilitation Nurses, published Standards of Rehabilitation Practice based on nursing process. The five professional standards are as follows[5]:

Standard 1. Data collection
The nurse continuously collects data that are systematic, comprehensive, and accurate. The nurse uses a data collection framework that facilitates an examination of the client's health status, incorporates information on the client's relationship to the environment and provides data for nursing diagnosis.

Standard 2. Nursing diagnosis
The nurse analyzes the data derived from the assessment to determine the nursing diagnosis.

Standard 3. Planning and goal setting
The nurse collaborates with the individual, family, significant others, and representatives of other disciplines to formulate a realistic plan that identifies goals, specific nursing actions, and resources to meet the individual's need.

Standard 4. Intervention
The nurse intervenes as guided by the individual care plan to prevent complications and promote, maintain, or restore the individuals physical and psychosocial function at a realistic, optimal level. Nursing actions are consistent with the total rehabilitation program to achieve patient goals.

Standard 5. Evaluation
The nurse evaluates the individual's responses to nursing actions. If the goals have not been attained, the data base is examined, further data are collected as needed, and nursing diagnoses and care plans are revised.

Each of these standards needs to be understood in more detail to truly appreciate the role of the nurse on the rehabilitation team.

Data Collection

The establishment of a data base is the first step, and this needs to be done using a structured format. The information gathered must reflect the perceptions of both the client and the nurse. Data collection must be systematic, comprehensive, accurate, and ongoing and include both history and physical assessment. Most institutions have a standard format for the collection of client information on admission to the rehabilitation facility (Fig. 3-1). This initial assessment is the first step to individualizing nursing care and allows the nurse to gain basic insight into the client's current problems and how the client perceives those

BRAINTREE HOSPITAL

Nursing Department
Nursing Admission Assessment

Date: _____   Arrival Time: _____

Admitted via: Ambulance _____   Private Car _____   Other _____

Allergies: _____

I.D. bracelet: (please specify type patient has on): _____

Orientation to unit routine: _____

I.   Health Perception/Health Management Pattern

Admitting diagnosis _____

Additional diagnosis/Past medical history: _____

_____

_____

_____

What does patient/family expect from this hospitalization: _____

_____

_____

Alcohol use: _____

What does patient know about his or her medications: _____

_____

_____

II.   Nutrition/Metabolic Pattern

Diet: _____   Height _____   Weight _____

History of weight gain or loss in the past six months: _____ Yes _____ No

(If yes, explain) _____

Has patient received any nutritional supplements while hospitalized? _____

_____

Results of first meal observation: _____

_____

Dentures: Yes _____   No _____   Upper _____   Lower _____   Partial _____

Condition of mucous membranes: _____

Skin integrity: Color _____   Temperature _____

Turgor _____   Edema _____   Lesions _____

Describe any alteration in skin integrity (Include incisions, pressure areas, decubiti, bruising or rashes.)

_____

_____

_____

_____

_____

_____

III.   Activity/Exercise Pattern

Transfers: _____   Bed mobility _____

Comments: _____

_____

MR-244

Fig. 3-1. A data collection tool based on functional health patterns. (Used with permission of the Braintree Hospital Nursing Department, 1989, unpublished, copyright pending.) (*Figure continues.*)

Nursing Admission Assessment
Page 2

Motor Function:

RUE: _____   RLE _____

LUE: _____   LLE _____

Patient's nurse's assessment of self-care abilities

	1	2	3	4	5	6	7
Bathing	___	___	___	___	___	___	___
Dressing	___	___	___	___	___	___	___
Grooming	___	___	___	___	___	___	___
Toileting	___	___	___	___	___	___	___

7 = Complete Independence (Timely, Safely)
6 = Modified Independence (Device)
MODIFIED DEPENDENCE
5 = Supervision
4 = Minimal Assist (Subject = 75%+)
3 = Moderate Assist (Subject = 50%+)
COMPLETE DEPENDENCE
2 = Maximal Assist (Subject = 25%+)
1 = Total Assist (Subject = 0%+)

IV. **Vital Signs**

Temperature _____   B/P _____   R ARM _____   L ARM _____

Pulse rate _____   AP _____   Rhythm _____   Resp. rate _____

Breath sounds _____

Comments _____

V. **Elimination Pattern**

Describe patient's usual bowel elimination pattern: _____

Changes in pattern?   Constipation _____   Diarrhea _____

Explain: _____

Actions taken/aids used: _____

Last BM _____   Bowel sounds _____

Describe patient's usual urinary elimination pattern: _____

Changes in pattern?   Frequency _____   Pain _____   Burning _____

Difficulty voiding _____   (Explain): _____

Last void: _____   ADM. U/A C/S sent: _____

VI. **Sleep/Rest**

Usual sleep-pattern: _____

Sleeping aids used: _____

Comments: _____

VII. **Cognitive/Perceptual Pattern**

Level of consciousness _____

Oriented to: Person _____   Place _____   Time _____

Comments: _____

If patient is not oriented or has altered level of consciousness, complete the following:

Able to follow 1 step commands: Yes _____   No _____

Remembers caregiver's name after   2 minutes _____   5 minutes _____

30 minutes _____

MR-244

Fig. 3-1 *(Continued).*

Nursing Admission Assessment
Page 3

Level of Attention:
Unattentive _____ Distractible _____ Restless _____ Agitated _____
Explain: _____
Pupils: Right _____ Left _____
Vision: _____
Hearing: _____
Glasses: _____ Contact lens _____ Hearing aid _____
Speech: Intact _____ Aphasia _____ Specify type: _____
Primary Language: _____
Comments: _____

Pain/Discomfort: No problem _____ Problem _____
If yes, please explain (describe location, type, intensity, onset, duration & what relieves pain)
_____
_____
_____

Safety: History of falls: Yes _____ No _____ Posey: Yes _____ No _____
Cleared for hot liquids: _____
_____

Does patient smoke? _____
_____
If yes is patient cleared for smoking independently? Yes _____ No _____
Comments: _____

VIII. Self-Perception/Self-Concept Pattern
How do you feel about being hospitalized or ill? _____
_____
_____
_____

IX. Role/Relationship Pattern
Marital Status _____ Occupation _____
Comments _____
_____

X. Sexual/Reproductive
Changes in sexual pattern/activities (if appropriate) _____
Breast self-examination: Yes _____ No _____ N/A _____
Testicular self-examination: Yes _____ No _____ N/A _____
Date of last menses _____ Comments _____

XI. Coping/Stress Tolerance Pattern
Experienced any recent major changes in your life (in addition to your illness or hospitalization)
Yes _____ No _____ If yes, explain _____
_____
_____

MR-244

Fig. 3-1 *(Continued).*

Nursing Admission Assessment
Page 4

Who/What helps you in coping with stress or problems? _____
_____
_____

XII. Value/Belief Patterns
Are there any religious practices that you would like to follow while in the hospital? _____
_____
_____

XIII. Other Patient Concerns
Educational Needs
  Patient identified: _____
  Nurse identified: _____
  Target person for teaching: _____
Additional comments: _____
_____
_____
_____
_____
_____
_____
_____

Assessment Summary
_____
_____
_____
_____
_____
_____
_____
_____
_____
_____
_____
_____
_____
_____
_____
_____
_____
_____
_____
_____

R.N. Signature _____
Date _____   Time _____

MR-244

Fig. 3-1 *(Continued).*

problems. Other sources of data available to the nurse include interviews with family, collaboration with other members of the team, and written medical records. The data collected during this initial encounter provide a basis for immediate care, facilitate the nursing diagnosis, and help in establishing priorities.

A popular method of organizing data uses Gordon's classification of functional health patterns.[6] As identified by Gordon, the functional health patterns are (1) health perception/health management, (2) nutrition/metabolic, (3) elimination, (4) activity/exercise, (5) cognitive/perceptual, (6) sleep/rest, (7) self-perception/self-concept, (8) role/relationship, (9) sexuality/reproduction, (10) coping/stress tolerance, and (11) value/belief. Under each pattern there is a list of possible nursing diagnoses to help the nurse identify actual or potential problems and plan appropriate nursing intervention. Although currently there are over 80 approved nursing diagnoses, certain ones appear more frequently and become a focus for rehabilitation nurses (Table 3-1).

Nursing Diagnosis

Nursing diagnosis is defined as "a statement, supported by valid data, of an actual or potential health problem whose etiology or significantly related condition or situation requires nursing intervention for effective and predictable management."[7] The nursing diagnoses are based on the client assessment and are chosen from the most recent list of nursing diagnoses currently accepted by the National Group for Classification of Nursing Diagnoses. There are three parts to each nursing diagnosis: title, related factors (etiology, medical diagnosis), and defining characteristics (cluster of signs and symptoms). Each diagnostic category comprises the assessment criteria, nursing interventions, and outcomes. Using nursing diagnoses grouped under functional health patterns gives the rehabilitation nurse a system for thinking about nursing care in a rational and scientific way rather than simply performing tasks mandated by tradition, intuition, or medical orders. An example of just one of the functional health patterns will reveal the benefits of organized information in identifying problem areas.

Table 3-1. Nursing Diagnoses Organized by Functional Health Pattern

Functional Health Pattern	Nursing Diagnosis
Health perception/ health management pattern	Potential for physical injury
Nutritional/metabolic pattern	Alteration in nutrition
	Potential impairment of skin integrity
	Impaired skin integrity
	Decubitus ulcer (specify stage)
Elimination pattern	Alteration in bowel elimination: constipation
	Alteration in bowel elimination: diarrhea
	Uninhibited bowel elimination
	Urinary retention
	Incontinence
Activity/exercise pattern	Activity intolerance
	Impaired physical mobility
	Self-care deficit
	Potential for joint contracture
	Ineffective breathing pattern (specify)
	Decreased cardiac output
	Deconditioning
Sleep/rest pattern	Sleep pattern disturbance
Cognitive/perceptual pattern	Alteration in comfort: pain
	Knowledge deficit (specify)
	Uncompensated sensory deficit (specify)
	Impaired memory
	Attention and concentration deficits
	Alteration in visual-spatial relationships
	Unilateral neglect
Self-perception/self-concept pattern	Fear
	Anxiety
	Reactive depression
	Body image disturbance
Role/relationship pattern	Impaired verbal communication
	Alteration in family process
Sexuality/ reproductive pattern	Sexual dysfunction
Coping/stress tolerance pattern	Ineffective individual coping
	Ineffectual family coping
Value/belief pattern	Spiritual distress

(Modified from Mumma,[8] with permission.)

Activity Exercise Pattern

Movement is one of the most important health patterns to both the client and the nurse working in rehabilitation. Movement allows people to control their immediate environment. The extent of a person's disability is often defined by existing mobility limitations. Several nursing diagnoses are included within the activity/exercise pattern in addition to those that deal with mobility including activity tolerance, self-care deficits, respiratory function, and cardiac function (Table 3-1). The screening assessment will reveal deficits in mobility, self-care, activity level, and activity tolerance. If the nursing diagnosis is impaired physical mobility, the nurse needs to be specific about the related factors. Examples of related factors (etiology) include the medical diagnosis (stroke, arthritis, neuropathies, amputation), psychological factors (depression, anxiety), perceptual or cognitive impairment, or prolonged bed rest. Including specific information about these factors is necessary so that appropriate care based on the client's specific disabilities can be planned. The defining characteristics of this nursing diagnosis further clarify the client's problem (e.g., limited range of motion, impaired perception of body parts, inability to purposefully move within the physical environment).[8] Once the specific nursing diagnosis has been established, all nursing intervention is directed toward resolving the client's identified problems. Because the number of nursing diagnoses for each client is not limited, it behooves the nurse to prioritize them so that those problems that affect basic physiologic functioning receive prompt nursing intervention. As certain problems are resolved, further assessment will identify new priorities.

Planning and Goal Setting

The practice of rehabilitation nursing is goal centered. Once problems are identified, the resolution of the problem becomes the desired outcome. Realistic short- and long-term goals (outcomes) are set with the client, the family, and representatives of the other disciplines. These goals are designed to optimize the client's residual function and prevent further complications. Each nursing diagnosis will have a specific goal or client outcome that is measurable and therefore easily evaluated.[1]

A care plan is established for each client that identifies nursing diagnoses in each of the previously noted functional health categories, desired outcomes, and the recommended independent and dependent nursing actions required to achieve these outcomes.

Intervention

Rehabilitation nurses working with a client who carries a diagnosis of impaired mobility can intervene in the following manner: perform and teach active and passive range-of-motion exercises during routine care; teach proper bed positioning, mobility, and transfer techniques according to the specific etiology of the mobility impairment; and help the client with activities of daily living by demonstrating the proper use of adaptive equipment. Other areas addressed by the nurse include pain assessments and the provision of enough time to accomplish self-care activities. All nursing interventions are carefully documented in the care plan so that other nurses caring for the client know which areas are being successfully addressed and how. Each nursing diagnosis is approached in this thorough and organized manner.

Evaluation

Once a care plan has been put into effect, there is continuing assessment of the plan and how it is working for the client. The implementation of a care plan frequently brings previously unrecognized problems to light. This may result in the need for more data, different nursing diagnoses, and a revised plan of care. A change in the client's functional or medical status also will result in a change of priorities and the addition or deletion of nursing diagnoses.

THE NURSE AS EDUCATOR

Rehabilitation is a learning process—one that requires a change in attitude and skills. The client and the family have much to learn and are constantly bombarded with new information from the entire team.[4] The rehabilitation nurse is with the client up to 24 hours a day and is the only member of the team who has this constant relationship with the client. Rehabilitation nurses are responsible for creating the warm, trusting, and therapeutic environment needed by clients in their efforts to accept their disabilities and achieve independence. Rehabilitation nurses have both the opportunity and the responsibility for teaching their clients and clients' families. This aspect of patient care must not be left to chance. Although everyone on the team is responsible for teaching certain skills and concepts to patients, it is the nurse who must be responsible for the outcome. The nurse is the team member most likely to have assessed the client's level of knowledge and to be able to diagnose specific knowledge deficits (Fig. 3-1).

Assessing areas in which learning must take place includes compiling a description of the client's sensory and cognitive capabilities. Rehabilitation nurses continuously assess their clients' levels of anxiety and their stage of acceptance of their disabilities. The nurses' awareness of clients' language skills, grasp of new ideas, attention span, level of consciousness, and need for communication aids allows them to determine learning readiness.[6] Nurses observe their clients as they struggle to practice what the therapists have taught and to reinforce these newly learned skills. Nurses are often called on to teach families and clients aspects of personal care that will be needed after discharge (see later). This may include decubitus ulcer prevention, bowel and bladder programs that ensure continence, use of adaptive equipment, medication instructions, and special techniques related to the administration of medication. General health education regarding nutrition, activity and exercise, sexuality, and general health promotion is included in the teaching plan.

Educational goals are developed with the patient or family, or both. These goals are based on ongoing physical and cognitive assessment as well as the nurse's knowledge of the client's home, role relationships, previous occupation, learning style, and readiness. Most teaching is done informally, during personal care, but the rehabilitation nurse will also teach certain skills to individual persons or groups in a more formal setting. The nurse will use audiovisual aids and printed material to reinforce learning whenever possible and appropriate. Goals are stated in measurable terms so that ongoing evaluation is possible. A nursing diagnosis of knowledge deficit carries with it a unique responsibility for ensuring that the specific learning needs of disabled clients are identified and met, in conjunction with the team and regardless of the extent of the client's disability.

DISCHARGE PLANNING

Discharge planning is an increasingly important aspect of nursing care, whether the nurse is a staff nurse, team manager, or continuing care nurse. With ever-increasing health care costs, shorter hospital stays, and sicker clients, careful discharge planning is often paramount in ensuring continuation of the rehabilitation process on an outpatient basis and successful reentry into the community. Every person who is hospitalized will need discharge planning. This planning should be started as soon as the client is admitted to the hospital so that adequate time is allowed for the process. The discharge planning process is similar to the nursing process. The six steps include assessment, goal setting, consultation with other team members, implementation, evaluation, and communication with community agencies.[9]

The initial nursing assessment should serve as a base for further planning (Fig. 3-1). Further detail regarding financial resources, disposition, and family relationships is obtained during the course of the hospitalization. In the rehabilitation setting, the nurse works closely with the client, the family, social services, and continuing care providers to assess these aspects of the client's premorbid life.

Goal setting is directly related to the client's educational needs (see earlier discussion), which are noted in the teaching plan or as specific goals for discharge.[9] For example, typical discharge goals for a diabetic client who has sustained a stroke might include (1) the client will demonstrate independence in safe transfers, or (2) the client's spouse will demonstrate correct injection technique for giving insulin.

Consulting with other members of the rehabilitation team during team meetings or on an informal basis allows the nurse to gain greater insight into client's needs as they relate to postdischarge living arrangements. As the client progresses through rehabilitation, the discharge plan is kept flexible to accommodate changing skill levels and emotional adjustment. The nurse must be aware of changes as they occur for the discharge plan to accurately reflect the client's needs. All members of the team are involved with decisions regarding discharge, none more so than the client and the family.

Implementation of the plan requires the active participation of the patient and family. For example, a diabetic stroke patient will agree to the following: (1) he will work with the physical therapist daily to learn correct transfer techniques, and (2) his wife will meet twice a week with the primary nurse to learn about insulin injections. It is absolutely imperative that the client agree to the goals and method of implementation or even the most careful planning is doomed to failure.

Team members must evaluate the progress being made toward the achievement goals for discharge. Careful documentation of positive or negative changes and of the client's reaction to the plan is required. This step in the process allows the nurse to make accurate assessments of the plan and to decide whether the goals are realistic or revision is necessary.[9]

The final step in the discharge planning process is direct communication with community agencies.[9] The rehabilitation nurse, along with other members of the team, needs to identify appropriate community resources for the client and family. These may include local visiting nurse associations, homemaker services, home health aides, outpatient rehabilitation facilities, and day care facilities. Telephone conversations, written referrals, and visits to the client's home or long-term care facility all help the team prepare the client for discharge. Sometimes the home will need structural changes, such as ramps or tub bars. Often the client will need special equipment. Frequently transportation to and from the clinic needs to be arranged. All too often families are not aware of the services available to them. The nurse can ensure that every effort is made to obtain all services needed by a client. Full utilization of available community resources can ease the transition from hospital to home and greatly improve the quality of life for the client and family.

The discharge plan should reflect the goal of continued progress toward the outcomes that are desirable and potentially achievable by the client.[1] Careful discharge planning can help to ensure the continuity of care that will be needed by disabled clients as they reenter the community and accommodate themselves to living with their disabilities.

WORKING WITH THE FAMILY

The family provides nurturing, growth, socialization, and caregiving functions. Serious physical disability creates a family crisis that may call for role changes in all family members. The success of the client in rehabilitation can depend on the reactions of close family members to the disability. The social worker or psychologist on the team carries the most responsibility for family assessment, but these evaluations often are not available to the nurse who begins discharge planning or teaching. The nurse must assume the responsibility for the initial family assessment. The purpose of this assessment is to identify genetic problems, communicable diseases, environmental problems, and interpersonal data that may influence the rehabilitation process.[8] Armed with a good understanding of the family, the nurse can then establish teaching and discharge goals (see earlier discussion) and develop appropriate interventions.[8]

The rehabilitation nurse needs to determine the client's role within the family as well as the nature of the spousal, parental, or sibling relationships.[10] The sudden disability of the primary decision maker, wage earner, driver, or primary caregiver significantly alters that family's function and role responsibilities. An impending divorce or recent loss of a close family member can profoundly affect family support during rehabilitation. Loss of employment, even if planned, can result in financial uncertainty and anxiety. A change in long-held plans because of the unexpected disability of one family member can cause feelings of loss, anger, resentment, and disappointment. The care requirements of a physically or cognitively impaired family member can strain the closest families, especially if one partner must give up a job (with resulting loss of additional income) to provide this care.

Although nurses should never attempt to counsel a dysfunctional family, their observations of the family will influence the entire team's approach to the client.

The nurse must identify the family member most likely to provide support and care to the client and assess that person's caregiving capacity. The previous relationship between these family members must also be assessed. How are family decisions made? Who was responsible for task delegation? Are there other family members with physical or psychological problems? Is the family able to express the grief, anger, and helplessness that unexpected disability can engender? How has the family handled previous stressful events? What financial and community resources are available to the family?[8]

Rehabilitation nurses are the team members with the most family contact. They are there during evening visiting hours and on weekends. They are most visible to families and most likely to observe the family structure and function. Their observations of the family are invaluable to the team members who have the professional skills to counsel families and clients to a fuller acceptance of disability and the life changes that must occur.

EDUCATIONAL PREPARATION AND PROFESSIONAL RESPONSIBILITIES OF THE REHABILITATION NURSE

Nurses working in the rehabilitation setting come from varied educational backgrounds and experiences. Primary nurses in most institutions are registered nurses with clinical experience in rehabilitation and specialized formal and informal education. Although the American Nurses' Association recommends the baccalaureate degree in nursing as entry-level educational preparation,[11] registered nurses in rehabilitation will come from all levels of the educational spectrum, including hospital-based diploma programs and associate degree programs. Working under the direction of these registered nurses are licensed practical nurses, rehabilitation technicians, and nursing assistants.

The Association of Rehabilitation Nurses, founded in 1974, initiated certification for specialty practice in 1984. The successful completion of this examination validates qualifications, knowledge, and practice in rehabilitation nursing on the basis of criteria defined by the professional group. To be eligible to take this examination the nurse, must have a current registered nurse license and 2 or more years of practice as a registered nurse in a rehabilitation setting. Certified nurses use the title Certified Rehabilitation Registered Nurse (CRRN). As of 1987, there were more than 1,800 certified rehabilitation registered nurses nationwide.[8]

Preparation for advanced practice in rehabilitation nursing requires a graduate degree in nursing, preferably a master's degree or higher in the field of rehabilitation nursing. The advanced practice roles of the rehabilitation nurse specialist (clinical specialist) include clinical practice, education, research, administration, and consultation — all of which require intradisciplinary and interdisciplinary collaboration.[1] Nurse practitioners are increasingly found in rehabilitation settings. These nurses possess advanced skills in the assessment of physical and psychosocial problems and work under protocol to independently diagnose and treat medical problems under the direction of a physician. Theory development and the development of research programs are most frequently directed by rehabilitation nurses who hold doctorates.[1]

The Association of Rehabilitation Nurses (ARN) was founded in 1974 for following purposes[1]:

- Advancing the quality of rehabilitation nursing service throughout the community.
- Offering educational opportunities that promote awareness of and interest in rehabilitation nursing and improve expertise of personnel on all levels.
- Facilitating the exchange of ideas in rehabilitation programs.

Membership in the Association of Rehabilitation Nursing is open to any nurse interested in rehabilitation nursing.

The ARN established the Rehabilitation Nursing Institute as its educational arm in 1976 and was formally recognized as a specialty nursing organization by the American Nurses' Association in that same year. Since then, the ARN has developed standards of practice and published a body of rehabilitation nursing knowledge in 1987 *(Rehabilitation Nursing: Concepts and Practice)*, which is now available in its second edition.[1]

Other professional organizations available to rehabilitation nurses are The American Nurses' Association, The National Association of Orthopaedic Nurses, and the American Congress of Rehabilitation Medicine (a multidisciplinary organization).

SUMMARY

The practice of rehabilitation nursing requires specialized knowledge and clinical skills to deal with the profound impact of disability on individual clients, their families, and significant others. This knowledge is essential because of the potential magnitude of the prolonged disruption to the client's physical, social, emotional, economic, and vocational status. Critical to rehabilitation nursing are the concepts of optimum wellness, socialization, sexuality, adaptation, change process, learning process, growth and development, and role theory. These concepts are the core of rehabilitation nursing in all health care settings.[1]

REFERENCES

1. Association of Rehabilitation Nurses: Scope of Rehabilitation Nursing Practice. Association of Rehabilitation Nurses, Evanston, IL 1988
2. Sorenson K, Luckmann J: Basic Nursing: A Psychophysiologic Approach. 2nd Ed. WB Saunders, Philadelphia, 1986
3. McHugh M: Nursing process: Musing on the method. Holistic Nurs Pract 1:21, 1986
4. Stryker R: Rehabilitative Aspects of Acute and Chronic Nursing Care. WB Saunders, Philadelphia, 1977
5. American Nurses' Association: Standards of Rehabilitation Nursing Practice. American Nurses' Association, Kansas City, KS, 1986
6. Gordon M: Nursing Diagnosis: Process and Application. McGraw Hill, New York, 1982
7. Henderson V: Nursing diagnosis: theory and practice. Adv Nurs Sci 1:1, 1978
8. Mumma C (ed): Rehabilitation Nursing: Concepts and Practice. 2nd Ed. Rehabilitation Nursing Foundation, Evanston, IL, 1987
9. DeRienzo B: Discharge planning. Rehabil Nurs 3:34, 1985
10. Gillies D: Family assessment and counseling by the rehabilitation nurse. Rehabil Nurs 12:65, 1987
11. American Nurses' Association: Educational Preparation for Nurse Practitioners and Assistants to Nurses. A Position Paper. American Nurses' Association, New York, 1965

4 Physical Therapy

KATHERINE S. BLACK
MARY KAY CAMPBELL

Physical therapy is a form of health care that prevents, identifies, corrects, and alleviates acute or prolonged movement dysfunction of anatomic or physiologic origin. The primary objective of physical therapy is to promote optimum human health and function. The physical therapist achieves this outcome through the assessment and treatment of the musculoskeletal, neuromuscular, and cardiopulmonary systems when these systems are dysfunctional as a result of illness, trauma, or congenital causes. The physical therapist provides this service to individuals across the life span in various practice settings. Physical therapists provide care to pediatric, adult, and geriatric individuals in settings that include hospitals, rehabilitation centers, outpatient clinics, school systems, and nursing homes. Often physical therapists will be found in the field, providing services in the home, on the athletic field, or at the work site. Since the body of knowledge in therapeutic approaches is growing, many therapists are involved in research activities that investigate the effects and efficacy of interventions. Active participation in research has increased, not only as required work for an advanced degree, but also to promote better understanding of the clinical applications of physical therapy.

The role of the physical therapist on the health care team is to evaluate the nature and origin of movement dysfunction. Since movement is the result of the functions of multiple systems, a physical therapy assessment will often reflect results related to aspects of the musculoskeletal, neuromuscular, or cardiopulmonary systems. The following sections discuss specific system assessments conducted by a physical therapist. The specific evaluations performed by a physical therapist establish a source of baseline information for comparing the patient's status on an ongoing basis and for assisting the physician in making a diagnosis or establishing a prognosis. In addition, the physical therapist provides assessment of functional abilities and limitations. This information provides clarification of the extent of an individual's physical disability and the impact it has on the individual's ability to function in daily activities.

HISTORY AND EMERGENCE OF THE PROFESSION

The physical therapy profession became solidly established in the United States at the time of World War I with the organization of the program for Reconstruction Aides. When war was declared in 1917, the Surgeon General instituted the Division of Special Hospitals and Physical Reconstruction for the physical rehabilitation, education, and vocational programs for the war injured. Several orthopaedic surgeons assigned to this division were responsible for organizing and developing the program for Reconstruction Aides in physical therapy. From the very beginning, it was the close collaboration and mutual respect between the orthopaedic surgeons and the Reconstruction Aides that led not only to the development of physical therapy but to its acceptance as a profession.

The occurrence of poliomyelitis of epidemic proportions in the United States during 1914 and 1916 also greatly influenced the growth of the physical therapy profession. The epidemics of poliomyelitis led to the establishment of the National Foundation for Infantile Paralysis in 1938. The foundation played an important part in continuing the profession's growth. Nearly 1,000 physical therapists participated in the emergency work provided by the Foundation between 1948 and 1960. During the Salk vaccine trials in the 1960s, 38 physical therapists performed more than 2,500 muscle tests and traveled more than 100,000 miles.

The practice of physical therapy changed a great deal, especially in the late 1940s, and particularly under the guidance of orthopaedic surgeons. Rehabilitation centers were established that emphasized the total rehabilitation of the patient. Emphasis was increasingly placed on functional exercises and activities. The scope of techniques in physical therapy also widened to include new treatment methods for strengthening muscles, regimens for treating peripheral vascular conditions, body mechanics exercise for posture and back conditions, and exercise for chest conditions.

THE PROFESSION TODAY

There are approximately 72,000 physical therapists practicing in the United States today. The physical therapy profession has become accountable for the quality and integrity of its practice through the activities of the American Physical Therapy Association (APTA), which has more than 38,000 members.[1] The APTA is now responsible for establishing educational standards and accrediting programs for physical therapists and physical therapist assistants. There are approximately 130 APTA-accredited entry-level professional programs for physical therapists, of which 80 offer a baccalaureate degree and 50 offer a master's degree. The APTA also accredits the 104 programs for physical therapist assistants. For physical therapists, there are now 40 advanced master and 10 doctoral degree physical therapy programs leading to higher education and research in the field. Many therapists have an advanced degree in related subjects, such as physiology, neurophysiology, neuroanatomy, education, anatomy, or hospital administration.

The qualifications to practice physical therapy are established by law in each state and include attainment of at least the bachelor's degree, graduation from an accredited program, and successful completion of a licensure examination. In 41 states, physical therapists can evaluate without physician referral and in 25 states they can provide treatment within

Table 4-1. Specialty Sections of the American Physical Therapy Association

Administration
Cardiopulmonary
Clinical electrophysiology
Community health
Education
Geriatrics
Hand rehabilitation
Neurology
Obstetrics/gynecology
Oncology
Orthopaedics
Pediatrics
Private practice
Research
Sports physical therapy
State licensure and regulation
Veterans' affairs

the scope of physical therapy without physician referral. Advanced degrees are usually needed to obtain administrative or faculty positions. In general, the physical therapist has a background in the biologic and physical sciences, the social and behavioral sciences, the humanities and liberal arts, and the science and art of physical therapy, plus clinical experience.

The APTA recognizes 17 specialty sections (Table 4-1) that represent clinical specialty areas as well as issues related to various practice settings. Through the efforts of the APTA and its specialty sections, physical therapists can become board-certified clinical specialists in orthopaedic, neurologic, cardiopulmonary, sports, geriatric, and electrophysiologic physical therapy. In addition, the APTA and many other specialty groups sponsor continuing education programs in the form of conferences, seminars, publications, workshops, and quality assurance activities.

PLANNING A TREATMENT PROGRAM

A physical therapy assessment provides information that identifies the primary problems contributing to movement dysfunction, as well as the current functional level. The physical therapist's knowledge of disease processes, psychosocial factors, and other variables that affect rehabilitation are used to estab-

Fig. 4-1. Function tasks incorporate strength and endurance gained in therapeutic exercise. The patient is working on concentric and eccentric control of the quadriceps through the functional task of stepping up and down.

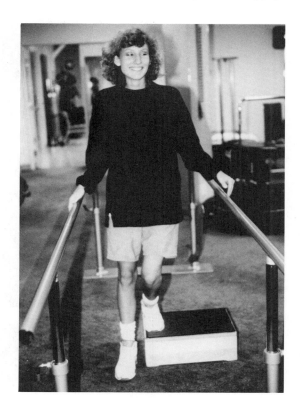

lish an individualized treatment plan. Treatment planning involves establishing long-term goals that reflect an individual's functional outcome and short-term goals that identify the components that are interfering with an individual's functional ability. For example, a tennis player who has sustained an ankle ligamentous strain may have long-term goals of returning to unassisted ambulation and competitive tennis and short-term goals related to decreasing swelling and pain, increasing strength and joint mobility, and independence in crutch walking.

Once goals are established, the physical therapist determines the most effective treatment intervention. A physical therapist is trained to provide treatment that includes therapeutic exercise (Figs. 4-1 and 4-2),[2] joint mobilization, application of physical agents (including the use of heat, cold, electricity, sound, traction, and water) (Fig. 4-3), training in activities of daily living, management of orthotics and prosthetics and other assistive devices (Fig. 4-4), the prescription

and procurement of equipment that contributes to functional independence, patient and family education, and prevention of deformity and disability.[3] The treatment interventions used by physical therapists are numerous and beyond the scope of this chapter to define in detail. The case studies presented at the end of the chapter provide examples of the types of assessment, goal setting, and treatment planning that are representative of a comprehensive physical therapy care plan.

By law in several states or because of reimbursement requirements, patients must be referred to the therapist by a physician. Physical therapists are professionals who need only a referral for evaluation and treatment that includes a summary of the diagnosis of the patient and any extraordinary precautions or complications. It is not only unnecessary but inappropriate for the referring physician to provide a specific prescription clarifying how to treat the patient. Physical therapists are independently able to deter-

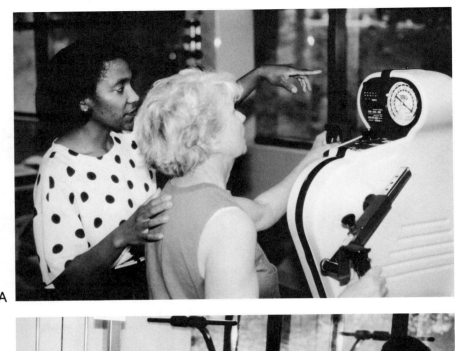

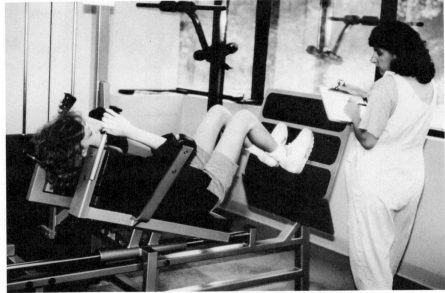

Fig. 4-2. (A & B) Physical therapists use equipment in planning upper extremity and lower extremity exercise programs. The therapist monitors repetitions, posture, and appropriate positioning during exercise progression.

Fig. 4-3. Functional electrical stimulation and biofeedback are examples of physical agents which can be used for muscle re-education during functional tasks.

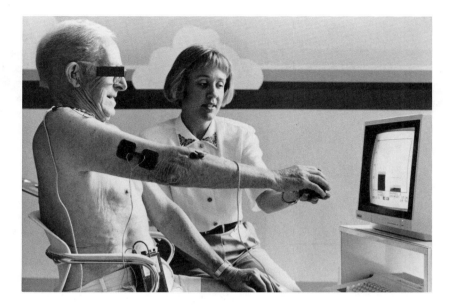

mine if the patient has a physical problem that can be ameliorated by physical therapy, estimate the time needed to achieve the treatment goal, know the most effective approach to solve the problem, determine when treatment is no longer effective or indicated, and recognize problems that need the attention of the physician. The physical therapist will keep the physician informed about the evaluation findings, treatment plans, and patient's response.

SYSTEMS APPROACH TO PHYSICAL THERAPY ASSESSMENT AND TREATMENT

Physical therapists use a systems approach to the assessment, treatment, and prevention of movement dysfunction. The musculoskeletal,[4] neuromuscular,[5] and cardiopulmonary[6] systems are the primary systems on which physical therapy has an impact. Each of these systems interrelate to result in normal movement and optimal function in the tasks of daily life. In this section we present an overview of the assessments usually provided by the physical therapist for each of these systems. In addition, we provide a review of functional assessment, since dysfunction of any of the major physiologic systems will ultimately have an impact on functional skills. A comprehensive physical therapy assessment integrates the contrib-

uting nature of each of the major systems and how they interact to interfere with the tasks of daily life.

Musculoskeletal System

Evaluation of the musculoskeletal system is especially important in the physical therapy profession.[7] Orthopaedic as well as neurologic, cardiac, and pulmonary dysfunction can involve disorders of this system.[8] The musculoskeletal system consists of soft tissue (muscles, fascial envelopes, tendons, tendon sheaths, ligaments, joint capsules, and bursae) and hard tissue (bone and cartilage). Appropriate consideration of these different tissue elements has a profound effect on the success or failure of the rehabilitation process.[9]

Radiologic examination of hard tissue can be helpful, but the soft tissue components of the musculoskeletal system provide most of the clues to determine effective treatment goals. Evaluation of soft tissue dysfunction is multifaceted.[10] Objective measurements of range of motion involve osteokinematic and arthrokinematic considerations. Osteokinematic movement occurs between two bones, and is usually determined at the starting point of movement. Once this movement begins, the range of motion measures the relationship of a moving bone relative to the stationary bone.

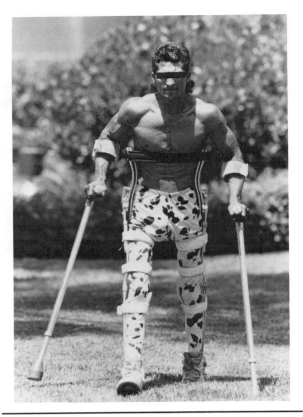

Fig. 4-4. Physical therapists provide gait training which includes the appropriate use and fit of an orthosis as well as functional training to achieve independent ambulation.

However, effective evaluation and treatment depends not only on accurate osteokinematics, but also on arthrokinematic movement, or what happens between joint surfaces during joint movement. In most movements in synovial joints, both "slide" and "roll" take place simultaneously. Restoration of restricted joint motion necessitates the use of techniques to restore the slide or roll to facilitate movement. Knowledge of these concepts is one of the first steps in effective assessment of musculoskeletal dysfunction.[11]

Because joint surfaces do not fit tightly, the capsule and ligaments remain somewhat lax. This creates joint "play" in most joint positions. Joint play is essential for normal joint function. Loss of joint play from some pathology, such as a tight joint capsule, will lead to alteration in function, usually involving restriction of motion and pain. In some cases, the entire joint capsule can be tight. This can be due to (1) joint effusion or synovial inflammation, or (2) capsular fibrosis. It is important to make the distinction between effusion and fibrosis since management and treatment will vary according to the cause of the restriction. Joint mobilization techniques are primarily used in cases of capsuloligamentous tightness or scar adherence. These techniques are specific to the restriction; manual therapists are well trained in mobilization skills (Fig. 4-5).[11]

Active, passive, and resistive movement tests assess the status of each of the component tissues of the physiologic joint. Findings yield specific information relating to the nature and extent of the pathology. Active movement tests relate primarily to the patient's functional status (cooperation or ability to move). Passive movement tests are generally more helpful; these determine overall mobility of the joint (normal, hypomobile, or hypermobile) as well as capsular or noncapsular patterns of movement. These tests also indicate cartilage displacement problems (loose bodies or cartilaginous lesions).

Resisted tests are designed to assess the status of musculotendinous tissue. Traditional muscle testing procedures are discussed under the neurologic system. In the musculoskeletal system, these strength tests determine whether there is some lesion or loss of continuity of the musculotendinous tissue itself. Tests are performed as maximal, isometric contractions. Pain associated with these tests signifies some pathology involving the muscle or tendon being tested.

Palpation of deep soft tissues, which include fat, fascia, muscles, tendons, ligaments, and joint capsules, can provide a wide range of helpful information. Tenderness is indicative of superficial lesions (e.g., medial ligament sprain at the knee).[8] Size and location of localized soft tissue swelling is helpful in determining articular or extra-articular lesions. Tenderness along bony sites may indicate problems at ligaments and tendons as well as structural deformities.

Posture evaluation is indicated because joint pathology may cause malalignment of body parts. Correction of abnormalities is considered in the long-term treatment goals. Poor posture encourages loss of soft

Fig. 4-5. Physical therapists are trained in manual assessment and treatment skills. This patient is receiving manual cervical traction for improved cervical and soft tissue mobility as well as relief from radiating pain symptoms.

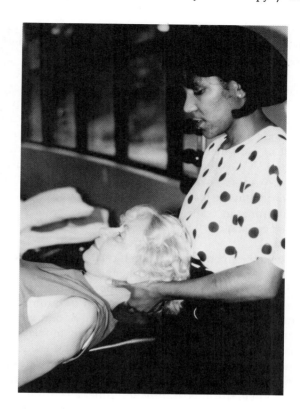

tissue mobility. Adaptive shortening on one side of the body can lead to lengthening on the other side. These compensatory changes can precipitate a secondary problem and further complicate successful healing.

Evaluation of gait pattern requires special study. Gait deviations can be caused by local and referred joint pain, altered muscle tone, decreased strength and range of motion, poor stability, structural or functional postural deformities, poor balance and coordination, and poor proprioception. Observation of gait in the clinic (or by videotaping or footprinting on paper) can measure velocity, cadence, ankle rotation, stride and step length, normal cadence, patterns of shoe wear, weight-bearing distribution, pressure areas, lateral or vertical pelvic shift, pelvic rotation, and center of gravity.

Taping of joints provides support to soft tissue. Many therapists, especially in sports medicine and outpatient clinics, are skilled in this technique, and it serves as a useful adjunct to prevention and care of orthopaedic injuries.

Musculoskeletal system disorders are far reaching and are affected by such neurologic dysfunctions as decreased sensation and altered proprioception. The physical therapist is trained to provide the most appropriate musculoskeletal evaluation, so that safe and effective exercise programs for patients with varied diagnoses is possible.

Neuromuscular System

Accurate assessment of the neuromuscular system is dependent upon a thorough musculoskeletal evaluation. The musculoskeletal assessment identifies problems caused by structural or mechanical dysfunction. The neuromuscular assessment provides the interface between the neurologic control that influences movement and the biomechanical system. The physical therapy neurologic evaluation provides information on the motor system, the sensory system, and the functions on which the integration of various neurologic systems have an impact.

The neurologic motor assessment includes a battery of evaluations that determine the cause of dysfunction of motor control. The manual muscle test can provide information that identifies weakness as a result of peripheral nerve, spinal root, or spinal cord injury.[12] Weakness can also be a result of disuse, which results in atrophy and loss of strength. The manual muscle test reflects a muscle's ability to generate force in relation to gravity and externally applied resistance.

Often movement dysfunction is related not to muscle weakness but to damage in other parts of the nervous system. Physical therapy evaluation can provide information on movement dysfunction by examining the patient's ability to perform isolated joint movement versus mass-patterned synergistic movement, coordination and speed of movement, and the presence of abnormal movement such as athetosis, ataxia, or dystonia. Therapists who are specially trained can perform electromyography and other electrophysiologic tests to determine nerve and muscle function.

Another aspect of motor control is the state of muscle tone. Muscle tone can range from hypertonic to hypotonic. Assessments done by a physical therapist to monitor muscle tone include deep tendon reflex assessment and assessment of abnormal reflexes resulting from postural changes of the head, neck, or trunk. Often, instances of severe muscle hypertonicity will result in contractures due to muscle shortening. In these cases, a physical therapist may use serial casting. Serial casting involves placing sequential casts every 3 to 7 days to inhibit a muscle by placing it on maintained stretch. Physical therapists are trained to cast the upper or lower extremities to achieve optimal positioning for reduction of tone and increased range of motion.

The neurologic assessment also includes a sensory evaluation. Sensory tests are done to determine the presence of light touch, and pain/temperature for peripheral, dermatomal, or cortical distributions. Results of the sensory test can be critical for accurate localization of a lesion or injury. Sensory testing also includes the assessment of proprioception and kinesthesia. Proprioceptive/kinesthetic sensation reflects the patient's ability to sense static joint or limb position; speed, direction, and amplitude of joint movement; and vibration. Patients can experience proprioceptive loss after injury of either the neuromuscular or musculoskeletal systems. Sensory loss can impair coordination and result in poor performance during tasks such as ambulation or other mobility skills. In addition, patients with sensory loss are at greater risk for complications such as skin breakdown.

Balance assessment is another component of the physical therapy evaluation. The physical therapist will assess static balance (the ability to balance while maintaining a position), and dynamic balance (the ability to balance while moving in a position). Balance is often assessed in various positions such as sitting and standing, and during functional tasks such as transfers or ambulation. Balance dysfunction can be a result of neurologic damage to the motor or sensory systems, or damage to the musculoskeletal system that causes joint limitation, weakness, or pain.

A thorough assessment of the neuromuscular system is integrated with results from the musculoskeletal system assessment to determine the primary cause of movement dysfunction and the impact it has on tasks of daily living. Physical therapy treatment is directed toward resolving or preventing the problems associated with these systems.

Cardiopulmonary System

Depending on the type of facility and the inpatient and outpatient programs offered, the role of the physical therapist is significant in the care and treatment of cardiac and pulmonary patients. Components of the cardiac and pulmonary system should be monitored in all patients with diagnoses ranging from joint arthroplasties to spinal cord injuries to chronic obstructive pulmonary disease. Following, recording, and checking vital signs is important with all patients in programs in which the emphasis is placed on maximal return to function. Increase in exercise programs or activities of daily living places a stress on the cardiopulmonary system. The long-term goal is to allow a person to return to whatever activity is compatible with the functional capacity of the heart.

Recognition of weaknesses in this system is important for goal setting as exercise levels are increased. The therapist's ability to recognize signs of cardiac stress by noting cyanosis, persistent unsteadiness, or angina during exercises, as well as to evaluate the chest (breathing patterns, auscultation of breath and heart sounds), can assist the physician in recognizing disproportionate responses to activities. Therapists specializing in cardiac care recognize electrocardiographic (ECG) arrhythmias and ischemic changes. Charting cardiopulmonary responses to exercise also assists the physician in stabilizing medications. Under the supervision of the therapist, the patient learns to recognize criteria for cessation of exercise. These criteria include, but are not limited to, changes in heart rate and blood pressure, marked dyspnea, S-T segment changes, angina, and presyncope.

Many hospitals and clinics offer inpatient and outpatient cardiac rehabilitation programs for patients who have either sustained a myocardial infarction or undergone open-heart surgery. Early physical therapy intervention is indicated in most cases under the supervision of the patient's prescribing physician. Exercise testing, prescription of an exercise program, and exercise progression are integral parts of a patient's rehabilitation program.[13]

The purposes of cardiac rehabilitation are (1) to reverse physical deconditioning; (2) to decrease anxiety and depression; (3) to assist the physician in recognizing disproportionate responses to activities (arrhythmias, hypotension, ischemic ECG changes); (4) to achieve patient self-sufficiency physically and emotionally; and (5) to maintain optimal functional capacity.

Education and experience enables the physical therapist to be a valuable member of a team responsible for the care of the patient with a pulmonary problem. These problems vary in patients with diagnoses that range from cystic fibrosis to chronic obstructive pulmonary disease to spinal cord injury to poor cardiovascular endurance (in the orthopaedic patient). Evaluation of breathing pattern and auscultation of breath sounds are important clinically in determining

which respiratory muscles are active and which inactive and what secondary muscles of respiration are being used.

The goals of treating patients with pulmonary dysfunction are (1) to improve the breathing pattern to provide tools for control of stressful symptoms; (2) to provide and maintain adequate bronchial hygiene and effective cough; (3) to improve and maintain the patient's work capacity; (4) to improve strength, range of motion, and posture as they relate to respiratory function; and (5) to teach the patient to coordinate breathing pattern with movement in activities of daily living.

Techniques for breathing retraining are important to teach the patient to coordinate breathing with body movement and daily activities. The therapist can determine if a patient is improving by noting the level of dyspnea. Subjective observation that the patient's level of breathing is less labored is a positive indicator of the success of rehabilitation. Appropriate training can effect change in respiratory muscular strength and endurance by increasing the efficiency of the breathing pattern.

Some patients require instructions in proper and effective coughing to mobilize secretions and promote pulmonary hygiene (e.g., the spinal cord injury patient with decreased lung volume). Assistive cough techniques are taught to achieve this goal.

Postural drainage is a treatment procedure that may be provided by physical therapy but is sometimes shared with nursing and respiratory therapy. Postural drainage is the sequential positioning of the patient in accordance with the segmental anatomy of the lung combined with percussion and vibration of the rib cage to facilitate the evacuation of secretions from the lungs.

There is a need for general reconditioning and progressive endurance activities in all patients. Developing cardiopulmonary fitness is a major goal of any rehabilitation program.

Functional Assessment

The functional testing done by the physical therapist is to determine the patient's highest level of independence in daily tasks that include bed mobility, wheel-

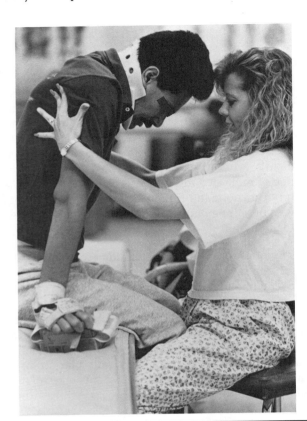

Fig. 4-6. Therapeutic exercise works on the components necessary to achieve independence in mobility skills. This individual with C6 quadriplegia is practicing a balance task in preparation for transfer activities.

chair mobility, transfers, and ambulation (Fig. 4-6). In preparation for teaching the patient these functional tasks, the therapist must know the physical requirements involved in the act, the degree of potential the patient has in meeting those requirements, and the assistive or adaptive devices that might be helpful. This analysis calls for an understanding of kinesiology, anatomy, biomechanics, and teaching techniques combined with knowledge of the patient's present and potential physical status. The therapist knows the tasks the patient needs to learn, the best sequence for learning, when the patient is ready for the next step, and the predicted amount of time it will take to learn the task.

Physical therapists specialize in knowing about the assistive and adaptive devices related to wheelchairs and ambulation. For example, therapists are able to select whatever crutch, walker, wheelchair, seat cushion, or orthosis a patient needs, teach the patient how to don or use the equipment, determine if the devices fit or need repair, and recognize when the patient no longer needs the device (Fig. 4-7). Therapists also determine if equipment is needed in the home. The therapist provides training in the use of the equipment to the patient, or to someone else who may be taking care of the patient at home.

In the area of function, physical therapists provide more than just a rehabilitative role. They also provide assessments in the community, workplace, recreational locations, and amateur and professional sport settings that address issues of accessibility, prevention of injury, and enhancement of performance.

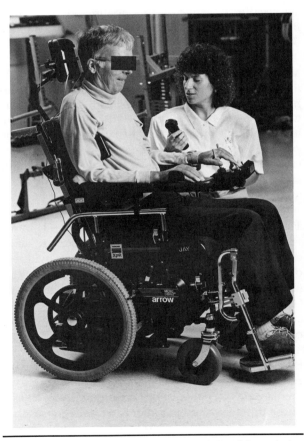

Fig. 4-7. Physical therapists have specialized knowledge in wheelchair and cushion options. For the patient with high quadriplegia, the physical therapist provides recommendations and training for powered mobility.

Physical therapists are involved in developing fitness programs, identifying potentially dangerous work sites, modifying tasks to prevent job-related injuries, performing postural and musculoskeletal screens in schools, and evaluating performance weakness and correcting physical deficiencies in athletes. The variety of assessments and interventions have one common goal: to promote optimum health and function.

FUTURE DIRECTIONS IN PHYSICAL THERAPY

The physical therapist's knowledge of the musculoskeletal, neuromuscular, and cardiopulmonary systems combined with an understanding of biomechanics, kinesiology, and functional implications of physical dysfunction defines a unique component within the healthcare team. This broad scientific and clinical base allows the physical therapist to provide service, in various settings, that is directed toward prevention as well as rehabilitation. The future direction of physical therapy will be influenced by both societal needs and the commitment of the profession to research and education. With the aging of the population at large, the demand for physical therapy in geriatric rehabilitation is increasing. In addition, health care in the 1990s will be directly affected by reimbursement trends; therefore, intervention must be directed toward individual functional outcomes that promote return to productive activity. The challenge for physical therapy will be to establish the efficacy of the scope of services provided by physical therapists.

The growth of the profession has been characterized by a commitment to quality care, clinical competency, and research activity. The movement of the profession toward a postbaccalaureate entry-level degree is made necessary by the in-depth scientific training and advances in the physical therapy knowledge base. The understanding of the clinical basis of physical therapy is increasing along with the development of new technologies. The profession's commitment to higher education, research that establishes the scientific foundation of physical therapy interventions, and the certification of clinical specialists is contributing to the growth and development of physical therapy as a primary source of health care within our society.

CASE STUDIES

Case Study 1

History

A 35-year-old man sustained a twisting and rotation injury to his lower back during his job working on an assembly line. He presented to the outpatient physical therapy clinic with a diagnosis of low back pain with lumbar disc injury ruled out. He is in a moderate amount of discomfort and is unable to sit or stand for long periods of time.

Physical Therapy Assessment

Physical findings are remarkable for left hip and buttock pain with intermittent left sciatica. He has pain with left straight leg raise and his plantar and patellar reflexes are decreased. Strength measures of the left ankle dorsiflexor and extensor hallucis longus are 4−/5 as compared with the right, which are 5/5. There is slight hypesthesia in the L4 dermatome. His posture is marked by a right lateral shift, elevation of the left shoulder and scapula, forward head and shoulders, and increased weight bearing on the right leg. He is tender to palpation at the L4-L5 spinous processes and has moderate lumbar paravertebral muscular spasm. Patellar reflex is slightly diminished. The lumbar spine is hypomobile. The skin in this area is warm to touch and there is minimal effusion at L3-L5.

Short-Term Goals

1. Improve soft tissue mobility along lumbar spine
2. Decrease localized swelling
3. Initiate home exercise program
4. Initiate instruction in appropriate posture
5. Monitor neurologic signs; if signs worsen, refer to physician

Long-Term Goals

1. Improve vertebral and soft tissue mobility
2. Continue exercise program to increase strength, coordination, balance
3. Education of body awareness
4. Work hardening program for return to work

Treatment Plan

1. Myofascial techniques for soft tissue mobility
2. Joint mobilization techniques for spinal mobility

3. Posture education and gait training
4. Exercises to promote trunk rotation and trunk stability/ progressive exercise program
5. Comprehensive exercises to lead to home exercise program

Case Study 2

History

The patient is a 21-year-old man who sustained a fracture-dislocation of T12–L1 in a motor vehicle accident, resulting in complete T12 paraplegia. He has been surgically stabilized and is currently in a Kydex thoracic-lumbar-sacral orthosis for the next 12 weeks. He has been admitted to a rehabilitation center with an expected length of stay of 4 weeks before discharge to home with parents.

Physical Therapy Assessment

Upper extremity strength and range of motion are within normal limits. Lower extremity strength is zero for all muscles. Lower extremities are flaccid with no deep tendon reflexes present bilaterally. Range of motion is within normal limits except for heel cord length, which is limited to 0° dorsiflexion with the knee extended, and hamstring length, which is at 45° on straight leg raise. Balance is good in long sitting and short sitting with upper extremity support, but poor without upper extremity support. He experiences orthostatic hypotension when being brought to full upright. Sensation is intact through the T12 dermatome and absent below.

Functionally, transfers require maximal assist to all surfaces. He is nonambulatory. Wheelchair propulsion is independent indoors but he requires maximal assist to negotiate ramps or curbs.

Short-Term Goals

1. Increase strength of upper extremities
2. Increase muscle length of heel cords and hamstrings
3. Increase tolerance to upright position
4. Increase sitting balance without upper extremity support

5. Prevent complications associated with immobility and sensory loss
6. Assess accessibility of home
7. Assess equipment needs, including wheelchair prescription, shower equipment, orthotic device

Long-Term Goals

1. Independent in all transfers
2. Independent in all wheelchair mobility
3. Independent in household ambulation with knee-ankle-foot orthoses and Lofstrand crutches
4. Independent in mobility and self-care within the home

Treatment Plan

1. Therapeutic exercise program for strength and mobility
2. Functional training in transfers, wheelchair skills, and ambulation
3. Patient education on prevention of contractures and decubitus ulcers
4. Home assessment to make recommendations regarding architectural barriers

Case Study 3

History

The patient is a 65-year-old woman who underwent a left total hip arthroplasty. The patient has a long history of heart disease; she underwent coronary artery bypass surgery 2 years ago. Her life-style has been sedentary because of hip pain and, since the surgery, she wishes to be more active and independent at home. She presented in the outpatient physical therapy clinic 6 weeks postoperatively. She is ambulating with a walker (partial weight-bearing on her left leg) and is in no apparent distress. She had physical therapy in the hospital for early gait training and transfer training instruction.

Physical Therapy Assessment

Physical findings are remarkable for 3+/5 strength throughout. Range of motion was normal, except for left hip flexion to 75° and adduction to 5°. Internal rotation was not tested. She is motivated, alert, and oriented. She is unable to walk long distances without shortness of breath and markedly increased heart rate. Resting heart rate is 100 beats per minute and blood pressure is 140/90 mmHg.

Short-Term Goals

1. Increase strength throughout all extremities, specifically the left hip, knee, and ankle
2. Continue gait training with walker, monitoring distance walked and vital signs
3. Initiate exercise program considering cardiac and pulmonary precautions
4. Instruct in independent transfers
5. Monitor pulmonary and vascular status

Long-Term Goals

1. Independent ambulation on stairs, various surfaces
2. 4/5 strength throughout
3. Independent home exercise program
4. Self-monitor heart rate/cardiac status
5. Improve endurance in activities of daily living
6. Stretching and strengthening program to maintain flexibility.

Treatment Plan

1. Begin low-level exercise program
2. Progressive gait training to independent on level surfaces, stairs
3. Educate patient in cardiac and pulmonary care during exercise

Acknowledgment. The authors wish to acknowledge Marilyn J. Lister, B.S., P.T., whose chapter in the previous edition provided reference for this revision.

REFERENCES

1. American Physical Therapy Association: The General Information Packet. American Physical Therapy Association, Washington, DC, 1989
2. Kisner C, Colby LA: Therapeutic Exercise: Foundations and Techniques 2nd Ed. FA Davis Company, Philadelphia, 1990
3. Scully RM, Barnes MR: Physical Therapy. JP Lippincott, Philadelphia, 1989
4. Gould JA: Orthopedic and Sports Physical Therapy. 2nd Ed. Mosby Year Book, St. Louis, 1990
5. Umphred DA: Neurological Rehabilitation. 2nd Ed. Mosby Year Book, St. Louis, 1990
6. Irwin S, Techlin JS: Cardiopulmonary Physical Therapy. 2nd Ed. Mosby Year Book, St. Louis, 1990
7. Hoppenfeld S: Physical Examination of Spine and Extremities. Appleton-Century-Crofts, New York, 1976
8. Spiegel P: Topics in Orthopaedic Trauma. University Park Press, Baltimore, 1984
9. Zohn D: Musculoskeletal Pain: Diagnosis and Physical Treatment. 2nd Ed. Little, Brown and Company, Boston, 1988
10. Rinehart M, Sutton T: Musculoskeletal Trauma. Aspen Publishers, Inc, Rockville, MD, 1987
11. Kesslere R, Hertling D: Management of Common Musculoskeletal Disorders: Physical Therapy Treatment and Methods. Harper & Row, Philadelphia, 1983
12. Kendall FP, McCreary EK: Muscles: Testing and Function. 3rd Ed. Williams & Wilkins, Baltimore, 1983
13. Dubin D: Rapid Interpretation of EKGs. 3rd Ed. Cover Publishing Company, Tampa, FL, 1978

5 Occupational Therapy

CAROL McGOUGH

Occupational therapy had its origins at the end of World War I, when many veterans returned from active military duty with new and complex rehabilitative needs. These veterans, too young to face a lifetime of hospitalization and yet too disabled to function outside an institution, required programs to maximize physical and occupational potential. Originally referred to as a period of "reconstruction," [1] this effort was renamed "rehabilitation," derived from the Latin word *rehabilitare*, meaning "to restore." [2] Early training of reconstruction aides has evolved into the specialized field of occupational therapy. Although the training of an occupational therapist has improved drastically over the past 70 years, the main focus of maximizing functional potential has remained unchanged.

The American Occupational Therapy Association (AOTA) was founded in 1917 with a group of six members and has grown to be the certifying body for over 30,000 Registered Occupational Therapists (OTR) and 6,000 Certified Occupational Therapy Assistants (COTA). The World Federation of Occupational Therapists was founded in 1952 and has supported development of educational standards for occupational therapists throughout the world.

The profession of occupational therapy has kept pace with advances in the fields of anatomy, physiology, injury, and repair processes, which has facilitated rehabilitation efforts and orthopaedic research. The past 10 years have witnessed specialization in rehabilitation in response to advances in emergency care and surgical techniques, which demand that therapists be more knowledgeable and demonstrate advanced clinical skills in their areas of expertise. In addition, changes in health delivery systems in the United States dictate that clinicians have effective and efficient treatment skills. These must be delivered in an environment of shrinking reimbursement and reduced patient days, with length of treatment often being determined by cost rather than need. Effective and efficient treatment can only be accomplished within the framework of specialization, wherein time, energy, and resources can be focused and channeled toward helping patients achieve maximum functional potential. By nature, rehabilitation efforts have been more comprehensive and personal than acute care medicine — "high-touch" rather than a *"high-tech"* approach[3] to patient care. As with all rehabilitation specialties, the "art" of occupational therapy in the future will lie in the therapist's ability to overcome "an approach to disease...with a dominance of procedures over patient sensitivities and a biomedical emphasis that disregards human meaning." [4] Occupational therapy is a high-touch profession whose mission is to help patients to regain the pride and self-fulfillment of independence.

Specialization is seen in inpatient rehabilitation with diagnosis-related programs in which specialists assess and establish treatment programs oriented toward the specific problems of patients. Great strides have been made in the care of stroke, brain injury, and spinal cord injury as a result of this specialized approach. Of late, programs to expedite the care of orthopaedic patients with hip fractures and lower extremity amputations have been developed, and functional outcome studies are demonstrating that patients achieve greater function much earlier after an intensive rehabilitation program.

Hand rehabilitation and return-to-work programs provide two excellent examples of how teamwork and focused resources in an outpatient setting can provide effective and efficient treatment programs for patients with orthopaedic disease and injury. Occupational therapists have played an important role in developing these specialized programs and will continue to contribute as more emphasis is placed on functional outcome.

ORTHOPAEDIC OCCUPATIONAL THERAPY

Successful therapy often depends on the occupational therapist's taking a role of supporter or motivator in addition to teacher. Patients who benefit the most from therapy are those who *adjust* to, even if they cannot fully accept, the problems for which they are being seen. An important part of adjustment is learning what is possible, versus focusing on what is impossible or impractical. Occupational therapy goals and treatment for the orthopaedic patient can be characterized as the three p's: *prevention* of deformity, *preparation* for function, and *promotion* of independence.

Prevention of Deformity

Prevention of unnecessary problems in rehabilitation is as important as the process of restoration itself and ensures that therapeutic efforts are geared toward rehabilitation rather than correction.

One problem to be prevented is joint stiffness. Clinical studies have shown that connective tissue subjected to immobilization or stress deprivation can lead to molecular cross-linking of the collagen, resulting in loss of soft tissue elasticity. Collagen deformation[5] can occur within a period of a few weeks, but it can take months of rehabilitation to correct. Clinically, prolonged immobilization leads to joint stiffness and eventual contracture, which may take many hours of therapy or even require surgical correction. Many times, severe contractures cannot be successfully reversed or corrected either through therapy or surgery, resulting in long-term functional impairment and additional potential complications.

Preventive treatment addresses proper body and extremity position, appropriate musculoskeletal alignment, and maintenance of passive mobility when active motion is not possible. Proper body and extremity position must be maintained at all times and can be accomplished through positioning techniques and posture supports at the bed, wheelchair, or ambulatory level.

Musculoskeletal alignment often can be maintained effectively by splinting or casting. An example is the patient with traumatic brain injury who exhibits severe spasticity, which may be exacerbated by a dominance of abnormal reflexes and hyperresponsive central and autonomic nervous systems (Fig. 5-1). Without appropriate therapeutic intervention, these patients will develop contractures and shortened muscle-tendon units. Management of spasticity must

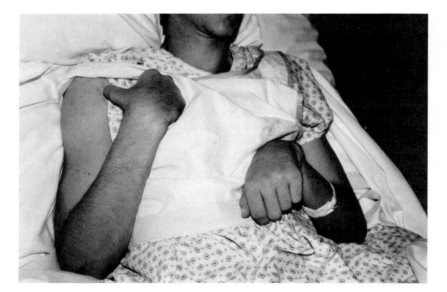

Fig. 5-1. Splints or casts are effective in maintaining musculoskeletal alignment.

Fig. 5-2. Motor nerve block injection is useful in selected patients.

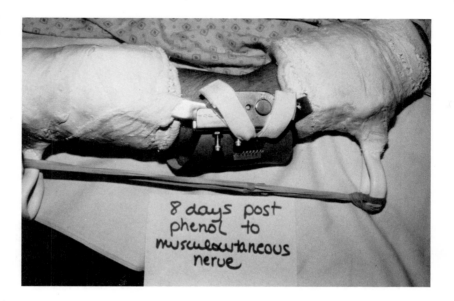

8 days post phenol to musculocutaneous nerve

be individual, with some patients being good candidates for local and surgical motor nerve block injection (Fig. 5-2). Others can be managed effectively by inhibitive casting. The important theme, whether managed therapeutically or surgically, is that a *preventive*, proactive approach to patient care is undertaken.

Splints can be used to support, protect, or immobilize joints, as in the case of the injured, diseased, or healing extremity (Fig. 5-3). In some cases, splints can provide support and gentle, prolonged stretch (Fig. 5-4). They may also be designed to prevent deformity by substituting for weak or absent muscle strength, as can be seen in ulnar nerve neuropathy, in which a

simple short opponens splint with lumbrical support can prevent unnecessary clawing of the hand.

In addition to appropriate position and alignment, prevention programs also have the goal of achieving and maintaining range of motion. Splints or casts can be used to transfer force dynamically from an immobilized joint to mobilize a stiff joint. For example, if the metacarpophalangeal (MCP) joints are stiff and the proximal (PIP) and distal (DIP) interphalangeal joints are mobile, when a patient attempts to flex the fingers, the interphalangeal joints will flex first, and the MCP joints may or may not move actively. Blocking exercises encourage movement of stiff joints, and splinting or casting can do the same (Fig. 5-5). In

Fig. 5-3. A dorsal hand resting splint will maintain good wrist and hand alignment in the presence of mild to moderate spasticity.

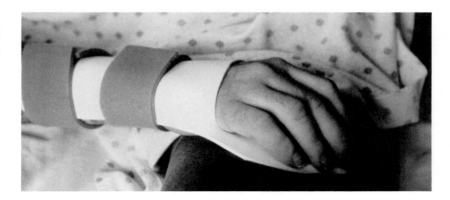

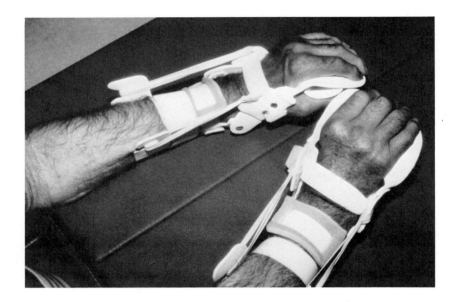

Fig. 5-4. This 75-year-old man with spinal cord injury lacked sufficient wrist extension for a functional tenodesis and required bilateral dynamic wrist extension splints.

cases in which there is a combination of soft tissue contracture coupled with tendon shortening, it may be necessary to use dynamic forces to attempt correction. A combination of casting and dynamic splinting is often required to provide gentle, controlled elongation of tissues (Fig. 5-6).

The introduction of continuous passive motion (CPM) devices as an adjunct to manual passive joint range-of-motion exercises has revolutionized therapy (Fig. 5-7). Occupational therapists are no longer limited by shortage of persons to perform the manual task or by the limitations of even the most "dynamic"

of splints. Formal and informal clinical studies are demonstrating the efficacy of CPM, and there is little doubt that this method is an important contribution to orthopaedic rehabilitation programs. Coutts[6] has shown that the use of CPM after total knee replacement improves venous dynamics and overall healing, resulting in earlier active motion. Gelberman and colleagues[7] reported that early mobilization promotes an intrinsic healing process that not only results in less scarring but also leads to tissues that ultimately may be stronger. Although specific parameters of intensity and duration are yet to be defined for some diagnoses, the success of CPM lies in

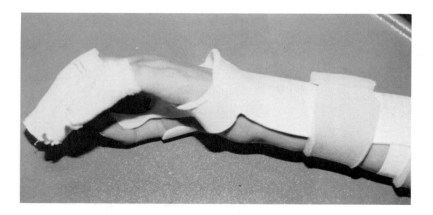

Fig. 5-5. A combination of splinting and casting was used to encourage active motion with these stiff MCP joints.

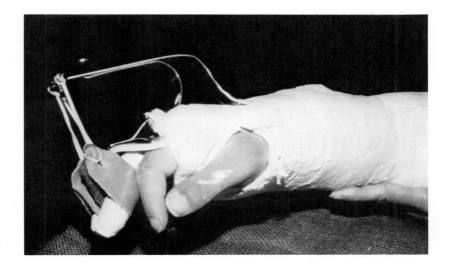

Fig. 5-6. Casting and dynamic splinting were used to provide gentle prolonged stretch after median nerve phenol block in this spastic head-injured patient.

the basic premise that early application promotes healing and prevents unnecessary problems associated with immobility.

Preparation for Function

Preparation for function may be the most challenging and critical goal of occupational therapy. With the orthopaedic patient, the role of the therapist is to be an evaluator of the problem, an engineer and artist, a teacher and motivator.

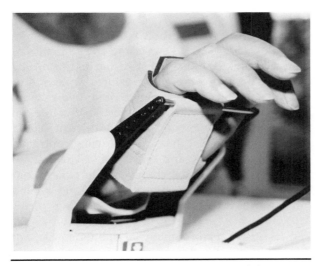

Fig. 5-7. Wrist CPM is helpful in treatment of this patient after Colles' fracture.

An occupational therapist must have an understanding of anatomy and physiology to be a good evaluator. To measure range of motion, the therapist should have both knowledge of the joint structures and an understanding of their relationship to movement. Knowledge of muscle innervation is important, as is knowing the various measures of muscle strength from manual muscle testing to gross grasp. At least a basic understanding of neuroanatomic structures and the afferent and efferent pathways that produce normal (and sometimes abnormal) motor responses also is necessary. Sensation is a very complex function, and the occupational therapist must be knowledgeable about peripheral nerve pathways and innervations, and also understand the role of the central nervous system in perception of pain, in kinesthesia, and in proprioception. A great deal of research is being done in the area of orthopaedics, and occupational therapists must keep current to ensure that proper evaluation techniques are being used. Current, objective evaluation tools are essential to record baseline information from which progress can be easily and readily measured; general and subjective observation of patient progress is not acceptable. Standard goniometer, dynameter, and pinch gauge measurements must be supplemented by measurable volumetric and sensory tests. The effectiveness of exercise programs can be measured by machines such as the Baltimore Therapeutic Equipment (BTE) work simulator.

Occupational therapists who design splints and equipment and analyze environmental conditions need the ability to conceptualize and create, and thus they must have a knowledge of engineering principles and the skills and finesse of an artist. The real "art" of therapy, however, is in making an identified problem into a working prop for functional recovery.

Positioning for Function

Positioning can be a very complex challenge with the patient who has low-level head injury. If the patient's posture is not in good central alignment, not only can premature uninhibited reflexes dominate, but in addition the patient is left in an unsupported and unbalanced position, which encourages deformity. Similarly, proximal stability is essential to encourage distal movement and control; therefore, all therapeutic intervention is depends on good central alignment.

Arm positioning devices, which provide support and mobility, often represent the difference between dependence and independence. Mobile and radial arm supports, originally designed for use with poliomyelitis patients, are excellent examples of proximal supports that allow poor to fair muscles to work in a gravity-free plane for functional activities such as eating.

Splinting for Function

Functional splints may be divided into three categories: those that *maintain position* of the hand or wrist; those that *substitute* for weak or absent muscle strength; and those that provide a *base of support for adaptive appliances.*

Splints can be designed to maintain position of the hand or wrist with the goal of providing stability for a weak, injured, or healing structure while allowing mobility and function. This type of splint is commonly used with the arthritic patient, as well as in conjunction with cumulative trauma disorder, in which the primary problem is tendinitis, tenosynovitis, or nerve compression. A functional splint that is commonly used with high median nerve problems is the long opponens splint (Fig. 5-8) and a splint used with low median nerve problems is the short opponens splint (Fig. 5-9). Both of these splints provide position and support for functional prehension by placing the thumb in apposition to the index and middle fingers.

A second category of functional splints includes those that substitute for weak or absent muscle strength. A classic example of this splint is a wrist-driven tenodesis splint, which uses wrist extension as the power source to drive the fingers into flexion to oppose a stabilized thumb (Fig. 5-10). This splint was originally designed for the poliomyelitis patient, and the technology was later used in caring for patients with cervical spinal cord lesions who had limited wrist extension but no distal hand function. Patients who sustain peripheral nerve damage also benefit from this type of splint. Patients who have a radial nerve lesion or palsy lose the ability to extend the wrist, fingers, or thumb volitionally. Although they have normal wrist and finger flexion, they may be unable to hold the wrist in a neutral position or release objects from the fingers and thumb volitionally. In this case, a dynamic extension splint maintains wrist position while allowing the fingers to "rest" in an extended position. Rubber bands allow the fingers to be flexed actively but will dynamically bring the fingers back into an extended position. The splint not only acts to maintain soft tissue structures in their proper alignment but also acts as a functional splint, allowing the patient to pick up, hold, and release objects.

Complex orthopaedic problems sometimes require complex splints (Fig. 5-11). During one patient's fall from a horse, the horse crushed her left arm. She sustained several compound fractures of the radius and ulna and faced a long period of immobilization. Rather than place her in a long arm cast after internal fixation, the hand surgeon ordered a thermoplastic splint with a hinge at the elbow allowing controlled motion at the elbow and wrist joints. This patient required no additional corrective surgery, her rehabilitation period was less than predicted, and her end function was excellent.

The last category of functional splints consists of those that provide a base of support for adaptive appliances. A splint can be as simple as a universal cuff providing support for feeding utensils or as complex as a ratchet-driven wrist tenodesis splint used

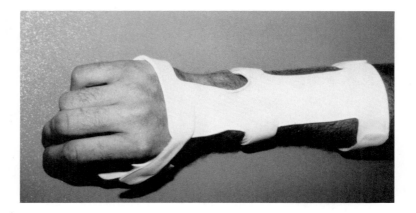

Fig. 5-8. Long opponens splint for high median nerve problems.

with high cervical spinal cord lesions. These orthoses take the specialized training of a orthotist to fabricate and require many hours of therapy for functional training.

A well-designed splint can stabilize structures while allowing freedom of movement in joints that do not require complete immobilization. The key to successful splinting is to provide stability when needed and to allow mobility when possible.

Patient and Family Education

Teaching and motivating are integral to the process of preparing a patient for function. A great deal of therapy is oriented toward preventive teaching (e.g., joint protection and energy conservation techniques for

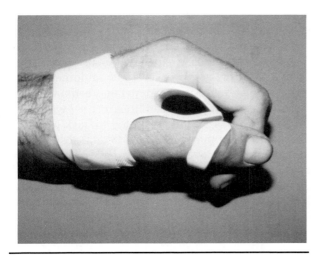

Fig. 5-9. Short opponens splint for low median nerve problems.

the patient with arthritis and hip fracture). Patient education is critical, ranging from simple wound care to the very complex problems associated with arthritis and diabetes. The key to promoting maximal health and independence is developing the patient's ability to be in control and take responsibility for self-care. This can only be done if there is knowledge of the "how to's" and a willingness to assume responsibility. Educating the family or caregiver also has become increasingly important as length of inpatient and outpatient treatment has decreased and patients are discharged at lower functional levels. Families must be taught the principles of prevention and functional enhancement to maximize rehabilitation potential.

Promotion of Independence

With maximal independence as an end goal of therapy, the occupational therapist sets the stage for the process to begin on day one. The props for functional recovery are very important, but they have their greatest impact within the context of a functional environment that is created by the therapist. A functional environment is realistic and meaningful rather than contrived, and it elicits interest, provides motivation, and rewards work well done. This is true whether designing treatment goals around self-care activities for a patient or working with an injured worker whose treatment goals will allow return to work.

Activities of daily living (ADL) is a phrase that is commonly associated with self-care tasks; in reality, it entails everything a person does from the time of

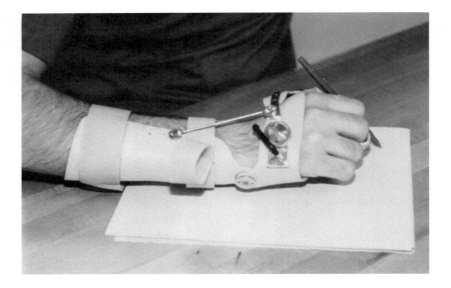

Fig. 5-10. Wrist-driven tenodesis splint used functionally.

waking up in the morning until retiring at night. Naturally, these activities vary from person to person, because life circumstances and demands are very different and activities are meaningful only if they relate to real-life situations. Designing realistic and meaningful treatment activities is the hallmark of occupational therapy, and this is where the skills and experience of the individual therapist are most evident.

Functional environments are the optimal place for therapy, whether a kitchen, a bathroom, a garden, the community, or the workplace. Driving rehabilitation is a good example of how specialized assessment and adaptation can provide a vital link to independence. Driving requires a challenging interaction among visual, cognitive, and perceptual systems, motor responsiveness, and control. It is a complex function that people tend to take for granted until it is no longer possible. A good driving assessment can screen out potentially dangerous drivers from those who can be safe and independent, either with specialized equipment or with instruction. The cost of providing this program is minimal in comparison to the price of having potentially unsafe drivers on the road or of public assistance for transporting people who could otherwise be independently mobile. Driver rehabilitation exemplifies realistic, meaningful, and functional therapy.

Another example of a realistic and meaningful therapy environment is found in work programs. Although occupational therapists have long been involved in evaluating an injured worker's physical status, it was not until the mid-1970s that return-to-work programs evolved. The term *work hardening* was first used at Rancho Los Amigos Hospital to describe a nontraditional therapy program that bridged the gap between acute therapy and return to competitive employment. Work injuries have claimed the attention of persons in industry administration and management, because large sums of money must be allocated to workmen's compensation and medical treatment. The social and economic consequences of workplace injuries are enormous, involving not only lost wages and medical expenses but also production delays, lost time of coworkers, and equipment damage. The National Safety Council has estimated that the total cost of workplace injuries in 1987 was $42.4 billion, with $14 billion attributed to back injuries.[8] Cumulative traumatic disorders take a close second and are posing an even greater threat as new, sophisticated technologic advances result in more biomechanical stress placed on the deconditioned musculoskeletal system. Some authors postulate that automation has relieved some of the physical labor, only to create a potentially more hazardous stress from static and constrained postures necessary to operate automated equipment. The concept of work

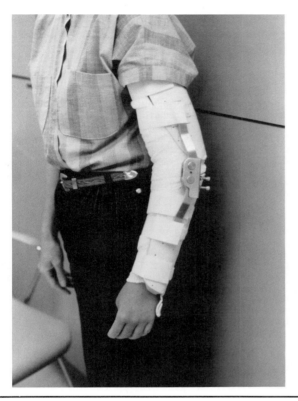

Fig. 5-11. Thermoplastic splint with hinge at elbow was used for complex orthopaedic injuries.

hardening recognizes the need for actual work or simulated work tasks to build physical endurance and tolerance to overcome the biomechanical stress associated with specific jobs. The graded, work-oriented treatment emphasizes improvement in the biomechanical, neuromuscular, cardiovascular, and psychological functions of the individual, because it is a combination of these factors that permits a return to work.

The therapist must consider all factors that influence a person's ability to work, not the least of which are the actual job methods and techniques. This often requires a job site visit to evaluate the work environment so that a therapy program can be designed or recommendations offered for job modifications. It is becoming more cost-effective for companies with large numbers of work-related injuries to offer therapy services on site, and this offers an ideal opportunity for therapists to work directly with the employer on developing prevention programs. Employers are also seeing the value in industrial consultations that offer techniques in stress management, back injury prevention, and education regarding cumulative trauma disorders in the workplace. Employers, especially those who are self-insured, are seeing a window of opportunity to save health care dollars by supporting prevention and wellness in the workplace.

Physical capacity evaluation (PCE) is used as an assessment tool after a work injury has occurred. Rather than being a generic evaluation, the PCE is designed to provide a realistic assessment of the injured worker's physical capacity in relation to specific work demands. Environmental factors, personal traits and attitudes, and specific work requirements are addressed and collectively represent the most limiting issues affecting return to work. For example, a patient may be able to perform a job physically, but not at the pace that is demanded by the employer expected by the employee who is paid by piecework. In some cases, it may be the worker's own fear that prevents return to work. The first step in helping a person return to work is to identify the problems and issues, and a PCE is invaluable in providing this type of information.

FUTURE ISSUES

The future of occupational therapy, and of all rehabilitation professions, will depend upon the ability to be responsive to changing health care needs and on proving the efficacy of treatment. There will be even more emphasis on specialization, to the extent that certifications in specialty areas will be encouraged and perhaps required. Occupational therapists must continue to explore and use objective evaluations that are valid and reliable and to apply scientific methods to examine treatment methods that are employed. Research and efficacy studies need to be completed to establish standards and treatment protocols for specific problems and to ensure that patients are treated on the basis of individual need rather than a general diagnosis only. Generic treatment protocols have become outdated, and occupational therapists need advanced, reasonable, and efficient treatment protocols to replace them. Functional outcome must be monitored closely to provide support for appropriate levels of therapeutic intervention and to aid in determining how health care dollars are best spent.

All professionals who contribute to the process of rehabilitation can learn to prevent, prepare, and promote: *prevent* the use of unnecessary and costly procedures that have no efficacy studies to support them: *prepare* for changes in the health care delivery system so that therapists are in a proactive position of stating what is needed, rather than constantly reacting to regulations based on dollars versus need; and *promote* an environment for patients that reinforces prevention, health, wellness, and functional independence. Above all, as the 21st century approaches in a technologically advanced society, it must be remembered that rehabilitation is a "high-touch" medical specialty that recognizes and reinforces human spirit and motivation as fundamental to successful rehabilitation.

REFERENCES

1. Gullickson G, Licht S: Definition and philosophy of rehabilitation medicine. p.1. In Licht S (ed): Rehabilitation Medicine. Elizabeth Licht, New Haven, CT, 1968
2. Nickel VL, McGough C: Model of a hand rehabilitation center. p.927. In Hunter JM, Schneider LC, Macklin EJ, Callahan AD (eds): Rehabilitation of the Hand. 2nd ed. CV Mosby, St. Louis, 1984
3. Naisbitt J: Megatrends. Warner Books, New York, 1984
4. Engel GL: The need for a new medical model: a challenge for biomedicine. Science 196:129, 1977
5. McGough C: Introduction to CPM. JBCR 9:494, 1988
6. Coutts RD: Continuous passive motion in the rehabilitation of the total knee patient, its role and effect. Orthop Rev 15:126, 1986
7. Gelberman RH, Vande Berg JS, Goran NL, Akeson WH: Flexor tendon healing and restoration of the gliding surface. J Bone Joint Surg [AM] 65:70,1983
8. National Committee for Injury Prevention and Control: Occupational injuries. p.177. In: Injury Prevention: Meeting the Challenge. Oxford University Press, New York, 1989

6 Speech-Language Pathology

ANN KOENEKE-VARLEY

Communication can be defined as: "to impart or transfer something intangible; an exchange of information through a common system of symbols."[1] By this definition, then, a person with a communication disorder has a decreased or limited ability to exchange information (e.g., facts). Perhaps more importantly, a communication disorder limits a person's ability to exchange thoughts and feelings. Communication disorders include speech, language, and hearing impairments. Speech-language pathologists diagnose and treat persons with communication disorders. They practice in varied settings, including schools, community clinics, hospitals, rehabilitation centers, skilled nursing facilities, and military and veteran facilities. Because of the variety and extent of communication disorders and their causes, speech-language pathologists must work with professionals in many other fields to ensure the optimal outcome for their clients.

Communication is the essence of people's existence. It gives them the control and purpose in their lives. It is, therefore, a speech-language pathologist's mission to help those with communication disorders to regain their ability to control their lives through communicating.

HISTORY AND EMERGENCE OF THE PROFESSION

Speech-language pathology is a relatively young field. The practice of speech pathology emerged in the United States in the early 1900s. At that time, the greatest amount of information and training came from speech pathologists in Europe. In 1925, a small group of professionals met and established the American Academy of Speech Correction. This group focused on the study of speech disorders and their treatment. The significance of the relationship between speech and hearing was recognized by the Academy in 1947. This resulted in a change of the organization's name to American Speech and Hearing Association. It was at this time that audiologists were included in the Association. Finally, in 1978, the Association adopted its present name, American Speech-Language-Hearing Association (ASHA). This change was intended to recognize that the profession was involved not only with speech and hearing deficits but also with communication problems that included language disorders. The changes in name were not the only ones made in the short history of communication disorders. The professionals themselves have had many name changes, from speech therapists and speech correctionists to speech clinicians and finally to speech-language pathologists.

QUALIFICATIONS AND PROFESSIONAL STANDARDS OF THE SPEECH-LANGUAGE PATHOLOGIST

The American Speech-Hearing-Language Association sets the standards of practice for speech-language pathologists. ASHA issues certificates of clinical competence in speech-language pathology to persons who have a master's degree or the equivalent with major emphasis in speech-language pathology, who have had 9 months of full-time professional experience (the Clinical Fellowship Year, or the equivalent), and who have passed the National Examination in Speech-Language Pathology.[2]

NATURE OF COMMUNICATION DISORDERS IN THE REHABILITATION SETTING

Speech-language pathologists treat a wide variety of disorders and persons of all ages in many different settings. For the purposes of this text, the discussion that follows illustrates more specifically the role of the speech-language pathologist in the rehabilitation setting. In this setting, the patient populations that most frequently have speech-language disorders are those who have incurred some form of neurologic injury, such as a cerebro-vascular accident (CVA) or a brain injury. Communication disorders that typically result from these injuries can be classified within the areas of language, speech, or cognitive disorders.

Language Disorders

Aphasia is "an impairment in language functioning following localized cerebral damage that results in a reduced likelihood that an individual involved in a communicative situation will understand or produce appropriate verbal formulations."[3] The term *aphasia* is broad, and frequently definitions do not provide a basis for differentiating aphasia from other communication disorders. It is important to know and understand the entities that are generally encompassed by the term to best assist the patient, family, and team working with that patient. "The aphasic patient's difficulty is in the processing of the language code, however received or expressed, whether by listening, reading, speaking, writing, or gesturing."[4]

Impaired Comprehension of Spoken Language: Auditory Comprehension Disorder

Patients with severe auditory comprehension disorders may not be able to understand the meaning of single words spoken to them. They can hear the words, but the words are just not meaningful. Less severe auditory comprehension deficits are manifested in an inability to understand lengthy or complex messages.

Impaired Comprehension of Written Language: Reading Comprehension Disorder

Patients with reading comprehension disorders may not be able to match a simple printed word to an object or picture, or they may be able to read words but cannot read sentences or paragraphs.

Impaired Formulation of Spoken Language: Language Expression Disorder

Disorders of language formulation are varied and often described with a number of different terms, such as anomia, Wernicke's aphasia, and global aphasia. Suffice it to say that the categorizations and descriptions of language expression disorders are not agreed on among speech-language pathologists owing to the intricate nature of language.

The severity and symptoms of an expressive language disorder are determined primarily by the cause, size, and site of the cortical lesion. A person may omit or misuse grammatical structures, may have difficulty recalling a specific word, may produce unintelligible sound combinations, or may not be able to say more than a single word—or even have no output at all. Perhaps the biggest difficulty in categorizing an expressive language disorder is that it is rarely, if ever, isolated or pure; rather, it most probably accompanies or is affected by cognitive, speech, or auditory comprehension disorders.

Impaired Formulation of Written Language: Written Expression Disorder

Written expression disorders can run the gamut from an inability to form letters to the production of meaningless word combinations and from forming incomplete sentences to forming complete sentences but with errors in spelling or syntax.

Speech Disorders

Dysarthria

The term *dysarthria* is used to describe speech disorders that are caused by central or peripheral neurologic damage. In contrast to aphasic patients, who have difficulty with symbolic coding of language, dysarthric patients have difficulty with the production aspect—that is, with speech execution. A patient with dysarthria may have difficulty in movement or coordination of any one or all of the systems of respiration, phonation, articulation, resonance, and prosody.

Apraxia

Speech production impairments, referred to as apraxia, result from a disturbance of the sensorimotor processes that initiate, execute, control, monitor, and adjust the selection and sequential ordering of speech muscle movements for the purposeful production of speech. Some characteristics that may be found in apraxic patients are visible and/or audible searching for target phonemes, greater ease or ability in production of automatic than volitional speech, difficulty with initiation of speech, and an ability to self-correct output errors.

Cognitive Disorders

The area of cognitive disorders is extremely complex and far too vast to describe here in any great detail. As an overview, general cognitive characteristics that may be seen in brain-injured patients or patients who have incurred a CVA, particularly a right-sided CVA, are poor memory, both short and long term; impaired reasoning and judgment; disorientation to time, person, and/or place; reduced recognition of, understanding of, and responsiveness to the environment; and inappropriate behaviors.

Dysphagia

In addition to the communication disorders mentioned previously, speech-language pathologists may also evaluate and treat patients with dysphagia, a dysfunction of the swallowing process. This disorder may result from neurologic or structural problems. Dysphagia can lead to inadequate nutritional intake or pneumonia.

SPEECH PATHOLOGY: CLINICAL MANAGEMENT

Speech-language pathologists perform a wide variety of services related to communication disorders. For the purpose of this text (i.e., explaining the role of a speech-language pathologist in a rehabilitation setting), the services can be classified as screening, evaluation, therapy, counseling, and consultation. Screening is the basic process of determining whether or not a communication disorder exists. An evaluation seeks to determine whether a communication disorder is present, and, if present, the degree of severity or the amount of impairment the communication disorder will cause the client. The evaluation should include recommendations, the therapy plan, and the prognosis or expected outcome. The evaluation also should provide information that will assist other professionals who will be communicating with or working with the client. Therapy services are those activities constituting the plan of treatment designed to ameliorate or compensate for the communication disorder. Counseling services are provided to help the client or family member, or both, deal most effectively with the communication disorder and with the problems that may result from it. Consultation services are provided by the speech-language pathologist to other professionals working with the client to make the best use of the time they spend with the client.

SPEECH-LANGUAGE PATHOLOGISTS: MEMBERS OF THE REHABILITATION TEAM

Traditionally, rehabilitation has been multidisciplinary, that is, a series of individual disciplines each evaluating and treating patients and, at varying points in time, informing the other team members of the focus of their treatment. The role of the speech-language pathologist on a multidisciplinary team, then, is to evaluate the nature and extent of a communication disorder in patients and to direct treatment toward remediation of that disorder. Although this may seem like a reasonable goal, because of the nature and extent of physical, cognitive, and emotional complications occurring after a stroke or brain injury, the process is not as efficient, as an interdisciplinary approach, nor does it have the far-reaching effectiveness of the latter approach.

An interdisciplinary approach provides the structure for the various disciplines to work together to discuss the goals of the patient, to plan jointly, and, therefore, work more effectively and efficiently toward the discharge outcomes. The speech-language pathologist's role in this interdisciplinary model is to see that all team members understand and use the best means possible to communicate with the patient. This ensures a greater understanding on the patient's part of the goals of the program, the patient's role and, most importantly, the patient's input in progressing toward the goals.

FUTURE DIRECTIONS IN SPEECH-LANGUAGE PATHOLOGY

As with all health care professions, the future of speech-language pathology is inextricably linked with governmental and insurance standards. As a profession, speech-language pathology must examine social, political, economical, and technological trends to ensure that it survives the uncertainties of an ever-changing industry. Speech-language pathologists must realize that the public is better informed and, therefore, more insistent on quality services. In seeming opposition to this trend, socio-economic conditions appear to be worsening and health care costs are rising. To ensure success, speech-language pathologists must face these issues head-on and act to bring about a brighter future.

REFERENCES

1. Webster's Seventh New Collegiate Dictionary. G & C Merriam Company, Springfield, MA, 1970
2. American Speech-Language-Hearing Association: Requirements for the Certificates of Clinical Competence. American Speech-Language-Hearing Association, Rockville, MD, 1990
3. Eisenson J: Adult Aphasia, Assessment and Treatment. Prentice-Hall, Englewood Cliffs, NJ, 1973
4. Darley FL: Aphasia. WB Saunders, Philadelphia, 1982

7 Social Work Services

HONORA K. WILSON
RUTH COX BRUNINGS

The social worker diagnoses and treats any of the patient's social and emotional problems that affect health and ability to benefit from medical care. The social worker by professional training is a specialist with expertise in helping individuals and families deal with personal problems that arise when they are faced with illness and disability. The psychosocial aspects of illness and disability are as profound as their physical symptoms.[1] The social worker's dual responsibility is to resolve the individual patient's psychosocial problems and at the same time to make changes in the health care delivery system to ensure that the psychosocial needs of all patients are met.[2]

HISTORY AND EMERGENCE OF THE PROFESSION

The specialty of medical social work in the profession of social work was inaugurated by a distinguished physician, Dr. Richard C. Cabot, Chief of Staff of the Massachusetts General Hospital in Boston. As the director of the Boston Children's Aid Society, he had observed social workers in action, sat in on case discussions, and studied case records. Later, when he saw some of the same children in the clinic, he realized how much better he understood them and their diseases through his knowledge of their psychosocial histories. He believed that, for a complete diagnosis, it was necessary to have information about a patient's home, diet, work, family, and personal problems.[3]

The realization of the close dependence of a person's physical well-being on his mental and socioeconomic condition resulted in the formation of the first social work department in the Massachusetts General Hospital in 1905. Ida Cannon was appointed by Dr.

Cabot as the first medical social worker in the United States.

From the beginning of this century, social work in hospitals expanded in a natural sequence from settings in public hospitals to university hospitals, nonprofit and sectarian hospitals, proprietary hospitals, and independent practice in the community. The expansion of social work in medical settings has occurred because of (1) increased knowledge in the behavioral sciences of the significance of social and emotional factors on physical health; (2) increased concern for medical care in the field of public welfare; (3) development of public health programs on local, state, federal, and international levels; and (4) development of special rehabilitation programs.

Today more than 80 percent of all United States hospitals have social work services. Moreover, the provision of social work services to patients is a standard for accreditation by the Joint Commission on Accreditation of Healthcare Organizations and for state licensure (Title 22 in California). The health care field employs the majority of all social workers in the United States.

SPECIAL QUALIFICATIONS

Formal professional education for social work dates from at least 1898.[5] Today the educational requirement for the professional social worker is a master's degree from an accredited school of social work. The master's degree takes 2 years to earn, and 99 accredited colleges and universities in the United States and four in Canada award it. Two-thirds to one-half of each semester's hours must be spent in clinical practice with supervision by a social worker with a master's degree. Education for the master's degree covers five major areas: human behavior and the social environment, social welfare policy and services, social work treatment modalities, research, and clinical practice. The social worker in a medical setting also takes specialized courses in the medical aspects of social work practice and has a clinical internship in a health care program. The social worker with a master's degree is the primary agent in the delivery of social work and carries responsibility for the provision of direct services to patients and families.

In California, a social worker can secure a license as a clinical social worker after 2 years of supervised practice followed by successful completion of written and oral examinations. There are now licensure laws in all but 6 states, where licensure bills are in process. These standards assure patients and the community that the clinical social worker has met professional educational requirements and has demonstrated clinical competence. Licensed clinical social workers can be expected to provide highly skilled, independent practice in psychosocial treatment of patients and families.

Forty-eight accredited colleges and universities in the United States and two in Canada now grant a doctoral degree in social work. Persons with such degrees are usually found in teaching, research, and administration. Numerous hospitals with large departments of social work have administrators with doctoral degrees.

Three hundred and sixty-five colleges and universities in the United States and two in Canada offer a bachelor's degree in social welfare. To meet accreditation standards, persons with such degrees must be supervised by social workers with master's degrees. Social work assistants are found more frequently in large departments of social work and their duties are largely confined to performing specific tasks for patients — tasks that require concern for patients and awareness of community resources, but not professional knowledge and skills. Sometimes small hospitals employ social workers with bachelor's degrees and contract for supervision by social workers with master's degrees. After a year or two of work experience, a social worker with a bachelor's degree tends to return to college or university to obtain a master's degree in social work.

In addition to the professional social work staff, social work assistants are trained on the job to perform concrete, specific tasks delegated by and under the supervision of the social worker. Increasingly, persons with a bachelor's degree in social welfare are being employed as social work assistants.

THE SOCIAL WORKER'S CONTRIBUTIONS AND FUNCTIONS IN REHABILITATION

The patient confronted by serious illness, particularly chronic illness, must undertake a variety of tasks to negotiate the process of rehabilitation. These have been described as illness-related and general adaptive tasks. Activities related to illness involve facing pain and incapacitation, dealing with the hospital environment and special treatment procedures, and developing adequate relationships with the professional health care staff. The general adaptations a patient must make include preserving a reasonable emotional balance, maintaining a satisfactory self-image, preserving relationships with family and friends, and preparing for an uncertain future.[6]

Social work services are directly involved with the general adaptive tasks. Sometimes the medical staff requests the social worker's participation in the illness-related tasks. The social worker intervenes with both the patient and the family to assist in difficulties or adjustments having to do with work, finances, living arrangements, social life, marriage, child care, and emotional life. The social worker recognizes that acquired or congenital disability may affect the person's self-esteem and relationships with other people, including the family. Chronic illnesses may also produce emotional, financial, and sexual problems that may retard recovery.

Psychosocial Assessment

The social worker's primary task is to make a psychosocial assessment,[7] that is, an evaluation of the patient as a person and the impact of the illness on the person's ability to cope with medical treatment and

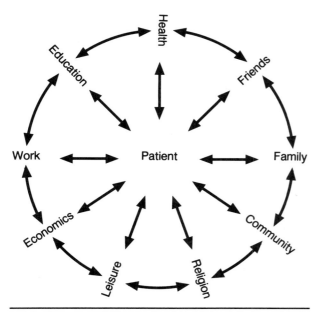

Fig. 7-1. Nine basic social systems interact with each other, influence a patient's social functioning, and together constitute a total social support system.

rehabilitation. In this role, social workers function in three areas of the treatment system. First, they use their knowledge and skill to assess the patients' social functioning and their capacity to cope with illness. Second, in assessing the impact of the patient's illness on the family, they determine where the family fits into the treatment system, particularly as part of the patient's support system (Fig. 7-1). Third, social workers share and interpret their assessments with the rest of the health care team. These assessments influence all questions of management and treatment procedures for the patient.

Studies in the field of chronic illness have suggested that specific and predictable phases of adjustment exist through which most patients must pass to achieve resolution of emotional trauma and successful rehabilitation. For most illnesses and disabilities, the phases seem to be as follows. First come confusion, doubt, and uncertainty. These emotions frequently are followed by denial, resulting in aggressive behavior, euphoria, and inappropriate defense mechanisms. This stage is followed by depression as the patient perceives reality. After the depression is worked through, the patient is able to reassess the

situation and move to some level of acceptance and adjustment.[8]

Just as the patient must go through several phases of adjustment until there is a restitution of self, so does the family experience the same evolution. For the family there is loss and grief, new roles, and change of status, followed by realignment of persons and social systems, and finally an adjustment to a new style of living. Family members also have pain over the guilt they experience. The guilt comes from unresolved anger, ambivalence, fears, and a desire to escape from the patient and the whole problem. When guilt is recognized, accepted, and worked through, the family is able to move to problem solving, to making necessary decisions, to participating with the health care team, and to remaining involved with the patient.

In rehabilitation facilities, all patients and their families are interviewed at the time of admission by the social worker. The social assessment made then consists of the following factors[9]:

1. Any adjustment problems prior to illness.
2. Social, emotional, and economic problems created or intensified by the illness.
3. The patient's goals in life and how they may need to be redirected.
4. People important to the patient.
5. The nature of interpersonal relationships.
6. Usual social roles and present role changes.
7. Emotional reactions to impaired physical condition and the hospital environment.
8. The nature of coping mechanisms.
9. Expectations of the rehabilitation program.
10. Social resources and personal strengths.
11. Specific behaviors and attitudes that suggest mental illness, such as severe anxiety, depression, excessive grief, or suicidal ideation.

With this outline as a guide, and with information from interviews with the patient, family, friends, community agencies, and other team members, the social worker makes a psychosocial diagnosis and treatment plan. The social worker then shares important information with the rest of the treatment team to help them understand the significant social and emotional factors of the person's health problem and assist in their total evaluation and individualized treatment of the patient.

Team Conference

This psychosocial diagnosis, although important to all team members, is of highest priority for the physician and the nurse. It is this knowledge that enables the physician to understand the patient's reaction to the medical environment, to the illness, and especially to surgical intervention. Knowledge of the patient's emotional status enables the surgeon to discuss an operation with an understanding of what it means to the patient. Thus, the surgeon can realistically explain the intervention to the patient in terms of who is giving support to the patient, what the surgery threatens in relation to economic survival, how the patient's family views disability, what the patient's fears are, and what the prospect of surgery stirs up in the patient's unconscious. All surgeons, but perhaps orthopaedic surgeons in particular, need to take pride in their own great skill in restoration, but also they must not be disappointed when the patient is less than enthusiastic or responsive to the proposed surgery. The literature is full of references to the repressed anger of patients at an operation that removes a limb or modifies it. This anger is aimed only indirectly at the surgeon. It primarily is the way in which many patients express their psychic pain of illness and disability. When the social worker shares with the surgeon some of the pain, some of the disappointment, some of the failures in the patient's life, the surgeon is better able to hear and understand the repressed anger when explaining surgery. Some patients can be identified as poor surgical risks because of acute or chronic psychosocial problems.

The same knowledge of the family, the major factor in the patient's support system, can reinforce the surgeon's ability to interpret to the family what can be expected from the operation. The family support system is the major force on which the health team can rely for successful rehabilitation. With knowledge of the family's hopes, fears, and disappointments, the physician can better deal with their expectations for treatment and rehabilitation.

The psychosocial assessment becomes important knowledge for the nurse in the daily care of the patient. Information from the social worker can help the nurse understand the patient better, know what approach to use for maximum cooperation, and maintain nonjudgmental attitudes.

The main vehicle through which the social worker shares the data from the psychosocial assessment is the team conference. As these data are shared, all members of the team look at their own specific assessment with new insights as to how the patient and family will go through the medical treatment system. The psychosocial diagnosis is discussed and interpreted in the team conference. Medical care as a comprehensive plan now includes a humanistic assessment of the patient's needs for psychosocial treatment.

Psychosocial Treatment

As the psychosocial diagnosis and assessment continue with the patient, the social worker offers treatment in the areas of identified need. The treatment modalities of social work include individual psychotherapy, environmental therapy, advocacy therapy, group therapy, conjoint and family therapy, sexual counseling, and play therapy.

The psychosocial treatment given in individual one-to-one interviews can be advice, information, counseling, or psychotherapy.[10] The social worker listens to the patients' fears about their bodies, their selves, their changes in role, and the unknowns of medical treatment. The social worker helps patients express their fears and anxieties and find emotional support for this experience.

As patients begin to feel relief from emotional tensions, the social worker intervenes in each area of need. If patients are concerned about money, help in securing financial assistance is given; if they are concerned about living arrangements, various housing alternatives are reviewed; if they worry about returning to work or change of work, referrals are made to vocational counselors. As the patients begin to deal with the physical and social limitations attendant on their illness, the social worker helps them if they are not able to do this themselves. Environmental therapy may include assistance with negotiating the bureaucratic requirements of the public financial assistance system, securing vocational counseling, appropriate housing, homemaker, and home health aide assistance, home nursing services, and transportation. The aforementioned services are also offered to the family, as a part of the patient's support system.

Advocacy for the patient is a traditional role of the social worker and has high priority in the social worker's arena of function. Advocacy becomes imperative as more and more social services are available and as the social systems become more complicated and more difficult to negotiate. The social worker also is an advocate for the patient in the medical system. As medicine becomes more complex and as the medical system adds more team members, the distance between the patient and the physician becomes broader and the risk of dehumanization becomes greater. The social worker continually intervenes to help the individual patient and to effect changes in the health care delivery system on behalf of human dignity.

Group treatment is a major tool in the social worker's armamentarium, and it can be offered at any time in the course of the patient's medical experience. The social worker offers a variety of group experiences and uses different group techniques. Group treatment can be educational or therapeutic or a combination of both. Group treatment can be given for patients, families, or patients and families. Peer groups are an important part of sharing experiences in chronic illness. The patient can be brought into a group at any time when the social worker ascertains the patient's need and readiness. Groups meet on a regular basis for 60 to 90 minutes. They are primarily for support, sharing of physical and psychic pain, problem-solving, and expression of feelings. The social worker shares with the rest of the treatment team any significant feelings expressed during the group sessions, but the content is kept confidential. Other groups that perform some of the foregoing and other functions are patient education groups. Usually the social worker organizes and plans these groups with all members of the team or individual team members throughout a series of meetings.

Social workers increasingly are offering group treatments for the families and significant others in the patient's life. These usually are planned for a certain number of meetings, primarily at night, when it is more convenient for those who work during the day. Family groups are for support, acquaintance with the medical team, sharing of information and knowledge, expression of feelings, and problem-solving. Such groups are particularly successful in helping parents of disabled children. More recently, groups for adults with elderly parents are being conducted. The social worker frequently schedules family groups with the patient and the entire family to verbalize conflicts and misunderstandings and to solve problems. On other occasions, the social worker has conjoint family therapy sessions with a husband and wife. Again, these groups focus on expression of feelings, clarification of misunderstandings, planning, and problem solving. Family conferences with staff to discuss the patient's condition, medical treatment, and discharge plans are led by the social worker. Many hospitals schedule weekly meetings to which different families are invited.

Sexual counseling is a well-established modality of treatment for the physically disabled. This treatment takes the form of individual counseling with the patient, conjoint counseling with the patient and sexual partner, and educational or therapeutic groups. The social worker, together with the physician, determine any areas of sexual dysfunction and provide the appropriate treatment, which may include education, information, or therapy to resolve discomfort with body image, fear of rejection, or emotional problems that interfere with sexual functioning. The disabled patient and partner frequently develop sexual dysfunction as a symptom of other problems inherent in the relationship. Sexual problems are not isolated and therefore can best be treated in the context of the total therapeutic experience with the social worker or other psychotherapist.

Play therapy is traditionally used with children as a medium of communication for the expression of problems, conflicts, and feelings. In working with physically disabled children with impaired speech, this method of treatment can assume added importance.

These psychosocial treatments are evaluated continuously and shared with the health care team for interaction with medical management.

Discharge Planning

The social worker's involvement in discharge planning varies with individual patients and families, depending on the personal strengths and weaknesses of both the patient and the family and their willingness to utilize assistance in working through their problems. Discharge planning is a total process that involves all aspects of the patient's medical problem and rehabilitaton. From the time of admission, much of the social worker's activity has been directed toward helping the patient come to a recognition, if not a resolution, of limited goals — of having reached a maximum level of physical functioning and of beginning the phase of living with the new self. This step includes awareness of physical limitations, of dependence on others for some part of personal care, of a new identity, of a new role, and, it is hoped, of a series of achievements and new abilities.

Four major factors must be considered in assisting a person to make plans for discharge.[11] The first factor is the degree of physical function that the patient will attain. If patients are fairly independent in activities of daily living and require little or no help with personal care, they may be able to live alone with a minimum amount of help from family, friends, or a part-time housekeeper. If they require considerable personal care and it is not feasible for them to live alone, they will need either a devoted family member or a live-in attendant for assistance.

A second consideration is the nature of patients' relationships with their families. The social worker assists patients and families in deciding if the patient will be cared for in the family home or in another living arrangement. This requires assessment of reality factors and the feelings of the patient and the family. To help the patient and family with the question of returning home or living elsewhere, weekend passes are encouraged to try out the plan for living. If the family can no longer care for the patient at home, then efforts must begin early in the hospital stay to work through the family's guilt and the patient's anger, disappointment, and feelings of rejection, and to make plans for other care.

A third factor to be considered is the emotional need of the patient for independence. If families cannot allow patients to dress or feed themselves or to struggle with this kind of physical independence at their own pace, conflicts arise. The social worker must work to reconcile patients' emotional needs for independence with their actual physical dependence. They must be helped to assert realistic independence even if they are physically different from before.

The fourth factor is the financial and social resources available in the community for the physically disabled. The financial resources include public assistance programs, social security disability insurance programs, and the Veterans Administration, to name a few major examples. Various agencies provide such specific services i.e., vocational counseling, recreation, transportation, housing, child care, family counseling, and psychiatric care. As part of discharge planning, the social worker coordinates referrals to community agencies or arranges to provide continued direct services on an outpatient basis. The physically disabled have developed their own national and local support organizations, furnishing a wide range of services. These organizations, such as the Association for the Physically Handicapped, make the able-bodied community aware of the needs of the physically disabled and have been increasingly effective in lobbying for legislative changes, removing architectural barriers, and bringing about changes in attitudes toward the physically disabled. Other organizations, such as the Centers for Independent Living, are self-help programs. They are staffed primarily by volunteers, with some paid professional staff (usually disabled). These centers have become a major resource for socialization, offer all kinds of services, have group programs, and are continually available to prevent people from retreating from the mainstream of living.

Finally, the patient must be helped emotionally to leave the total support system of the hospital. This process is eased somewhat by follow-up care as an outpatient provided by the same inpatient rehabilitation team whom the patient has come to know and trust.

RELATIONSHIP OF THE SOCIAL WORKER TO REHABILITATION TEAM MEMBERS

An understanding of the interrelationships of the physical, social, and emotional factors in illness and disability has become a cornerstone of contemporary medical practice. Increasingly, the orthopaedic surgeon, who treats some of the most disabling illnesses and disabilities, finds it impossible any longer to limit involvement to the patient's skeletal structure. As the orthopaedic surgeon increasingly becomes a team partner and relies on the knowledge of internists, so does the surgeon in turn heed the counsel and expertise of the nurse, physical therapist, occupational therapist, vocational counselor, and social worker. The primary medium of communication is the team conference, in which information is shared by all professional disciplines. At this conference the social worker may take the lead in encouraging the team to include the psychosocial aspects in the formulation of the total medical treatment plan.

RELATIONSHIP TO THE COMMUNITY

In recent years the hospital setting has come to be seen as a community. This philosophy is related to the concept of preventive medicine and to the hospital in the broadest sense as part of health services. This health service, of which prevention is a major part, demands that the medical caregivers move to share their knowledge and expertise with the total community. Social workers play a part in this design. Social workers participate in medical symposia for doctors, nurses, and all allied health professionals to share their knowledge of psychosocial factors in health care and the humanity of the patient. They are on faculties of medical schools and allied health schools. Social workers are on boards of the major voluntary health agencies across the country, such as those for heart disease, cancer, and lung disease.

FUTURE DIRECTIONS

The practice of social work in health services is predicted to show continued expansion and improvement. More and more hospitals will comply with the standards of social work services for accreditation and licensing. As social workers demonstrate competence and effectiveness in more and more facilities, the demand for their services from both patients and hospital staff will increase.

Social work services can be billed on a fee-for-service basis, as insurance companies and Medicare make direct payment for psychotherapy given by licensed clinical social workers. Now that social work services are revenue-producing, there is an opportunity for further expansion in health care facilities and in independent practice, with social workers accepting referrals from community physicians.

In addition to this predicted quantitative change, the quality of social work services in health care should improve as well, as more and more social workers with master's degrees and training in medical settings are employed to provide direct services. This increased use of professional social workers will occur as the standards for social work services are upgraded by the Joint Commission for the Accreditation of Healthcare Organizations to require licensed clinical social workers.

Another change in the future will concern access to social work services. The revisions in the welfare system in the United States away from social work services and toward concentration on financial assistance have occurred at the same time as the expansion of social work services in the health care system. A person needing comprehensive social work services will increasingly obtain them in relation to health care rather than in relation to financial assistance. As health care facilities become the primary social system providing social work services to the community, the population served will increase to include all socioeconomic classes.

SUMMARY

The goal of social work is to maintain or restore each patient to his or her highest level of personal, social, and economic functioning. The factor determining whether or not persons have been successfully rehabilitated is the degree to which they adapt to their environments or their environments can be adapted to them. Social work with patients is directed toward the difficult transition between functioning in a hospital setting and returning home to assume responsibilities in the community. To achieve this readjustment and return to the community, social workers assist patients and their families in resolving personal and social problems. Social workers also use and develop community resources and serve as the liaison with community social agencies.[9]

REFERENCES

1. American Hospital Association: The Hospital's Responsibility for the Psychosocial Aspects of Health Care (pamphlet). American Hospital Association, Chicago, 1970
2. Bartlett HM: Social Work Practice in the Health Field. p. 51. National Association of Social Workers, New York, 1966
3. Lurie HL: Encyclopedia of Social Work. p. 114. National Association of Social Workers, New York, 1965
4. National Association of Social Workers and the American Hospital Association: Standards for hospital social work services. Health Soc Work 3(2):3, 1978
5. Kahn E: The Dynamic Social Work Department. p. 3. American Hospital Association, Chicago, 1972
6. Moos RH: Coping with Physical Illness. p. 9. Plenum Press, New York, 1977
7. Bartlett HM: The Common Base of Social Work Practice. p. 139. National Association of Social Workers, New York, 1970
8. Dunham OC: Phases of adjustment of the rehabilitation patient. Presented at the Institute on Rehabilitation and Chronic Disease for Faculty of Schools of Social Work, Rancho Los Amigos Medical Center, Downey, CA, February 1966
9. Brunings RC: Social Work Policy and Procedure Manual. Section II, Part 1. Rancho Los Amigos Medical Center, Downey, CA, 1979
10. About Hospital Social Work Services (pamphlet). p. 6. Channing L. Bete, Greenfield, MA, 1978
11. Nickel VL, Stauffer ES, Wilcox NE, Erickson ER: Final Report, Regional Spinal Cord Injury Rehabilitation Center SRS Grant 13-P-55279/9. p. 217. Attending Staff Association of the Rancho Los Amigos Medical Center, Downey, CA, 1972

8 Vocational Rehabilitation

MARY LOU HARRIS

Vocational rehabilitation is helping people, with a disability which handicaps their capacity for work, to remain or become employable. It is a process that integrates people, disabilities, and work. Vocational rehabilitation is designed to help persons with disabilities to (re)enter the work force. Generically it is practiced by people in a broad range of areas, including (but not limited to) physicians, nurses, therapists, teachers, employers, and family members. Professionally the vocational rehabilitation counselor working within a wide range of settings and with various professionals is the person responsible for managing the process. Vocational rehabilitation is (or should be) an integral part of the practice of orthopaedic rehabilitation, which treats the majority of the nation's disabled citizens of working age — those with repetitive injuries and chronic low back problems.[1]

Although helping a person with a disability find suitable work sounds uncomplicated, the actual process is a great deal more complex. The process involves people, with all their individual differences; their environment, with its particular support network; the handicapping effect(s) of the disability; and "work", that cornerstone of our identity that takes up the major portion of our lives and provides a spectrum of psychological, social, and economic benefits.[2]

Vocational rehabilitation is best practiced as an integral component of a person's total rehabilitative effort, not as a separate and distinct segment. Although the focus is on resolving work and disability problems, when an injury or other disability occurs, emotional, family, financial, and legal difficulties can affect the patient's recovery and return-to-work

planning. Transportation, mobility aids and devices, job training, and motivation are frequently involved.[3] A standard quality of care for rehabilitation requires a team effort of medical, vocational, and community resource personnel working in cooperation with the individual patient and the family within the boundaries of their particular environment(s).

Actual vocational rehabilitation activities take place after acute medical concerns are addressed. However, early contact with patients whose disability may constitute a permanent functional limitation can reduce their anxiety about working options by making them aware of the services available for future planning, thereby facilitating the patients' recovery.[3] As medical treatment decreases, vocational rehabilitation activities should increase. This coordinated medical-vocational case management is important to a timely, cost-efficient, and effective return-to-work outcome.

WORK AND DISABILITY

In the not too distant past *work* and *disability* were antithetical terms. Technology, legislation, changes in workers and in the concept of work itself, and a raised social awareness have altered this view and the attitudes toward disability and occupation.

Advances in technology have changed the face of disability, not only by increasing the numbers of the persons who survive after sustaining severe disability but also by allowing people to be helped to function independently and productively at home and at work. Computers, robotic aids, and other adaptive devices have helped to eliminate or decrease many of

63

the handicapping effects of severe disability, such as occur in injury to the spinal cord.[4,5] Principles of ergonomics, biomechanics, and industrial engineering are being combined to influence people's abilities to work productively with the most efficiency and the least physical and mental stress. The effects of legislatively mandated equal employment opportunities are beginning to be noticed in the labor market. The rise in the social (and legal) conscience of employers and the reality of having fewer workers have increased the retention and hiring of qualified employees with disabilities by accommodating their needs. Employment and disability are no longer antithetical, however, adults of working age with disabilities continue to have an inordinately high rate of unemployment.[6]

An important distinction within the field of vocational rehabilitation and work disability is that of *disability* versus *handicap*. The general assumption is that having a disability puts a person at a disadvantage (or produces a handicap). This is true for many activities. However, all people, with or without a diagnosed disability, have a spectrum of abilities; they excel in some activities and are disadvantaged in others. Sometimes this "disadvantage" comes from their own attitudes or motivation and other times it can be caused by a concrete limitation or obstacle. This is the difference between disability and handicap as used in the field of vocational rehabilitation. Disability is that diagnosed medical condition or impairment that restricts a function, such as walking, lifting, seeing, or hearing. Handicap is the environmental or personal restriction placed on the disability through architectural barriers, attitudes, invalid job requirements, or motivation. The disability is usually not correctable. The handicap is what vocational rehabilitation aims to reduce.

Another assumption is that the more severe the disability the more difficult it is to remove the vocational handicap. This may or may not be true. The extent of the disability or handicap is set by the dynamic interaction of the disability and the vulnerability (or psychological makeup) of the person, combined with the social and vocational environment within which that person must function.[7,8] Therefore, a medically defined mild disability can be aggravated by the personality of the patient and produce a major vocational handicap to be resolved. Usually it is the psychosocial and environmental factors that are more complex and more difficult to work with than the medical factors and that have the greatest impact on return to work.[9] Some additional factors that have been shown to influence the level of disability and return to work are the following:

- The physician[3]
- Receipt of disability compensation[1,10]
- Attorney involvement[1,11]
- Extended time away from work[1]
- Relationship with supervisor or low job satisfaction[9]
- Substance abuse[1]
- Employer policies, job availability, lack of information or resources regarding accommodation, and disbelief of employers regarding capabilities[6]

In summary, work disability results from a combination of factors, not the least of which is the vulnerability of the person to the change precipitated by the disability. For all people living in this era of change, the ability to adapt to daily stresses is the essence of personal stability. People's continued ability to remain in control of their lives and to achieve organization, structure, and a sense of purpose is founded on this capacity to respond positively to ongoing change. This is taxing even for the least vulnerable. How would people react if, tomorrow, they were forced to cope with a sudden onset of physical or mental impairment that interfered with their well-ordered existence, that changed how the outside world responded to them, and that required them to redefine their personal, social, and work realities? What would be the extent of their work disability or handicap? Although this is a rhetorical question, it is important to remember that anyone can become a member of this minority group at any time. People need to be aware of their own attitudes, stereotypes, and actions that place unnecessary handicaps on persons with disabilities.

HISTORY AND DISTRIBUTION OF DISABILITIES

Vocational rehabilitation as a specialty emerged from crises created by the two world wars, and federal laws were enacted to provide basic job retraining to World War I soldiers who returned with physical disabilities. The shortage of workers created during World War II spurred additional federal legislation that broadened the eligibility criteria for services to include mental retardation and mental illness. Later, during the Vietnam conflict, as a result of attempts to solve national economic problems, vocational rehabilitation came to be used by public assistance recipients, public offenders, and other persons who were job handicapped—that is, those who were not necessarily physically or mentally disabled but were socially handicapped. The birth of the professional vocational rehabilitation counselor came through the Rehabilitation Act Amendments of 1954. This legislation allowed for allocation of research and training monies for all aspects of medical and vocational rehabilitation, creating many jobs and resulting in increased bureaucracy.

Types of Disabilities

In 1987 the Social Security Administration paid approximately $32 billion in cash benefits to 7.5 million (of the projected 36 million) people with disabilities and to the families of workers with disability. Of these, it is claimed that only 10 to 15 percent have realistic prospects for rehabilitation, primarily because of age and severity of disability.[10] (Fewer than 2 percent are actually referred and accepted for service by the state vocational rehabilitation agency.)

Nationwide, injuries resulting from repetitive trauma to the upper extremities and chronic low back ailments are causing disability to workers at an increasing rate. Reportedly 83 percent of worker's compensation claimants have orthopedic injuries. According to the National Safety Council, 29 percent of all job-related injuries are to the back. In fact, severe back injuries represent half of all worker's compensation injuries classified as serious. Fifty-six percent of beneficiaries receiving Social Security or long-term disability compensation have a back injury.[1] A 1988 report to the Rehabilitation President's Council of California indicated that people with industrial injuries to the wrist, hand, or finger have only a 50 percent chance of returning to work; this is the same as the percentage reported for head injury. Back and neck injuries were almost equally represented in the "did return to work" and "did not return to work" categories. The impact of disability on work and correspondingly on the economy is substantial, particularly in terms of medical expense, lost work days,

and reduction of earning capacity. Consequently, the provision of vocational rehabilitation to reduce the handicapping effects of disability and return the worker to work takes on great significance.

SETTINGS

Professionals in vocational rehabilitation may be employed in a variety of settings: public agencies, workers' compensation system, and private practice, including medical settings and self-insured corporations.

Public Agencies

Public agencies for vocational rehabilitation exist in every state and territory. These agencies are supported by both federal and state funds. Government-funded agencies employ the largest number of vocational rehabilitation counselors. Eligibility for services is 2-fold: a diagnosed disability that creates a vocational barrier and the ability to benefit from services. The type and extent of services are policy directed and include medical as well as vocational services. In public agencies persons with severe disabilities have selection priority. The Rehabilitation Act of 1973, with major amendments in 1978 and 1986, forms the basis for the current program of federal and state vocational rehabilitation services and also sets the stage for the "rights" era for persons with disabilities. (Title V of the 1973 Act prohibits employers who receive monies from federal sources from failing to hire or from terminating the employment of qualified disabled individuals on the basis of disability.) With the recently passed Americans with Disabilities Act of 1990, prohibition of discrimination on the basis of handicap now parallels in scope that afforded to persons on the basis of sex, race, national origin, and religion.

Workers' Compensation

The first workers' compensation laws were enacted in the United States in the early 1900s. Rehabilitation services have been associated with workers' compensation since its inception, but the emphasis, until recently, has been medical. It was not until the 1970s, when the option of vocational rehabilitation was added as an insurance benefit, that vocational rehabilitation took its rightful place as integral to the recovery process.[12] In some states, the employer is required by law to offer vocational rehabilitation when the injured person is unable to return to the job held at time of injury but is not so severely disabled that employment in the general labor market is precluded. Once offered, vocational rehabilitation can be accepted or rejected by the injured worker; thus, the reality that vocational rehabilitation must be a cooperative, agreed-on process is recognized.

Workers with industrial injuries make up 15.5 percent of the nation's disabled (in contrast, 64 percent of serious worker disability is caused by acute and progressive non–work-related illnesses).[13] The majority of injured workers have chronic low back or other orthopaedic problems.[14] In theory, the workers' compensation system is a no-fault system designed to pay all costs associated with job-related employee injuries and return the injured employee to work as soon as possible. For the majority of workers, this is accomplished. However, for many other workers the complexities and adversities within the system increase their disabilities and reduce their chances of successful return to work. For employers, workers' compensation insurance costs have escalated significantly. Dollars spent for medical and vocational rehabilitation have risen substantially over the past 5 years, as have litigation costs. Across the country, legislative changes are occurring to attempt to lower the costs of workers' compensation and increase the benefit to workers. In many states, this is directly affecting or has already affected the benefits of vocational rehabilitation.

Private Practitioners

Private, for-profit practitioners of vocational rehabilitation have essentially taken over the workers' compensation vocational rehabilitation service delivery from the state agencies, which originally bore the responsibility.[12] The state Departments of Vocational Rehabilitation, supported by tax dollars, had heavy caseloads of severely disabled persons who may have had no previous work history. Service delivery could be delayed and then extended over a long period of time. Additionally, rehabilitation in the public sector, as practiced by many state agencies, is (unfortunately) viewed as a social program. In contrast, in private practice rehabilitation is viewed as a business

and possesses a degree of accountability not characteristic of most state agencies.[3] The cost-conscious employer wants an expedient return to employability with the use of transferable skills, short retraining programs, and job placement assistance. The private rehabilitation companies direct their marketing efforts toward this need, espousing expedient return-to-work counseling and planning within the appropriate legal framework. Failure to provide the advertised services will quickly put the private practitioner out of business.

The private vocational rehabilitation counselor has been recognized by legal, medical, and insurance representatives as a professional with the requisite of quality standards and ethics. The growth of the private market has been nationwide and includes private evaluation centers, job analysis consultation, rehabilitation engineering, work hardening, and expert testimony services. Other expanding opportunities for private sector vocational rehabilitation counselors include work within medical settings and self-insured corporations.

Medical Settings

The role of vocational rehabilitation within the medical rehabilitation setting is an important one. No longer can medical specialists treat only the injury, without looking at how that injury affects the person's earning capacity. Additionally, with the change in health care delivery and reimbursement, hospitals are being forced to diversify their services and are looking at how they can help to return the patient to independence within the community more quickly —with marketable skills.[15] Acute rehabilitation and industrial medical settings can provide the best opportunity for a medical-vocational rehabilitation team approach. Integrated therapies, physical capacity evaluations, work hardening, and vocational assessment and planning, under physician direction, are coordinated with efficient and timely case management. This directly benefits the individual patient and provides more successful return-to-work outcomes.[16,17]

Self-Insured Corporations

Employer-based rehabilitation is another area (albeit as yet small) for the vocational rehabilitation counselor. With the escalation of health care and disability benefit costs and the need to comply with state and federal legislation, the larger (and more often self-insured) employer attempts to contain costs through the development of disability management programs.[18,19] The rehabilitation counselor working within such an organization (as opposed to a state agency counselor or private rehabilitation consultant) can use the organization's policies and structure more effectively to retain the experience and knowledge of the worker who is or has become disabled. The rehabilitation counselor working within an organizational setting needs additional capabilities and knowledge including basic business and management skills and the ability to use mediation and negotiation principles. These skills and abilities are needed to promote the resolution of conflicts and cooperation within the organization for successful integration of disabled workers.[20] The counselor's job responsibilities are usually expanded to include injury prevention activities, guidance to supervisors on reasonable accommodation and disability management of workers, policy development related to disability, and light duty management, an effective program paralleling the concept of work hardening by using graded work activities within medical restrictions as a conditioning agent for return to usual work, while maintaining regular wages.

In-house rehabilitation is a positive development in our society. Employers generally have created their own handicapped workers; therefore, controlling the rehabilitation of those workers makes sense both in monetary terms and in benefits to employees. Ignoring responsibility for the workplace and its effect on the health of employees is no longer possible for the employer who wants to contain health care and compensation costs and retain productive workers.

Summary

Historically, vocational rehabilitation services have developed from legislative initiatives and economic need. These factors will continue to affect the delivery of services. In a depressed economy, budgetary reduction will occur in federal and state programs. Private industries reduce manpower and social conscience tends to be overshadowed by concerns over profit and loss. In periods of high unemployment, untrained workers and those who have never been employed before are last to be hired. Our system of private enterprise works on the theory of supply and demand and depends on competitive production levels for success. When faced with rising costs associated with injury, absenteeism, employee turnover, and a diminishing workforce, employers are forced to look at how their workplaces can be adjusted to better fit the worker and at the worker's fitness to perform the job.

SERVICES

Theoretically the services of vocational rehabilitation constitute a system of disability management within the workplace. This may include employee health promotion, both physical and psychological; risk management, including work site safety and preplacement screenings; career development, to increase job satisfaction; and employment policy development, to promote equal employment treatment. Ideally, vocational "rehabilitation" should begin before injury—that is, there should be a comprehensive analysis of the interactive elements of the work environment, equipment, tasks, and personnel within an organization. Paying attention to these activities may prevent injury (or reinjury) or reduce the extent of disability that may be caused by an injury.

More commonly, however, vocational rehabilitation services take place after injury or illness have affected the person's ability to work and are grouped into three main areas: (1) evaluation, (2) rehabilitation plan development and implementation, and (3) job analysis, placement, or restructure.

The primary competencies required by practitioners of vocational rehabilitation to perform these functions satisfactorily have been established as follows: counseling, knowledge of human behavior, case management, client assessment, medical aspects of disability, information management, and job analysis, placement, or restructure.[21] Educationally, the vocational rehabilitation professional holds a graduate degree (or has equivalent experience) and is certified by the Commission on Rehabilitation Counselor Certification (accredited by the National Commission for Health Certifying Agencies).

Evaluation

After medical eligibility for vocational rehabilitation is established by the physician, the disabled person is referred to a vocational rehabilitation counselor for an evaluation of vocational feasibility. The initial assessment takes place as an interview and can be the single most important contact for the success of the vocational rehabilitation plan. The vocational counselor gathers pertinent information to assess the client's present physical, cognitive, emotional, and motivational status from a comprehensive compilation of data, derived not only from medical and legal reports but also from the client's self-report of injury and psychosocial and work histories. It is in this initial interview that the client is informed about the process of vocational rehabilitation and the professional and personal responsibilities required for a successful outcome. The feasibility of using rehabilitation services to benefit the client is decided and the first steps of developing the rehabilitation plan are taken. If the client is still employed, job restructuring and accommodation are seriously researched. The importance of the counseling function, as practiced by the counselor in the first meeting, cannot be overemphasized; it can be the single most important factor in the success of vocational rehabilitation. The counselor must be able to establish a bond of trust, empathy, and support while helping clients face the reality of the labor market and their own capacities and motivation to compete within it. The counselor must be able to understand the medical aspects of the client's disability and be able to translate these into understandable vocational terms to the client — and to current or future employers.

Often the rehabilitation counselor will need additional information to make a vocational diagnosis of rehabilitation potential. In this case, authorization from the agency supervisor or payer is obtained and the client is referred for work evaluation.

Work evaluation centers are most often found in agencies funded by state or federal monies, private rehabilitation settings, or medical settings. Personnel employed will ideally include physical and occupational therapists in addition to the vocational evaluator (a specialist within the vocational rehabilitation field). A comprehensive program will offer the following [6,9,22]:

- Standardized psychometric testing of work interests, aptitudes, and temperaments
- Worker trait assessment (e.g., the ability to get along with co-workers, respond to supervision, adhere to work rules and safety practices, and productivity
- Work tolerance screening (e.g., the measuring of the physical work performance factors basic to work output, including strength, mobility, endurance)
- Work simulation activities using work samples or actual work tools or environments, or both
- A work hardening screening and treatment program, incorporating individualized graded work activities for symptom control and a progressive increase in physical tolerances, stamina, endurance, and productivity through work pacing techniques, modified work tools, and compensatory work methods
- An exit conference at the conclusion of any selected service to clarify the results and what they mean in terms of rehabilitation potential to the participating client and referring or paying parties

Some evaluation programs offer the opportunity for clients to try out modified tools, assistive devices, and adjusted work stations to determine whether an accommodation can offset their particular physical limitation or restriction; in addition, computerized evaluations, when available, can significantly shorten the evaluation period.

A note of caution about computerized testing should be introduced. Cumulative research findings have shown that aptitude tests alone are poor predictors of performance on the job. Unless computerized testing models incorporate individual observation of the patient's performance on real or simulated work activities, scores may be invalid for assessing future performance on a job. Even though time is costly, it may continue to be the best ally in the clinical prediction of future work performance.[23] Controversy about testing in general and its application to vocational potential is of long standing and will not be discussed fully here. However, some points to consider are the following: (1) tests are not the final solution, (2) tests can be misused and are subject to error; and (3) scores, even if "accurate," cannot reliably be used in isolation.

Nevertheless, standardized tests and work evaluations administered by competent professionals can

- give a basis for comparison with workers in the field
- give the client a sense of what is involved in different work activities
- provide the client with a positive knowledge of abilities or skills
- provide an excellent transition period for the individual from "patient" to "worker"
- provide an observation period of consecutive days to more accurately assess worker stamina and motivation
- be of invaluable assistance to physicians who are required to make return-to-work decisions;
- objectively describe to employers what can be expected in terms of the ability of the worker to perform required job tasks safely and productively[9,19,24]

Theoretically, predictive validity is strongest when the testing activities most closely replicate the tasks demanded by the previous, current, or potential job and the environment within which it is performed. Progressive evaluation programs will therefore require that a job analysis accompany the referral for an evaluation of the person's capacity to perform a specific type of work or for development of a work hardening program.

Written evaluation reports conclude the work evaluation and are directed toward the information requested, summarizing the current mental and physical worker strengths and limitations as observed and tested within the period of evaluation. Reports usually include recommendations regarding potential work options. Increasingly, evaluation reports are being used in courtrooms for personal injury settlements, wrongful discharge complaints, and determinations of disability. Therefore, emphasis in the testing arena must be placed not only on validity, reliability, norm data, and test selection, administration, and interpretation but also on the credentials of the professional(s) involved.[23]

Rehabilitation Plan Development and Implementation

After the client has completed the initial evaluation interview or work evaluation period, an individualized rehabilitation plan is designed, written, and executed. The successful outcome of the plan depends on the accurate analysis of information obtained and the client's participation in its design. Factors that can either facilitate or complicate rehabilitation outcome include motivation, age, education, medical problem(s), transferable skills, geographic area, and, in cases of industrial injury and long-term disability, the status of claim liability.[1] Again the rehabilitation counselor's ability to understand human behavior, motivation, and medical and vocational information, and to coordinate it all into a realistic return-to-work plan is essential for success.

The rehabilitation plan identifies a suitable vocational objective along with its labor market availability and outlines the steps and costs necessary to achieve employability. It can include additional medical or psychological treatment if necessary, physical or behavioral conditioning, vocational training, remedial education, or—with identified transferable skills—direct job placement activities. (The total cost is a function of plan type and duration.) The rehabilitation plan usually covers a period of 3 months to 1 year, with the client maintaining disability compensation for the plan period, and sometimes for a trial work period.

For qualified injured workers (worker's compensation claimants who are deemed medically eligible by the physician and vocationally feasible by the rehabilitation counselor for the vocational rehabilitation benefit), types of rehabilitation plans include return to a modified job with the same or another employer, return to a different job with the same or another employer, schooling or training, on-the-job training, direct placement, or self-employment. It has been demonstrated by numerous studies that modified work with the same employer offers the best chance for successful rehabilitation, and at the least cost. Conversely, schooling to enter a different line of work (the plan most often selected) has been demonstrated to be the most expensive and the least successful.[4]

Although the types of plans are comparable, the average state agency individually written rehabilitation plan (IWRP) can extend for a considerably longer period than the workers' compensation insurance rehabilitation plan. This is due primarily to the preponderance of severely disabled clients, the absence of work history, the length of time away from work, and the use of public education and training opportunities rather than the shorter term private schools.

Ongoing counseling support and case management by the vocational rehabilitation counselor are required throughout the rehabilitation plan. Regular reports describing the client's progress (or lack of it) are required by the payer source (insurance company, employer, public agency, and so forth). A rehabilitation plan can be suspended or terminated if medical exacerbation, legal difficulties, or lack of motivation prevents progress toward the vocational objective.

Job Placement, Analysis, or Structure

A much misunderstood idea about vocational rehabilitation is that the provision of service guarantees a job. Although the anticipated outcome is competitive employment, the stated objective is employability. A significant difference in the degree of personal responsibility is implied by this distinction.[3] Part of becoming employable is learning to find and keep a job. The job development activities of résumé development, securing job leads, filing an employment application, and interviewing are important components of placement. Often these are accomplished in a structured group environment so that job lead information can be shared and peer support given. Job search can be a time of high anxiety and self-doubt (as anyone who has looked for work knows). Daily rejections over an extended period of time can reduce the enthusiasm of the most motivated job seeker. The vocational rehabilitation counselor's positive reinforcement at this time is essential.

A new type of job placement for adults with severe disability that has been promoted by government funding is *supported employment* . Whereas traditionally job training or schooling has preceded placement in the workplace, the objective of supported employment is to place a client within a competitive employment situation and then train that person to do the required job tasks using techniques and technology necessary for satisfactory performance. This applies the belief that all persons, no matter how severely disabled, can work—provided that training strategies and aids are designed to fit that person's needs[25] and supportive services are continued throughout their employment.[2] Originally developed for persons with severe mental retardation, this type of placement is gaining as a rehabilitation option for patients with brain injury and other severe disabilities. Currently supported employment is funded only by public agencies.

Job analysis has an important role in all areas of vocational rehabilitation. It is an assessment process that analyzes the actual requirements to perform a job in a productive, safe manner. It provides a detailed and systematic analysis of physical and mental work demands, work skills, functions, the equipment, tools, or materials needed, and the environment of a specific job. It is most accurately completed at the job site by interviewing those who actually perform the work. A job analysis is of inestimable assistance to physicians in making objective return-to-work decisions or in designing job simulation activities for work capacity evaluation and work hardening.[17] Job analysis is a tool that can be used to determine the medical eligibility for workers' compensation vocational rehabilitation services. (For instance, if after review of an injured worker's job analysis, the physician finds no medical reason that would prevent the worker from returning to the usual work, the insurance company will not deem that person a Qualified Injured Worker or eligible for vocational rehabilitation.) A job analysis also is necessary to document the suitability of the vocational objective within a rehabilitation plan. Many times it is a job analysis that allows an employer to "legally" terminate a disabled worker who can no longer perform the essential functions of the job and for whom no reasonable accommodation is available. Formats of job analyses are many and can range from long narrative reports to one-page checklists. The reason for the job analysis request will usually dictate the type of report to be completed. In some instances, descriptions of occupations from the *Dictionary of Occupational Titles* will be used to substantiate rehabilitation decisions. Although this is a valuable resource for comparison and general knowledge of job requirements, the value of a job analysis lies in its specificity to the individual person performing the job.

Job restructure is an exciting trend in vocational rehabilitation, which focuses on keeping the worker on the job through worksite modification when physical limitations or medical restrictions threaten the person's ability to meet performance standards. Often a modification precipitated by a disabled worker's need will be used to redesign the production method for the entire workforce. Job restructure has come into favor with the passage of federal and state legislation requiring that employers reasonably accommodate qualified handicapped workers. (*Reasonable accommodation* is a somewhat undefinable term that must be applied to individual situations and can include the provision of assistive devices, substitution of duties, flexibility of hours, worksite modifications, or job transfer.) Again the job analysis is vital to individual job restructure. Until recently, job modification was usually done informally by the rehabilitation counselor and the disabled worker. Now, with the availability of advanced technology and a new profession (rehabilitation engineering), theories of ergonomics, industrial engineering, and biomechanics are applied to design more expansive job restructure using scientific knowledge to increase productivity and safety while lowering the functional requirements to perform the job. The worker with the disability is still the primary participant in the development of the job restructure and, because complicated design and intricate devices can be both expensive and difficult to maintain, the favored approach continues to be one of "keeping it simple".

It is important to keep in mind that not every person with a disability will require all (or perhaps any) vocational rehabilitation services. The selection, timing, extent, and intensity of these described services are most effective when situationally determined by the individual circumstance of the consumer(s), their medical care provider(s), and insurance payers, under the professional expertise of a vocational rehabilitation counselor. Unfortunately, in many instances appropriate early intervention and provision of vocational rehabilitation services are prevented or unduly delayed by old-line attitudes of employers, health care or insurance reimbursement policies, medical practitioners with limited knowledge of employment requirements or available resources, or basic questions about the costs or benefits of services.

Studies have shown the cost of these services is a fraction of the cost of worker's compensation and continuing long-term disability compensation. The average worker can receive $76,602 in long-term disability compensation over a 6-year period.[5] The average rehabilitation plan, excluding compensation for the plan's duration, costs 10 to 15 percent of this. Numerous studies of costs and benefits related to state agencies have demonstrated the greater benefit of tax monies gained from wages earned compared to the cost of rehabilitation services.

SUMMARY

Vocational rehabilitation exists within a changing environment. The changes in funding, legislation, workplace design, worker satisfaction needs, health care reimbursement, and the present proclivity for litigation have created both opportunities and barriers for the provision of services. Roles of the vocational rehabilitation practitioner have expanded into areas of expert testimony, employee health and counseling, risk management and safety, and legislative consultation for employment discrimination. A number of advances — "reasonable accommodation" requirements of state legislation (the federal 1973 Rehabilitation Act, as amended, and the Americans with Disabilities Act of 1990); complex and changing workers' compensation rules and regulations; and the escalation of employers' health care costs — have made the competency requirements of vocational rehabilitation counselors expand beyond counseling and placement. Successful rehabilitation practitioners must now be able to use and coordinate the languages of business, insurance, law, psychology, and medicine — in addition to their own jargon — with that of the client into a rehabilitation plan that will help the person return to a productive job, providing financial stability and personal satisfaction. A close alliance with allied health professionals is essential to achieve this challenging objective of total rehabilitation.

REFERENCES

1. Menninger Clinic: A Comprehensive Analysis of Private Sector Rehabilitation Services and Outcomes for Workers' Compensation Claimants. Publication No. TMF-1016-41. The Menninger Clinic, Topeka, KS, 1989
2. Ellamy GT, Rhodes L, Mank D, Albin J: Supported Employment: A Community Guide. Paul H. Brookes, Baltimore, 1988
3. Deutsch PM, Sawyer HW: A Guide to Rehabilitation. 5th Ed. New York, Matthew Bender, 1989
4. Brody H: The great equalizer: PCs empower the disabled. PC/Computing, July 1989, p.83
5. Rehabilitation Brief: Bringing research into effective focus. Vol. X. PSI International, Falls Church, VA, 1988
6. Rehabilitation Brief: Bringing research into effective focus. Vol. IX. PSI International, Falls Church, VA, 1988
7. Howerton PS, Osborne-Fryman M: Vocational assessment in hand rehabilitation. p.83. In Fry R (ed): Third National Forum on Issues in Vocational Assessment — The Issues Papers. Materials Development Center, University of Wisconson – Stout, 1988
8. Stolov WC: Comprehensive rehabilitation: Evaluation and treatment. p.1. In Stolov WC, Clower MR (eds): Handbook of Severe Disability. US Government Printing Office, Washington, DC, 1981
10. Disability Advisory Council: Final Report to Congress on Medical and Vocational Aspects of Disability Programs. Department of Health and Human Services, Social Security Administration, Washington, DC, 1988
11. Jones K: The effect of attorney involvement in the worker's compensation system on time, benefits cost and return to work. p.39. In Fry R (ed): Second National Forum on Issues in Vocational Assessment — The Issues Papers. Materials Development Center, University of Wisconsin – Stout, 1987
12. Tebb A: Getting the injured worker back in the labor market. Risk Management, June 1988, p.12
13. Hester E: Vocational assessment of workers who become disabled. p.209. In Fry R (ed): Third National Forum on Issues in Vocational Assessment — The Issues Papers. Materials Development Center, University of Wisconsin – Stout, 1988
14. Virgil RM: Physical capacity evaluation and work hardening programming: the Carle Clinic association model. p.233. In Smith C, Fry R (eds): National Forum on Issues in Vocational Assessment — The Issues Papers. Materials Development Center, University of Wisconsin – Stout, 1985
15. Baum CM: Competing in a changing marketplace. p.63. In Fry R (ed): Third National Forum on Issues in Vocational Assessment — The Issues Papers. Materials Development Center, University of Wisconsin – Stout, 1988
16. Frank S: Vocational assessment of people with severe physical disability. p.53. In Fry R (ed): Second National Forum on Issues in Vocational Assessment — The Issues Papers. Materials Development Center, University of Wisconsin – Stout, 1987
17. Tyler S, Blaine J: Work hardening: A bridge to return to work. p.153. In Fry R (ed): Second National Forum on Issues in Vocational Assessment — The Issues Papers. Materials Development Center, University of Wisconsin – Stout, 1987
18. Lesher CL: Rehabilitation practice in business and industry. Rehabil Educ 1:119, 1987
19. Pati GC: Economics of rehabilitation in the workplace. J Rehabil, Oct-Nov-Dec 1985, p.22
20. Hoeffel J: In-house rehabilitation. Rehabil Educ 1:111, 1987
21. Harrison L, Chia CL: Rehabilitation counseling competencies. J Appl Rehabil Counseling 10:135, 1979
22. Smith P, McFarlane B: Work hardening model for the 80s. p.227. In Smith C, Fry R (eds): National Forum on Issues in Vocational Assessment — The Issues Papers. Materials Development Center, University of Wisconsin – Stout, 1985
23. McDaniel R: Vocational evaluation: What direction? p.227. In Fry R (ed): Second National Forum on Issues in Vocational Assessment — The Issues Papers. Materials Development Center, University of Wisconsin – Stout, 1987
24. Fairhurst P, Halstead L: Late effects of poliomyelitis: implications for vocational assessment and rehabilitation. p.71. In Fry R (ed): Second National Forum on Issues in Vocational Assessment — The Issues Papers. Materials Development Center, University of Wisconsin – Stout, 1987
25. McLoughlin C, Garner JB, Callahan M: Getting Employed, Staying Employed: Job Development and Training for Persons with Severe Handicaps. Paul H. Brookes, Baltimore, 1987

9 Clinical Psychology

DOUGLAS CAIRNS

All that the title of clinical psychologist indicates is that the person has had 4 years of graduate training in the study of human behavior followed by 2 years of internship, possesses a doctoral degree, and helps people achieve or maintain a healthy adjustment. The practice of this discipline — including the manner of approaching the patient and using specific skills — can vary tremendously. In part this results from the differing philosophies in graduate programs of different schools. Some are strongly oriented toward the behaviorist viewpoint, which focuses on understanding the factors that influence directly observable behavior. Others place more emphasis on internal events, such as thoughts and feelings, as the key to understanding a patient's difficulties in adjustment. Most programs require participants to develop skills in the areas of psychological testing, research design, statistics, neurophysiology, psychotherapy techniques, and psychopharmacology, but the degree to which these are emphasized differs.

Some difficulties may arise in the team setting because the clinical psychologist's role has not been understood. Another member of the team, for example, may make a request for a specific test or function (e.g., a Minnesota Multiphasic Personality Inventory or a behavior modification program for weight loss) without realizing that the clinical psychologist is really best able to judge what programs or techniques would be most appropriate for a particular patient. Members of the rehabilitation team generally should specify what information is needed or what changes they wish to see in the patient's emotional status, leaving the psychologist free to determine the best method of carrying out this request.

The material in this chapter tends to focus on behavioral approaches to rehabilitation.

DISABILITY

The Behavioral Viewpoint

Understanding factors governing human behavior and attempting to promote behavior change are the primary tasks of the clinical psychologist. Considering the complex nature of human behavior and the many forces exerting influence on it, these tasks appear quite formidable. In an attempt to establish some rational framework within which human behavior might be examined, psychologists have always sought a model suitable for objective study.

For many years the clinical psychologist practiced within the medical model, in which abnormal behavior was seen to represent an underlying emotional pathologic condition. A pathologic state was viewed as unconscious desires, unresolved childhood conflicts, weak egos, strong superegos, and other hypothetical constructs that, unless treated, would not permit return to "normal" behavior. In the field of psychology, the medical model has not proved to be satisfactory; numerous difficulties have been encountered in attempting to measure the hypothetical constructs assumed to cause symptons. Moreover, symptoms can be altered directly without treating the assumed underlying pathologic condition. If symptomatic abnormal behavior can be eliminated without treating the underlying abnormal state, the medical model has questionable application at best. The past 25 years have been devoted to a lage extent to developing and testing alternative models.

One such model evolved from behavioral science laboratories has been the "operant learning model." Stated simply, this model assumes that human behavior is dependent on consequences it produces in the environment. That is, if a particular behavior leads to a reinforcement, there is increased likelihood that the behavior will occur again under similar circumstances.

The learning model does not assume that behavior is the function of an underlying unitary personality structure and its dynamics. Instead of seeking to explain behavior by theorizing about assumed intrapsychic causes the focus for examination becomes environmental consequences for expressing behaviors. Understanding why a person does or does not behave in a particular way requires knowledge of reinforcers specific to the individual. The process of ascertaining what is and what is not reinforcing for a given person is termed a *behavioral analysis.*

Reinforcement is defined as anything that strengthens a behavior. Common examples of reinforcers are food and water, money, attention or approval from others, power, and prestige (it would be interesting to see how many books and articles would be written if the author's name were routinely omitted). Behavior is also strengthened if it produces an avoidance of punishment. Avoidance of unpleasant situations or people is an extremely powerful reinforcer, exerting influence over people's behavior on a daily basis. Speed limits and traffic signals are obeyed to avoid traffic fines. We say "yes" when we would rather say "no" to avoid rejection and interpersonal difficulties.

Developing a Disability

Injuries or tissue pathology resulting in chronic illness significantly alter individual behavior. Changes in behavior that occur when the *person* becomes a *patient* range from taking medication, requesting help from others, and using assistive devices to total dependence devoid of self-responsibility.

Changes also occur in the patients' environments. Family and friends minister to them, expecting little in terms of independent function and offering much sympathy and support. If the patient enters the hospital, illness behavior is the norm. Typically, the hospital staff interacts with patients only if there is a problem. When the doctor makes bedside rounds, patients are asked to report their status. Often, the doctor responds to expressions of problems with a reassuring lengthy discussion. Statements of improvements usually result in less reinforcement — an inattentive smile and a perfunctory "that's good" as the doctor moves on the next bed.

Expressions of illness behavior can produce a disability beyond what would be expected from the degree of tissue pathology. For example, continued expressions of disability may remove patients from intolerable work situations; provide them excuses for avoiding responsibility ("don't be upset by the fact that he slapped the child; after all, he *is* in a lot of *pain,*" or "not tonight, dear; I have a headache/backache/chest pain/asthma attack"); offer the opportunity to avoid unpleasant social situations ("as soon as I get well my mother-in-law will move in with us — and I am not fond of my mother-in-law"); or provide much needed attention and support ("so long as I'm unable to care for myself, my daughter will stay with me — after that I'll be alone again"). Under such circumstances, expressions of illness instead of well behavior are strongly reinforced.

The major concern related to reinforcement factors in chronic illness is that of time. The more time required for tissue healing the more opportunity there is for illness behavior to be reinforced. If such a situation develops, treatment of tissue pathology alone may have little or no impact on altering the level of disability. It is therefore necessary for the clinical psychologist to determine if reinforcement factors are at work. If they are, they must be dealt with in the rehabilitation process.

PREREQUISITES TO REHABILITATION: DETERMINING NEEDS

Prior to treatment, the psychologist determines the needs of the patient and staff. The most common need expressed by staff members is that patients cooperate with the treatment regimen. They are expected to arrive promptly at the treatment area and participate fully in therapy activities. They are expected to perform these activities often without understanding the rationale and without seeing progress for weeks or even months.

On the ward, medication is to be taken as prescribed without questions as to content and side effects. During bedside rounds, patients are expected to listen attentively and agree to "doctor's orders." They are expected to understand explanations of the disease process even when they involve such complex statements as "you have a defect in the pars interarticularis—you were born with it," or more simple-minded statements as "you have rusty pipes" or "you've slipped a disc." Much nodding of the head occurs on the part of the patient during these lectures and everyone assumes all is understood. Experience suggests that head-nodding is highly correlated with a complete lack of understanding. Furthermore, it can be assumed with some degree of validity that patients remember only about 20 percent of what is said to them at any given time.

Very often when patients' responses to treatment do not satisfy the needs and expectations of the staff, they receive labels such as "unmotivated," "uncooperative," "combative," "manipulative," "a crank," and "flaky." In a few cases these may be apt descriptions. For the most part, however, they reflect an inadequate understanding of the patient's needs.

Many patients experience difficulty with a lengthy rehabilitation process because they need to understand their disability more completely. Others may need more frequent reinforcement than is typically available in therapy. Usually the only reinforcement for participation in therapy activities is an increase in functional ability. If improvement is not likely for several weeks at best, patients may give up in frustration.

Some patients require firm direction in their treatment program, whereas others need a close, supportive relationship with staff. There are some, however, with whom such a relationship may foster dependency or self-pity. Still others may require support during early stages of rehabilitation and a push toward independence later on, and there are patients for whom the opposite sequence is better. The psychologist is often the only member of the rehabilitation team fully aware of the needs of patients *and*

staff. Being aware of these needs serves to avoid misunderstandings and maintain communication. Once these needs are established, the rehabilitation program begins.

THE REHABILITATION PROCESS

Psychological Factors Affecting Rehabilitation

Rehabilitation is a most complex and comprehensive process, requiring coordinated efforts of surgical and allied health specialists in addition to those of the patient. Each individual enters this process with personal expectations and goals for the treatment's results. In general, the overall goals are to restore function or maintain existing function and improve the quality of life. If these aims are to be accomplished, there must be no conflict among the goals of each rehabilitation team member and they must be consistent with those of the patient.

Having evaluated the patient, the psychologist gains an understanding of the emotional aspects of the disability, readiness for the program, and goals for treatment results. Emotional aspects of the disability can dramatically affect rehabilitation. Patients involved in orthopædic rehabilitation who have lost significant function or have lost an extremity from trauma or disease often progress through the stages of emotion usually seen with the terminally ill. Basically, these stages are denial, anger, bargaining, depression, and acceptance. This sequence of emotions is associated primarily with *loss* and is quite natural and in fact, according to some, necessary for eventual healthy adjustment.[1]

Patients who are depressed—that is, those who do not have access to reinforcement—may have no goals for treatment, appear passive, and receive a label of "unmotivated." Those who are angry or are attempting to fix blame for their condition may appear uncooperative, causing the staff to become impatient and request a discharge for disciplinary reasons. Patients in the denial phase might *appear* well adjusted and accepting of the loss, but they may express unrealistic goals. For example, with one of the most devastating losses of all, the upper extremity amputation, the patient may wish to be fitted with a cosmetic hand rather than with the more functional hook.

Careful discussion with the patient about personal goals for treatment is conducted by each team member. The psychologist's advice regarding these goals usually is in response to requests from patients for a clear understanding of implications for future function and concerns about physical appearance. The psychological portion of rehabilitation, then, focuses on at least two major points: (1) ensuring that patients have an adequate understanding of their disability and what they must *do* in the rehabilitation process, and (2) helping them cope with demands of physical rehabilitation and, if necessary, adjustment to permanent loss of function or disfigurement and acceptance of assistive devices.

Because the patient's emotional status affects participation in all aspects of treatment on a day-to-day basis, the psychologist maintains daily contact with other members of the team. Close contact enables the psychologist to receive information about the patient's progress in therapy as well as apprise members of the rehabilitation team of relevant psychological information. For example, patients might experience difficulty understanding and implementing self-care aspects of the therapy program for several interrelated reasons. They may wish to maintain a dependency relationship with family members; they may not adequately understand or may want to deny the permanent aspects of their disability and thus feel that self-care is irrelevant; they may have difficulty paying attention because of worries or anxieties related to other matters; they may fear that too much progress will decrease the settlement of a pending litigation; or they may not like the therapist.

Often a great emphasis is placed on the need for understanding what implications disability has for the patient. This is certainly an appropriate and even necessary part of rehabilitation. Also important is determining the implications for improving function. People tend to assume that consequences for improved function can be nothing but positive. In some cases, however, improvement may have extremely negative consequences that far outweigh any gains made in rehabilitation. One patient, for example, had suffered separate injuries to his hand and lower back.

Although he was progressing satisfactorily in his hand therapy program, he was resistant to low back treatment. It was revealed that his low back injury was work related and compensable under worker's compensation. His hand injury was not work related. If he were to progress with therapy for his low back injury, he would eventually be rated as fit for work with regard to his back problem and compensation benefits would be discontinued. However, he would remain disabled from his job as a sheet-metal worker because of his hand disability, which was expected to require several additional months of rehabilitation. During this time, he could not receive adequate income. He saw as his only alternative, then, a continued low back disability until his hand had regained enough function to permit return to work.

Another patient noted to have difficulty following through with his rehabilitation program indicated that once he recovered and was able to return to work, he would be required to resume alimony payments. So long as he remained on disability income, he was able to make more money than if he returned to work.

Careful monitoring of the patient's response to treatment places the psychologist in a position to deal with problems as they arise. To be effective, the psychologist's role must never be one of a consultant on the periphery, to be called in after problems have become unmanageable. Otherwise the psychologist enters the scene as a stranger, having little impact until a therapeutic relationship with the patient and a working relationship with the staff can be developed.

Techniques for Promoting Function

Having a thorough understanding of the patient's emotional reactions to disability and implications for improving, the psychologist is able to determine if certain behavioral techniques for promoting function would be worth including in the therapy programs. These techniques would involve application of the learning model defined earlier in the chapter. Behavioral techniques for promoting function have been well presented and documented elsewhere.[2] They are referred to only briefly here.

The Therapist as a Behavioral Engineer

Viewing physical disability as a collection of behaviors subject to the influence of learning makes the distinction between physical and psychological disability less important than might be expected, provided that the patient has the physical capacity for improved function. Virtually all rehabilitation can be seen as behavior modification even though it is performed by professionals in fields other than psychology. The power of social reinforcement in terms of the therapist's responses to the patient must never be underestimated. Often unknowingly, therapists produce significant change in the patient's level of disability simply by their reactions during treatment sessions. Because these reactions will occur regardless of a therapist's awareness of them, the psychologist assists therapists in recognizing their effect on the patient so as to ensure change in the desired direction.

Biofeedback

A behavioral technique that has received considerable attention lately is biofeedback.[3] Advances in electrical instrumentation have made possible the manufacture of relatively inexpensive devices for measuring the physiologic activity of body processes. Levels of activity are then displayed to the patient visually or auditorily. Feedback is then used by the patient to learn voluntary control over the system being monitored. For example, if it is believed that the patient is suffering from muscle tension headaches, surface electromyograph electrodes are placed over the frontalis muscles. Minute changes in muscle activity are measured and displayed on a meter. The patient then seeks to lower the meter reading, resulting in lower levels of muscle tension, in hopes of decreasing headache pain. Although it is extremely difficult to reduce muscle activity when simply instructed to do so, appreciable decreases are achieved when the patient is able to see small changes that have occurred.

Using a blood pressure cuff, the same principle has been employed to teach patients with essential hypertension to lower their blood pressure. Other disorders that appear to be treated successfully with biofeedback include migraine headaches, bruxism, epilepsy, insomnia, phobic reactions, and anxiety.

Biofeedback has been applied as well to muscle reeducation. Stroke victims have been taught successfully to strengthen muscles by a procedure opposite that of muscle relaxation. Instead of decreasing muscle activity, these patients learn to increase, in small increments, the activity of muscles affected by the stroke.

If it is possible to determine the underlying physiologic process associated with a disorder and if small changes can be measured, it is then theoretically possible to treat the problem with biofeedback. Biofeedback, although currently finding wide applications, remains in the research stage. Any application of biofeedback requires a carefully planned protocol and evaluation of treatment results if it is to become a rational treatment procedure.

Contracts

Behavioral contracts offer an additional technique for promoting function when the patient is not progressing sufficiently.[4] Staff concerns about the patient's slow progress are presented to the patient and, with the patient's cooperation, a contract is established whereby access to reinforcers is made dependent on specific amounts of improvement. The patient identifies the reinforcers and, by signing a contract, agrees that they are to be delivered only after specified behavior has been achieved. For example, a 12-year-old boy with juvenile rheumatoid arthritis scheduled for bilateral total hip joint replacement surgery was experiencing difficulty assuming the prone position and ambulating because of pain. He refused to participate in physical therapy, spending most of his time in his room assembling model airplanes supplied by recreational therapy. With his cooperation, a contract was devised that required him to purchase model kits *and* gain access to them using tokens (poker chips) earned in physical therapy. The more progress he made, the more tokens he earned, and the more time he could spend working on his models in the evening. The result was improved participation and progress.

Progress in rehabilitation typically is quite gradual. Patients work for weeks and sometimes months before improvement is evident. Under these circumstances, reinforcement of participation by obvious signs of improvement is delayed. Psychologists know that if reinforcement is to strengthen behavior efficiently, it must occur assoon as possible after that behavior. To accomplish this more effectively, progress can be measured, recorded, and, in some cases, graphically displayed. Small gains can then be presented, thereby providing the patient with reinforcement to continue. These gains can also be recognized by staff members through giving attention and approval, providing additional reinforcement. All too often, attention from staff members occurs only if the patient is not improving and serves to strengthen the wrong behavior — that is, lack of progress.

REHABILITATION OF CHRONIC SPINAL PAIN

Behavioral approaches to rehabilitation provided the basis for the Spinal Pain Service at Ranchos Los Amigos Hospital in Downey, California.[5-7] Between 1971 and 1982, more than 4,000 patients were admitted to the program, and results have been encouraging. The behavioral approach, embracing as it does the concept of operant conditioning, directs psychologists to evaluate the consequences of pain behavior. Patients gain attention, sympathy, and suppport from significant others after complaints of pain — the patient's spouse exhibits concern, friends and relatives visit more frequently, and children become more helpful. Reinforcement continues so long as expressions of pain continue.

In most cases, family and friends eventually tire of this routine. If they stop providing reinforcement, however, pain behavior typically increases in strength and frequency. A normal gait becomes a limp. A limp now requries a cane or crutches. More time is spent in bed, and emergency room visits are more frequent. Under these conditions, it becomes increasingly difficult to withhold attention and sympathy.

As pain behavior increases, the resulting inactivity may cause joints to become stiff and muscles to weaken. Pain becomes the primary focus of attention and topic of conversation. Medication intake increases and aspirin is discarded in favor of narcotic analgesics. Behavior associated with what was once an acute pain evolves into a disability strengthened by continued reinforcement.

Although social reinforcement in the form of attention and concern plays a role in the learning and maintenance of pain behavior, it is by no means the most important variable. Disability associated with low back pain appears to develop more frequently under conditions in which expressions of pain remove unpleasant stimuli, provide time out from stress, and relieve the person of responsibilities.Distasteful or dangerous work duties are avoided; and, if difficulties in selfassertion exist, expressions of pain provide greater control in social interactions.

After the initial injury, activities that aggravate pain become less frequent. Close examination may reveal these to have a low reinforcing value or they may even be aversive. For example, riding in a car to and from an unpleasant job may be painful, or sitting long enough to perform the job may increase pain. This pain may be endured, however, while riding in a car to visit friends or sitting to watch a good movie. In a sense, the patient may be saying, "If I am going to hurt, I might as well hurt while I am doing something I like." Unfortunately, family members, employers, and insurance companies will rarely tolerate such an attitude. A husband may ask his wife why she is able to work in the garden, visit friends, and go shopping, but cannot wash clothes, clean the house, and prepare meals. The insurance company may wish to know why the patient can play golf and go fishing but cannot work. Not surprisingly, the inquiries begin to acquire an aversive nature and to avoid them the patient becomes increasingly inactive. Under such circumstances, then, pain behavior originally associated with tissue pathology comes under the control of the patient's environment.

Evaluation

On admission to the Spinal Pain Service, the patient routinely underwent psychological testing, including the Minnesota Multiphasic Personality Inventory (MMPI). Testing is not designed to determine if pain is "real" or "imaginary," because this is an artificial distinction and is most always an unproductive pursuit. Instead, testing attempts to illustrate the degree to which pain complaints and perception may be influenced by reinforcing environmental factors and how the patient is likely to respond to treatment. A behavioral analysis is also conducted to determine further the role of environmental factors affecting expressions of pain by examining the consequences they produce in terms of attention, sympathy, and avoidance of unpleasant situations.

Results of the evaluation are then presented to rehabilitation team members for planning the treatment. Because the problem of chronic spinal pain cannot be treated solely medically or soley psychologically yet it does involve a considerable amount of psychological assessment, the psychologist serves as the coordinator of the treatment program, consulting with patients and team members daily.

Target Activities

Target activities or goals take two forms: those identified by the treatment staff and those identified by the patient. Staff goals usually involve increasing muscle-strengthening exercises and functional ability, decreasing medication, returning the patient to work and recreational activity, and reducing the pain. Unless these are also the patient's goals, treatment will be unsuccessful. Patients are required to specify in behavioral terms activities they wish to perform. For example, "I would like to be able to stand 30 minutes for shopping and washing dishes, sit for 60 minutes, and walk for 15 minutes."

Almost any activity limited by pain may be measured objectively in time or frequency. Activity baselines may be obtained for walking distance and velocity, sitting time, time spent out of bed, standing time, exercise repetition, and time and distance on an exercise bicycle.

Precise measures are essential, in some cases requiring counters or timers, so any initial slight change in the desired direction can be reinforced. For example, a switch similar to that which operates an automatic door may be placed beneath a chair and attached to an electric clock to measure sitting time. A similar apparatus can be used to measure time out of bed. The physical therapist establishes the patient's tolerance for mat exercises, walking, exercise bicycle, and quadriceps strengthening and provides instruction in posture and basic spinal anatomy. The occupational therapist establishes tolerance for sitting and standing time and provides instruction in relaxation, time management, body mechanics, and assertion skills to learn alternatives to using pain as an excuse for avoiding responsibility.

Medication

Medications are measured or categorized by frequency, dosage, and type. Because the patient typically is inaccurate when recording intake, the spouse may be recruited to make these recordings at home. Hospital baselines are obtained from the nurse when medication is initially prescribed on an "on-demand" basis.

Subjective Pain Level

Baseline pain levels are determined by asking the patient to rate pain on a daily basis, using a scale of $0 =$ no pain to $100 =$ worst possible pain. The accuracy of this measure of pain is not a concern in the present setting, because pain ratings over time are more an indication of willingness to admit improvement than of actual intensity.

Time Out of Bed

Amount of time spent out of bed is most easily measured by an up-time recorder. This device consists of a pressure-activated switch placed under the mattress and connected to a clocklike apparatus mounted on the headboard. The clock only runs if the patient is out of bed, measuring this time cumulatively.

Health Care Utilization

The number of doctor's visits, emergency room visits, and hospitalizations and the amounts of money spent for treatment and medication are measures of health care utilization. Baselines can be obtained prior to admission from the patient, the spouse, or, in some cases, the insurance company. Continued recordings after discharge provide some indication of the effects of treatment.

Behavioral Treatment

Providing praise and attention for well behavior while remaining unresponsive to pain behavior appears to be an effective method of treatment for chronic low back disability. At the outset, procedures are initiated to shift the focus of attention from pain sources and behavior to well behavior. Patients are informed that discussing their pain in daily conversation is counterproductive. Such talk does not reduce pain but instead provides a focus for attention. They are informed that staff members will avoid engaging in pain-related conversations. Instead, attempts are made to elicit other reinforceable conversation by responding to pain complaints with: "Let's not talk about your pain; let's talk about the progress you're making." Although this seldom eliminates all complaints, it does seem to reduce them appreciably.

Reluctance to stop *all* pain references probably reflects the caution with which most patients approach change. Treatment, for many, means a radical change in the way they conduct their lives. Most patients continue expressing pain simply in order to communicate their wariness: "I may be improving, but don't expect too much too soon. I'm not sure I'm ready to deal with what is expected of me when I get well."

Increasing amounts of each activity are prescribed daily by the therapists. The use of a publicly displayed performance graph is a particularly effective means of recording and reinforcing desired changes in target activities. A large graph (60 × 90 cm) is placed above the bed, and walking distance, sitting time, standing time, and other factors are plotted on it daily by staff members making bedside rounds. If the plotted level represents an increase in activity, time is spent at the bedside praising the patient and engaging in non–pain-related conversation. If no improvement is noted, the graph is simply plotted and returned to its position over the bed.

Behavioral treatment also involves individual and group sessions in which techniques of pain management are presented and discussions are held about identifying sources of stress and reinforcers for pain behavior.

Medication

The frequency of narcotic usage found in treating chronic low back pain is of such magnitude as to require a drug detoxification plan. First it is necessary to discontinue medication on a pain-dependent basis. Under these conditions, medication serves as a reinforcer for pain complaints. All narcotics, then, are mixed in a liquid masking agent and administered orally every 4 hours regardless of pain complaints. The amount of liquid is held constant at 15 ml while the active ingredients are gradually withdrawn. Eventually medication consists solely of the masking agent. The patient is informed that the medication will be decreased but will not be told when reduction occurs.

Family Education

If changes in target activities are to persist after discharge, the spouse or relatives must be willing and able to continue an atmosphere reinforcing these activities. To accomplish this, the patient and principal relations meet with staff for instructions in reinforcement techniques. The staff emphasizes the importance of identifying and reinforcing well behavior. Videotaped examples of a patient expressing pain behavior and well behavior are presented. Instruction in the application of reinforcement techniques follows. Weekend passes are provided and then the patient and family attempt to apply these techniques in practice. Difficulties encountered are discussed with staff members during frequent contact with the spouse or relatives throughout treatment.

When patient and family become actively involved in the rehabilitation process, they assume a major portion of the responsibility for improvement. Accomplishing this step early in treatment makes the transition from hospital to home much smoother at discharge. For many patients, the rehabilitation process is lifelong, and only a small portion of this process occurs in the hospital. If progress is to continue, the family must be supportive in the proper direction.

SUMMARY

The role of the clinical psychologist is perhaps the most comprehensive compared with other members of the rehabilitation team. To understand the patient's emotional reaction to disability, the psychologist must have a thorough understanding of both tissue pathology and the demands of physical rehabilitation. She/he must be able to monitor the patient's reaction to each aspect of the therapy program, maintaining close contact with both patient and staff. The psychologist also must know the patient's family so as to understand the interpersonal dynamics that may affect therapy and postdischarge follow-up.

Perhaps one of the most important functions of the clinical psychologist is to be able to communicate psychological information to the members of the rehabilitation team. Care must be taken to avoid useless esoteric terminology in written and verbal reports because psychological information is often used to alter the treatment approach or to understand patient reactions to particular aspects of therapy.

Examining the results of treatment by way of applied research represents the psychologist's contribution to the future of orthopaedic rehabilitation. This future depends on using rational treatment approaches of demonstrated effectiveness. By virtue of background and training, the clinical psychologist is often the member of the rehabilitation team called on to design

research and analyze data. In the rehabilitation setting, where the goal of treatment is to improve the quality of life, the psychologist views all treatment as applied research to determine whether, in fact, this goal is accomplished. Research, then, does not necessarily take the form of testing hypotheses in carefully controlled laboratory settings. It involves careful evaluation of the patient's progress with various treatment approaches and an examination of follow-up results. These data, then, provide a rational basis for modifying the treatment furnished by all members of the rehabilitation team.

REFERENCES

1. Kubler-Ross E: On Death and Dying. Macmillan, New York, 1969
2. Fordyce W: Behavioral Methods for Chronic Pain and Illness. CV Mosby, St Louis, 1976
3. Brown BB: Biofeedback — New Directions for the Mind. Harper & Row, New York, 1974
4. Kanfer FJ, Phillips JS: Learning Foundations of Behavior Therapy. John Wiley & Sons, New York, 1970
5. Cairns D, Pasino J: Comparison of verbal reinforcement and feedback in the operant treatment of disability due to low back pain. Behav Ther 8:621, 1977
6. Cairns D, Thomas L, Mooney V, Pace J: A comprehensive treatment approach to chronic low back pain. Pain 2:301, 1976
7. Mooney V, Cairns D: Management in the patient with chronic low back pain. Orthop Clin North Am 9:543, 1978

10 Orthopaedic Surgery

MICHAEL J. BOTTE

The specialty of orthopaedic surgery is defined by the American Academy of Orthopaedic Surgeons as "the medical specialty that includes the preservation, investigation, and restoration of the form and function of the extremities, spine, and associated structures by medical, surgical, and physical methods"[1] (American Academy of Orthopaedic Surgeons, personal communication, 1991). Few other medical or surgical specialties place as much emphasis on the anatomy, physiology, function, and biomechanics of the extremities and spine. Orthopaedic surgeons not only perform operative intervention of bones and joints, but can also repair or reconstruct tendons, muscles, skin, nerves, arteries, and veins of the extremities. With this background, the orthopaedic surgeon is equipped to evaluate, treat, and restore or maximize function in chronic neuromusculoskeletal afflictions and thus is an integral member of the rehabilitation team.

The purpose of this chapter is to summarize the development of this specialty, review recent changes, and to discuss the role of the orthopaedic surgeon in rehabilitation. The chapter is divided into three sections: (1) historical aspects of orthopaedic surgery, (2) orthopaedic organizations and the further establishment of the specialty, and (3) orthopaedic rehabilitation as a subspecialty.

ORTHOPAEDIC SURGERY: HISTORICAL ASPECTS

Evidence of musculoskeletal disorders or disease has been found from the skeletal remains of primitive humans. Afflictions include fractures, osteomyelitis, degenerative arthritis, rheumatoid arthritis, periostitis, and bone tumors (Fig. 10-1).[1] The femur of Java man, *Pithecanthropus erectus*, dated approximately half a million years ago, demonstrates a mass of bone in its proximal portion that had been designated an osteochondroma, but may in fact be reactive bone formed in response to local soft tissue injury and periosteal injury.[2] The Neanderthal skeleton was suggestive of a man with advanced osteoarthritis, accounting for the bent knees and rounded (kyphotic) spine.[3] Satisfactory bone union and alignment of fractures were also found in the Neanderthal skeletons.[4] Neolithic skeletons (circa 7000 to 3000 B.C.) show spinal deformity consistent with tuberculosis.[3] Bone injuries from flint arrowheads have been discovered, some of which have shown bone healing while others did not, suggesting that death probably occurred shortly after injury.[1,2,5] Other ancient remains show skulls with depressed and fissured fractures and deep furrows, thought to be caused by some type of axe or knife, and skeletons with evidence of limbs having been hacked from the trunk.[2]

Egyptian mummies (circa 1300 to 1000 B.C.) were commonly found to have skeletal abnormalities. Spinal defects suggestive of tuberculosis, limb wasting consistent with poliomyelitis, foot deformities resembling clubfoot, and skeletal evidence of arthritis, gout, and bone tumors have been discovered.[3]

Bone splints were used in early civilized cultures. Primitive bone setters were thought to have played a role in evolving civilizations,[1,6] Specimens of primitive art such as pottery, mural decorations, and carvings show figures with apparent fractures.[7,8]

With the development of knives and crude saws, primitive operative procedures were devised. Limb amputation was one of the earliest major operative procedures. Finger amputations were thought to have religious symbolism, as shown by mural drawing in caves at La Tene in France.[9] Egyptian papyri dating from about 1600 B.C. are among the earliest

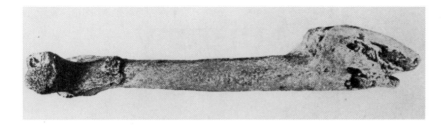

Fig. 10–1. Prehistoric femur with healed fracture.

written materials on surgery of the musculoskeletal system.[2,3,10]

The Hippocratic writings from Greece dating from between 400 B.C. and A.D. 100 depict impressive advancements on the understanding of extremity injuries (Fig. 10-2).[1–3,6,7] Among these are the works entitled *On Fractures* and *On Articulations,* which contain discussions of diagnosis and treatment of fractures. Methods of traction and splinting for the reduction and immobilization of long bone fractures were explained.[6] Tools that were used to manipulate fracture fragments are described. These writings demonstrated an appreciation of the problems of joint ankylosis, spinal deformities, clubfeet, congenital hip dislocation, and traumatic shoulder dislocation (Fig. 10-3). Wine was used as an antiseptic for open fracture management,[1,6] and cautery was a popular way to treat wounds, infections, and tumors. The careful and extensive use of operative surgery with the knife

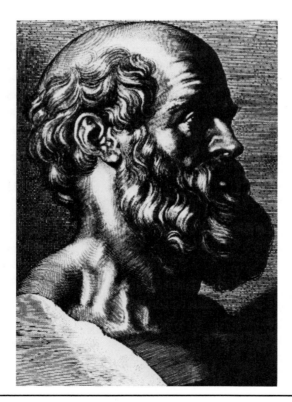

Fig. 10–2. Hippocrates. Engraving by Paul Ponce (1603–1658) after drawing by Peter Paul Rubens (1577–1640). (Antwerp [?], 1638.)

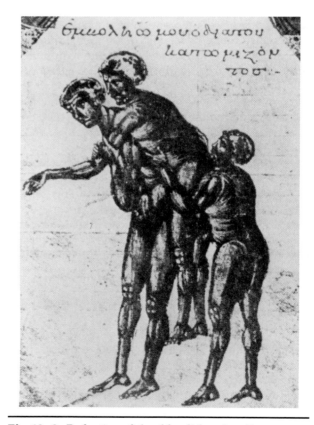

Fig. 10–3. Reduction of shoulder dislocation. From an ancient Greek codex.

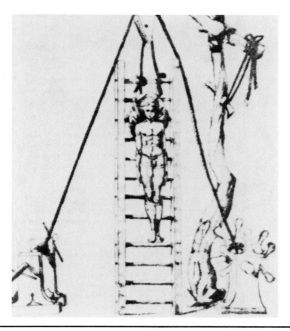

Fig. 10-4. Mechanics and mathematics in the form of levers and pulleys of Archimedes were employed in Alexandrian orthopaedics. (From Bettman,[11] with permission.)

and effective techniques for bandaging the extremities were explained.[3,6] The writings describe the need for immobilization of open fractures and the benefits of joint mobilization for rehabilitation of injured limbs. The healers of that time appreciated that exercise strengthened extremities and inactivity resulted in wasting.[3]

Between 323 and 285 B.C., Alexandria became established one of the capitals of medicine.[11] Alexandrian influences include systematic training of physicians, emphasis on observation and measurements in research, the need to study anatomy through dissection, and the application of mathematics and mechanics to medicine. Archimedes was one of the great scientists of this time (Fig. 10-4).

Galen A.D. 131–201 was one of the first notable clinical investigators.[3,6,7,11,12] He was the first to use the terms *kyphosis, lordosis,* and *scoliosis.* Galen described amputations, resection of bone tumors, and the drainage of abscesses, and he produced a number of writings on skeletal anatomy (Figs. 10-5 and 10-6).[3,6,7]

Progress was slower during the Middle Ages (5th to 15th centuries). Paul of Aegina (625–690) discussed management of patellar fractures, osteotomy of long bones for malunion, and laminectomy. He also recognized the malleability of soft callus. Salves and plasters were employed by the Arab civilizations. During the 12th and 13th centuries, Western civilization was emerging and renewed efforts were made in the study of human anatomy and surgical techniques. Appreciation of cleanliness in the operating room, the use of simpler splints and braces, the use of weights and pulleys for continuous traction, and the use of surgical cauterization were addressed.[6,7]

Further strides were made during the Renaissance period (15th and 16th centuries).[3,6,7] Studies on human anatomy were performed by cadaver dissection. Leonardo da Vinci (1452–1519) portrayed muscles of the body and of the osseous skeleton accurately and in detail (Fig. 10-7). Because of the many

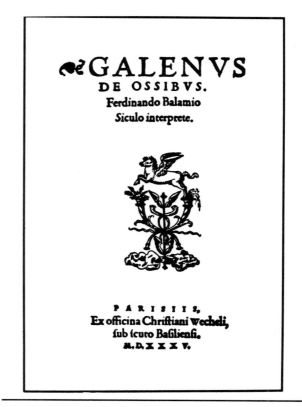

Fig. 10-5. Galen's book on bones, printed for the first time in 1535.

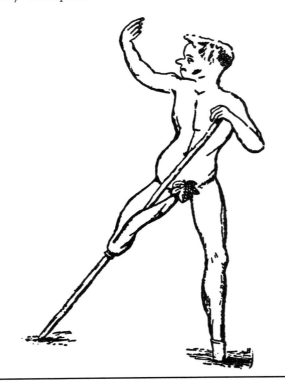

Fig. 10–6. Prosthesis of the right leg and left foot. (From an Italian vase of the fourth century B.C.)

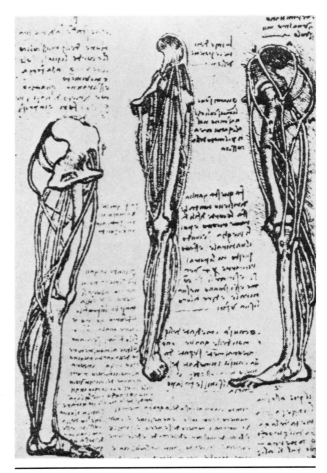

Fig. 10–7. The anatomy of the lower extremity by Leonardo da Vinci. The bones are joined by cords to indicate the lines of muscular traction. (Quaderno V. folio 4r.)

armies in action during this period, additional attention was directed toward skeletal trauma (Fig. 10-8). The Spaniards introduced the concept of field hospitals.[13]

The modern era in medicine is considered to commence with the publication of *De humani corporis Fabrica* by Vesalius in Basle in 1543. Vesalius, who was both an anatomist and a surgeon, stressed the need for objective research and education. His text on anatomy became a classic[11,12,14] (Figs. 10-9 and 10-10).

The following year, the *Chirurgia e graeco in latinum conversa* was published by Guido Guidi (Vidius) in Paris. In this work Guidi presented multiple illustrations dealing with the treatment of fractures and dislocations[11,12] (Figs. 10-11 to 10-13).

Numerous contributions were made by Ambroise Paré (1510–1590), including the use of ligatures in amputations, the first arthoplasty of the elbow, im-

provements in fracture care (including vertebral fractures), descriptions of motor-sensory deficits and incontinence after spinal cord injury, and an operative approach to the vertebral column for spinal cord decompression (Figs. 10-14 and 11-15).[1-4,6] Early prostheses were devised, and Paré provided series of illustrations of mechanical artificial upper extremity devices made of metal.[3] During this period, Hans von Gersdorff, a wartime surgeon, advocated applied pressure to stop heavy bleeding.

Through the 17th and 18th centuries, modern methods of scientific investigation were applied to physiology, histology, and skeletal tissue. Fabry discussed

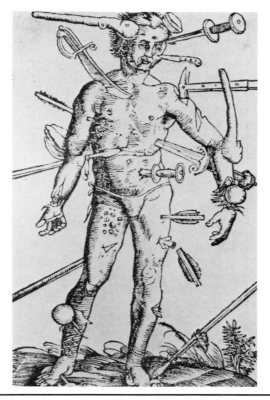

Fig. 10-8. The "wound man," indicating various injuries from different weapons. (From the Grosse Wundartzney, 1536, of Paracelsus.)

proximal amputation in the management of gangrene, described astragalectomy, introduced improved methods of treatment for clubfoot, and published the first pictorial description of scoliosis. Further contributions by Sydenham, Leeuwenhoek, Havers, Stenson, and Harvey marked the beginning of orthopaedics as a medical specialty.[1,7]

In 1741, the term *orthopaedia* was coined from its use as the title of a treatise published by Nicholas Andry.[1,2,7] The word was derived from the Greek roots *orthos* (straight) and *paidios* (child) to express Andry's belief that many musculoskeletal deformities begin in childhood. He stated:

As to the title, I have formed it of two Greek words, vis, orthos, which signifies straight, free from deformity and paidios, child. Out of these Two Words I

have compounded that of orthopaedia, to express in one Term the Design I propose, which is to teach the different methods of preventing and correcting the Deformities of children.[7]

During the 18th, 19th, and 20th centuries, studies on bone growth and repair were undertaken. With the advent of anesthesia and asepsis, operative intervention in many musculoskeletal disorders became possible.[6,7] William Ditmold (1808–1894) has been identified as "the first American orthopaedic surgeon."[15] A student of the German surgeon Stromeyer, Dimold was recognized for his operative treatment of clubfeet and established a public clinic for the treatment of crippled children in New York at the College of Physicians and Surgeons.[1] Lewis Sayre was another recognized early American orthopaedic surgeon, who organized the orthopaedic clinic at Bellevue Hospital. With his interest in scoliosis and tuberculosis, he was the first American to receive the title "Professor of Orthopaedic Surgery."

Hugh Owen Thomas (1834–1891) was another of the most respected early American orthopaedic surgeons[6,9,11,12] (Fig. 10-16). He emphasized the use of rest for the relief of pain and inflammation and stressed the importance of careful clinical examination of the musculoskeletal system. Sir Robert Jones (1857–1933), a nephew of Thomas, popularized the earlier techniques that Thomas had advocated. Jones gained international recognition as he headed the orthopaedic service of the British Army during World War I.[1,2,6,15]

Many other persons have been influential in the development of modern orthopaedics, and their achievements have been summarized by Enneking and coworkers[2] and Evarts.[1] James Knight (1810–1887), and his successor Virgil Gibney (1847–1927), served as founders and Surgeons-in-Chief, Hospital for The Ruptured and Crippled; Charles F. Taylor (1827–1888) founded the New York Orthopaedic Dispensary and Hospital. Newton M. Schaeffer (1846–1928), Edward H. Bradford (1848–1926), DeForrest Willard (1846–1910), H. Winnett Orr (1877–1956), Jose Trueta (1897–1977), and Reginald Watson-Jones (1902–1972) provided countless contributions in books and scientific reports.[6] Reginald Watson-Jones advocated the involvement of the

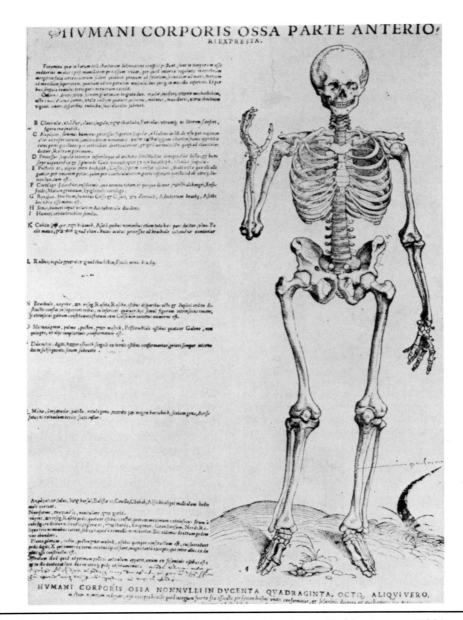

Fig. 10-9. The skeleton, designed by Calcar. (From Vesalius' Anatomical Tables, Venice, 1538.)

allied health professions in chronic care, which paved the way for the team approach and a more modern organization to rehabilitation.

Sir John Charnley (1911–1982) deserves special mention for his contributions. His early writings discussed fracture healing, the methods of closed treat-ment of fractures, and the principles of joint arthrodesis using compression. He later pioneered the development of low-friction total joint arthroplasty for hip arthritis. Charnley emphasized the role of airborne bacterial wound contamination in the operating room and studied the influence of clean-air systems.[6]

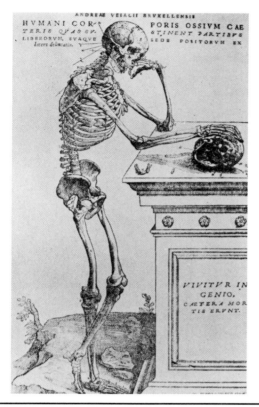

Fig. 10–10. The skeleton in meditation. (From Vesalius' *Fabrica*.)

ORGANIZATIONS OF ORTHOPAEDIC SURGERY AND THE FURTHER ESTABLISHMENT OF A SURGICAL SPECIALTY

By the late 19th century, the specialty of orthopaedic surgery was gaining interest and popularity as a separate area of medicine. In 1884, the *Archivio di Ortopedia*, among the earliest of the specialty orthopaedic journals, was established. Three years later, the first and oldest of the major United States orthopaedic organizations, the American Orthopaedic Association, was founded. The first *Transactions* were published in 1889, and the journal continued until 1903. At that time, the *American Journal of Orthopaedic Surgery* was published. In 1922, this journal became the *Journal of Bone and Joint Surgery*. The American Academy of Orthopaedic Surgeons was established in 1932 and held its first annual meeting the following year. Since then, the organization has grown to be the largest orthopaedic organization in the world, with 12,094 members and 1,926 emeritus fellows as of 1991[1,2] (American Academy of Orthopaedic Surgeons and American Board of Orthopaedic Surgery, personal communication, 1991).

The American Board of Orthopaedic Surgery was founded in 1934. It has had the responsibility of examining and certifying voluntary candidates. The Board has standing committees on Eligibility, Examinations, Finance, Graduate Education, Planning and Development, and Recertification. The Board establishes minimum educational requirements in the specialty, conducts the certifying examinations, issues certificates, stimulates education, and aids in the evaluation of educational facilities in the best interest of the public and the medical profession.[1,2] (American Academy of Orthopaedic Surgeons and American Board of Orthopaedic Surgery, personal communication, 1991).

An increase in the interest, training programs, and positions for graduate training in orthopaedic surgery occurred after World War II. To maintain minimum standards of education, these programs came under scrutiny of the Joint Review Committee of the American Medical Association and the American Board of Orthopaedic Surgery.[2] The Residency Review Committee of Orthopaedic Surgery was founded in 1953. Its purpose is to maintain the standards of residency education in the orthopaedic programs throughout the United States.[1,2]

Additional scientific and regional organizations have been established during the last 60 years. Among these are the Western Orthopaedic Association (1932), the Association of Bone and Joint Surgeons (1947), the Orthopaedic Research Society (1954), the Orthopaedic Research and Education Foundation (1955), the Eastern Orthopaedic Association (1970), the Mid America Orthopaedic Association (1982), the Central States Orthopaedic Society, the Advisory Council for Orthopaedic Resident Education (1975), the Academic Orthopaedic Society (1971), and the Ruth Jackson Orthopaedic Society (1983). Organizations representing areas of subspecialization within orthopaedic surgery have also been established. These include the American Society for Surgery of the Hand (1946), the Scoliosis Research Society

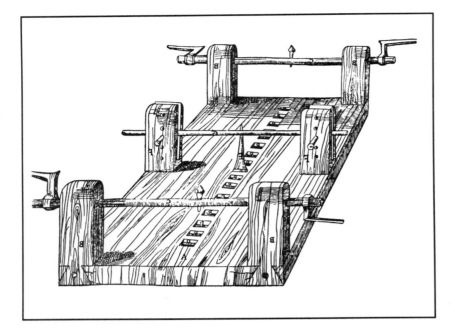

Fig. 10–11. The *scamnum,* or fracture table of Hippocrates. Woodcut probably after Francesco Primaticcio. From Guido Guidi, *Chirurgia e graeco in latinum conversa* (Paris, Gaultier, 1544, p. 519).

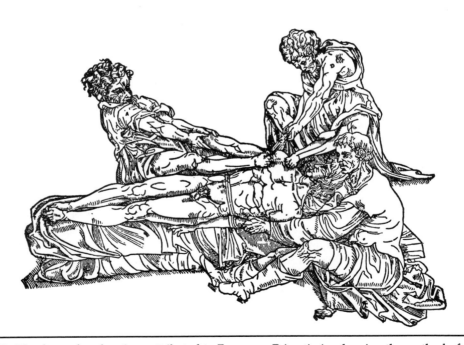

Fig. 10–12. Woodcut, after drawings attributed to Francesco Primaticcio, showing the method of reducing a dislocation of the shoulder. From Guido Guidi, *Chirurgia e graeco in latinum conversa* (Paris, Gaultier, 1544).

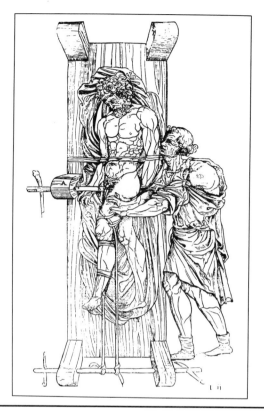

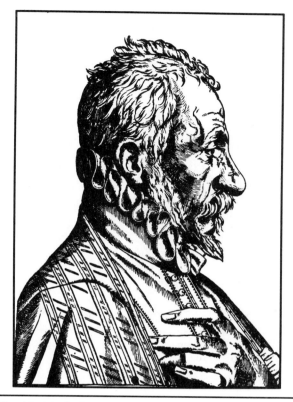

Fig. 10–13. The *scamnum* used to reduce a posterior dislocation of the hip. From Guidi, *Chirurgia e graeco in latinum conversa* (Paris, Gaultier, 1544, p. 527).

Fig. 10–14. Ambroise Paré (1510–1590). Woodcut from the first edition of his collected writings, *Les oeuvres de M. Ambroise Paré, consieller, et premier chirurgien du Roy* (Paris, Gabriel Buon, 1575).

(1966), the American Orthopaedic Foot and Ankle Society (1969), the Hip Society (1969), the Sports Medicine Society, the Spine Society, the Cervical Spine Research Society (1973), the Orthopaedic Trauma Association (1974), the International Arthroscopy Association (1974), the International Society of the Knee, the Knee Society (1983), the Association of Children's Prosthetic and Orthotic Clinics (1980), the American Shoulder and Elbow Surgeons (1982), the Pediatric Orthopaedic Society of North America (1984), the North American Spine Society (1985), the Federation of Spine Associations, the Association for Arthritic Hip and Knee Surgery (1991), and the Council of Musculoskeletal Specialty Societies. Among the most recent of the recognized orthopaedic subspeciality societies is the Orthopaedic Rehabilitation Association, founded in February 1990.

All of these organizations have played a role in the establishment of orthopaedic surgery and in the promotion of knowledge, teaching, and research of the musculoskeletal system. Through these organizations, education of members and the sharing of ideas continues to assist increase the quality of the specialty.

Because of the expansion and complexity of orthopaedic surgery, a recent trend toward further subspecialization has been noted. Many orthopaedists now tend to emphasize or restrict their practices to the subspecialities. These include spine surgery, hand and microvascular surgery, adult reconstruction (total joint replacement), orthopaedic trauma surgery, pediatric orthopaedics, foot and ankle surgery, sports medicine, tumor surgery, orthopaedic re-

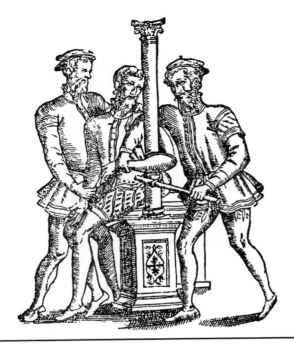

Fig. 10-15. Reduction of an elbow dislocation. (From Paré's *Chirurgia,* 1573.)

ognized separate area of study for the orthopaedic in-training examination (an examination given annually to orthopaedic surgery residents during each year of their training), further emphasizing its recognition and importance to orthopaedic surgery.

Fellowships in rehabilitation are available at rehabilitation centers such as Rancho Los Amigos Medical Center, Downey, CA; the Santa Clara Valley Medical Center, San Jose, CA (affiliated with Stanford University); and Craig Hospital Swedish Medical Center, Englewood, CO. However, a background for rehabilitation subspecialization can be gained with general orthopaedic training combined with an interest and experience in clinical and research issues. Other fellowship areas also will further prepare the orthopaedist for specializing in rehabilitation. For example, fellowships in hand, foot, spine, or pediatric orthopaedic surgery can provide a solid foundation for rehabilitation care in these areas.

search, and rehabilitation. Although rehabilitation is now considered a subspeciality, all orthopaedic subspecialties are involved in rehabilitation. Section IV of this text, which discusses generalized disorders, provides an example of the subspecialization within orthopaedics. The authors of these chapters were selected because of their specialized training, interest, and recognition in these areas.

ORTHOPAEDIC REHABILITATION: A RECOGNIZED SUBSPECIALTY

Interest in rehabilitation as an orthopaedic subspecialty and as an area of clinical and research emphasis has increased in recent years. The American Academy of Orthopaedic Surgeons now recognizes rehabilitation as an official subspeciality, and in February of 1990, the Orthopaedic Rehabilitation Association (ORA) was formed in New Orleans, Louisiana. David F. Apple, Jr., M.D., served as the first president. The first official annual research meeting of the ORA subsequently followed in San Antonio, Texas, in November 1990, hosted by John D. Hsu, M.D., and David F. Apple, Jr., M.D. Rehabilitation is also a rec-

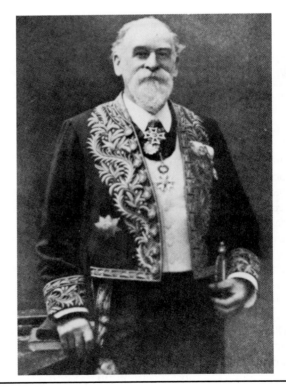

Fig. 10-16. Hugh Owen Thomas (1834-1891) exerted an enormous influence on the treatment of fractures.

Rehabilitation should now be considered a *surgical* as well as medical subspecialty. A multitude of surgically treatable extremity problems can develop in patients with chronic neuromuscular disorders. Surgery in rehabilitation can offer limb reconstruction in cases of brain injury, stroke, spinal cord injury, cerebral palsy, myelomeningocele, muscular dystrophy, or peripheral nerve dysfunction. Surgical release of refractory contractures, resection of heterotopic bone, tendon transfers to restore function, open nerve blocks or neurectomy to decrease spasticity, and débridement and/or local or free tissue transfers to cover chronic wounds or ulcers are a few examples. Surgical placement of implantable electrodes for electrical stimulation of muscle is gaining merit. Spine stabilization will promote rehabilitation after injury and will preserve pulmonary function in neuromuscular diseases the lead to compromised vital capacity from thorocolumbar deformity. Multiple trauma patients with fractures can undergo much earlier and aggressive rehabilitation if extremity injuries are stabilized surgically. For the patient with chronic arthroses or arthritis, surgery can offer arthroscopy, synovectomy, osteotomy, joint arthrodesis, or arthroplasty to improve function or obliterate pain. In the diabetic patient or peripheral vascular disease patient, management of dysvascular or infected extremities includes surgical débridement, incision and drainage of infections, and, when necessary, amputation of avascular or gangrenous limbs followed by prosthesis fitting and early rehabilitation.

It should also be emphasized that, in many cases, rehabilitation can optimally start very early, often when the patient is still in the acute phase of the injury or affliction. Rehabilitation planning can commence when a patient with brain or spinal cord injury is still in the trauma unit or intensive care facility. Fractures are stabilized aggressively to promote limb mobilization and assist rehabilitation. Splinting or casting of spastic limbs is instituted as soon as possible, ideally within the first few days of acute hospitalization, and while the patient is still in the intensive care unit. Consultation with the rehabilitation team members, such as rehabilitation nurses, physical and occupational therapists, and social workers, can be obtained when the patient is still in the early or acute phase of treatment, and therapy is instituted as soon as the patient's medical condition permits. Discharge planning can rarely be started *too early*. Rehabilitation is a team approach, and early awareness and involvement of the entire team will optimize patient care.

SUMMARY

From prehistoric times to the present, humans have been afflicted with acute and chronic neuromusculoskeletal diseases. As a result of efforts to treat these conditions, orthopaedic surgery has emerged as a medical and surgical specialty. Rehabilitation is an area of subspecialization, and the orthopaedic surgeon, along with the rest of the rehabilitation team, plays an active role in helping to ameliorate these problems and in restoring or improving function and comfort in the patient with chronic neuromusculoskeletal problems.

REFERENCES

1. Evarts CM: Historical highlights of orthopaedics. p. 1. In Surgery of the Musculoskeletal System. Churchill Livingstone, New York, 1983
2. Enneking W, Brower T, Ralston E, Hughston J: The history of orthopaedic surgery. p. 1. In Manual of Orthopaedic Surgery. American Orthopaedic Association, 1972
3. Lyons AS, Petrucelli RJ (eds): Medicine: An Illustrated History. Abradale Press, Harry N Abrams, New York, 1987
4. Packard RR: Ambroise Paré. Hoeber, New York, 1921
5. Orr HW: On the Contributions of Hugh Owen Thomas, Sir Robert Jones, John Ridlon to Modern Orthopaedic Surgery. Charles C Thomas, Springfield, IL, 1949
6. Peltier LF: Fractures: A History and Iconography of Their Treatment. Norman Publishing, San Francisco, 1990
7. Bick EM: Source Book of Orthopaedics. Hafner Publishing, New York, 1968
8. Dawson WR: Pigmies, dwarfs, and hunchbacks in ancient Egypt. Am Med Hist 9:315, 1927
9. Garrison FH: History of Medicine. WB Saunders, Philadelphia, 1929
10. Breasted JH: The Edwin Smith papyrus. NY Hist Soc Q Bull 6:5, 1922
11. Bettmann OL: A Pictorial History of Medicine. Charles C Thomas, Springfield, IL, 1956
12. Castiglioni A: A History of Medicine. 2nd Ed. Alfred A. Knopf, New York, 1958
13. Billings JS: History of Surgery. In Dennis FS (ed): System of Surgery. Lea Brothers, Philadelphia, 1895–1896
14. Lasky II: The martyrdom of Dostor Vesalius. Clin Orthop 259:304, 1990
15. Shands AR Jr: The Early Orthopaedic Surgeons of America. CV Mosby, St. Louis, 1970

11 Trauma Surgery and Trauma Nursing

DAVID B. HOYT
PEGGY HOLLINGSWORTH-FRIDLUND

Improvements in trauma care mean that more persons are surviving major injuries. These injuries often have severely disabling effects, which require intense rehabilitation efforts that are tailored for a specific diagnosis. Most trauma patients require some degree of rehabilitation, which may be as simple as wound care instructions after the repair of a laceration in the emergency room.

In 1985 approximately 9 million disabling injuries occurred in the United States, 340,000 of which were associated with some degree of impairment.[1] Permanent disabilities occur at least twice as frequently as fatalities, but only about 10 percent of patients have access to rehabilitation services. A general awareness of the need for rehabilitation, the resources required, and the accessibility to service is largely undeveloped among health care systems in the United States.

This fact places new demands on health care providers, particularly those involved *early* in the care of injured patients. The challenge has become to ensure that the trauma patient not only survives but also achieves the best possible restoration of physical, psychological, social, and vocational function. Deciding on methods to deal with this problem is somewhat hindered by the unavailability of information, in part because the trauma patient population tends to be young, single, and mobile, with poor compliance with follow-up care.

Some evidence does exist that specific injuries are the most important predictors of disability.[2] Table 11-1 shows the three major injury categories among the

1,022 patients requiring rehabilitation over a five-year period at University of California at San Diego Medical Center, a Level I hospital in a trauma system. Head injury, spine injury, and combined pelvic and long bone injury accounted for 788 of these patients, or more than 75 percent of patients needing rehabilitation services. The need for rehabilitation can be directly related to the Abbreviated Injury Scale (AIS) groups (AIS-3, moderate; AIS-4, severe; AIS-5, critical). Predictive factors influencing return to work include age, level of education, prior work experience, a strong social support system, and access to a rehabilitation program.[3]

Of equal importance is ensuring that primary care initiated at the time of resuscitation is integrated with a successful rehabilitation program. The trauma surgeon and trauma nurse are in the unique position to recognize this need and to initiate the process of identifying rehabilitation needs, which are then integrated into definitive treatment and long-term planning.

ANTICIPATING THE NEED FOR REHABILITATION: A STATE OF AWARENESS

The foundation of any rehabilitation program rests on the premise that the consequences of injury must be minimized, preventable complications avoided ("do no harm"), and the permanent loss of function limited. Of equal importance is the maintenance and development of remaining function to full capacity to achieve maximal functional independence.

Table 11-1. Patients from UCSD, a Level I Trauma Center Requiring Rehabilitation by Major Diagnostic Category and Abbreviated Injury Score (*N* = 1,022 total)

	Total	Abbreviated Injury Score[a]		
		AIS-3	AIS-4	AIS-5
Head	448	63	186	198
Spine	276	55	69	145
Pelvis or long bone	64	64	—	—
	788			

[a] AIS-3, moderate; AIS-4, severe; AIS-5, critical.

Recovery of a trauma patient can be divided into four phases: the resuscitation and critical care phase, the intermediate phase, the rehabilitation phase, and the reintegration phase. The focal point for team members taking care of the trauma patient during each of these phases changes dramatically. During the resuscitation and critical care phase, life saving is a priority. The primary role of the trauma surgeon in this phase is to lead all team efforts and deal with acute injury sequelae. During the intermediate phase, prevention of complications of injury and immobility become additional priorities. The rehabilitation and reintegration phases have traditionally been considered the domain of the physiatrist and other rehabilitation team members.

Interaction between the physiatrist and the trauma surgeon as a team in the resuscitation and critical care phase allows for initial identification of common problems, needs, and goals. This has been formalized into mandatory rehabilitation consultation by some trauma systems.[4]

Complete assessment and evaluation of the rehabilitation potential is the goal of this interaction. Although it is difficult to predict a final outcome after trauma, certain parameters aid in determining the extent and the rate of the patient's recovery. These strengths and weaknesses fall into the areas of physical, intellectual, and psychosocial functioning. Accurate understanding of the rehabilitation goals early in the care of these patients allows the trauma surgeon to have realistic interaction with the family, the patient, and the other people involved in the patient's care. Table 11-2 demonstrates an example of reasonable rehabilitation goals for patients after spinal cord

Table 11-2. Spinal Cord Injury Level and Potential for Rehabilitation

C4	Environmental controls with mouth
C5	Feed self, use electric wheelchair
C6	Manual wheelchair with rim lugs
C7–C8	Independent transfers, independent bowel and bladder management
T1–T10	Wheelchair independent, stand with support
T10–L2	Exercise ambulation
L3–S1	Community ambulation

injury and identifies the limits of physical abilities that are potentially achievable.

Although rehabilitation is often viewed as an isolated period in a patient's recovery it is really what provides momentum as a patient moves throughout the recovery period. Maximized patient function should be a common goal for patient and physician, although patients should be aware of recovery limitations in the acute phase of illness. The focus of this chapter is to identify those areas in the early resuscitative and critical care phase with which the trauma surgeon and nurse are specifically involved. During these phases the patient is completely dependent on medical professionals to anticipate complications and plan future progress.

RESUSCITATIVE AND ACUTE CARE PHASE

Although different injuries have distinct rehabilitation needs, the majority of patients requiring long-term rehabilitation will fall into the categories of head injury, spinal cord injury, and multiple trauma with multiple fractures. The following discussion therefore focuses on these areas. The injured patient's condition is obviously made more serious by comorbid disease, extremes of age, and combinations of injuries.

The introduction of trauma systems with organized prehospital and integrated intrahospital care has reduced immediate mortality and morbidity by efficient management of life-threatening injuries.[5,6] Although life-threatening injuries must be the primary concern in the emergency setting, unattended injuries that are seemingly minor may ultimately be the most devastating for the patient's long-term rehabilitation. Delays in treatment, failure to treat unidentified injuries, and iatrogenic injuries from emergency procedures can create additional morbidity, resulting in lengthened or complicated rehabilitation processes.

INITIAL PRIORITIES

Because the trauma surgeon's initial priorities are to prevent mortality, the emphasis is placed on early treatment of acute head injury and respiratory distress, and the identification and control of continued hemorrhage. Systematic protocols for management have been adopted as nationwide standards.[7] This phase usually involves multiple diagnostic procedures and may involve intubation and paralysis or prolonged surgical intervention. Concentration on these priorities may initially interfere with thorough assessment of rehabilitation requirements.

As soon as the patient is hemodynamically stable, within the first 24 hours after injury, reevaluation for obvious injuries requiring rehabilitation can be done. Treatment of a head injury with paralysis and sedation may mask some injuries. Bone surveys and careful reexamination should be done to reassess for any possible additional injury. A missed fracture or unnoticed brachial plexus injury can hinder a rehabilitation plan unless detected early.

Understanding of potential physical complications related to the injury itself and immobility-related complications is useful in highlighting acute-phase goals. In this area, the patient, trauma surgeon and physiatrist can have the greatest impact by working together.

INTEGRATION OF REHABILITATION INTO THE CRITICAL CARE UNIT

It is essential to maintain a rehabilitation team presence in the intensive care unit. Critical care nurses and trauma surgeons should be involved with the physiatrist and the occupational and physical therapists as early as the first 24 hours after injury.

An effective means for integrating rehabilitation into the critical care unit is by rehabilitation rounds. Personnel participating in rounds should include the trauma physician and nurse team members, nursing supervisors, and social workers. The process of rehabilitation rounds emphasizes the need to institute an early plan of therapy. It also replaces the inefficient "piecemeal" ordering of physical or occupational therapy and provides a guided approach to the total needs of the patient.

These rounds are intended to establish exercise and positioning regimens and institute splinting, skin care, prothesis needs, and bowel and bladder training programs. Discussions on levels of functional recovery and plans for posthospitalization placement also are initiated. Physical and occupational therapists are in a position to report on patient progress. The rehabilitation service then follows patients from the beginning of their hospitalization, which gives them a personal, long-term history of each patient's specific needs and response to therapy.

Most intensive care specialists have limited knowledge of the details of rehabilitation efforts, the length of time required for each phase of rehabilitation, the long-term effects of rehabilitation on daily living, or the training techniques the patient might need once discharged from the hospital. Often the trauma surgeon and nurse are the first persons to be asked about these aspects by the family. These questions arise once the initial shock of traumatic injury is resolved as they try to assimilate any subsequent effects the situation will have on their lives. Accurate early information through rehabilitation team involvement with a physiatrist creates a means by which these questions will be answered consistently as the entire team counsels the family.

Acute care providers also tend to lack awareness of how critical care influences long-term functional recovery. This may be due to the high-technology atmosphere of the intensive care units (ICUs) today. More likely, ICU health workers rarely have a routine system of obtaining follow-up information on patients transferred out of the specialty care unit. The information that patients have contractures of upper extremities as a result of poor positioning or lack of range-of-motion exercise may never reach the critical care physician or nurse. ICU nurses must be taught an understanding of a "critical pathway" to be able to direct patients on the path to total fulfillment of their rehabilitation potential.

The rehabilitation rounds also help establish the professional competence of physical (PTs) and occupational therapists (OTs) and increase other team members' familiarity with their roles. For example, rehabilitation personnel frequently urge ICU staff members to examine the patient's ability to tolerate any kind of exercise daily. Cooperation among ICU nurses, PTs, and OTs is important so that the respective roles of nurses and rehabilitation therapists in the acute phase are better delineated.

Gaining a consistent understanding of what anatomic structures can be mobilized on a polytraumatized patient makes every team member aware that the patient with uninjured extremities should be placed in an exercise program immediately. This maintains good limb function and places the patient at an advantage in later stages of recovery.

Early use of occupational and physical therapy even in unconscious patients helps nurses in creating a specific set of goals. Reevaluations on a daily basis help them become accepted as an integral part of the patient's critical care. For example, although nurses in an ICU normally would consider passive range-of-motion exercises a nursing function, these are frequently a low priority because of the many demands at the bedside. Instituting a weekly range-of-motion measurement of the major joints by a PT may prove to be very beneficial. It gives both nurses and the therapist a progress measurement and leads to serial assessment graphs, which can be maintained at the patient's bedside. These simple interventions and documentation prevent what in the past has been left to a matter of convenience and give it the equivalent priority of good pulmonary toilet or the initiation of enteral feeding.

TRAUMA SURGEON INTENSIVIST: SPECIFIC ROLES BY BODY SYSTEM

The initial evaluation and intraoperative control of hemorrhage is not the end of the injury process. The concept of secondary injury suggests that hypoxia, metabolic abnormalities, or immunosuppression and infection can subsequently cause further damage. It is the trauma surgeon intensivist's role to prevent further secondary injury on a system-by-system basis.

Central Nervous System and Spine

Initial head injury assessment is done using the Glasgow Coma Scale.[8] Patients who are unconscious and have abnormal motor function will generally be treated aggressively with paralysis and hyperventilation for a severe brain injury and intracranial hypertension. In addition, they will undergo computed tomographic scanning for diagnosis and subsequent operative intervention if appropriate. Seventy percent of these patients have no operative lesion and will be managed with control of intracranial pressure to prevent secondary injury, maintenance of hemodynamic stability, and avoidance of hypoxia. Rehabilitation teams must work closely with the clinician because control of high intracranial pressures (ICPs) may be the limiting factor in carrying out vigorous exercise activities, even in paralyzed patients. The team should be aware of the need for immediate splinting and positioning techniques during this phase of care. When ICP is not adversely affected by exercise regimens, these regimens should be instituted immediately.

If a patient has fractures requiring fixation to facilitate early mobilization, the critical decision to be made is whether the patient's head injury is too severe to tolerate surgery. If a patient can tolerate surgery, fractures should be stabilized internally as early as possible because there is good evidence that fixation within 24 hours leads to decreased nitrogen excretion, allows earlier mobilization, and simplifies nursing care.[9]

Spinal cord injury can be complicated by the increased risk of respiratory dysfunction. This may require immediate treatment with intubation and ventilation. Patients can have loss of sympathetic tone and associated hypotension but this also mandates consideration of sources of hemorrhage. If no obvious bleeding source is found, treatment with systemic vasopressors to maintain mean arterial pressure should be done to avoid secondary injury from hypotension. These patients may become poikilothermic owing to lack of sympathetic control and loss of the shivering response. Temperature control and regulation need to be carefully monitored.

A mechanism of injury that produces head and spinal cord injury usually mandates rapid diagnostic decisions regarding a thorough assessment for cavitary hemorrhage, ventilatory status, and associated fractures. Failure to control bleeding sources or permitting patients to become hypoxic or hypoventilatory adds a significant component of secondary injury to head and spine injuries from decreased perfusion, decreased oxygen delivery, and intracranial hypertension.

Respiratory System

Any patient with head injury, spinal cord injury, or multiple fractures with decreased respiratory movement is less able to mobilize secretions and may have significant alteration in respiratory function. It should be anticipated that these patients may have compromised respiratory status. The presence of an endotracheal tube is associated with the development of pneumonia in approximately 70 percent of patients undergoing mechanical ventilation for more than 5 days.[10] Aggressive pulmonary toilet, including turning, coughing, and nasotracheal suctioning of intubated patients, should be routine. Kinetic bed therapy may be of use. Early fevers, infiltrates on chest radiographs, or change in sputum should be treated with antibiotics selected to cover the flora endemic in the hospital. Lobar collapse or failure to resolve a pneumonia should be treated with bronchoscopy. Patients with multiple rib fractures may require pain control measures that facilitate not only respiratory therapy but also exercise and activity tolerance.

Cardiovascular System

In addition to the potential for hemodynamic instability owing to sympathectomy after spinal cord injury, patients can demonstrate continued hemodynamic instability from bleeding that is not treatable with surgery (fractures, retroperitoneal hematomas). Cardiovascular assessment by measurement of cardiac output may be necessary to optimize oxygen delivery. Volume resuscitation should be guided by precise hemodynamic measurements. If hypotension occurs as a result of sympathectomy, decreased peripheral vascular resistance may require treatment with vasopressors.

Loss of supporting muscle tone and resulting venous stasis may lead to venous pooling and orthostatic changes as a patient is mobilized in the first few days after injury. Patients who have been at bed rest and demonstrate orthostasis in the upright or sitting position can be placed on a tilt table to gradually improve tolerance. Leg wraps and compression hose will also help.

All patients immobilized from head injury, spinal cord injury, or multiple fractures have a significant potential for thrombophlebitis, deep venous thrombosis (DVT), and pulmonary embolus as late complications. These should be anticipated immediately after injury. Patients should be treated with lower extremity venous compression hose and subcutaneous heparin. They should be monitored carefully with serial plethysmography or echography. In the event that they develop DVT they should be treated with systemic heparin or vena caval interruption. Because one of the leading causes of late death in trauma patients after immobility is pulmonary embolus, routine prophylaxis should be part of normal acute care.[11]

Gastrointestinal System: Nutrition, Catabolism, and Gastrointestinal Function

The multiply traumatized patient undergoes a general stress response produced by circulating catecholamines, glucagon, insulin, interleukin-1 (IL-1), interleukin-6 (IL-6), and tumor necrosis factor (TNF), which leads to hypercatabolism, negative nitrogen balance, and protein-calorie malnutrition.[12] This contributes to muscle weakness and causes severe muscle atrophy, which further hampers potential for rehabilitation.

Increasing evidence suggests that patients without enteral nutritional supplementation are potentially at risk for secondary injury as a result of bacterial translocation and sepsis. Early initiation of enteral feeding seems to be warranted.[13] If enteral feeding cannot be initiated for 5 to 7 days, parenteral hyperalimentation has demonstrated efficacy in preventing protein-calorie malnutrition and subsequent infection.

Access for feeding can be accomplished either by placement of a feeding gastrostomy in patients with significant head injury or by duodenal feeding tubes. Delayed gastric emptying can be treated with intravenous metoclopramide hydrochloride. Recognizing a patient's need for intervention is the critical feature so that the hypercatabolic state can be supported.

Upper gastrointestinal bleeding from stress ulceration is a preventable complication. All patients should have nasogastric tubes and monitoring of nasogastric aspirate pH. pH should be titrated with either H_2 blockers or antacids to keep the pH at 5.0. The optimal pH is still a source of debate.

The anticipation of return of gastrointestinal function and early attention to a bowel program in patients with severe head or spinal cord injury are essential. All patients should undergo digital examination to make sure there is no fecal impaction. Tube feedings must be adjusted to avoid constipation and diarrhea. The provision of stool bulking agents is essential for the development of an effective nutritional supplementation program and its acceptance by the nursing staff. Spinal cord injury patients should be started on a bowel program while in the intensive care unit. Cathartics can be used to stimulate evacuation.

Urinary System

The loss of effective gravity in patients who are bedridden and the resulting urinary stasis leads to increased urinary calculi and sediment in both the renal pelvis and the bladder. Acutely, urinary tract infection is also a problem because of indwelling catheters. Passive turning, either through log rolling or through use of kinetic beds, can aid in the effective emptying of the bladder early after injury, particularly with head injury and spinal cord injury. Frequent urine cultures in anticipation of infection should allow early treatment with appropriate antibiotics. Indwelling Foley catheters in patients with spinal cord injury should be replaced with intermittent catheterization programs as quickly as possible.

Musculoskeletal System

Evidence suggests that early fracture fixation decreases negative nitrogen balance and decreases respiratory complications.[9] The primary advantage of early fixation is to allow passive and active assisted range-of-motion exercises to begin early after injury. These exercises should be started as early as the patient is able to be assessed for unappreciated injuries, usually within 24 hours. Appropriate positioning and body alignment in bed and chair are important for immobilized extremities.

Contraction deformity is one of the most serious preventable complications that occur during the acute phase. Appropriate attention must be paid to positioning. Pillows should not be placed behind the patient's head. Debilitated patients or patients paralyzed with pharmacologic agents will develop "swan-neck" contracture, which will lead to significant deformity and ultimately interfere with ambulation. Uninjured shoulders, elbows, wrists, hips, knees, and ankles should be placed through a range of motion while patients are immobilized or paralyzed. It is easy and convenient to measure and record the range of motion to set both nurses' and therapists' goals.

In patients sustaining above-knee or below-knee amputations, early hip joint stiffening can occur, hindering long-term rehabilitation. This can be counteracted by turning the patient in the semiprone position toward the unaffected side and gently stretching the hip joint on the affected side. This "partial pronation" can be coordinated with other aspects of routine care so it is not overlooked.

Each patient's full rehabilitation potential should be specifically calculated and anticipated in the earliest phases of care, because it may influence the decisions in management of other injuries. For example, a paraplegic with bilateral humerus fractures should be considered for aggressive intramedullary rodding because the patient's upper extremities will be the weight-bearing surfaces for self-transfer. Nonjudicious placement of humeral plates with inadequate weight-bearing strength for transfer may affect a patient's timely rehabilitation. These are the type of situations that can be avoided by careful planning.

Osteoporosis and heterotopic ossification should be anticipated, and resistance exercises and active weight-bearing should be started as soon as possible to prevent abnormal calcification and bone fragility. Calcium supplementation should be avoided.

Integumentary System

Prolonged pressure to skin diminishes capillary blood supply and stops nutrient flow, leading to cell necrosis, subsequent infection, and delayed rehabilitation. In addition, trauma patients frequently have open wounds and abrasions that can become infected. Assessment should include evaluation of skin integrity, attention to nutritional status, and determination of risk status for breakdown. Patients should be repositioned at least every 2 hours and more often in the presence of previous hypotension or increased weight. Kinetic beds may aid in the maintenance of skin integrity but must be used correctly because skin lesions can result from their misuse.

All the areas at risk should be massaged to promote circulation, and patients should be taught to inspect their own skin and shift weight frequently in areas that are insensate. In general, skin breakdown, subsequent infection, and its complications — which can prolong hospital stay — should be entirely preventable by avoiding inappropriate positioning and by frequent turning of the patient.

Host Defense System: Infection and Immunosuppression

After the initial complications of bleeding and uncontrollable intracranial hypertension, the next most important determinant of morbidity and mortality is infection. This is partly the result of injury-induced immunosuppression, which has been the topic of much research in the last decade. The immunosuppression that occurs after trauma is initiated by injury itself. It is also thought to be aggravated by bacterial translocation due to mucosal breakdown after injury, which can be partially prevented by enteral feeding. Furthermore, nutritional deficiencies have been shown to compound the immunosuppressed state. Early alimentation is an attempt to promote normal host defense.

General principles to follow in treating the immunosuppressed state include timely changing of all invasive devices, such as intravenous lines and Foley catheters, adequate tissue débridement, drainage of all infected sources, and aggressive institution of nutrition, preferentially by the enteral route. All of these have been associated with decreased infection.

Infection should be anticipated in patients with open fractures, open dura, and open enteric wounds, and prophylactic antibiotics should be started. Patients

whose normal host defense barriers have been violated should be monitored on an expectant basis for developing nosocomial infection. Intubation for longer than 3 to 5 days leads predictably to pneumonia, which should be anticipated.

The possibility of induction of resistance by the antibiotics selected should be appreciated. Patients with infections should have serial specimen cultures every other day, and antibiotic therapy should be guided by the results.

In addition to nutritional deficiencies and breakdown in host barriers, the injury-induced inflammatory state is immunosuppressive. Current evidence suggests that inflammatory cell–based cytokines IL-1, TNF, and Il-6 are some of the significant mediators of the hypermetabolic response to injury. They can aggravate the initial injury by causing secondary injury.

No specific forms of modulation or control of these processes currently exists. They are intimately related to a patient's muscle atrophy and wound healing and affect ultimate rehabilitation fulfillment. Attempts to characterize the other deficiencies that occur after injury tend to involve virtually every aspect of inflammation and healing. These include failure to process new antigens, decreased effectiveness of phagocytic inflammatory cells, and abnormalities in various aspects of specific and nonspecific immunity. These are in part generated by the injury itself and sustained by ongoing infection and in part aggravated by nutritional deficiencies that accompany injury. Attentiveness and an understanding based on ongoing research of these processes will allow the trauma surgeon increasingly to influence the rehabilitation process, by lessening the secondary injury due to these factors.

Psychological Factors and Pain Control

Given the complexity of treatment of acutely injured patients, who are often head injured, hypoxic, or paralyzed for several days, it is understandable that often little attention is paid to their immediate psychological well-being.

Pain control should be maintained with careful dosing. As many as 50 percent of trauma patients are known to have intoxicating levels of either alcohol or drugs. Their premorbid alcohol and drug history is usually unknown. It is possible for these patients to go through toxic withdrawal, which should be anticipated. This condition is usually evidenced by a fever in the first 48 hours that cannot be explained by an infected source.

The desensitization of the ICU patient resulting from constant stimulation and lack of restful sleep must be appreciated. Patients should be appropriately sedated so that they do not have excessive anxiety. Once the acute phase has passed, every attempt should be made to reestablish the sleep cycle of patients who are still ventilator dependent but are awakening. When these patients work on range-of-motion exercises or weaning from the ventilator they are better rested and have an improved attitude.

Sensitivity to pain, particularly during range-of-motion exercises (active or passive), should be part of ongoing assessment so that the patient's attempts are not met with unnecessary pain, frustration, and failure. Posttraumatic stress syndrome should be given consideration. This can lead to significant depression and ultimately affect a patient's rehabilitation potential.

Finally, after injury, patients need specific neuropsychiatric evaluation and a program of cognitive rehabilitation that is practical and focused. Mental impairment is the most frequent cause of disability in patients with moderate or severe head injury.[14]

INJURY-SPECIFIC PROBLEMS

Head Injury

Most patients with severe head injury who survive will become rehabilitation candidates. Ninety percent will have achieved their maximum recovery within 6 months. Duration and depth of coma may assist in the prediction of survival and the length of memory deficit. Patients with posttraumatic amnesia of less than 14 days' duration generally have a good recovery 1 year following injury. Amnesia of greater than 28 days' duration is associated with a high degree of moderate to severe disability.[15]

Several other problems also affect the ultimate rehabilitation potential of head-injured patients. These are alterations of neuromuscular control that result in weakness, loss of sitting and standing balance, and development of spastic contractures. Spasticity occurring after head injury is attributable primarily to loss of abnormal inhibition over spinal and superspinal reflexes. These can be aggravated by stress and anxiety, and the initial attempts to control spasticity should be to modulate aggravating factors and maintain range of motion. Dantrolene sodium and diazepam may be helpful in some patients.

Posttraumatic epilepsy occurs in some patients who have sustained a head injury. This cannot be directly anticipated, from the initial injury but must be treated if it develops.

Behavioral abnormalities that may affect recovery potential after head injury are a function of the patient's premorbid personality and the social environment to which the patient returns. Frontal lobe injuries often cause deficits that include decreased initiative, impaired self-identity, and disregard for social standards. Temporal lobe lesions may result in episodic violent behavior without an accompanying seizure disorder. These emotional outbursts must be anticipated and not attributed to personality per se because they can be controlled with medications. If not appreciated and appropriately treated, these abnormalities can become a major impediment to rehabilitation and resocialization.

Spinal Cord Injury

The main goal after spinal cord injury is to minimize the functional deficit as soon as possible. In addition to establishing a stable bowel and bladder routine and avoiding decubitus ulcers and heterotopic ossification, the prevention of spasticity is essential. Muscle relaxants may be beneficial.

Autonomic dysreflexia may occur in patients with thoracic cord injuries above the T6 vertebral level and can be associated with distention of the bladder, rectal stimulation, and a number of other visceral stimuli. The syndrome is attributed to autonomic nervous system dysfunction and is characterized by severe hypertension and headaches. Treatment should be aimed toward removing the noxious stimulus, which will usually stop the problem. Diazoxide or hydralazine (Apresoline) may occasionally be required to control the hypertension.

Major Fractures

Once the patient's condition is stabilized, the goal of rehabilitation is to increase mobility. If rigid stabilization or immobilization has been achieved through external or internal fixation, early passive range-of-motion exercises can be started even in comatose patients. Continuous passive motion devices can be used in the ICU.

Once the patient is more alert, isometric exercises can be used to increase normal strength and tone. Muscle stimulation can retard the development of disuse atrophy and should be encouraged. Functional bracing can be an important adjunct to internal fixation in a complex unstable fracture to enable the patient to be up and moving. Patients with braces should have their skin condition serially assessed and the braces adjusted or padded.

SUMMARY

The trauma surgeon's job is to evaluate all life-threatening injuries and initiate therapy to stop the primary injury process. Of equal concern, anticipation of the potential for secondary injury and its effects on the ultimate rehabilitation outcome for a patient needs to be part of admission evaluation and treatment during the critical care phase.

Whether the patient has a severe head injury, spinal cord injury, or multiple fractures after polytrauma, neurologic, respiratory, cardiovascular, gastrointestinal, urinary, musculoskeletal, integumentary, and host defense needs are important. All are affected by the injury process, and prevention of complications in each of these systems can improve the ultimate rehabilitation results for the patient.

Emphasis on rehabilitation potential immediately after injury is essential. This should be accomplished through the coordinated efforts of a physiatrist and rehabilitation team, including acute care nurses, physical therapists, occupational therapists, and social workers. A strategy that calculates initial rehabilitation potential and appropriate therapy toward mobilization and prevention of contractures, skin breakdown, and infection should be planned as early as 24 hours after injury. Enlistment of help from the patient's family should start early and be based on knowledge of the patient's rehabilitation potential.

REFERENCES

1. Rice D, MacKenzie E et al: Cost of Injury in the United States: A Report to Congress. Institute for Health and Aging, University of California, San Francisco, and Injury Prevention Center, The Johns Hopkins University, Baltimore, 1989
2. MacKenzie E, Siegal J, Shapiro S et al: Functional recovery and medical costs in trauma: an analysis by type and severity of injury. J Trauma 28:281, 1988
3. MacKenzie E, Shapiro S, Smith R et al: Factors influencing return to work following hospitalization for traumatic injury. Am J Public Health 77:329, 1987
4. 1989–90 Standards for Trauma Center Accreditation. Pennsylvania Trauma Systems Foundation, Mechanicsburg, PA, 1989
5. Shackford SR, Mackersie RC, Hoyt DB: Impact of a trauma system on outcome of severely injuried patients. Arch Surg 122:523, 1987
6. Hoyt DB, Shackford SR, McGill T et al: Impact of in-house surgeons and operating room resuscitation on outcome of traumatic injuries. Arch Surg 124:906, 1989
7. Advanced Trauma Life Support Program: 1988 Instructor Manual. American College of Surgeons, Chicago, 1988
8. Jennett B, Teasdale G, Braakman R: Predicting outcome in individual patients after severe head injury. Lancet 1:1031, 1976
9. Bone L, Johnson K, Weifelt J, Scheinberg R: Early vs. delayed stabilization of femoral fractures: a prospective randomized trial. J Bone Joint Surg [Am] 71:336, 1989
10. Rodriguez J, Gibbons K, Bitzer L et al: Pneumonia: incidence, risk factors and outcome in the injured patient. J Trauma 30:928, 1990
11. Shackford SR, Davis JW, Hollingsworth-Fridlund P et al: Venous thromboembolism in patients with major trauma. Am J Surg 159:365, 1990
12. Bessey PQ, Watters JM, Aoki TT, Wilmore DW: Combined hormonal infusion simulates the metabolic response to the injury. Ann Surg 200:264, 1984
13. Moore FA, Moore EE, Jones TN et al: TEN versus TPN following major abdominal trauma—reduced septic morbidity. J Trauma 29:916, 1989
14. Heident J, Small R, Catou W, et al: Severe injury and outcome: a prospective study, p. 238. In Popp AJ, Bourke RS, Nelson CR, Kennelberg HK (eds): Neural Trauma. Raven, New York, 1979
15. Jennett B: Scale and scope of the problem, p. 127. In Rosenthal M, Griffin ER, Bond MR, Miller JD (eds): Rehabilitation of the Head Injured Adult. FA Davis, Philadelphia, 1983

12 Anesthesia for Rehabilitation Surgery

CLAIRE M. STILES
MEENAL PATEL
MARY ANN E. KEENAN

This chapter is not intended to provide a detailed account of all types of anesthesia used in the rehabilitation settings. Instead, it focuses on certain points the authors have judged to be important from their years of experience in this field. The description of services follows the structural organization at Rancho Los Amigos Medical Center, Downey, California.

ADULT BRAIN INJURY PATIENTS

Patients with head trauma who are to undergo rehabilitation procedures range from persons in coma vigil to those who are ambulatory with minimal residual effects from the injury. The majority fall into the middle range of the spectrum and tend to be combative or uncooperative. Generally this is a transient phase during recovery, although it can sometimes be permanent. Extra care must be taken with patients in the combative phase (who may kick, bite, hit, yell, and so forth) to prevent injury to patients and personnel. Soft restraints and padded bed rails are sometimes helpful.

Because the sympathetic and pain responses are intact in patients in coma vigil, these patients need an anesthetic. Generally, anesthesia is induced in brain injured patients for procedures performed to facilitate rehabilitation or nursing care. Examples of the types of procedures these persons undergo are multi-

ple tendon transfers on three of the four extremities, open phenol nerve blocks to relieve spasticity for 6 to 8 months, and resection of heterotopic ossification involving major joints, such as hip, shoulder, and elbow.

Preoperation Evaluation

The past medical history of adult patients with brain injury frequently is unobtainable, so all medical decisions are made on the basis of current evaluation and data. If there is any indication of chest injury at the time of the head trauma, a baseline electrocardiogram (ECG) and chest radiograph should be obtained. These patients, particularly in the early stage of rehabilitation, may have recurrent aspiration secondary to cranial nerve injury or atelectasis and pneumonia owing to inability to cough.

Medications that should be continued in the perioperative period include antihypertensive and anticonvulsive preparations.

Types of Anesthesia

Because of contractures, spasticity, and the length and extent of the rehabilitation procedure, general anesthesia usually is indicated, even in patients in coma vigil who are unresponsive. Both inhalation and narcotic anesthetics are well tolerated if given in small doses. In addition, Bier blocks may be done in patients with reflex sympathetic dystrophy to facilitate occupational therapy. If they are successful, serial Bier blocks may be beneficial.

Special Problems

Frequently the first problem encountered is locating a site for intravenous access. If the extremities are in casts or are the site of the current surgical procedures, the external jugular vein may be the only alternative. Problems that occur with intraoperative monitoring must be solved by mutual agreement with the surgeon. Often a blood pressure cuff may need to be moved from one extremity to another as the operation proceeds.

Enough staff members must be available to be able to control combative patients. Only after adequate sedation has been achieved should intravenous access be attempted. If sedation cannot be accomplished preoperatively, methohexital sodium (Brevital) can be given intramuscularly in the operating room, where ventilatory equipment is readily available.

Muscle relaxants should be chosen carefully. During the first year after injury, depolarizing agents should not be used. A single minimal dose of vecuronium bomide or atracurium besylate is suggested for procedures requiring the intraoperative use of a nerve stimulator, such as open phenol nerve blocks. Generally, such nerve blocks pose no problem for the surgeon but, if necessary, they can be reversed intraoperatively.

Blood loss may be rapid and substantial during operations for resection of heterotopic ossification. Use of a cell saver may reduce the need for transfusions with bank blood.

Patients with severe head trauma have poor temperature control, possibly of central origin. Frequently they are hypothermic preoperatively and, once under anesthesia, their temperatures may drop at an alarming rate. Active warming measures must be taken at the beginning of the procedure.

Recovery

Generally patients with head trauma emerge slowly from anesthesia. Therefore, the anesthetic agent should be lowered to a minimal concentration well before the end of the procedure. Criteria for extubation of such patients, especially those in coma vigil, include satisfactory expiration time, CO_2, tidal volume, and oxygen saturation on room air. If there is any doubt, the patient should be placed on a T tube with oxygen in the recovery room and extubated only when these values are within satisfactory limits.

Labile hypertension may appear first in the recovery room. Antihypertensive medications may be required after ruling out hypoxia, hypercarbia, and pain. Those patients who have not had a tracheostomy must be monitored carefully for upper airway obstruction. Frequent suctioning of secretions often is required.

Because of the patient's inability to cooperate or control secretions, atelectasis, pneumonia, or aspiration is a frequent unavoidable complication. Incentive spirometry should be encouraged if patient cooperation is even minimal.

STROKE PATIENTS

Most stroke patients belong to the geriatric group and have multiple medical problems, including cardiac disease, hypertension, and diabetes. They may be classified by the cause of the cerebrovascular accident: hypertensive bleed, thrombosis, or rupture of berry aneurysm. Most patients are first seen for surgical rehabilitation procedures several months after the initial injury. As with all diseases, patients exhibit varying degrees of involvement, from minimal residual effects in one extremity to total body involvement in massive or multiple strokes.

The surgical procedures for these patients involve mainly releases of contractures to facilitate nursing care and tendon transfers to improve mobilization.

Preoperative Evaluation

A detailed history of medical problems is essential. Most patients are taking several medications, including anticoagulants, antihypertensives, cardiac medications, and antidiabetic agents. Anticoagulants are discontinued preoperatively, whereas the other medications are maintained in the perioperative period.

The chest radiograph should be evaluated carefully for atelectasis and pneumonia secondary to repeated aspiration, a possible complication of strokes involving cranial nerves.

Types of Anesthesia

In medically stable patients, general anesthesia is acceptable so long as the patients are monitored carefully. Because these patients are more cooperative than those with head trauma, regional anesthesia can be used. A femoral-sciatic nerve block may be used for procedures below the knee. The tourniquet is generally well tolerated, and any minimal discomfort is easily treated with small amounts of sedatives or narcotics.

An ankle block is sufficient for distal foot and toe procedures. An anklet of subcutaneous lidocaine about 4 inches above the malleoli allows a sterile Esmarch tourniquet to be applied just above the ankle with no discomfort. Spinal and epidural blocks may be used if the patient's condition is stable and 6 months have elapsed since the injury. However, we favor the use of femoral or sciatic and ankle blocks.

Special Problems

The blood pressure is frequently labile despite apparently adequate perioperative control. It is essential to avoid more than a 25 to 30 percent drop in blood pressure. Even though the patient appears to do well throughout the remainder of the procedure, a significant hypotensive episode may result in an ischemic cerebrovascular accident in the perioperative period.

Hypovolemia may be another preoperative problem, particularly in the more severely involved patients coming from chronic care facilities. These patients may need to be hydrated in the preoperative or early intraoperative period. This must be done carefully, especially in cardiac patients, to avoid congestive heart failure. In addition, electrolyte imbalance resulting from use of diuretics must be corrected prior to surgery.

Administration of succinylcholine for intubation is avoided for at least 1 year after the cerebrovascular accident because of the possibility of hyperkalemia and cardiac arrest. With the introduction of the newer nondepolarizing muscle relaxants, however, this should no longer be a problem.

Recovery

Blood pressure may remain labile in the immediate postoperative period. A hypertensive crisis is treated with supplementation of antihypertensive drugs, such as nifedipine, provided that hypoxia, hypercarbia, and pain are first ruled out. Patients who have received regional anesthesia usually require minimal postoperative pain medications for the first 8 to 10 hours. In diabetic patients this period may be extended to 12 to 18 hours.

POSTPOLIOMYELITIS PATIENTS

The group of patients with postpoliomyelitis syndrome is relatively healthy and seeks treatment mainly for procedures involving the extremity. The respiratory tract is not involved, and associated medical problems usually are minimal. Common procedures performed on this group of patients include multiple tendon transfers, osteotomies, and occasionally abdominal fascial transplants.

Preoperative Evaluation and Types of Anesthesia

The preoperative work-up and anesthesia course in these patients present no specific problems. Because of the length of the procedures, general anesthesia is chosen most commonly.

Special Problems

Patients undergoing abdominal fascial transplants should be extubated while still fairly deeply anesthetized because bucking and coughing may weaken or tear the newly constructed struts.

Recovery

The patient may breathe shallowly because of pain or decreased vital capacity. Incentive spirometry should be used routinely. In general, these patients present no special anesthetic problems.

CONNECTIVE TISSUES DISEASE PATIENTS

Patients of all age groups with connective tissue diseases such as arthritis or ankylosing spondylitis, lupus erythematosus, scleroderma, and dermatomyositis may require surgery. With the exception of patients with juvenile rheumatoid arthritis, most are adults. They range from ambulatory patients with minimal systemic involvement to those with multisystem disease or an unstable cervical spine in traction. Patients with erosive rheumatoid arthritis may have eroded cervical facets, causing the odontoid process to project cephalad through the foramen magnum. Such patients are a surgical and anesthetic challenge.

The most common procedures performed on these patients in our hospital are total joint arthroplasties involving the hip, knee, and occasionally shoulder. In later stages of these diseases, arthroplasties of the phalangeal joints may be undertaken. Some patients, especially those with juvenile rheumatoid arthritis, have such marked limitation of motion of the temporomandibular joint that an arthroplasty is indicated for this joint as well. Cervical spine fusions are performed for stabilization, and spinal osteotomies may be done in an attempt to correct the severe kyphosis in ankylosing spondylitis. In addition, patients with any of the connective tissue diseases may need relatively minor procedures on one or more extremities.

Patients with far advanced scleroderma or dermatomyositis may develop an esophageal stricture that will require repeated esophageal dilatation on a routine basis. Although these procedures are not orthopaedic ones, they may be required in orthopaedic patients and present unique and difficult problems for the anesthesiologist.

Preoperative Evaluation

A careful, detailed medical history must be obtained, including any history of neck pain or cervical neurologic symptoms. Previous anesthesia history may involve a difficult traumatic intubation or even a failed intubation resulting in loss of the airway, emergency tracheostomy, or cancellation of the procedures.

Arthritis patients are often taking multiple medications, which require careful evaluation. Most commonly, long-term steroid, immunosuppressive, and anti-inflammatory drugs are used. All patients who have received steroid medications within the previous year should be given a preoperative steroid preparation. In addition, these patients may give a history of drug-induced hepatitis.

Laboratory values almost always show chronic anemia. The policy at our institution is not to demand a hemoglobin value of 10.0 g to proceed with elective surgery, but rather to evaluate each case on an individual basis.

Routine chest radiographs may show rheumatoid nodules, which must not be mistaken for neoplasm. Cervical spine radiographs, including lateral views, should be obtained from any patient with cervical symptoms. Any irregularity in the cervical radiograph is an indication for a fiberoptic intubation.

Types of Anesthesia

Patients with connective tissue disease usually are scheduled for general anesthesia for several reasons. Their joints—including shoulder, hip, and back—are immobile or extremely painful to move, thus making the use of regional anesthesia impossible. In addition, these patients are so uncomfortable lying in one position for any length of time that even if regional anesthesia were possible, they would require such large doses of narcotics or sedatives merely to tolerate the position that the airway might be compromised. Thus, general anesthesia with a fiberoptic intubation results in better control of the airway and fewer additional drugs to complicate the immediate postoperative course.

A moderate hypotensive technique is used when indicated to minimize blood loss, especially in total hip arthroplasties.

Special Problems

Patients with connective tissue disease may develop problems beginning in the preoperative room. They have very fragile veins that move excessively in the subcutaneous tissue because of lack of connective tissue integrity. Frequently it is necessary to insert a very small-bore catheter for induction and then start a second large-bore line in the operating room, preferably before intubation.

Care must be taken to use minimal tape to secure the intravenous line. Even paper tape has been known to tear the skin when it is removed. If necessary, a small piece of paper tape can be used at the site of insertion, followed by additional stabilization with Kerlex wrap.

The major problem during induction is maintenance of the airway. Careful assessment for possible airway problems must be made preoperatively and repeated just prior to inducing anesthesia. Induction drugs are slowly titrated, and the patient's ability to ventilate is verified before any muscle relaxants are given. If assisted ventilation becomes difficult or impossible, the patient is allowed to awaken immediately. Fiberoptic intubation is then accomplished with the patient awake by having the patient first gargle with viscous lidocaine. While an assistant holds the tongue forward and places a bite block between the molar teeth, the fiberoptic endoscope is passed to the level of, but not between, the vocal cords. A second assistant can inject 2 percent lidocaine through the suction port of the endoscope, thus anesthetizing the vocal cords and upper trachea. The endoscope is removed and after about 30 seconds gentle intubation using a fiberoptic laryngoscope is performed.

Assuming the airway is not compromised in any way during induction, a muscle relaxant is administered. In most arthritic patients, fiberoptic intubation is indicated because the larynx is usually very anterior and, in patients with erosive disease, may demonstrate a triplane deviation that would make a blind oral or nasal intubation impossible.

In addition, the epiglottis is often flush with the posterior pharyngeal wall, necessitating extra maneuvering of the endoscope despite anterior jaw thrust by an assistant. We routinely use fiberoptic intubations in patients with neck pain, cervical neurologic symptoms such as tingling of the hands, abnormal cervical spine radiograph, small mandible, inability to extend the neck, temporomandibular joint involvement, or any stabilizing device such as a halo-vest. Frequently, the patient will have a combination of these factors.

Many patients with chronic disease are hypovolemic on admission to the hospital. Because they are now admitted on the day of operation, there is no opportunity to correct this preoperatively. Therefore, adequate replacement fluids are given intravenously

early in the course of administering the anesthetic, before positioning, especially when the patient must be turned to the lateral or prone position.

Positioning patients with connective tissue diseases for any procedure must be done with care. All pressure points are well padded with egg-crate foam to prevent decubitus ulcers, which can develop in a very short time. Even seemingly light pressure from a surgeon's arm resting on an unpadded leg can cause skin sloughing requiring grafting.

Recovery

The main problem during the recovery period is again maintenance of the airway. The patient must be fully awake before extubation. Any loss of airway at this point can be much harder to handle than at the beginning of the procedure. Secretions are usually copious and obscure vision through the fiberoptic endoscope despite vigorous suctioning. Pharyngeal or glottic structures may be somewhat edematous, making a previously difficult intubation now impossible.

In general, patients with scleroderma, dermatomyositis, and systemic lupus erythematosus may have diffusion problems with restrictive lung disease as a result of a stiff chest wall and replacement of lung tissue by fibrous tissue. There may also be cardiac and renal involvement and vasospastic disease (Raynaud's phenomenon). Baseline arterial blood gas levels should be determined routinely and the patient should not be extubated until the physician is certain the patient is capable of adequate spontaneous respiration. This is probably best accomplished by following serial arterial blood levels. Postoperatively, the patients need to have aggressive pulmonary therapy, usually under the direction of a pulmonologist.

SPINAL DEFORMITY PATIENTS

Patients with spinal deformity range from those with idiopathic scoliosis, who are usually healthy teenagers whose curvature has been discovered during a school screening program, to those with scoliosis secondary to a congenital malformation or a neuromuscular disease, who may be seen at any age and with any degree of involvement. The deformity may be relatively localized, as with a hemivertebra, or it may involve most of the spine with a thoracolumbar curve.

The patients almost always are scheduled for spinal fusions. If the curve is severe, the patients frequently come for an anterior transthoracic fusion to be followed in 2 weeks by posterior stabilization.

Preoperative Evaluation

Previous anesthesia history, if available, is extremely important, especially in muscular dystrophy patients, some of whom are at increased risk of developing malignant hyperthermia. Any significant medications, particularly anticonvulsive therapy, should be continued in the perioperative period.

Laboratory work includes a routine ECG and chest radiograph. In patients with severe idiopathic scoliosis and in all others whenever possible, baseline arterial blood gas determinations and pulmonary function tests should be done. Those persons unable to cooperate owing to severe cerebral palsy or mental retardation should have arterial blood drawn immediately after induction for blood gas determination.

Types of Anesthesia

All patients on the spinal deformity service require general anesthesia. To facilitate surgery and minimize blood loss, a hypotensive technique usually is employed. This requires an arterial line, which is inserted in the preoperative room and placed on a heparin lock, to be activated in the operating room after the patient is positioned. A sodium nitroprusside (Nipride) drip is prepared and given via a Harvard pump, if necessary, to maintain moderate hypotension from the onset of the procedure. An intravenous β blocker may be used during the anesthesia to assist in maintaining hypotension without exceeding the toxic dose of Nipride.

Because evoked potentials are employed routinely, the anesthesia is mostly nitrous oxide or narcotic. However, the addition of 0.25 to 0.50 percent isoflurane (Forane) does not significantly dampen the waveform and therefore Forane in this strength is an acceptable ancillary agent.

Although the cell saver is routinely set up in these cases, the amount of blood retrieved varies markedly from patient to patient.

Special Problems

Fluid balance and blood loss must be closely monitored throughout these lengthy procedures. Patients with muscular dystrophy are prone to excessive oozing and blood loss, possibly as a result of poor tissue tone.

Perhaps the most important problem is that of maintaining adequate ventilation postoperatively. Patients having an anterior spinal fusion routinely receive a nasal intubation, so that the tube may be left in place overnight. Assisted or controlled ventilation, if required, becomes quite simple, and pulmonary toilet is markedly enhanced. The patients generally are extubated the following day, but occasionally a patient with severe cerebral palsy will require 2 days or more of assisted ventilation. Timing of extubation is determined by monitoring serial arterial blood gas levels.

The majority of patients having posterior spinal fusions do considerably better in the postoperative period. They are usually intubated orally and extubated in a routine manner in the operating room. Only those patients with pulmonary involvement or severe mental retardation require nasotracheal intubation and ventilator support postoperatively.

If the preoperative vital capacity is less than 30 percent of that predicted, consultation with the pulmonary or pediatric service is advisable. An elective prefusion tracheostomy should be considered. If performed, the tube should remain in place until the patient has recovered after the final stage of the procedure. The tracheostomy may then be plugged and the patient decannulated as tolerated.

Recovery

A pneumothorax that occurs during a posterior spinal fusion may first be recognized in the recovery room. If it is suspected postoperatively, a chest radiograph should be obtained immediately because a pneumothorax of 30 percent or greater necessitates placement of a chest tube. With smaller pneumothoraces, however, the patient's vital signs, oxygen saturation level, and respiratory status may remain clinically stable, giving no clue as to the underlying pathologic state.

Blood loss via drains may be considerable in the immediate postoperative period. The loss must be monitored closely and replaced with either blood or crystalloid as necessary.

Because of the length and extent of the procedure, the patients are usually hypothermic in the recovery room despite warming measures taken in the operating room. Use of the Bair Hugger patient warming system seems to be the most effective means of rewarming patients. This is a lightweight air-filled blanket that warms more rapidly than the older, heavy, water blankets, which are prone to develop holes and thus to soak patients and their surroundings.

SPINAL INJURY PATIENTS

Patients on the spinal injury service can be grouped in two different ways: by time span since the injury and by level of spinal cord lesion. The former group includes patients with relatively recent injuries and unstable cervical spines and those with long-standing injuries and multiple joint contractures. Patients classified by the level of spinal cord lesion may be subdivided into three additional groups: (1) those with high quadriplegia who are ventilator dependent; (2) those with lesions of T12 and above but not respirator dependent; and (3) the group with low paraplegia. The first two groups are prone to develop autonomic dysreflexia (see Special Problems). Included also in this service are patients with a herniated disc, the majority of whom are ambulatory and have no major medical problems.

Procedures commonly performed in the early postinjury phase involve spine stabilization, such as a cervical or thoracolumbar fusion. In late phases of treatment, procedures involve releases, tendon transfers, and resection of heterotopic bone. Patients with disc disease usually are scheduled for a percutaneous diskectomy, laminectomy with disc removal, or occasionally a posterior spinal fusion.

Preoperative Evaluation

A detailed medical history must begin with the date of injury and documentation of any multisystem involvement. History of aspiration pneumonia or frequent atelectasis in high quadriplegics must be established. Patients must be questioned carefully regarding any history of autonomic dysreflexia or involuntary spasms.

A single baseline ECG is necessary to rule out cardiac injury. A chest radiograph is checked for signs of atelectasis or pneumonia.

Types of Anesthesia

A moderate number of spinal injury patients easily tolerate local anesthesia with intravenous sedation for procedures such as postcervical fusion, certain hand procedures during which it is necessary for the patient to move the fingers, and percutaneous diskectomies. If the spinal cord injury is complete, almost any procedure below the sensory level may be carried out with monitored anesthesia care. However, patients scheduled for obturator neurectomy may require a general anesthetic to abolish the involuntary spasms that might interfere with the surgical procedure.

General anesthesia is required for all anterior cervical fusions, some posterior cervical fusions, all thoracolumbar fusions, and procedures in patients with incomplete spinal cord injuries. Fiberoptic intubation must be used if a cervical injury is involved.

Special Problems

Because of the resulting hyperkalemia and possible cardiac arrest, depolarizing muscle relaxants must not be administered within the first year after injury. If a rapid-sequence induction is necessary, a nondepolarizing muscle relaxant may be administered after use of a priming dose.

Autonomic dysreflexia usually occurs with injuries at the level of T5 and above. However, it has been reported to occur with lesions as low as T12. Should the patient develop autonomic dysreflexia, it may be treated easily with trimethaphan camsylate intravenously, titrated to effect. This may be used with general anesthesia or monitored anesthesia care. We do not use spinal anesthesia to abolish dysreflexia because it can be handled easily with trimethaphan. A Foley catheter is advisable in all but the shortest procedures to avoid bladder distention, a frequent trigger of dysreflexia.

Patients with spinal cord injury frequently have low blood pressures preoperatively. Blood pressure drops even further with anesthesia and positioning, thus setting the stage for profound hypotension. Therefore, it is advisable to consider fluid loading before induction.

Any patient with a history of cervical injury or surgery at any time in the past should be intubated with the help of the fiberoptic endoscope. To prevent any flexion or extension of the cervical spine, intubation is performed with the head either in the neutral position or in any form of external stabilization device.

A hypotensive technique occasionally is requested for lumbar laminectomies and posterior spinal fusions. This requires placement of an arterial catheter to titrate the dose of Nipride administered. Moderate hypotension (60 mean arterial pressure) is usually achieved easily with an inhalation anesthetic and positioning on the Andrews frame. Therefore, even with healthy patients, Nipride is needed only occasionally. All patients to be placed on the Andrews frame should have their legs wrapped with elastic bandages and should be given extra fluids prior to positioning to prevent extreme hypotension.

Recovery

Ventilation is carefully monitored in the recovery room, especially in patients undergoing anterior cervical fusions. These patients are prone to develop edema of the neck, which may result in airway obstruction. It is therefore important to monitor arterial saturation overnight.

Because ventilation is easily depressed, smaller doses of sedatives or narcotics should be used. The effects of even these small doses appear to be greater in quadriplegic persons.

PEDIATRIC PATIENTS

Patients on the pediatric service have a wide variety of medical problems and vary in age from neonates to adults. Most commonly seen are patients with cerebral palsy; they, in turn, range from children with minimal apparent involvement to those who are noncommunicative and severely mentally retarded. Other diseases seen are a variety of muscular dystrophies, arthrogryposis, osteogenesis imperfecta, spina bifida, and congenital dislocation of the hips. In addition, many of these patients, especially those with muscular dystrophy, are more prone to develop malignant hyperthermia. These patients are candidates for a wide variety of orthopaedic procedures, most commonly those involving the extremities. Spinal fusions have already been discussed.

Preoperative Evaluation

A careful medical and family history must be obtained from these patients, especially those with Duchenne's muscular dystrophy, who have a markedly increased propensity for malignant hyperthermia. Any airway management problems during previous inductions of anesthesia must be noted carefully.

Special medications should be continued in the perioperative period. Blood levels of anticonvulsants should be checked on all patients taking such agents and the dosage regulated appropriately to achieve the therapeutic range. Anesthesia premedication dose is decreased in most severely involved patients with cerebral palsy, muscular dystrophy, or arthrogryposis.

Any patient with a cardiomyopathy secondary to muscular dystrophy must have an ECG and cardiology consultation preoperatively.

Types of Anesthesia

All of these children require general anesthesia, with the rare exception of an occasional patient with spina bifida who has decreased sensation and is scheduled to undergo a minor lower extremity procedure. Those with muscular dystrophy or a questionable history of malignant hyperthermia receive a trigger-free anesthetic, i.e., one not employing an agent known to initiate the hyperthermic response. In addition, those patients with a definitive diagnosis of malignant hyperthermia receive dantrolene, 2.5 mg/kg intravenously, 30 to 60 minutes preoperatively.

Special Problems

Because of the wide variety of diseases encountered on the pediatric service, numerous anesthetic problems must be considered. For instance, children with osteogenesis imperfecta easily become hyperthermic during the procedure. Atropine is avoided in the premedication, and cooling measures are begun early. Extreme care must be taken with handling and positioning because even a tourniquet for laboratory work may fracture the humerus. In contrast, although in osteogenesis imperfecta the head is large and almost always appears to have frontal bossing, intubation and maintenance of the airway are not a problem.

Patients with muscular dystrophy present multiple problems for the anesthesiologist. Intravenous access is difficult to impossible in the later stages of the disease. Intubation becomes progressively more difficult because of a large tongue and immobility of the neck. During the procedure, especially if performed in the prone position, the tongue can swell, producing upper airway obstruction postoperatively. These patients must remain intubated overnight with a T tube and are extubated only when the integrity of the airway is assured. As the disease progresses, the children may need ventilatory assistance in the postoperative period. They are slow to resume breathing, and respirations are shallow even after full reversal of muscle relaxants. In addition, while appearing to be breathing satisfactorily in the recovery room, they may fatigue over a period of time. Therefore, they should be extubated with caution and watched closely in an intensive care setting overnight. In the last stages of the disease, they require a permanent tracheostomy with full ventilatory support.

The main problems in patients with arthrogryposis are intravenous access and maintenance of the airway. Intubation will become progressively more difficult with time, eventually requiring the use of a fiberoptic endoscope.

Patients with cerebral palsy, severe mental retardation, and Down's syndrome have similar problems and may be considered together. Their temperature regulation is poor (i.e., it is low at the beginning of the procedure and drops rapidly thereafter, especially if the surgical area is extensive). Therefore, extra precautions are taken to warm the operating room, warm the intravenous fluids and preparation solutions, and use a warming blanket from the onset. If the temperature still continues to drop, heating lamps are added to the regimen.

Emergence from anesthesia is slow even after minimal procedures. Therefore, it is not wise to perform operations on these children late in the day, especially as outpatients, unless special arrangements are made for postoperative monitoring. Extubation must not be performed until the patient has returned to the preoperative level of consciousness. These children frequently vomit on emergence, another good reason for delaying extubation. A nasogastric tube or a suction catheter may be passed to empty the stomach just prior to extubation. Patients are then transferred to the recovery room in the lateral position if possible.

Recovery

Temperature trends for the patient that began in the operating room may continue in the recovery room and should be treated appropriately. Because of the special problems noted earlier, the airway and ventilation must be monitored carefully in the recovery room. Each patient is assessed individually prior to transfer to the room or the intensive care unit.

ORTHOPAEDICS-DIABETES AMPUTEE

The patients on this service usually are somewhat older patients with diabetes mellitus who have multiple medical problems, often including heart disease, severe peripheral vascular disease, hypertension, and renal failure. Occasionally the young patient with brittle diabetes will require an amputation, in which case the attendant medical problems are few but the diabetes is more difficult to control.

The vast majority of these patients are scheduled for amputation of the lower extremity. The level varies from removal of a toe to an above-knee amputation.

Also frequently seen are patients who need incision and drainage, skin grafts, or various revisions or second-stage procedures (e.g., stage II Syme's amputation).

Preoperative Evaluation

As with any patient with multiple problems, a detailed medical history is essential. Antihypertensive and cardiac medications are continued in the perioperative period. The insulin is withheld the morning of surgery until an intravenous infusion is started with 5 percent dextrose in water, after which one-half to two-thirds of the regular morning dose is administered subcutaneously.

Preoperative laboratory studies are routine, but special attention must be paid to the fasting blood sugar level. Our protocol is to recheck the sugar concentration in the preoperative room by means of a fingerstick. All patients above the age of 40 years have a baseline ECG and any of them with a significant history of cardiac problems receive a further work-up, including echocardiogram and determination of ejection fraction as necessary.

Types of Anesthesia

We prefer to use regional anesthesia for most of these patients for two reasons: first, because of their poor medical status, and second, because they frequently undergo multiple procedures during their hospital stay. An ankle block is performed for any procedure at the midfoot level or distal to it. A femoral-sciatic block is used for through-knee amputations and below. A spinal or general anesthetic is used for above-knee amputations, and a general anesthetic for any patient who refuses a regional technique.

Blocks with 1 percent lidocaine and 0.25 percent bupivacaine (Marcaine) in equal volumes should be instituted 45 minutes prior to the expected time of incision. These blocks will, however, last up to 12 hours in the diabetic patient, and therefore provide good postoperative analgesia.

Special Problems

Occasionally an incomplete block can be supplemented by the surgeons. Narcotics or tranquilizers are given intravenously in small doses for the comfort of the patient. All blocks are done in the preoperative room and must be monitored throughout with an ECG. Oxygen and ventilatory support must be immediately available.

Recovery

Pain usually is not a problem if the patient has received a regional anesthetic. These patients are usually in the hospital for the first few postoperative days, so complete return of sensation in the recovery room is not necessary. However, for outpatients, long-acting blocks would not be appropriate.

DECUBITUS ULCER MANAGEMENT

Patients undergoing procedure for decubitus ulcer management are mainly those with spinal injury involving any level. Occasionally patients with severe rheumatoid arthritis or multiple sclerosis will have a decubitus ulcer. The procedures almost exclusively involve the use of skin grafts or various flaps to cover the decubitus ulcer.

Preoperative Evaluation

A careful history must be taken to determine if the patient has ever had autonomic dysreflexia. Otherwise a routine preoperative work-up is done.

Types of Anesthesia

Because the patient usually has a spinal cord lesion, monitored anesthesia care often is sufficient. General anesthesia is required for patients who have no loss of sensation or whose spinal cord injury is minimal.

Special Problems

Autonomic dysreflexia is the most common problem and is treated with a trimethaphan camsylate (Arfonad) drip titrated to effect. This can be used during general anesthesia, with monitored anesthesia care, or in the recovery room. Placement of a Foley catheter in the preoperative room in patients with cervical or thoracic spinal cord injury avoids distention of the bladder and thereby eliminates one cause of autonomic dysreflexia. Using this protocol, we have not found it necessary to perform spinal anesthesia to control this problem.

Patients with spinal cord injury frequently have a systolic blood pressure in the 90s and accompanying bradycardia of 45 to 50 beats per minute even with adequate fluid replacement.

Recovery

If the blood pressure drops in the recovery room to between 70 and 80 mm Hg systolic, a fluid challenge is given. This usually will bring the blood pressure back to the preoperative level.

CONCLUSION

Patients undergoing rehabilitation surgery may receive the same anesthesia regimen as any other patient with three caveats: drugs must be titrated because small amounts are usually effective; drugs must be administered slowly; and patients must be monitored closely because minor changes may precede the onset of a major decline in the patient's condition.

SUGGESTED READINGS

Biddle CJ, Hernandez S: Perioperative control of diabetes mellitus—revisited. AANA J 51:138, 1983

Botte MJ, Waters RL, Keenan MA et al: Approaches to senior care #3. Orthopaedic management of the stroke patient. Part II. Treating deformities of the upper and lower extremities. Orthop Rev 17:891, 1988

Davis FM, Laurenson VG, Gillespie WJ et al: Deep vein thrombosis after total hip replacement. A comparison between spinal and general anesthesia. J Bone Joint Surg [Br] 71:181, 1989

Katz J, Kadis LB: Anesthesia and Uncommon Disease. WB Saunders, Philadelphia, 1973

Keenan MA, Stiles CM, Kauffman RL: Acquired laryngeal deviation associated with cervical spine disease in erosive polyarticular arthritis. Anesthesiology 58:441, 1983

Messick JM, Newberg LA, Nugent M, Faust RJ: Principles of neuroanesthesia for the neurosurgical patient with CNS pathology. Anesth Analg 64:143, 1985

Reginster JY, Damas P, Franchimont P: Anaesthesia risks in osteoarticular disorders. Clin Rheumatol 4:30, 1985

Roelofse JA, Shipton EA: Anaesthesia in connective tissue disorders. S Afr Med J 67:336, 1985

Stiles CM: A flexible fiberoptic bronchoscope for endotracheal intubation in infants. Anesth Analg 53:1017, 1974

Stiles CM: Anesthesia for the mentally retarded patient. Orthop Clin North Am 12:45, 1981

Stiles CM, Stiles QR, Denson JD: A flexible fiberoptic laryngoscope. JAMA 21:1246, 1972

Zambricki CS: Perioperative care of the patient with traumatic brain injury. AANA J 51:85, 1983

13 Orthotics

JEFFREY SUTHERLAND

Orthoses are external devices that supplement function or are used to treat pathologic conditions of existing parts of the body. Orthoses have been used for centuries, although some of the historical evidence reveals ineffective techniques and concepts. For example, Hippocrates suggested that scoliosis is a dislocation of the spinal vertebrae that can be forcibly reduced as a fracture is reduced.[1] However, many other techniques are little changed from the originals and are still being used today. Elsewhere in his writings, Hippocrates described resin and wax bandaging of fractured limbs. Over the centuries the practice of orthotics has followed, and is dependent on, contemporary medicine. An understanding of biomechanics, kinesiology, and skeletal, muscular, and neural anatomy on the part of the practitioner has increased the effectiveness of orthotic treatment plans.

NOMENCLATURE

In the 1960s, orthotic nomenclature underwent significant changes. It had become apparent that the terminology used to communicate among rehabilitation teams needed to be clarified. In the past different types of orthoses tended to be identified with specific pathologic conditions. Although this was useful in some instances, it limited perspectives. Instead of prescribing an orthosis strictly on the basis of the patient's pathologic condition, it is more logical to consider the biomechanical deficit and then address that problem directly. Many pathologic conditions create similar or even identical biomechanical symptoms. In addressing these deficits directly, the prescriber and orthotist can more successfully treat patients.

The present nomenclature allows greater flexibility and greater precision, identifying the orthosis by the segments of the body included in the device. Thus, a long leg brace is called a knee-ankle-foot orthosis (KAFO). A bivalved body jacket is called a thoracic-lumbar-sacral orthosis (TLSO); a wrist gauntlet is a wrist-hand orthosis (WHO), and so forth. Further definition is provided by describing permitted or blocked motion and assistive motion—for example, wrist-action wrist-hand orthosis (WAWHO), with extension assist and adjustable flexion-extension stops.

PRINCIPLES AND APPLICATIONS

It is not feasible to describe every possible orthosis in this chapter; therefore, examples have been selected that illustrate important principles of orthotic treatment. The principles selected represent a broad cross-section and can be adapted to many other patient problems.

The medical team evaluating a patient for rehabilitation must determine the patient's biomechanical needs and then, if an orthosis is to be included in the treatment plan, the role of the orthosis must be defined clearly. Different indications demand different functions of orthotic devices. These different functions can be divided into four groups: (1) prevention of deformities, (2) enhancement of function, (3) relief of pain, and (4) limitation of motion to allow healing. An orthosis might serve only one or any combination of functions. An example of a device with only one role is a custom-molded Uvex face mask applied to patients with healing second- and third-degree burns. The even pressure of the smooth contours of the face mask prevents hypertrophic scarring of the skin. The only purpose of this orthosis is to prevent skin deformity, which it does by compressing the damaged tissue.[2] Other orthoses, such as the cock-up wrist splint used on arthritic patients, serve multiple roles, such as immobilizing the carpal joints to pre-

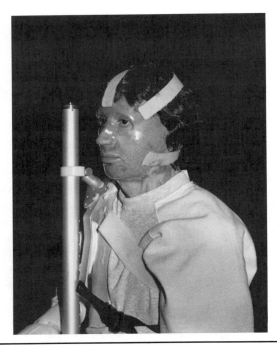

Fig. 13-1. Custom molded Uvex face mask used to treat facial burns.

mities usually require surgical correction. Sometimes an orthosis is used before surgery to give the surgeon more to work with or to prevent continuing deformation while awaiting surgery. An example is a burn patient unable to undergo immediate surgery who can benefit from an orthosis to arrest or improve contractures of a limb. If limbs are maintained by orthoses in extended positions while scar tissue is forming, problems relating to range of motion are minimized.[2]

Another example is the use of orthotics in treating a patient with a humeral fracture complicated by radial nerve paralysis. The fracture is reduced and can be immobilized with a humeral fracture orthosis. The associated lesion of the radial nerve will create a muscle imbalance that, if not treated, will deform the hand. If the nerve heals spontaneously after a period of time but soft tissue contractures have deformed the hand, function of the hand will remain impaired; however, if the potential for deformity is anticipated and the appropriate preventive measures are included in the treatment program, the chance of successful rehabilitation is greatly enhanced (Fig. 13-3).

In the absence of surgical correction, orthoses can provide accommodation. Only flexible deformities can be improved by orthoses.

Idiopathic scoliosis is in a class by itself. Orthotic treatment attempts to direct growth rather than force immediate correction. A scoliotic orthosis uses three-point pressure systems to encourage more symmetrical posture.[4-6] These three-point systems do not, by

vent pain; positioning the wrist for prehension, thereby enhancing function; and preventing flexion deformity[3] (Figs. 13-1 and 13-2).

Prevention of Deformities

Preventing deformities should not be confused with correcting deformities. It is easier to prevent than to correct deformities with orthoses; major rigid defor-

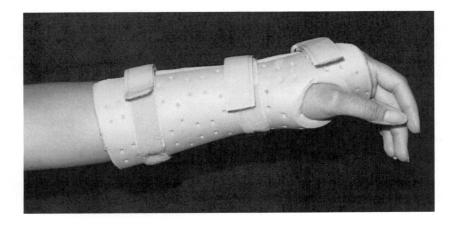

Fig. 13-2. Wrist-hand orthosis (Plastazote cock-up splint).

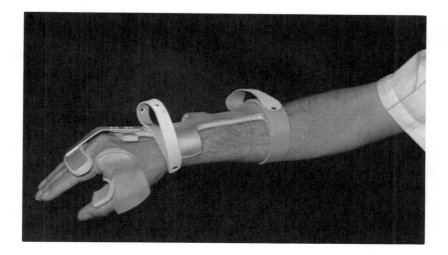

Fig. 13-3. WHO with metacarpophalangeal extension stop.

themselves, force the spine into the desired position; rather, they depend on the active assistance of the trunk muscles to pull away from the prodding of the pads. Although this concept is widely accepted,

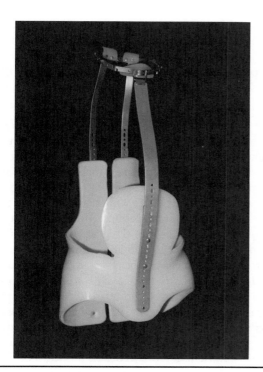

Fig. 13-4. Milwaukee thoracic-lumbar-sacral orthosis used for lumbar-thoracic scoliosis. Note: Thoracic pad (not shown) is needed to treat thoracic curve.

doubt has been cast on the active role of the muscles by Wynarsky and Schultz.[7] It is important to recognize that these systems cannot be used successfully on patients with paralytic spinal deformities because of their inability to actively pull away from the strategically placed pads. It is also important to note that these systems are ineffective after bone growth has ceased, when the only means of correction is surgical (Fig. 13-4).

It is obvious that angulation or rotation of bones cannot be corrected by applying the necessary forces to skin surfaces because of the likelihood of tissue breakdown. Rotational control of the extremities with orthoses is difficult if not impossible. The extremities, which are roughly cylindrical, have no points of advantageous leverage needed to control rotation. One orthosis that has been used to correct internal rotation of the femur (the twister cables) has fallen into disfavor with many physicians. This twister cable orthosis uses bilateral cables attached to a pelvic band at one end and shoes at the other. The shoes are fixed in a toe-out alignment. The cables act as torsion springs to resist toe-in of the feet, which is meant to translate to external rotation of the femur. The problem with this system is that the great torsional force translates through the articular tissues of the feet and knees to the femur. Even though the alignment of the feet is improved, the femoral rotation remains unchanged and the improved foot alignment is achieved at the expense of the ligaments of the knee or ankle and foot, or both.

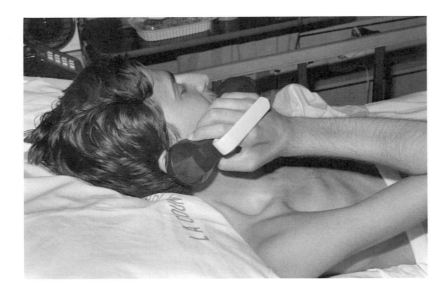

Fig. 13-5. Clip used to facilitate grasp of telephone receiver.

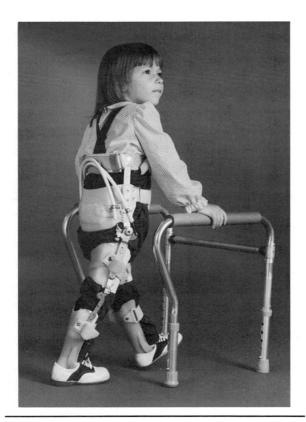

Fig. 13-6. Reciprocating gait orthosis. (Courtesy of Durr-Fillauer Medical, Inc.)

Enhancement of Function

Enhancing function can be as simple as providing a utensil holder for an impaired hand or as complicated as adapting a reciprocating orthosis to a paraplegic child's body, or providing prehension to the patient with paralyzed finger and thumb flexors (Figs. 13-5 to 13-7).

Limitation of Motion

The challenge to the orthotist is greatest when limited motion is desired, which is often the case when an orthosis is utilized to enhance function, such as in a patient with paralysis or spasticity. A patient with weak ankle plantar flexors, full range of ankle motion, and good proprioception benefits from an ankle-foot orthosis (AFO) that only restricts dorsiflexion. A patient with weak ankle dorsiflexors benefits from an AFO that only restricts plantar flexion (Fig. 13-8). A patient with a flail ankle and intact proprioception can be given an AFO that both prevents excessive dorsiflexion during stance and assists dorsiflexion in swing. The same patient with deficient proprioception and adequate quadriceps strength can benefit from a locked-ankle AFO (Figs. 13-9 and 13-10). The reaction of the AFO to the floor during loading response gives position sense stimuli

Fig. 13-7. Wrist-driven wrist-hand orthosis.

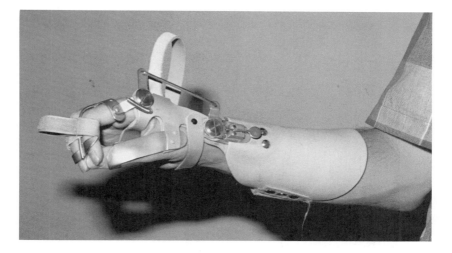

to the region of the knee. A locked-ankle AFO creates a flexion moment during loading response, which will destabilize a knee with inadequate quadriceps strength, and a KAFO may be required[8] (Figs. 13-11 to 13-13).

Prevention of Pain

How can an orthosis prevent pain? Usually it is easier to design and construct an orthosis that limits most or all motion. Many materials and methods are avail-

able to encase articulations, effectively preventing motion and thereby relieving pain[3] (Fig. 13-14).

Side Effects

When an orthosis is to be used in a treatment plan, the prescriber should be aware of the possible adverse side effects. These side effects can be grouped as follows: (1) psychological dependency, (2) physical de-

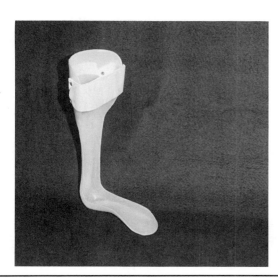

Fig. 13-8. Polypropylene leaf-spring ankle-foot orthosis, which provides restricted plantar flexion and dorsiflexion assist).

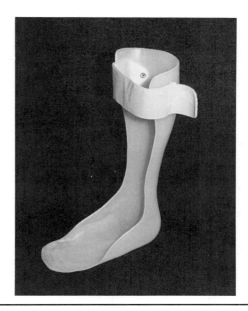

Fig. 13-9. Polypropylene ankle-foot orthosis locked in neutral (stops both dorsiflexion and plantar flexion).

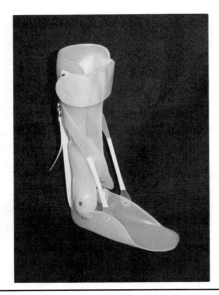

Fig. 13-10. Polypropylene ankle-foot orthosis with adjustable dorsiflexion stop and dorsiflexion assist.

pendency (muscles of the affected area atrophy and function becomes wholly dependent on the orthosis), and (3) increased endpoint stresses (Fig. 13-12). A painful arthritic subtalar joint might be helped by a rigid plastic AFO, which would strictly limit ankle motion; however, this could aggravate the next proximal joint, the knee. By reinforcing one region a neighboring region's weakness becomes more pronounced. The patient has the potential to develop a second chronically painful joint if an orthosis to relieve the first joint of pain is prescribed.

Fracture Bracing

Fracture bracing, as an alternative to rigid cast immobilization in the treatment of closed fractures of the long bones, has been developed and popularized by Sarmiento.[9-15] This method of treatment offers substantial benefits when applied appropriately. By allowing controlled movement or weight bearing during the healing phase, soft tissue contractures and muscle atrophy are minimized and bone healing is enhanced.

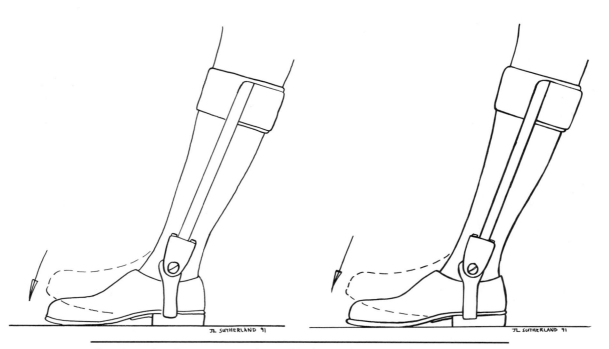

Fig. 13-11. Loading response of an ankle-foot orthosis with free plantar flexion.

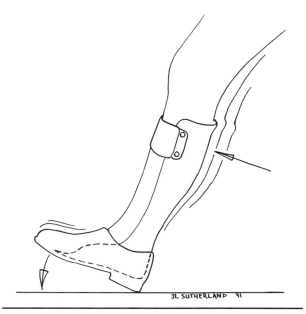

Fig. 13-12. Loading response of a locked ankle-foot orthosis.

Postoperative Use of Orthoses

The use of orthoses to facilitate healing postoperatively is also expanding. It has been demonstrated that motion enhances healing after surgery; therefore, it has become common practice for orthopaedic surgeons to order orthotic devices rather than rigid plaster immobilization. After reconstructive surgery of a joint, some motion in a single plane prevents the formation of adhesions or muscle contractures.[16] This practice has greatly reduced both postsurgical rehabilitation time and the occurrence of postsurgical permanent contractures. Devices such as an adjustable flexion-extension knee orthosis and a continuous passive motion machine are good examples of this category. The knee orthosis is static and allows limited motion (Fig. 13-15). It can be used in conjunction with a continuous passive motion machine.[17]

Everted plastic AFOs are often used postoperatively for congenital clubfoot to maintain the surgical

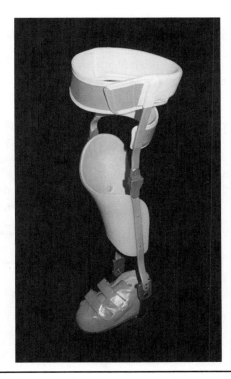

Fig. 13-13. Knee-ankle-foot orthosis with drop lock knee joints.

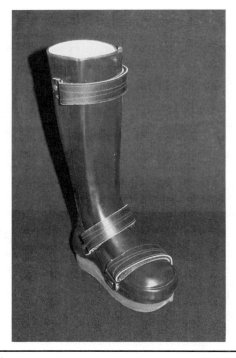

Fig. 13-14. Bivalved polypropylene ankle-foot orthosis with rocker bottom used by patients with rheumatoid arthritis or Charcot joint.

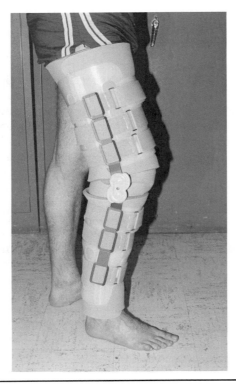

Fig. 13-15. Adjustable flexion-extension knee orthosis.

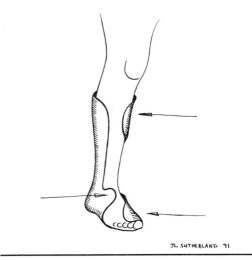

JL SUTHERLAND 71

Fig. 13-16. Polypropylene clubfoot ankle-foot orthosis.

correction while remodeling of the bones is occurring (Fig. 13-16). Bivalved plastic body jackets (TLSOs) protect healing after spinal fusion surgery (Fig. 13-17). An elbow orthosis protects tendon transfers as range of motion is regained in a controlled manner, (Fig. 13-18). An AFO with the ankle set at 90° to the tibia helps prevent retightening of the tendo calcaneous after surgical lengthening.

Prefabricated Orthoses

Modern manufacturing techniques and newer materials that interface with the skin in a friendly manner have increased the use of prefabricated complete orthotic systems. The advantages of prefabricated orthoses are decreased production costs, consistent quality, and rapid application. The disadvantage is that prefabricated systems are inherently designed to fit people in the median group of characteristics. Unfortunately, patients with long-standing pathologic conditions are often unlike the median group. Con-

sequently, prefabricated systems have found more success in the treatment of normal persons with new conditions, as in the use of a femoral fracture orthosis (Fig. 13-19). Another example is the use of a leaf-spring orthosis for the management of paralytic drop foot (Fig. 13-8). In the case of peroneal nerve injury with drop foot and normal anatomy, a prefabricated leaf-spring AFO might be sufficient; however, a post-

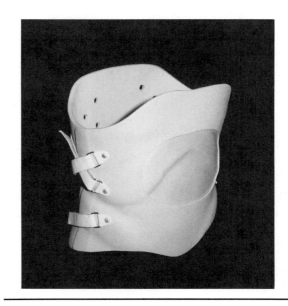

Fig. 13-17. Thoracic-lumbar-sacral orthosis body jacket.

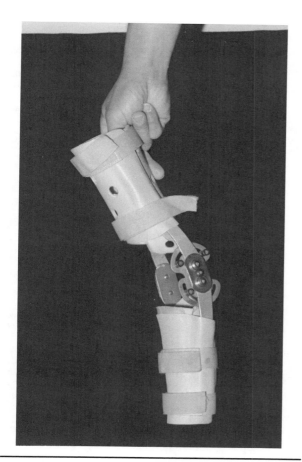

Fig. 13-18. Elbow orthosis with adjustable flexion and extension stops.

More efficient electrical cells will allow longer lasting or more powerful assists to externally powered orthoses. Pressure transducers, accelerometers, and miniaturized computer circuitry will allow more input to be read, analyzed, and used to direct movement.

Some notable directions currently under study include hybrid ambulation systems composed of a hip-knee-ankle-foot orthosis (HKAFO)[18] or reciprocating gait orthoses guiding lower extremity movements provided by functional electrical stimulation of muscles.[19] Another area of related research is the development of KAFOs with smart systems that lock the knee joint during the stance phase of gait but hinge freely during the swing phase.[20,21] Another notable research project, still unpublished, is the "Rancho

poliomyelitis patient with paralytic drop foot, pes cavus, and pes varus deformity needs to be accommodated with a custom-molded orthosis.

PREDICTIONS

The future of orthotics will be influenced by the use of new materials and techniques developed by chemists and engineers. Of course, the applications of these materials and techniques will be directed by clinicians. New materials and techniques will allow more selective limitation on the movements of the body. An increasing array of interchangeable prefabricated components will permit the orthotist and physician to precisely tailor systems to individual patient needs in a cost-effective manner.

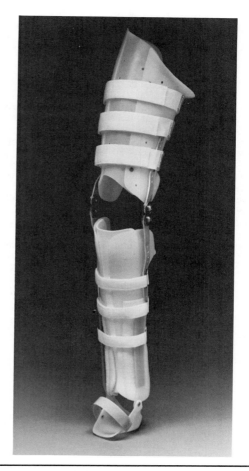

Fig. 13-19. Femoral fracture brace. (Courtesy of Orthomedics—O.S.I.)

CRO'' a dynamic orthosis that ranges a joint to preset levels of tension. The CRO ranges motion using the tensioning feedback to determine the range-of-motion (ROM) limit. By challenging the ROM limit with each cycle, joint rehabilitation is accelerated. It is utilized to prevent or correct the formation of soft tissue contractures.

An area that particularly needs development is an ankle-foot orthosis that more nearly approximates the control offered by normal musculature. This type of orthosis would automatically adjust its range of motion to accommodate varying inclines and use some of the energy absorbed during loading response to progressively resist dorsiflexion during late stance. This orthosis cannot be just a simple spring because it must provide or allow toe clearance during preswing and swing, and it must not return energy during double-limb support because this could be detrimental to efficient walking gait.

REFERENCES

1. The Genuine Works of Hippocrates. Translated from the Greek by Francis Adams. William Wood & Company, New York, 1886
2. Rivers EA: Rehabilitation management of the burn patient. Adv Clin Rehabil 1:177, 1987
3. Hicks JE, Leonard JA Jr, Nelson VS, et al: Prosthetics, orthotics, and assistive devices. 4. Orthotic management of selected disorders. Arch Phys Med Rehabil 70:S210, 1989
4. Blount WP, Moe JH: The Milwaukee Brace. 2nd Ed. Williams & Wilkins, Baltimore, 1980
5. Lonstein JE, Winter RB: Adolescent idiopathic scoliosis. Orthop Clin North Am 19:239, 1988
6. Chase AP, Bader DL, Houghton GR: The biomechanical effectiveness of the Boston brace in the management of adolescent idiopathic scoliosis. Spine 14:636, 1989
7. Wynarsky GT, Schultz AB: Trunk muscle activities in braced scoliosis patients. Spine 14:1283, 1989
8. Perry J, Hislop HJ: Principles of Lower-extremity Bracing. American Physical Therapy Association, Washington, DC, 1973
9. Sarmiento A: A functional below-knee brace for tibial fractures. J Bone Joint Surg [Am] 52:295, 1970
10. Mooney V, Nickel VL, Harvey JP Jr, Snelson R: Cast-brace treatment for fractures of the distal part of the femur. J Bone Joint Surg [Am] 52:1563, 1970
11. Sarmiento A: Functional bracing of tibial and femoral shaft fractures. Clin Orthop 82:2, 1972
12. Connally JF, Dehne E, LaFollette B: Closed reduction and early cast-brace ambulation in the treatment of femoral fractures. J Bone Joint Surg [Am] 55:1581, 1973
13. Sarmiento A, Latta L, Zilioli A, Sinclair W: The role of soft tissues in the stabilization of tibial fractures. Clin Orthop 105:116, 1974
14. Latta L, Sarmiento A, Tarr R: The rationale of functional bracing of fractures. Clin Orthop 146:28, 1980
15. Zych G, Zagorski J, Latta L, et al: Modern concepts in functional fracture bracing: the lower limb. Instr Course Lect 36:403, 1987
16. Odenbring S, Lindstrand A, Egund N: Early knee mobilization after osteotomy for gonarthrosis. Acta Orthop Scand 60:699, 1989
17. Salter RB: Clinical application of basic research on continuous passive motion for disorders and injuries of synovial joints; a preliminary report of a feasibility study. J Orthop Res 1:325, 1984
18. Andrews BJ, Baxendale RH, Barnett R, et al: Hybrid FES orthosis incorporating closed loop control and sensory feedback. J Biomed Eng 10:189, 1988
19. Phillips CA: Electrical muscle stimulation in combination with a reciprocating gait orthosis for ambulation by paraplegics. J Biomed Eng 11:338, 1989
20. Malcom L, Sutherland DH, Cooper L, et al: A digital logic controlled electromechanical orthosis for free knee gait in muscular dystrophic children. Orthop Trans 5:90, 1981
21. Chen D: An automatic electrically controlled leg brace for knee joint instability. Master's Thesis, Department of Electrical Engineering, Ohio State University, March 1972

14 Prosthetics

KEVIN E. CALVO
JOHN W. MICHAEL

HISTORY

Prosthetics is the art and science of fashioning mechanical replacements for missing limbs. The world's first prosthetists were amputees who survived trauma or disease and fashioned crude crutch-like replacements for themselves.[1] Prior to the Middle Ages, little had been done to compensate for missing limbs. During medieval times, however, highly skilled armorers were sometimes called on to fashion an iron replacement for limbs lost in battle. From these beginnings emerged prosthetics as a profession.

In the mid-1800s, surgical advances included the discovery of asepsis, antisepsis, and anesthetics. This allowed significant numbers of persons to survive amputation surgery without succumbing to infection or shock. After the end of the Civil War, an American amputee named J. E. Hanger improved on the prostheses of the day[2] and helped launch the fledgling field of prosthetics into a viable occupation.

For the next 100 years, the field evolved slowly as a skilled craft, often handed down from father to son. Little had changed in terms of materials or design. Immediately following World War II, however, Congress focused much attention and money on the task of rehabilitating returning soldiers, and prosthetic advancements were devised rapidly. In cooperation with leading orthopaedic surgeons of the day, a national program was established to certify the competence of properly trained practitioners.[3] The materials used in the Civil War era — wood, leather, and iron — were gradually replaced by lighter and stronger modern plastics and alloys. Socket designs and component options have become increasingly precise and sophisticated, making ongoing education a prerequisite for modern practice.

Formal education in the field increased rapidly during the years after World War II. From the initial training courses offered in the 1950s, which lasted a few weeks, accredited education available has progressed so that there are several 4-year baccalaureate degrees in prosthetics and orthotics, a number of postgraduate certificate programs, and at least one master's degree program. Over the years the American Board of Certification in Orthotics and Prosthetics (ABC) gradually raised its standards as the complexity of the field increased. Current entrants into prosthetic practice must possess at least a baccalaureate degree and complete a 1-year supervised internship prior to taking comprehensive national Board examinations. Successful candidates are awarded the title of Certified Prosthetist (C.P.).

An overwhelming majority of ABC certified prosthetists belong to the American Academy of Orthotists and Prosthetists, which is patterned after the American Academy of Orthopedic Surgeons. The Academy is the primary source for continuing education in the field. Since 1988, regular continuing education has been a prerequisite for active membership in the Academy as well as for recertification by the ABC.

Commensurate with the increased complexity, responsibility, and education that marks modern prosthetic practice, the field is making the transition from a manual craft to a true profession. Education and practice standards are expected to increase further as the field continues to advance. However, prosthetic rehabilitation remains a team effort, requiring the interdisciplinary cooperation of physician, prosthetist, therapist, and amputee. Despite significant technical advances, the most important ingredient for rehabilitation success remains the individual effort contributed by each member of the team.

Table 14-1. Distribution of Upper and Lower Extremity Amputations by Age, Cause, Level, and Sex[a]

Causes	Average Age		Percentage	
	Lower	Upper	Lower	Upper
Causes				
Congenital	12.2	8.9	2%	18%
Trauma	38.2	34.8	22.5%	70.4%
Tumor	36.1	37.1	6%	6%
Vascular	62.2	43.4	69.5%	5.6%

Level[b]
AE—35.4% }
BE—64.6% } UPPER   16%

AK—37.1% }
BK—62.9% } LOWER   84%

Male—73.6%
Female—26.4%

[a] There are slightly more than 1.5 amputees per 1,000 people in the United States and Canada.

[b] AE/BE, above/below elbow; AK/BK, above/below knee.

DEMOGRAPHICS

Very few hard data exist on the frequency of amputation in the United States. The National Center for Health Statistics estimated in 1981 that approximately 900,000 citizens will have sustained a major amputation by the year 2000.[4] Compared to estimates of similar countries in Europe, these figures may be somewhat low.

Table 14-1 summarizes the results of a national study conducted by New York University in 1979. The ratio of male to female amputees remains at about 3:1, and the proportion of upper to lower limb amputees is about 15 to 85 percent. These figures are similar to the distribution in previous decades.

However, two significant trends are noted. The percentage of lower level amputation continues to increase. This is believed to reflect more accurate techniques to determine the lowest viable amputation level and widespread recognition that rehabilitation rates are significantly higher for lower amputation levels. The second trend noted is a steady increase in the percentage of amputees with vascular disease. The elderly dysvascular amputee now constitutes the majority of all prosthetic patients, and this percentage is expected to increase as the population ages.

Terminology used to describe levels of amputation is illustrated in Figures 14-1 and 14-2. The level is referenced to the nearest proximal joint. It should be noted that extremely short amputations (within 1 or 2 cm of the proximal joint) are the functional equivalents of a higher level disarticulation. That is to say, a 1-cm above elbow amputation will be treated functionally as if it were a shoulder disarticulation.

As a general rule, it is worthwhile to save all functional length when selecting an amputation level. A functional residual limb requires smooth bone terminations, some muscle padding, and intact, sensate skin. Although disarticulation is a special case, this is the preferred method of amputation because in a growing child, it effectively avoids the recurrent problem of bony overgrowth. In addition, disarticulation is quicker and is a less traumatic operation than alternatives, and it offers the prosthetic advantages of inherent suspension, end weight bearing, and improved rotational control. However, in the skeletally mature person, disarticulation restricts the component options available to the patient and requires a somewhat bulky and cosmetically unattractive pros-

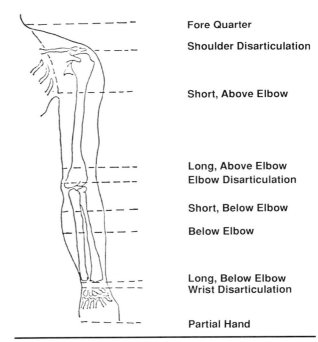

Fig. 14-1. Amputation types for the upper extremity by functional level of amputation.

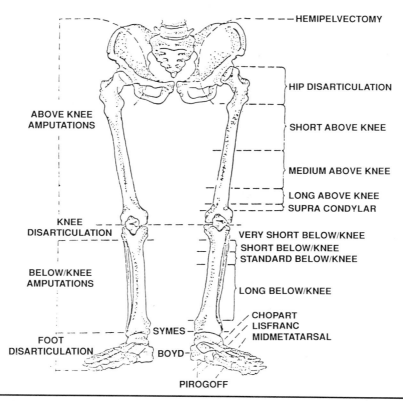

HEMIPELVECTOMY

HIP DISARTICULATION

SHORT ABOVE KNEE

MEDIUM ABOVE KNEE

LONG ABOVE KNEE
SUPRA CONDYLAR

VERY SHORT BELOW/KNEE
SHORT BELOW/KNEE
STANDARD BELOW/KNEE

LONG BELOW/KNEE

CHOPART
LISFRANC
MIDMETATARSAL

ABOVE KNEE AMPUTATIONS

KNEE DISARTICULATION

BELOW/KNEE AMPUTATIONS

FOOT DISARTICULATION

SYMES

BOYD

PIROGOFF

Fig. 14-2. Types of amputations for the lower extremity. The longer the stump the greater the efficiency.

thesis. For these reasons, disarticulation in the adult remains a controversial topic.

LOWER LIMB REHABILITATION

Because below-knee amputation is the most common type performed in the United States, prosthetic rehabilitation management is reviewed in some detail here. The same principles apply to higher levels of amputation, but the complexity increases with the loss of each additional joint.

Preoperative preparation for the amputation, when it is possible, offers a distinct advantage for the patient. Physical factors such as range of motion, muscle tone, and presence of flexion contractures can be evaluated and sometimes improved prior to surgery. Visits from members of a recognized amputee support group can provide a significant psychological boost. A brief ex-

planation of the surgical procedures and postoperative care will help minimize the patient's fears.

The optimum postoperative management would be some form of rigid dressing (Fig. 14-3). Although several types can be identified in the literature, they all offer the following advantages[5,6]:

- Protection of the residual limb from additional trauma
- Prevention of knee flexion contractures
- Prevention of gross postsurgical edema
- Enhanced wound healing
- Speeding of residual limb maturation

Nursing staff should monitor the amputee who has been treated with a rigid dressing to be certain it remains firmly in contact with the residual limb. Atrophy is normal, and a cast change is normally required after 10 days. If the cast becomes loose prematurely it should be changed immediately, because there is risk of damage to the skin. Moderate discomfort and fluid staining of the cast are normal. However, nursing staff should be alert for any unpleasant

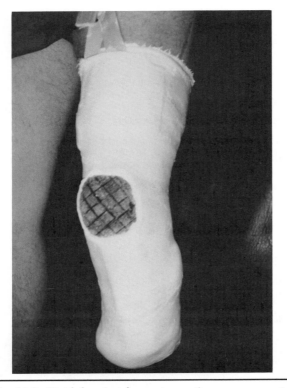

Fig. 14-3. Rigid dressing for postoperative management.

odors or sudden increases in the patient's temperature, which could indicate the presence of infection and require immediate cast removal.

In selected cases, a prosthetic foot may be attached to the rigid dressing (Fig. 14-4), allowing limited ambu-

lation 24 hours after the amputation. Although this procedure carries some risk, it is the most psychologically positive approach. With proper supervision, immediate postoperative fitting improves the patient's balance and reduces wound discomfort.

Many surgeons, however, are reluctant to permit immediate ambulation for patients with a dysvascular residual limb. For this reason, interest has focused on an early preparatory prosthesis, defined as one received within 30 days of amputation. It now appears that so long as the prosthesis is provided within 1 month of amputation, the long-term rehabilitation outcome is virtually identical to that for an immediate postoperative prosthesis.[7]

The initial preparatory prosthesis may be made of a variety of materials, including plaster, Fiberglas casting tape, and various plastic materials (Figs.14-5 and 14-6). So long as the socket is carefully fitted to provide total surface contact with the residual limb and the suspension is secure, the material itself is of secondary consideration. Most authorities believe that the intermittent pressure of the total-contact socket enhances wound healing and thereby residual limb maturation. Because rapid limb atrophy is to be expected, the fit of the prosthesis needs to be inspected at frequent intervals and adjusted as necessary.

Whether an immediate prosthetic fitting is undertaken or early preparatory fitting is recommended, all patients begin with "touch-down" weightbearing initially. By initially using the prosthesis only within

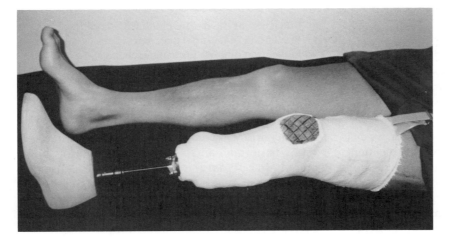

Fig. 14-4. Some patients may benefit by attachment of a prosthetic foot to the rigid dressing.

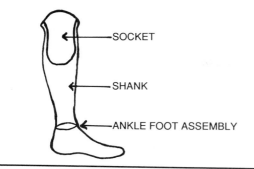

Fig. 14-5. Components of a below-knee (BK) prosthesis.

the safety of parallel bars and limiting weight bearing to less than 10 pounds of pressure, damage to the residual limb can be avoided. The patient increases the weight bearing gradually, over a period of weeks, as tolerated. The patient should never be permitted to bear weight to the point of pain. Uncooperative patients, unreliable patients, and those with insensitive residual limbs cannot use an immediate or early prosthesis safely. Their prosthetic fitting should be deferred until full wound healing has occurred, and it should be closely supervised to minimize the risk of skin breakdown.

Patients' motivation and psychological outlook are usually significantly improved when they are encouraged to ambulate as soon as possible with a prosthesis or with crutches or a walker. Particularly for elderly amputees, an aggressive early rehabilitation program minimizes the effects of prolonged immobilization. If residual limb hypersensitivity is a problem, referral to physical therapy for desensitization exercises is often useful.

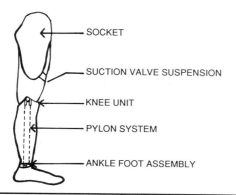

Fig. 14-6. Components of an above-knee (AK) prosthesis.

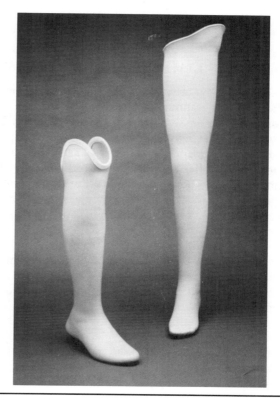

Fig. 14-7. Endoskeletal BK and AK prostheses with prosthetic skin covering.

Numerous alternative methods of postoperative prosthesis care are possible, including elastic bandaging, the use of specially knitted shrinker sleeves, and pneumatic sleeves. Although these techniques offer immediate access to the residual limb for wound inspection, controlled studies have shown that they delay prosthetic rehabilitation compared with immediate and early fittings. Ideally, these techniques would be reserved for uncooperative or unreliable patients.

Patients who successfully ambulate with a preparatory prosthesis have an excellent prognosis for using a definitive device (Fig.14-7). Although numerous studies have attempted to predict which patients will do well with a permanent prosthesis, a more effective screen than success with a preparatory device has yet to be identified. The definitive prosthesis is often similar in design to the preparatory one, but it differs in that it offers a more intimate fit about the residual limb and generally has more sophisticated components.

UPPER LIMB REHABILITATION

Because the majority of upper limb amputations are the result of trauma[8] or are required because of a congenital anomaly, wound healing is much less troublesome than in the lower limb. Immediate postsurgical fittings and rigid dressings are possible, but they do not offer as much benefit as for the lower limb. Except when lying down, the upper limb is above the heart; therefore, simply elevating the extremities allows rapid resolution of much postoperative edema.

Neuromuscular control is a key factor for the upper limb amputee, who must use the prosthesis for relatively fine activities. This is in contrast to the lower limb amputee, who simply needs to make gross repetitive movements to be able to ambulate. With the widespread availability of electromyographically controlled prostheses, precise muscular control has taken on increased importance. For that reason, many prosthetists suggest myodesis to help stabilize muscle sites, particularly for the high-level amputee, such as the shoulder disarticulate.

Although a limb amputated at virtually any level can be fitted with a prosthesis, the lower the levels the higher the percentage of successful rehabilitation. It has been estimated that approximately 50 percent of all upper limb amputees choose not to wear an artificial limb.[9] Externally powered (myoelectric) fittings are now expected to increase the acceptance rate somewhat, but the rejection rate remains far higher than for the lower limb. This seems to be attributable, in large part, to the limitations in current prosthetic technology. No prosthesis can restore the lost sensation, and fine grasp requires both concentration and practice.

A preoperative visit from someone with an amputation at a similar level can be very helpful. An increasing number of consumer support groups are being formed around the country to offer this service.

The most common postoperative dressing is an elastic bandage. In general, range-of-motion therapy should begin as soon as possible after amputation. Motion—particularly pronation and supination—quickly becomes restricted in the inactive upper limb.

Once again, the concept of a 30-day "golden period" for rehabilitation has been noted. Those upper limb amputees who had been provided with a prosthesis within 1 month of amputation had a far higher rehabilitation rate than those fitted 3 or 4 months later.[7] This is probably due to preservation of two-handed skills when fitting is undertaken early. Patients who are not fitted quickly will devote their postoperative energies to becoming more proficient at doing tasks one-handedly. Prosthetic training then becomes more frustrating, because the patient must learn yet another technique for accomplishing a given task.

A variety of mechanical components are available for the upper limb prosthesis.[9] They are selected, in consultation with the patient and the prosthetist, to offer the best possible function. At present most American amputees receive a body-powered prosthesis. This is typically suspended by a lightweight webbing harness and is powered by shoulder motion transmitted via a metal cable.

The most common terminal device in the United States is a voluntary opening hook. Although its appearance is distasteful to some, it is an extremely efficient grasping tool. Its lightness, simplicity, reliability, and versatility make it a practical choice for many amputees, particularly those with bilateral upper limb involvement. Mechanical hands also are available, but these offer a limited grip force and tend to be clumsy in comparison to the hook. For that reason, most amputees who desire a hand prefer the externally powered versions.

Currently these prostheses are powered by small electric motors and offer much stronger pinch force than their mechanical equivalents. The simplest version is controlled by a switch, but many amputees develop sufficient coordination to use electromyographically controlled devices. These "myoelectric" prostheses offer a good combination of attractive appearance and function and are preferred by many patients. Although the initial cost is significantly higher than the body-powered alternatives, the long-term cost is less prohibitive because most of the expensive components can be reused during subsequent fittings.

For an increasing number of amputees, a passive cosmetic restoration is a good choice. Passive does not necessarily mean "nonfunctional," because the psychological sense of being "whole" may assist amputees in returning to a fully active life-style.[10] In addition, passive prosthetic devices can be used for bimanual gasping, can help stabilize objects being manipulated by the remaining hand, and often may be positioned to hold lightweight objects such as cocktail glasses. Because the cosmetic devices contain no sophisticated internal mechanism, they are generally significantly lighter in weight than alternatives.

The higher the amputation level the lower the percentage of successful prosthetic use, and the more difficult it becomes to create a practical active prosthesis. For example, only a very small percentage of scapular-thoracic amputees choose to wear a prosthesis for a long time. Most of these patients are best served by provision of a lightweight shoulder cap, which restores torso symmetry and permits wearing of normal clothing. The added weight of a cosmetic arm restoration is seldom found to be advantageous for persons with amputations at this level.

The most important criterion for success in upper limb prosthetic fitting is to create a device that meets the needs of the particular patient. Careful consideration of the amputee's vocations, avocations, and goals is critical to successful prosthetic rehabilitation.

PEDIATRIC PROSTHETICS

In contrast to the skeletally mature amputee, the pediatric patient is constantly growing and changing. Successful prosthetic rehabilitation must take into account the patient's developmental readiness, and as a result the process must become more complex as the child grows.[11]

The child born with an absent limb is, technically, not an amputee; the child simply has a physical difference. Although a number of children with such conditions are successfully fitted with prosthetic devices, many choose not to wear a prosthesis, and this option should always be available. Particularly for the child with high-level, bilateral, congenital missing limbs, prosthetic devices may not significantly enhance overall functioning. Most child amputees become very adept at performing activities of daily living with compensatory motions in their remaining limbs, particularly by using their feet and toes. Such activities should always be strongly encouraged.[12]

One of the primary prosthetic considerations in fitting patients in this age group is durability, because the child's world includes such environments as sand boxes. In addition, most children will outgrow the prosthesis within a year or two. Removable inner sockets can be provided, allowing for both circumferential and longitudinal growth, and thus extending the useful life of the prosthesis. Overall length should be checked frequently, particularly for the lower limb amputee, and adjustments for growth should be made at regular intervals.

The recommended age to fit infant amputees remains controversial. There appears to be no practical limit to how young a child can be successfully fitted with a prosthesis. However, most authorities recommend upper limb fitting when the child begins to attain sitting balance (at about 6 months) and lower limb fitting when the child begins to pull to stand (at about 9 months). Myoelectric fittings in children remain controversial, primarily because of the cost involved. However, long-term data from Canada and Europe indicate that many children readily become successful users of electrically powered prostheses, regardless of their age at fitting.

Functionally, most pediatric amputees do well with lower limb prosthetic devices. In part, this is because children are so adaptable and energetic. The emotional impact of pediatric amputation falls on the parents' shoulders. Referral to a pediatric amputee support group can be helpful for the parents of child amputees in dealing with their situation effectively.

Adolescence is a time of great psychosocial tumult and growth, and amputee are not excepted. Peer pressure and body image are particularly important at this time, and many amputees develop a strong interest in cosmetic refinement of their prosthetic devices.[14] The patient's acceptance of the prosthesis increases when the clinic team listens carefully to the desires of the adolescent amputee and encourages active participation in clinic decisions.

BIOMECHANICS AND GAIT

The goal of every lower limb prosthesis is to allow as normal a gait as possible. The higher the amputation level the less completely can this goal be met.

For the below-knee amputee, almost no gait deviations should be perceptible to the eye. For the above-knee amputee, a somewhat slower cadence and slight lateral trunk leaning is common. The shorter the residual limb the more pronounced the limp becomes. For the patient with hip disarticulation and the hemipelvectomy amputee, a very slow gait with a noticeable limp is virtually inevitable.

Formal physical therapy training enhances the use of lower limb prosthetic devices. Although basic ambulation is easily learned by many amputees, specific instruction in the proper methods of falling, ascending and descending stairs, and negotiating ramps or uneven ground greatly expands the usefulness of the prosthesis. Proper use of external aids such as canes or walkers, proper donning and doffing of the prosthesis, and correct adjustment of limb socks all add immeasurably to the practical usefulness of the prosthetic device. Specific details on physical therapy gait training are available in several sources.[15,16]

It is now well documented that the amount of oxygen consumption per meter of distance traveled is increased in all amputees. Furthermore, the higher the amputation level the greater the amount of energy required to walk. Therefore, a fundamental goal in lower limb prosthetics is to allow the most efficient gait possible.[17] In general, this is accomplished by aligning the prosthetic components so they are stable during the stance phase but can be readily flexed during the swing phase. Adjustments are made in dynamic alignment when the amputee ambulates in the prosthetic laboratory using the prescribed components. The prosthetist makes small angular and linear changes at the foot, ankle, knee, and hip to achieve the best "balance" for that person. The final alignment is influenced by such variables as level of amputation, weight and height of the amputee, and cadence of the gait. As a general rule, the narrower the distance between the feet during gait the more energy-efficient the prosthesis.

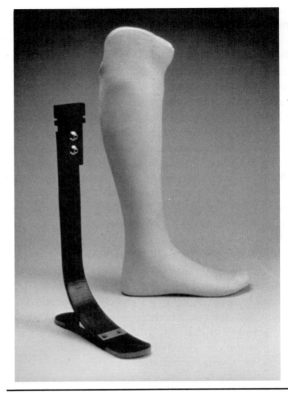

Fig. 14-8. Graphite energy-storing flex foot assembly.

Newer components are constantly being developed in an effort to improve gait efficiency. A variety of so-called energy storing feet (Fig.14-8) have been developed over the past 10 years in an effort to add some measure of propulsion during the push-off phase. Fluid-controlled knee mechanisms, which were developed in the 1960s, have been demonstrated conclusively to provide the smoothest knee motion and allow a variable cadence.

The upper limb amputee also will benefit from formal training in prosthesis use. Occupational therapy helps make the transition from simply opening and closing the device to using it in a practical manner for activities of daily living. Electrically powered prostheses, although heavier and more expensive, generally are less restrictive and offer a wider range of functional options for the upper limb amputee. The more complex the prosthetic device, the more beneficial formal occupational therapy training becomes.

Fig. 14-9. Athletes competing in sports activities may use a prosthesis especially designed for their sports.

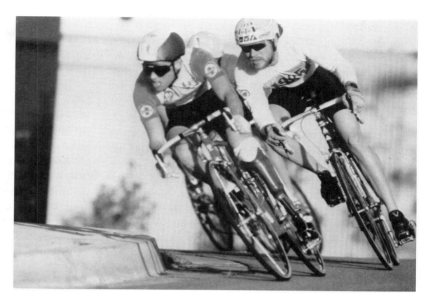

RECREATIONAL PROSTHESES

Although special adaptations for sports and recreational activities have always been available from a small cadre of creative and dedicated prosthetists, today's vigorous amputees increasingly demand prostheses that permit physically active life-styles.[18] Several unilateral below-knee amputees have successfully completed full 26-mile marathons; others are competitive triathletes or cyclists (Fig. 14-9). The current world record for the 100-yard dash with a prosthesis is less than 2 seconds different from the nonamputee record! A number of amputee athletic associations have been formed, many under the auspices of the United States Olympic Committee. They provide a competitive environment, graded classes of competition, and organized instruction for the committed athlete.

Recent developments in flexible sockets,[19] resilient feet, and related components have dramatically increased the degree of prosthetic restoration that is possible. Many nationally ranked amputee athletes use a specialized prosthesis designed solely for their sport activities (Fig. 14-9). However, for the majority of recreational athletes, a specialized limb is not necessary. Meticulous attention to detail during the initial fitting plus application of sophisticated components currently available will allow many amputees to jog, play court sports, or ride a bicycle with their regular prosthesis.

It should be noted that not every recreational activity requires the use of a prosthesis.[20] Many swimming and water sports activities are readily accomplished without a prosthesis, although some patients prefer prosthetic devices for specific tasks. With care and creativity, simplified devices that are salt water resistant can be designed.

For activities on very rough terrain or under muddy or sandy conditions, some amputees prefer a variation on the old-fashioned "peg-leg." The simplicity and reliability of such a basic prosthesis makes it useful for fishing, hiking, hunting, and similar recreations.

Snow skiing is another activity that has attracted many amputees, who ski either with or without prosthetic devices. As a general rule, the lower level or unilateral amputee will generally use the prosthesis in snow skiing, whereas the higher level or bilaterally involved person often will do better with adapted skiing equipment.[21]

Numerous specialized adaptations are available for the upper limb amputee as well. Many use the same basic prosthesis and simply connect special items in lieu of the terminal device. Examples include a connector for camera operation, a baseball mitt adaptation, and bowling attachments. Other possibilities include golfing adaptations, fishing reel attachments, and a swimming mitt. Numerous articles have been published detailing specifics of such recreational designs.[22,23] As stated by Fouchheimer, *"The most advanced application of technology is not necessarily the same as the application of the most advanced technology."*[24]

One recurrent problem relating to sports and recreational prosthetics is securing adequate funding. In the current cost containment environment, it is becoming increasingly difficult to secure third-party coverage for advanced prosthetic designs. However, in many cases, the same techniques that are used for today's competitive athlete will become incorporated into conventional practice as enhancements for all amputees in the future, as the state of the art advances. Amputees are increasingly considering active participation in society as a prerequisite for successful rehabilitation, rather than a luxury.

THE FUTURE

As in many medically related fields, prosthetics is currently facing a number of conflicting forces. The overall quality of care available in the United States is envied by other countries of the world. Increasingly, American prosthetists are being invited to lecture, teach, or practice in developing countries throughout Central and South America, the Soviet Union, and elsewhere.

At the same time, the high cost of the latest and most sophisticated technology strains our ability to fund such care. Availability of services for the indigent varies widely from state to state. Increasingly, cost containment pressures inadvertently encourage less than adequate prosthetic devices. The emphasis seems to be shifting from "What's best?" to "What's tolerable?" Understandably, amputee self-help groups are much alarmed by these trends and are becoming increasingly vocal with their concerns.

As the federal budget has been cut, support for prosthetic research and education has been decreasing rapidly. Unless this trend reverses quickly, it is projected that half the accredited prosthetic education programs in the United States will close their doors within a few years. If this is allowed to occur, the inevitable result will be an increased shortage of

practitioners, long delays in providing care, and higher costs. The ultimate outcome of these disturbing trends will be a drastic reduction in the quality of care for amputees.

On a more positive note, the current state of the art permits a more complete restoration to levels of preamputation function than ever before. Particularly for lower limb devices, the degree of comfort, stability, and mobility afforded by prosthetic restoration has never been greater. Advances in electronic components have expanded upper limb options as well, but more effective methods of control and perceptive feedback are necessary to allow precision prehension. Cosmetic appearance and durability are acceptable, but they should be improved.

SUMMARY

Prosthetic rehabilitation has advanced significantly over the past decades. With the availability of more sophisticated plastic and alloy materials, prosthetic devices have become progressive lighter and more responsive. As our understanding of the finer points of biomechanics has improved, so too has the precision with which prosthetic sockets can be fitted, resulting in increased comfort and control for the amputee.

A dazzling array of mechanical joints are available for virtually every level of amputation. When selected according to the amputee's goals and carefully aligned dynamically by the prosthetist, mobility can be very effectively restored in most cases.

The least successful prostheses are those for the most difficult challenges: the high-level amputation or bilaterally involved person. Although research continues, loss of each higher joint results in a greater percentage of unsuccessful prosthetic rehabilitation efforts. In the upper limb, use of the remaining limb or development of foot dexterity may be easier than mastering a complex prosthetic device. In the lower limb, wheelchair mobility may consume far less energy than ambulation with bilateral above-knee prostheses.

For the moment, it is necessary to accept that prosthetic restoration is impractical for some high-level amputees and encourage alternate methods of rehabilitation. As scientific advances continue, more effective solutions may be developed for these challenges.

REFERENCES

1. Putti V: Historic artificial limbs. Am J Surg 6:111,1929
2. American Association of Orthopaedic Surgeons: Orthopedic Appliance Atlas. JW Edwards, Ann Arbor, MI, 1960
3. Wilson AB: Limb Prosthetics. 6th Ed. Demos Publications, New York, 1989
4. National Center for Health Statistics: Prevalence of Selected Impairments, United States — 1977. US Department of Health and Human Services, Publication (PHS) 81-1562, Hyattsville, MD, 1981
5. Golbranson F: Prosthetics and Rehabilitation. p. 1724. In Rutherford RB (ed): Vascular Surgery. 3rd Ed. Vol. 2. WB Saunders, Philadelphia, 1989
6. Kay H: Wound dressings: soft, rigid, or semi-rigid? p. 41. In Mastro and Mastro (eds): Selected Reading: A Review of Orthotics and Prosthetics. American Orthotic and Prosthetic Association, Washington, DC, 1980
7. Malone JM, Fleming LL: Immediate, early, and late post-surgical management of the upper-limb amputation. J Rehabil Res Devel 21:33, 1984
8. Baumgartner RF: The surgery of arm and forearm amputations. Orthop Clin North Am 12:805, 1981
9. Muilenburg A, LeBlanc M: Body-powered upper-limb components. p. 29. In Atkins D, Meier R (ed): Comprehensive Management of the Upper-Limb Amputee. Springer-Verlag, New York, 1989
10. Beasley RW: General considerations in managing upper limb amputations. Orthop Clin North Am 12:743, 1981
11. Setoguchi Y, Rosenfelder R: The Limb Deficient Child. 2nd Ed. Charles C Thomas, Springfield, IL, 1982
12. Marquardt E: The Heidelberg experience. p. 241. In Atkins D, Meier R (eds): Comprehensive Management of the Upper-Limb Amputee. Springer-Verlag, New York, 1989
13. Lamb D, Law H: Upper-Limb Deficiencies in Children. Little, Brown, Boston, 1987
14. Blakeslee B: The limb deficient child. University of California Press, Los Angeles, 1963
15. Mensch G, Ellis P: Physical Therapy Management of Lower Extremity Amputations. Aspen, Rockville, MD, 1986
16. Karacooff L: Lower Extremity Amputation: A Guide to Functional Outcomes in Physical Therapy. Aspen, Rockville, MD, 1986
17. Supan T, Thomas S: Comparison of current biomechanical terms. J Orthot Prosthet 2:107, 1990
18. Michael J, Gailey R, Bowker J: New developments in recreational prostheses and adaptive devices for the amputee. Clin Orthop 256:64, 1990
19. Kinstinson O: Flexible sockets. J Orthot Prosthet 37:25, 1983
20. Michael J: New developments in prosthetic feet for sports and recreation. Palaestra 5:21, 1989
21. Kegel B: Sports for the Leg Amputee. Medical Publishing Co, Redmond, WA, 1986
22. Radocy B: Upper-extremity prosthetics: consideration and designs for sports and recreation. Clin Prosthet Orthot 11:131, 1987
23. Viau A: The Viau-Whiteside swimming attachment. The fragment. War Amputations of Canada, Ottawa 141:41, 1983
24. Fouchheimer F: Prosthetics and Orthotics International 11:9, 1987

15 Orthopaedic Technologist

THOMAS P. BYRNE

A technologist is defined as one who applies the technology of a particular field. Therefore, an orthopaedic technologist is a health care provider who has a strong understanding of the apparatus and materials employed in the care of orthopaedics patients. Furthermore, an orthopaedic technologist must be knowledgeable in the methods used to apply these materials properly, as ordered by the orthopaedic surgeon.

Modern orthopaedic patient care is affected by the vast and ever-changing array of new and updated materials and devices. To deal not only with the new materials but also with the tremendous amount of detail regarding the proper indications, contraindications, and idiosyncracies of these materials, the profession of aorthopaedic technology has evolved.

HISTORY

Although most of the established health care professions can trace their origins at least to the turn of the century — some much farther than that — the formal term *orthopaedic technologist* was slow in evolving and came into use after World War II. It was in the military that the "cast technicians" or even "cast room technicians" first carried out the duties related to the application of casts. These responsibilities expanded rapidly to include traction and even operating room assisting.

Over the next 20 years the profession changed and grew, and finally in 1981 a group in the Midwestern United States began efforts to formally establish a professional national association for orthopaedic technologists. The purpose of this association would be the pursuit of excellence through education. A formal charter and bylaws marked the beginnings of this the National Association of Orthopaedic Technologists, which is still the primary source of education and political effort for the furthering of the profession.

In 1982 the National Board of Certification for Orthopaedic Technologists was established, and, through the diligent efforts of this board, in June of 1983 the first board examination was administered. The board increased support for the test further in 1986 when all military technologists were permitted to sit for the examination through their Base Education Office and under the guidance of the D.A.N.T.E.S.

This board examination is offered to qualified applicants annually at sites throughout the United States. It is a means to define standards and measure the fundamental knowledge of those who take the test. Certification is maintained through formal continuing education programs and re-examination.

In August of 1986 the National Association of Orthopaedic Technologists met with representatives from Canada, Great Britain, and Sweden to form the International Association of Orthopaedic Technologists. Annual conventions, newsletters, communication, and assistance to local chapters have been developed and maintained by the national group.

EDUCATION

One of the basic requirements for any health care profession is a formal education base. To that end, formal curricula have been developed to provide students with the didactic classroom education on theory, laboratory practical training, and clinical site supervised training. This system teaches the theory of "why" and develops the manual skills needed to learn "how" and finally the clinical experience to convert theory to actual patient care.

In 1982 the Grossmont Community College of San Diego, CA, through funding by the San Diego County Regional Occupation Program, instituted the type of program that established formal education for Orthopaedic Technologists. This format includes a combination of classroom, laboratory, and clinical training modalities. Cook County Hospital, San Jose School of Orthopaedic Technology, and other programs provide alternative means to accomplish the goal of educating and standardizing the knowledge of orthopaedic technologists.

Today there are over 2,500 certified orthopaedic technologists in the United States who are also members of the National Association of Orthopaedic Technologists.

IMPORTANCE OF COMMUNICATION

Orthopaedic technologists carry out the direct orders of the orthopaedic surgeon whenever they treat a patient. The relationship with the surgeon must include a strong communications system to ensure that precise orders and specific parameters are understood by the physician and the technologist carrying out the orders. The technologist must be as accurate and effective in communication with the surgeon as with the patient. Observations, theories, or just simple questions should be shared in a professional manner, usually out of the patient's hearing, whenever they arise.

Communicating with other health care professionals is yet another area where accuracy and a strong knowledge of the terminology of orthopaedics is critical. Physical and occupational Therapists, radiologic technologists, and nursing staff will interact with the technologists.

SPLINTING AND CASTING

The most traditional function of the technologist is that of splint and cast application and removal. It was in this particular area that the profession emerged,

when physicians realized that ancillary health care professionals could be trained to apply specific types of casts and splints, thereby freeing up the surgeon for more efficient patient care.

Splints

Splints are noncircumferential supports for extremity injuries. They are the most appropriate means of treating musculoskeletal injuries within 48 hours of the injury. The risk in applying a cast early is related to the great chance for volume changes of the limb. Edema, ecchymosis, and other factors make a circumferential support dangerous. Compartment syndrome or Volkmann's ischemic contracture can result from the cast, which is really another compartment. Therefore, splints are appropriate when these risks are present.

Basic first aid training teaches the axiom "Splint the injury where it lies." This basic premise is the standard for patient care whether it be in the ambulance or the operating room or wherever definitive care cannot be established. This initial or emergency splinting usually is just a very temporary means of immobilizing and protecting an injured part. An emergency splint may be made from virtually any object that will support the affected limb.

The next stage in splinting is definitive splinting. In this phase, a formal, conforming device is applied in a specific position to the affected limb. In this stage the fracture is reduced or the soft tissue injury addressed.

The basic materials used by orthopaedic technologists to make definitive splints are plaster, Fiberglas, or aluminum. The old standard, plaster ($Ca_2SO_4 \cdot 2H_2O$) is inexpensive, forgiving, and quite malleable. Plaster comes in two basic forms, as rolled bandages ranging in width from 2 to 6 inches, and as "splints," which actually are slabs of the same material that the rolls are made of. These flat splints are available in 3×15-inch, 4×15-inch and 5×30-inch dimensions.

A third form, less widely used, is the "roll form" splint. In this form, 14 to 20 layers of plaster are sewn into a tubular stockinette and one side is padded with foam. This roll form comes in 25-foot lengths. The user simply measures the length needed to treat the

Table 15-1. Specific Splint Applications

Splint Type	Materials	Indications
Upper extremity		
Palmar (volar)	4 × 15 splint	Carpal tunnel
		Secondary wrist support
Ulnar gutter	5 × 30 splint	Fourth or fifth metacarpal fracture
Radial gutter	5 × 30 splint	Second or third metacarpal fracture
Thumb spike splint	3 × 15 splint	Thumb metacarpal or to rule out scaphoid fracture
Sugar tong splint (coaptation)	3 × 30 splint	Radius and ulna fractures
		Humeral fracture
Lower extremity		
Sugar tong splint (coaptation)	4 × 40 splint	Tibia and fibula fractures
Robert Jones dressing	4 × 40 splint	Acute fractures of tibia and fibula
	1 lb cotton roll	

limb involved and cuts the appropriate length of splint material. It is then a simple matter of dipping the roll form splint into the water and molding it to the limb with the padded side toward the patient. An elastic wrap or bias-cut cotton stockinette holds the splint in place. Table 15-1 describes some specific splint applications.

The setting time for plaster is indicated by the color of the packaging. Blue packaging denotes "fast setting," or 5 to 8 minutes, and green packaging indicates "extra fast setting," or 3 to 4 minutes. This setting time is basically the time available for applying the cast or splint from the moment it is dipped in water to the time of final molding. Any pressure applied to the cast after it sets only destroys the crystals as they form. Plaster requires a full 32 hours of setting time before it can support weight. Furthermore, plaster is by nature not durable, especially when moisture is present.

For these reasons, synthetic materials have been introduced. The primary synthetic splint and cast material today is Fiberglas. Fiberglas is actually a combination of polyurethane and a glass fiber substrate. The polyurethane is water activated and then acts as the catalyst for the glass fiber. Modern products have evolved to a very impressive state, and synthetic casts and splints are preferred by both patients and staff.

One myth that should be exposed regarding Fiberglass is that while Fiberglass splints and casts will not deteriorate when exposed to moisture, the patient's skin most certainly will if the exposure is of long enough duration. Skin maceration is a major compli-cation if splints or casts are exposed to water or moisture. Notably, normal sweat does not lead to skin breakdown, because the salinity of sweat is similar to that of the skin. Plain water will, result in skin maceration, however, and for that reason all current manufacturers of synthetic splint and cast materials state that these materials should not be exposed to water.

Materials have been developed recently in the area of padding for cast and splints. Goretex and foam with special holes designed to keep water away from skin have been produced and marketed. However, these products are still improved as of this writing.

Casts

A cast is a rigid, circumferential support that is conformed to an extremity to support a fracture or soft tissue injury. As with splints, the materials of casts consist basically of plaster bandages or Fiberglas. The primary difference between a cast and a splint is that the cast is rolled on the patient's limb and molded to conform to the dimensions of that limb. Again, the difficulty comes when the effects of trauma are present. A conforming cast applied to a very swollen limb will be loose and nonfunctional within days. Conversely, a well-molded cast applied to an acutely injured limb that may increase in volume can lead to serious problems.

Once the initial 48 hours of high risk have passed and the limb edema has resolved, a cast can be applied using the technique that has evolved over the years and actually still varies regionally. The following description is a reasonable guide to the application of a cast; however, it is only a guide. Few modern, definitive publications on cast application are available.

Initially, a tubular stockinette of an appropriate diameter and approximately 2 or 3 cm longer than the intended cast is placed on the limb. This layer is followed by a minimum of two and a maximum of five layers of rolled padding. This material is available in various widths and as a cotton or rayon base. It is my belief that the use of 100 percent cotton under cast padding has advantages over the use of synthetic padding material. Primarily, the cotton is less likely to be constricting, is more absorbent, and is less irritating to skin. A standard guideline during application of casts is to use slight tension when applying the padding, but never to use tension when applying or rolling the actual cast material.

Examples of some types of casts that are common in rehabilitation patients follow.

Serial Casts

The serial cast, a specific adaptation of a standard cast, may be used to counter muscle or soft tissue contracture. The basic concept is to apply a well-padded, rigid cast that allows the technologist to maintain a counter-pull or stretch on the affected joint and connective tissue. This must be done in such a way that it will not cause decubitus ulcers—a difficult challenge, considering the amount of force needed to stretch the equinus contracture of a near-drowning victim. Neurologically compromised patients also exhibit this contracture, and it is quite difficult to push against this force and not injure the patient further.

The serial casting technique allows for reasonable counterforce and 2- to 3-week interval cast changes. The concept behind this type of cast is that the trauma of the stretch is applied in limited stages with regular repetition. Changing the cast more often than every 2 or 3 weeks leads to problems with pressure and may even aggravate the contracture.

Another means for preventing the pressure of the procedure from causing difficulties is to use advanced techniques in cast padding. The use of articulated $\frac{1}{4}$ inch, open cell foam as a complete layer under the cast can allow for molding yet decrease the occurrence of pressure necrosis seen with standard cast padding techniques.

Diabetic Foot Casts

The diabetic patient requires special considerations when a cast is applied for any reason. A diabetic limb with an open ulcer presents definite problems. In the past the standard for care of a patient with an ulcer was a technique referred to as "total contact." In this method, the cast is applied using only two layers of stockinette and felt pads over the malleoli. The rationale behind this technique was to disperse pressure by spreading that pressure over the entire surface of the lower extremity.

Use of this method requires a thorough understanding of the materials and methods of casting because there is no margin for error. Even a slight fold or tuck could lead to development of an open sore. In addition, these casts are not designed to allow weight bearing. For these and other reasons an alternative method is now employed for diabetic foot ulcers. In this plan the ulcer is first débrided to remove dead tissue. A dry, 4×4-inch sterile gauze pad is the only dressing. Standard stockinette and padding methods are then used, with the exception that the foot and toes are completely covered by the cast padding.

A more recent change in casting technique is the use of the $\frac{1}{4}$ inch foam known as Sifoam to completely cover the limb where the cast is to be applied. A single layer of plaster is then employed as an absorbent, astringent layer. This is followed by four 4-inch rolls of Fiberglas. Fiberglas is used because this cast allows weight bearing, even with an open ulcer. Again, the cast incorporates the entire foot and covers the toes.

The casts are changed every 2 weeks. Admittedly the cast (and the contents) can become somewhat malodorous, causing the patient some distress if there is a lot of drainage; however, the ulcer will do well.

Dropout Casts

Hemophilia casts or dropout casts are designed to allow for limited joint motion. Specifically, the casts are cut away to allow the patient's contracted joints to be manipulated by the patient, physician, or physical therapist. For example, in the case of a child with Achilles tendon shortness, a short leg cast can be cut out over the dorsum of the foot and just proximal to the ankle joint. The cast is applied with the foot in maximum dorsiflexion as tolerated by the patient. Once the edges have been smoothed, the patient will be able to dorsiflex but not plantar flex the ankle, allowing the parents or therapists to manipulate the ankle and foot.

Dropout casts are changed every 2 weeks.

Patellar Tendon – Bearing

Augusto Sarmiento's patellar tendon–bearing (PTB) cast is an innovative technique that has changed the way orthopaedists think about applying a cast. Sarmiento proposed applying a below-the-knee cast that is able to control the rotation of the tibia yet allow for knee flexion and extension. This is possible because this cast is formed superior to the femoral condyles and with direct pressure on the patellar tendon. The cast is then trimmed superior to the molds. The result is a cast that allows early motion and increased blood supply in acute tibial fractures. Weight bearing is another positive aspect of PTB cast.

Delbet Cast

Sarmiento's application of hydraulics and similar theories in the PTB cast led orthopaedic technologists to rethink how and why casts and braces are used. One step further was a rethinking of control of the tibia in a cast (the Delbet cast). Actually this is an old idea that has been redeveloped into a below-knee cast that, because it is formed over both malleoli, allows motion at the ankle. The patient wears a shoe and ambulates normally. The cast is most appropriate for patients with clinically healed lesions who may lack full radiologic evidence of healing. Because the cast does not limit the range of motion of the knee or the ankle, it can sometimes help the stubborn fracture to heal. The Delbet cast is not appropriate for proximal or distal third fractures, however.

CONCLUSION

The evolution of the profession of orthopaedic technology is an ongoing process. The rapid changes in splinting and casting methodologies will demand that orthopaedic technologists continually increase their knowledge in the proper application of this type of patient care. Local and national associations geared toward this education will expand, and those who wish to remain professionals will have to assimilate this information.

16 Rehabilitation Engineering and Assistive Technology

KENNETH P. KOZOLE

Technology affects all people in every walk of life. Computers have changed the future for everyone, as we now handle information processing at rates and in quantities beyond comprehension. We research, design, manufacture, and sell more efficiently with the aid of electrical pulses streaming through complex circuits and tiny silicon chips. It is very apparent that both the world and the universe continue to become smaller as a result of technology applications such as sophisticated communication networks and ventures into outer space.

In an effort to capture and apply the benefits of modern technology, and to enhance the lives of others, a group of professionals known as rehabilitation engineers and rehabilitation technologists have begun to emerge. The varying definitions of rehabilitation engineering can be summarized as, *the systematic, practical application of engineering principles and modern technology to meet the needs of persons with disabilities.*[1,2] In the last decade, this diverse group has begun to formalize the application of assistive technology for the purpose of improving the quality of life for persons who have physical, sensory, or cognitive disabilities.

In recent years a number of states have received federal grant funding as a result of Public Law 100-407, the Technology Related Assistance for Individuals with Disabilities Act of 1988. The Act set aside federal funds to establish consumer-responsive statewide programs that promote assistive technologies for persons with disabilities. *The Technology Related Assistance Act defines an assistive technology device as: "Any item, piece of equipment, or product system · · · that is used to increase, maintain, or improve functional capabilities of individuals with disabilities."* An assistive technology service "directly assists an individual with a disability in the selection, acquisition, or use of an assistive technology device."

Assistive technology developments have expanded significantly in the last decade. They have found applications in a number of areas. ABLEDATA,[3] a data base distribution network consisting of comprehensive information, lists over 18,000 commercially available products for rehabilitation and independent living. This information can be accessed by contacting an ABLEDATA searching service, or by subscribing to the Hyper-ABLEDATA program. Hyper-ABLEDATA is available to any organization, individual, or facility, and can be installed in an office on a personal computer for unlimited use at no hourly charges. Updates from ABLEDATA are sent semiannually to subscribers. ABLEDATA categorizes types of assistive technology as indicated in Table 16-1.

BACKGROUND OF REHABILITATION ENGINEERING

Since World War II, practitioners in the field of orthotics and prosthetics have helped shape the futures of many people who have benefited from orthoses and

Table 16-1. ABLEDATA Assistive
Technology Categories

Ambulation
Architectural elements
Communication
Computers
Controls
Home Management
Mobility
Orthotics/prothetics
Personal care
Recreation
Seating
Sensory aids
Therapeutic aids
Transportation
Vocational/educational

artificial limbs used to support or replace body parts. Many of those who pioneered applications in orthotics and prosthetics combined modern materials and technologies in their creative and functional designs. Yet the benefits of technology have reached far beyond the applications of orthotics and prosthetics in rehabilitation. Modern medical technology and improved resuscitative procedures are allowing more people to survive life-threatening situations, therefore, increasing the demand for assistive technology. For instance, many World War II soldiers did not

survive life-threatening injuries, whereas the Vietnam veteran survived and returned, requiring rehabilitation and assistive technology.

Consumers, rehabilitation engineers, therapists, physicians, teachers, counselors, and technologists, to name a few, have realized the powers of technology and have focused on blending technology with rehabilitation, health care, and education. From newborn to senior citizen, assistive technology has found a wide spectrum of applications. Communication devices and computers help people with physical disabilities and speech impairments (Fig. 16-1); new manual and power-propelled wheelchairs offer mobility to those who have severe physical involvement; and attention to seating and body positioning needs has resulted in a variety of seating systems designed to prevent life-threatening and costly pressure sores and orthopaedic deformities (Fig. 16-2). Electrical stimulation has been shown to have beneficial functional and therapeutic value for persons with spinal cord injury and other disabilities.[4] Lifts and hand controls fitted into tractors and combines have enabled a number of farmers who have limited function of their lower extremities to return to work (Fig. 16-3). Today's challenge is to extract the useful technology and match it to the needs of those who may gain functionally.

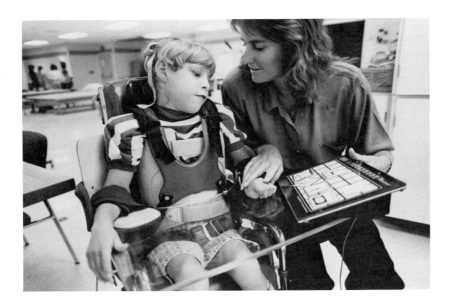

Fig. 16-1 Computerized communication devices allow access via single switch and use synthesized speech and printed outputs to communicate. (Courtesy of Sharp Rehabilitation Center, San Diego, CA.)

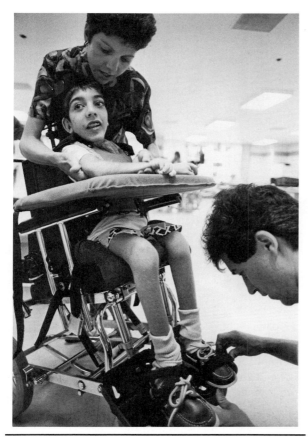

Fig. 16-2. A custom molded seating system allows for safe and functional, independent sitting for a person with severe spinal deformity. (Courtesy of Sharp Rehabilitation Center, San Diego, CA.)

The Rehabilitation Engineering Society of North America (RESNA) was founded in 1980. A few years later it was defined as the Interdisciplinary Association for the Advancement of Rehabilitation and Assistive Technologies to "more accurately reflect the broad array of interests and skills within the organization. RESNA is concerned with transferring science, engineering, and technology to the needs of persons with disabilities. Its members are rehabilitation professionals from all pertinent disciplines, providers and consumers."[5]

The mission of RESNA is "to contribute to the public welfare through scientific, literary, and educational activities by supporting the development, dissemination, and utilization of knowledge of rehabilitation and assistive technology in order to achieve the highest quality of life for all citizens."[6] Annual national and regional RESNA conferences offer persons interested in assistive technology, from consumer to engineer, the opportunity to share state-of-the-art technology research and applications. "RESNA brings together individuals whose credentials, activities, and interests vary widely but all of whom are committed to designing, developing, evaluating, and delivering the appropriate technology to disabled persons."[5]

RESNA continues to grow yearly, and is striving to define the roles of those professionals involved in the broad range of assistive technology applications through the activities of Special Interest Groups (SIG) and Professional Specialty Groups (PSG). Each of the sixteen SIGs provides a forum for exchanging information related to its area of specialty and offers opportunity for cross-fertilization of ideas between the various disciplines. These groups comprise:

Service delivery and public policy issues (SIG 1)
Personal transportation (SIG 2)
Augmentative and alternative communication (SIG 3)
Prosthetics and orthotics (SIG 4)
Quantitative functional assessment (SIG 5)
Special education (SIG 6)
Technology transfer (SIG 7)
Sensory aids (SIG 8)
Wheeled mobility and seating (SIG 9)
Electrical stimulation (SIG 10)
Computer applications (SIG 11)
Rural rehabilitation (SIG 12)
Robotics (SIG 13)
Job accomodation (SIG 14)
Information networking (SIG 15)
Gerontology (SIG 16)

The efforts of the Rehabilitation Engineering PSG (RE PSG), and the RESNA Quality Assurance (QA) committee are presently being directed at establishing criteria related to qualifications, education, and role definition for persons emerging as rehabilitation engineers. The purpose of the QA program includes assuring the highest quality of service and products, fostering continued professional growth and guidance, creating an accountable system that assures payment for services and equipment, and facilitation of professional recognition for those involved in service delivery.[7] As the field of assistive technology

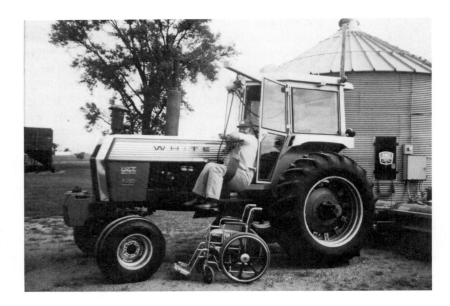

Fig. 16-3. A powered lift enables this farmer to independently transfer from his wheelchair to the tractor seat. (Courtesy of the Easter Seal Society of Iowa, Farm Program, Des Moines, IA.)

service delivery grows, so will the demand for qualified rehabilitation engineers and accredited programs. Quality assurance and quality improvement will need to be closely linked to the growth of this field as it continues to develop professionally.

THE ASSISTIVE TECHNOLOGY TEAM

Assistive technology applications have gone beyond the clinical team, and it is recognized that there is a need for cooperation among varying disciplines in order to make technology work.[8] Although members may vary depending upon the situation, the assistive technology team may include any or all of the following individuals[8]:

Person with a disability/consumer
Family and/or caregiver
Physician
Occupational therapist
Physical therapist
Nurse
Speech pathologist
Rehabilitation engineer
Rehabilitation technologist
Psychologist
Teacher
Rehabilitation technology supplier
Social worker or case manager
Vocational counselor

Employer
Orthotist prosthetist

Essential components of any comprehensive rehabilitation technology service delivery program have been defined as[9]:

Knowledgeably trained, available service providers
Consumers who are informed and understand the benefits technology offers and know where to find services
Professionals who understand the benefits technology offers their clients, and who can make appropriate referrals
Financial resources available to pay for products and services
Information that links these other components together

WHAT DOES THE REHABILITATION ENGINEER BRING TO THE REHABILITATION TEAM?

A postion paper has been drafted by the RE PSG, and accepted by RESNA, as a working document, or first draft, from which more specific and consistent criteria will evolve related to the role of rehabilitation engineers. As the benefits of technology continue to be realized in the field of rehabilitation, the need for rehabilitation engineers as members of the rehabilitation team will help rehabilitation facilities, assistive technology teams, research programs, and manufacturers as they strive to remain progressive by keeping pace with technological developments and their applications. As stated by the RE PSG[1]:

Rehabilitation Engineers have specific training and background which uniquely qualify them to play an important role on the rehabilitation team. For example:

— For device access the rehabilitation engineer can employ knowledge of input/output processing, ergonomics, human factors engineering, human/machine interface design, component compatibility, electronics and programming.

— In providing an interface to various technologies, the rehabilitation engineer can utilize expertise in design, and knowledge of a wide variety of electromechanical components.

— In assessment of body positioning and stability the rehabilitation engineer can employ knowledge of static mechanics, dynamics, kinematics, and materials in relation to body mechanics and function.

— For systems integration the rehabilitation engineer can utilize knowledge of digital and analog interfaces together with the relationship to requirements for signal conditioning, logic, or computing.

— For assessment of component and system alternatives the rehabilitation engineer has unique qualifications needed for obtaining and interpreting product design information and operation characteristics from a manufacturer or other sources.

The engineer's training and design and problem solving combined with wide ranging knowledge of rehabilitation and assistive technologies then permit analytic consideration of alternatives, including custom design and modification when appropriate.

The primary difference between a rehabilitation engineer and other engineers, such as mechanical or electrical engineers, is that the rehabilitation engineer must understand not only engineering principles but also the applications of technology with respect to the needs of persons having physical, sensory, and/or cognitive disabilities. This involves an in-depth understanding of a myriad of disabilities, and the implications of how a condition affects a person's functional performance. Also, the rehabilitation engineer must be able to communicate effectively with the person who has a disability, other members of the rehabilitation team, and engineering or technical

support staff, in order to facilitate a match between technology and human needs.

NEED FOR CREDENTIALING

The rehabilitation engineer has been trained in a formal engineering discipline, and has gained additional knowledge through experience. These skills are then applied via assistive technology to the needs of persons with disabilities. As a result, the rehabilitation engineer brings engineering and scientific skills to the problem-solving process of the rehabilitation team, enhancing the solution options. Credentialing of rehabilitation engineers will continue to be a primary focus of the RESNA RE PSG because it will help resolve current issues related to identity, education, third party reimbursement, quality control, and liability insurance.

As assistive technology has become more commercially available, members of other disciplines have become well versed in the assessment, selection, and appropriate application of this technology. In other words, therapists, teachers, technologists, vocational counselors, and others are becoming more specialized in technology applications, including computers, controls, communication devices, wheelchairs, seating and positioning, driving, and work site assessment and modification. Also, there are many existing assistive technology practitioners with a strong background in design and fabrication skills who have been providing effective assistive technology solutions. As quality assurance issues continue to arise they tend to be a driving force for accountability, affecting practitioners across many disciplines. Consequently, it is also necessary to have credentialing for these specialists. Credentialing will result in defining the roles of rehabilitation and education professionals who have become specialists in assistive technology applications.

THE PROBLEM-SOLVING PROCESS

It is important that the whole picture be considered when assessing a person with a disability for technological solutions (Fig. 16-4). Ideally, a variety of technologies and strategies should be incorporated to meet the person's needs without interfering with other functions. For example, an individual who has

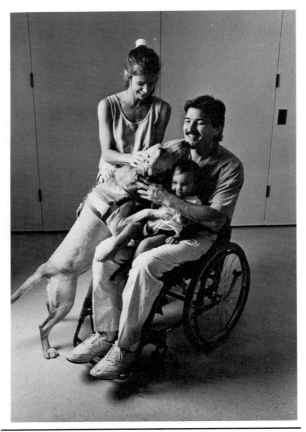

Fig. 16-4. All aspects of the person's lifestyle must be considered when recommending assistive technology. (Courtesy of Sharp Rehabilitation Center, San Diego, CA.)

cerebral palsy may require the use of an electrically powered wheelchair. Functional placement of the joystick controller may require the controller to be located directly in front of the client; however, the controller may interfere with an electronic communication system to be placed on a laptray directly in front of the person. By combining use of a swing-away joystick control arm and communication device mounting bracket, a functional system is provided. The assistive technology team considers pros and cons of technology mixtures such that optimal performance can be obtained.

"Gadget tolerance" has become a common issue in recent years. Some people have a low tolerance for assistive technology, such that any devices provided for them spend most of the time on a shelf whereas others may utilize assistive technology to its fullest. The assistive technology team must involve the person with a disability from the beginning to avoid nonuseable recommendations. Trial use of assistive technology prior to pruschase will help sort out acceptable solutions. Recommending assistive devices based on a picture in a catalog, without trial use first, often results in disappointment and lost time and money. Many assistive technology programs have a large variety of commercially available devices for use in the assessment process and for demonstration. A good relationship, and inclusion of the rehabilitation technology supplier on the team, will often provide easy access to many devices for trial use. Manufacturer representatives are excellent resources and have also been known to supply equipment for trial use.

Simulation is another means to assess the appropriateness of assistive technology application. Simulation has been a powerful tool in determing the effectiveness of seating systems ranging from planar to custom-molded contoured shapes.[10] A person can be positioned in the simulator and "hands-off" observations can be made by the team. A variety of functions and activities, such as power wheelchair control or communication and computer access, can then be performed by the person seated in the simulator, and assessed. Simulation is also available to assess functional abilities in work-related activities, control access, range of motion, strength, and endurance (Fig. 16-5).

When assessing and recommending assistive technology, the following guidline should generally be considered to achieve the most cost effective solution [2,8]:

1. Does the person need a device, or is there a technique that can be incorporated to accomplish the same goal just as effectively?

"Compensatory strategies," or restructuring of tasks, activities, and the environment, may offset the functional limitations experienced by the individual. This could involve occupational or physical therapy techniques, attendant care arrangements, or environ-

Fig. 16-5. Simulated work situations help define needs and solutions. (Courtesy of Sharp Rehabilitation Center, San Diego, CA.)

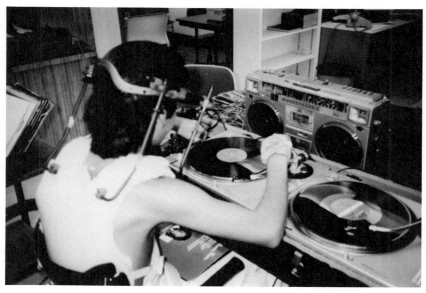

mental modifications.[2] For example, rearranging most frequently used items in one's office or home may eliminate the need for a person with limited upper extremity range of motion to use a reacher device. Refining wheelchair transfer techniques may eliminate the need for lifts or transfer boards.

2. Is there an assistive device commercially available that meets the person's needs?

Volumes of rehabilitation technology catalogs and equipment data bases exist offering the consumer many choices of commercially available "off-the-shelf" equipment. It should be noted that assistive devices also include nonmedical equipment. Many devices are being developed with attention to universal design or accessibility considerations for persons without disabilities that may also be helped for persons with disabilities. General consumer and industrial goods should always be considered when determining assistive technology solutions.

Whenever possible, trial use of assistive devices before purchase is recommended. Compare cost, function, portability, compatibility with other equipment, durability, warranty period, safety features, size, weight, repair history, maintenance, power requirements, "user friendliness," and availability. *High tech, low tech, light tech,* and *no tech* are terms

currently used to define types of technology. Regardless of the terminology, knowledge of how, when, and where to blend "low tech" with "high tech" equipment is a valuable skill that is only gained through experience. For example, a person with a C4 spinal cord injury may prefer using a "low tech" mouthstick to access a very powerful "high tech" computer system instead of using the variety of available computer input technologies, such as speech recognition or ultrasonic and optical target pointing systems.[11] Although considered "low tech" by some, a mouthstick is easily manipulated by the user as an extension of the body, providing effective access to other conventional devices, appliances, and controls in the home and office. The mouthstick in this case is a simple device offering very high function. "Low tech" should not be confused with low function; often it proves to be the contrary, because simplicity has merit in most assistive technology designs. The seasoned rehabilitation engineer and assistive technology specialist know the importance of listening to the client throughout the problem-solving process, assessing with trial use of equipment whenever possible, and carefully scrutinizing sophisticated technological solutions.

3. If the commercially available device does not fully meet the person's needs, can it be modified?

Several concerns must be considered before modifying a device. First, safety should not be compromised by a modification. Anyone providing the modification will be liable should a safety concern arise. Second, the modification should not alter the product durability or warranty if possible; contacting the manufacturer may clarify this concern. Finally, additional cost and time for modification of the original device must also be considered. As a member of the assistive technology team, the rehabilitation engineer's training in design and problem solving allows for practical, safe, and efficient solutions regarding modifications.

4. If a commercially available device cannot be modified to meet the person's needs, could a custom device be designed and fabricated to provide the necessary function?

Design-to-delivery time, durability, reliability, maintenance, safety, warranty, compatibility with existing equipment, and cost are primary concerns when providing a custom-designed assistive device. These need to be confirmed with the consumer and assistive technology team prior to project initiation.

Through the application of sound engineering principles and an organized problem-solving process, the rehabilitation engineer can sort out the most appropriate technique, materials, components, and mechanisms in a minimum of time to arrive at a safe, practical, and functional device. Experienced engineers adhere to the "keep it simple" premise and involve the consumer and team throughout the problem-solving and design process.

In all cases, training should be considered a priority before the equipment is issued, and a follow-up program should be integrated into the delivery process. The "no news is good news" approach is not a reliable indicator of *successful* technology application. The importance of this critical issue is currently being addressed in the federally funded project "Implementation and Follow-up of Rehabilitation Technology."[12] By providing (1) verbal training regarding use of the device(s), (2) written instructions and information when the device(s) is issued, (3) follow-up after use, and (4) feedback to manufacturers and researchers, the implementation and follow-up system will increase the overall acceptance and use of devices, increase user satisfaction, and Initiate a feedback loop to product manufacturers.

MODELS OF ASSISTIVE TECHNOLOGY SERVICE DELIVERY

Assistive technology services are now available in a variety of areas. In *Rehabilitation Technology Service Delivery: A Practical Guide,*[13] Smith presented seven models of service delivery. Each model has its own character and personality.

Rehabilitation Equipment Supplier

This supplier was previously known as the Durable Medical Equipment (DME) supplier because, over 20 years ago, MediCare defined reimbursable equipment, including certain wheelchairs, walkers, and other medically related equipment, as durable medical equipment. As home care has expanded over recent years, and assistive technology became more diverse and sophisticated, the rehabilitation equipment supplier has evolved away from the local drug store to larger supply facilities. Some have hired therapists and encouraged sales staff to receive specialized training and education. To ensure a smooth transition from assessment to delivery of equipment, the rehabilitation equipment supplier is encouraged to be an active member of the rehabilitation team. Because of the close relationship to the manufacturers of assistive technology, the rehabilitation equipment provider can offer important information and feedback to the team and manufacturers. The majority of products issued by these suppliers consist of commercially available devices.

Department within a Comprehensive Rehabilitation Program

This service delivery program may or may not be based within a hospital setting; however, the primary focus of such a program would be to support the comprehensive rehabilitation service, which is multidisciplinary. The rehabilitation engineer and rehabilitation technologists working in this model are part of a team that provides technology services to help the consumer reach a common goal. Modifications, custom design, and fabrication capabilities are frequently available in this model. Funding related to this model is usually based on a fee-for-service reimbursement to third-party payers.

University Based Rehabilitation Engineering Center

The university based rehabilitation engineering centers (RECs) are presently funded by the National Institute of Disability and Rehabilitation Research (NIDRR). The main focus is research and development related to assistive technology and dissemination of information. Research and development is a critical factor in keeping assistive technology in pace with the benefits of modern technology. REC staff is composed of not only clinical, but also highly technical, engineering personnel.

Other University settings may have a separate affiliated clinical service delivery program. Service delivery offered in a university clinical setting may be funded through contractual agreement or fee-for-service to third-party payors.

State Agency–Based Program

Some state governments support and administer this type of service delivery system. The state agency works to provide an organized state-wide delivery system providing both metropolitan and rural areas with a wide range of services. Funding in most cases is provided through federal funds or state-matched federal funds for vocational rehabilitation programs. In some settings, the state agency acts as an information source referring those in need of assistive technology services to private service delivery providers in the state.

Private Rehabilitation Engineering/ Technology Firm

In addition to family-run businesses, a number of individuals have set up consultation firms offering services. They include computer applications, van modifications, orthotics, prosthetics, job and work site accommodations, seating, and general rehabilitation engineering. Service is usually based on fee-for-service reimbursement or contractual agreement payment.

Local Affiliate of a National Nonprofit Disability Organization

Rehabilitation technology services are being provided through national nonprofit organizations such as the National Easter Seal Society, the Muscular Dystrophy Association, the United Cerebral Palsy organization, the Association for Retarded Citizens, the American Association for the Blind, the American Heart Association, and the Arthritis Foundation. Both the functional service categories and the population served tend to be relatively specific to the disability organization itself. The majority of funding for these services is provided through monies solicited through donations and special fund-raising events.

Miscellaneous Programs

A variety of volunteer organizations are available to provide services, including the Telephone Pioneers of America and the Volunteers for Medical Engineering. Information sources related to assistive technology, such as ABLEDATA, have been developed to assist consumers, researchers, and rehabilitation practitioners in their search needs. The Job Accommodation Network (JAN)[3] is a free information service whereby the caller explains the problem to an information specialist who has access to a computerized data base of possible solutions. Information is provided related to work site modifications, products, and other job accommodations. Funding for such services usually is partially provided through grants, large institution sponsorship, or fee-for-service.

Annual trade shows such as the Abilities Expo and the National Home Health Care Exposition offer "hands-on" opportunities to explore the vast realm of assistive technology. Examples of additional seminars and conferences include those sponsored by the American Occupational Therapy Association, the American Physical Therapy Association, RESNA, California State University at Northridge, the American Speech and Hearing Association, the International and United States Societies for Augmentative and Alternative Communication, and Closing the Gap. These gatherings offer workshops, lectures, exhibits, and the opportunity to network, for those in-

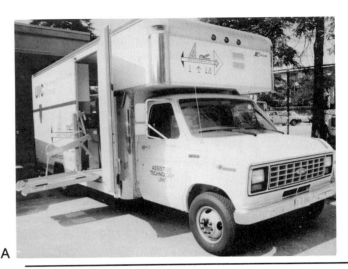
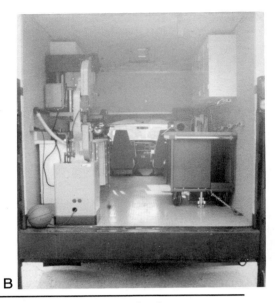

Fig. 16-6. (A & B) A mobile service delivery unit outfitted to provide on-site assistive technology assessment, fabrication, and modifications. (Courtesy of the University of Illinois at Chicago UAP Assistive Technology Unit, Chicago, IL.)

terested in staying abreast of the rapidly growing field of assistive technology.

ASSISTIVE TECHNOLOGY MOBILE SERVICE DELIVERY

Although assistive technology services are becoming increasingly available, there are persons who cannot receive services at the above-mentioned facilities. Therefore, a recent trend has been the provision of assistive technology services via mobile service delivery units (Fig. 16-6). A variety of vehicles have been incorporated into the mobile service delivery approach, ranging from 18-wheelers to vans to pickup trucks pulling trailers. The majority of mobile units contain fabrication equipment, including large power tools (drill press, sander, band saw, welder, etc.), small hand tools, and materials and supplies.[14] Often, assessment equipment is on board so that on-site evaluation, design, fabrication, and fitting can all be provided efficiently.[15]

The mobile units not only act as an outreach system, bringing technology where it may be otherwise unavailable, but also act to identify problems and bring referrals to the main facility. An example would be

assessing a client in a rural school for an electric-powered wheelchair and discovering severe scoliosis, which may not be addressed appropriately through the use of a custom-molded seating system. In this case, the client would be referred back to the main facility for further assessment by appropriate specialists and require possible orthopaedic intervention.

Another example would be the application of assistive technology at the work site for a farmer who had a spinal cord injury. After acute hospitalization and rehabilitation, the farmer returns home and can no longer access his tractor and other equipment because of lower extremity paralysis. The question becomes: has this person realized all the benefits of the rehabilitation process? The rehabilitation engineer and assistive technology team would be able to visit the farmsite via the mobile service delivery unit. They would then work with the farmer to provide the necessary modifications, such as lifts and hand controls, throughout the farm to enable the farmer to return to work.

Types of assistive technology provided by mobile service delivery units have included seating and positioning, computer access, wheelchairs, work site/

tool modification and accommodation, controls, augmentative communication devices, and orthotics and prosthetics. This approach is proving to be an effective means of building an awareness of the benefits of assistive technology.

REHABILITATION ENGINEERING CENTERS

Research has always been a strong component in the growth and development of the rehabilitation engineering field. Federal funding in the 1970s encouraged centers to develop assistive technology and promoted commercial manufacturing and availability of these devices. During the 1980s additional emphasis was focused on funding the development of assistive technology service delivery programs. There was a need to bring the technology to the consumer. The next decade will bring an emphasis on the combination of developing new technologies and refining the delivery system. There is now an awareness that assistive technology service is not limited to the device and equipment; of equal importance is the means by which the device obtained by the intended persons.

The National Institute of Disability and Rehabilitation Research (NIDRR), through the U.S. Department of Education, provides grant funding to support Rehabilitation Engineering Centers (RECs). Each REC is assigned a "priority area" so that research and development activities can be focused without duplication of effort. A primary NIDRR objective is the dissemination of information regarding developments and applications of new assistive technology in an accessible format to persons with disabilities, clinicians, independent living programs, counselors, third-party payers, researchers, and manufacturers.

Childress (personal communication) has described five important ways in which NIDRR REC's and related research are mechanisms for advancements in the rehabilitation field:

1. Continued activity related to device development is crucial to the needs of persons with disabilities in the next decade.
2. NIDRR support has had a big impact on the field through the attraction and direction of professional

people into the commercial sector, the clinical sector, and into the research and development sector.
3. Continued research support will allow the rehabilitation engineering field to go beyond the empirical phase and to develop the basic foundation of principles and theories that are necessary for the field to reach its true potential.
4. Research has had a powerful impact on a field's development and can substantially alter methods of rehabilitation practice. Research will force or drive the rehabilitation technology field in new directions and point out current shortcomings.
5. Information dissemination, agenda setting, and consensus methods regarding rehabilitation engineering technology and techniques is an important way that engineering centers impact the lives of disabled persons and the field of rehabilitation practice.

An exhaustive overview of the REC activities is not within the scope of this chapter; however, a brief overview of the priority areas and their RECs follows. Additional current information can be obtained by contacting NIDRR.[3]

Augmentative Communication Devices

(REC: A.I. Dupont Institute, Applied Science and Engineering, Wilmington, DE)

This REC's activities have been focused on improving access to communication devices for a wide range of disabled users. Current assistive technology techniques and developments are increasing printed output. For example, abbreviations can be used as a technique in accelerating vocabulary generation of an individual using a communication aid. Research is being conducted on more efficient generation of personalized abbreviation schemes, and reducing the selection demands (e.g., number of keystrokes) on the user.[16] Another project goal was to increase the communication rate of physically disabled individuals via Natural Language Processing techniques. A compressed message containing mainly the content words spoken by a disabled person was interpreted by a system that had the potential to generate a syntactically and semantically well-formed sentence.[17] The REC will disseminate their research results to clinicians, manufacturers, educators, and persons with disabilities.

Modifications to Jobs, Work Sites, and Educational Settings

(REC: Cerebral Palsy Research Foundation of Kansas, Inc., Wichita, KS)

Rehabilitation engineering research and development at this REC are focused primarily on providing work opportunities for persons with disabilities. All aspects of employment are considered, including independent living, mobility, seating and positioning, advocacy, transportation, speech and language development, and computer/work station access. Development of computer training programs is being investigated to facilitate employment. A current project has shown that the cognitive load required by a computer input device, such as a trackball, a voice input system, and a two-degree-of-freedom keyboard accessed with headsticks, can have a significant effect on task performance.[18]

Technologies to Promote "Hearing" in Deaf and Hearing-Impaired Individuals

(REC: City University of New York Center for Research in Speech and Hearing Sciences, New York, NY)

This REC is currently developing new and markedly improved hearing aids to provide superior performance by matching the incoming speech signals to the limited dynamic range of the impaired auditory system and reducing the interference from background noise. Alerting or alarm systems and improved assessment tools and techniques are also being researched and developed. Establishment of a resource center and training programs will offer information and techniques to service delivery professionals

Prosthetics and Orthotics

(REC: Northwestern University Rehabilitation Engineering Program, Chicago, IL)

Research and development at this REC are focused on improving orthotic and prosthetic assessment techniques, instrumentation, and design criteria. Applications and standards of new materials will be established. A current research program is being conducted applying computer-assisted design/computer-assisted manufacture (CAD/CAM) technology to produce orthotic and prosthetic devices. Dissemination of information is provided through workshops and training/educational materials available at the Information and Education Resource Unit. The unit is known as a national resource center for information on orthotics and prosthetics.

Technology for Children with Orthopaedic Disabilities

(REC: The Rancho Los Amigos Medical Center, Rehabilitation Engineering Center, Downey, CA)

The mission of this REC is to develop appropriate technology and assessment procedures in the field of orthopaedic rehabilitation and assure their availability to children with disabilities. It will employ a total approach to rehabilitation, combining medicine, engineering, and related sciences. Research will include improved grip strength in body-powered terminal devices for children; new lightweight and cosmetic ankle-foot orthoses; an orthosis to treat neonates and infants with congenital hip dislocations; and a powered orthosis to reduce joint contractures. Published guidelines, a consumer's guide, and a resource library will be methods of information dissemination.

Access to Computers and Electronic Equipment

(REC: University of Wisconsin–Madison, Trace Research and Development Center on Communication, Control, and Computer Access for Handicapped Individuals, Madison, WI)

Research and development at this REC are aimed at improving computer and electronic device access for persons of all ages and disabilities. Systems and devices studied include standard microcomputers, microcomputer operations systems, special rehabilitation/education software; electronic office equipment, telecommunication devices, emergency control systems, teletransaction systems, electronic information systems, electronic directories, electronic shopping systems, and emergency systems and devices. Activities include blind user access to popular graphics-user interface (GUI) systems. Computers such as the Apple Macintosh and operating systems such as Microsoft Windows use the GUI approach.

Multisensory, multiaccess techniques such as vibro-tactile displays, tones, stereo sound imaging, and voice control navigation are being investigated to solve this access problem.[19]

Improved Wheelchair and Seating Design

(REC: University of Virginia Rehabilitation Engineering Center, Charlottesville, VA)

This REC's activities involve the many aspects of wheelchair design and seating/positioning development. Total function of manual and powered wheelchairs and seating systems will be investigated to identify malfunction type and frequency, reliability, durability, safety, and function. The expected outcome will be improved wheelchairs, wheelchair components, and seating systems. The REC has been conducting research and development on computerized methods of prescribing and manufacturing seating systems. The electrical shape sensor (ESS) defines contour and force when a person is seated in an assessment chair that has an array of acrylic balls mounted on springs and connected to the sensor. Information is sent to a computer, where an image is charted both graphically and numerically. The clinician can then adjust the information to allow for proper cushion pressure distribution. The image and the chart can be sent by modem to a commercial central fabrication facility (Pin Dot Products), or to the center's own fabrication facility, and the cushion can be molded immediately.[20]

Low Back Pain

(REC: University of Vermont Rehabilitation Engineering Center, Burlington, VT)

Activities at this REC are directed at investigating the causes of and successful rehabilitation of persons with low back pain. Projects focus on all facets of low back pain, from assessment techniques and instrumentation to potential solutions, including orthotic systems, functional electrical stimulation, and tool and work site modifications. Video instructional tapes, training, and written materials provide access to research information. Projects have included lifting strength testing using an isokinetic strength testing machine, and a system for measuring three-dimensional trunk motion in the workplace.[21]

Quantification of Human Physical Performance

(REC: Harvard-MIT Rehabilitation Engineering Center, Cambridge, MA)

Research activities at this REC involve quantitative assessment of functional electrically stimulated grasp devices, posture and balance abnormalities, movement disorders, human motor system adaption, and the ability of upper extremity amputees to use hand tools. Assessment instrumentation will be developed and refined. Computer techniques will be utilized to help teach methods of analysis in objective ways. A data registry will be developed to help define a variety of diseases and their effect on function. A recent study has shown that forces on joints estimated from gait analysis studies underestimate the forces actually experienced. The researcher stated that "knowledge of joint forces is essential for safe specification of joint-replacement prostheses, for understanding joint deterioration in osteoarthritis, and for understanding the contribution of individual muscles to movement."[22]

Evaluation of Rehabilitation Technology

(REC: National Rehabilitation Hospital Rehabilitation Engineering Center, Washington, D.C.)

This REC's goal is to identify factors influencing selection and long-term use of products. Product comparative and performance testing will be conducted at the REC laboratory, and by a private testing firm. Product testing results will be available for dissemination in a series of published reports. The usefulness of this research will be realized by users and assistive technology providers in making informed decisions related to appropriate technology choices. Various models will be developed for product demonstration and in-service training, as well as multimedia modules and human factors design criteria.

Development and Evaluation of Sensory Aids for Blind and Deaf-Blind Individuals

(REC: The Smith-Kettlewell Eye Research Institute Rehabilitation Engineering Center, San Francisco, CA)

This REC develops sensory aids that either enhance the use of residual vision or substitute auditory and/or tactile information for missing visual input. Employment of blind individuals is being enhanced through the development of many job-related instruments with auditory and tactile output. Also, new developments by this REC are facilitating access to computers, communication devices, and educational devices for this population. The REC acts as a national information resource on sensory technology and produces the *Smith-Kettlewell Technical File*, which is a periodical for visually handicapped persons interested in current technology.

Innovative Models for Cost-Effective Rehabilitation Engineering

(RECs: The Center for Rehabilitation Technology Resources, Institute for Human Resource Development, Glastonbury, CT; and The Rehabilitation Engineering Center, South Carolina Vocational Rehabilitation Department, West Columbia, SC)

Rehabilitation technology service delivery models will be identified and evaluated by this REC. The resulting information will be available through publications, newsletters, statewide technology provider data bases, and continuing education and training programs. The REC will define information requirements of various user groups encompassing the areas of service, maintenance and repair resources, and available technological devices. The South Carolina Vocational Rehabilitation Department REC will provide training for rehabilitation personnel in the delivery of service and will disseminate information about the effectiveness of that technology. Areas of emphasis include driver training and vehicle modification, job site modification, custom seating, and orthotic and orthopaedic procedures.

Functional Electrical Stimulation for Restoration of Neural Control

(REC: Case Western Reserve Rehabilitation Engineering Center, Cleveland, OH)

This REC will provide research and development regarding clinical systems employing functional electrical stimulation (FES) technology, which provides control of the upper and lower extremities, stabilization of the trunk, and function of the respiratory and urinary systems. Projects include lower extremity FES and hybrid systems for standing and walking, upper extremity FES and hybrid systems for manipulation and grasp, FES/orthotic systems to provide trunk stabilization and to correct trunk deformities, control of spasticity in stroke and head injury, control of respiration in central respiratory insufficiency, and control of micturition in the neurogenic bladder. Information on FES will be provided through an information center in conjunction with the Services for Independent Living Program.

Rehabilitation Technology Transfer

(RECs: Electronic Industries Foundation (EIF) Rehabilitation Engineering Center, Washington, DC; and the Rancho Los Amigos Medical Center Rehabilitation Engineering Center, Downey, CA)

Research activities at EIF are intended to facilitate the transfer of modern technology to people with disabilities by addressing problem areas that may affect the intended market. These areas include needs assessment of persons with disabilities, alternative financing strategies, safety and liability issues, and models of universal accessibility designs. Information dissemination will include providing guidelines for design considerations and educational seminars held at industry and professional conferences.

The Rancho Los Amigos group is concerned with facilitation of commercial product development, training programs and materials on delivery of assistive technology, and measuring the effects of training methods, product information, and follow-up on user satisfaction. Results will be disseminated to providers, consumers, and third-party payors.

CONCLUDING REMARKS

Rehabilitation engineering and applications of assistive technology will continue to touch the lives of many in the future. The Americans with Disabilities Act (ADA, Public Law 101-336) prohibits discrimination against individuals with disabilities in four areas: employment (Title I), public services and transportation (Title II), public accommodations (Title III), and telecommunications (Title IV). The ADA and future legislation will have considerable impact on society to encourage successful integration of persons with disabilities. Rehabilitation engineers and assistive technology specialists will be an integral part of the team to assure these provisions are met. *In order to offer the most effective technology, those professionals in the various areas of research, service delivery, and manufacturing must continue to maintain open lines of communication with each other and the people who will ultimately use the technology.* Technological developments and human needs will continue to define and establish the evolution of rehabilitation engineering and assistive technology.

Acknowledgments. The author wishes to thank the following for their information and editorial contributions: Dudley Childress, Ph.D.; Glenn Hedman, B.S.B.E., M.E.M.E.; Alicia Hunt; Anna Kozole, B.S.N.; Simon Levine, Ph.D.; Jessica Presperin, O.T.R., M.B.A.; David Sulier, M.B.A.; Monica Sulier, M.S.R.D.; Gerald Warren, M.P.A.; and Jerry Weisman, M.S.M.E.

REFERENCES

1. Levine SP: Position on qualifications and credentialing of rehabilitation engineers. In Proceedings of the 13th Annual conference of the Rehabilitation Engineering Society of North America. RESNA Press, Washington, DC, 1990
2. Corthell DW, Thayer T: Rehabilitation technologies. p. 1. In Thirteenth Institute on Rehabilitation Issues. Publisher, Little Rock, AK, 1986
3. Enders A, Hall M: Assistive Technology Sourcebook, RESNA Press, Washington, DC, 1990
4. Rodgers MM, Hooker SP, Figoni SF et al: Training responses of SCI individuals to FNS-induced knee extension exercise. p. 365. In Proceedings of the 13th Annual Conference of the Rehabilitation Engineering Society of North America. RESNA Press, Washington, DC, 1990
5. Rehabilitation Engineering Society of North America Membership Brochure. RESNA Press, Washington, DC, 1990
6. Rehabilitation Engineering Society of North America, Board and Committe Handbook. p. B1.1. RESNA Press, Washington, DC, 1991
7. Warren GC: Quality assurance, the challenge. RESNA News 2(6):1, 1990
8. Hedman G: Rehabilitation Technology. Haworth Press Inc, Binghamton, NY, 1990
9. Enders A: Overview. p. 3. In Rehabilitation Technology Service Delivery, A Practical Guide. RESNA Press, Washington, DC, 1987
10. Bergen AF, Presperin J, Tallman T: Positioning for Function. Valhalla Rehabilitation Publications, Ltd, Valhalla, NY 1990
11. Burnett JK, Klabunde CR, Britell CW: Voice and head pointer operated electronics and computer assisted design workstations for individuals with severe upper extremity impairments. p. 48. In Proceedings of the 14th Annual Conference, of the Rehabilitation Engineering Society of North America. RESNA Press, Washington, DC, 1991
12. Mortola PJ, Kohn J, LeBlanc M: Implementation and follow-up of rehabilitation technology. p. 202. In Proceedings of the 12th Annual Conference of the Rehabilitation Engineering Society of North America. RESNA Press, Washington, DC, 1989
13. Smith RO: Models of service delivery in rehabilitation technology. p. 9. In Rehabilitation Technology Service Delivery, A Practical Guide. RESNA Press, Washington, DC, 1987
14. Willkomm TM: Mobile rural assistive technology unit p. 183. In Proceedings of the 14th Annual Conference of the Rehabilitation Engineering Society of North America. RESNA Press, Washington, DC, 1991
15. Whitmeyer JJ: Mobile delivery services—taking rehab on the road. Team Rehab Report, June, p. 52, 1990
16. Stumm GM, Demasco PW, McCoy KF: Automatic abbreviation generation. p. 97. In Proceedings of the 14th Annual Conference of the Rehabilitation Engineering Society of North America. RESNA Press, Washington, DC, 1991
17. Jones M, Demasco P, McCoy K et al: Knowledge representation considerations for a domain independent semantic parser. p. 109. In Proceedings of the 14th Annual Conference of the Rehabilitation Engineering Society of North America. RESNA Press, Washington, DC, 1991
18. Klien M, Malzahn D: The effects of physical ability on the working memory requirements of computer input devices. p. 115. In Proceedings of the 14th Annual Conference of the Rehabilitation Engineering Society of North America. RESNA Press, Washington, DC, 1991
19. Ford K: A user's perspective on blind access to graphical user interfaces. p. 330. In Proceedings of the 14 Annual Conference of the Rehabilitation Engineering Society of North America. RESNA Press, Washington, DC, 1991
20. University of Virginia: A prototype computerized seating system. Homecare Magazine, Autumn, p. 69, 1989
21. Weisman G, Baumhauer J, Pope M: Isokinetic strength testing: full body lifts vs segmented lifts. p. 119. In Proceedings of the 12th Annual Conference of the Rehabilitation Engineering Society of North America. RESNA Press, Washington, DC, 1989
22. Mann RW: Agonist-antagonist muscle co-contraction: ubiquitous but unappreciated. p. 57. In Proceedings of the 13th Annual Conference of the Rehabilitation Engineering Society of North America. RESNA Press, Washington, DC, 1990

Section II
REHABILITATION FACILITIES

17 The Rehabilitation Center

MICHAEL J. BOTTE

EARLY REHABILITATION CENTERS

The concepts of rehabilitation and rehabilitation centers arose formally after World War I from society's interest and compassion for severely injured veterans. Training schools, hospitals, and various institutes were founded for the sole purpose of maximizing functional deficits in chronic neuromusculoskeletal problems. The term *rehabilitation* first appeared in 1922 in a paper by E. M. Law, M.D., in which an account of the care of amputees after World War I appeared.[1]

Although the hospital and ward facilities after World War I seem to constitute some of the first formal "rehabilitation centers," the treatment of chronic neuromusculoskeletal diseases and the need for rehabilitation was appreciated long before, and the specialty of orthopaedic surgery had been providing this type of care for many years previously (see Chapter 11). Egyptian papyri dating from about 1600 B.C. are among the earliest written material on surgery of the musculoskeletal system,[2-4] including limb amputation. The discussions in the Hippocratic writings from Greece, dating from between 400 B.C. and A.D. 100 depicted a later but impressive understanding of extremity afflictions and the need for rehabilitation.[4-6] These writings discuss joint ankylosis, spinal deformities, clubfeet, congenital hip dislocation, and traumatic shoulder dislocation. The need for immobilization of open fractures and the benefits of joint mobilization to rehabilitate injured limbs were explained. Healers of that era appreciated that exercise strengthened extremities and inactivity resulted in muscle wasting.[4]

Use of baths and mineral springs as a means for rehabilitation became popular during the Hippocratic, Alexandrian, and Roman Empire periods, and in a sense these may have been among the earliest "rehabilitation" centers. Hydrotherapy, special exercises, massage, and sweat baths were important methods of medical treatment for chronic afflictions. Natural baths and mineral waters were believed to have special therapeutic powers. The temples of Aesculapius were built near healing springs, and the Romans were enthusiastic about the therapeutic qualities of the waters of Tivoli.[3]

In addition to hydrotherapy, heat therapy as a form of medical treatment has been employed in rehabilitation settings since ancient times. From the earliest methods using heated stones wrapped in blankets or jugs filled with hot water, to the more recent hot water bottles, hot towels, heating pads, and electrical devices, forms of thermotherapy have been used for comfort, decreasing pain, and promoting circulation.[3]

Further efforts were made in the treatment of chronic neuromusculoskeletal diseases by Galen (A.D. 131–201), who was one of the first notable clinical investigators.[4,5] He defined kyphosis, lordosis, and scoliosis and discussed amputations, resection of bone tumors, and drainage of abscesses.[4,5] Additional advances were made by Paul of Aegina (625–690), who described laminectomy, osteotomy of long bones for malunion, and management of patellar fractures. During the 12th and 13th centuries, simple but effective splints and braces were fabricated from wood, leather, and metal.[5]

Ambroise Paré (1510–1590), among the earliest "rehabilitation" physicians, provided detailed descriptions of spinal cord injury. He was cognizant of motor and sensory deficits and incontinence after spinal cord injury. He described an operative approach to the vertebral column for spinal cord decompression and provided a rationale for treatment of vertebral fractures.[4,6–8] Paré also addressed problems of limb amputation and produced a series of illustrations depicting mechanical prosthetic upper extremity devices made of metal.[4] Fabry, in the 17th century, discussed proximal amputation in the management of gangrene, described astragalectomy, introduced improved methods of treatment of clubfoot, and published the first pictorial description of scoliosis.

Sir Hugh Owen Thomas (1834–1891) and his nephew, Sir Robert Jones (1857–1933), developed newer methods for treating tuberculosis and fractures. Reginald Watson-Jones (1902–1972), another great contributor, advocated the involvement of allied health professionals in chronic care, which paved the way for the team approach and a more modern organization to rehabilitation.[6,7,9–12]

After World War I, rehabilitation hospitals and various training institutes were founded on a relatively modest scale. Programs were slow to develop despite legislation and efforts by volunteer organizations. The devastation of World War II and the numbers of injured veterans prompted governments, especially in the United States, to develop facilities and programs for rehabilitation of persons with amputations, paralysis, blindness, deafness, and "shell shock" disease. Howard Rusk, head of the American Air Force Convalescent Training Program, was a strong leader in organizing these programs and extended their scope beyond the restoration of disabled persons to reconditioning military personnel suffering from any illness or injury.

In the 1950s, the poliomyelitis epidemic resulted in the formation of large poliomyelitis wards, clinics, and rehabilitation units, thus expanding the concept of specialization in rehabilitation. Newer methods of surgical limb reconstruction were devised. The first cervical spine fusion and the halo skeletal fixator were developed as a result of the need for neck stabilization in the poliomyelitis patient with cervical muscle paralysis.[13]

Today, most major medical school and hospitals have a department or division devoted to rehabilitation. These departments are increasingly becoming organized into teams that concentrate on rehabilitation of specific physical afflictions or specific anatomic regions, such as amputation, spinal cord injury, stroke, traumatic brain injury, and hand rehabilitation. In addition to specialized teams of physicians and allied health professionals, entire hospital wards are becoming limited to certain areas (e.g., the traumatic brain injury ward) to meet the complicated needs of the different types of rehabilitation patients. Rehabilitation techniques also have been applied to disabilities occurring after ablative surgery, such as laryngectomy, colostomy, ileostomy, and breast excision, and rehabilitation now extends to systemic medical illnesses such as cardiac rehabilitation.

Self-help groups have sprung up through the efforts of disabled patients and have assisted in the restoration and adjustment of patients to a fuller, more satisfying life. These organizations, along with the efforts of the rehabilitation team members, have been helpful in altering the previously negative attitudes of the public to the rehabilitation patient. Over the last decade Americans in general have become more appreciative of the needs of the patient with disabilities and have taken steps to address them, including the increased use of wheelchair ramps, elevators, reserved parking spaces, preboarding of airplanes, and alterations of public rest rooms to accommodate wheelchairs.

MODERN REHABILITATION CENTERS

The rehabilitation center today is the main meeting and working place of the rehabilitation team, where the most comprehensive and intense rehabilitation efforts are carried out. The rehabilitation center usually is organized as a facility or wing within a hospital or stands as a separate building. Quite a variety of facilities exist, with some centers performing only outpatient services and others having inpatient beds, specialized wards, full laboratory services, operating and recovery rooms, and 24-hour staff coverage.

An example of a comprehensive rehabilitation medical center is the Rancho Los Amigos Medical Center in Downey, California. This facility is the rehabilitation center for Los Angeles County–University of Southern California (USC) Medical Center and is a separate, free-standing hospital whose grounds cover approximately 210 acres. It has 735 inpatient beds, seven operating rooms, many outpatient clinics, full blood, chemistry, and microbiology laboratory facilities, a comprehensive pathokinesiology evaluation and research laboratory, and a medical library. It is staffed by approximately 255 physicians and surgeons, 480 rehabilitation nurses, 84 physical therapists, 62 occupational therapists, 29 speech pathologists, 20 social workers, 9 orthotists, and 3 prosthetists. Approximately 4,269 inpatients and 83,381 outpatients are seen per year (based on 1990 statistics). This facility also conducts continuous research in multiple areas of rehabilitation and provides a setting for the teaching of physicians, surgeons, and allied health professionals.

Common to most rehabilitation centers or services are the medical-surgical services, occupational therapy services, physical therapy services, vocational rehabilitation services, social work services, speech and communication services, psychology services, patient evaluation area (clinics), and meeting area where the rehabilitation team can discuss strategy and formulate goals. Since a trend has emerged toward subspecialization, separate "teams" often are formed within the rehabilitation center to treat a particular type of patient or affliction. These include such subspecialties as stroke, traumatic brain injury, spinal cord injury, peripheral nerve injury, amputation, and pediatrics. Each team optimally has the full complement of team members from the various disciplines that make up the rehabilitation team, including the rehabilitation nurse, occupational therapist, physical therapist, speech therapist, social worker, vocational rehabilitation therapist, orthopaedic surgeon, internist, neurologist, physiatrist, psychologist, psychiatrist, orthotist, and prosthetist.

Because of the needs and benefits of subspecialization, entire rehabilitation centers themselves are now becoming subspecialized into spinal cord injury centers, traumatic brain injury and stroke centers, hand rehabilitation centers, sports medicine rehabilitation centers, pain management rehabilitation centers, back schools, and work hardening program centers (see following chapters). In the future, subspecialization will probably produce separate facilities for foot rehabilitation, arthritis and joint replacement rehabilitation, pediatric rehabilitation, and major fracture rehabilitation.

PROCESS OF PATIENT EVALUATION AND TREATMENT

Patients usually are evaluated first through referral to the outpatient clinic or as an inpatient for suitability for transfer to the rehabilitation center or ward. It is desirable that the decision to accept or reject a patient be made by a team and evaluation be done by multiple members of the rehabilitation team. The concept of triage is important, and only patients believed to be suitable candidates should undergo attempts at rehabilitation. The limited resources available for rehabilitation emphasize the need to select the appropriate candidates. Patients considered to be candidates for rehabilitation are admitted to the rehabilitation center for a specified number of weeks. Patients whose appropriateness for rehabilitation is in question may be admitted to the facility for a short trial (e.g., 2 weeks). If they prove to be reasonable candidates, a time extension is granted and rehabilitation continues; if not they are returned to the previous facility or to the home. Thus, goals and timing are addressed early. Time extensions are granted if a patient continues to benefit from a comprehensive rehabilitation program.

The incoming patient requires a thorough medical work-up prior to the initiation of therapy or rehabilitation efforts. Although serious medical problems such as pneumonia and cardiac failure are deterrents to acceptance to the center, patients with minor problems can be treated at the center. Patients admitted to the rehabilitation center tend to have numerous coexisting medical problems or complications, including decubitus ulcers, fracture malalignment, unhealed or unrecognized fractures, urinary tract infections, reflex sympathetic dystrophy, fixed contractures, anemia, and malnutrition. Obviously, attention must be paid to obtaining as much information as possible on the patient's past medical history, medications, and allergies.

Once a patient is selected for treatment at the rehabilitation center, the day is carefully divided up between therapy sessions, social activities (when appropriate), meals, rest, and medical management of concomitant problems. A master time schedule for each patient that is visible to the ward central desk makes locating the whereabouts of a patient a rapid process. Ample time for family visits, group therapy, and patient-team conferences should be provided. Surgery, as needed, is planned accordingly, and the team is informed so as to adjust daily activities and treatment plans to accommodate the surgery.

Plans and timing for discharge are decided on early, optimally at the time of admission, so that the team maintains its set goals, time is maximized, and there are no placement problems at the time a patient has finished inpatient rehabilitation. Outpatient rehabilitation is continued as necessary and patients are readmitted at a later date if their condition changes or if they require further inpatient care.

REFERENCES

1. Law EM: Problems in rehabilitation of victims of wars. J Fla Med Assoc, p 152, 1922
2. Breasted JH: The Edwin Smith papyrus. NY Hist Soc Q Bull 6:5, 1922
3. Castiglioni A: A History of Medicine. 2nd Ed. Alfred A Knopf, New York, 1958
4. Lyons AS, Petrucelli RJ (eds): Medicine: An Illustrated History. Abradale Press, Harry N Abrams, New York, 1987
5. Bick EM: Source Book of Orthopaedics. Hafner Publishing, New York, 1968
6. Evarts CM: Historical highlights of orthopaedics. p 1:3. In Surgery of the Musculoskeletal System. Churchill Livingstone, New York, 1983
7. Enneking W, Brower T, Ralston E, Hughston J: The history of orthopaedic surgery. p 1. In Manual of Orthopaedic Surgery. American Orthopaedic Association, Chicago, 1972
8. Packard RR: Ambroise Paré. Hoeber, New York, 1921
9. Peltier LF: Fractures: A History and Iconography of Their Treatment. Norman Publishing, San Francisco, 1990
10. Shands AR Jr: The Early Orthopaedic Surgeons of America. CV Mosby, St. Louis, 1970
11. Watson-Jones R: Dame Agnes Hunt. J Bone Joint Surg [Br] 30:709, 1948
12. Watson-Jones R: Death and growth of bones. J Bone Joint Surg [Br] 30:736, 1948
13. Perry J, Nickel VL: Total cervical spine fusion for neck paralysis. J Bone Joint Surg [Am] 41:37, 1959

18 The Injured Worker Program: Evaluation and Work Hardening

CINDY DOWDY
MARGARET CULLEN
SHELLI L. DELLINGER

. . . no country has been so work-oriented as the United States.

Walter S. Neff, *Work and Human Behavior*[1]

Work and the ability to work is an integral part of American society. Historically, the United States derived its passion for work from the masses of immigrants entering the country beginning in the 1840s, who sought to escape the political and economic inequities prevalent in Europe at the time. The structure of European society, with its sharp divisions between the aristocracy and the working class, afforded limited possibilities for the working class to advance economically or socially.

The chance to immigrate to America afforded European laborers the hope of elevating themselves to a status of wealth and social prestige that was virtually unattainable in European society. The poor immigrant was able to gain economic success in America through hard work. As wealth increased, social advancement followed. A cause-and-effect relationship developed between this newfound wealth and social status, prompting enrichment of self-esteem. American society began to emphasize work to gain social stature and economic security.

Today in the United States, Americans identify themselves through their occupation. This identity is threatened once a work injury is sustained. Physical, mental, social, and economic aspects of a worker's life are affected following an injury. The injured worker faces a complex rehabilitation process that involves dealing with the bureaucracy of the worker's compensation system, interaction with a fragmented medical delivery system, and disruption of personal life-style and daily rhythms.[2]

The injured worker program is a systematic approach of case management, evaluation, and treatment that prepares and directs the worker for successful work re-entry. This chapter defines an injured worker program and describes evaluation of an injured worker and the treatment process of work hardening. Additionally, this chapter addresses planning and implementing an outpatient program.

HISTORICAL PERSPECTIVES

The development of injured worker programs and occupational therapy are closely linked, dating back to the early 1900s. Occupational therapy emerged as a result of the need for patients to engage in purposeful activity (occupation) and develop proficiency in all aspects of daily living, including physical, psychological, social, and economic issues.[3] Historically, the occupational therapist's role has been to provide "opportunities to learn those skills needed for adaptation in educational, work, home and community environments."[3]

In the early 1920s there was an increase in the disabled population in America as a result of several factors: World War I, a severe polio epidemic in 1916, a rise in industrial accidents, and the expanded availability and use of the automobile.[4] With the advancement of both technology and medicine, those who once died in devastating accidents were now living with residual disabilities. Concurrently, Congress passed the Vocational Rehabilitation Act, which defined rehabilitation as "return to remunerative employment." The act granted "training in existing schools, industry and commercial establishments, or by a tutor."[5] As a result of this landmark legislation, the need for new therapeutic techniques in treatment and vocational retraining of the disabled populations arose.[6] This "treatment process involves the use of selected activities, assistive devices, and educational techniques to restore the client to the highest level of independent function."[3]

During the 1930s, curative workshops became popular; their purpose was to return the industrial worker to gainful employment by way of "work-related activity as the treatment."[7] Specifically, one program in Canada aimed its treatment at shortened rehabilitation time, with obvious cost containment. The program included occupational, physical, and recreation therapies. This was one of the first programs to use job simulation: "For example patients built brick walls, painted buildings, laid railroad ties and repaired plumbing."[7–9]

In the United States, Liberty Mutual Insurance Company, during the 1940s, became the first such company to establish rehabilitation workshops. Disabled workers were provided rehabilitation with the goal of swift return to their jobs.[10]

A resurgence of interest in the treatment of the injured worker emerged during the 1970s as a result of the rising costs of health care. In addition, objective data collection was needed because of the "discrepancy between the patient's report of symptoms and disability and his [physician's] objective evaluation data."[11]

With the acceleration of development in this field, the industrial rehabilitation process has grown to encompass a multidisciplinary approach. "At no other

time in the history of rehabilitation has such a multitude of professionals been so involved in the management of the injured worker."[2] As a result of this growth, the Commission on Accreditation of Rehabilitation Facilities (CARF) has established guidelines to assure the quality of services provided to the injured worker.[12]

DESCRIPTION OF AN INJURED WORKER PROGRAM

Injured worker programs provide outpatient services for those persons who have sustained work-related injuries and have completed acute medical and therapeutic treatment. The evaluation and treatment process uses work, real or simulated, as the focal point for service delivery.

The primary function of the program is to assess the patient's ability to return to work safely. If treatment is warranted, a 4- to 8-week therapy program is established and implemented based on the evaluation results. Finally, the program outcome directs the return to work recommendations. Case management and recommendations are generated by a multidisciplinary team that may include a physician, occupational therapist, physical therapist, psychologist, vocational counselor, rehabilitation nurse, and rehabilitation engineer. The on-site clinical staff are delineated by the structure of the organization and needs of the patient population. Providing assessment and treatment may involve the use of allied health professionals such as occupational therapists, physical therapists, certified occupational therapy assistants, physical therapy assistants, and trained aides. Contracts are frequently retained for the services of physicians, psychologists, vocational rehabilitation counselors, rehabilitation nurses, and rehabilitation engineers.

Injured worker programs are outpatient in nature and may be located in a free-standing clinic or within an institution. The ideal location for such programs is the ground floor of an industrial warehouse with an open space of several thousand square feet. The programs are supported by private or institutional funding.

ESTABLISHING AN INJURED WORKER PROGRAM

Developing a Task Force

Programs are often designed via committee or task force. Members of the task force include allied health professionals, vocational counselors, and psychologists. In addition, it is beneficial to have a physician involved in the early planning stages to provide a perspective regarding the medical needs of the patient population. The program supervisor or manager may be a physician, allied health professional, or vocational counselor and is accountable for all administrative areas.

Task Force Goals

After the task force has been created, weekly meetings are scheduled. The focus of the first meeting is to define the purpose of the program and to set long-term and short-term goals. Such goals should address the business plan, budget, clinic size, location and floor plan, staff education, form development, equipment purchase, marketing, and networking strategies. Some of these goals are discussed in more detail in this section.

Staff Education

The importance of staff education must be recognized for the program to develop successfully. It is recommended that each staff member attend different training seminars to give the program a well-rounded approach.

Defining the Target Population

Clients best suited for an injured worker program include any workers unable to return to their usual and customary occupation following a work-related injury. The diagnostic categories may include, but are not limited to, cumulative trauma injuries, severe burns, orthopaedic injuries, spine injuries, and neurologic impairment.

Selection of a Clinic

Factors to consider when choosing a clinic include location, space, design, and environment. The location of the clinic should be easily reached by public transportation. The building should be wheelchair accessible. Space and design should allow for storage and safe operation of multiple pieces of equipment. The design should also allow each patient the freedom to perform work tasks and allow for ongoing assessment of interpersonal skills by the evaluator. Environmental factors should be considered when simulating physical and psychosocial work demands. The environment should provide good lighting and ventilation and moderate temperature to promote the patient's optimal level of function (Fig. 18-1).

Form Development

The task force should develop or modify the various forms necessary for the efficient functioning of an injured worker program. These may include some or all of the following forms.

Referral Form. The referral form should be thoroughly filled out by the referral source. Forms that briefly describe the type of service offered are helpful to the referral source (Fig. 18-2).

Intake Form. The intake form is completed by the primary therapist during the patient interview (Fig. 18-3).

Daily Notes. Documentation should note the client's progress or change in status. Client behaviors (i.e., worker traits) are described, subjective symptoms are recorded, and future treatment plans are documented (Fig. 18-4).

Pain Questionnaire. Suggested pain questionnaires to be utilized include the Visual Analog Scale (VAS), the McGill Pain Questionnaire,[13] the Quantified Pain Drawing by Ransford (also known as the body chart),[13] and The Borg Pain Scale.[13]

Consent Form. The consent form should be read aloud with the client during the intake process. This contractual form involves a description of expected client participation and program parameters, including compliance with work precautions or restrictions. This form must be signed by the client prior to treatment.

Evaluation Form. The evaluation form will contain results specific to the client's level of function. It will include musculoskeletal evaluation, cardiovascular

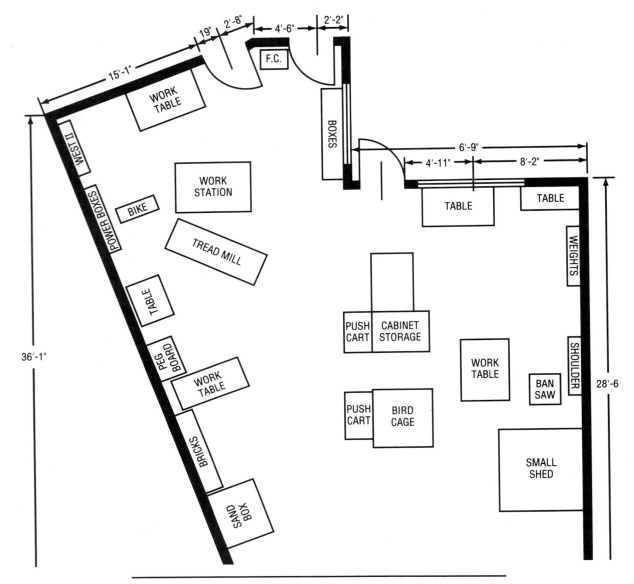

Fig. 18-1. Floor plan allowing for open design and multiple work tasks.

assessment, type and location of pain, isokinetic strength testing results, lifting tolerance, and results of standardized testing specific to job requirements. Evaluation is addressed in detail in the case study later in the chapter.

Patient Schedule Board. A large (usually 4 feet by 6 feet) erasable board is used by clients to structure their work activity program each day (Fig. 18-5).

Daily Work Schedule Form. Client activities are listed, specifying resistance, repetitions, and time required to complete each work task (Fig. 18-6).

Exercise and Home Program Forms. These forms include but are not limited to cardiovascular fitness, musculoskeletal strengthening, and range of motion exercise.

INJURED WORKER REFERRAL FORM

Name of Client:_____

Client Mailing Address:_____

_____

Telephone Number:_____ Date of Birth:_____

Social Security No.:_____

Diagnosis:_____

Date of Injury:_____

Precautions/Work Restrictions:_____

_____

_____

Referral Source:_____

Address:_____

Telephone Number:_____

Insurance Company:_____

Address:_____

Telephone Number:_____

Claims Adjuster:_____

_____

SERVICE REQUESTED

_____   **Work Tolerance Screening** (2-8 hour evaluation): This evaluation is a base line assessment of musculo-skeletal, strength, endurance, dexterity and functional capabilities.

_____   **Work Capacity Evaluation** (2-10 days): This evaluation measures potiential to sustain work over an extended period of time. ____Job Specific ____Non-Job Specific

_____   **Work Hardening** (2-8 weeks): A rehabilitation program consisting of job simulation in preparation for return to work.

_____   **Work Site Evaluation**

_____   **Tool Modification**

Please attach the **most recent** medical information. This material **must be received before** the evaluation can be conducted.

Physician Signature:_____ Date _____

Fig. 18-2. Referral Form. Typically used as physician prescription for evaluation and/or treatment.

```
                        INTAKE INTERVIEW FORM


Name:_____Referral Source:_____
Date of Injury:_____
Insurance Company:_____
Insurance Claim Number:_____

Personal Data
Age:_____ Height:_____ Weight Pre-Injury:_____ Current Weight:____
Hand Dominance:_____Glasses: Yes_____ No_____
Home Address:_____
Home Telephone Number:_____
Resides With:_____
Current Driver's License:Yes:_____ No:_____ License Number:_____

Occupational Information
Job Title:_____
Employer:_____
Employer Address:_____
Employer Telephone Number:_____
Years of Employment at Present Job:_____
Brief Description of Injury:_____
_____
_____
Previous Work Injuries:_____
Client's Return to Work Efforts:_____
_____

Medical Information
Diagnosis:_____
Past Surgeries:_____
_____
Physical Restrictions or Preclusions:_____
_____
Splints or Braces:_____
Past Therapy:_____
Current Medication:_____
Chief Complaint:_____
Pain Description and Location:_____
_____
Past Medical History:_____
_____
_____

Miscellaneous
Level of Education: _____
_____
Activity of Daily Living Status(list most difficult or unable
activities):_____
_____
_____
```

Fig. 18-3. Intake Form. Basic background information is collected during initial client contact.

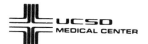

WORK EVALUATION PROGRESS RECORD

Source   Date

Patient Identification

DATE						
EVALUATION: WTS/WCE/OT/PT/DC						
FLEXIBILITY/STRETCHING:						
Upper Body						
Lower Body						
Spine						
Response						
Endurance						
CONDITIONING:						
STRENGTHENING:						
WORK SIMULATION:						
Task Time						
Response						
Endurance						
Task Time						
Response						
Endurance						
Task Time						
Response						
Endurance						
Task Time						
Response						
Endurance						
SPLINTING/POSITIONING						
BODY MECHANICS TRAINING						
JOINT PROTECTION						
ENERGY CONSERVATION						
PATIENT EDUCATION/TRAINING ATTENDANCE						
TREATMENT TIME						
INITIALS						

CODES

I = independent
S = supervised
CS = constant supervision
OS = occasional supervision

Evaluation
WTS = work tolerance screening
WCE = work capacity evaluation
OT = occupational therapy
PT = physical therapy
DC = discharge evaluation

Endurance
G = good
F = fair
P = poor

Response Codes
C = physical complaints
NC = no physical complaints
HP = high productivity
LP = low productivity

Treatment Time
HD = half day
FD = full day

Attendance Code
T = treatment given
C = treatment cancelled
F = failed

COMMENTS:

_____

_____

_____

_____

_____

_____

_____

_____

INITIALS	PRINT NAME	SIGNATURE	INITIALS	PRINT NAME	SIGNATURE

B334(1-90)6   WHITE - Medical Record   YELLOW - Work Evaluation Center Chart

Fig. 18-4. Daily Progress Record. Check list format used to document daily treatment.

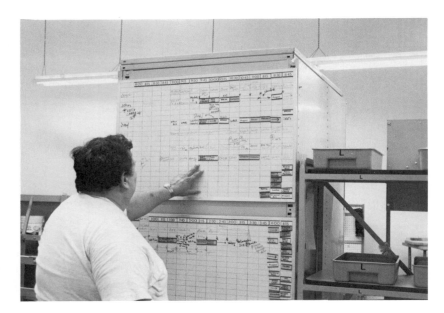

Fig. 18-5. Schedule Board. Lists specific work hardening activities in a chronological order.

After initial form creation, several weeks of trial usage should follow before permanent typesetting. Form development is a dynamic process, and forms must be continually updated to meet the changing needs of the clinic.

Equipment Purchase

An injured worker program requires equipment that can closely assess the client's physical capacity or level of function as well as progress the client through a graded level of job simulation tasks. Industrial rehabilitation equipment may be commercially purchased and/or constructed in the clinic. According to Niemeyer and Jacobs,[14] therapists may be pressured to purchase high-tech and high-cost equipment "by administrators or insurance companies because of the lure of scientific validation and quantification." However, they believe equipment "should be used to complement, not substitute for, professional skills. Treatment is a combination of art and science."[14]

Suggested equipment to be utilized for assessment and treatment in an injured worker program may include the following items.

Equipment Costing Less Than $500

Goniometer: a tool used to measure joint motion.
Jamar dynamometer: a tool used to measure the strength of grasp in pounds or kilograms.
Pinch gauge: a tool used to measure the strength of pinch in pounds.
Volumeter: evaluates any change in edema in an extremity from the fingertips to the elbow through water displacement.
Semmes-Weinstein Monofilament Test: objective sensory evaluation used to determine cutaneous sensibility, including that to light touch and deep pressure.
Purdue Pegboard Test: timed fine motor test that assesses unilateral and bilateral manipulation of small pins, collars, and washers.
Jebson Taylor Hand Function Test: uses functional tasks to evaluate prehension and manipulation skills; allows for comparison between nondominant and dominant hands.
Crawford Small Parts Dexterity Test: timed fine eye-hand coordination test used to evaluate manipulation of small objects with fingers and small tools (screwdriver and tweezers).
Minnesota Rate of Manipulation Test: timed test assessing unilateral and bilateral manipulation of small discs.
Pennsylvania Bimanual Test: combines gross movements, finger dexterity, and eye-hand coordination; requires bilateral hand use and evaluates ability to integrate a number of prehension patterns.

DAILY WORK SCHEDULE

Client Name _____

Date _____

Time	Min	Activity	Position	Comments	Modification

Fig. 18-6. Daily work schedule is completed by the client documenting specific tasks and subjective feedback.

Bennett Small Tools Test: timed gross motor assessment that evaluates bilateral use of tools with ordinary mechanic's tools.

O'Connor Test: timed test of dexterity focusing on precision and steadiness in the use of small tools.

The Dictionary of Occupational Titles (The DOT): outlines over 12,000 job profiles.[15]

Equipment Costing Greater Than $500

Computerized work simulator: simulates work tasks with isometric, isotonic, or isokinetic modes of exercise; allows for a variety of work positions; examples: B.T.E. and Loredan Work Set.

Computerized lifting assessment: assesses lifting capability with isometric, isotonic, or isokinetic resistance in various positions and heights; examples: Loredan Lift and B.T.E.

Computerized isokinetic extremity assessment: used for assessment and treatment of extremity strength with isometric, isotonic, or isokinetic resistance; example: Loredan Lido Extremity (Fig. 18-7).

Computerized back assessment: used for assessment and treatment of the back with isometric, isotonic, or isokinetic resistance; examples: Cybex T.E.F. unit, Isotechnologies B-200 (Fig. 18-8).

Valpar Component Work Sample 1: Small Tools (Mechanical): measures ability to work with assorted small mechanical tools; test demands work in small, confined spaces using both hands and tools; work is often performed with visual obstruction.

Valpar Component Work Sample 4: Upper Extremity Range of Motion: measures the upper extremity range of motion, which requires manipulation of nuts and bolts.

Valpar Component Work Sample 5: Clerical Comprehension and Aptitude: measures ability to perform and comprehend a variety of clerical tasks, including telephone answering, mail sorting, filing, bookkeeping, and typing.

Valpar Component Work Sample 8: Simulated Assembly: measures a prolonged assembly line activity; equipment consists of an adjustable-speed rotary wheel, pegs, and two sizes of discs.

Valpar Component Work Sample 9: Whole Body Range of Motion: measures the agility of a person's gross body

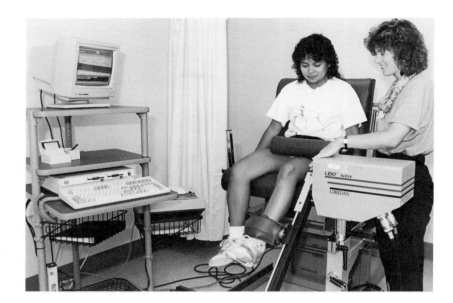

Fig. 18-7. Lido Extremity Equipment used for isokinetic assessment and strengthening of upper and lower extremities.

movements; assesses overhead and shoulder reaching, bending, stooping, and squatting while performing prehension activities (Fig. 18-9).

Valpar Component Work Sample 19: Physical Capacities and Work Tolerance: measures lifting and carry tolerances as defined by the DOT (Fig. 18-10).

Vocational Interest, Temperament and Aptitude System (VITAS): standardized work samples that assess performance time and quality of a variety of job-specific skills.

WEST (Work Evaluation Systems Technology) 1, 2, 4, and 7: multistation system that addresses lifting capacity, upper extremity strength, torque, bilateral upper extremity dexterity, and assembly.

Force gauge: measures resistance in pounds of force exerted during various work tasks.

Weights and weight training system: used for extremity strengthening (Fig. 18-11).

Vocational tests: measure general interests, aptitude, and academic ability; examples: Microcomputer Evaluation and Screening Assessment.

Miscellaneous Treatment Equipment

crates
stationary bicycle
upper body exerciser
stair and/or ladder climbing simulator
treadmill
trampoline
shovel and sand bin

mechanical tools and work bench
sled and hand truck (Fig. 18-12).
power tools (i.e., woodworking)
calculator
blood pressure cuff and stethoscope
desk clerical station
pipe tree
rolling carts
concrete bricks
bird cage (Fig. 18-13).

REFERRAL SOURCES

Referral occurs because a multitude of issues arise regarding the worker's return-to-work status. Patient referral to an injured worker program is generated by one or more of the following sources: (1) a physician, (2) a worker's compensation insurance claims adjuster, (3) a vocational rehabilitation counselor, (4) an allied health professional, (5) a rehabilitation nurse, and (6) an attorney. The question most often asked by a referral source is "Can the injured worker return to work?"

Each referral source has a different motivation for referring the injured worker to a program, based on that professional's relationship with the patient. For

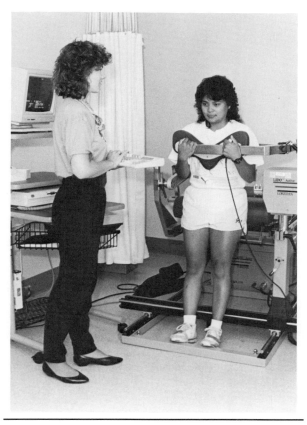

Fig. 18-8. Lido Extremity Equipment developed for interchangeable spine evaluation and treatment.

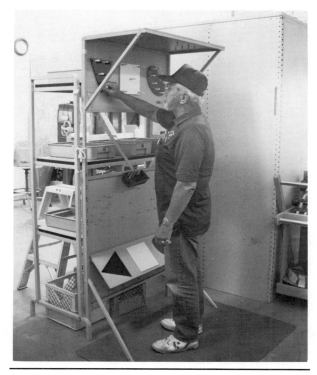

Fig. 18-9. Valpar Component Work Sample 9 allows for assessment of whole body movement.

example, Matheson and Niemeyer suggested that physicians who are seeking "objective findings greatly prefer to have a short trial of work hardening available before they set the work restrictions or before they clear the injured worker to return to work."[16] The worker's compensation insurance carrier is seeking objective behavioral and physical data to substantiate treatment of the work injury.[11] Vocational rehabilitation counselors use the information generated by the injured worker program to assess employment options and to guide the patient through the rehabilitation process. Allied health professionals facilitate referrals through a physician following acute-care treatment of the worker. Rehabilitation nurses request services in fulfilling their role as case managers for complex claims. An attorney will request referral for plaintiff or defendant cases to establish facts pertinent to case settlement.

EVALUATION AND TREATMENT TERMINOLOGY

Within the industrial rehabilitation field there is a lack of universal terminology regarding evaluation and treatment. Instead, each facility chooses the terms specific to their training. To provide clarity, the various terms and sources used most often in clinical treatment are defined and discussed in this section.

Baseline Evaluation

The baseline evaluation is a 2- to 8-hour assessment that provides an overview of the patient's current physical and functional capabilities. It provides objective data from which goals and a treatment plan may be established. This type of evaluation is also known as *work tolerance screening* ("intensive short term (usually 1 day) evaluation that focuses on major physical tolerance abilities related to musculoskeletal strength, endurance, speed, and flexibility"),[16] and the *functional capacity evaluation process* ("consists of evaluation procedure, questionnaires and observa-

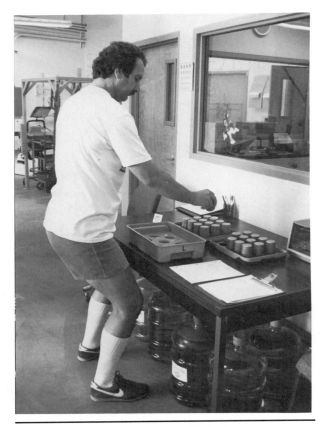

Fig. 18-10. Valpar Component Work Sample 19 assess maximum safe lifting tolerances.

tion which documents the patient's ability to perform work from a physical, behavioral, and ergonomic perspective").[11]

Physical Endurance Capability Assessment

The physical endurance capacity assessment measures a patient's potential to dependably sustain work. It is a 2- to 10-day assessment that can determine a patient's potential for competitive employment as well as provide recommendations for further services. Such assessment is also known as *work capacity evaluation* ("systematic process of measuring and developing an individual's capacity to dependably sustain performance in response to broadly defined work demands"),[16] and *work tolerance assessment* ("is designed specifically for one client and one job and gives very specific answers to specific questions . . . it is an evaluation of a worker struc-

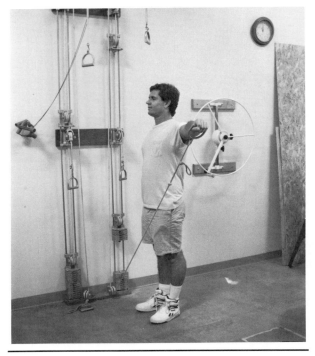

Fig. 18-11. A variety of weight training equipment may be used for strengthening and endurance training.

tured toward a particular job description. It requires knowledge of the job and simulation of specific work activities").[17]

Work Conditioning

Work conditioning prepares the patient to return to competitive employment. It is a structured program lasting 2 to 8 weeks and utilizing real and simulated work activities specifically designed for each client. This is accomplished through duplication of the client's typical work schedule. The program's design is to gradually improve cardiovascular, musculoskeletal, biomechanical, and psychosocial functioning.

Another term for work conditioning is *work hardening.* Isernhagen defined work hardening as "a work oriented treatment program that has outcome which is measured in terms of improvement of the client's productivity. This is achieved through increased work tolerances, improved work rate, mastery of pain (through the effective use of symptom control techniques), increased confidence and proficiency,

Fig. 18-12. Sled and hand truck: Push/pull equipment used for work simulation.

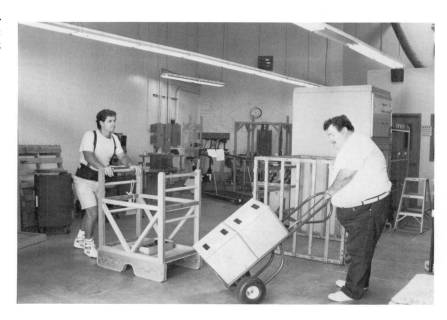

with work adaptations or assistive devices. Work hardening involves the client in highly structured, simulated work tasks, and an environment where expectations for basic worker behaviors (e.g., timeliness, attendance, and dress) are in keeping with work place standards."[2] Other terms for such programs include *work readiness, work reconditioning,* and *work capabilities.*

Job Site Evaluation

Job site evaluation has a twofold purpose: gathering of information for work simulation in the clinic setting and assessment of risk factors present in the client's job. Chronologic on-site assessment of the daily, weekly, and monthly physical parameters and tasks specific to the performance of the job are noted. An actual site visit will encompass measuring, weighing, and calculating force and repetition of critical work demands to provide data that will be used for clinical simulation. As outlined in *Cumulative Trauma Disorders: A Manual for Musculoskeletal Diseases of the Upper Limbs,*[18] "checklists may be used to itemize undesirable worksite conditions or worker activities that contribute to injuries." The checklist used should encompass (1) physical stress, (2) force, (3) posture, (4) workstation equipment, (5) repetiveness, and (6) tool design.[18] After the completion of a job site evaluation, outcome recommendations

that encompass task or workstation redesign, reduction of load, force, and/or repetition, tool modification, and body positioning are determined. Job site evaluation is also known as *work site analysis, work site consultation, work site evaluation,* and *ergonomic assessment.*

Job Analysis

Job analysis is a systematic categorization of job tasks. It is a descriptive process involving documentation of what the worker does, how the work is done, results of the work, and the skills, knowledge, and abilities needed to accomplish the tasks.[19] This information is gathered through interview, questionnaire, work diaries, and observation.[19] Typically a job analysis is provided by a vocational rehabilitation counselor as a basic categorization and description of job duties.

CASE STUDY: THE MECHANICS OF AN INJURED WORKER PROGRAM

In this section, the components of an injured worker program are illustrated with the case of client Y.P. A case study format is utilized to provide specific clinical examples inclusive of evaluation, treatment planning, documentation, and recommendation. This case study chronologically describes the transformation of an acute medical patient to a productive worker.

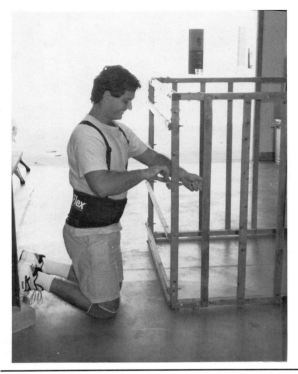

Fig. 18-13. Birdcage: Work simulation task to develop endurance for varied work.

The initial process involves the transition of the "patient" to a "client." The term *patient* is indicative of illness and disability. A patient who progresses to a postacute level of function after injury "graduates" from "patient" to "client" status, a change that signifies the transformation from a "sick individual" to a "injured worker." The injured worker program provides a transition between acute care and return to work while addressing the issues of work productivity, worker characteristics, physical tolerances, and proper body mechanics.

Work Tolerance Screening

Y.P. is a 35-year-old, right hand–dominant female employed as a food service worker at an institutional cafeteria. She sustained a right arm strain/lateral epicondylitis when placing a large tray on a rack at an overhead height. Y.P. was referred by an orthopaedic physician for a 1-day baseline assessment known as a Work Tolerance Screening (WTS), to be followed by a job-specific work hardening program, if indicated.

Y.P. had been out of work for a total of $4\frac{1}{2}$ months. She completed her acute medical treatment, and surgery was not performed. During that time, Y.P. had received physical therapy for 6 weeks, consisting of ultrasound and range of motion exercises, and was seen by an occupational therapist for splinting and stretching exercises for the right upper extremity. Y.P. had been partially compliant with her home exercise program; however, she indicated a fear of "overdoing" and limited herself to light activities of daily living (ADLs). She indicated other family members were now performing the heavier work tasks at home, such as laundry, yard work, and minor household repairs.

Intake Interview

The WTS commenced with an intake interview involving information collection from the client. Prior to the evaluation, pertinent medical records corresponding to the work-related injury and past medical history were acquired. Additionally, Y.P.'s usual and customary job of food service worker was described via telephone interview with her supervisor and a written job description was provided by her employer. All information was reviewed and discussed during the intake interview process. Notation was made concerning sitting tolerance, dress, grooming, and general demeanor.

Musculoskeletal Assessment

Following the intake interview, a musculoskeletal examination was performed and the following information was noted.

1. *Appearance of injured area:* client had no visible scars; no swelling over the lateral epicondyle was observed.
2. *Edema:* volumetric and circumferential measures of the injured and noninjured extremities were recorded, and both morning and afternoon measurements were taken to assess any soft tissue changes resulting from the evaluation process; no significant differences were noted.
3. *Sensation assessment:* Semmes-Weinstein Monofilament testing was performed on both upper extremities; all findings were within normal limits.
4. *Active range of motion specific to injury:* client's right wrist motion was noted to be limited in extension only.
5. *Manual muscle test:* Weakness of the right wrist extensor muscles were noted.
6. *Grip and pinch strength:* right hand grip and pinch were

moderately impaired; the client scored within the 25th percentile for her age and sex.

7. *Whole body flexibility:* right elbow extension flexibility was limited because of a subjective pain complaint.

Standardized Testing of Physical Capacities

Standardized tests were used to assess the client's physical capacities in order to obtain normative data for comparative scoring (50th percentile scoring is considered average performance). Documentation concerning physical complaints or observation were recorded during all such testing.

The Purdue Pegboard was used to evaluate fine motor manipulation.[20] Right and left hand speed and accuracy data were recorded. Y.P. scored in the 10th percentile with the right hand and the 50th percentile with the left hand. To make the evaluation procedure job specific, an additional standardized fine motor manipulation test was performed. The Crawford Small Parts Dexterity Test Parts I and II was administered. Testing results placed Y.P. in the 30th percentile in both Part I and Part II. She offered a complaint of right wrist pain during this test.

Standardized gross motor assessment was performed with the Valpar Component Work Sample 4: Upper Extremity Range of Motion. Valpar normative data are based on methods, time, measurement (MTM) standards for both time and errors. The MTM process analyzes a manual operation in terms of basic movements that are required to perform the task. An MTM score of 100 is considered entry-level performance.[21] Y.P. scored at 80 MTM percent.

Finally, standardized testing was performed to evaluate Y.P.'s lifting tolerances. The lifting requirements, as described by her employer in the written job description, were frequent lifting and carrying of items up to 10 pounds and occasional lifting and carrying of items up to 20 pounds. This placed Y.P. job in the light work category, as described by the DOT. To return to work, it was necessary for her to attain lifting tolerances at a light work, entry-level production speed.

The Valpar Component Work Sample 19: Physical Capacity and Work Tolerance was used to assess Y.P.'s lifting capabilities for strength and endurance.

In part I, she was able to perform strength lifting at 75 MTM percent in the light work category. Light work is described in the DOT as lifting 20 pounds maximum with frequent lifting and/or carrying of objects weighing up to 10 pounds. Notations were made regarding verbal and nonverbal (e.g., facial grimacing) responses, body positioning, lift and carry style (body mechanics), and changes in position during testing.

Part II of the lifting assessment involved endurance lifting. Y.P. was tested at her safest, most symptom-free tolerance with repetitive material handling. She was able to tolerate continuous lifting at 70 MTM percent in the sedentary work category. The DOT describes sedentary work as lifting 10 pounds maximum and occasionally lifting and/or carrying objects weighing 10 pounds or less.

It should be emphasized that Y.P. was asked after each portion of the lifting assessment if she could continue testing. Furthermore, she was asked to report physical symptoms after the testing was completed. She reported right elbow and wrist pain following endurance testing.

Job Simulation

Finally, job simulation was performed based upon the written job description and Y.P.'s subjective description of her working environment. This assessment consisted of the most critical physical demands of her job as food service worker. Simulation was performed to her tolerance. Y.P. identified tray loading and dish scraping as the two most demanding tasks; replication was performed in the clinic setting.

Task I

Y.P. was required to load full trays of food and dishes onto a cart at a range of 12 to 55 inches from the floor for 30 minutes. Trays ranging from 3.5 to 10 pounds were to be lifted repetitively for 30 minutes. She performed repetitive tray loading for 12 minutes and 43 seconds before stopping because of reported right forearm pain and weakness. Y.P. was observed to have less bilateral upper extremity control when handling trays at the 45- to 55-inch heights. She was also noted to rub her right forearm and lateral epicondyle with her left hand intermittently during the last 2 minutes of her task simulation.

Task II

Dish scraping was required on a daily basis for 45 minutes. The task required tray disassembly and dish cleaning with a gloved hand. The working range was between Y.P.'s waist (approximately 30 inches from the floor) and her shoulder (approximately 50 inches from the floor). Repetitive shoulder and elbow flexion and extension were required throughout this task. Weights handled varied from 1 ounce to 1 pound. Y.P. was able to perform this task repetitively for 20 minutes and 10 seconds before reaching her tolerance. She cited increased right forearm pain and right are fatigue as the primary factors for ending the task. She was observed intermittently rubbing her right forearm after 5 minutes and using her left arm when reaching from chest to shoulder level.

Summary

Y.P. completed testing after 6.5 hours and was found to display the following deficits:

1. Limited active range of motion, right wrist/elbow
2. Diminished right wrist and hand strength
3. Diminished lifting capacity (as required for entry level of usual and customary job)
4. Poor endurance with repetitive right upper extremity use
5. Limited application of independent symptom control methods

Y.P. indicated motivation and desire to return to her usual and customary position as a food service worker. Furthermore, she described her frustration with her inability to control her right arm pain and weakness.

A 6-week, job-specific work hardening program was recommended to address Y.P.'s deficits and ascertain if she was capable of returning to her previous employment. A physician prescription and insurance authorization was obtained prior to the commencement of her program.

Work Hardening Program

Once the evaluation process has been completed and the specific client deficits and goals are identified, an individualized job-specific program should commence as soon as administrative arrangements can be made. The commencement of a work hardening program should be initiated without delay to prevent further decondition of the client.

Y.P. had become accustomed to sleeping late in the morning and having little or no time constraints on her daily schedule. She indicated that returning to a structured work schedule would be challenging. Work hardening offers a structured program 5 days a week that provides the psychosocial framework to begin the return-to-work process.

Week 1

Typically, clients who have remained out of work for greater than 3 months begin work hardening on a half-time basis and advance as tolerated. Y.P.'s schedule began on a half-day basis for the first week, from 8:30 A.M. to 12:00 P.M. She was given a daily 15-minute break at 10:15 A.M. to 10:30 A.M. Y.P.'s attendance was recorded through the use of a time card. Her unscheduled breaks resulting from increased symptoms were noted on her daily work schedule.

The initial schedule developed for Y.P. contained the following activities:

8:30 A.M.: check in
8:35 A.M.: circumferential and volumetric measurement, both upper extremities
8:40 A.M.: aerobic conditioning: treadmill for 20 minutes
9:00 A.M.: flexibility exercise, emphasis on right forearm and wrist (Fig. 18-14)
9:30 A.M.: isotonic and isokinetic strengthening
10:15 A.M.: break
10:30 A.M.: work simulation: (1) tray loading, (2) dish scraping, (3) dishwasher unloading, (4) condiments dispenser, and (5) tray carrying
11:55 A.M.: reassess circumferential and volumetric-measurements, both upper extremities
12:00 P.M.: check out

Y.P. was allowed to perform each task to her maximum symptom-free tolerance. She was asked to change to a different task with the onset of any right arm symptoms (i.e., fatigue, weakness, pain), and to record her performance time for each task. Individual instruction was provided regarding proper handling techniques, alternation of hand use, neutral upper extremity and spine positioning, body mechanics, and pacing techniques.

Fig. 18-14. Stretching: Daily flexibility exercises to prepare muscles for daily work tasks.

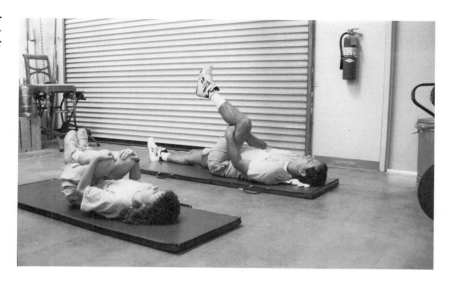

Counterforce bracing was initiated at this time. Over the course of treatment, a variety of tennis elbow braces were assessed for comfort, fit, and effectiveness.

Weeks 2 and 3

During the second and third weeks, Y.P.'s program was increased to 5 hours daily Monday through Friday. She continued aerobic conditioning with a 30 to 45-minute treadmill program, 45-minute stretching program, and 1-hour strengthening program, with emphasis on improving muscular endurance. Control of symptoms was accomplished through icing and stretching of her right dorsal forearm. Stretching was performed intermittently throughout work simulation and icing was accomplished during lunch and scheduled breaks. Independence with alternation of right and left hand use became inherent during work simulation and functional activities. However, Y.P. continued to require individual instruction with neutral forearm and wrist positioning, intermittent stretching, and body mechanics during lift-and-carry simulation.

Weeks 4 and 5

During weeks 4 and 5, full-time work hours (8:30 A.M. to 4:00 P.M. daily) began. Y.P. now required icing only during her morning and afternoon breaks. She was advised to rest her right upper extremity during lunch. Y.P. was able to walk on the treadmill for 45 minutes (Fig. 18-15). Stretching time was increased to 1 hour daily. The strengthening program was now modified to improve both muscular endurance and strength. A full afternoon of work simulation was tolerated by Y.P. She progressed to a maximum lift and carry at 20 pounds, but continued to require cuing for neutral positioning of her upper extremities. Y.P. had mastered upper extremity material handling, alternation of right and left hand use, and intermittent upper extremity stretching regarding symptom control. She was able to continue to alternate her critical work tasks as needed, and her recorded tolerances were nearing her work requirements.

Y.P.'s upgraded daily schedule was as follows:

8:30 A.M.: check in

8:35 A.M.: circumferential and volumetric measurement, both upper extremities

8:40 A.M.: aerobic conditioning: treadmill for 45 minutes

9:25 A.M.: flexibility exercises, emphasis on right forearm and wrist

10:25 A.M.: break: ice right forearm

10:40 A.M.: isotonic and isokinetic strengthening

12:00 P.M.: lunch: rest right forearm

12:30 P.M.: work simulation: (1) tray loading, (2) dish scraping, (3) dishwasher unloading, (4) condiments dispenser, and (5) tray carrying (alternate activity as needed; 30-second intermittent stretches as needed)

2:45 P.M.: break: ice right forearm

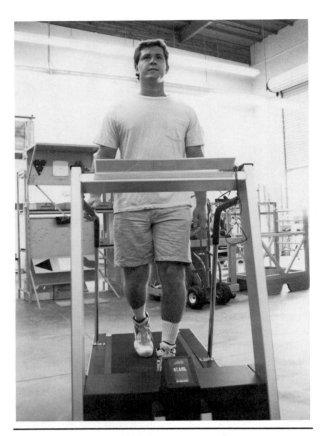

Fig. 18-15. Treadmill: Daily aerobic conditioning program that develops physical endurance.

3:00 P.M.: continue work simulation as above
3:50 P.M.: reassess circumferential and volumetric measurements, both upper extremities
4:00 P.M.: check out

Week 6

After 5 weeks of graded activity, Y.P. was prepared for a trial of full-time work simulation. Using the employer's job description as a guide, the actual time required to complete each task was established for a full-time work simulation trial.

At the start of the sixth week, instructions in positioning, handling techniques, use of a tennis elbow brace, icing, and lift-and-carry instruction were reviewed. Y.P. had mastered many prevention techniques since beginning her program and was independent in her application of symptom control techniques.

During day 2, Y.P. reported a dull ache in her dorsal right wrist and forearm after completing tray loading for 30 minutes. Task analysis noted symptoms with tray loading above shoulder level. To alleviate this problem, Y.P. stood on a footstool to load the trays; decreased symptoms were reported shortly thereafter. The footstool eliminated overreaching; however, to safely load the trays, work time was increased by 15 minutes. The increased time and the use of the footstool altered the usual and customary job requirements. (Any change in the worker's usual and customary job creates a need for job modification. Modification must be prescribed by the referring physician and addressed with the employer prior to return to work.)

Y.P. was able to successfully complete her trial work and perform within the production times required in her job description with the use of the elevated platform as the only physical modification. She was able to control her pain symptoms by means of several techniques:

> The use of ice during her regularly scheduled breaks
> Rest of her right arm during lunch
> Intermittent stretching of her right forearm and wrist
> The use of her right tennis elbow brace (as a final measure)
> The use of an elevated platform to reduce end-range reaching at chest and shoulder levels.

The physician received the final Work Hardening Report and immediately released Y.P. to full-time work as indicated above.

Y.P.'s successful return to work was achieved by: (1) her motivation, (2) the employer's willingness to modify the work environment, and (3) the physician's adoption of program recommendations and expedient release to work.

CONCLUSION

The potential loss of a job through a work-related injury represents more than lost wages. The individual's identity, which is directly linked to the occupation, is threatened. The expedient progression from injured worker to gainfully employed worker reduces the loss of self-esteem and economic hardship.

Injured worker programs are a cost-effective method that rapidly evaluates the client's ability to return to the usual and customary job. It affords the client an arena to prepare for return to work in a safe environment with the guidance of a professional staff of health care providers.

REFERENCES

1. Neff W: Work and Human Behavior. Aldine Publishing Company, New York, 1985
2. Isernhagen S (Ed): Work Injury Management and Prevention. Aspen Publishers, Inc, Rockville, MD, 1988
3. Ad Hoc Committee of the Commission of Practice: The role of occupational therapy in the vocational rehabilitation process: Official position paper. Am J Occup Ther 34:881, 1980
4. Woodside HH: Occupational therapy—a historical perspective: The development of occupational therapy—1910–1929. Am J Occup Ther 25:226, 1971
5. Cromwell FS: Vocational readiness programming in occupational therapy: Its roots, course, and progress. In Competency-Based Curriculum in Vocational Readiness. American Occupational Therapy Association, Baltimore, 1984
6. West WL: The role of occupational therapy in work adjustment: Work adjustment as a function of occupational therapy. p. 1. In Proceedings of the Third International Congress of the World Federation of Occupational Therapists. Vol 5. Wm. C. Brown, Dubuque, IA, 1964
7. Jacobs K: Occupational Therapy: Work Related Programs and Assessments. Little, Brown and Company, Boston, 1985
8. Smith HV: Workmen's Compensation Board, occupational therapy workshop. Can J Occup Ther 7:26, 1940
9. Lomey MB: Rehabilitation under the Workman's Compensation Act. Can J Occup Ther 8:25, 1941
10. Cromwell FS: The world of industry: Arena for OT skills. Presented at the National Occupational Therapy Association Conference, Philadelphia, May 1982
11. Blankenship K: Industrial Rehabilitation. A Seminar Syllabus. American Therapeutics, Inc, 1990
12. National Advisory Committee of Work Hardening Program Standards: CARF National Advisory Committee meets to review work hardening program standards. Indust Rehabil Q 4:1, 1991
13. Reading AE: The McGill Pain Questionnaire: An Appraisal. Raven Press, New York, 1983
14. Niemeyer L, Jacobs K: Industrial rehab: Fast growing specialty. O. T. Week 4(34):4, 1990
15. U.S. Department of Labor: Dictionary of Occupational Titles, 4th Ed. U.S. Government Printing Office, Washington, DC, 1977
16. Matheson LN, Niemeyer LO: Industrial Rehabilitation Resource Book 1989. Publication Division of Roy Matheson and Assoc, Inc, CA 1989
17. Isernhagen S: Isolated testing, functional capacity evaluation and work tolerance assessment differences, similarities, and purposes. Indust Rehabil Q 4(2);7, 1991
18. Putz-Anderson V (Ed): Cumulative Trauma Disorders: A Manual for Musculoskeletal Diseases of the Upper Limbs. Taylor and Francis Inc, Cincinnati, 1990
19. Materials Development Center, Stout Vocational Rehabilitation Institute, University of Wisconsin–Stout: A Guide To Job Analysis: A "How To" Publication for Occupational Analysis. Division of Occupational Analysis, United States Employment Training Administration, U.S. Department of Labor, Washington, DC, 1982
20. Tiffin J: Purdue Pegboard Examiner Manual. Science Research Assoc Inc, Chicago, 1968
21. Valpar International Corporation: Manual of Valpar Component Work Samples, 1, 4, 5, 8, 9, and 19. Valpar International Corporation, AZ, 1986

19 The Hand Rehabilitation Center

MARY PATRICIA DIMICK

Hand rehabilitation centers are designed and structured to meet the challenge of providing complete treatment for the intricate, fragile, and essential human hand. They provide comprehensive services so that patients with hand or upper extremity trauma and disease may achieve a maximum level of function in a minimum amount of time. Services are designed to help the patient regain lost function, mobility, confidence, and independence. In a hand rehabilitation center, all components of upper extremity rehabilitation are offered, from providing acute care to preparing patients to return to work and their individual life-styles. Hand therapy involves the entire upper extremity and the entire person. Therapy is determined by the specific injury, the individual patient, and the demands the patient makes on the hand. The underlying philosophy of hand rehabilitation centers is that the patient must be actively involved for rehabilitation to be successful.

Injuries and diseases affecting the hand and upper limb cause very complex problems. The hand consists of 27 bones with supporting ligaments, tendons, muscles, nerves, and blood vessels. The hand's multiple joints are susceptible to a variety of abuses, which result in lost mobility and therefore lost function. The hand is also subject to dysfunction as a result of indirect upper body or neurologic injuries and to a variety of diseases. In addition to its numerous specific functions, the hand is responsible for dexterity, precision, sensitivity, and expressiveness. Therapy must aim for recovery of all elements of functional utility—sensitivity, mobility, flexibility, coordination, muscular strength, and endurance.

FEATURES AND BENEFITS

The hand rehabilitation center offers a unique blend of features and benefits that distinguishes it from traditional occupational therapy and physical therapy programs. This is possible because of the advantages that specialization affords to centers of this nature. Staff, space, equipment, operations, and policies are focused and designed for only one patient population and therefore the depth of services provided to this group can be greater. Protocols, treatment techniques, educational aids, and home programs can be standardized and used efficiently. The volume and similarity of conditions treated at a hand rehabilitation center lead to a refinement of hand therapy skills by the staff. In turn, the staff's experience and expertise in treating hand injuries frequently leads to the development of new and better treatment techniques. Patients treated at hand rehabilitation centers are often the first to benefit from state-of-the-art treatment and equipment.

Another advantage of a hand rehabilitation center is its ability to provide continuity of care from the time of initial injury or surgery until discharge. Individualized treatment plans are designed through the combined efforts of the referring physician, therapist, patient, and rehabilitation nurse or counselor. All aspects of care are attended to in one setting, and when changes are needed the entire team participates in making them. Communication among the team members and early therapy, skilled medical management, and patient participation are the critical elements that lead to greater vocational success and to higher levels of functional recovery than seen with the patients discharged from traditional settings.[1]

Perhaps the greatest benefit of the hand rehabilitation center is the opportunity for patients to see other persons with similar conditions. The hand rehabilitation center provides a professional, psychological, and social milieu that encourages healing. During therapy sessions patients have the opportunity to interact with other patients and staff members in an informal way, which facilitates support, encouragement, and psychological adjustment to the injury or disease.

A final benefit of hand rehabilitation centers is the role they play in advancing state-of-the-art hand therapy. Hand therapists are frequently involved in teaching and research. The hand rehabilitation center provides an ideal setting for clinical research and advanced training fellowships for therapists interested in becoming specialists in hand therapy. In addition, hand rehabilitation centers often provide consultation to patients, community groups, other professionals, and employers.

HAND THERAPY

Hand therapy has developed as a specialty of occupational therapy and physical therapy in response to advances in surgical techniques that permit greater functional restoration of injured and diseased upper extremities. The foundation of hand therapy treatment is derived from the traditional skills and knowledge of both occupational therapy and physical therapy, combined with innovative approaches to treatment that have been developed empirically. The theory and foundation of hand therapy are based on a comprehensive understanding of upper extremity anatomy and how it is altered by pathologic conditions; the histologic aspects of tissue healing and the effects of immobilization on connective tissue; muscle, sensory, vascular, and connective tissue physiology; kinesiology and biomechanics of the upper extremity; the effects of temperature and electrical

currents on tissue; and surgical procedures for the upper extremity.[2] The purpose of hand therapy is to prevent dysfunction, restore function, or reverse the progression of pathologic conditions in the upper extremity resulting from trauma, disease, or congenital or acquired deformity.[3]

Hand therapy is perhaps the fastest growing area of occupational and physical therapy. This specialty has been officially recognized since the incorporation of the American Society of Hand Therapists (ASHT) in 1977. The ASHT was organized to promote continuing education, research, publication of related information, and standards of practice in rehabilitation of the upper extremity. In recent years the body of knowledge of hand therapy has grown significantly. Hand therapists have contributed to this through publication, research, and teaching. A number of books on hand rehabilitation are now available, and *Journal of Hand Therapy*, which began quarterly circulation in 1987, is filled with original research and clinical articles relating to this specialty.

HAND THERAPISTS

Hand therapists are occupational therapists or physical therapists who have become proficient in the application of advanced skills to treat upper extremity dysfunction. They have gained a comprehensive body of knowledge and skills related to upper extremity rehabilitation through advanced continuing education, clinical experience, and independent study. Hand therapists employ therapeutic techniques derived from both occupational therapy and physical therapy. The merger of traditional skills from these two professions in combination with innovations evolving from practice has produced a specialized field.[2]

The demand for qualified hand therapists by physicians, employers, and consumers has led to an increased number of practitioners entering the field of hand therapy. As a result, standards for the provision and quality of care had to be established to ensure competence and to protect patient welfare. The first certification examination in hand therapy was given in 1991. The content of this examination is based on the results of a role delineation study of hand therapy that was conducted in 1985 by the ASHT and the

American College Testing Program.[3] This study surveyed occupational therapists and physical therapists in the United States who were likely to be practicing hand therapy. The respondents provided information about themselves and their practices. They also rated a variety of professional activities, estimated how frequently those activities were performed in their practices, and gauged how important they thought these were to the practice of hand therapy. This information led to the development of an official definition and scope of practice of hand therapy[2] and provided the foundation for the certification examination.

DIAGNOSTIC CONDITIONS TREATED

Patients with acute upper extremity injuries or conditions usually attain the most benefit from hand therapy intervention. Persons with chronic conditions, however, may be treated at a hand rehabilitation center if realistic rehabilitative goals can be established. The following conditions are most appropriate for treatment in a hand rehabilitation center: amputations, arthritis, brachial plexus injuries, burns, congenital deformities, crush injuries, Dupuytren's contracture, fractures, dislocations, sprains, multiple systems trauma, peripheral nerve injuries, reflex sympathetic dystrophy, cumulative trauma disorders, replantations, secondary upper extremity reconstruction, shoulder injuries, soft tissue injuries, and tendon injuries. Patients with these conditions can be referred to a hand rehabilitation center at any time but the best results occur when referral is made early.

Most hand rehabilitation centers are outpatient facilities because most of the conditions treated do not require lengthy hospitalization. For hospitalized patients, hand therapy can be performed either at bedside or at a hand rehabilitation center if the patient can be transported easily.

DIVERSITY OF SERVICES

A wide range of services are typically performed by personnel in hand rehabilitation centers. These range from providing acute care to injured patients to providing injury prevention programs to industry. Acute care services include performing comprehensive upper extremity evaluations. These evaluations utilize standardized tests and measuring techniques for objective assessment of range of motion, strength, sensibility, wound healing, pain, edema, dexterity, hand function, and the ability to perform activities of daily living and work skills. Patients also receive individualized therapy programs to treat upper extremity dysfunction. This treatment may be provided on a one-to-one basis, in a group, or by consultation. Treatment may include wound and scar management, edema control, pain control, sensory re-education, range of motion exercises, strengthening, dexterity training, orthotic fabrication and training, prosthetic training, work conditioning, and activities of daily living training. A variety of techniques may be used to augment treatment, including therapeutic heat and cold, manual therapy, electrophysiologic techniques, neuromuscular techniques, purposeful activities, and the provision of adaptive equipment. In addition, patient and family education and home exercise, splinting, and activity programs are used extensively to promote the patient's active participation in the therapy process.

In addition to acute care many hand rehabilitation centers also provide work evaluation and conditioning programs for their patients with work-related injuries. Formal patient education programs and industrial injury prevention programs are also services frequently provided by hand rehabilitation centers.

PHYSICAL SPACE REQUIREMENTS

Adequate physical space is critical for a successful hand therapy program. There must be enough room to treat several patients at the same time, supervise them while they are performing their independent therapy programs, and provide them with the range of services necessary to treat complex upper extremity disorders. A floor plan that has a large, open space surrounded by specialty rooms will allow for maximum efficiency and safety and for optimum patient flow (Fig. 19-1). This is because the majority of patients can be observed by all staff members. This design can also facilitate interaction among the patients and with the treatment team.

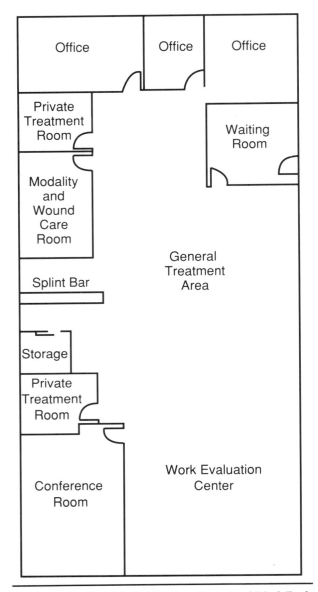

Fig. 19-1. The Hand Rehabilitation Center and Work Evaluation Center, University of California, San Diego, is 44 feet × 91 feet, equaling 4,004 square feet. This floor plan has large open area surrounded by specialty rooms.

The sizes and designs of hand rehabilitation centers vary depending on the nature and size of the referral base. The recommended minimum amount of space needed to develop a hand rehabilitation center is 1,600 square feet. A successful program is possible in a smaller area, but with less space some of the effi-

ciency and special features of the hand rehabilitation center will be compromised.

The hand rehabilitation center is best organized so that activities with similar requirements and functions can take place in the same area. The following functional environments are necessary to provide comprehensive services to this patient population.

General Treatment Area

The largest area of the center should be designed for general treatment. It can be divided into functional treatment areas by the subtle arrangement of furniture and equipment (Fig. 19-2). Space for individual hands-on treatment sessions with the therapists should be located in an area that provides the best vantage points for viewing the rest of the room. It is also helpful if this area is away from the most distracting activities. This area should be furnished with treatment tables. A popular design in hand rehabilitation centers is a table that is no more than 24 inches wide. The therapist uses proper body mechanics by sitting directly across from the patient. It is also helpful to pad the edge of the table where the therapist rests the elbows to prevent repeated compression to them (Fig. 19-3).

In close proximity to this area should be regular tables where patients who require close supervision can sit. Here, they can use equipment, perform functional activities, and work on refining prehensile patterns. The rest of this general area should be set up for strengthening and endurance building. Here, weights and special equipment such as the work simulator are located. If work evaluation and work hardening are to be performed, a much larger area is recommended.

Private Treatment Area

A quiet, private, distraction-free room is needed for sensibility evaluations, shoulder treatment, sensory re-education, patient consultation, and some aspects of activities of daily living training. Depending on the size of this room, it could be used for small conferences and staff meetings. This room should be furnished with a small evaluation table, a treatment

Fig. 19-2. The general treatment area of the Hand Rehabilitation Center, University of California, San Diego, is divided into functional treatment areas. Specialty rooms have windows, which allow viewing of patients in the general treatment area.

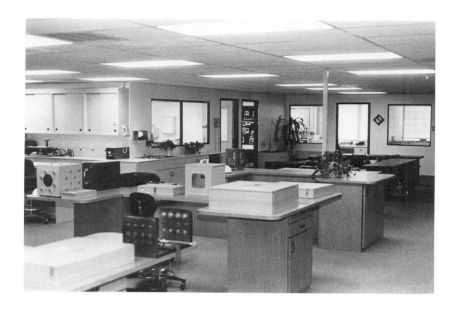

plinth, and equipment necessary to perform evaluations and activities of daily living assessments.

Wound Care Area

A semiprivate, clean area with a sink is needed for wound care. The hydrotherapy equipment is ideally near this area. This is also a good place to store equipment and supplies such as hot packs and paraffin

because this is typically not an area where patients are left unattended.

Splint Area

Because orthotic fabrication is a major component of treatment plans, the splint area should be well designed and stocked for maximum efficiency. Splinting equipment and materials should be organized in an easily accessible, functional work space. This area

Fig. 19-3. Specially designed tables encourage good body mechanics. Pads are used to prevent compression on elbows and forearms.

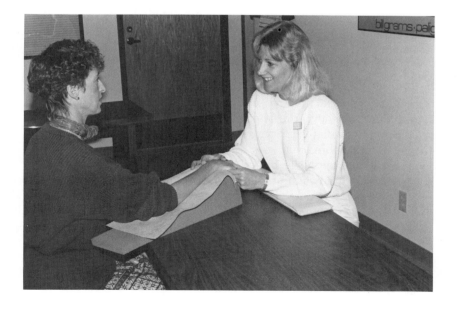

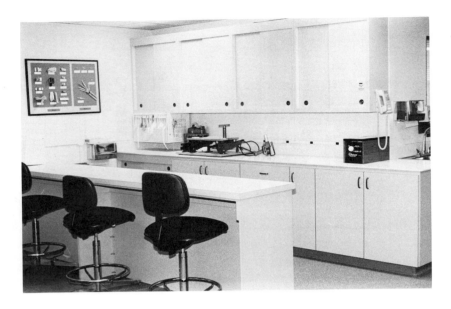

Fig. 19-4. A splint bar allows for great efficiency while fabricating splints and requires a minimal amount of space.

can be located near the general treatment area so that the therapists can supervise other patients while fabricating splints. A very useful design is a splinting bar. This allows for great efficiency while splinting and requires a minimal amount of space (Fig. 19-4).

Support Areas

In addition, space needs to be allotted for support functions such as staff offices, reception areas, and storage. If necessary these areas need not be in immediate proximity to the rest of the hand rehabilitation center, but efficiency will be enhanced if they are nearby.

Additional Considerations

A number of special features in room design can enhance the efficiency and safety of treatment and maximize the available space. Installing windows in the peripheral rooms that look into the main treatment areas will allow for better observation of patients. These windows can be covered with blinds to provide privacy when needed. Instead of using valuable wall space for storage, treatment stations can be designed with storage areas so that the needed equipment is readily available where it is used (Fig. 19-5). The hand rehabilitation center should have as many sinks as possible, not only for hygiene purposes but also for use as treatment stations.

DAILY OPERATIONS

Two common features of a hand rehabilitation center are that patients are treated in groups and therapy sessions are longer than in traditional settings. Therapy sessions typically include a modality, hands-on work with a therapist, and supervised activity to improve function. Although this method of treating is ideal in a theoretical sense, in reality much can go awry. Great care must be taken to ensure that the patient is performing activities correctly and that the plan of progression is appropriate. Hand rehabilitation centers must be carefully structured so that the needs of individual patients are not compromised by allowing them to fall into rote schedules without a clear treatment plan or concrete goals. A number of policies and procedures can be developed to help ensure that the quality of patient care is never compromised.

Primary Therapists

The ideal is to have each patient seen by only one therapist throughout the rehabilitation, but often this is unrealistic in actual practice. Staff schedules, which include part-time employees, vacations, sick leave, and non–patient care responsibilities, will frequently conflict with this ideal practice. It is more important that patients be on a consistent daily schedule so that they can devote the necessary time

Fig. 19-5. Centrally located treatment stations have built-in storage so that needed equipment is readily available.

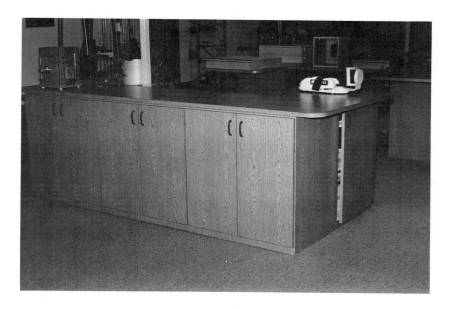

to their recovery. The primary therapist system represents a good compromise to the ideal situation. Each patient is assigned a primary therapist at the time of the initial therapy appointment. This therapist is responsible for the patient's evaluations, treatment planning, and insurance paperwork. This therapist sees the patient at each visit until the initial evaluation is complete, the treatment plan and the short-term and long-term goals have been discussed with the patient, the initial splints are fabricated, and a home program is assigned. After this, the primary therapist sees the patient as much as possible, but at a minimum of once a week, to upgrade the program and reevaluate progress. This therapist is also responsible for communicating all changes in the treatment plan to the rest of the staff.

Patient Schedules

Scheduling hand rehabilitation center appointments is sometimes quite difficult because of the volume of patients and the length of the therapy sessions. Not only therapist slots but also equipment, rooms, and modalities must be allocated to prevent time and equipment conflicts with other patients (Fig. 19-6). This greatly smooths patient flow throughout the day. It is also a good idea to schedule patients for a full week of appointments in a single time slot so that they can have as much consistency in their schedules

as possible (Fig. 19-7). Special treatments such as re-evaluations and splint modifications also should be scheduled in advance so that they will not be deferred because of schedule conflicts.

Levels of Activity

Another way to ensure quality care is to classify all of the activities performed independently by the patients into levels of difficulty. This will help prevent random selection of an activity and should provide consistency to most patient programs. A proposal for a five-level plan follows.

Level I: activities that promote early motion or purposeful use of the injured hand.
Level II: activities that promote progressive prehension and coordination and initiate strengthening.
Level III: activities that provide moderate resistance to improve dexterity and increase strength and endurance.
Level IV: activities that provide moderate to heavy resistance to encourage maximum strengthening and to improve work tolerance.
Level V: activities providing moderate to heavy resistance that simulate the demands of the patient's job and prepare the patient for return to work.

Forms

The use of forms will greatly improve paperwork efficiency, encourage uniformity in recording the results of treatment, and facilitate communication

	8:00	8:30	9:00	9:30	10:00	10:30	11:00	11:30
Whirlpool								
Fluido								
Hot packs								
Hot packs								
Paraffin								
Jobst								
Other								
Eval room 1								
Eval room 2								
THERAPISTS 1								
2								
3								
4								
5								
6								
BTE								
Activities								
Notes:							Day	Date

Fig. 19-6. This daily schedule form is designed to facilitate a smooth flow of patients. Patients are scheduled according to the availability of therapists, equipment, space, and modalities.

among the treatment team and with the patients. Standard forms for evaluations, progress notes, splint wear and care, home exercise programs, and patient education can be developed to meet the needs of the facility and the patient population. It is recommended that duplicates of all forms be made so that a copy can be kept in the patient's medical record.

Meetings

Regularly scheduled meetings should be held to discuss the center's caseload. At these meetings new patients, problems, and changes in treatment orders should be discussed. Policies on how all information affecting patient care is communicated to the staff should be consistent.

ADMINISTRATIVE ISSUES

The organizational structure of a hand rehabilitation center will vary depending on the ownership of the center. Hand rehabilitation centers are usually connected with a hospital or clinic, are part of a hand surgery office, or are privately owned by a therapist. Staffing patterns may vary in these settings depending on whether or not the staff is involved with issues such as billing, payroll, insurance, and licensing.

Regardless of ownership, a minimum number of staff members is needed to run a comprehensive program and still be able to respond to growth opportunities. This minimum staff requirement includes a full-time lead hand therapist, a half- to full-time staff therapist, a three quarter– to full-time occupational ther-

University of California, San Diego, Medical Center

Hand Rehabilitation Center

3969 Fourth Avenue, Suite 105
San Diego, California 92103
(619) 294-3744

Source	Date

Patient Identification

DAY	MONDAY	TUESDAY	WEDNESDAY	THURSDAY	FRIDAY
DATE					
TIME					

Comments_____

_____

_____

B160(5-87)3

Fig. 19-7. Patients are scheduled for at least 1 week of appointments at a time. This encourages consistency in their daily schedules.

apy or physical therapy assistant, and a half- to full-time secretary. The daily operation of a hand rehabilitation center should be directed by the lead therapist regardless of ownership because this person is closest to the issues and can best handle situations as they arise. Assigning the responsibility for program development to this therapist will likely lead to increased enthusiasm and motivation and result in a better program. Management personnel have a tendency to think that money can be saved by not hiring support staff and that the therapists can perform all support functions. This thinking is unwise because the support staff will ensure program growth by allowing the professional staff the time to provide direct patient care and the time to market the center's services. Therapy job descriptions should include only tasks that utilize professional skills. This excludes activities such as typing, cleaning whirlpools, and maintaining the inventory.

In recent years the health care market has become quite competitive. A hand rehabilitation center must develop a plan so that it can maintain a share of this market. The marketing plan should include strategies to meet the needs of the center's customers — the patients, referring physicians, and insurance companies. The most obvious need of these customers is quality patient care provided in an efficient and timely manner. The marketing plan should focus on strategies to meet this need and policies should be developed to support it.

The quality of patient care is directly related to the knowledge and skills of the staff members. The therapists are the most visible of the staff members. It is their skill and the rapport between them and the customers that will have the greatest influence on referral patterns. To ensure that the staff is well trained, hand rehabilitation centers should have in-service programs, thorough new employee orientation, and funds for continuing education.

It is important to remember that the hand rehabilitation center is marketing a service. This means that all policies and procedures must support customer relations. Front-line employees must have the attitude and the independence to do whatever is reasonable for the customer. To do this, the administrative staff of the center must have flexible policies related to the availability of appointment times, hours of operation, staff overtime, and report writing turnaround times. A true customer-oriented approach to patient care means that the center is constantly listening to the needs of the clientele that makes up its market and changing its policies to meet those needs.

A number of other ways to market hand rehabilitation center services exist. The staff can network with other therapists, physicians, and insurance representatives by becoming involved in professional organizations. Giving lectures and seminars will increase the credibility and visibility of the staff. Brochures, stationery, educational pamphlets, and home programs should be well designed and should display the name and logo of the center prominently. When-

ever possible, representatives of referral sources should be invited to the center to discuss patients. The more familiar these individuals are with the staff and the services, the more likely they will be to continue to use the center for their patients.

THE HAND REHABILITATION CENTER MODEL

This chapter has presented a model for the development of a hand rehabilitation center. Although quality hand therapy can be given in a variety of settings, therapy for patients with complex upper extremity involvement is best provided in a specialized center where comprehensive services are available. The goal of this model hand rehabilitation center is to be a center of excellence where quality care is required and quality outcomes are standard. To achieve this, all aspects of the center must be designed with this underlying philosophy, and the center must foster an environment in which the staff and patients can work together to achieve the best possible results.

REFERENCES

1. Nickel VL: The model of a hand rehabilitation center. p. 665. In Hunter JM, Schneider LH, Mackin EJ, Bell JA (eds): Rehabilitation of the Hand. CV Mosby, St. Louis, 1978
2. American Society of Hand Therapists: Definition and scope of practice of hand therapy. J Hand Ther 1:16, 1987
3. Chai SH, Dimick MP, Kasch MC: A role delineation study of hand therapy. J Hand Ther 1:7, 1987

20 The Spinal Cord Injury Center

DAVID F. APPLE, JR.

Prior to World War II, spinal cord injury was a lethal problem, with a survival rate of less than 15 percent. In 1944, Sir Ludwig Guttman established the first spinal cord injury center devoted exclusively to this problem at Stoke-Mandeville, England. The ensuing years have seen a steady decrease in the mortality rate, and at the present time the death rate is less than 15 percent in those patients who reach the hospital setting alive. The Stoke-Mandeville unit was established with a single physician in charge of patient management and a multidisciplinary team responsible for coordinating the patient's care. The team consisted of nurses, physical therapists, occupational therapists, social workers, recreational therapists, and vocational counselors. The focus was to return the patient to the highest level of function consistent with the neurologic deficit.

At the same time, in the United States, Dr. Donald Munro, at the Boston University Medical Center, with help from Liberty Mutual Insurance Company, developed a dedicated spinal cord injury unit. As World War II was coming to an end, the Veterans Administration, under the leadership of Drs. Estin Comar, Ernest Bors, and William Talbot, recognized the necessity for establishing units to handle the spinal cord–injured soldiers. Dr. John Young implemented the spinal unit concept, first at Craig Hospital in Englewood, Colorado, and subsequently at the Good Samaritan Hospital in Phoenix, Arizona.

The federal government first became involved in the problem of spinal cord injury in 1968. A study group was organized by the Rehabilitation Services Administration. The recommendation that resulted from this study was that a model of care should be developed that allowed for early recognition and referral of spinal cord–injured patients to a rehabilitation center that had a designated area for such patients. These patients would there be managed by an expert team charged with identification and utilization of all the community agencies and existing services to augment the patients' rehabilitation. Finally, the spinal center had to commit to long-term follow-up to monitor the gains obtained through the rehabilitation process.

In 1970, the unit developed at the Barrow Neurological Institute and the Good Samaritan Hospital under the directorship of Dr. John Young became the first federally designated model spinal cord injury system. Over the ensuing 20 years, 21 other centers have been similarly designated (Fig. 20-1). Results of the 20 years of the system of care are documented in a publication entitled "The Spinal Cord Injury Model".[1] Review of that document indicates a clear advantage for managing a spinal cord injury in a center that is part of a total system of care.

DEVELOPMENT OF A SPINAL CORD INJURY UNIT

In the initial phase of establishing a spinal cord injury unit or center there are four absolutely essential requirements. A knowledgeable, committed *physician,* surgeon or non-surgeon, must assume the role of providing the impetus for establishing the unit. Working in concert with the physician must be an *administrator*[2] who understands rehabilitation concepts and how they require different approaches from the usual acute hospital management principles. The administrator should also have reasonable

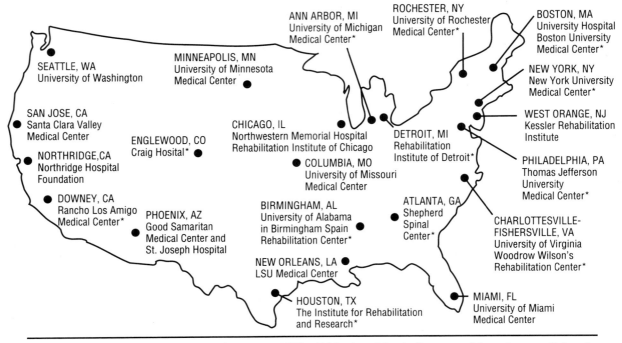

Fig. 20-1. Model spinal cord injury system, 1970–1990. Asterisks indicate model system participants, 1985–1990.

autonomy in the decision-making process as the unit is established.

The next essential is a *catchment area* that will provide a patient population sufficient to support a categorical unit. Statistics on incidence indicate that approximately 30 new injuries per 1 million population occur each year. The average length of stay for a patient in an efficient spinal cord injury center is approximately 90 days. Therefore, a population of 1 million would support an eight-bed unit. From a therapy management standpoint, a physical therapist or occupational therapist assisted by a technician can manage approximately eight patients at a time. Therefore, from a functional standpoint, the smallest reasonable unit would also be eight beds. However, from a practical standpoint this does not work because of vacation time, sickness, and general fluctuation of the patient population.

The American Spinal Injury Association, in a monograph on spinal cord administration,[2] suggested 20-bed units as the ideal situation. However, a 16-bed unit will function satisfactorily and provide the

American Spinal Injury Association's recommended minimum of 50 new patients a year as a requirement for maintaining team expertise. A 16-bed unit can be coordinated well by a single physician whose primary responsibility is spinal cord patient management.

A 16-bed unit could be developed in a population area of 2 to 2.5 million, could function well, and would be able to provide sufficient numbers of patients to justify not only physical therapists, occupational therapists, nursing, and social work staff but also education, recreational therapy, and vocational counseling. Speech, therapy, respiratory therapy, psychological services, and nutritional support can be provided on a consultative basis.

The final requirement is *space*. Ideally the space should be a designated area within a general rehabilitation center, or a separate facility that is connected to an acute care hospital. Because of the complexity of managing spinal cord–injured patients and the various medical problems they may have, it is necessary to have a diversified consulting staff. Included are internists with a special expertise in respiratory problems. Other medical specialties for which there is frequently need are neurology, cardiology, and gastroenterology. The urologic needs of spinal cord–injured patients are significant. Thus, having at least one physician with a primary interest in the neurogenic bladder is absolutely necessary. If the spinal cord injury unit is run by a physiatrist, both an orthopaedist and a neurosurgeon with expertise in the management of trauma to any level of the spine must be involved.

The American Spinal Injury Association has delineated minimal requirements for spinal cord physicians.[3] If the spinal cord injury unit is to be managed by an orthopaedist or a neurosurgeon, that physician must have the commitment not only to manage the spinal cord and spinal column injury but to direct the care as the patient proceeds through the rehabilitation process. This necessarily will take significant time and thus reduce the amount of time available for operating. Finally, the unit must have access to all the modern radiology techniques with a commitment by that department to provide the services on a very timely basis.

TEAM FUNCTIONING

Physician/Team Manager

In most centers, the team leader or manager is a physician; in a few centers, however, a knowledgeable nonphysician becomes the team or program manager. It is the responsibility of the team manager to not only coax the maximum effort from the patient but also to lead the team in a goal-oriented, efficient, individualized program for each patient. The physician manager is in charge of monitoring the day-to-day medical progress and requesting timely, appropriate consultation. The physician manager must involve both the patient and the family by imparting knowledge that allows full understanding of the injury and the consequences, in addition to the expectations of the therapy program. Thus, more time will need to be spent with the patient in family conferences than is customary in the usual surgical practice.

The physician will be required to make patient visitations at least four times a week and will need to lead the Commission on Accredited Rehabilitation Facilities (CARF)–mandated team conference, during which the patient's progress from the previous week is reviewed and the goals for the coming week are set. In this manner, the physician can delegate portions of the patient's care to the various team professionals. The manager has the ultimate responsibility for the outcome, including coordination of the patient's discharge so that the necessary services the patient requires in the community are obtained.

Nurse

Nursing staff assigned to the patient will be responsible primarily for management of bowel and bladder function and maintenance of the skin. Additionally, they will carry out traditional nursing roles in the acute care setting, managing the patient's medications and various comfort items. The nurse will need to be knowledgeable about bowel and bladder programs, specifically as they relate to spinal cord injury. Early in the patient's course, bladder care will mean understanding the use of the Foley catheter. After the switch is made to an intermittent catheterization program, the nurse supervises sterile technique for insertion and also is involved in teaching patients, if they are capable, to master their own intermittent catheterizations. The nurse must understand the mechanisms of a reflex bladder and know when to exploit the reflex voiding as it develops in the passage of time from the initial spinal cord injury.

Likewise, the nurse will need to understand thoroughly the development of a good bowel program, starting first with daily bowel evacuation done in the evening and progressing to an every-other-night fully functional reflex bowel program. The third primary area for spinal cord responsibility for the nurse is the maintenance of the skin. The insensitive skin must be protected by increasing the turn times at night and lengthening weight shift times during the day. The nurse not only needs to teach the patient why and how this should be done but also must be able to instruct care providers or significant others in all these programs when patients are incapable of doing them on their own.

Physical Therapist

The physical therapist has the responsibility for helping the patient with all mobility skills. This includes transfer activities (getting out of bed into the wheelchair and from the wheelchair to the toilet, bathtub, car, chair, or other pieces of furniture). Paraplegic patients will need wheelchair skills that are more advanced, including capabilities to perform special maneuvers ("wheelies"), to get up and down curbs and to get back into the wheelchair from the floor. All patients, whether quadriplegic or paraplegic, need to know the maintenance and basic repair techniques for their wheelchairs. If they are not physically able to perform these tasks themselves, they should be able to verbally instruct someone else in what is required. If the patient can walk, the physical therapist has the responsibility for gait evaluation, gait training, and prescribing appropriate brace and crutches.

Occupational Therapist

The occupational therapist is responsible for teaching the patient alternative methods for performing activities of daily living. These activities include all of those things which people routinely do, such as grooming, shaving, feeding, dressing, undressing, and communicating. All of these are basically upper extremity functions, but dressing does involve lower extremity function as well.

Respiratory Therapist and Speech Pathologist

For special needs, the occupational therapist may need to call on two other types of therapists: respiratory therapists and speech pathologists. For example, the respiratory therapist is valuable especially in the therapy of high quadriplegic patients. In such cases the respiratory therapist is responsible for initiating and progressing through a weaning process that frees the patient first from the respirator and then from the tracheostomy tube if the patient's neurologic condition warrants. As this procedure is progressing, very close cooperation between the occupational therapist and the respiratory therapist is required with respect to sitting and weaning, because often it is not possible to get patients in an upright position and wean them from a ventilator at the same time. For some patients, the goal will first be to get them sitting upright as the accessory respiratory muscles are strengthened; only then can they be successfully weaned from the ventilator. For other patients, it may be necessary to wean them from the ventilator before being able to fully accomplish sitting to 90°.

During the time the patient remains on a ventilator and with the tracheostomy, a speech pathologist can assess the patient's swallowing function and help with communication until the tracheostomy tube has been removed and normal speech resumed.

Social Worker

The social worker must be involved with the patient from the beginning to help the patient cope with the implications of the injury as it will affect marriage and other relationships, home, and productivity. This will require working not only with the patient but with the family to ascertain any problems in the funding for the patient's care, identifying governmental and community resources, and developing a good discharge plan. The social worker will be able to identify problem areas, which can be relayed to the rehabilitation team and help the rehabilitation plan proceed smoothly.

Psychologist

The psychologist works in conjunction with the social worker with regard to adaptation and coping mechanisms that will need to be used as the patient progresses through the grieving process. The psychologist will be able to identify how the patient managed problems prior to injury and help focus those same strengths and qualities on the alterations brought about by the spinal cord injury. Additionally, a psychologist with special interests in sexuality and sexual therapy will need to be involved. The sexual issue is best addressed during the injury phase because it is an area of high concern for the spinal cord–injured patient, who is usually young. The patient will obtain a more positive feeling if sexuality is approached scientifically and forthrightly with compassion, in the same way that alterations of other functions (e.g., bowel and bladder) were approached.

Recreational Therapist

Therapeutic recreation should be a part of each program. Most persons who sustain a spinal cord injury have been injured while partaking in some activity.

The patient's recreational interests before the injury should be ascertained and, if possible, adaptations made so that the patient can continue in those spheres of interest. However, if this is anatomically impossible, satisfactory substitutes should be identified and encouraged. Additionally, at least in the early months after injury the patient has more leisure time, and keeping that time filled with meaningful activity provides a very positive benefit. Patients who can utilize their leisure time constructively and can become involved in a rewarding activity that coincides with general fields of interest are more likely to return to a productive life-style, including return to work.

Vocational Counselor

The vocational counselor should be involved early to assess the patient's work history, interests, and skills. With this information, planning can start with early intervention leading to training for the appropriate job, especially if it involves a job or career change. The counselor should foster the idea that the spinal cord–injured patient is supposed to return to work rather than imply that it is unusual if such a patient does return to work.

Education Specialist

Much of the education about the injury and its consequences that must be imparted to the patient and family is provided by nursing staff; however, if the center population is large enough, education specialists can be very effective. Initially patients need to be evaluated for their vocational level, intelligence quotas, and best learning mode. With these determinations, the patient's education can be approached in the optimal fashion for their particular learning spectrum. The patient must have a thorough understanding of how the nervous system works and what alterations have taken place with the spinal cord injury. The patient might also benefit from teaching on problem-solving skills. The patient's care providers or significant others should also have a similar level of understanding of the implications of the spinal cord injury, know when the patient needs help, and, equally, know when help is not required.

Nutritionist

One other staff member who is important is a nutritionist to evaluate the patient's nutritional status during the acute recovery period and to make sure there is adequate intake of both liquids and solid food to augment a good bowel and bladder program. During the early phase immediately after injury, the patient is in a marked catabolic phase and may lose 30 percent of body weight. The caloric requirements during this early phase may reach 4,000 to 5,000 kcal/day. When the patient is maintained on intravenous fluids only, caloric needs will not be met, and ultimately the body draws on fat and protein stores. In this malnourished state complications are more frequent and the ability of the patient to participate in a vigorous rehabilitation program is diminished.

Working to a Successful Outcome

The physician, as the team manager, has the responsibility for coordinating all of these professional activities to provide an effective rehabilitation program that leads to a successful outcome. What is a successful outcome? It is one in which the patient has learned the skills necessary to have maximum function for the level of injury that has been sustained, and one in which the patient has in-depth knowledge of all areas of care. Additionally, the family should be educated similarly. At the time of discharge, the patient's home living situation should be fully accessible. All of the necessary equipment should be available and appropriately individualized. Finally, the patient should have a firm postdischarge care plan, all of which facilitates the patient's return to a productive life-style.

THE REHABILITATION PROCESS

Case History

A. A., a 20-year-old man, dove into a river near his home, striking his head on the bottom, and floated to the top. He was removed from the river by his friends, one of whom had summoned an ambulance. On arriving at the scene, the Emergency Medical Technicians ascertained that the patient was unable to move his legs and was only weakly moving his upper extremities. He was immobilized in a cervical collar, placed carefully on a spine board, and carried to the ambulance. During this time, the patient's respirations were monitored.

Upon arrival at the Emergency Room, the patient was transferred on the spine board to the examining table, where the Emergency Room physician performed an evaluation. Neurologic examination revealed sensation was normal to the lateral aspect of the forearm, and altered at the level of the base of the thumb and index finger, and absent below. Motor examination revealed the biceps muscle to be grade 3 (i.e., able to move through the full range of motion without resistance) with no function distally. Rectal examination revealed a flaccid sphincter and an absent bulbocavernosus reflex. There was no obvious bony malalignment. The remainder of the examination was unremarkable. Radiographs demonstrated displacement of vertebral body C5 on C6 by 50 percent, with 6 mm of soft tissue swelling anterior to the inferior body of C3.

The Emergency Room physician consulted the orthopaedist, who repeated the evaluation, confirming the findings. He placed the patient in tong traction, applying 35 pounds of weight. Concomitently, the patient was given prednisolone in a dose of 30 mg/kg of body weight and was started on an hourly dose of 5.4 mg/kg body weight of the same medicine. Radiographs did not demonstrate any change in the vertebral position. With the orthopaedist attending, additional weights were added, up to 50 lb. At that juncture, radiographs demonstrated that the forward subluxation was reduced to about 25 percent. Further attempts to improve the alignment were unsuccessful.

The patient was admitted to the intensive care unit. On repeat evaluation in 4 hours there was no change, but at 8 hours the patient had developed deep pressure sensation rectally and the bulbocavernosus reflex had returned. Repeat radiographs showed no change in vertebral position. The patient was taken to the operating room thereafter, and both an open reduction with restoration of normal alignment and a posterior wiring and fusion were accomplished. By the first postoperative day the patient had developed deep pressure sensation in the ankles and 48 hours later there was a trace of wrist extensor activity.

The orthopaedist, as leader of the rehabilitation team, involved the physical therapist, occupational therapist, social worker, and nurse in this early phase. This team began strengthening the muscles that were present and started measures to prevent contractures, skin breakdown, and other problems from developing. Particularly important during this early phase was prevention of contractures of the shoulder, which was accomplished by appropriate positioning in bed and by early attention to range-of-motion exercises.

On the seventh day after injury, the Foley catheter was removed and the patient was begun on an intermittent catheterization program with the ultimate goal of developing reflex bladder emptying. Between the seventh and 10th days the remainder of the rehabilitation team joined the original group. A psychologist, recreational therapist, educational specialist, respiratory therapist (since the patient was having respiratory difficulties), and speech pathologist were added to the team. All of these professionals became involved with the patient's day-to-day care. About this time, the first team conference was held with all of the rehabilitation disciplines represented. Long-term goals were developed for the patient. In subsequent weekly conferences, short-term goals were developed and their attainment monitored through the team conference process.

Variations of the Team Approach

In the classic sense, the team function is a multidisciplinary effort. This means that each therapeutic area of expertise is monitored by a professional so trained. However, in the more advanced concepts of rehabilitation, an intradisciplinary approach — or, if possible, a transdisciplinary approach — will achieve better results. In these instances, the particular members of the team are more functionally oriented and do not adhere strictly to the traditional roles of nurse, occupational therapist, physical therapist, and so forth. For instance, in developing a bladder program, generally it is the nurse's role to determine the times that the intermittent catheterization needs to be performed and to perform this task. As the program proceeds, the occupational therapist becomes involved and is responsible for teaching the patient how to manipulate and insert the catheter. In an intradisciplinary or transdisciplinary approach, the nurse could proceed with teaching the insertion techniques in addition to determining the time. If the time for catheterization should occur when the patient is in an occupational therapy program—or for that matter during any therapy program—the particular professional would take care of the catheterization rather than having the patient go to the nursing service for that interval, only to return to the therapy area once the intermittent catheterization is completed.

For the patient described in the case history above, who has a C5-C6 quadriplegia, the long-term goals are achieving independence in doing weight shifts during the day in the wheelchair. Some assistance at night would be required for turning while asleep. Patients with this level of injury can learn to do intermittent catheterization and can learn a bowel program with the aid of a brace with minimal, if any, assistance. The activities of daily living would largely be done independently, with assistance being required for dressing the lower extremities and in setting up for the more difficult tasks in grooming. The patient would require a wheelchair with standard rims for transportation for short distances. However, in a work or school situation a power wheelchair would be necessary. The patient could be taught to drive but would require a van with a power lift and appropriate hand controls for maneuvering. A list of general activity goals and degrees of functional ability for injuries at different neurologic levels is given in Figure 20-2.

Rehabilitation Program Phases

From the program standpoint, the patient's hospitalization can be divided into three phases. In phase I, the patient is not only injured but also is still sick from the injury. It is during this phase that determinations are being made about management of the spinal column and the exact extent of the damage to the spinal cord is being assessed.

When the patient is able to be out of bed for approximately 3 hours each day and to be involved in some type of therapy program, phase II begins. During this phase, the nursing staff continues with skin, bowel, and bladder management. The physical therapist be-

comes more involved with teaching wheelchair skills, which include transfers, manipulation of the wheelchair, and wheelchair maintenance. The occupational therapist proceeds with instructions in activities of daily living—that is, feeding, grooming, dressing, and communication skills. The social worker will continue to monitor the patient's progress on a social as well as an environmental level, with a large amount of effort being focused on discharge planning. Therapeutic recreation specialists will be assessing the patient's premorbid recreational and leisure time interests. The intent is to try to develop a program that not only will arouse the patient's interest in these recreational and leisure pursuits but also, it is hoped, lead to a positive outlook about resuming employment after discharge.

The educational specialist will teach the patient about the injury and its consequences and involve the family so that there is a uniform level of understanding of the meaning of spinal cord injury. The psychologist will monitor the patient as the grief reaction develops and guide the recovery from this necessary but painful process. The psychologist will counsel the patient regarding issues of sexuality and sexual functioning. In uncomplicated cases of paraplegia, phase II will take 6 to 8 weeks; in uncomplicated cases of quadriplegia, it will take 8 to 10 weeks.

Phase III is entered when there appear to be about 4 weeks left until discharge. During this phase, the patient is weaned from much of the help formerly given in many of the activities and encouraged to be as independent as possible. The patient should also know what medications are being taken and be aware of both the desired and adverse reactions.

The patient should go home on a pass during this time to assess any particular problems the home environment will cause and communicate these to the rehabilitation team, who will help solve problems. As the patient approaches the discharge date, appropriate steps should be taken to transfer the patient to effective outpatient care, whether at the same center or in the community from which the patient comes. If possible, the patient's home should have been made wheelchair accessible by this time. All of the patient's equipment should have been obtained and be appro-

Functional Activities

	Eating	Dressing	Grooming	Toileting	Homemaking	Driving	Public Transportation	Wheelchair Transfers	Ambulation	Communications	Bed Transfer	Vocational	Sexual Functioning
C1	A	A	A	A	A	NP	A	NP	NP	A	A	PA	PA
C2	A	A	A	A	A	NP	A	NP	NP	A	A	PA	PA
C3	A	A	A	A	A	NP	A	NP	NP	A	A	PA	PA
C4	A	A	A	A	A	NP	A	NP	NP	A	A	PA	PA
C5	A	A	A	A	A	A	A	A	NP	A	A	PA	PA
C6	A	A	A	A	A	A	A	A	NP	A	A	PA	PA
C7	A	A	A	A	A	A	A	N	NP	A	N	PA	PA
C8	N	N	N	N	N	A	A	N	NP	N	N	PA	PA
T1	N	N	N	N	N	A	A	N	NP	N	N	PA	PA
T2	N	N	N	N	N	A	A	N	NP	N	N	N	PA
T3	N	N	N	N	N	A	A	N	NP	N	N	N	PA
T4	N	N	N	N	N	A	A	N	NP	N	N	N	PA
T5	N	N	N	N	N	A	A	N	NP	N	N	N	PA
T6	N	N	N	N	N	A	A	N	NP	N	N	N	PA
T7	N	N	N	N	N	A	A	N	A	N	N	N	PA
T8	N	N	N	N	N	A	A	N	A	N	N	N	PA
T9	N	N	N	N	N	A	A	N	A	N	N	N	PA
T10	N	N	N	N	N	A	A	N	A	N	N	N	PA
T11	N	N	N	N	N	A	A	N	A	N	N	N	PA
T12	N	N	N	N	N	A	A	N	A	N	N	N	PA
L1	N	N	N	N	N	A	A	N	A	N	N	N	PA
L2	N	N	N	N	N	A	A	N	A	N	N	N	PA
L3	N	N	N	N	N	A	A	N	A	N	N	N	PA
L4	N	N	N	N	N	A	N	N	A	N	N	N	PA
L5	N	N	N	N	N	A	N	N	A	N	N	N	PA
S1	N	N	N	N	N	A	N	N	N	N	N	N	PA
S2	N	N	N	N	N	N	N	N	N	N	N	N	PA
S3	N	N	N	N	N	N	N	N	N	N	N	N	PA
S4	N	N	N	N	N	N	N	N	N	N	N	N	PA

N	Normal or near-normal function.
A	Needs some type of personal or mechanical assistance.
PA	Partially available but options need to be discussed.
NP	Not practical or not probable.

Fig. 20-2. Patient functional ability according to level of spinal cord injury.

priately customized and ready for use. On arrival home, there will be a variable length of time for adjustment to the home situation. The patient should be encouraged to get back into either work or school as soon as possible.

During these phases, the physician acts as the team manager and coordinates not only the medical care but also the rehabilitation effort. This will involve the judicious and appropriate use of consultants who have the knowledge and capability to treat the more

Table 20-1. Frequency of Complications in Spinal Cord Injury Patients by Early Versus Late Admission

Complication	Early Admission (Day 1) (%)	Delayed Admission (Days 2 to 60) (%)	P Value
Contractures	3.3	5.3	.03
Heterotopic ossification	3.3	6.1	.004
Gastrointestinal hemorrhage	3.4	4.1	.45
Atelectasis	19.7	25.5	.002
Pneumonia	16.5	19.7	.06
Deep vein thrombosis	16.3	13.3	.06
Pulmonary embolus	4.0	5.5	.06
Cardiac arrest	4.0	6.5	.02
Chills and fever (urosepsis)	23.7	27.3	.07
Abnormal renal function	0.2	1.4	.004
Decubitus ulcers (any grade)	35.2	46.0	.0001
Decubitus ulcers (grade 2, 3, or 4)	21.7	25.9	.02

common secondary complications (Table 20-1). Many, and sometimes all, of these complications occur in any one patient. However, the occurrence as well as severity can be minimized by appropriate aggressive early management of the spinal cord injury, so that in essence the rehabilitation process starts within the first day or two after injury.

Because many of these patients are going to require some type of assistance at home, it is necessary to involve the family. The most effective way to accomplish this is to conduct an admissions conference soon after the injury in which the injury is discussed with the patient and family. The expectations and an outline of the program that will be undertaken in the rehabilitation center should be discussed. Additional training must be given to the care providers or significant others prior to any pass home so that these individuals understand the areas in which the patient needs help or may need help. They must also be able to recognize the more acute complications that can occur in a 24- or 36-hour period while the patient is on the pass. Toward the conclusion of the rehabilitation program, another session with the care providers or significant others is helpful to review the basics of the patient's program to be sure that there is a good level of understanding by all concerned.

If this general outline is followed for the spinal cord–injured patient treated in a center that is part of a system of care, the average length of stay for a paraplegic person should be 80 to 90 days from time of

Table 20-2. Length of Stay in Treatment Centers in a System of Care Versus Nonsystem Hospitals

	Length of Stay (Days)	
	System	Nonsystem
Paraplegia		
Incomplete	71	78
Complete	88	98
Quadriplegia		
Incomplete	92	98
Complete	129	129

Table 20-3. Five-Year Survival Rates for Spinal Cord–Injured Patients

	Model System	North California Residents
C1-C3	75	30
C4–T1 complete or C1–T1 incomplete	78	70
T2–L3 complete	96	84
All	87	82

injury to discharge, and for a quadriplegic person, 95 to 105 days (Table 20-2). If the patient is managed in a hospital outside a system of care the length of stay is increased (Table 20-2). High quadriplegia with the attendant problems of respiration and ventilation dependence significantly increases the stay—by another 6 to 8 weeks on the average.

Concluding Remarks

Spinal cord injury is a catastrophic problem, but the damage can be minimized by effective early referral into a system of care that has a rehabilitation team whose responsibility it is to return the patient to as high a level of function as is consistent with the remaining neurologic function in a reasonable amount of time. In such a setting, the complications can be reduced and the length of hospital stay is decreased. In addition, the mortality rate is less (Table 20-3), with the overall 10-year survival for system-treated patients being 77 percent.

REFERENCES

1. The Spinal Cord Injury Model: Lessons Learned and New Applications. Proceedings of the National Consensus Conference on Catastrophic Illness and Injury. [Publisher?], Washington, DC, 1990
2. Spinal Cord Administration. American Spinal Injury Association, Chicago, Ill, 1982
3. Training Guidelines for Spinal Cord Injury Physicians. American Spinal Injury Association, Chicago, Ill, 1982
4. Spinal Cord Injury: The Facts and Figures. The University of Alabama at Birmingham, Birmingham, AL, 1986

21 The Sports Medicine Rehabilitation Center

CHRISTOPHER JOBE
FRANK W. JOBE
MARILYN PINK

Rehabilitation has been defined as "a therapeutic program designed to minimize the consequence of a permanent or protracted disability." To an athlete, "disability" may mean a level of functioning that would be normal for a non athlete. The uniqueness of sports medicine rehabilitation is the high baseline of necessary and normal function. An uninjured athlete is already engaged in a routine of strengthening and conditioning for optimization of performance, a program that might be called "prehabilitation." The athlete's body has made specific adaptations for the performance of that athletic activity. Determining what is normal activity for the athlete is the key to understanding sports medicine rehabilitation. A successful sports medicine rehabilitation program must consider the level of performance required by the athlete, the specific mechanics of the sport, and the response of tissues to the inherent stresses and demands placed on the athlete.

The mechanics of sport are sport specific and complex. Various sports have in common increased velocity of body part(s), increased joint forces, excessive joint range of motion (ROM), transfer of energy from one body part to another, and a repetitive event (or events). The increased joint velocities, joint forces, and excessive joint ROM stress the joint and have the potential to break down the static stabilization if the activity is not performed in a mechanically sound fashion or if it is performed with insufficiently conditioned tissues.

Athletic activities involve the transfer of high kinetic energy across the joints rather than use of the muscles of a single isolated joint to generate the motion. An example of this is the baseball pitch (Fig. 21-1). The energy for the pitch comes from a falling forward onto the leg contralateral to the pitching arm and then a directing of the derived energy into progressively smaller body segments. As the mass of the rotating segments decreases, the velocity increases. The energy is transferred through the trunk, delivered to the shoulder, elbow, and hand, and finally imparted to the ball. This chain of events, or whiplike action, is vital to the generation of power. The accuracy of timing of the chain of events and complexity of rotations and derotations is imperative to the prevention of injury.

The energy remaining in the body must be dissipated by muscles in a follow-through motion. The power produced by one joint moved by a single muscle could not approach that which is accumulated and transferred through coiling and uncoiling of the body. This use of the falling body to generate energy and high muscle forces is common to many athletic activities. Running, for example, is a series of controlled falls. This natural motion in sport activities is

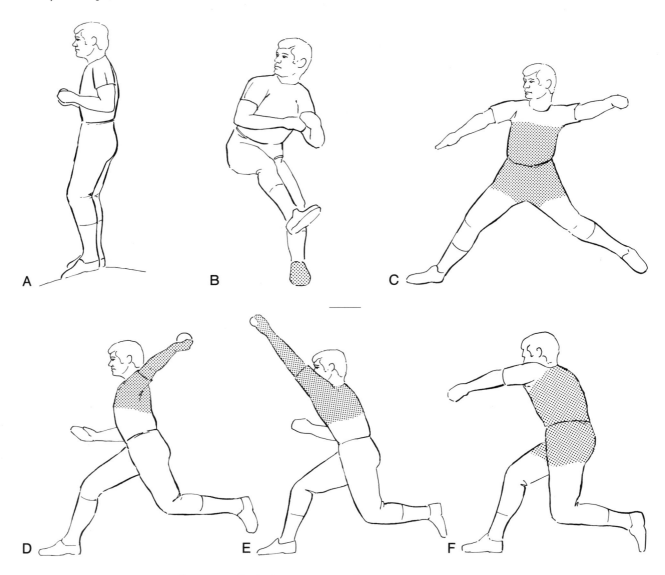

A B C

D E F

in sharp contrast to the usual pattern of rehabilitation exercises, in which the motion is produced at a single joint by the adjacent musculature without dealing with the other body parts or sources of power. Athletic motions also do not follow the simple pulley-and-hinge arrangement that rehabilitation machines use, but rather consist of a complexity of rotations and derotations.

The final common denominator of sports activities, the repetitive nature of the event, brings into consideration all of the loads and demands over the length

of time it took the athlete to learn and practice the sport.

The musculoskeletal tissues adapt in varying fashions to imposed demands and applied loads. Obviously, the more akin the rehabilitative activity is to the sport, the more specific the resulting adaptation is to the athlete's needs. However, after an injury, healing tissues need to be protected, and a graduated approach must be taken in returning to activity. Thus, the rehabilitation program takes into consideration the specificity of the sport as well as the tissues that

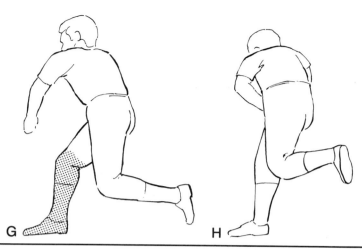

Fig. 21-1. An 8-frame sequence prepared from high-speed cinematography of a major league baseball pitcher. The stippled areas in each of the frames indicates the region of the body in which the most rapid motion is about to take the place. For example, between frames 2 and 3, the most rapid motion occurs in the joints of the foot and ankle as the pitcher falls toward the catcher. Between frames 3 and 4, the most rapid motion occurs in the hips and torso. This illustration shows how in the throwing motion, as in many athletic endeavors, the athletes uses a controlled fall to generate kinetic energy. If we assume an average weight and height for the pitcher and a downward slope on the pitching mound, the thrower would generate about 300 joules of energy by falling onto his opposite foot. This energy is then directed by a series of motions into a smaller and lighter portion of the body—that is, the throwing arm. Because this portion of the body is smaller and lighter, its velocity is tremendously increased—actually it is far faster than the athlete would be able to achieve with muscle use alone. The baseball of average weight traveling at 90 mph would only take away 88 joules of energy from the thrower, leaving him with approximately 212 joules of energy to dissipate with his follow-through motions in order to prevent injury. This figure illustrates the tremendous forces that are generated by athletic endeavors and the rehabilitation of the muscles that would be necessary to control these motions and—perhaps more importantly—the importance of restoring the proper patterns of motion to prevent reinjury or new injury.

are injured. The rehabilitation activities then begin at the maximum level that will not damage an injured or surgically treated structure and progress to a full athletic endeavor.

These rehabilitation activities are the focus of this chapter. We begin by discussing the musculoskeletal soft tissues and the rehabilitation activities used for each of the individual tissues. We then give an example of two rehabilitation protocols: one for the anterior cruciate ligament reconstruction at the knee and one for the anterior capsulolabral reconstruction of the shoulder. These two protocols are given as examples rather than as a recipe to be followed strictly. The protocols are subject to change as more is learned about the responses of tissues to healing and to rehabilitation. This chapter is intended as an outline for the reader of the thought process used in designing

rehabilitation programs. By following this thought process, readers will be able to develop their own rehabilitation protocols, integrate the constant influx of new information, and understand and evaluate new rehabilitation programs as they appear in the literature.

MUSCULOSKELETAL TISSUES

The building blocks for musculoskeletal tissue are extracellular and intracellular macromolecules, such as collagen, proteoglycans, and actomyosin (Fig. 21-2). When the tissue is called on to perform its particular function, production of these macromolecules is stimulated. For example, myocytes are stimulated when producing force, fibrocytes when resisting tension, and osteoblasts when resisting compression, tension, and shear. If the stimulus is diminished, pro-

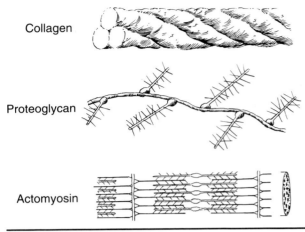

Fig. 21-2. There are three important groups of macromolecules in the musculoskeletal system. First there is collagen, which is the tension-bearing element found throughout the soft tissue matrix. Collagen is made up of small neutral amino acids and assumes a tightly coiled, rope-like form, which is ideal for its function. A triple helix is the natural form that the most abundant types of collagen assume. Because it is so tightly coiled on itself, it occupies a rather small space in comparison with proteoglycan. The second macromolecule is proteoglycan, which is a combination of charged sugar molecules in small proteins. Because of their heavy negative charges these molecules assume an extended position occupying 10,000 times the volume of a collagen molecule of like weight. These molecules provide soft tissue lubrication between tissue layers and in cartilage because of their extended position and tendency to imbibe water. They provide the stiffening of the turgor of the cartilage in which they are encased. The third molecular combination is made up of actin and myosin. These molecules form an intracellular matrix that functions to produce force. One of the ways in which muscles respond to applied demand is to produce more actin and myosin within each cell.

duction of the large macromolecules decreases, and thus muscular disuse atrophy sets in, or tendons become thinner and stiffer, or bone becomes weaker. If the stimulus is increased, muscular hypertrophy occurs, ligaments become thicker and more flexible, or bone becomes stronger. Along with the desirable production of these macromolecules during stimulation, the cells also produce metabolic by-products. The metabolic breakdown or destruction needs to be balanced by production of the macromolecules—a condition of homeostasis. When loading a structure too much, too fast, or too often, destruction surpasses the cellular production, and fatigue failure or sudden

traumatic failure in the extracellular or intracellular matrix results (Fig. 21-3).

On a day-to-day basis, an athlete's tissues function at a very high level. Because of the high baseline, the athlete's tissues have experienced this "hypertrophy" and are maintaining a status quo. However, the athlete may upset the status quo by moving too much, too fast, or too often and thus increase the rate of destruction over production, with concomitant injury. Once the primary injury occurs, secondary losses of strength and flexibility occur from edema and immobilization. The sports medicine rehabilitation program must balance the desire to stimulate the tissue to perform a function with the avoidance of reinjury and destruction of healing tissue. This again is the recurring theme in sports medicine rehabilitation.

Human tissue can be categorized in numerous ways. Because the focus of this chapter is rehabilitation of sports injuries, the categories of connective tissue and muscular tissue that were selected for discussion are the most common sites of injury. Among the connective tissues are bone, cartilage, and soft tissues, such as bursa, capsule, skin, tendon, and ligament. Although muscular tissue can be categorized as soft tissue, it is discussed separately because it is so specific and variable in its rehabilitation.

REHABILITATION BY TISSUE

Connective Tissue

Bone

Bone is designed to be a load-bearing element. The macromolecules form an extracellular mineralized matrix of collagen with some proteoglycans. The function of bone is to bear stresses, the most important of which is compression, but also some shear and tension stresses. Bone is constantly turned over (renewed) and rearranged to reflect applied stresses. The vascularity and metabolic rate of bone are higher than those of cartilage and are actually higher than in many of the surrounding soft tissues. Thus, bone is among the tissues that recover most quickly after injury.

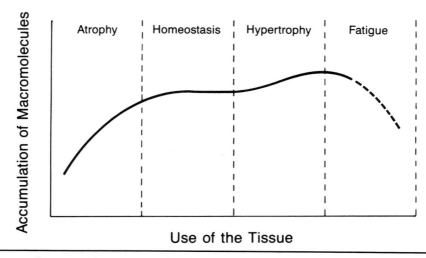

Fig. 21-3. Diagram illustrating the response of the musculoskeletal tissues to use. In the natural course of events there is a turnover of macromolecules. They are produced and destroyed under events of disuse or immobilization. Production of new macromolecules is not stimulated, and so destruction outpaces production resulting in an overall loss of macromolecules. Under activities of daily living a homeostasis occurs, with production equaling destruction. Athletic activities lead to a condition wherein production of macromolecules exceeds their destruction, and so there is a net accumulation. Because of the hypertrophy of collagen or muscle cells, the stimulated structure becomes broader; therefore, although the overall applied forces are greater they are spread over a greater cross-sectional area of the stimulated structure and a new level of homeostasis is achieved. On the far right of the graph is the effect of overuse, whether because of total load or because of increased frequency of use of a particular structure. Microscopic defects accumulate at a rate more rapid than the newly stimulated tissue remodeling can repair, and microscopic or macroscopic failure occurs with inflammatory response to the tissue injury. In their regimens for recovery the physician and therapist try to keep the patient's tissues operating in the hypertrophy level of stimulus without falling into fatigue (by overstimulus) or into atrophy (by excessive prolongation of immobilization).

Treatment for disuse osteopenia is basically graduated loading of the bone. In practice, the limiting considerations on the patients' activities usually are those of the surrounding and attached soft tissues, because the bone recovers its physical properties earlier in the course of treatment than do the ligaments and tendons. By the time the patient returns to physical performance, the bone usually has recovered its strength. An exception to this occurs when there are residual stress raisers in the bone from previous surgical procedures. This occurs, for example, in the forearm after removal of plates and screws.

Cartilage

Cartilage was once considered an inert tissue but is now recognized as having an ongoing metabolism. Because this tissue is avascular, nutrients are brought into it and waste products are removed by cyclical loading and unloading. The functioning macromolecules produced by the chondrocytes are proteoglycans and collagen. In cartilage, the proteoglycans are grouped into highly compressed "sponges" contained within a complex and tight collagen wrapper. The constraint of these compressed proteoglycan molecules produces the stiffness of the cartilage. Metabolic loss of proteoglycans or their constraining collagen, or both, results in the loss of cartilage stiffness (chondromalacia) and fissuring. In addition to the loss of cartilage nutrition, immobility can lead to direct growth of adhesions from the synovium to the cartilage.

The treatment of cartilage consists of motion and loading. Surgical considerations may limit the range of motion or loading. Compromise is often achieved by using a brace to limit the patient to a safe range of motion; thus, the only load on the cartilage may be from adjacent muscle rather than the higher load of weight-bearing. Continuous passive motion (CPM) machines can also be used to produce motion within a safe range, if the use of the muscles is proscribed.

Because cartilage has a slow metabolic rate, the effect of various therapeutic manipulations is difficult to study. It therefore is difficult to know how much loading or motion is the necessary minimum, or the effect of medicines such as nonsteriodal anti-inflammatory drugs (NSAIDs). This is an area that future studies will address.

Soft Tissues

The soft tissues considered here include bursa, capsule, skin, tendons, and ligaments. The principal cell in all of these tissues is the fibroblast, which produces collagen. Collagen is a major structural protein that forms strong, flexible, inelastic structures. In general, soft tissues are composed of layers of collagen, arranged according to applied stresses, with interposed fat cells or layers of proteoglycans. A decrease in motion leads to decreased collagen strength, loss of fiber orientation, and loss of proteoglycans. Cross-binding between layers of collagen occurs and cause stiffness of the tissues (Fig. 21-4). Corticosteroids decrease collagen production. The effects of NSAIDs are unknown.

Immobilization (which is a decrease in the applied stress) leads to a decreased synthesis of the functioning macromolecules. In addition, there is a loss of proper orientation of collagen molecules and bridging between layers. This decrease in strength and increase in stiffness may be compounded by trauma or a reaction to a surgical procedure with associated edema. In addition, wounds have a tendency to heal in continuity—that is, a single layer of healing tissue from the skin down to the deepest portion of the wound. This continuity of healing decreases the mobility of the soft tissue.

Perhaps the simplest, most thoroughly studied, and among the most frequently injured of the soft tissues are the ligaments and tendons. Tendons are parallel arrays of collagen fascicles that are designed to efficiently transmit forces generated by muscle to bone. Ligaments are designed to maintain and guide the

1. Stiffness effect of adhesions

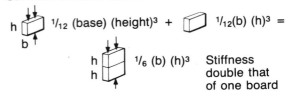

2. With adhesions

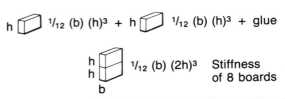

Fig. 21-4. Diagram illustrating how small losses in tissue lubrication produce large increases in stiffness. In 1, two rectangular load-bearing elements resembling boards that might be used in carpentry are used to illustrate the point. When placed one on top of the other the boards produce a stiffness double that of either board alone. However, if the two boards become adherent to each other (as in 2), so that one board has twice the height, instead of doubling the stiffness this stiffness really becomes 8 times as great under the same loading conditions.

alignments of articulations. Tendons and ligaments exemplify the weakness-stiffness response to immobility. They have a slow response (months) to restored activity, in comparison to the quick decline (weeks) in material properties in response to immobility (Fig. 21-5).

Tendons and ligaments are attached to tissues with a higher rate of metabolism (i.e., muscle and bone). This becomes another limiting factor in rehabilitation because transition points between different materials are frequent sites of failure. Therefore, the limitations on the ligaments may delay the rehabilitation of the muscles.

Treatment of soft tissue consists of several modalities, the most important of which is motion. Motion tends to promote the production and orientation of collagen and the production of proteoglycans. In addition, motion guides the healing of the various layers so that they are able to move independently of each other. Types of motion include active motion within a protected range of motion, intermittent passive motion, or CPM. Motion is particularly important for

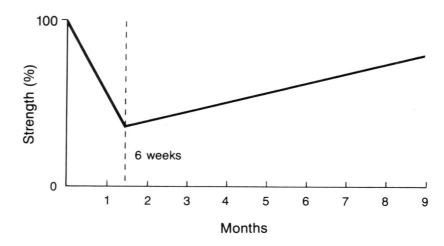

Fig. 21-5. Response of musculoskeletal tissues to applied stimuli. Six weeks of immobilization produces such a large loss in strength of tissues that even at 9 months after restoration of activities the strength has not been fully recovered.

tendons and ligaments. CPM may be more effective than intermittent passive motion to maintain or increase the rate of motion. This is an area currently undergoing investigation.

Stretching or joint mobilization may be necessary if there is tightness of, or adhesions in, the soft tissues. Stretching is done by applying constant pressure at the end of the ROM, and the stretched position is held for a period of 15 to 30 seconds. Joint mobilization is typically directed toward capsular or ligamentous tissue. The goals of joint mobilization can be to stretch the tissue, increase the range of motion, decrease pain, or alleviate adhesions. There are many schools of thought for joint mobilization, which offer slightly different techniques.

Techniques used in the treatment of soft tissues include the local application of heat or cold, electrical stimulation, massage, compression, and elevation.

Heat can be applied superficially or deeply. The simplest way is to heat the surface of the involved area; the underlying structures are then heated in proportion to their proximity to the skin. The other form is deep heating, which uses either electromagnetic heating or sound waves (ultrasound). The goals of heat are to increase local metabolism, local circulation, and the elasticity of fibrous material, and to produce a local analgesia. Unfortunately, heat also increases the formation of edema. Thus, heat is only used once the acute injury phase has subsided. Increased local metabolism produces local consump-

tion of oxygen, activity of leukocytes and other phagocytes, and axonal reflex activity. Increased circulatory effects involve the arteries, capillaries, veins, and lymphatics, with the subsequent delivery and removal of metabolic materials. This also includes an increase in capillary permeability. Heat is contraindicated in cases of poor sensation, poor thermal regulation, or malignancy.

Cold can be used in the first 48 hours after surgery or trauma and after the acute phase of injury. Cold is administered superficially and has an effect similar to that of heating in terms of being a local anesthetic. However, it has effects opposite those of heating in many other ways. It decreases the local metabolic rate, probably through its effect on enzyme kinetics. The blood vessels become constricted, collagen becomes stiffer, and inflammation is delayed, which is the reason cold is used instead of heat in the acute phase of injury.

Electrical stimulation is used to resolve edema, stimulate healing, decrease pain, and drive ions into the tissues (iontophoresis). The effects of electrical stimulation on soft tissues can be physiologic, chemical, or thermal. The tissue responds to the electrical current similarly to the manner in which it normally functions and grows. The degree of benefit of electrical stimulation depends on the intensity, duration, waveform, modulation, and polarity of the current as well as the specific physiologic response characteristics of the individual tissue.

Compression, massage, or elevation of the involved limb may be therapeutically indicated for soft tissues. Postoperative or postinjury compression helps to limit edema and may provide some comfort. Adherent soft tissue may be massaged to restore the movement between tissue layers. The extremity is elevated to help drain fluid centrally.

Muscular Tissue

Muscular tissue can be categorized as a soft connective tissue and treated as such. However, because of its importance in sport and the specificity of its rehabilitation, it is treated separately here.

Muscle tissue is designed to contract and thereby move other tissues and organs. Skeletal muscle differs from smooth muscle in that it is striated and moves the bony levers. The cellular units of the muscle (called the muscle fibers) are grouped into bundles called fasciculi. The amount of strength, the fatigability, and the blood supply vary for different types of fibers. The two basic categories, at either end of the spectrum, are slow twitch and fast twitch. The slow twitch fibers are of low intensity and high endurance, with high oxidative and low glycolytic characteristics. The fast twitch fibers are of high intensity, with rapid fatigability and high glycolytic and low oxidative properties. The slow twitch fibers are most receptive to endurance training, which produces an increase in mitochondrial numbers; the fast twitch fibers are responsive to strength or power training, which increases the amount of actin and myosin in the cells. A given muscle will have many different types of fibers, yet different muscles will have different proportions of high and low oxidative characteristics. Thus, sometimes a muscle is referred to as a endurance muscle or a strength muscle.

Muscle contraction adapts to (1) the speed of motion, (2) the ROM over which it is exercised, (3) the direction (muscle shortening versus lengthening), (4) the amount of external resistance, (5) the need for endurance, and (6) the coordination and timing with other joints and muscles. All of these adaptation characteristics must be taken into consideration when developing a rehabilitation program.

When the muscle is the injured tissue, some bleeding may occur into the tissue. If it is a mild contusion or strain, the damage is kept to a minimum because there has been no actual derangement of the fibers, and the elasticity of the fibers is maintained. If the injury is severe enough that fibers are destroyed, proliferation of new fibers and regeneration of tissue occurs to some degree. If the tissue is actually severed, healing occurs from ingrowth of granulation tissue. Frequently, however, reinjury occurs with additional hemorrhage. Thus, the rehabilitation program needs to protect the tissue while still stimulating the healing process. Methods such as heat, cold, electrical stimulation, massage, and compression can be used therapeutically in muscular injuries. In addition, because skeletal muscle has a specific response to exercise and because it is the only voluntarily contractile tissue in the body, exercise plays a large role in the return to function.

EXERCISES IN SPORTS MEDICINE

Four basic types of exercise are employed in sports medicine rehabilitation: stretching, strengthening, endurance, and sport-mimicking.

Stretching Exercises

A stretching program takes into consideration the ROM required by the specific athletic activity, the vulnerability of the joints involved with the stretch, and the inherent hyperelasticity or tightness in the individual patient's tissues. For example, a baseball pitcher requires extremes of humeral external rotation during the late cocking phase of the pitch. It is normal to see pitchers with ROM levels of external rotation that are above, and ROM levels of internal rotation that are below, those of the nonoverhand athlete population. Yet the total arc of motion is similar in the two populations. Because of the functional need for external rotation in the pitcher, the therapist and athlete would want it maintained. In addition, the therapist would not stretch in the direction of internal rotation because there is no need for the extra motion.

This brings up the second consideration in stretching: the vulnerability of the joints involved in the stretch. The example of the baseball pitcher is retained, because it focuses on the shoulder. The shoulder is very vulnerable to hypermobility at the expense of stability. Thus, a stretching program would consider this crucial balance. When stretching the shoulder joint, caution must be exerted not to overstretch, and the therapist must also be aggressively involved with strengthening the muscular component of stability.

The inherent hyperelasticity or tightness of the individual patient's tissues is the third consideration in a stretching regimen. An example here is a swimmer. Swimmers are thought to exhibit joint laxity throughout the body. The posture of a swimmer is that of a forward head, forward shoulders, and genu recurvatum. Swimming also requires extremes of shoulder ROM in a repetitious motion. To further stretch the shoulder of a swimmer with inherent hyperelasticity is to ensure an offset of the stability-mobility balance, with ensuing injury. It is not surprising that approximately half of all competitive swimmers will report shoulder discomfort at some point in their careers. Thus, a shoulder stretching program for a swimmer with hyperlax muscles and joints may need to be dropped.

Strengthening Exercises

Strengthening exercises can be done isometrically, isotonically, or isokinetically. The word isometric means "same length"; an isometric contraction is one in which the muscle length does not change, and the limb does not move. Patients in a cast or brace can still perform isometric exercises. Also, isometric exercises may be done safely by persons with an irritated joint because the joint does not move. A common example of this would be a patient with chondromalacia of the patella, for which the isometric exercise is a "quad set." Isometric exercises are often the first kind of exercise in a rehabilitation program. The strength gains with isometric exercise are specific to isometric contractions, and at only a given position with little spillover into other types of activity.[1]

If a patient can move through a ROM, isotonic exercises may begin. Isotonic means "same tone or force." These are exercises done against a constant resistance. An example is lifting free weights, such as in the forearm curl. The external force (the weight) is constant. The exercises can be done eccentrically (while the muscle is lengthening) or concentrically (while the muscle is shortening). Eccentric contractions produce greater muscle forces than do concentric contractions and therefore have a greater potential for

causing soreness and possibly injury.[2] Thus, concentric contractions may be the desired form early in rehabilitation. However, it is not known how much carryover there is from concentric training to eccentric strengthening. Research is currently being done on this question.

Muscle is most effective at generating force when there is optimum overlap of the actin and myosin. When the muscle is elongated maximally, this overlap and the ability to generate force are lost. In this case, some measured muscle force is actually tension in the collagen framework of the muscle. When the muscle is completely shortened there is little room for further complexing of the actin and myosin, and strength is lost. Also, the line of application of the external weight relative to the joint changes throughout the ROM, which in turn changes the extension moment that must be resisted (Fig. 21-6). In effect, this is changing the resistance throughout the ROM; likewise, the muscle effort needed changes throughout this range. In addition, the maximum external force that can be moved (i.e., the weight) is only that which is allowed by the weakest part of the range. Thus, the greatest strength gain will be at the weakest part of the range. If there is a portion of the ROM that is painful, the pain will limit the amount of external weight and thus the strength gains. To accommodate for this, "variable resistance" forms of isotonic exercise have been developed. Companies such as Nautilus and Universal have built machines on this concept. However, even the variable resistance machines are specific to isotonic exercise — that is, the maximum benefit is in the performance of isotonic exercise.[1] There is little replication in these exercises of the high speed, timing, and coordination of muscle firing as is seen in athletic events.

Isokinetic means "same speed." An isokinetic contraction is one in which the joint moves through the ROM at a constant speed, and the resistance varies. Proprioceptive neuromuscular facilitation (PNF) patterns are a manual way of doing isokinetic exercise. Companies such as Cybex, Biodex, and Kin-Com have developed machines that are used for isokinetic exercise. By keeping the speed constant and the resistance variable with the patient's effort, the patient is able to get through the painful or weak parts of the range with a relatively small amount of resistance,

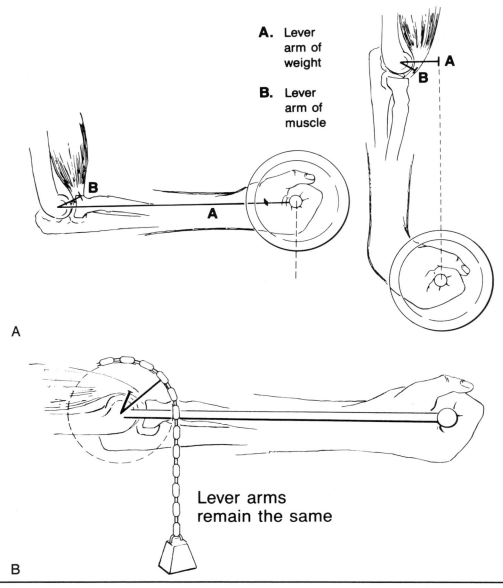

Fig. 21-6. (A) The use of free weights does not apply a constant load to the muscle being stimulated (in this case the brachialis muscle). Although the amount of weight does not change and the lever arm of the muscle changes relatively little in going from the position shown on the left to the position on the right, there is a tremendous change on the lever arm of the free weight. It is this effect that is removed by the pulley system. **(B)** In this case, the patient moves a lever arm that is attached to a wheel with a resistance applied by a weight. Because of the constant radius of the wheel to which the weight is applied, the applied external resistance remains the same. Even in this situation, there is some variability. However, it is all specific to the muscle (i.e., any changes in the lever arm of the muscle and changes in the muscle strength relative to its length-tension curve). The alterations in strength related to the muscle factors have been addressed in some exercise systems by making specific alterations on the lever arm of the applied weight to try to match up the external force to the specific force-generating abilities of the muscles.

and the stronger parts of the range with heavier resistance. In this fashion, the muscle can be strengthened throughout the ROM. Through isokinetic exercise, a patient also can more closely mimic the speeds of the athletic event. However, it must be remembered that even isokinetic exercises of isolated joints do not generate the speeds used in sports.

Endurance Exercises

Once the athlete has adequate strength in the injured muscles, muscular endurance training must commence. By understanding the mechanics of the sport, the health care professional knows which muscles are called on to contract repeatedly. Development of slow twitch fibers is then the goal. For example, during the freestyle swimming stroke, the subscapularis and serratus anterior muscles are constantly active at high levels.[3] Thus, endurance training specific to these muscles is critical. For the serratus anterior, this may consist of using an upper limb ergometer for up to 15- or 20-minute sessions. For the subscapularis muscle, it may consist of isokinetic training on isokinetic equipment for humeral rotation at high speeds. Endurance training on isokinetic equipment is typically quantified by the number of repetitions performed at 30 revolutions per minute (180°/s) before the muscle drops to 50 percent of the original peak torque.[1]

Sport-Mimicking Exercises

After adequate flexibility, strength, and endurance in the muscles are restored, the athlete can return to gentle sport-mimicking exercises. For a runner, this may mean slow jogging over short distances. The health care professional observes the first stages of return to sport to ensure that the timing, coordination, and synchrony of the activity are normal. Any abnormal patterns in the motion necessitate a recall to the training room to develop the deficient component. The road through the rehabilitation process at this point takes much patience; the competitive athlete is returning to a well-loved sport and is zealous to charge forward. The words of Robert Frost must be the quide at this point in the rehabilitation process: "you must learn to work easy in the harness" (Fig. 21-7).

SUMMARY

The continuum of exercises and modalities used in sports rehabilitation was outlined to show the complexities and considerations in developing a program. The appendices of this chapter provide two templates, one for an anterior cruciate ligament reconstruction of the knee, and one for an anterior capsulolabral reconstruction of the shoulder. These are only guides, to demonstrate how these exercises and modalities are blended with the natural history of the patient's healing into a program design. By having the background understanding of the mechanics of sport and the response of tissues, a health care professional can both modify and enhance the rehabilitation programs to the specific needs of the athlete and incorporate new scientific information. The end result is a thought process approach to an effective and efficient rehabilitation program, with the goal of optimal return to the athlete's prior level of functioning.

APPENDIX 1

Rehabilitation Protocol for the Anterior Cruciate Ligament Reconstruction of the Knee

Surgical procedures and rehabilitation protocols for anterior cruciate ligament (ACL) reconstructions have vastly improved in the past few years as the result of intensive research. The focus of this research has been on the graft fixation and failure. In the laboratory, grafts fail at the attachment site at 2 weeks after surgery and fail in the substance at 8 weeks. Thus, in the early phase of rehabilitation, the patient would want to avoid stretching the graft and not use the quadriceps in the first 60° of flexion. The exception would be at full extension, where other structures such as the posterior capsule and menisci resist forward translation of the tibia on the femur. This leg extension is not ballistic, and the tension produced in the graft is a fraction of what good fixation should withstand.

Cartilage, bone, and nonoperated ligaments are not limiting factors in an ACL reconstruction. These tissues must continue to be stimulated by motion throughout the rehabilitation process. The only limi-

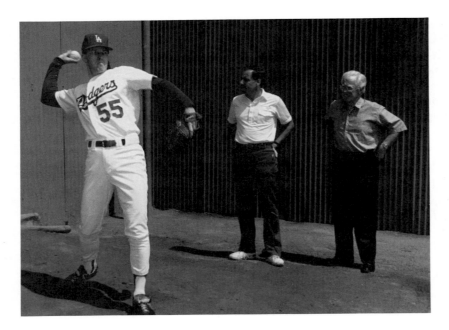

Fig. 21-7. " . . . You must learn to work easy in the harness."

tations to motion are those defined by the graft, swelling, effusion, and patient comfort.

Muscle suffers more quickly than other tissues from lack of use. In addition, the quadriceps mechanism is weakened when the graft is taken from the patellar tendon. The most important limiting consideration in retraining the quadriceps muscle is the potential for repeated stress on the ACL replacement graft.

The following protocol takes into consideration the constraints imposed by the graft, the needs of the nonoperated tissues, and the retraining progression of muscular strength and coordination.

Day 1 to Day 10

- Continuous passive motion (CPM)
  Days 2 to 4 (hospital): While in the hospital, the patient will be instructed in the use of the CPM machine
- Days 4 to 10 (home): 8 to 10 hours per day at the slowest speed (e.g., 1 to 2 cycles/min)

Day 10 to 2 Weeks

- Wall slides
- Isometric hip adduction
- Isometric knee extension ("quad sets") with support
- Isometric knee flexion
- Continue use of CPM 6 to 8 h/day

2 to 6 Weeks

- Hamstring curls
- Hip adduction
- Hip abduction, if there are no patellofemoral tracking problems
- Hip extension
- Heel slides, if there is 120° to 125° of knee flexion
- If the patient is non–weight-bearing or partial weight-bearing, begin ankle plantar flexion with surgical or rubber tubing
- Discontinue CPM at 2 to 4 weeks if able to reach and maintain the maximum available CPM range
- Weight-bearing to tolerance at 2 to 3 weeks with brace locked in 0° extension or as prescribed by physician. Patient gradually progresses in weight-bearing status (e.g., partial weight-bearing with two crutches to single crutch to full weight-bearing)
- Begin stationary bicycle exercises if patient has 115° to 120° of knee flexion
- Short arc quadriceps (with co-contraction of the quadriceps and hamstrings). May be added at 4 to 6 weeks after surgery

1 ½ to 3 Months

- Joint mobilization techniques as needed
- Extension lock is released, allowing flexion during weight bearing
- May begin hip abduction if not started earlier
- Toe raises

3 to 4 Months

- Eccentric quadriceps exercise
- Resisted tibial internal and external rotation, if necessary
- Standing hip flexion

4 to 5 Months

- Step-ups, beginning with 45° to 65° of knee flexion
- May begin isokinetic strength and endurance training
- Running program: Patient should be able to lift 15 lb during short-arc quadriceps exercises prior to beginning the running program; may begin by jogging in place on a trampoline

5 to 6 Months

- May add knee extension from 90° if continuing a progressive resistive weight program (weight is determined by the amount the patient is able to lift in the 0° to 40° range)
- Progress to treadmill running
- First isokinetic strength and endurance test. First stability test

6 to 7 Months

- Continue running program:
  Progress to treadmill running for 10 to 15 minutes at 6 to 8 min/mile and 3 to 5 percent grade; progress to outdoor running

7 to 8 Months

- Progress in running program. Begin agility drills when able to run 2 to 3 miles; agility drills include lateral and backward running, vertical jumping, jumping rope, stair climbing, high knee drills, and figure-eight running

8 to 9 Months

- Begin practicing the drills of the sport
- Second isokinetic strength and endurance test; second stability test

APPENDIX 2

Rehabilitation Protocol for the Anterior Instability of the Shoulder

Two features of shoulder anatomy are essential to keep in mind in planning a rehabilitation protocol, whether it be after chronic injury or after surgery.

The first is the tremendous reliance of the glenohumeral joint on its rotator cuff musculature for joint stability. All protocols should stimulate the rotator cuff early. The second feature is the wide range of shoulder positions in which there is no passive tension on the capsular structures. This has two important implications for shoulder rehabilitation: (1) much of the range of motion of the shoulder can be used by the therapist without applying traction to an injured or surgically manipulated joint capsule; and (2) the patient also has a tremendous capacity for developing contracture, because the full range of motion of the capsule may not be used after injury or operation. The very existence of this available range demands that it be used.

Overstretch of the capsular structures without sudden trauma is a common source of shoulder pain in the young athlete. This overstretch results from fatigue of the muscles of the rotator cuff during sports activity. The athlete then comes to rely on the capsule for stability, and this reliance produces the stretch on the capsule. Continued activity such as this leads to subluxation of the joint. This in turn will cause pain and irritation of the rotator cuff, especially in the abduction–external rotation position, and, if it is allowed to continue, may lead to rotator cuff tear. In daily routines the athlete walks the narrow line between loss of range of motion and overstretch of the capsule. This is the same narrow range goal sought by the therapist who is rehabilitating a shoulder after the anterior capsulolabral reconstruction (ACLR).

In the ACLR the surgeon has sought to reattach the ligament to the glenoid and reduce the "capacitance" of the anterior inferior capsule (i.e., its ability to accept a volume of humeral head) without shortening the ligament, which would limit range of motion. In addition, dissection is carried out between muscles (e.g., deltopectoral groove) or in a muscle-splitting fashion (e.g., subscapularis). No muscle or attachment is divided. As a result only three areas of healing are of concern: (1) healing of ligament and labrum to underlying bone, (2) healing of capsule to itself where it is overlapped, and (3) healing of capsule to the overlying subscapularis muscle to re-establish the correct connection between muscle and ligament.

The postoperative rehabilitation begins with early mobilization through a large range of motion that will not produce tension in the repair, and a resting position in a splint that allows attachment of the subscapularis muscle to the anterior capsule in an noncontracted position. The patient progresses with healing from this protected rest position and range-of-motion exercises to greater range of motion as healing progresses. As the dynamic protection of the shoulder proceeds the muscle exercises advance in resistance, speed, and need for coordination.

0 to 2 Weeks

- Splint: Patient is immobilized in an abduction splint at 90° of abduction in the scapular plane and 45° of external rotation
- Active shoulder range of motion (ROM): The abduction splint should be removed twice a day for active shoulder ROM exercises with the help of a physical therapist; external rotation is performed in 30° of horizontal adduction; do not force external rotation beyond tolerance; abduction in the scapular plane can be done above 90° to tolerance with external rotaton
- Isometric shoulder exercises and ball squeeze
- Active resistive elbow, forearm, and hand exercises
- Aerobic conditioning, such as the exercise bicycle

2 to 5 Weeks

- Omit splint at 2 weeks
- Active ROM exercises: Continue with emphasis on protecting the anterior capsule
- Active assistive ROM exercises: Progress to wand exercises and wall climbs
- Mobilization: Gentle mobilization of the shoulder as needed; watch for posterior capsule tightness
- Active resistive exercise: Shoulder flexion, extension, abduction to 90°, scapular plane abduction (arms in 30° of forward flexion, thumbs down) above 90°
- Active resistive exercise to the scapular rotators
- Continue with aerobic conditioning

6 to 8 Weeks

- Continue with progressive resistive exercises: Emphasis on the rotator cuff, but including the scapular rotators (such as the trapezius and serratus anterior), positioning muscles (the deltoids), and gentle resistance for the power muscles (pectoralis major and latissimus dorsi). Full ROM should be attained by the end of 8 weeks.

- Scapular synchrony: Observe bilateral scapular motion during planar and functional movements; if any asymmetrical motions are noted, reinforce the exercises to strengthen the deficient motion; do not progress to more advanced motions until symmetrical and synchronous scapular motion is achieved
- Isokinetics: May begin upper extremity internal and external rotation isokinetic exercise at speeds of 90°/s and 120°/s with the arm in 15° to 20° of forward flexion to protect the anterior joint capsule
- Posterior and inferior capsule stretching: Check the posterior and inferior capsule to ensure that it allows adequate excursion of the humerus; if the posterior capsule is tight, it can push the humerous too far forward, thus damaging the anterior components; if the inferior capsule is tight, it can cause scapular winging as the arm is raised

2 to 4 Months

- Continue with progressive resistive exercises
- Continue with aggressive aerobic conditioning
- Continue with exercises for scapular synchrony
- Isokinetics: May progress to faster speeds (e.g., 200°/s or more) for shoulder internal and external rotation (the shoulder is still positioned in 15° to 20° degrees of flexion); may also begin shoulder flexion and abduction at speeds of 90°/s and 120°/s
- Push-up with a plus: Add push-ups, lowering the body until the arms are level with the trunk; begin with wall push-ups, progressing to modified (on the knees) and then military push-ups (on the toes); at the top of the push-up, and extra "push" is given, thus causing scapular protraction (an excellent exercise for the serratus anterior); the arms are positioned at 80° to 90° of abduction; do not lower the body so much that the arms go past the body, which would stress the anterior capsule

4 to 6 Months

- Continue with progressive resistive exercise: Emphasis on the muscles needed for sport-specific activity
- Continue with aerobic conditioning
- Continue with isokinetics: At both low and high speeds (i.e., 90°, 120°, and 200°/s)
- Isokinetic strength test: Each plane of movement (i.e., rotation, abduction, flexion) is tested on a different day
- Sport-specific activity: Begin with gentle velocities if isokinetics test indicates adequate strength and endurance (80 percent or more as compared with the uninvolved shoulder); once again, watch for smooth scapular motion during the sport activity

REFERENCES

1. Drez DJ (ed): Therapeutic Modalities for Sports Injuries. Year Book Medical Publishers, Chicago, 1989
2. Strauber WT, Clarkson PM, Fritz VK, Evans WJ: Extracellular matrix disruption and pain after eccentric muscle action. J Appl Physiol 69:868, 1990
3. Pink M, Perry J, Jobe FW et al: The normal shoulder during freestyle swimming: an EMG and cinematographic analysis of eight muscles. Presented at the American Academy of Orthopaedic Surgeons Annual Meeting, AOSSM Specialty Day, 1991

SUGGESTED READINGS

Adeyanju K, Crews TR, Meadors WJ: Effects of two speeds of isokinetic training on muscular strength, power and endurance. J Sports Med 23:352, 1983

Arendt EA: Strength development: a comparison of resistive exercise techniques. Contemp Orthop 9:67, 1984

Berger RA: Effect of varied weight training programs on strength. Res Q 33:168, 1962

Campbell DE, Glenn W: Rehabilitation of knee flexor and knee extensor muscle strength in patients with meniscectomies, ligamentous repairs, and chrondromalacia. Phys Ther 62:10, 1982

Costill DL, Coyle EF, Fink WF et al: Adaptations in skeletal muscle following strength training. J Appl Physiol 43:96, 1979

Costill DL, Fink WJ, Habansky AJ: Muscle rehabilitation after knee surgery. Phys Sports Med 5:71, 1977

Coyle EF, Feiring DC, Rotkis TC et al: Specificity of power improvements through slow and fast isokinetic training. J Appl Physiol, 51:1437, 1981

DeLorme TL: Restoration of muscle power by heavy resistance exercises. J Bone Joint Surg 27:645, 1945

DeLorme TL, Watkins AL: Techniques of progressive resistance exercise. Arch Phys Med 29:263, 1948

Dickinson A, Bennett KM: Therapeutic exercise. Clin Sports Med 4:417, 1985

Fischer E, Solomon S: Physiological responses to heat and cold. p. 126. In Licht S (ed): Therapeutic Heat and Cold. E Licht Publisher, New Haven, 1965

Foran B: Advantages and disadvantages of isokinetics, variable resistance and free weights. NSCA J 7:24, 1985

Frank C, Akeson WH, Woo SL-Y et al: Physiology and therapeutic value of passive joint motion. Clin Orthop 185:113, 1984

Gelberman RH, Vande Berg JS, Lundborg GN, Akeson WH: Flexor tendon healing and restoration of the gliding surface. J Bone Joint Surg [Am] 65:70, 1983

Gettman LR, Cutler LA, Strathman TA: Physiologic changes after 20 weeks of isotonic vs isokinetic circuit training. J Sports Med 20:265, 1980

Grimby G: Progressive resistance exercise for injury rehabilitation: special emphasis on isokinetic training. Sports Med 2:309, 1985

Kellet J: Acute soft tissue injuries: a review of the literature. Med Sci Sports Exerc 18:489, 1986

Knapik JJ, Mawdsley RH, Ramos MV: Angular specificity and test mode specificity of isometric and isokinetic strength training. J Orthop Sports Phys Ther 5:58, 1983

Knight KL: Guidelines for rehabilitation of sports injuries. Clin Sports Med 4:405, 1985

Knowlton GC, Bennett RL: Overwork. Arch Phys Med 38:18, 1957

Lander JE, Bates BT, Sawhill JA et al: A comparison between free-weight and isokinetic bench pressing. Med Sci Sports Exerc 17:344, 1984

Lehmann SF, deLateur BJ: Therapeutic heat. p. 404. In Lehmann JF (ed): Therapeutic Heat and Cold. 3rd Ed. Williams & Wilkins, Baltimore, 1982

Lehmann SF, deLateur BJ: Cryotherapy. p. 563. In Lehmann JF (ed): Therapeutic Heat and Cold. 3rd Ed. Williams and Wilkins, Baltimore, 1982

Lehmann SF, Warren CG, Scham SM: Therapeutic heat and cold. Clin Orthop 99:207, 1974

Lind M: Increase of muscle strength from isometric quadriceps exercises at different knee angles. Scand J Rehabil Med 22:33, 1979

MacConaill MA, Basmajian JV: Muscles and Movements: A Basis for Human Kinesiology. p. 421. Williams & Wilkins, Baltimore, 1969

McMaster WC, Liddle S: Cryotherapy: an influence on posttraumatic limb edema. Clin Orthop 150:283, 1980

McMorris RO, Elkins EC: A study of production and evaluation of muscular hypertrophy. Arch Phys Med 35:420, 1954

Meeusen R, Lievens P: The use of cryotherapy in sports injuries. Sports Med 3:398, 1986

Michlovitz SL, Wolf SL: Thermal Agents in Rehabilitation. FA Davis, Philadephia, 1986

Moffroid MT, Whipple RH: Specificity of speed of exercise. Phys Ther 50:1692, 1970

Noyes FR, Torvik PJ, Hyde WB et al: Biomechanics of ligament failure. J Bone Joint Surg [Am] 56:1406, 1974

Paulos L, Noyes FR, Grood E, Butler DL: Knee rehabilitation after anterior cruciate ligament reconstruction and repair. Am J Sports Med 9:140, 1981

Prentice WE: Therapeutic Modalities in Sports Medicine. CV Mosby, St. Louis, 1986

Rosentsweig J, Hinson E, Hinson M: Comparison of isometric, isotonic and isokinetic exercise by electromyography. Arch Phys Med Rehabil 53:32, 1972

Rozier CK, Elder JD, Brown M: Prevention of atrophy by isometric exercise of a casted leg. J Sports Med 19:191, 1979

Salter RB, Bell RS, Keeley FW: The protective effect of continuous passive motion on living articular cartilage in acute septic arthritis. Clin Orthop 159:223, 1981

Salter RB, Simmonds DF, Malcolm BW et al: The biological effect of continuous passive motion on the healing of full-thickness defects in articular cartilage. J Bone Joint Surg [Am] 62:1232, 1980

Seitz LM, Kleinkort JA: Low-power laser: its applications in physical therapy. p. 217. In Michlovitz SL (ed): Thermal Agents in Rehabilitation. FA Davis, Philadelphia, 1986

Smith MJ: Muscle fiber type: their relationship to athletic training and rehabilitation. Clin Sports Med 4:179, 1985

Smith MJ, Melton P: Isokinetic versus isotonic variable-resistance training. Am J Sports Med 9:275, 1981

Yacksaw L, Adams C, Francis KT: The effects of ice massage on delayed muscle soreness. Am J Sports Med 12:159, 1984

22 Motion Analysis: Lower Extremity

DAVID H. SUTHERLAND
KENTON R. KAUFMAN

Musculoskeletal function cannot be fully understood without studies of movement. The modern motion analysis laboratory that has evolved from this realization now has the potential of opening new avenues of progress in the treatment of disorders of the musculoskeletal system. Every health professional dealing with such disorders must evaluate and treat the patient on the basis of assumptions made about the relative contributions of central nervous system malfunction, weak or spastic muscles, joint contractures, and bony deformities in gait. If methods to make measurements were not available, the time-honored arts of visual gait observation, physical examination, and manual muscle testing would have to suffice and professionals would, of necessity, have to act on what they have learned from their own observations or follow treatment algorithms handed on by others. Many centers now have laboratories and skilled personnel to carry out scientific study rather than rely on intuition and assumptions. If scientific progress is to continue, the already existing gait facilities should be utilized and others should be developed so that the majority of patients who could profit from a quality study can be accommodated. At the same time, it is imperative that these laboratories be staffed by trained professionals whose skills are constantly honed by regular clinical studies, research activities, and interlaboratory collaboration. Is it unreasonable to anticipate that the data and videos of complicated gait cases will be reviewed in several centers, just as the slides of pathologic tissue are often sent to multiple pathologists for interpretation? This is already occurring to some degree. Rapid transmis-

sion of data is made possible by linking computer terminals by modem.

EQUIPMENT AND METHODS

The necessary ingredients for a successful motion analysis laboratory are institutional support, committed space, trained personnel, and proper equipment. Institutional support is required for the expenses of establishing and maintaining the laboratory until patient revenues and grant support offset operating expenses. The cost of establishing our laboratory and the first updating of equipment was provided by individual donors, organizations, and charitable foundations. This has been the most common initial funding means throughout the United States, because few hospitals or universities have capital equipment budgets with sufficient flexibility to incorporate major acquisitions of the magnitude involved. To this time, few, if any, of the gait laboratories have directly produced revenue over costs from clinical studies alone. However, if the referral of patients to the institution and the income from related services are considered, the financial impact has been offset. Current improvements in computer hardware and software are reducing the labor requirements for processing data, which, in turn, allows greater efficiency and permits accommodation of more patients. These factors improve the financial viability of a clinical laboratory.

Committed space is required to house the equipment so that unnecessary setup time is not consumed in performing studies. This space can be partitioned into an examining room, the laboratory itself, a repair room, and office space for personnel. The examining room for patients needs to be located close to a hallway where clinical observations of gait may be made. The laboratory should be wide enough so that cameras can be placed on either side of the walkway. This is necessary for the conduction of bilateral studies. A separate repair room is needed for routine maintenance of equipment and storage of supplies. Dedicated office space is required for personnel to perform data reduction and analysis and write patient reports.

To be successful, gait analysis requires an interdisciplinary approach, employing personnel with expertise in orthopaedics, engineering, physical therapy, and kinesiology. An engineer (or more than one) is needed to set up and maintain the equipment, since many of the applications are custom designed. The engineer also is required to establish new methodologies and validate the integrity of the data. A physical therapist is needed to perform clinical assessments of the subject and to assist in the gait study and interpretation of the data. Kinesiologists collect data and carry out data reduction processes. An orthopaedic surgeon, with special skills in gait analysis, interprets the data and makes clinical recommendations. A secretary is needed for patient intake, information, patient billing, and typing of gait reports.

The decision regarding proper equipment is continually changing. Rapid advances are occurring in the technical equipment available, which makes decisions about the purchase of equipment difficult. To make these decisions, a thorough review of current products is necessary. The remainder of this section outlines the major components required for establishment of a gait laboratory.

Movement Measurements

In the biomechanical analysis of motion skeletal segments are studied as rigid links moving through space, which are interconnected through a series of frictionless joints. Measurement systems that are aimed at capturing the spatial trajectories of body segments usually involve a camera system that tracks a series of body-fixed markers. Using stereophoto-grammetric principles, the planar projections of markers at each camera are used to reconstruct the spatial coordinates of each marker. The derivation of segmental kinematics (i.e., linear position and angular orientation) necessary to document the motion of the body segments has been done in most cases by attaching the markers to anatomic landmarks and using geometric assumptions to characterize the spatial motion of given limbs.

A typical kinematic analysis consists of four distinct phases — data collection, tracking, computation, and presentation of the results. Data collection is the only phase that is not computerized. In this phase, video recordings of an activity are made using two or more cameras. We currently use five cameras (Fig. 22-1) to obtain bilateral movement measurements. A few restrictions apply: (1) all cameras must record the action simultaneously to provide synchronization, (2) the cameras must not move between the recording of calibration points and the recording of the activity, and (3) the activity must be clearly seen throughout its duration from at least two cameras. Prior to the gait study, the measurement volume must be calibrated by accurately establishing the location of at least six fixed, non-coplanar points visible from each camera view (calibration points). These points need not be present during the activity as long as they can be seen before the activity. Usually they are provided by some object or apparatus of known dimensions that is placed in the general area of the activity, recorded, and then removed.

These rules for data collection allow great flexibility in the recording of an activity. Information about the camera location and orientation, the distance from camera to subject, and the focal length of the lens is not needed. The image space is "self-calibrating" through the use of calibration points that do not need to be present during the actual performance of the activity. A method commonly applied to obtain high precision three-dimensional object space reconstruction is the conventional direct linear transformation approach.[1,2] "Two modified DLT algorithms also have been presented that improve the accuracy of three-dimensional object space reconstruction by almost an order of magnitude when compared with conventional methods."[3]

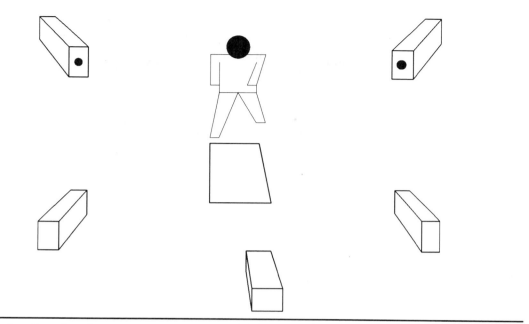

Fig. 22-1. Location of motion measurement cameras in laboratory. There are two cameras on each side and one in front to permit bilateral motion measurements.

Tracking of the spatial trajectories of the markers is the second phase of the analysis. In the past this was done by hand digitizing the location of each of the subject's body-fixed markers in each frame of a video image through the use of a digitizing monitor. More recently, two-dimensional (2-D) marker identification has been used to identify the stored marker image points as seen by each camera. In this method, each labeled 2-D image point corresponded to a valid "ray" from each camera. Frame by frame, photogrammetric software then calculated the point of closest proximity of rays from different cameras with the same label. These points were then stored as the three-dimensional (3-D) coordinates of the labeled markers. The disadvantages of this procedure were that the markers had to be identified for each camera in turn, which was time consuming. Second, the 2-D marker image trajectories frequently crossed or passed very close to each other. Although the physical markers were generally well separated in three dimensions, wrong labels could be applied to the markers. Consequently, the 3-D coordinates could be reconstructed erroneously. Currently, several companies have software available that automatically computes 3-D target marker trajectories from 2-D trajectory segments with the target markers. In this

implementation, marker identification in two dimensions is not necessary. The software searches for 3-D ray intersections. The entire process is fully automatic. The 3-D marker trajectories are labeled only once, and points on different trajectories cannot coincide because the data are three-dimensional. Thus, erroneous calculations owing to user misidentification are not possible.

Two types of systems have been used for tracking the 3-D location of these markers in space. The first method uses computer-controlled optical detectors.[4,5] The optical detector is capable of locating reference points (infrared light-emitting diodes [LEDs] pulsed sequentially, miniature incandescent light bulbs, or light reflectors) on an analog photodetector or on an image detector in the sensing unit through a standard television camera lens. The image field can then be scanned by a computer so that the point locations can be digitized and time multiplexed for data reduction. The second system uses retroreflective markers mounted on the subject. This system uses video cameras interfaced to a host computer. The cameras use charge couple device (CCD) image sensors. The CCD components offer highly linear, stable imaging geometry. Thus, simultaneous multimarker sampling at standard to elevated speeds is possible. Furthermore, the relaxing of earlier ambient and background light constraints plus the inherent freedom from errors by spurious marker reflection is possible.

The computation phase of analysis is performed after the 3-D marker trajectories have been calculated. Three or more markers are attached to each limb segment, which is estimated as a rigid object. These markers are located within a coordinate system embedded in each limb segment. Subsequently, the 3-D position of each marker allows for estimation of the position in three dimensions and the angular orientation of each limb segment. Velocities and accelerations are calculated from the displacement data once these data have been suitably smoothed by digital filtering techniques.

The presentation phase of the analysis allows computed results to be viewed and recorded in a number of different formats. Body position and motion can be presented in both still frame and animated stick figures in three dimensions. Multiple stick figures can be displayed simultaneously for comparison purposes (Fig. 22-2). Results can also be reported graphically (Fig. 22-3). Plots of body segment linear and angular displacements, velocities, accelerations, forces, and moments can be produced in a number of format options. In addition, results may also be reported in numerical form.

Forces Platforms

The study of forces involved in human walking (and other motions) is known as kinetics. Force platforms can be used to define the magnitude and direction of the resultant ground reaction force (GRF) applied to the foot by the ground. The measured GRF is the superimposition of two components: (1) the support of the weight of the body, and (2) the forces required for the horizontal, vertical, and lateral accelerations of the body. A piezoelectric force plate contains four piezoelectric triaxial transducers whose output indicates the force exerted by the subject's foot in contact with the plate.[6] The GRF vector is three dimensional and consists of a vertical component plus two shear components acting along the force plate surface. The shear forces are applied parallel to the ground and require friction. These shear forces are usually resolved in the anterior-posterior and medial-lateral directions (Fig. 22-4). Vertical force and shear forces are combined to give a force vector originating at the center of pressure.

Force platforms measure the resultant force applied by the ground to the foot, but they do not describe how the force is distributed across the base of the foot. An additional variable is needed to define the location of this GRF vector. The center of pressure is defined as the point about which the distributed force has zero moment when applied to the foot (Fig. 22-5). It is found by determining the line of action of the forces measured by the platform and calculating where that line intersects the surface of the force platform. The foot is supported over a varying surface area with different pressures at each part. Even if the individual pressures under every part of the foot were known, there would still be the expensive problem of calculating the net effect of all these pressures as they change with time. Attempts have been made to develop suitable pressure measuring shoes, but these devices have been expensive and are capable of measuring vertical forces only.

When the position of this force line with respect to joint center has been established by combining force and movement data, the extrinsic joint moment, which is the product of lever arm and force, plus gravity and inertia can be calculated. This moment is of great importance because in the case of lower extremity muscles acting during load bearing, it determines the requirements for intrinsic force (muscle). For example, when the force line falls behind the knee joint center, quadriceps muscle action is required to prevent knee collapse, and when the force line falls in front of the knee, extension muscle force is not needed.

Electromyography

A tracing of the electrical signal associated with the contraction of a muscle is called an electromyogram (EMG). A biologic amplifier of certain specifications is required for recording of the EMG. The major considerations to be made when specifying the EMG amplifier are (1) gain in dynamic range, (2) input impedance, (3) frequency response, and (4) common

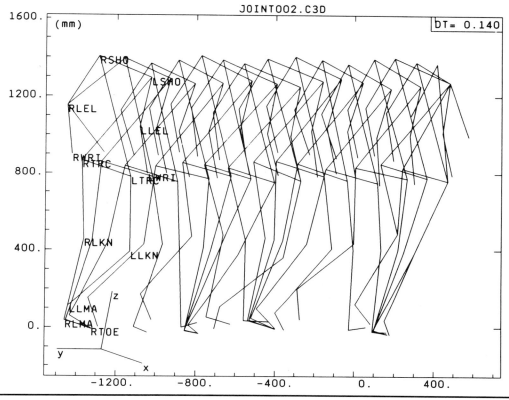

Fig. 22-2. A stick figure diagram of a normal subject walking in the laboratory. Both legs and arms are displayed.

mode rejection ratio. The technical details of these specifications are discussed by Basmajian and De-Luca[7] and by Loeb and Gans.[8]

The two main types of electrodes used in EMG studies are surface electrodes and intramuscular wire electrodes. Surface electrodes usually consist of pairs of metal pads. These are attached to the skin over the muscle to be studied. In some cases, the pads are built into a holder, which ensures consistent spacing between pads and which sometimes contains an amplifier to increase the signal strength (Fig. 22-6). Wire electrodes are made of pairs of fine wire, 50 μm in diameter, and introduced through a single 25- or 27-gauge needle, which is then withdrawn.[7] The wires are insulated except for the tip, which is bare and bent into a hook (Fig. 22-7). When the needle is withdrawn, the electrodes remain hooked in the muscle tissue. The free ends of the fine wires are then connected to the EMG amplifier.

Each type of electrode has its advantages and disadvantages. Surface electrodes are convenient, are easy to apply to the skin, and do not cause pain, irritation, or discomfort to the subject. However, they pick up signals from active muscles in the general area of application. This feature makes surface electrodes the ideal choice for analysis of global activity in superficial muscle or muscle groups. However, surface electrodes are sensitive to movement of the skin under the electrodes and have poor specificity. They are influenced by significant muscle "cross-talk," in which the electrode signals of one muscle interfere with the signals from another.[9] Thus, the activity of adjacent muscle groups can interfere and lead to false results. The major advantage of needle electrodes is selectivity. Needle electrodes can be used to measure the activity of specific muscles in isolation. The influence of electrical activity of nearby muscles is greatly reduced. Nonetheless, a number of disadvantages are associated with needle electrodes. Pain on insertion, the difficulty of accurate placement, wire move-

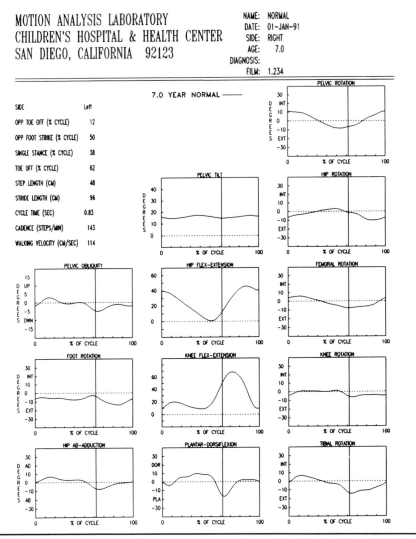

Fig. 22-3. Average dynamic joint angles for the left lower extremity of 46 normal seven-year-old children. The time-distance parameters for this age group are shown in the upper left-hand corner.

ment with muscle contraction, and the need for licensure to utilize wire electrodes are some of the drawbacks. Furthermore, subjects with indwelling electrodes walk more slowly after insertion of the electrodes.[10] Because they are to be inserted into a subject's body, needle electrodes must be sterilized and sufficiently strong to resist breakage.

How are these advantages and disadvantages of surface versus fine-wire electrodes weighed to select the choice of electrodes, and how are the number of

muscles chosen for clinical studies? A study of all of the muscles in the lower extremities by fine-wire electrodes would be optimal but clearly impractical. Commonsense considerations, such as time, expense, pain experienced during a long study, the tolerance of the subject to multiple needle insertions, and the influence of indwelling electrodes on walking, necessitate a selection of the muscles most relevant to the specific movement abnormalities. Large muscles near the surface can be studied well with surface electrodes, whereas small muscles and those surrounded

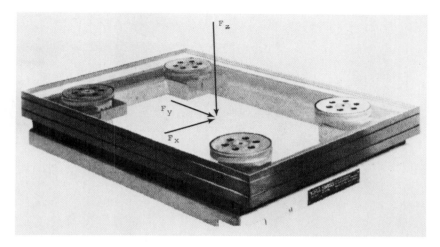

Fig. 22-4. A piezoelectric force plate with a clear top. It is used to measure the ground reaction force and visualize the weight bearing surface of the foot. The triaxial Piezoelectric transducers are located in the four corners of the plate. The ground reaction forces are divided into three components, F_x, F_y, F_z. F_x and F_y are shear forces and F_z is the vertical force.

by other muscles require insertion of fine-wire electrodes, of electrical stimuli must be given to confirm the accuracy of placement. In the authors' laboratory, fine-wire electrodes are seldom used in children under 4 years of age.

The EMG is recorded throughout the gait cycle. The gait cycle is indicated either with synchronization of the kinematic data or with foot-switch information to indicate each foot strike and toe-off. Analysis of the EMG is done by a phase-time plot of the activity of the muscle against events of the gait cycle. There are many difficulties in correlating the EMG signal am-

plitude with muscle force magnitude. Both linear and nonlinear relationships between the force level and skeletal muscles and the EMG signal have been reported.[11-19] Consequently, the EMG is commonly used in clinical practice in gait analysis to determine phasic patterns for individual muscles or muscle groups. It is possible to examine simple on/off patterns,[20] or the EMG can be processed to find a graduation of signal level, after which EMG patterns are examined as defined by the level of activity over the gait cycle.[21-23] In the latter process, it is common to normalize the signal as a percentage of voluntary maximum muscle contraction. The process of detecting when a muscle is "turned on or off" is usually one of testing whether the average level of the signal is above some predefined limit. This limit is often defined as a percentage of the maximum voluntary muscle contraction. The determination of on/off time is often done by calculating the EMG level and then testing for occasions when the level exceeds some threshold value. EMG on/off times are generally more variable from step to step than either kinematic or kinetic gait measurements. A typical EMG pattern for the vastus lateralis is shown in Figure 22-8.

Energy Expenditure

The measurement of energy expenditure is another important function of a motion analysis laboratory. A number of ways of making this measurement are available; however, the method of measuring the oxygen consumed in performing a task sets the standard for comparison of the other methods of

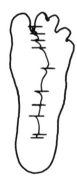

7 y.o.
NORMAL

Fig. 22-5. Progression of the center of pressure for a normal seven-year-old. Each horizontal cross-hatch is drawn by a computer plotter from force plate data at 5 percent intervals in the walk cycle.

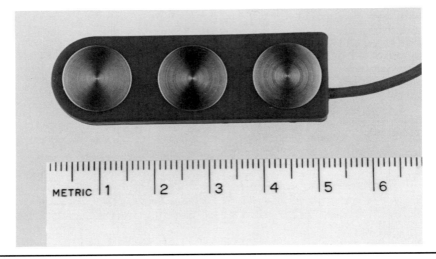

METRIC 1 2 3 4 5 6

Fig. 22-6. Surface EMG electrode. The center disk is the ground and the other two disks are active recording sites.

study.[24,25] Some of these alternative methods include measuring the heart rate, which tends to parallel oxygen consumption,[26] and Cavagnas' technique of measuring work output from force data.[27]

Gait Analysis Flow Chart

Several steps are necessary to conduct a successful gait analysis. These are shown in Figure 22-9. The preanalysis phase consists of two distinct tasks. First, the cameras are calibrated before each study, and certain diagnostic tests are performed on the force plate and EMG equipment to verify that they are operating properly. Next, a pregait study is conducted by a physician and a physical therapist to determine the patient's physical impairments, determine which muscles will be studied with electromyography, and decide whether surface or fine-wire EMG techniques will be utilized. During phase II, anthropometric data are collected from the subject. These data are used to calculate mass and inertial characteristics of the subject. The information is also used in algorithms to locate the true joint centers. Static data acquisitions may also be performed to account for fixed deformities in a subject mathematically. Phase III is the portion of the study in which the patient is asked to walk within the calibrated measurement volume to collect a kinematic, kinetic, and

EMG profile. Many trials are required to achieve at least five runs in which the subject strikes the force plate without altering stride characteristics. Additional trials are also performed for various conditions, such as barefoot walking, shoes, and braces. At the completion of phase III, all raw data have been collected. At least one set of data should be viewed before the patient leaves to determine that the data collection has been successful.

Phase IV is performed after the subject has left. During this phase, the raw data from each camera view are tracked and combined with other camera views to yield the 3-D trajectories of each marker on the subject. The markers are also identified for subsequent analysis. The analog data are synchronized with the marker data. Phase V consists of extensive mathematical calculations to produce the kinematic, kinetic, and EMG data on the subject as a function of the gait cycle. This information is printed out in the form of charts and tables in phase VI and collated into a binder. The physician is then notified that the gait study is ready to be reviewed; review and interpretation of the results of the gait study constitutes phase VII. Recommendations are included with the interpretation. The patient's data and the interpretation are distributed to the patient's chart, the business office, and the referring physician in phase VIII. The

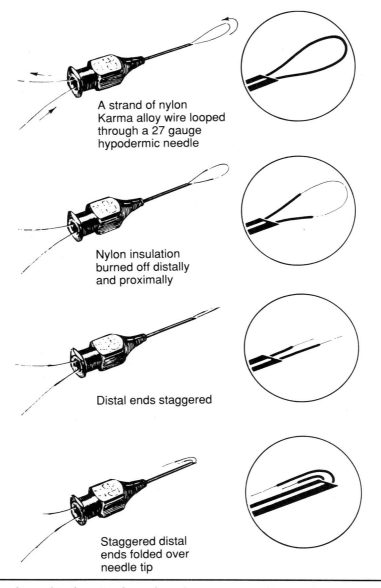

A strand of nylon
Karma alloy wire looped
through a 27 gauge
hypodermic needle

Nylon insulation
burned off distally
and proximally

Distal ends staggered

Staggered distal
ends folded over
needle tip

Fig. 22-7. Steps in making a bipolar wire electrode with its carrier needle used for insertion (From Basmajian,[7] with permission.)

patient data are also archived in a data base for future retrieval and comparison with subsequent studies.

NORMAL VALUES

Normal gait must be clearly understood to appreciate the special features that characterize gait disorders. The basic requirements for walking are as follows:

bones to support the body and to provide attachment to muscles, joints to allow movement between bones, muscles to move the body segments, ligaments to stabilize the joints and guide their movements, sense organs and a central control system to coordinate the action of muscles, and gravity to provoke ground reaction force. Human bipedal walking consists of alternately advancing one lower extremity while

232 / Orthopaedic Rehabilitation

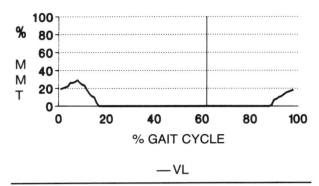

—VL

Fig. 22-8. Myoelectric activity of the vastus lateralis displayed as a function of the gait cycle. The activity is normalized to a maximum manual muscle test. (From J. Perry and the Pathokinesiology Laboratory, Rancho Los Amigos Hospital, Downey, CA.)

supporting the body weight on the other; thus there are two periods of double support in each gait cycle. The center of the mass of the body oscillates minimally as the body is cyclically supported on one limb while the other leg is advanced, due to exquisite energy-conserving mechanisms that have been classically described.[28] The center of mass of the body rises to its highest point near the middle of single-limb stance and falls to its lowest point during double-limb support. In this process, kinetic and potential energy are exchanged.

Kinetic energy is at its lowest level when potential energy is at its highest level (near the middle of single-limb stance). An analogy can be drawn to the action of a pendulum in which kinetic energy is greatest at the bottom of the pendulum swing; in the case of human walking, this is at the initiation of

double support. If walking were entirely energy efficient, potential and kinetic energy levels would be equal over one or many gait cycles. The difference between the two represents the energy expended by the action of muscles, and this principle forms the basis of determining the work output of walking by the method of Cavagna.[27] In the normal mature child or the normal adult, walking at a self-selected pace, the pattern is smooth and energy efficient.[24-26]

A brief list of definitions of terms used in the description of gait will be helpful before normal data are presented.

The *gait cycle* is defined as the movements and events that occur between successive steps with the same foot. In normal subjects the gait cycle begins with heel contact and ends with heel contact of the same foot. Because in pathologic gait the forefoot may make the initial floor contact to begin the gait cycle, the term *foot strike* is used, instead of heel strike, to designate the first event of the gait cycle. *Stance phase* ends with *toe-off*, which initiates the *swing phase*. The *swing phase* ends with foot strike. *Opposite toe-off* and *opposite foot strike* are the other significant gait events, which separate the stance phase into periods of *initial double support, single-limb stance,* and *second double support*. The swing phase is separated into three periods (*initial swing, midswing,* and *terminal swing*) by two events: first, movement of the swinging ankle beyond the opposite standing tibia, and, second, vertical alignment of the swinging tibia. To allow comparisons among subjects, all measurements of the events, phases, and periods of the gait cycle are given as percentages of the total gait cycle.
Phasic muscle activity is the period during the walking cycle when there is EMG activity of a muscle (percentage of gait cycle).

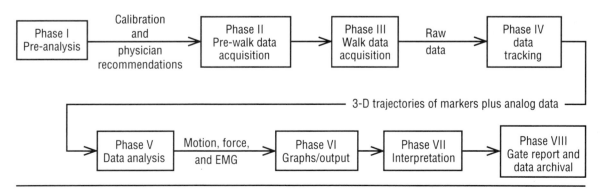

Fig. 22-9. Gait analysis flow chart indicating the steps necessary for completing a gait study.

Step length is the distance between two points, each at the same location on the foot, during double-limb support. *Stride length* is the distance traveled by the same point on the same foot during two successive steps. Therefore, each stride length is composed of one right and one left step length.

Cadence is the number of steps per minute.

Walking velocity is defined as the average distance traveled per second (in centimeters). It is determined by dividing stride length by cycle time or by measuring the time required to walk a measured distance (the latter method is the more accurate).

Joint moment (extrinsic joint torque) is defined mathematically as *force* times the *perpendicular distance* from the action line of the force to the center of rotation of the joint. The moment is composed of gravitational, inertial, and ground reaction forces.

Mean normal values of dynamic joint angles and time-distance parameters (stride characteristics) for age 7 years are shown in Figure 22-3. At age 7 years the joint angles are indistinguishable from those of the adult; in fact, the transition from immature to mature pattern is largely complete by 3 years of age.[20,29] However, stride length, cadence, and walking velocity change with growth beyond 7 years. It is obviously of great importance to compare children's gait measurements with age-related normal values.

APPLICATIONS

Now that some of the principal measurement techniques used in the modern motion analysis laboratory have been outlined briefly, some examples of the application of these methods of study in a rehabilitation setting are given here.

Case 1   Guillain-Barré Syndrome (Beneficial Effects of Bracing)*

Patient C. M. became quadriplegic after having had symptoms of Guillain-Barré syndrome at age 14 years. Over a 19-month period, muscle strength gradually returned to all muscle groups except those below the knees. At the time of the gait study, walking was difficult without ankle support, but with bilateral polypropylene ankle-foot orthoses the patient could walk fairly well. No contractures were present.

---

* From Sutherland,[30] with permission.

Table 22-1. Leg Muscle Strength in Patient C.M.

Muscle	Right Leg[a]	Left Leg[a]
Hip flexors	4+	4+
Gluteus maximum	4+	4+
Gluteus medius	4+	4+
Quadriceps femoris	4+	4+
Hamstrings	4	4
Triceps surae	2	2
Toe extensors	0	0
Tibialis anterior	0	1
Peroneals	0	0

[a] Muscle strength is graded: 0 = Nothing, 1 = Trace, 2 = Can move joint with gravity eliminated, 3 = can move joint through a full range of motion against gravity, 4 = can hold joint against moderate resistance, 5 = normal.

Examination of motor power revealed minor weakness of hip and thigh muscles, but major paralysis was present below the knees (Table 22-1). Gait analysis was done to compare walking with and without propylene ankle-foot orthoses. The goal in the study was to determine the effectiveness of the braces.

Tracings of film from the right-side camera without orthoses (Fig. 22-10A) showed flat foot strike, extended knee during single-limb stance, drop foot, and exaggerated hip flexion in early swing phase. This exaggeration of hip flexion, a compensatory movement for foot drop, is commonly referred to as steppage gait. Film tracings from the right camera with the patient wearing orthoses (Fig. 22-10B) exhibited the following gait improvements: restoration of heel strike, increased step length, and reduction of hyperflexion in the swing phase. Extension of the knee in the stance phase persisted. Film tracings from the front camera of the walk cycle without orthoses (Fig. 22-10C) showed abnormally wide ankle spread. Film tracings from the front camera with the patient wearing orthoses demonstrated diminished ankle spread (Fig. 22-10D).

Significant improvement in walking velocity, cadence, and stride length occurred when orthoses were worn (Fig. 22-10E). Stride length increased from 73 to 106 cm, cadence from 85 to 101 steps/min, and walking velocity from 52 to 89 cm/sec. Pelvic rotation was restored to normal with the orthoses, which also improved anterior pelvic tilt,

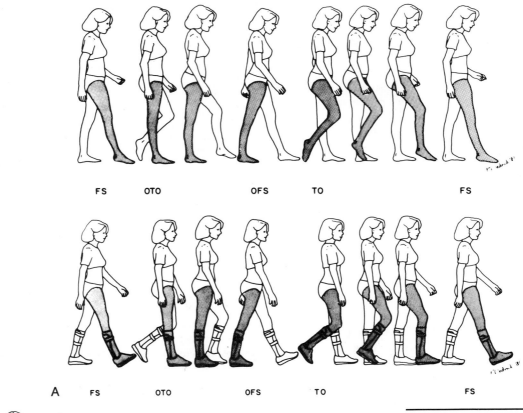

A FS   OTO   OFS   TO   FS

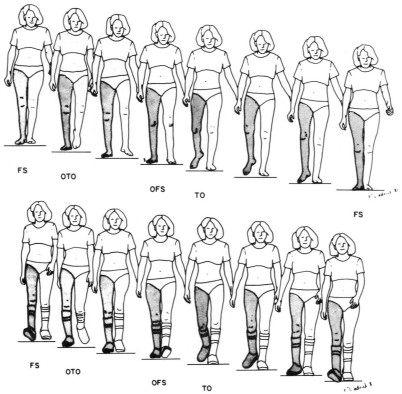

Fig. 22-10. Patient C.M.: Guillain-Barré syndrome. **(A)** Tracings of film from right-side camera, and **(B)** with bilateral ankle-foot orthosis. *(Figure continues.)*

B

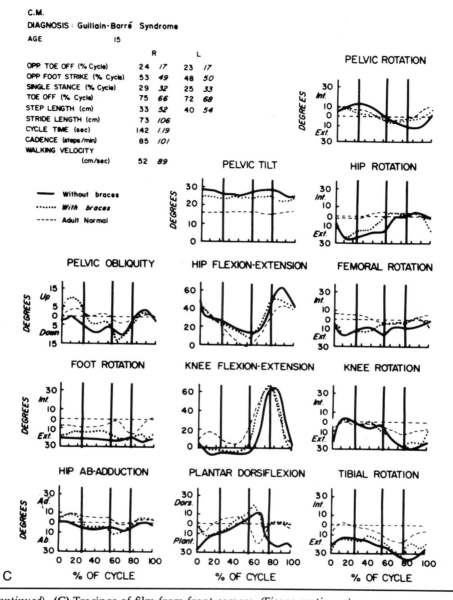

Fig. 22-10 *(Continued).* **(C)** Tracings of film from front camera. *(Figure continues.)*

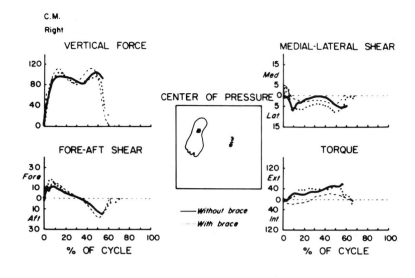

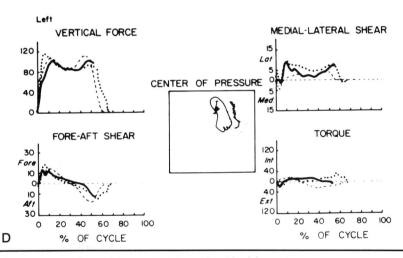

Fig. 22-10 *(Continued).* **(D)** Tracings of film with bilateral ankle-foot orthoses.

corrected hyperflexion of the hip in swing phase, and improved ankle motion. The use of orthoses likewise led to improvements in floor reaction measurements for both lower extremities, (initial loading, forward shear, and lateral shear). The calcaneal pattern of center of pressure progression improved slightly (Fig. 22-10F).

To summarize the findings, this patient with Guillain-Barré syndrome benefited markedly from wearing bilateral ankle-foot orthoses. Drop foot was well controlled, but calcaneal weakness still dominated the pattern and explained her relatively slow gait. The patient's walking velocity and stability might be improved by arthrodesis of the ankle joints. However, she did not find her disability sufficient to consider surgical treatment. She also believed that she was still recovering strength. The recommendation was to continue observation and orthotic management and to change to a more rigid type of ankle-foot orthosis.

Case 2   Proximal Weakness Owing to Limb Girdle Dystrophy*

Patient A. A., a 19-year-old youth with limb girdle dystrophy, had marked weakness and atrophy of the upper arms, hips, and thighs. His abdominal muscles were strong enough to permit him to do multiple sit-ups, but stair climbing and running were difficult. Minimal hip abduction contractures were present. Muscle testing demonstrated gluteus maximum strength of 2+/3 and quadriceps strength of 4−/4−. Film tracings from the side camera showed increased lordosis and posterior alignment of the trunk (Fig. 22-11A). The knee was held in full extension throughout single-limb stance. The increase in lumbar lordosis and the posterior alignment of the trunk maintained the GRF line behind the hip joint, preventing flexion torque (which the weak hip extensors could not resist). The force line was maintained in front of the knee, except in the last portion of single-limb stance, preventing knee flexion torque (which the quadriceps could not resist).

The front camera view showed mild increase in shoulder sway (Fig. 22-11B). Hip, knee, and ankle torque measurements from this subject compared

with normal subjects are shown in Figure 22-11C. In the normal pattern, hip torque begins in flexion and passes to extension at 30 percent of the gait cycle. This subject had a short period of flexion torque, followed by hip extension torque throughout the remainder of the walk cycle. The normal pattern of knee torque begins as flexion, passes to extension at approximately 22 percent of the cycle, and then returns to a final slight flexion torque near 50 percent of the cycle. Note that torques have been plotted only for the period of single-limb stance. In this subject, the extension torque (force line in front of the knee) persisted through the majority of single-limb stance, only changing to flexion torque at the end of the period. This demonstrated a postural adaptation to relieve stress on the weak quadriceps. The principal movement abnormalities, evident in joint angle measurements (Fig. 22-11D) were flat foot strike, rapid hip extension after foot strike, hyperextension of the hip in stance phase, and full knee extension throughout all of the early portion of single-limb stance. Comparison is made with average adult values.

This patient's impairment did not require bracing for quadriceps insufficiency. His weakness had progressed, but the rate of progression was slow. No treatment measures were contemplated at that time, but a baseline status for further observation was established and long-leg braces may be needed in the future. Although attempts to get this patient to return for a repeat gait study have not been successful, his friends state that he is having increasing difficulty with falls and is avoiding physician contact because he is unwilling to consider wearing braces.

Case 3   Stiff Knee Gait in Cerebral Palsy (Effects of Surgical Treatment by Transfer of the Rectus Femoris)*

Patient J. A. was born at 30 weeks' gestation and weighed 1,500 g. The first 2 months of life were spent in the neonatal intensive care unit for complications related to neonatal asphyxia, hypothermia, respiratory distress syndrome, and pulmonary interstitial emphysema. The diagnosis of cerebral palsy and spastic quadriparesis with intellectual and psychomotor delay was made. The patient was seen for or-

---

* From Sutherland,[30] with permission.

* From Sutherland et al,[31] with permission.

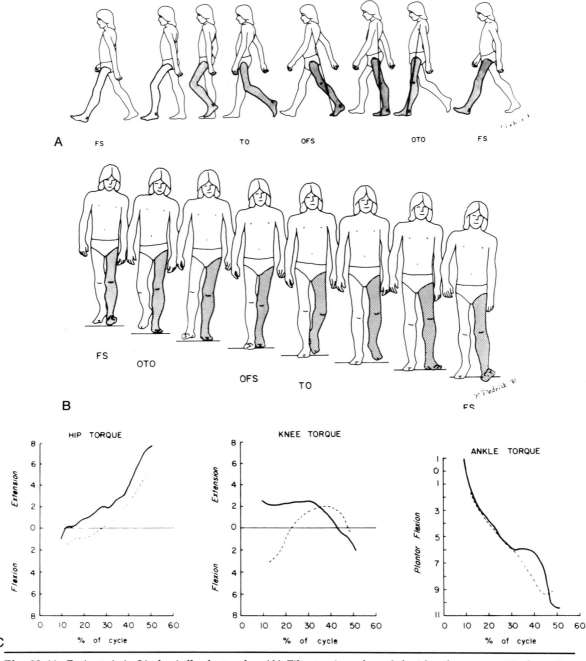

Fig. 22-11. Patient A.A. Limb girdle dystrophy. **(A)** Film tracings from left side of camera with force line superimposed during single limb support. **(B)** Film tracings, frontal view. Cycle proceeds from left to right. **(C)** Hip, knee, and ankle moment compared with mean of normal subjects. Moment values are normalized by adjustment for body weight and height. Thus moment values are unitless. Solid lines = patient A.A. Broken lines = adult normal values. *(Figure continues.)*

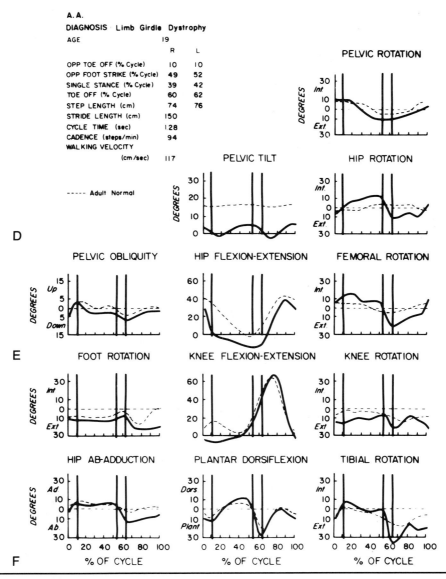

A.A.

DIAGNOSIS Limb Girdle Dystrophy

AGE   19

	R	L
OPP TOE OFF (% Cycle)	10	10
OPP FOOT STRIKE (% Cycle)	49	52
SINGLE STANCE (% Cycle)	39	42
TOE OFF (% Cycle)	60	62
STEP LENGTH (cm)	74	76
STRIDE LENGTH (cm)	150	
CYCLE TIME (sec)	1.28	
CADENCE (steps/min)	94	
WALKING VELOCITY (cm/sec)	117	

----- Adult Normal

Fig. 22-11 *(Continued).* **(D)** Linear measurements and joint angles at 19 years of age. **(E)** Patient C.M. Linear measurements and joint angle measurements with and without braces. Adult normals are given for comparison. **(F)** Patient C.M. Floor reaction forces for right and left lower extremities with and without braces. Adult normal force plate values are given for comparison (broken lines).

thopaedic consultation at age 4 years. Flexion and adduction contractures of the hips were treated with bilateral iliopsoas lengthenings and bilateral adductor transfers. He began to walk with the aid of a rolling walker after surgery. Subsequently, he developed hamstring and equinus contractures that were treated by bilateral distal hamstring lengthenings and tendo Achillis lengthenings at age 5 years.

Stiff-knee gait characterized by circumduction and toe dragging appeared after the hamstring and heel cord operation. The prone rectus test was positive bilaterally, with buttock rise and knee flexion of 65°. Gait analysis was performed to obtain objective data and plan additional treatment. Motion analysis data demonstrated reduced time spent in the swing phase, delayed timing of peak knee flexion, and decreased

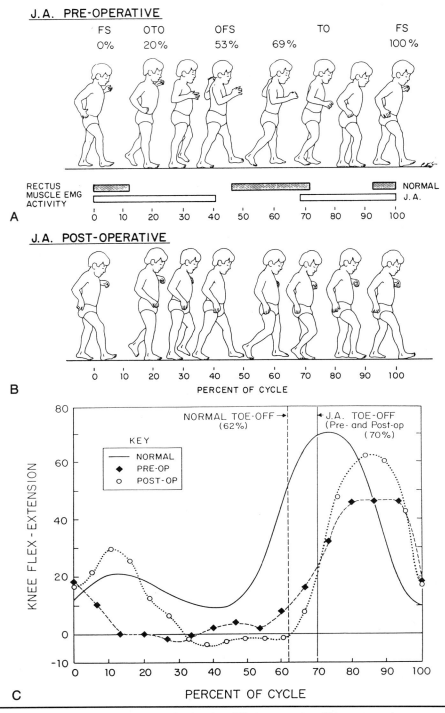

Fig. 22-12. Patient J.A. Stiff knee gait in cerebral palsy. **(A)** Preoperative film tracings from camera at right of right gait cycle. **(B)** Postoperative film tracings from camera at right of right gait cycle 9 months after bilateral transfer of distal rectus to sartorius. **(C)** Knee flexion-extension of right knee before and after surgery with the normal knee for comparison.

magnitude of flexion in the swing phase. These abnormalities were present bilaterally and accompanied by prolongation of rectus femoris EMG activity on the left and abnormal rectus EMG activity on the right in swing phase. Figure 22-12A shows preoperative film tracings of body alignment during right gait cycle and dynamic EMG. Bilateral transfer of the distal rectus to the distal sartorius was performed to improve swing phase knee flexion[31-34] and the postoperative gait was analyzed 9 months after operation. The improvement in right knee flexion in the swing phase after rectus transfer is evident in the postoperative film tracings (Fig. 22-12B) and in the knee flexion-extension joint angle measurements (Fig. 22-12C).

RATIONALE

Although many orthopaedic surgeons have been enthusiastic in referral of patients to gait analysis laboratories, some other surgeons have reacted negatively to the idea of formal studies of individual patients in a laboratory setting, perhaps fearing loss of autonomy in decision making. If this is their objection, it is unwarranted unless their unwillingness to learn the discipline of gait analysis prevents them from making full use of the information or unless the gait studies are interpreted by persons lacking the necessary clinical background to bridge the disciplines of bioengineering, orthopaedic surgery, rehabilitation, physical therapy, and kinesiology.

Another objection sometimes raised by physicians, but seldom by patients, is that the studies are too costly. Such an objection raises the question of "costly compared to what"? The cost is less than that of one day in the hospital or slightly more than a CT scan. It is approximately the same as the cost of a CT scan with 3D reconstruction. The gait study now routinely offered in the most advanced laboratories is not only three-dimensional but dynamic, with measurements of force and EMG included. It takes an average of 2 hours of laboratory time to collect the data and 4 to 8 hours of technician time to prepare the data for analysis. In terms of cost-benefit ratio, the most compelling consideration is the high cost of inappropriate treatment. Is it necessary to be reminded that an operation that is unsuccessful may require subsequent procedures to deal with the original problem, or with unfavorable changes in function

brought about by the surgery? The risk of inappropriate surgery is particularly relevant in treatment of cerebral palsy. There is, of course, no assurance that gait studies prior to operative intervention will always ensure favorable outcome, but careful planning, based on objective data, will provide a foundation for decision making, and postoperative studies will give the information required for objective evaluation of treatment results.

REFERENCES

1. Marzan GT, Karara MM: A computer program for direct linear transformation solution of the colinearity condition and some applications of it. p. 420. In: Proceedings of the Symposium on Close Range Photogrametric Systems. American Society of Photogrametry, Falls Church, VA, 1975
2. Miller NR, Shapiro R, McLaughlin TM: A technique for obtaining spatial kinematic parameters of segments of biomechanical systems from cinemagraphic data. J Biomechan 13:535, 1980
3. Hatze H: High-precision three-dimensional photogrametric calibration and object space reconstruction using a modified DLT approach. Biomechan 21:533, 1988
4. Tandon S, Marsalais EB: Three-dimensional stroboscopic gait analysis. J Bone Joint Surg 57A:574, 1975
5. Conati FC: Real time measurement of three-dimensional multiple rigid body motion. MS Thesis, Massachusetts Institute of Technology, Cambridge, MA, 1977
6. Hawthorne JR, Keller CW, Hagy JL et al: A dynamic force plate. Bone Joint Surg [Am] 55:653, 1973
7. Basmajian JV, DeLuca CJ: Muscles Alive: Their Functions Revealed by Electromyography. p. 223. Williams & Wilkins, Baltimore, 1985
8. Loeb GE, Gans C: Electromyography for Experimentalists. University of Chicago Press, Chicago, 1986
9. Perry J, Easterday CS, Antonelli DJ: Surface versus intramuscular electrodes for electromyography of superficial and deep muscles. Phys Ther 61:7, 1981
10. Young CC, Rose SE, Biden EN et al: The effect of surface and internal electrodes on the gait of children with cerebral palsy, spastic diplegia type. J Orthop Res 7:732, 1989
11. Woods JJ, Bigland-Ritchie B: Linear and nonlinear surface EMG/force relationships in human muscles. Am Phys Med 62:287, 1983
12. Matral S, Casser G: Relationship between force and integrated EMG activity during voluntary isometric and isotonic contraction. Eur J Appl Physiol 46:185, 1977
13. Bigland-Ritchie B, Kukulka CJ, Woods JJ: Surface EMG-force relationships in human muscles of different fibre composition. J Physiol (Lond) 308:103P, 1980
14. Maton B, Bouisset S: The distribution of activity among the muscles of a single group during isometric contraction. Eur J Appl Physiol 37:101, 1972
15. Zuniga EN, Simons DG: Nonlinear relationship between averaged electromyogram potential and muscle tension in normal subjects. Arch Phy Med Rehabil 50:613, 1969
16. Komi PV, Buskirk ER: Effective eccentric and concentric muscle conditioning on tension and electrical activity of human muscle. Ergonomics 15:417, 1972
17. Moritani T, deVries HA: Reexamination of the relationship

between the surface integrated electromyogram (IEMG) and force of isometric contraction. Am J Phys Med 57:263, 1978

18. Lippold OCJ: The relation between integrated action potentials in a human muscle and its isometric tension. J Physiol (Lond) 117:492, 1952

19. Messier RH, Duffy J, Litchman HM et al: The electromyogram as a measure of tension in the human biceps and triceps muscles. Int J Mech Sci 13:585, 1981

20. Sutherland DH, Olshen RA, Biden EN, Wyatt MP: The Development of Mature Walking. MacKeith Press, Oxford, England, 1988

21. Limbird TJ, Shiavi R, Frazer M, Borra H: EMG profiles of knee joint musculature during walking: changes induced by anterior cruciate ligament deficiency. J Orthop Res 6:630, 1988

22. Shiavi R, Green N: Ensemble averaging of locomotor electromyographic patterns using interpolation. Med Biol Eng Comput 21:573, 1983

23. Wooten ME, Kadaba MP, Cochran GUB: Dynamic electromyography. II. Normal patterns during gait. J Orthop Res 8:259, 1990

24. Bard G, Ralston HD: Measurement of energy expenditure during ambulation, with special reference to evaluation of assistive devices. Arch Phys Med Rehabil 40:415-420, 1959

25. Waters RL, Hislop HJ, Thomas L, Campbell J: Energy cost of walking in normal children and teenagers. Dev Med Child Neurol 25:184-188, 1983

26. Rose J, Gamble JG, Medeiros J et al: Energy cost of walking in normal children and in those with cerebral palsy: comparison of heart rate and oxygen uptake. J Pediatr Orthop 9:276, 1989

27. Cavagna GA: Force platforms as ergometers. J Appl Physiol 39:174, 1965

28. Inman VT, Ralston HJ, Todd F: Human Walking. Williams & Wilkins, Baltimore, 1981

29. Sutherland DH, Olshen R, Cooper L, Woo SL: The development of mature gait. J Bone Joint Surg [Am] 62:336, 1980

30. Sutherland DH: Gait Disorders in Childhood and Adolescence. Williams & Wilkins, Baltimore, 1984

31. Sutherland DH, Santi M, Abel MF: Treatment of stiff-knee gait in cerebral palsy: a comparison by gait analysis of distal rectus femoris transfer versus proximal rectus release. J Pediatr Orthop, V 10:433, 1990

32. Sutherland DH, Larsen LJ, Mann R: Rectus femoris release in selected patients with cerebral palsy: a preliminary report. Dev Med Child Neurol 17:26, 1975

33. Perry J: Distal rectus femoris transfer. Dev Med Child Neurol 29:153, 1987

34. Gage JR, Perry J, Hicks RR et al: Rectus femoris transfer to improve knee function of children with cerebral palsy. Dev Med Child Neurol 29:159, 1987

tials in a human muscle and its isometric tension. J Physiol (Lond) 117:492, 1952

23 Motion Analysis: Upper Extremity

MARY ANN E. KEENAN
JACQUELIN PERRY

Persons who have sustained damage to the central nervous system from stroke, traumatic brain injury, or anoxia frequently are left with residual spasticity and impaired motor control.[1-19] In the upper extremity the most common pattern of spasticity is one of flexion. The unmasking of primitive patterning reflexes may further contribute to the motor impairment. Spasticity (hyperactive response to quick stretch), rigidity (resistance to slow movement), or movement dystonias may be present. The extent of motor control in the upper extremity often is not obvious by clinical examination alone.

In addition to the variable combinations and patterns of upper motor neuron lesions, other types of local pathologic conditions may coexist. Static or dynamic limb deformities may result from spastic paralysis. Myostatic contractures, heterotopic ossification, or other bony deformities may be present. Heterotopic ossification is seen in 11 percent of patients with traumatic brain injury and restricts joint motion.[20] Because brain injury frequently occurs in combination with multiple trauma, fractures and dislocations are common. These injuries, however, are missed in 11 percent of cases.[21] Radiographs should be obtained whenever joint movement is limited to detect bony deformities or heterotopic ossification.

Peripheral neuropathy is a second class of impairment to be considered when evaluating motor control.[21,22] A prospective study conducted at Rancho Los Amigos Medical Center revealed that 34 percent of brain-injured patients admitted for acute rehabilitation had one or more peripheral nerve injuries that had not been previously diagnosed.[22] The most common nerve injuries in the upper extremity involve the brachial plexus, the ulnar nerve at the elbow, and the median nerve at the wrist. Brachial plexus injuries are most commonly seen in victims of motorcycle accidents. Any flaccid paralysis in the upper extremity should raise the possibility of a traction injury to the brachial plexus. An associated fracture of the clavicle may also be seen.

Compression of the ulnar nerve within the cubital canal at the elbow most frequently arises as a complication of the flexor spasticity in the upper extremity.[22,23] The elbow is held in tight flexion, resulting in excessive traction on the nerve as it passes behind the medial epicondyle of the humerus. Direct pressure also is placed on the nerve as the patient constantly leans directly on the nerve. Indeed, it is not uncommon to see a decubitus ulcer form directly over the nerve at the elbow. When heterotopic ossification is present at the elbow, the intense inflammatory response and soft tissue induration result in ulnar nerve compression. In many cases the heterotopic bone will completely encase the nerve, but ulnar neuropathy can occur regardless of the location of the heterotopic bone in relation to the elbow joint. Atrophy of the intrinsic muscles of the hand often is the initial presenting sign of the neuropathy.

Compression of the median nerve against the proximal edge of the transverse carpal ligament secondary to a severe spastic wrist flexion deformity is a frequent finding. The spastic finger flexor tendons

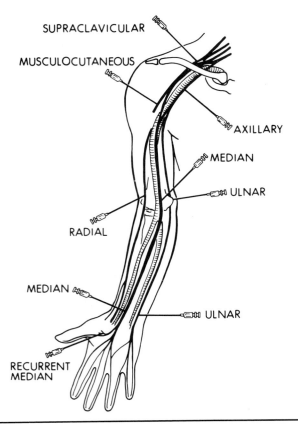

SUPRACLAVICULAR

MUSCULOCUTANEOUS

AXILLARY

MEDIAN

ULNAR

RADIAL

MEDIAN

ULNAR

RECURRENT
MEDIAN

Fig. 23-1. Location of commonly performed anesthetic nerve blocks in the upper extremity. (From Keenan,[12] with permission.)

create additional pressure on the nerve by pushing it against the ligament.[24]

Severely increased muscle tone can mask underlying volitional control. By selectively eliminating or reducing specific muscle forces using anesthetic nerve blocks, a more accurate assessment can be obtained of the degree of control and the extent of contractures (Fig. 23-1). Judgments about motor control based on the position a limb assumes at rest or during an activity can be misleading because position is often the result of multiple muscle forces. Dynamic, multichannel electromyography (EMG) has been shown to be a useful supplement to clinical examination when evaluating muscle function in both normal and spastic persons.[17,19,25-33] It is important, however, to differentiate between cause and effect with prudence when evaluating muscle activity patterns on EMG.[19]

GENERAL PRINCIPLES OF ASSESSMENT

Upper extremity function depends on complex and highly sophisticated mechanisms working in concert. Clinical examination is the starting point and mainstay of evaluation. For the complex situation of spasticity, nerve blocks and laboratory techniques are required. General principles of patient assessment include an appraisal of cognition and communication skills. Ideally the patient should be capable of following simple commands given verbally or by gesture. The more complex the evaluation techniques used, the greater the patient cooperation required.

Sensory Evaluation

Intact sensation is essential to upper extremity function. The basic sensations of pain, light touch, and temperature must be present to utilize motor control for functional activities. Two-point discrimination is a very useful test. A patient will rarely use the hand for functional activities if two-point discrimination is greater than 10 mm.[1,13,15,17,18] In addition, proprioception and kinesthetic awareness of the limb in space are important for function. Kinesthetic awareness can be tested in a hemiplegic patient by placing the spastic limb in a position and asking the patient to duplicate this position with the sound limb while keeping the eyes closed. Stereognosis, although useful in other patient populations, is not a practical test of sensation in spastic patients because they lack the fine motor control necessary to manipulate an object in the hand.

Observation of a patient's spontaneous use of the upper extremity is extremely useful in assessing both sensation and motor control. A patient with impaired sensation may use the hand to perform an activity when requested by the examiner, relying on visual feedback, but may not routinely use the extremity even as a functional assist. Visual perceptual deficits can add more problems involving awareness and motion of the limb.

Clinical Evaluation of Motor Control

Flexor spasticity is the predominant pattern seen in the upper extremity (Fig. 23-2). The result is an adducted, internally rotated shoulder, a flexed elbow,

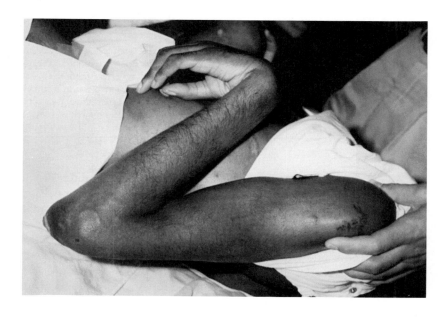

Fig. 23-2. A flexor pattern of spasticity is most commonly seen in the upper extremity. The shoulder is held adducted and internally rotated. The elbow, wrist, and fingers are held in flexion.

and a clenched fist with the thumb in the palm. Passive range of motion of each joint should be established first. This is tested by slow extension of the joint to avoid the velocity-sensitive response of the muscle spindle. When spasticity is significant and passive joint motion is incomplete, it is necessary and advisable to perform an anesthetic nerve block to assess whether a myostatic contracture is present. To evaluate passive joint motion in the entire upper extremity, a brachial plexus block using lidocaine or bupivacaine is performed. The axillary approach to the brachial plexus, familiar to most physicians, often is not feasible in patients with severe spasticity and an adducted shoulder. In this situation the brachial plexus is injected either using the supraclavicular approach or where the plexus passes below the coracoid process of the scapula.

The degree of spasticity within selected muscles can be graded clinically in response to a quick stretch as mild, moderate, or severe. There is surprising consistency between observers using this simple grading system. Another method of quantifying muscle tone, which is easily performed at the bedside, is to measure the amount of intramuscular pressure generated by a passive quick stretch or during functional use of the limb. Intramuscular pressure can be measured using a wick or slit catheter technique. The pressure

generated within the muscle is proportional to the force of contraction.[34]

Motor control can be graded in the extremity using a clinical scale (Table 23-1). The extremity may be hypotonic or flaccid and without any volitional movement (grade 1). A spastic extremity may be held rigidly without any volitional or reflexive movement (grade 2). Patterned or synergistic motor control is defined as a mass flexion or extension response involving the entire upper extremity. This mass patterned movement may be reflexive in response to a stimulus but without volitional control (grade 3). The mass patterned movement also can be initiated volitionally by the patient (grade 4). However, this is a neurologically primitive form of motor control and of no functional use in the upper extremity. Selective motor control with pattern overlay is defined as the ability to move a single joint or digit with minimal movement in the adjacent joints when performing an activity slowly (grade 5). Rapid movements or physiologic stress makes the mass pattern more pronounced. Finally, selective motor control is defined as the ability to move a single joint or digit volitionally independently of the adjacent joints (grade 6).

Spasticity can mask underlying volitional control. Blocks of selected peripheral nerves using a local anesthetic are useful to reduce or eliminate muscle ac-

Table 23-1. Clinical Scale of Motor Control

Grade	State	Control
1	Flaccid	Hypotonic, no active motion
2	Rigid	Hypertonic, no active motion
3	Reflexive mass pattern (synergy)	Mass flexion or extension in response to stimulation
4	Volitional mass pattern	Patient-initiated mass flexion or extension movement
5	Selective with pattern overlay	Slow volitional movement of specific joints; physiologic stress results in mass action
6	Selective	Volitional control of individual joints

tion temporarily for more accurate clinical assessment. For example, when severe spasticity is present in the extrinsic finger flexor muscles, no volitional control of grasp may be detected. An injection of the median and ulnar nerves at the elbow using a dilute solution of lidocaine will partially block the nerves and relax the finger flexors without causing complete paralysis. The hand can then be re-examined for evidence of volitional motor control. Using a stronger concentration of local anesthetic, the median and ulnar nerves can be completely blocked to more effectively evaluate the motor control of the antagonist extensor muscles.

Laboratory Assessment of Motor Control

When more detailed information is required about the activity of specific muscles during a functional activity, dynamic EMG provides the most useful information. Dynamic EMG testing is performed using the techniques previously described from our laboratory (Fig. 23-3).[17,19,28,33,35,36] Each muscle's electrical activity is registered through paired 50-μm diameter, nylon-shielded wire electrodes inserted into the muscle and transmitted by telemetry to be recorded on a multichannel analog tape. A printed record is used for visual interpretation of the dynamic EMG. The patient is seated during the testing procedure with the head upright. Position is standardized because it influences the vestibular input to muscle tone and control.

Initially, to determine accurate electrode placement and to provide baseline data for quantification of the electrical signals, recordings are made at rest, during quick stretch, and during maximal contraction in a manual muscle test. Volitional muscle activity is tested with the patient actively moving the extremity through its available arc of motion during a func-

tional task. Elbow and wrist range and speed of motion are recorded simultaneously using single-axis, double-parallelogram electrogoniometers. Grasp and release of the hand are marked on the EMG record by the therapist's pressing a button when finger flexion is seen (Fig. 23-4). An alternative method of displaying information about finger motion and grip strength is to use an instrumented bulb dynamometer, which records the timing and force generated with grasp and release. When evaluating thumb function, we use an instrumented pinch gauge to record the timing of thumb motion and the amount of pinch force generated.

The EMG data are digitized at 2,500 samples/s and can be quantified as reported previously.[37] Baseline noise is removed, as determined by the level of electrical activity at rest. The quantified, dynamic EMG values are then compared to and expressed as a percentage of that value obtained during a maximal effort manual muscle test. This percentage of maximal EMG is then expressed on 0.02-second intervals for each muscle tested. Accurate quantification is difficult in the spastic patient owing to the difficulty of obtaining an accurate baseline measurement during manual muscle testing. Several measurements are required during manual testing and activities to determine the true "maximal effort." If this is not done, the values obtained during functional activities may be in excess of the values seen during the manual muscle test.

After the findings in several previous studies of spastic patients from our institution were combined, the following classification of EMG activity was devised to standardize terminology and may be used for either the upper or the lower extremity (Table 23-2).[17,19,33,35,36] Class I constitutes a normal phasic pattern with appropriate on/off EMG activity. Class II

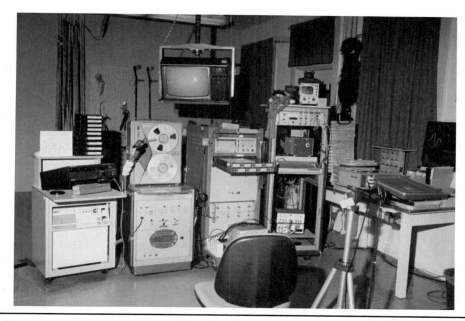

Fig. 23-3. The Pathokinesiology Laboratory at Rancho Los Amigos Medical Center, where dynamic electromyography and gait studies are performed.

consists of EMG activity that, although phasic, begins prematurely and continues for a short period beyond the normal duration of activity for that muscle. This is more commonly seen in the lower extremity.[35,36] Class III consists of phasic activity with prolongation beyond the normal timing of the muscle; this class can be further subdivided into three patterns, depending on the degree of prolongation. Class IIIA consists of phasic activity with a short period of low-intensity EMG activity extending into the next phase

Fig. 23-4. A therapist records the timing of hand grasp by pressing an event marker button.

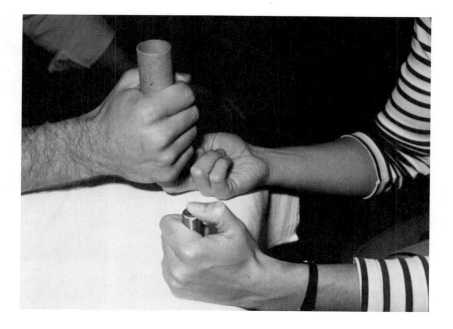

Table 23-2. Classification of Electromyographic Activity

Class I	Normal phasic activity
Class II	Premature prolonged activity
Class III	Phasic prolonged activity
IIIA	Mild
IIIB	Moderate
IIIC	Severe
Class IV	Continuous activity
Class V	Stretch response activity
Class VI	Absent activity

of the flexion-extension cycle as a result of mild spasticity. Class IIIB consists of phasic activity with prolongation extending for at least half of the next phase of motion; this is indicative of a moderate amount of spasticity. Class IIIC represents a severely spastic muscle and consists of phasic activity with severe prolongation, in which EMG activity is continued throughout the next phase of motion at a high intensity, but the underlying phasic nature of the muscle activity is still distinguishable. Class IV consists of continuous EMG activity without phasic variations. Class V consists of EMG activity seen only in response to a quick stretch by the antagonist muscles; there is no volitional activation of the muscle. This pattern is common in the finger extensors.[19] Class VI consists of absent EMG activity.

ASSESSMENT OF SPECIFIC FUNCTIONS

Hand Placement

Control of limb placement depends on both shoulder and elbow control. Active forward flexion of the shoulder generally is not a major problem in the upper extremity with potential for function. Smooth control of elbow flexion and extension, however, is frequently impaired and limits the patient's ability to perform activities of daily living even when good hand control is present.

The usual clinical picture is one of cogwheel motion on attempted extension of the elbow (Fig. 23-5). Elbow extension is markedly prolonged and frequently incomplete. Dynamic EMG combined with electrogoniometric measurement of elbow motion defines the pattern of muscle activity responsible for

this clinical picture (Fig. 23-6) (Table 23-3). The pattern most commonly seen is that all three heads of the triceps muscle are operating in a normal phasic pattern (class I). The brachioradialis muscle, being the most spastic elbow flexor, frequently shows continuous EMG activity (class IV). Both heads of the biceps muscle show an intermediate degree of spasticity with class IIIB or IIIC activity. A mild degree of spasticity is observed in the brachialis muscle with class IIIA activity. No significant change in EMG activity of these muscles is seen with the more complex movement of reaching forward.[33]

Hand Grasp and Release Function

The fingers are generally held in a clenched-fist position. This is often accompanied by wrist flexion as well. The degree of motor control may be masked by the severe amount of tone present in the finger flexors. Passive range of motion should be established first. After this, the patient is asked to open and close the fingers and to flex and extend the wrist. If no active wrist or finger extension is seen, it is still important to assess whether active control of finger flexion appears to be present. In the continuum of neurologic impairment and recovery, control of wrist and finger flexion is seen prior to active control of extension. A finger is placed in the patient's palm and

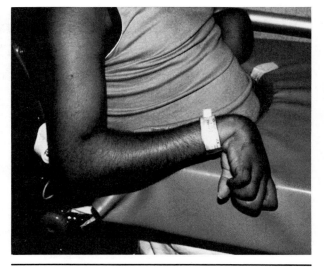

Fig. 23-5. Elbow flexor spasticity results in difficulty in hand placement. Elbow extension is slow and often incomplete.

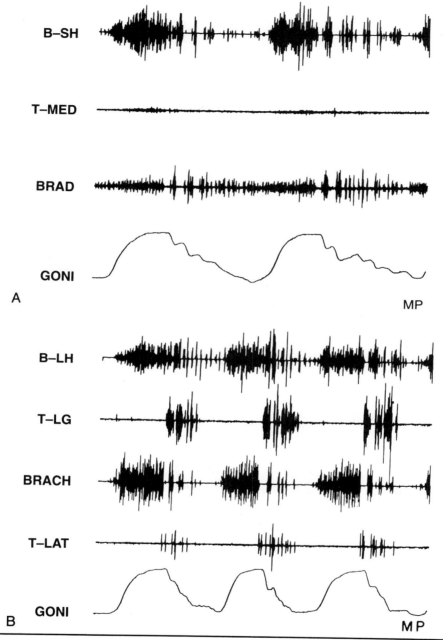

Fig. 23-6. **(A)** The dynamic EMG obtained during elbow flexion and extension shows a smooth upward tracing of the goniometer (GONI), indicating rapid elbow flexion. The downward tracing of the goniometer is uneven and prolonged, indicating a cogwheel type of elbow extension. The short head of the biceps (B-SH) shows class IIIB EMG activity with phasic firing during flexion but a moderate prolongation of activity extending throughout elbow extension. The medial head of the triceps (T-MED) shows no activity (class VI). The brachioradialis (BRAD) shows continuous firing (class IV EMG activity). **(B)** The elbow goniometer shows rapid flexion (upward tracing), but extension is prolonged (downward tracing). The long head of the biceps (B-LH) exhibits moderate spasticity (EMB class IIIB). The long (T-LG) and lateral (T-LAT) heads of the triceps show normal phasic activity (EMG class I). The brachialis (BRACH) muscle is only mildly spastic, with class IIIA EMG activity.

Table 23-3. Electromyographic Activity Patterns During Elbow Flexion and Extension

Muscle	EMG Class (Percent)							
	I	II	IIIA	IIIB	IIIC	IV	V	VI
Biceps								
Short head	5	0	10	40	30	10	0	5
Long head	10	0	5	35	40	5	0	5
Brachioradialis	5	0	10	10	20	50	0	5
Brachialis	10	0	35	30	10	15	0	0
Triceps								
Medial head	80	0	0	0	0	0	0	20
Lateral head	75	0	0	0	0	0	0	25
Long head	75	0	0	0	0	0	0	25
Coracobrachialis	25	0	10	10	20	10	0	25

the patient is asked to grasp. Often an increase in the pressure of the grasp can be felt, indicating underlying muscle control. The proximal interphalangeal joints of the fingers rapidly develop severe flexion contractures because of the severe spasticity seen in the flexor digitorum superficialis muscles (EMG class IIIC or IV), as opposed to the flexor digitorum profundus muscle, which is often normal (class I EMG activity) (Figs. 23-7 and 23-8).[19]

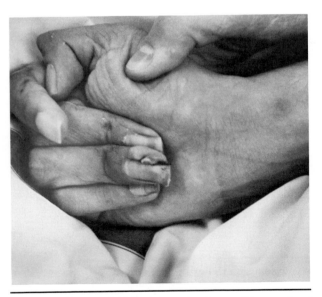

Fig. 23-7. Severe, rigid flexion contractures of the proximal interphalangeal joints occur secondary to the severe spasticity present in the flexor digitorum superficialis muscles. The distal interphalangeal joints show minimal or no flexion deformity because the flexor digitorum profundus muscle shows normal activity on dynamic EMG.

Next an anesthetic block of the median nerve should be performed in the antecubital space as well as a block of the ulnar nerve within the cubital canal to eliminate flexor tone temporarily. With the flexor muscles relaxed, the activity of the extensor muscles can be evaluated more accurately. When extensor control returns, it is generally seen in the wrist extensor muscles and extensor indicis proprius muscle first. Dynamic EMG studies are useful in obtaining more detailed information regarding patterns of motor control. These studies also give clues to the phylogenetic development of the brain and the organization of motor control pathways. The flexion pattern of spasticity seen after damage to the cerebral cortex is reminiscent of the flexed posture of the forelimbs of many birds, flying mammals, and quadruped animals. When the advanced areas of the brain have been damaged, the more primitive patterns of muscle activity become dominant.

Active finger extension will not be detected by dynamic EMG if it is not seen on clinical examination or after an anesthetic block of the forearm flexor muscles. However, it is not possible to determine accurately the exact timing of each muscle by clinical evaluation alone. Dynamic EMG studies yield information regarding the specific timing of each muscle that cannot be elicited clinically.

Dynamic EMG analysis of grasp and release, performed on 48 upper extremities of adults with spasticity from a brain injury, revealed that 80 percent of the finger flexors exhibited volitional motor control[19]

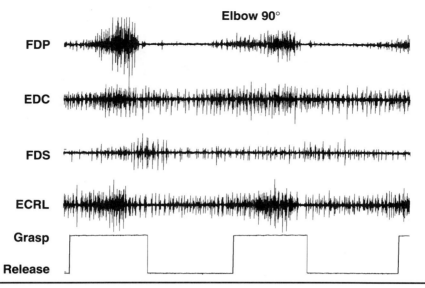

Fig. 23-8. The dynamic EMG obtained during hand grasp and release shows normal phasic activity (EMG class I) in the flexor digitorum profundus (FDP) muscle. In contrast, the flexor digitorum superficialis (FDS) muscle exhibits severe spasticity with continuous firing (EMG class IV). The extensor digitorum communis (EDC) muscle shows class IV activity and the extensor carpi radialis longus (ECRL) muscle exhibits class IIIC activity.

(Table 23-4). Despite the high percentage of patients with volitional control (EMG class I, II, or III) of the flexor digitorum superficialis, this muscle often showed an increased intensity of the EMG signal when compared with the flexor digitorum profundus muscle in the same patient (Fig. 23-8). This disparity in EMG intensity correlates clinically with the excessive flexion deformity of the proximal interphalangeal joint so commonly seen (Fig. 23-7).

Why should such a significant difference exist between the amount of spasticity seen in the superficial and deep finger flexor muscles? One explanation could be the evolutionary development of motor control pathways in the brain. The flexor digitorum profundus is a more primitive muscle. Although individual tendons go to each finger, they share a common muscle belly and must act together in gross grasp. The control of this relatively primitive muscle

Table 23-4. Electromyographic Activity Patterns in the Hand

Muscle[a]	EMG Class (Percent)					
	I	II	III	IV	V	VI
EPL	30	0	20	30	5	15
EIP	45	0	15	25	10	5
EDC	45	0	20	20	5	10
ECRL	25	0	60	10	5	0
FPL	40	0	35	15	0	10
FDP	50	0	35	5	5	5
FDS, ring	55	0	20	15	5	5
FDS, index	70	0	15	20	0	5

[a] Key: EPL, extensor pollicis longus; EIP, extensor indicis proprius; EDC, extensor digitorum communis; ECRL, extensor carpi radialis longus; FPL, flexor pollicis longus; FDP, flexor digitorum profundus; FDS, ring, flexor digitorum superficialis of the ring finger; FDS, index, flexor digitorum superficialis of the index finger.

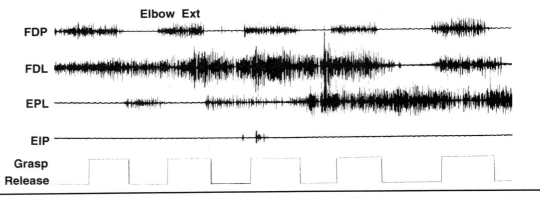

Fig. 23-9. The flexor pollicis longus (FPL) muscle shows some degree of volitional control in 75 percent of cases. An EMG signal of high intensity as seen here in the FPL indicates significant underlying spasticity.

is less dependent on the motor cortex and less likely to develop spasticity with cortical injury. The flexor digitorum superficialis, however, is a more sophisticated muscle with individual muscle bellies, allowing for independent finger motion. Having developed at a later time, the flexor digitorum superficialis is more dependent on the cerebral cortex for control. Brain injuries that disrupt pathways of cortical control therefore result in more pronounced spasticity in the superficial finger flexor muscles.

The intensity of the EMG signal is greatest in the flexor digitorum superficialis muscles of the long and ring fingers. This is clinically apparent as a more severe flexion deformity in the fingers on the ulnar aspect of the hand seen in all patients. It may also be the result of phylogenetic development. The power of grip strength comes primarily from the ulnar fingers of the hand. This power of grip is important in arboreal primates living in the forest canopy.

The flexor pollicis longus muscle shows volitional control (EMG class I, II, or III) in 75 percent of cases. A high intensity of EMG signal is seen, indicative of significant underlying spasticity (Fig. 23-9).

The extensor muscles of the thumb and fingers show less volitional control than the flexor muscles. Only 50 percent of patients demonstrate volitional thumb extension. Out-of-phase activity in the extensors appears to be a stretch response elicited by finger flexion (EMG class V). The extensor indicis proprius muscle displays volitional control in 60 percent of hands. The extensor digitorum communis muscle also ex-

hibits volitional action in 60 percent. The extensor carpi radialis longus manifests normal phasic activity (EMG class I) in 25 percent of hands and prolonged phasic activity (EMG class III) in 60 percent. Volitional control of this important wrist stabilizer is therefore present in 85 percent of hands.

Analysis of the EMG data on each muscle with the elbow flexed 90 degrees and with the elbow completely extended reveals that arm position causes a mild change on the intensity of muscle EMG activity but has no significant effect on the classification of the timing of EMG activity.

Intrinsic Function

Extension of the fingers at the metacarpophalangeal (MCP) joints may be blocked by spasticity of the interossei and lumbrical muscles of the hand (Fig.23-10). Another manifestation of intrinsic spasticity is the tendency to either boutonnière or swan-neck positioning of the fingers. The amount of tone in the extrinsic finger flexors determines the final position of the fingers in the presence of intrinsic spasticity. When severe spasticity is present in the flexor digitorum superficialis muscles, a boutonnière deformity is favored.

The degree of tension caused by the intrinsic muscles can be demonstrated by comparing the amount of proximal interphalangeal joint (PIP) flexion obtained with the MCP joints flexed to that obtained while the MCP joints are extended. If there is less PIP flexion with MCP extension, the intrinsic tendons are con-

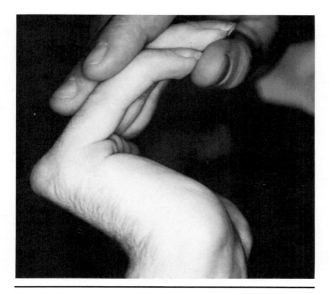

Fig. 23-10. Extension of the fingers at the metacarpophalangeal (MCP) joints may be blocked by spasticity of the interosseous and lumbrical muscles of the hand. Swanneck or boutonnière deformities are also common when intrinsic spasticity is present.

sidered to be tight. This test should be performed both before and after a lidocaine block of the ulnar nerve at the wrist to distinguish between intrinsic tone and contracture. The amount of active MCP extension before and after block also should be observed.

Thumb Function

The thumb-in-palm deformity, frequently seen in the spastic hand (Fig. 23-11), generally occurs secondarily to spasticity of the flexor pollicis longus muscle and the median- and ulnar-innervated thenar muscles. Because the spastic thumb-in-palm deformity is a manifestation of the combined activity of several muscles acting on the thumb, it is therefore heterogeneous in its appearance.[38] The offending muscles causing impaired thumb function may be suggested by the position of the thumb. If a flexion deformity of the interphalangeal (IP) joint of the thumb is present, the flexor pollicis longus muscle is spastic. Adduction of the thumb indicates spasticity of the adductor pollicis muscle and possibly the first dorsal interosseous muscle.[39] A quick stretch of the thumb into abduction often will elicit a clonic response.

Distinguishing the activity of different intrinsic and extrinsic thumb muscles on the basis of physical examination alone can be difficult and misleading. Selective pharmacologic block of the median and ulnar nerves can help to identify spastic muscles.[1,40] An anesthetic block of the ulnar nerve in Guyon's canal at the wrist will eliminate intrinsic tone temporarily. This will demonstrate the presence of any myostatic contractures and also will confirm that the adductor pollicis was one of the muscles involved in the deformity.

If the thumb metacarpal remains flexed after the ulnar nerve block, spasticity of the opponens pollicis, flexor pollicis brevis, and abductor pollicis muscles is present also. These muscles are innervated by the recurrent motor branch of the median nerve. A median nerve block in the carpal tunnel using a local anesthetic will eliminate the spasticity in these muscles temporarily and establish whether or not a contracture is present. However, the thenar musculature shows significant variation in the distribution of median and ulnar innervated segments, limiting the usefulness of nerve blocks.[41]

Dynamic EMG provides a more precise method to investigate muscle function. As indicated by the heterogeneous appearance of the thumb-in-palm deformity, there is a wide variability of thumb function in spastic patients. Twenty-five percent of patients with some useful upper extremity function use the hand only as a minimally assistive stabilizer; the remaining 75 percent use the upper extremity as an active assist.

By integrating the EMG signal during functional tasks and comparing this to the electrical activity obtained during a maximal contraction of the same muscle, the EMG can be quantified and expressed as a percentage of maximal effort. Muscle function has been evaluated during lateral pinch using an instrumented pinch gauge and quantitated EMG. When pinch force is plotted against the quantitated EMG signal for individual muscles, 75 percent of patients exhibit good motor control during a gradual pinch, with a linear relationship between pinch force and EMG activity (Fig. 23-12). This indicates a pattern of normal recruitment of muscle fibers. Twenty-five percent of patients show an unsynchronized recruitment, often with an all-or-none pattern of muscle

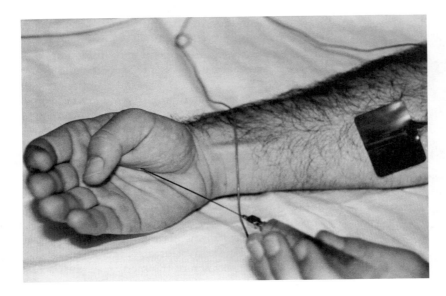

Fig. 23-11. A spastic thumb-in-palm deformity is caused by spasticity of both the median and ulnar innervated thenar muscles and spasticity of the flexor pollicis longus muscle.

activity (Fig. 23-13). Regardless of the degree and quality of motor control, all spastic muscles are weak, with significant reduction of pinch force. Maximum pinch force was less than 15 pounds in all patients, and 50 percent of the patients had a pinch force of less than 10 pounds. Pinch strength was 25 to 30 pounds in age- and sex-matched controls.

The EMG signal is difficult to quantify in spastic patients owing to the problems in obtaining an accurate baseline measurement of EMG activity during a

maximal contraction. The lack of normal fine motor control restricts the patient's ability to perform manual muscle tests. The EMG signal obtained during a functional activity is frequently in excess of the 100 percent value obtained during the manual muscle test (Fig. 23-12). Despite this limitation, valuable information regarding motor control is obtained by comparing the maximal activity during a controlled

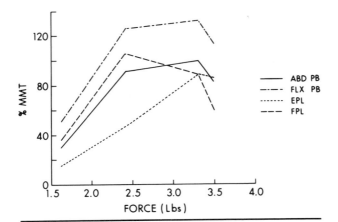

Fig. 23-12. When pinch force is plotted against the quantitated EMG signal for individual muscles, 75 percent of patients exhibit good motor control during a gradual pinch with a linear relationship between pinch force and EMG activity. This indicates a pattern of normal recruitment of muscle fibers.

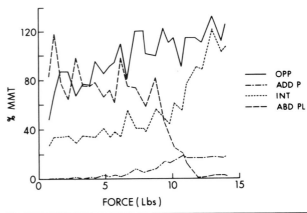

Fig. 23-13. Twenty-five percent of patients show an unsychronized recruitment, often with an "all-or-none" pattern of muscle activity, during pinch, indicating inability to recruit motor units in an organized manner. The EMG signal is difficult to quantify in spastic patients owing to the problems in obtaining an accurate baseline measurement of EMG activity during a maximal contraction. The signal is frequently in excess of the 100 percent value obtained during the manual muscle test.

manual muscle test with the excess activity seen during a physiologically more stressful functional task. Indeed, this value is an indication of the amount of pattern overlay to selective motor control present in the muscle.

Studies of thumb function using dynamic EMG have revealed that the flexor pollicis brevis, opponens, flexor pollicis longus, first dorsal interosseous, and adductor pollicis muscles are most active during pinch. No particular muscle was overwhelmingly spastic or out of phase during the grasp-and-release study. The opponens muscle showed the most prolonged activity indicative of spasticity. The extensor pollicis longus, abductor pollicis longus, and abductor pollicis brevis muscles exhibit the most prolonged activity consistent with their function of stabilizing the thumb during functional use. The pinch graphs did not demonstrate any statistically significant pattern of muscle function in brain-injured patients. These findings suggest that a cookbook surgical approach cannot be used for treatment of the thumb-in-palm deformity.

The complexity of the thumb muscles is such that physical examination, anatomic knowledge, and intuition together are not sufficient to define their action. Using EMG to identify spastic muscles, quantifying preoperatively the muscle weakness, and identifying the primary and secondary muscles used for pinch may be useful in planning appropriate muscle releases or tendon transfers.

The patterns of muscle activity in patients with brain injury and impaired thumb function are diverse. Dynamic EMG during lateral pinch, grasp, and release can demonstrate selective control and identify muscles that are inappropriately active. This knowledge can be used to individualize surgical treatment and achieve a better functional result.

SUMMARY

The assessment of limb motion and motor control is complex. More diverse patterns of movement are seen in the upper extremity than in the lower extremity. This is especially true for movement of the thumb and fingers. The variance can be attributed to the functional use of the hand requiring more precise and independent movement of adjacent structures or digits. The diversity of upper extremity motion requires the careful combination of clinical assessment and laboratory investigation for accurate understanding of function. Treatment strategies in the spastic hand based on such detailed investigation lead to improved function.

REFERENCES

1. Botte MJ, Keenan MAE: Reconstructive surgery of the upper extremity in the patient with head trauma. J Head Trauma Rehabil 2:34, 1987
2. Braun RM, Hoffer MM, Mooney V et al: Phenol nerve block in treatment of acquired spastic hemiplegia in the upper limb. J Bone Joint Surg [Am] 55:580, 1973
3. Braun RM, Vise GT, Roper B: Preliminary experience with superficialis to profundus tendon transfer in the hemiparetic upper extremity. J Bone Joint Surg [Am] 56:466, 1974
4. Caldwell CB, Braun RM: Spasticity in the upper extremity. Clin Orthop 104:80, 1974
5. Garland DE, Rhoades M: Orthopedic management of brain-injured adults. Clin Orthop 131:111, 1978
6. Garland DE, Thompson R, Waters RL: Musculocutaneous neurectomy for spastic elbow flexion in non-functional upper extremities in adults. J Bone Joint Surg [Am] 62:108, 1980
7. Garland DE, Lucie RS, Waters RL: Current uses of open phenol nerve block for adult acquired spasticity. Clin Orthop 165:217, 1982
8. Garland DE, Keenan MAE: Orthopedic strategies in the management of the adult head-injured patient. Phys Ther 63:2004, 1983
9. Garland DE, Lilling M, Keenan MA: Phenol blocks to motor points of spastic forearm muscles in head-injured adults. Arch Phys Med Rehabil 65:243, 1984
10. Hoffer MM, Waters RL, Garland DE: Spastic dysfunction of the elbow. p. 616. In: Morrey BS (ed): The Elbow And Its Disorders. WB Saunders, Philadelphia, 1985
11. Katz J, Knott LW, Feldman DJ: Peripheral nerve injections with phenol in management of spastic patients. Arch Phys Med Rehabil 48:97, 1967
12. Keenan MAE: The orthopaedic management of spasticity. J Head Trauma Rehabil 2:62, 1987
13. Keenan MAE, Abrams RA, Garland DE, Waters RL: Results of fractional lengthening of the finger flexors in adults with upper extremity spasticity. J Hand Surg [Am] 12:575, 1987
14. Keenan MAE, Korchek JI, Botte MJ, Garland DE: Results of transfer of the flexor digitorum superficialis tendons to flexor digitorum profundus tendons in adults with acquired spasticity of the hand. J Bone Joint Surg [Am] 69:1127, 1987
15. Waters RL, Keenan MA: Surgical treatment of the upper extremity after stroke. p. 1449. In Chapman M (ed): Operative Orthopaedics. JB Lippincott, Philadelphia, 1988
16. Meals RA: Denervation for the treatment of acquired spasticity of the brachioradialis. J Bone Joint Surg [Am] 70:1081, 1988
17. Keenan MAE: Surgical decision making for residual limb deformities following traumatic brain injury. Orthop Rev 27:1185, 1988
18. Keenan MAE: Management of the spastic upper extremity in the neurologically impaired adult. Clin Orthop 233:116, 1988
19. Keenan MAE, Romanelli RR, Lunsford BR: The use of dynamic electromyography to evaluate motor control in the hands of adults who have spasticity caused by brain injury. J Bone Joint Surg [Am] 71:120, 1989

20. Garland DE, Blum C, Waters RL: Periarticular heterotopic ossification in head-injured adults. Incidence and location. J Bone Joint Surg [Am] 62:1143, 1980
21. Garland DE, Bailey S: Undetected injuries in head-injured adults. Clin Orthop 155:162, 1981
22. Stone L, Keenan MAE: Peripheral nerve injuries in the adult with traumatic brain injury. Clin Orthop 233:136, 1988
23. Keenan MAE, Kauffman DL, Garland DE, Smith C: Late ulnar neuropathy in the brain-injured adult. J Hand Surg [Am] 13:120, 1988
24. Orcutt SA, Kramer WG, Howard MW et al: Carpal tunnel syndrome secondary to wrist and finger flexor spasticity. J Hand Surg 15A:940, 1990
25. Boivin G, Wadsworth GE, Landsmeer JMF, Long C: Electromyographic kinesiology of the hand: muscles driving the index finger. Arch Phys Med Rehabil 50:17, 1969
26. Close JR, Todd FN: The phasic activity of the muscles of the lower extremity and the effect of tendon transfer. J Bone Joint Surg [Am] 41:189, 1959
27. Hoffer MM, Perry J, Garcia M, Bullock D: Adduction contracture of the thumb in cerebral palsy. J Bone Joint Surg [Am] 65:755, 1983
28. Hoffer MM, Perry J, Melkonian DVM: Dynamic electromyography and decision-making for surgery in the upper extremity of patients with cerebral palsy. J Hand Surg [Am] 4:424, 1979
29. Long C: Intrinsic-extrinsic muscle control of the fingers. Electromyographic studies. J Bone Joint Surg [Am] 50:973, 1968
30. McFarland GB, Weathersby HT: Kinesiology of selected muscles acting on the wrist: electromyographic study. Arch Phys Med Rehabil 43:165, 1962
31. Pinzur M, Wehner J, Kett N, Trilla M: Brachioradialis to finger extensor tendon transfer to achieve hand opening in acquired spasticity. J Hand Surg [Am] 13:549, 1988
32. Samilson RL, Morris JW: Surgical improvement of the cerebral palsied upper limb. Electromyographic studies and results of 128 operations. J Bone Joint Surg [Am] 45:1203, 1964
33. Keenan MAE, Haider TT, Stone LR: Dynamic electromyography to assess elbow spasticity. J Hand Surg 15A:607, 1990
34. Baumann JU, Sutherland DH, Hanggi A: Intramuscular pressure during walking: An experimental study using the wick catheter technique. Clin Orthop 145:292, 1979
35. Keenan MA, Creighton J, Garland DE, Moore T: Surgical correction of spastic equinovarus deformity in the adult head trauma patient. Foot Ankle 5:35, 1984
36. Waters RL, Frazier J, Garland D et al: Electromyographic gait analysis before and after treatment for hemiplegic equinus and equinovarus deformity. J Bone Joint Surg [Am] 64:284, 1982
37. Perry J, Barnes G, Gronley JK: The postpolio syndrome. Clin Orthop 233:145, 1988
38. House JH, Gwanthmey FW, Fidler MO: A dynamic approach to the thumb-in-palm deformity. J Bone Joint Surg [Am] 63:216, 1981
39. Matev I: Surgical treatment of spastic "thumb-in-palm" deformity. J Bone Joint Surg [Br] 45:703, 1963
40. Botte MJ, Keenan MA, Gellman H et al: Surgical management of spastic thumb-in-palm deformity in adults with brain injury. J Hand Surg [Am] 14:174, 1989
41. Rowntree T: Anomalous innervation of the hand muscles. J Bone Joint Surgery [Br] 31:505, 1949

Section III

BASIC SCIENCE ASPECTS OF REHABILITATION

24 Neuromuscular Physiology, Function, and Plasticity

RICHARD L. LIEBER

SKELETAL MUSCLE STRUCTURE AND FUNCTION

Skeletal muscle represents a classic biologic example of a structure-function relationship; therefore an understanding of muscle function requires an understanding of its structure.[1] Whole muscles are composed of single muscle fibers (Fig. 24-1). As is discussed later in this chapter, the physical *arrangement* of these fibers is critical in determining a muscle's contractile properties. Interestingly, although muscles are found in a variety of sizes and shapes, the size of the component muscle fibers is relatively consistent. Mammalian muscle fibers range from 20 to 80 μm in diameter.

Muscle fibers are multinucleated cells composed primarily of a parallel arrangement of myofibrils with an average diameter of 1 μm (Fig. 24-1). (For the purposes of this chapter anatomic discussion is limited to cellular components involved in the generation of force.) Myofibrils are composed of units called sarcomeres arranged in series (Fig. 24-1). The structural hierarchy continues at the molecular level with sarcomeres composed of myofilaments, which appear ultrastructurally as "thick" and "thin" filaments. The filaments are themselves polymeric structures composed of monomers of actin (thin filament) or myosin (thick filament). Myofilaments are responsible for the generation and regulation of muscle force.

In addition to the components that generate force, muscle cells contain a complex membrane system that is responsible for excitation of the contractile filaments.[2] The membrane system originates as surface membrane invaginations, extending transversely from the long axis of the muscle fiber into the interior, and is therefore known as the transverse tubular system, or T system. The second component of the membrane system surrounds the myofibril and is known as the sarcoplasmic reticulum (SR). The SR is responsible for release and uptake of calcium during contraction and relaxation, respectively.

Excitation-Contraction Coupling

Together, the membrane and force generating systems are responsible for initiation and generation of muscle force. The process by which a nervous impulse ultimately ends in muscle contraction is known as excitation-contraction coupling.[3] In this process, a nervous impulse travels from the peripheral nerve to the neuromuscular junction. At the neuromuscular junction, the neurotransmitter acetylcholine diffuses across the neuromuscular cleft and depolarizes the muscle fiber surface membrane, which is itself an excitable membrane. The impulse propagates along the muscle fiber and then dives deep into the fiber via the T system. At intervals along the T system, the impulse is relayed to the SR, which releases calcium

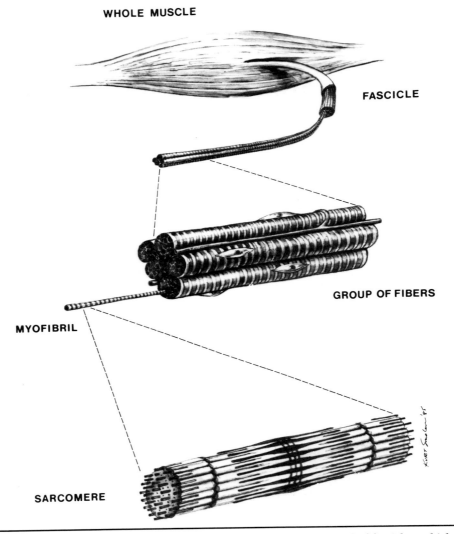

WHOLE MUSCLE

FASCICLE

GROUP OF FIBERS

MYOFIBRIL

SARCOMERE

Fig. 24-1. Structural hierarchy in skeletal muscle. Whole muscles are composed of fascicles, which in turn are made up of single muscle fibers arranged in series and in parallel. Single muscle fibers are composed of myofibrils arranged in parallel. Myofibrils are composed of sarcomeres arranged in series. Sarcomeres are composed of interdigitating thick and thin filaments. Thick and thin filaments are composed of contractile and regulatory proteins. (From Lieber,[9] with permission.)

in the vicinity of the myofilaments. Calcium binding to regulatory proteins on the actin filament then releases the inhibition on actin and permits actin-myosin interaction, which results in force generation (Fig. 24-2, rising portion of twitch). As long as calcium levels are elevated above threshold, force generation occurs. When the nervous impulse stops, the calcium concentration drops as calcium is pumped back into the SR. The decrease in calcium concentration results

in muscle fiber relaxation (Fig. 24-2, falling portion of twitch). If repeated impulses are delivered to the muscle, calcium release-uptake cycles result in cyclic force generation and relaxation (Fig. 24-2, 10 Hz). As stimulation frequency increases, force increases because the impulses are delivered faster than the calcium is removed. This results in tetanic contraction owing to fusion of individual pulses (Fig. 24-2). Variation of stimulation frequency is actually one method

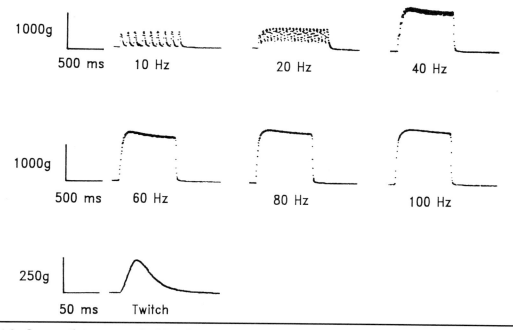

Fig. 24-2. Contractile response of rabbit tibialis muscle to stimulation at different frequencies. **(Lowest record)** Twitch contraction in response to a single electrical impulse. Force generation followed by relaxation reflects calcium release and sequestration by the SR. **(Upper records)** Tetanic contractions in response to stimulation at different frequencies. Note the compressed time scale and expanded force scale for the twitch contraction.

used by the nervous system to alter skeletal muscle force.

Length-Tension Relationship

The length-tension relationship states that conractile force is directly proportional to myofilament overlap. Figure 24-3, illustrates the classic length-tension curve that was elucidated in single frog muscle fibers by Gordon and co-workers.[4] At intermediate sarcomere lengths muscle force is maximum (Fig. 24-3, 2.0 to 2.25 μm), whereas shorter or longer lengths result in decreased force. For example, at very long lengths it can be seen that no muscle force is generated, because there is no potential for interaction between actin and myosin myofilaments (Fig. 24-3, 3.65 μm). As muscle length decreases from this long length, force increases owing to the increasing number of force generators that interact between the actin and myosin filaments. When all possible interactions between actin and myosin are made, the muscle generates maximum tension. As further shortening occurs, the thin filaments from one side of the sarcomere

actually begin to interfere with cross-bridge formation on the opposite side of the sarcomere, resulting in decreased force (Fig. 24-3, 1.3 to 2.0 μm). Finally, the thin and thick filaments collide with the Z line, resulting in a further decrease in force owing to this "supercontraction" (Fig. 24-3, 1.05 μm). Such a condition probably cannot occur physiologically because of restrictions imposed by the skeleton. However, it is possible to cause supercontraction intraoperatively or experimentally by activation of an unloaded muscle.

The interdigitation of the actin- and myosin-containing filaments gives rise to the well-known muscle striation pattern observable on electron micrographic longitudinal sections (Fig. 24-4). The light-dark striation pattern is due to the periodic overlap and nonoverlap of actin and myosin filaments.[5] The A band represents the sarcomere region containing the myosin filament, and, depending on muscle length, may also contain actin filaments. The I band contains only the actin filament and is therefore optically much lighter. The H band represents the central region of

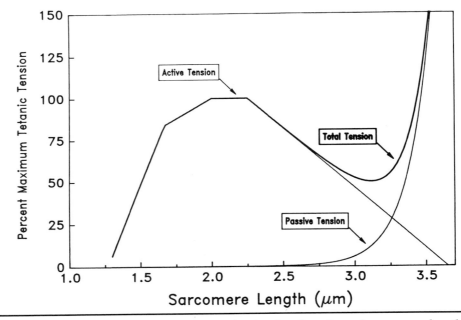

Fig. 24-3. Sarcomere length-tension curve. Active tension is a function of muscle sarcomere length and results from interdigitation of actin and myosin filaments as described in the text. Passive tension results from elastic structures within the sarcomere.

the A band, which contains only myosin filaments. The M band is a specialized region of the A band where the myosin filaments are thought to be anchored. Thus, examination of a skeletal muscle electron micrograph in longitudinal section reveals the

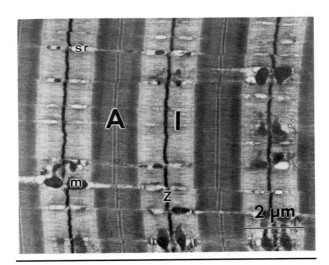

Fig. 24-4. Ultrastructural appearance of the mammalian sarcomere in longitudinal section. A, A band; I, I band; z, Z disk; m, mitochondrion; sr, sarcoplasmic reticulum.

level of muscle shortening by virtue of the relative sizes of the A and I bands. In this way, it is possible from such structural information to deduce the relative tension-generating capacity of that muscle sample. The Z band represents the boundaries of the sarcomere. Although its specific function and properties have not been fully elucidated, it has a number of unique features. First, Z band width varies as a function of fiber type (see later discussion). Second, the Z band (actually, the anatomically defined Z disk) seems to represent the "weak link" in muscle injury due to high-tension exercise.[6]

Force-Velocity Relationship

The force-velocity relationship states that contractile force is a function of muscle velocity.[7] For shortening (concentric) contractions, muscle force decreases rapidly as muscle shortening takes place (Fig. 24-5, right). This general type of contraction would occur, for example, in the quadriceps during leg extension exercises as the weight was lifted. For lengthening (eccentric) contractions, muscle force rapidly rises as a muscle is stretched (Fig. 24-5, left). This type of contraction is very common physiologically and

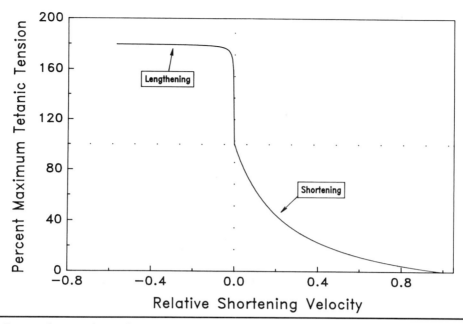

Fig. 24-5. Force-velocity relationship. For shortening (concentric) contractions, skeletal muscle force drops rapidly as shortening velocity increases. For lengthening (eccentric) contractions, muscle force increases rapidly and then plateaus.

occurs, for example, during running, as eccentric contraction of the quadriceps decelerates the body after foot strike. Thus, a muscle generates more force during an isometric contraction than in concentric contraction. Also if a muscle is forced to lengthen, it sustains even greater forces than in shortening. This may provide insight into why eccentric contractions are very useful in strengthening skeletal muscle during exercise. (High muscle tensions are thought to be a potent strengthening stimulus.)

Skeletal Muscle Architecture

Skeletal muscle architecture refers to the arrangement of component muscle fibers relative to the axis of force generation. The significance of the arrangement of these fibers is twofold: (1) muscle force is proportional to the total muscle fiber cross-sectional area, and (2) muscle velocity is proportional to muscle fiber length.[8,9] For example, consider the situation shown in Figure 24-6. In *A* the muscle is composed of long muscle fibers oriented along the axis of force generation. However, in *B* the muscle is approximately the same size as the muscle in *A*, but it is composed of short muscle fibers oriented at a 30° angle to the force generation axis. Because muscle *A* is composed of fibers that are approximately twice as long as those in muscle *B*, muscle *A* will contract at twice the velocity of muscle *B*. However, because muscle *B* contains approximately three times the number of muscle fibers as muscle *A*, it will generate approximately three times the force. Thus, it is not sufficient to simply know the entire quantity of contractile material (i.e., the muscle mass) to predict functional properties. It is the *arrangement* of the contractile material that is of greatest importance. Interestingly, muscles in different parts of the body have dramatically different architectures. Because muscle architecture influences skeletal muscle function and adaptive capacity, surgeons need to consider donor muscle architectural properties when transferring or transplanting muscle. In addition, it is clearly inappropriate to use measures such as muscle mass or muscle cross-sectional area as determined from computed tomography scans as indices of "atrophy" or "strength," because these parameters may or may not be related to the total muscle fiber cross-sectional area.

Overall, skeletal muscle structural complexity (i.e., different architectures) permits a decrease in the complexity of the neural control signal required to

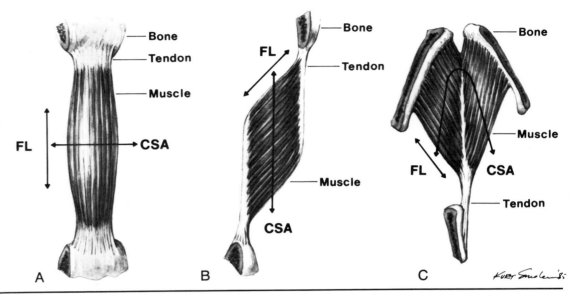

Fig. 24-6. Example of whole muscle architecture demonstrating different fiber arrangements. Average fiber length is shown by the line labeled FL. Average fiber cross-sectional area is shown by the line labeled CSA. Muscle contraction velocity is proportional to the length of line FL, whereas contraction force is proportional to the length of line CSA. **(A)** Longitudinal muscular architecture designed to provide high contraction velocity. **(B)** Pennated architecture with the fibers oriented at a fixed angle relative to the axis of force generation to provide high contractile force while conserving space. Note that this muscle would generate more force and contract at a slower velocity than the muscle shown in **A**. **(C)** Pennated architecture with the fibers oriented at varying angles relative to the axis of force generation. This muscle would generate more force than the muscles in either **A** or **B**, but would contract at a lower velocity than either muscle. On inspection, all three muscles appear to be of similar size but normalization of force or velocity to gross muscle size would be misleading. (From Lieber,[9] with permission.)

perform a task. In other words, the neuromusculo-skeletal system is composed of very specific "motors" at remote sites, which receive general information from the nervous system and "decode" it by virtue of their intrinsic structure to perform a specific task. (This is analogous to the increased use of "smart" peripheral devices in various computer systems.)

A colleague and I performed a detailed architectural study of the rabbit hind limb.[10] The properties of 26 muscles were measured and then subjected to a statistical method, which was able to determine the "typical" properties of the various functional groups (i.e., quadriceps, hamstrings, plantar flexors, and dorsiflexors). For example, the quadriceps muscles

are characterized by their large pennation angle and moderate size, generally designed for force production (Fig. 24-7). The hamstrings, in contrast, are very large, long muscles composed of longitudinally arranged fibers, designed intrinsically for excursion but, owing to their size, also able to generate large forces. In the shank, dorsiflexors are small muscles with relatively long, longitudinally arranged fibers, designed for excursion. The plantar flexors, like the quadriceps, are highly pennated, albeit smaller, with short fibers. Thus, the plantar flexors clearly are designed for force production, whereas the dorsiflexors clearly are designed for excursion. The thigh muscles appear less extremely adapted, with the hamstrings possessing a tendency toward excursion but retaining

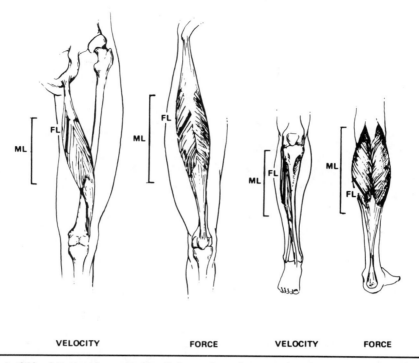

VELOCITY   FORCE   VELOCITY   FORCE

Fig. 24-7. ''Typical'' architectural properties of the various functional muscle groups. These properties were obtained by discriminant analysis of architectural data from 26 muscles of the rabbit hindlimb (see Lieber and Blevins[10] for details). Generally, muscles with long fibers were designed for velocity whereas muscles with short, pennated fibers were designed for force production. FL, fiber length; ML, muscle length.

a good deal of size for adequate force production. Similarly, the quadriceps maintain a tendency toward force production and are less well adapted for excursion. Of course, complete explanation of design tendency must ultimately include information on muscle moment arms. Such studies are currently underway in our laboratory.

Skeletal Muscle Fiber Types

Skeletal muscle fibers can be classified into three types.[11] This classification scheme is based on contractile speed (during isotonic contraction), muscle fiber oxidative capacity (ability to generate adenosine triphosphatase [ATP] with oxygen), and muscle fiber glycolytic capacity (ability to generate ATP without oxygen). It should be noted that there is actually a nearly continuous range of muscle fiber speeds and of oxidative and glycolytic capacities. However, generally speaking, muscle fibers can be classified into one of three categories: (1) slow-contracting fibers

with high oxidative capacity and low glycolytic capacity (type SO); (2) fast-contracting fibers with high oxidative and glycolytic capacities (type FOG); and (3) fast-contracting fibers with low oxidative and high glycolytic capacity (type FG). In normal muscle, approximately 90 percent of the fibers can be classified into one of these three categories by qualitative histochemical staining. However, it should be remembered that muscle fibers vary continuously on these scales and that classification into discrete types is simply a matter of convenience.

Demonstration of muscle fiber type distribution is accomplished by staining serial muscle sections for enzymes related to speed (myofibrillar ATPase), oxidative capacity (succinate dehydrogenase), and glycolytic capacity (α-glycerophosphate dehydrogenase) (Fig. 24-8). Note that this is not the same procedure as is typically used in pathology laboratories to discriminate between fiber types based on myofibrillar ATPase activity under various pH con-

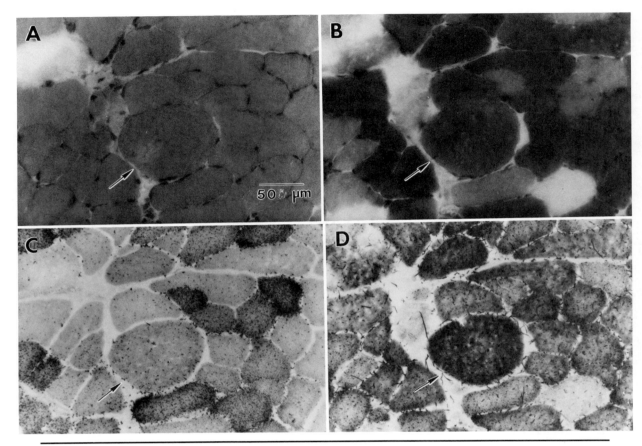

Fig. 24-8. Histochemical classification of muscle fiber types based on differential staining of serial sections of a rabbit tibialis anterior muscle. **(A)** Conventional hematoxylin and eosin stain. Note the tightly packed polygonal fibers with peripherally placed nuclei. **(B)** Same fibers as in A stained for routine myofibrillar ATPase activity (pH = 9.4), which differentiates between fast-contracting and slow-contracting muscle fibers. **(C)** Same fibers as in A stained for a mitochondrial oxidative enzyme, succinate dehydrogenase. Note the spectrum of oxidative capacity present in the various muscle fibers. Note that the S fibers from B all stain dark, whereas the F fibers stain either light or dark, suggesting that oxidative capacity of fast fibers can be high or low. **(D)** Same fibers as in A stained for an enzyme associated with glycolysis, α-glycerophosphate dehydrogenase. Generally, the F fibers stain dark while the S fibers stain light. Taken together, these micrographs suggest that muscle fibers can be classified into three types: SO, FOG, and FG.

ditions. We prefer the metabolic classification scheme using multiple stains of serial sections because the presence of enzymes is observed directly and not simply inferred on the basis of their putative relationship to ATPase activity.

SO muscle fibers generally predominate in muscles required to perform low-level contractions for a prolonged period of time (i.e., postural muscles). Thus, it is not surprising to observe a high proportion of these fibers in muscles involved in standing (soleus, vastus intermedius, and erector spinae muscles). Conversely, types FG and FOG fibers are found throughout the body in muscles required to generate high forces for a relatively short period of time. Most mammalian muscles contain all three fiber types; however, their proportion is roughly tailored to the particular needs of that muscle. (It should be mentioned that the influence of muscle fiber type proportion on performance has been grossly overstated in the literature. For example, although it is true that many sprinters' muscles contain a large proportion of fast fibers, it can be shown that the actual influence of this increased proportion on performance is quiet small.)

The various skeletal muscle fiber types also have distinct structural properties at the ultrastructural level.[5] For example, the width of the Z band, the amounts of T system and SR, the mitochondrial density, the capillary density, the amount and distribution of glycogen, and the amount of lipid also vary considerably between muscle fiber types. Most of these structural specializations make intuitive sense in relation to the general functions described earlier. For example, muscle fibers that are required to contract rapidly and relax rapidly (i.e., types FG and FOG fibers) have a large proportion of T system and SR. However, in muscles that need not contract rapidly but are required to generate tension for long periods of time (i.e., type SO fibers), the T system and SR are sparse but a large number of mitochondria are present to supply ATP aerobically — a more efficient method of energy production. An adaptation whose role is not clear is variance in the width of the Z disk. This width allows fair discrimination between fiber types at the ultrastructural level, but the specific reason for its difference among the three fiber types is not clear.

The Motor Unit

Whereas the functional unit of force generation is the sarcomere (actually the half-sarcomere owing to sarcomere symmetry), the functional unit of movement is the motor unit. The motor unit is defined as the alpha motoneuron and the muscle fibers that it innervates. Motoneurons exit the spinal cord at the ventral root, where they travel to the muscle and innervate a number of muscle fibers. Skeletal muscle fibers of a particular motor unit are distributed throughout the muscle. The number of muscle fibers innervated by a particular axon (i.e., the innervation ratio) varies among motor units. Similarly to muscle fibers, motor units can be classified on the basis of their contractile properties (Fig. 24-9). Early experiments by Burke[12] demonstrated that, by measuring the twitch contraction time, a fatigue index, and the presence or absence of ''sag'' (a phenomenon whereby the tension level of a partially fused tetanic contraction slowly decreased), motor units could be classified into three categories: (1) fast fatigable (FF)

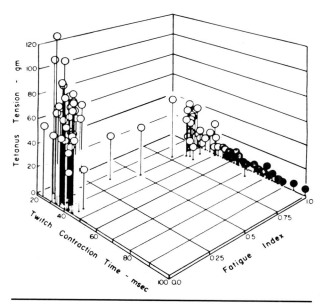

Fig. 24-9. Three-dimensional representation of motor unit types from the cat medial gastrocnemius muscle. The vertical axis represents the maximum tetanic tension of the motor unit. The horizontal axes represent the twitch contraction time (time required to reach peak twitch tension) and fatigue index (the ratio of tension after 2 minutes of stimulation compared to the initial tension). Note that, on the basis of these three parameters, motor units can be classified into three types, much like muscle fibers: fast fatigable (FF) units, fast fatigue-resistant (FR) units, and slow fatigue-resistant (S) units. (From Burke RE, Levine DN, Tsairis P et al: Physiological types and histochemical profiles in motor units of the cat gastrocnemius. J Physiol (Lond) 243:723, 1973, with permission.)

units, which have a short contraction time, a low fatigue index, and sag; (2) fast, fatigue-resistant (FR) units, with a short contraction time, a relatively high resistance to fatigue, and sag; and (3) slow, fatigue-resistant (S) units, with a long contraction time, high resistance to fatigue, and no sag. FF units were found to be composed of FG fibers, FR units were composed of FOG fibers, and S units were composed of SO fibers.

Many investigators have shown that the different motor unit types generate different absolute tensions, with FF units generating the highest tension and S units the lowest tension. It has been determined that the FF units generate these high tensions, based primarily on the fact that they are composed of a greater number of fibers of a larger size than either FR or S units.[13]

Motor units occupy specific regions within a muscle. Burke[12] demonstrated that, owing to the high fiber pennation angle, muscle fibers from a particular unit may be found at different levels along the muscle proximally to distally. In addition, more recent work by Bodine and coworkers[13] demonstrated that motor units occupy specific territories within a whole muscle cross-section. This information is particularly important for investigators interested in measuring the "representative" electrical activity of a muscle by electromyography. It is obviously possible to insert electrodes into muscles and selectively record muscle activity that may not be representative of the entire muscle.

The Size Principle

How are motor units activated physiologically? Considering the variety of motor units and fiber types, how are smooth contractions generated voluntarily? In the early 1960s, Henneman and colleagues[13a] performed the classic experiments that addressed these questions, elucidating the so-called size principle (see discussions of the many implications of the size principle in Binder[14]). The size principle states that axons are recruited in an orderly fashion according to their size. Henneman and coworkers demonstrated that, as a muscle was slowly stretched and tension slowly increased, electrical activity was recorded first from the very small axons, which generated small action potentials (Fig. 24-10A, middle trace, number 1). With increasing stretch, a second unit was recruited of slightly higher amplitude (Fig. 24-10A, right trace, number 2), and as stretch increased subsequent units were recruited, which generated action potentials of even higher voltage. Conversely, as the tension level was decreased (Fig. 24-10B), fibers were "de-recruited" in the opposite order to the one in which they were recruited. Because it was known that action potential voltage is related to axon size, these data suggested that the first units to be recruited in normal contraction were those composed of small axons.

It is known that S units (with the smallest axons) innervate slow muscle fibers. Thus, during a physiologic contraction, motor units are recruited in the

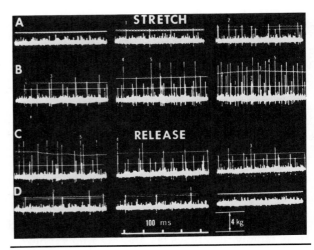

Fig. 24-10. Demonstration of the size principle. The cat soleus was stretched and the electrical activity of the muscle recorded. Note that early in the stretch a small action potential (labeled 1) is generated. As stretch progresses and tension increases, action potentials of increasing amplitude are recruited (labeled 2, 3, 4, and 5). These data suggest that axons are recruited in order from smallest to largest. (From Henneman E, Samjen G, Carpenter DO: Functional significance of cell size in spinal motoneurons. J Neurophysiol 28:560, 1965, with permission.)

order S, then FR, then FF. In other words, first slow-contracting fibers (type SO), and then fast fatigue-resistant fibers (type FOG) are recruited. Only in all-out efforts are the fast fatigable fibers (type FG) recruited. In summary, at the neuromuscular level motoneuron size distribution determines the distribution of muscle fibers activated during physiologic contractions.

The size principle is also consistent with the observation of Bodine and colleagues[13] that the FF units have the highest innervation ratio. This is because the large axons would be expected to provide sufficient axoplasm to support the many branches that innervate the muscle fibers. Finally, the size principle predicts that the fibers that are part of motor units innervated by small axons (i.e., the SO fibers) are active a much greater proportion of the time than other fibers belonging to other units. This may explain their relatively high oxidative capacity.

Another demonstration of the orderly recruitment of muscle fibers was assembled by Saltin and Gollnick,[15] who showed that, at low exertion levels, only slow fibers were recruited (Fig. 24-11). As exertion

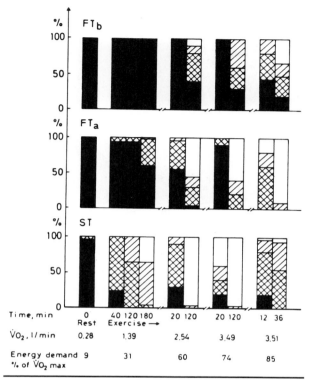

Fig. 24-11. Schematic illustration of the relationship between muscle fiber recruitment (as evidenced by muscle fiber glycogen depletion) and exercise intensity and duration. Dark bars represent fibers filled with glycogen, and therefore not recruited, whereas hatched and light bars represent fibers partially or fully recruited, respectively. Exercise intensity is expressed relative to the subject's maximum aerobic capacity (VO_{2max}). Note that as exercise intensity and duration increase, fiber type recruitment proceeds from ST (similar to SO) to FT_a (similar to FOG) to FT_b (similar to FG). This is presumably a manifestation of the size principle. (From Saltin and Gollnick,[15] with permission.)

level and duration increased, FOG fibers and then FG fibers were recruited. Thus, in exercise at lower intensities, selective activation of slow-contracting, highly oxidative, and fast-contracting oxidative fibers was seen. It was only during near-maximal efforts (actions such as power lifting and sprinting) that the FF units (and therefore the FG muscle fibers) were activated.

Interestingly, there is evidence that during external electrical stimulation of skeletal muscle such as that used in rehabilitation, motor units are activated in the reverse sequence. From the previous discussion, it should be clear that this is an undesirable result in rehabilitation, in which the stimulation is used for strengthening. This happens because muscle fibers that are used least often (FF units composed of FG fibers) will be activated most often and therefore receive the greatest training stimulus. Although it may be possible to measure an increase in a person's maximum voluntary strength after electrical stimulation therapy, such strengthening might be useless in normal activities of daily living, during which the "trained" FG fibers are not used at all.

SKELETAL MUSCLE PLASTICITY

Skeletal Muscle Response to Immobilization

The previous discussion describes the "typical" organization and function of the neuromuscular system. However, all of the characteristics of the system can be changed, given the appropriate stimulus. Thus, muscle fiber size, fiber type distribution, motor unit distribution, and even architecture are all "plastic." Numerous models have demonstrated that muscle adapts to the functional demands placed on it.[16] One of the most common models used to study plasticity is limb immobilization, which is designed to elucidate the factors that cause muscle atrophy. Clearly, this model is of interest to both basic scientists and clinicians. However, although most investigators agree that chronic immobilization of a muscle in a shortened or neutral position causes atrophy, not all muscles atrophy to the same extent. Why is it that one muscle atrophies to a different extent than another?

Investigators have demonstrated that muscles composed mainly of type SO fibers (i.e., "slow" muscles) atrophy to a greater extent than muscles composed mainly of type FG and FOG fibers (i.e., "fast" muscles). Additionally, antigravity muscles atrophy to a greater extent than their antagonists. This has been demonstrated experimentally by comparing the atrophy of slow muscles (e.g., soleus) to that of fast muscles (e.g., gastrocnemius, tibialis anterior, plantaris, extensor digitorum longus) after a period of limb immobilization. However, several difficulties arise in making comparisons between these two muscle types. First, the two muscles are immobilized at different lengths, which dramatically affects the atrophic response.[17] Second, the two muscle types normally have different activity levels. Thus, the *change* in level of use after immobilization differs. Third, the muscle fiber lengths, fiber length/muscle length ratios, and number of joints crossed differ among these different muscles, precluding definitive determination of the cause of atrophy. Thus, the relative influences of architecture, function, and fiber type distribution have not been clearly determined.

My colleagues and I performed a study on three heads of the dog quadriceps muscles (vastus lateralis [VL], vastus medialis [VM], and rectus femoris [RF]), which permitted the sorting out of these various factors.[18] The dog is uniquely suited for this type of study in that the three muscles mentioned have nearly identical architecture and fiber length but differ in fiber type percentage and number of joints crossed. (The RF acts both as a knee extensor and as a hip flexor and is composed of about 50 percent type SO fibers. The VM and VL both function as knee extensors only, but the VM contains about 50 percent type SO fibers and the VL contains only about 20 percent type SO fibers.) This model thus allowed comparison between the VM and VL, which can be immobilized at precisely the same length but contain different percentages of types SO and FOG fibers (to determine the influence of fiber type distribution). Similarly, comparisons between the RF and VM, which have similar fiber type percentages but cross different joints, could be made. Because dog muscles contain no type FG fibers, unequivocal identification of fiber types could be made from a single histochemical stain for myofibrillar ATPase activity. Finally, the external fixation procedure in this study permitted more reproducible setting of joint angle between animals than did simple cast immobilization and produced a more rigid fixation (Fig. 24-12).

Muscle fiber size and fiber type distribution were measured in the three muscles after 10 weeks of external fixation. In general, specimens from the immobilized side displayed muscle fibers with a variable distribution of size, shape, and staining intensities relative to the nonimmobilized side (Fig. 24-13). Neither necrotic nor inflammatory cells were observed. The oxidative activity of the immobilized muscles, as evidenced by histochemical staining intensity, de-

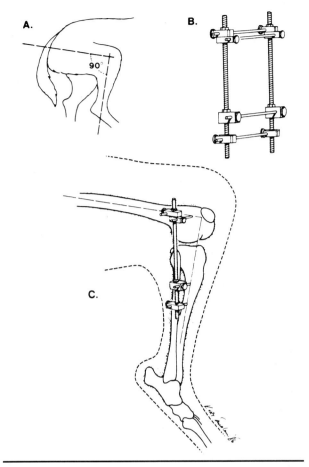

Fig. 24-12. Method used for immobilization of right knee at 90° **(A)** with an external fixator **(B). (C)** Device in the desired position. (From Lieber et al,[18] with permission.)

creased. However, the FOG fibers retained their normal oxidative staining pattern, with the highest mitochondrial staining density being on the fiber periphery. Qualitatively the VM atrophied to the greatest extent whereas the RF atrophied the least. The VL atrophic response was intermediate between that of the VM and that of RF (Fig. 24-14).

No difference in type SO or FOG fiber areas was observed between any muscles on the control side. However, the 10 weeks of immobilization resulted in significant decreases in both type SO and type FOG

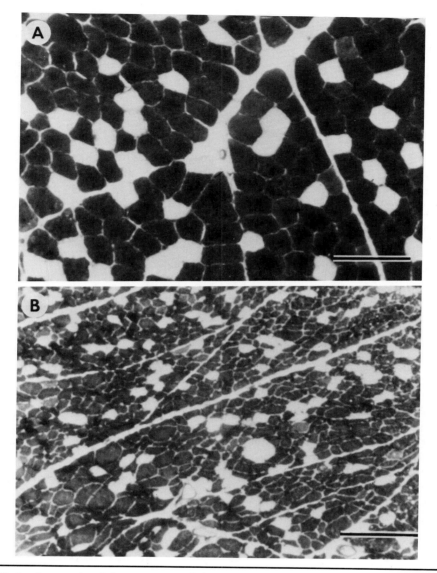

Fig. 24-13. Photomicrograph of dog vastus medialis muscle stained for myofibrillar ATPase activity after preincubation at pH 10.0. Fast fibers stain black. **(A)** Control muscle from "normal" leg. **(B)** Immobilized muscle. Calibration bar = 60 μm. This muscle demonstrates the greatest degree of atrophy. (From Lieber et al,[18] with permission.)

muscle fiber area. Although no significant difference was found among the type SO areas of the three immobilized muscles, a significant difference was observed among the type FOG areas of the immobilized muscles. Specifically, the type FOG fiber areas of the immobilized VM and VL were significantly smaller than the type FOG area of the immobilized RF.

Immobilization caused proliferation of endomysial and perimysial connective tissue relative to the control leg, perhaps contributing to the increase in joint stiffness after immobilization. In addition, a significant increase in fast fiber percentage after immobilization was observed in the VM. The atrophic response for type S fibers was thus, in order from most to least atrophied, VM > VL > RF (Fig. 24-14),

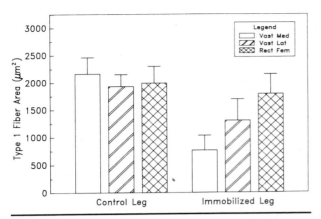

Fig. 24-14. Slow muscle fiber area from the three heads of the quadriceps muscle. Note that all muscles from the immobilized leg demonstrate atrophy. However, the degree of atrophy is greatest for the VM and least for the RF.

whereas for type F fibers the corresponding order was VM = VL > RF.

This study thus established the relative influence of two factors that contributed to immobilization-induced atrophy. The most significant factor was the degree of immobilization (number of joints crossed), and next was the change in use relative to normal function. The initial percentage of slow muscle fibers was a fair indicator of the normal use of the muscle and a good predictor of the relative degree of atrophy that could be expected. These data also indicated that a blanket concept of "slow fiber atrophy" did not apply to all muscles. Rather, it was a *combination* of factors that determined the muscular response to decreased use.

Relative Vulnerabililty of Muscles to Atrophy

Given the structure and fiber type distributions of the various human muscles, it is possible to predict which muscle will be most vulnerable to immobilization-induced atrophy: those that function as antigravity muscles, cross a single joint, and contain a relatively large proportion of slow fibers. This description fits the soleus, vastus medialis, and vastus intermedius muscles. The next class of muscles susceptible to immobilization-induced atrophy would be muscles that are antigravity, predominantly slow, and cross multiple joints — namely, the longissimus and transverso-

spinalis (erector spinae), gastrocnemius, and rectus femoris muscles. These muscle groups should be immobilized conservatively to avoid severe loss of strength. Conversely, phasically activated, predominantly fast muscles (e.g., tibialis anterior, extensor digitorum longus, biceps) could be immobilized with less loss of strength. This hierarchy of susceptibility to immobilization is supported by the data of Edgerton and colleagues,[19] who measured morphologic, biochemical, and physiologic properties of immobilized hindlimb muscles from *Galago senegalensis* (bush baby) and found that muscles atrophied in the following order (from most to least atrophy): soleus > plantaris > vastus intermedius = vastus lateralis > gastrocnemius > tibialis anterior = rectus femoris. This order agrees well with the principles stated earlier.

Skeletal Muscle Response to Electrical Stimulation

As another example of skeletal muscle plasticity, the response of muscle to chronic electrical stimulation is discussed briefly here. The chronic stimulation model has long been used by basic scientists to investigate the time course and nature of muscle adaptation. The clinical implications of such studies have been described elsewhere.[20]

The best documented effects of electrical stimulation on skeletal muscle are those that occur after chronic, low-frequency stimulation of a predominantly fast muscle during normal cage activity. In this setting, a well-defined progression of changes is observed whereby the muscle changes first its metabolic and then its contractile properties to become a slow muscle. This has been documented in the rabbit tibialis anterior and extensor digitorum longus, the rat extensor digitorum longus, the cat intertransversarii, and the cat peroneus longus and flexor digitorum longus muscles, so that effects observed are probably not species or muscle specific. The fast-to-slow transformation is detectable by measuring muscle contractile, ultrastructural, histochemical, biochemical, and morphologic properties. In all cases after transformation, the new slow fibers are completely indistinguishable from normal slow skeletal muscle fibers. It is also clear, from the results of time-series studies and single fiber biochemistry, that the changes result

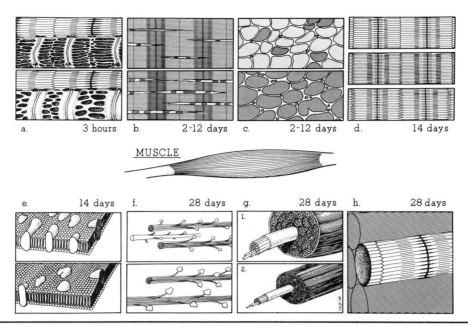

Fig. 24-15. Schematic representation of the time coruse of muscle fiber transformation. **(A)** The SR begins to swell after 3 hours of stimulation. **(B)** After 2 to 12 days of chronic stimulation, an increase in the volume percentage of mitochondria is observed. **(C)** After 2 to 12 days of chronic stimulation, an increase in capillary density and increase in type FOG fibers (represented as dark staining in this simulated succinate dehydrogenase are observed. **(D)** After 14 days the Z band begins to increase in width. **(E)** After 14 days a decrease in the amount and activity of calcium ATPase is observed. **(F)** After 28 days the myosin light chain profile is altered (this figure is schematic and actual structural changes associated with differences in light chains are not known). **(G)** After 28 days muscle mass and fiber area are decreased. **(H)** After 28 days the Z band extends the full width of a normal slow-contracting muscle and the density of the T system has increased. At this point the transformed fast-contracting muscle in indistinguishable from a normal slow-contracting muscle. (From Lieber,[21] with permission.)

from transformation at the level of the single fiber and not from fast fiber degeneration with subsequent regeneration of slow fibers.

Time Course of Muscle Fiber Transformation

If low frequency stimulation is applied 24 hours/day, the total process of transformation requires only about 30 days.[18] The earliest observed changes occur within a few hours after the onset of stimulation as the SR begins to swell (Fig. 24-15A). Within the next 2 to 12 days, increases are measured in the volume percentage of mitochondria, oxidative enzyme activity, number of capillaries per square millimeter, total blood flow, and total oxygen consumption, reflecting the increased metabolic activity of the muscle (Fig. 24-15B&C). Histochemically, this is reflected in an increased percentage of FOG fibers at the expense of

FG fibers (Fig. 24-15C). At this point, the width of the Z band begins to increase toward the wider value observed for normal slow muscle (Fig. 24-15D). The calcium transport ATPase decreases in amount and activity and its particle distribution changes within the SR bilayer (Fig. 24-15E). This decrease in the amount and activity of calcium ATPase can be detected physiologically as a prolonged time to peak twitch tension and a prolonged relaxation time of a muscle twitch, or as a decrease in the fusion frequency. The increases in oxidative enzymes and capillary density are manifested as a decrease in muscle fatigability. Finally, after about 4 weeks of continuous stimulation, an alteration in the myosin light chain profile is observed whereby the normally fast muscle, containing only light chains LC1F, LC2f, and LC3f, now contains light chains characteristic of slow fibers (i.e., LC1s and LC2s) (Fig. 24-15F). By this time, muscle fiber cross-sectional area, maximum tetanic tension, and muscle weight have significantly decreased (Fig. 24-15G). The Z band is now as wide as that normally observed in a slow fiber and the density of the T system is greatly decreased (Fig. 24-15H). The muscle is now indistiguishable from a normal slow skeletal muscle in every respect.[21]

Two basic conclusions were reached on the basis of this well-established time course of transformation: (1) muscle metabolic enzymes, capillaries, SR, and T system are much more easily altered than contractile proteins, and (2) although chronic stimulation does increase muscle endurance capacity, it is not automatically an effective means for strengthening normal muscle. (This second conclusion may be due, however, to the fact that most basic science studies have been performed while the limb is allowed to move freely. In accordance with the well-known force-velocity relationship [see previous discussion], this would result in very low force contractions, which is usually not the case in clinical application of stimulation.)

The chronic stimulation model illustrates the intimate relationship between muscle structure and function. For example, the early changes in the SR and T system are reflected in altered twitch contraction kinetics. Similarly, the decrease in myofibrillar area is manifested as a decreased muscle tetanic tension.

Neural Adaptation to Exercise

Results from the chronic stimulation model presented earlier suggest that alterations in muscle force-generating capacity require several weeks of prolonged training. How then is it possible to explain dramatic performance increases observed after only a few days of training? The answer lies in the nature of the voluntary contraction itself. It is possible to separate the effects of muscular adaptation and neural adaptation by measuring the activation signal that is sent to the muscle — the electromyogram (EMG). Although there are a number of limitations in methods used for obtaining EMGs and in EMG interpretation, under certain conditions the EMG provides a reliable indicator of the number of motor units activated during a certain task.

In a classic study (see review by Sale[22]), Moritani and DeVries measured the EMG and joint torque in a

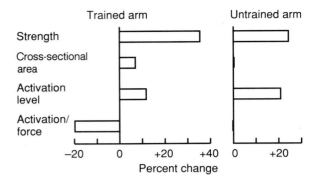

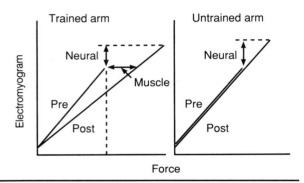

Fig. 24-16. Proportion of strength increase due to neural or muscular factors following 8 weeks of elbow flexion training in exercised (left) and contralateral control (right) limbs. Note that the increase in strength observed for the experimental limb (45 percent) was due partially to an increase in electromyographic (EMG) activity and partially to increased muscular strength. However, the significant increase observed in the control limb (25 percent) was due only to an increase in EMG activity.

number of subjects who performed elbow flexion exercises at relatively high intensities, twice per day for 8 weeks (Fig. 24-16). These investigators showed that the exercised arm increased in strength by about 40 percent after 8 weeks. At the end of 8 weeks, they demonstrated that the increase in strength was due primarily to an increase in muscle mass. However, they also observed a 20 percent increase in strength after only *1 week* of training. They demonstrated that this early change was due to an increased level of muscular activation, not to intrinsic changes in the muscle itself. Similarly, at the end of the 8-week training period the contralateral, nonexercised arm also increased in strength by 25 percent. Almost all of this was shown to be the result of increased muscle activation, not of changes in the muscle. It is thus clear that alterations in central drive may be partially responsible for the rapid increase in strength observed after training.

Other investigators have demonstrated more subtle changes in the EMG that can also alter muscle force output. For example, increasing the degree of synchronization of the various motor units leads to increased muscle force. Similarly, increases in motor unit firing rates result in increased muscle force in the absence of intrinsic changes in the muscle itself. Finally, decreased coactivation of a muscle antagonist results in an increase in strength for the agonist movement. All of these changes have been observed in training programs and may lend credence the concept of "central nervous system training" to increase performance levels.

SUMMARY

Skeletal muscle is exquisitely tailored at both macroscopic and microscopic levels to perform its task. Muscles themselves are highly specialized in terms of architecture, fiber type, and motor unit distribution. Thus, the specialized muscle is able to convert generalized activation information from the neural system and perform the appropriate external task. Skeletal muscle demonstrates a remarkable degree of plasticity, which may be exploited in the rehabilitation setting to strengthen muscle or decrease atrophy. An understanding of muscle plasticity may also be used in the diagnostic setting to elucidate a muscle's activation history.

REFERENCES

1. Squire J: The Structural Basis of Muscular Contraction. Plenum Press, New York, 1981
2. Peachey LD, Franzini-Armstrong C: Structure and function of membrane systems of skeletal muscle cells. p. 23. In Peachey LD, Adrian RH (eds): Handbook of Physiology. Section 10. Skeletal Muscle. American Physiological Society, Bethesda, MD, 1983
3. Ebashi S: Excitation-contraction coupling. Annu Rev Physiol 38:293, 1976
4. Gordon AM, Huxley AF, Julian FJ: The variation in isometric tension with sarcomere length in vertebrate muscle fibers. J Physiol (Lond) 184:170, 1966
5. Eisenberg BR: Quantitative ultrastructure of mammalian skeletal muscle. p. 73. In Peachey LD, Adrian RH (eds): Handbook of Physiology. Section 10. Skeletal Muscle. American Physiological Society, Bethesda, MD, 1983
6. Friden J, Kjorell U, Thornell L-E: Delayed muscle soreness and cytoskeletal alterations. An immunocytological study in man. Int J Sports Med 5:15, 1984
7. Hill AV: First and Last Experiments in Muscle Mechanics. Cambridge University Press, New York, 1970
8. Gans C: Fiber architecture and muscle function. Exercise Sport Sci Rev 10:160, 1982
9. Lieber RL: Skeletal muscle adaptability. I. Review of basic properties. Dev Med Child Neurol 28:390, 1986
10. Lieber RL, Blevins FT: Skeletal muscle architecture of the rabbit hindlimb: functional implications of muscle design. J Morphol 199:93, 1989
11. Edgerton VR: Mammalian muscle fiber types and their adaptability. Am Zool 18:113, 1978
12. Burke RE: Motor units: anatomy, physiology, and functional organization. p. 345. In Brooks VB (ed): Handbook of Physiology. Section1. The Nervous System. Vol. II. American Physiological Society, Bethesda, MD, 1981
13. Bodine SC, Roy RR, Eldred E, Edgerton VR: Maximal force as a function of anatomical features of motor units in the cat tibialis anterior. J Neurophysiol 57:1730, 1987
13a. Henneman E, Somjen G, Carpenter DO: Functional significance of cell size in spinal motoneurons. J Neurophysiol 28:560, 1965
14. Binder M: The Segmental Motor System. Oxford University Press, New York, 1989
15. Saltin B, Gollnick PD: Skeletal muscle adaptability: significance for metabolism and performance. In Peachey LD, Adrian RH (eds): Handbook of Physiology. Section 10. Skeletal Muscle. American Physiological Society, Bethesda, MD, 1983
16. Pette D (ed): Plasticity of Muscle. Walter de Gruyter, New York, 1980
17. Simard CP, Spector SA, Edgerton VR: Contractile properties of rat hindlimb muscles immobilized at different lengths. Exp Neurol 77:467, 1982
18. Lieber RL, Friden JO, Hargens AR et al: Differential response of the dog quadriceps muscle to external skeletal fixation of the knee. Muscle Nerve 11:193, 1988
19. Edgerton VR, Barnard RJ, Peter JB et al: Properties of immobilized hind-limb muscles of the Galago senegalensis. Exp Neurol 46:115, 1975
20. Lieber RL: Skeletal muscle adaptability. III. Muscle properties following chronic electrical stimulation. Dev Med Child Neurol 28:662, 1986
21. Lieber RL: Time course and cellular control of muscle fiber type transformation following chronic stimulation. ISI Atlas of Science: Animal and Plant Sciences 1:189, 1988
22. Sale DG: Neural adaptation to resistance training. Med Sci Sports Exercise 20:S135, 1988

25 The Biological Basis of Musculoskeletal Rehabilitation

WAYNE H. AKESON
DAVID AMIEL
JEAN-JACQUES ABITBOL
STEVEN R. GARFIN

This chapter addresses rehabilitation from the standpoint of relevant biologic, pathophysiologic, and biomechanical effects of altered stresses on the musculoskeletal system. Emphasis is placed on describing the effects of stress deprivation on synovial joints, the biochemical events occurring in connective tissue matrices underlying those changes, and the resulting biomechanical distortion of the joint composite.

One of the crucial goals of rehabilitation is to prevent or at least minimize the myriad events set in motion when cells no longer respond to external physical forces above some threshold level. Therapeutic decisions must be made with this goal constantly in mind. Whether the modalities used are medical, surgical, physical therapeutic, orthotic, or prosthetic, the goal remains clear: The patient must be engaged in a dynamic process of mobilization at the earliest possible time.

Cells adapt to environmental conditions. Of the many influences to which cells must respond, none are more universal than mechanical forces. Yet until recently the importance of mechanical forces for tissue homeostasis has received relatively little attention. Virtually nothing is known about the mechanisms of signaling by which mechanical forces induce cellular responses. A recently described array of cell membrane receptors called integrins has been found to be employed by cells to achieve adherence to other cells or to adjacent extracellular matrices.[1] The integrins provide the linkage between the cytoskeletal components within the cell and the adjacent extracellular matrix. Integrins probably also are an element in the communication system of the mechanoreceptor complex. Details of this complex remain to be described, but the technologies of cellular biomechanics, molecular biology, and immunohistochemistry offer opportunities to develop a better understanding of the manner by which cells interact with their physical environments.

These issues have practical value; therapeutic choices of use versus rest must be made daily in management of the disorders of the musculoskeletal system. The rapid deterioration of synovial joint tissues under conditions of stress deprivation has been described in detail over the past two decades. Moreover, the slow recovery from these effects also has become painfully clear. Consequently, the need for active motion to maintain synovial joint homeostasis has been well accepted as the means of preventing stress deprivation effects. These concepts have been incorporated into virtually every aspect of management of injuries and disorders of the spine and appendicular skeleton. Examples of such applications abound, including early mobilization of extremities via aggressive stabilization of fractures in the multiply injured patient, aggressive rehabilitation of the anterior cruciate ligament reconstructed knee, the widespread use of braces rather than casts, early passive motion of repaired tendon lacerations, and the whole concept of continuous passive motion. Shortened hospitalization times and consequent decrease in health care costs have been an important by-product of this approach.

STRESS DEPENDENCE OF CONNECTIVE TISSUE

The interrelationship of skeletal form and function has long been accepted. The most explicit expression of the relationship has been Wolff's law, which states that bone adapts to the applied stresses. This law has been found to apply equally importantly to the joint composite, including articular cartilage, ligament, tendon, capsule, and synovial membrane.[2-16] This broader expansion to include other tissues than bone suggests this law also is "Wolff's law of connective tissue," although other "laws" also govern relationships between form and function of fibrous connective tissue and the joint composite.[6]

The following material summarizes present understanding of the effects of stress enhancement and stress deprivation on synovial joints. Generalizations are possible to a certain extent, but it is important to remember that specialized connective tissues retain unique characteristics, which modulate responses to mechanical influences. As is pointed out later, even fibroblasts may not respond uniformly from site to site. However, the basic principle is clear: prevention of stress deprivation effects is the key to success, as it is in most of medical therapeutics.

ANATOMIC PATHOLOGY

Reviewing the protean manifestations of stress deprivation on synovial joints will allow therapeutic decision making to be placed into perspective. Experimental animal and human changes are closely similar. These changes are conveniently divided into (1) periarticular and synovial tissue changes, and (2) articular cartilage and subchondral bone changes.

Periarticular and Synovial Tissue Changes

Grossly, the periarticular and synovial tissues of immobilized joints consistently reveal a fibrofatty connective tissue proliferation within the joint space.[7,8] In knee immobilization models, this phenomenon is seen prominently in the intercondylar notch but is also observed in other joint recesses. The proliferative fibrofatty connective tissue covers exposed intra-articular soft tissue structures such as the cruciate ligaments and the undersurface of the quadriceps tendon. It also blankets the nonarticulating cartilage surfaces. With the passage of time, adhesions develop between the exposed tissue surfaces as the fibrofatty connective tissue is transformed into more mature scar. The proliferation of this type of tissue is essentially the same in such diverse species as the rabbit, rat, dog, and primate. Similar changes are also prominent in human posterior intervertebral and knee joints.[8]

Articular Cartilage Changes

The changes that occur as a result of immobility of articular cartilage can be separated into those in noncontact areas and those in contact areas. The changes in noncontact areas are thought to result in part from the fibrofatty connective tissue proliferation described earlier. The ingrowth of connective tissue, which fills the joint space, soon covers the joint surfaces. In the rat model studied by Evans and colleagues,[7] the articular surfaces became covered by 30 days. The connective tissue became more dense and adherent during the subsequent month and remained relatively constant thereafter. The surface cartilage cells gradually became confluent with the overlying connective tissue. By 60 days the tangential layer of cartilage cells was lost in many of the animals. There was consistent evidence of gross thinning of the cartilage beginning peripherally, where the adhesions first occurred. Fibrillation of the cartilage and variable loss of staining of matrix also were observed. Staining changes were described by Baker and coworkers,[9] in human spinal facet joints after anterior spine fusion. These changes included first a zone of loss of staining around the cells peripheral to the cellular lacunae. Ultimately, loss of definition of lacunae occurred, and the cartilage cells became stellate, with poorly defined margins. Such change in staining characteristics of cartilage matrix had been described much earlier by von Reyher in 1874.[10] Baker and associates[9] described similar changes and termed them "Weichselbaum's space."[9,11] Parker and Keefer observed this process in cartilage beneath rheumatoid pannus and proposed that it represented a metaplastic process of cartilage cells transformed into fibroblasts,[12] a view that Baker and colleagues endorsed.

In the contact areas of opposed articular surfaces, mild to severe changes of articular cartilage are observed, depending on the rigidity of immobilization, the position of immobilization, and, most important, the degree of compression. Typically, mild changes consist of loss of staining intensity of the matrix. Areas with greater compressive forces may show varying degrees of destruction, up to and including full-thickness ulceration of cartilage with cellular distortion and necrosis, fibrillation of matrix, and erosion of the matrix down to subchondral bone.[13,14]

The major areas of alteration in the subchondral bone occur beneath cartilage lesions in joints immobilized 60 days or longer. Hyperemia in the subajacent marrow spaces is noted, with proliferation of connective tissue. In some areas this tissue has penetrated the subchondral plate and has entered the calcified layer of articular cartilage. Trabecular atrophy and resorption in the areas subajacent to cartilage lesions also are seen. Subchondral cysts sometimes develop in this location in animals followed for longer periods.

Not surprisingly, such profound alterations in gross and microscopic architecture are associated with significant biomechanical and biochemical changes.

EXPERIMENTAL MODELS OF THE FIBROUS CONNECTIVE TISSUE RESPONSE TO STRESS ALTERATION

Considerable interest has been expressed in the underlying processes involving the capsular and ligamentous changes in immobilized limbs, and in the possibility of modifying the responses through the use of drugs of hormones. In an experimental model designed to evaluate the soft tissue response to immobility in our laboratory, the hind limbs of dogs[2] and rabbits[15] were immobilized for up to 12 weeks using internal fixation procedures, and periarticular connective tissues were examined.

Casts and internal fixation of the flexed knee with a threaded pin placed through the tibia and femur well posterior to the knee joint give similar results. The latter technique has generally been preferred to prevent ulcer formation from cast compression and friction.

Biomechanical Changes of the Knee Composite

The knee contracture can be assessed immediately after the animals are killed through an apparatus called an arthrograph.[16] The arthrograph measures the joint stiffness in knees in terms of a torque-angular deformation (T-0) diagram. The experimental and control knees from each animal were mounted on the arthrograph and cycled at a frequency of 0.2 Hz. Two ranges of motion, five cycles each, were used in sequence: the first was 50° to 80° and the second 45° to 95° of knee angles. Each cycle of flexion and extension was recorded on the X-Y recorder. Recording of the first cycle of the contracture knee is particulary important because subsequent cycles required substantially less energy. In addition, the amount of torque required to extend the knee from 50° to 65° from acute flexion during the first cycle also is significantly higher than that of subsequent cycles. The increases in torque and area of hysteresis are used as measures of increase in joint stiffness or severity of joint contracture. A progressive increase in the strength of contracture is observed on serial evaluations between 2 and 12 weeks. Detailed descriptions of the apparatus and technique are given in earlier papers.[15,16] The arthrograph permits evaluation of the efficacy of therapeutic modalities such as drug or hormone injections on the process. Interestingly, hyaluronic acid has been shown to inhibit contracture development significantly under stress deprivation conditions.[17]

Biomechanical Changes in Ligaments

After 9 weeks of immobilization, the linear slope, ultimate load, and energy-absorbing capabilities of the rabbit medial cruciate ligament (MCL)–bone complex during tension decrease to approximately one-third those of the contralateral nonimmobilized control knee. The load-strain characteristics of the MCL substance deteriorate. Further immobilization of up to 12 weeks causes additional degradation of the MCL substance.[4] These data are obtained with the aid of the video dimensional analyzer system, in which the mechanical properties of ligament substance and structural properties of the bone-ligament complex can be evaluated simultaneously[18].

The failure mode is altered in this model, as are reduction in the failure load and reduction in modules of elasticity. The bone resorption at the ligament insertion site causes failure by avulsion at the insertion site, a problem noted by several investigators.[19–21]

These mechanical alterations occur after a relatively brief stress deprivation period compared to common clinical treatment programs for fractures and joint injuries. They have important implications for the rationale for selection of treatment options and, as is seen, equally dramatic implications for rehabilitation after recovery from the initial injuries.

Exercise Effects on Specialized Connective Tissue Structure

An animal model has been used to evaluate effects of exercise on bone, tendon, and ligament in normal subjects. In one study, miniature swine were exercised at intervals on a track over 1 year on a schedule that created cardiac hypertrophy and increased cardiac output.[22] At the end of 1 year, cortical bone showed improved structural properties of about one-third, indicative of cortical hypertrophy. The material properties were unchanged, indicating that the changes observed were entirely due to bulk change rather than qualitative improvement. Similar changes were observed for digital extensor tendons. The cross-sectional areas 12 months after onset of the exercise period were increased 21 percent, and the load to failure increased 62 percent.[23] It is important to observe that, at 3 months after onset, changes in bone and extensor tendon were not significant, indi-

cating that a long time and large effort are required for improvement in structural properties. Furthermore, site and tissue-specific factors are involved, because digital flexor tendons and ligaments were less responsive to the exercise program than were bone and extensor tendon.

Recovery from Stress Deprivation

Interestingly, the recovery of the MCL properties after immobilization may be quite rapid. The load-strain curve properties of the MCL from the experimental knee of animals immobilized for 9 weeks recover to those of the control after 12 weeks of cage activity. The recovery curve for the knees immobilized for 12 weeks remains slightly inferior after a cage-activity recovery period of 12 weeks.[24] The experimental knee ligaments continue to have inferior structural properties as compared to those of the control knees. The P_{max} and the A_{max} for the experimental knees are approximately two-thirds those of the controls. The slower recovery of strength of the bone-ligament junction confirms findings obtained by other investigators.[19,21,25]

The surprising finding, however, is that after remobilization a rapid recovery of properties of the MCL substance occurs in the functional range (up to 5 percent ligament strain), although the ultimate load and energy-absorbing capability of the MCL-bone complex are still considerably inferior.[24] The tibial insertion sites continue to be the weakest link. These results are consistent with the earlier conclusion of Noyes and colleagues,[25] who showed that up to 1 year of reconditioning is required to regain the strength of anterior cruciate ligament–bone complex after 8 weeks of immobilization. Additionally, our data indicate that the ligament substance will recover rapidly during remobilization and the ligament itself can function normally in the physiologic range.

The implications for treatment are that prevention of stress deprivation effects are paramount to the success of rehabilitation efforts. This conclusion forms the central basis of the scientific rationale supporting rehabilitation therapies at the earliest possible juncture.

Biochemical Events Consequent to Stress Deprivation

The biochemical changes of periarticular connective tissue matrix are manifold. Space does not permit a detailed description of those changes. However, a summary follows, along with key references to the literature on the subject. An important point, which has evolved from our laboratory, is that there are notable differences between cellular and biochemical matrix characteristics of ligaments and tendons and, furthermore, differences occur between particular ligaments. The functional implications of these differences are not yet entirely clear and require further study.

Extracellular Fluid Volume Changes

The water content of fibrous connective tissues is in the range of 65 to 70 percent. Because the population of cells is relatively sparse in this tissue, the majority of this water is necessarily in the extracellular space. On gross inspection, the dissected tissues from the immobilized limb appear less glistening and more "woody" in texture. Chemical analysis shows a significant decrease in water content of 4 to 6 percent as compared to the control side.[26] It seems likely that this amount of water loss is functionally significant. Fluid movement, which plays such an important role in articular cartilage load bearing and lubrication, is equally important in fibrous connective tissue in imparting viscoelastic properties. It has been established that hyaluronic acid and its attached or entrapped water is the principal fibrous connective tissue lubricant.[27]

The interstitial fluid in a densely fibrous "connecting" anatomic structure is presumed to serve as a spacer between individual collagen fibers or fibrils, permitting discrete movement of one fiber or fibril past the adjacent fibers. The importance of interstitial fluid to tissue rheology is obvious because the concept of viscoelasticity of connective tissue rests on the dual fluid and solid nature of these systems.

Glycosaminoglycan Changes

The largest change found in the composition of the stress-deprived periarticular connective tissue is reduction in the concentration of glycosaminoglycans (GAGs).[28] The decreases in chondroitin 4-sulfate and chondroitin 6-sulfate (30 percent) and hyaluronic acid (40 percent) are statistically significant, whereas the percentage of change of dermatan sulfate thought to be associated with fibers is smaller. Decreased concentration of GAGs and water would be expected to alter the plasticity and pliability of connective tissue matrices and to reduce lubrication efficiency. Biochemical analyses of articular cartilage and meniscus from the immobilized knees also show a reduction of 24 percent and 31 percent, respectively, of GAG content in these tissues.[28]

Water content appears to parallel the GAG ranges, which is in agreement with known high water-binding capacity of GAGs. The preferential loss of GAGs also is consistent with known facts about their rapid turnover half-life (1.7 to 7 days)[29] as compared with collagen (half-life of 300 to 500 days).[30] Turnover studies utilizing tritium-labeled acetate show that the decrement in specific activity of hyaluronic acid with time after preliminary labeling is the same for control and immobilized limbs. The conclusion therefore is that the mechanism is not acceleration of degradation but rather a reduction in the synthesis of hyaluronic acid in the immobilized extremities. The fibroblasts of the fibrous connective tissue matrix apparently respond to physical forces by a homeostatic feedback loop to maintain the proper balance of connective tissue constituents.

That a gel-like structure is created by the interaction of water and GAGs is currently well accepted by physiologists working with interstitial fluid flow questions.[31] Clearly, the gel structure is severely compromised in the connective tissue deprived of mechanical stimulation. It is postulated that the GAG and water changes are permissive insofar as qualitative changes in collagen are concerned, because fiber-fiber distances must be reduced when water and GAG volumes are reduced.

The lubricating and volume-separating effects provided by hyaluronic acid and water are presumed to allow the independent gliding of microfibrils past one another, facilitating the tissue adaptation to motion permitted by the particular connective tissue weave pattern. Loss of this volume-separating and lubricating property provides for fibril-fibril friction and makes possible adhesions or cross linking between adjacent collagen fibrils. Newly synthesized collagen tends to be randomly dispersed and to create interference with the functional gliding between fibers necessary for normal mobility, particularly because, in the stationary attitude, maturation processes may encourage growth in fibril diameter by including these newly synthesized random fibrils within the fiber structural units. Such mismatch with respect to functional elongation needs and weave without regard to the usual physical force and motion probably is central to the pathomechanics of joint stiffness.

Collagen Changes

The processes seen in the studies described earlier, which rely on the techniques of anatomic pathology, suggest that connective tissue proliferation or simple granulation tissue production is the basis of joint contractures. However, collagen turnover studies are difficult to reconcile with this concept at first examination. For example, the studies by Brooke and Slack[32] showed that collagen precursor uptake was actually reduced in denervated rat limbs compared to controls. However, the collagen synthesis did proceed, but at a reduced level. Peacock[33] used saline solubility of collagen to estimate the amount of new collagen synthesized and found no differences in immobilized and control joints except in the posterior capsular area, which showed increased collagen solubility. However, because Peacock used pin fixation with a placement proximate to the posterior capsule, the signficance of finding total collagen mass changes became uncertain. Investigators in our laboratory were able to demonstrate reduction in total collagen of only 10 percent by total joint mass evaluation using the whole periarticular connective tissue unit.[34] Studies of Klein and associates[35] using long-term labeling techniques (which are more sensitive for this purpose) found small increases in collagen mass in denervated limbs.

We believe, however, that strategic placement of anomalous cross links of newly synthesized collagen fibrils in the contracture process is of importance. These cross links can act as bridges between existing functionally independent fibers with divergent tracking patterns. Using a simplified model (i.e., the Chinese finger trap mechanism), it can be seen that fixed contact at just a few nodal points defeats the functional gliding of the whole apparatus. Demonstration of such changes within the weave of the joint capsule is quite difficult because of right-to-left variability in microarchitecture and the small degree of change necessary to effect a mechanical impediment. However, it is easy to be convinced that such a process must play a role in the synovial joint contracture process. Disorganization in the cruciate ligament of a rabbit after 9 weeks of immobilization has been demonstrated in our previous work.[36] The pattern of cellular alignment becomes distorted as well, almost certainly reflecting a more random matrix organization.

Collagen Cross Link Alterations

The studies of quantitative changes in the cross linking of collagen from the immobilized rabbit knee periarticular connective tissue show significant increases in the sodium borohydride–reducible intermolecular cross links.[37] A typical radioactive elution profile from column 1 of a $3N$ p-toluene sulfonic acid hydrolysate of [3H]NaBH$_4$ reduced periarticular connective tissue from control and immobilized joints, and the rechromatography results on an extended basic column of the aldolhistidine dihydroxylysinonorleucine peaks show a twofold increase in dihydroxylysinonorleucine (DHLNL) on the immobilized side. It was shown that DHLNL, hydroxylysinonorleucine (HLNL), and histidinohydroxymerodesmosine (HHMD) are the major cross links that increase following immobilization. No change in hydroxylysine-lysine ratio between the immobilized and control periarticular connective tissue collagen was detected.

It can be speculated that the increased intra- and intermolecular collagen cross links are important in the contracture process. How do such cross links interact at a molecular level? To begin with, it is unlikely that a fiber-to-fiber distance is bridged by a lysine-lysine or lysine-hydroxylysine reaction. The distances are much too great and the forces too small to create the nodal fiber-to-fiber cross link that is proposed to hamper joint motion. Rather, it is presumed that the nodal fiber-to-fiber cross links are brought about by aggregation of new fibrils with preexisting fibers of the matrix. The process may proceed in the usual manner of aggregation of fibrils into fibers, followed by incorporation of bridges of newly synthesized collagen fibril elements into pairs of existing fibers. Such structures become mechanically constraining at the time when the joint is freed from constraining devices.

Collagen Type Changes

Because the formation of reducible cross links follows collagen synthesis,[38] and because the presence and relative amounts of these cross links may, in part, depend on the type of collagen being synthesized,[39] it is important to examine the type or types of periarticular connective tissue collagen synthesized during the period of immobilization. Examination of the densitometric scans of the sodium dodecyl sulfate (SDS) gel of the cyanogen bromide (CNBr)–cleaved peptides from control and immobilized tissue reveals no alteration in the type of collagen being synthesized during the period of immobilization.[34] The peptides α_1[III] CB3 and CB6 characteristic of type III collagen are absent in the CNBr digest of the control and immobilized periarticular connective tissue collagen. Furthermore, these results are confirmed by amino acid analysis and SDS gel electrophoresis performed on intact components separated by CM cellulose chromatography. These results provide additional supportive evidence that only type I collagen is found in the dense fibrous structures of normal and contracture knees.

The changes in collagen type ratios and cross-linking patterns observed as a consequence of stress deprivation probably reflect the effects of increased collagen turnover. The altered mechanics, in turn, most probably result from the random orientation of newly synthesized fibrous matrix constituents. These new fibrils are disposed without regard to mechanical requirements because of the lack of input from the mechanical signals that are normally operative.

DEVELOPMENT OF CONCEPTS OF PASSIVE MOTION

The events described earlier indicate a disturbing and very harmful outcome of stress deprivation on synovial joints, which threatens the success of rehabilitation after treatment with casts or splints for trauma or other disorders requiring immobilization. It was not unexpected, therefore, to observe the development of new concepts of treatment emphasizing early motion. The controversy about early motion had, in fact, erupted earlier still. The archetypical protagonists commonly identified as providing leadership for the motion versus rest camps in the century past were Hugh Owen Thomas, called "Hugh the rester," and J. Lucas-Championniere, whose philosophy of treatment was exemplified by his phrase "in motion there is life." These advocates of rest versus motion relied almost entirely on empirical observation and appeals to authority for the basis of therapeutic decisions. It remained for the effects of stress on synovial joints to become clarified before the therapeutic decision- on rehabilitation could be properly prioritized. Equally important in the evolution of modern rehabilitation philosophy were fundamental studies on the influence of stress and motion on repair of bone, tendon, ligament, and cartilage. Furthermore, studies on stress and motion effects on disorders of the synovial joint composite have provided a foundation for musculoskeletal management decisions that are approaching a more logical construct. Technological advances have occurred that, hand in hand with these observations, have provided new avenues for treatment that could be coupled with the early-motion philosophy of rehabilitation.

In fracture management, for example, it has been possible to achieve improved fracture stability with biomechanically sound internal fixation devices. These devices, applied very early in the post-injury period, have permitted not only early joint mobility[40] but also mobilization of the total patient. The ability to mobilize patients after multiple trauma has resulted in a marked improvement in the survival rates in the critically injured patient—a tribute to the modern trauma management system and to the philosophy of early mobilization.

This philosophy of early mobilization has adapted passive motion in several forms (occasional, interrupted, and continuous, with various combinations thereof) to the early postinjury or postoperative state, in which patient compliance with active motion programs cannot reasonably be expected because of postoperative pain or weakness.

For successful application of passive motion to the post-injury state, the integrity of the repair—bone, ligament, or tendon—must be maintained. Details of specific applications await further contributions from basic and clinical science. However, enough is known that it is possible to develop an understanding of some of the general principles of application that should find universal utility in musculoskeletal rehabilitation for the foreseeable future. What follows is a brief outline of the evidence that passive motion is effective in a variety of clinical applications and a summary of the scientific basis of those applications.

Synovial Joint Space Clearance during Continuous Passive Motion

Studies on clearance rates from synovial joints have demonstrated the value of passive motion in facilitating transport of intrasynovial contents. Cyclical changes in intra-articular pressure during CPM have been documented.[41-43] The clearest example of this application is the paper of O'Driscoll and colleagues[44] on the clearance of blood from the joint space. These data demonstrated convincingly that a hemarthrosis in a model system treated by continuous passive motion (CPM) was cleared more rapidly than in contralateral mobilized joints. The clearance rate of indium[III] oxine–labeled erythrocytes was double that seen in the immobilized joints. After 1 week significantly less blood remained in the joints treated with CPM. These results were supported by Danzig and associates.[45]

This effect was seen indirectly in a study by Skyhar and colleagues on nutrition of anterior cruciate knee ligaments under conditions of CPM and rest using $^{35}SO_4$.[46] They demonstrated that in knees exercised with CPM less $^{35}SO_4$ uptake occurred than in a cage-activity group. The effect of CPM on synovial fluid clearance was so large that the uptake of $^{35}SO_4$ in the CPM-treated knees was less than that in the immobilized knees, suggesting, at first, poor diffusion under conditions of CPM, but actually indicating that clearance of isotope occurred before diffusion into the ligament could occur.

These experiments demonstrate the importance of the convection effect of activity to the nutritional support of synovial joint components, especially ar-

ticular cartilage and ligaments. Furthermore, the clinical application of CPM in the postoperative state is emphasized as a practical step in improved patient care postoperatively or after trauma. The clearance of blood from the joint space is of undisputed advantage considering the harmful effects of chronic hemarthrosis in states such as hemophilia.

Continuous Passive Motion in Treatment of Septic Arthritis

The use of motion to favorably influence the outcome of septic arthritis has been demonstrated in papers by Salter and coworkers[47,48] in a model system. The beneficial effect was seen most prominently in articular cartilage, in which the damage of the septic process from proteolytic enzymes was reduced by the imposition of a passive motion program. Presumably, clearance of the deleterious lysosomal enzymes that accumulate in joint fluid in septic arthritis was facilitated by motion-induced convection effects. The articular cartilages of joints treated by the activity protocols presumably were spared exposure to high levels of matrix-destroying enzymes by the acceleration of clearance of those products from the joint space by CPM. Clinical support for this application has been presented by Mooney and Stills.[40]

Passive Motion Effects on Repair

Several repair models have been studied under the influence of one of the passive motion modalities. In several applications the quality of repair appears to be improved under motion conditions in comparison to immobility. These applications require stability of the repair line for healing to proceed successfully. This is seen most clearly in flexor tendon repair, in which failure of the suture line in the early postoperative state can result in tendon disruption. However, if the suture line is maintained, improved outcome has been observed in several respects.[49] In certain circumstances intermittent passive motion has resulted in a successful outcome. In the case of ligaments, cage activity has been shown to be superior to the immobilized condition.[50] In still other circumstances, especially in cartilage healing, CPM was shown to provide a superior outcome.[51] Generally speaking, the experimental models have indicated improved healing rates of bone, tendon, ligament, and cartilage under motion conditions and also improved quality of repair. Indeed, in the case of the flexor tendon within the flexor tendon sheath, healing has been shown to proceed by different mechanisms under motion conditions (intrinsic healing) versus immobilization conditions (extrinsic healing — the one-wound concept).[49] The available data are insufficient to describe optimum clinical protocols of frequency, intensity, or duration of passive motion. We have spoken of the problem as analogous to the drug dose-response curve. In fact, the optimum values for passive motion may be found to vary in the spectrum of specific applications. Until such data are available, empirical rules will apply.

The examples that follow, however, will provide insights into the range of potential applications of passive motion to the problems of specialized connective tissue healing and the broad principles that underlie these uses.

Continuous Passive Motion Influence on Cartilage Healing

Early concepts of cup arthroplasty recognized that conversion of the new arthroplasty surface to fibrocartilage after débridement of the degenerative hip and reaming to a concentric sphere of bleeding bone required motion. Without motion the surface would contain only fibrous tissue. In a few instances the opportunity arose to observe bone surfaces in patients who had not been able to move the hip for unrelated medical reasons. In these patients, conversion of fibrous tissue to fibrocartilage had not occurred. Mooney, and Ferguson showed this effect in the rabbit metatarsophalangeal joint, in which immobilized segments did not develop fibrocartilaginous surfaces as well as did mobilized joints.[52] Hohl and Luck were able to demonstrate superior healing than was seen in immobilized knees in drill hole defects in femoral cartilage of primates if motion occurred.[53] Convery and associates studied various sized drill hole defects of femoral condyles of horses on pasture grazing activity and observed that relatively small defects ($\frac{1}{8}$-inch diameter) healed readily, but larger defects ($\frac{1}{4}$-inch to $\frac{7}{8}$-inch diameter) did not heal.[54] The dimensional aspect of cartilage healing is important to recognize, because with or without motion regimens, large defects ($\frac{1}{4}$-inch or larger) simply do not heal by restoration of hyaline cartilage, nor do

arthroplasty surfaces heal with hyaline cartilage. The composition of the articular surface replacement matrix is fibrocartilage, not hyaline cartilage. This conclusion has been demonstrated convincingly by histologic and biochemical methods. These factors have obvious functional and clinical implications, which must temper the interpretation of CPM effects on cartilage healing.

Salter and colleagues have been important contributors to the studies of facilitation of cartilage healing under the influence of CPM. They have shown convincingly that small defects of rabbit femoral articular cartilage of the order of magnitude of $\frac{1}{8}$-inch diameter will heal with hyaline cartilage in a significant percentage of knees mobilized by CPM. This is an important observation, which relates to several clinical circumstances in which small defects in hyaline cartilage of the joint surface occur, such as cracks in articular surfaces seen commonly in fracture patterns. It is important to note that the facilitation of repair of primitive mesenchymal cells to hyaline cartilage occurs *only* in the very small defects, not in large defects or full-surface defects.

Continuous Passive Motion Influences on Periosteal and Perichondrial Grafting of Cartilage Defects

The fact that only very small cartilage defects heal with a satisfactory extracellular matrix of hyaline cartilage has led several investigators to search for improved techniques of treating such defects. Ohlsen[55] and Engkvist[56] studied rib perichondrial tissue as a potential source of primitive cells with chondrogenic potential for this purpose. The work was later confirmed by Coutts and associates,[57] Salter and coworkers,[58–60] and Mooney and colleagues.[61] Because experimental studies offered considerable promise, pilot clinical perichondrial arthroplasty studies for small joints of the hand were performed soon thereafter with some success.[62] Poussa and colleagues[63] showed similar chondrogenic potential of periosteal grafts. O'Driscoll and Salter confirmed this work in a rabbit knee joint model.[48] They were able to improve the result from 8 percent success in immobilized knees to 59 percent success in knees managed by CPM. Fixation of the periosteal or perichondrial membrane is crucial to the successful outcome of periosteal or perichondrial grafting. O'Driscoll and Salter and their colleagues developed a method of stretching the periosteal membrane over a bone plug sized to fit the defect to be filled. This technique has worked effectively in the experimental application,[48,58-60] but different methodology will probably be required for clinical application.

Continuous Passive Motion Influence on Fracture Healing

The development of modern biomechanical devices and modern principles of application of such devices to fracture fixation permits the use of CPM early in the postinjury state.[40] CPM is applied most effectively in intra-articular fractures, in which fracture lines through subchondral bone and articular cartilage are commonly observed. In accordance with the observations of Salter,[59] the width of the gap between fracture fragments after reduction frequently is less than $\frac{1}{8}$ inch. If congruence of the joint is established and the cartilage fracture gaps are narrow, CPM may facilitate the cartilage healing process. Additional benefits should be anticipated in terms of facilitation of the rehabilitation program by lessening stress deprivation effects and by providing stress enhancement to guide deposition of matrix components in an orderly and functionally desirable alignment.

Intermittent Passive Motion Effects on Tendon Healing

The application of passive motion to flexor tendon healing in the "no man's land" of the flexor tendon sheath has been slow to evolve, for two reasons: (1) concern about integrity of the suture line and (2) concern about the mechanism of tendon healing requiring ingrowth of connective tissue from the flexor tendon sheath. The paradox of the latter process, termed the "one-wound concept" by Peacock,[33] is that the very tissue ingrowth that caused healing also caused the tendon to be locked against the flexor sheath, thus limiting the functional tendon excursion. Indeed, the major failures in tendon surgery are not with tendon healing but with tendon adhesions, which markedly reduce the range of motion of the tendon and affected joints. The fundamental studies of Gelberman and colleagues[49] reversed this thinking by demonstrating clearly that tendon healing could occur by an intrinsic mechanism of proliferation of

epitenon and endotenon cells when the extrinsic mechanism is blocked by intermittent passive motion. The canine forepaw model was used for these flexor tendon studies. Not only did the tendon heal by the intrinsic route with passive motion application, but in addition healing occurred more rapidly and with greater mechanical strength while simultaneously preserving mobility of the tendon and the joints of the affected finger.

It is important to note that the motion required for this effect is not of great duration. The mobilization schedule used in the studies mentioned earlier was only 5 minutes of careful manual passive motion conducted by a technician twice a day. The remainder of the time the limb was immobilized in a Fiberglas cast. This "mini" passive motion schedule recognized the concerns about possible rupture of the suture line if a more aggressive passive motion protocol were used.

In this instance, passive motion therapy was able to convert the healing mode from extrinsic to intrinsic, while providing improved healing strength and improved mobility—a string of therapeutic bonuses of a type that are seldom so clearly identified after modification of a postoperative treatment protocol.

Salter and colleagues have shown, in the patellar tendon laceration model, similar effects of improved healing associated with continuous passive motion. In this case, repair involves both extrinsic and intrinsic mechanisms owing to the anatomic differences between patellar and flexor tendons.

Intermittent Active Motion Effects in Ligament Healing

The discussion of ligament healing is confounded by the unique anatomic and physiologic features of the diverse structures classified with the ligaments. For example, the anterior cruciate ligament (ACL) of the knee will not heal for reasons not precisely known, although the "hostile" synovial environment in which the ACL resides is widely presumed to be an important or even decisive factor in that outcome. The ACL receives significant nutrition from synovial fluid but that nutritional source may not be adequate to support fibroblastic proliferation (although it will support a healing response in the case of flexor tendon). We have demonstrated in our laboratory that the cells of the ACL have fibrocartilaginous characteristics.[64] Failure of fibrocartilaginous structures to heal is well known. However, whether the cellular morphology of the ACL is the explanation for its poor healing is unproved. The enigma remains. Nevertheless, CPM is used by many clinicians in the postoperative period after replacement of the ACL by a grafting technique in which a tendon or a bone-tendon-bone unit is employed. Burks and colleagues have cautioned that CPM can cause failure of the tendon graft if the graft is not isometric and is not firmly secured[65]; indeed, in such cases the graft is unlikely to survive in a rehabilitation setting whether CPM is used or not. Clinical studies by Noyes and coworkers support the conclusion that CPM is a safe modality when surgery is performed properly.[66] Tendon grafts actually become very weak structurally 3 to 6 weeks after insertion. Nevertheless, the best clinical successes have occured with early and aggressive rehabilitation protocols.

Experimental studies have shown that tendon cells of the ACL graft undergo autolysis in the intrasynovial environment[67] and are replaced by cells from synovial sources. The matrix of the graft is gradually remodeled and assumes the matrix characteristics of ACL.[67] In none of the animal studies has the ACL graft substitute recovered the degree of mechanical strength and structural properties of the original tissue.

Better experimental and clinical results can be reported for most other ligaments. The medial collateral ligament (MCL) of the knee, for example, has an abundant surrounding soft tissue blood supply, which offers ample nutritional and cellular support for the needed fibroplasia. The work of Inoue and colleagues in this area has provided strong evidence supporting early active motion of the knee.[50] When compared with knees immobilized for the entire postoperative period or knees immobilized for the first half of the postoperative period, the early activity group clearly showed superior mechanical and structural strength at the end of 12 weeks. Other authors have shown a favorable effect of CPM on reorganization of the fibrils of the scar into parallel arrays.[68] It is to be emphasized that in these models

the cruciate ligaments are intact, thus providing the stability necessary for early ambulation or CPM.

Continuous Passive Motion after Total Knee Replacement

The total knee replacement procedures now frequently performed for degenerative or rheumatoid arthritis have provided a challenging problem for the application of CPM. Early achievement of a nearly full range of motion postoperatively is important in the rehabilitation of these patients. Slow recovery of flexion is commonly observed postoperatively, sometimes requiring forceful manipulation under anesthesia.

A multiinstitutional study of over 100 total knee replacement cases treated traditionally and compared to similar cases treated with CPM has provided data that clarify the effectiveness of CPM in a clinical rehabilitation setting.[69,70] The patients treated with CPM had a more rapid gain in knee motion and had a shorter hospital stay than patients treated traditionally, a finding supported by other studies.[71-73] Data in Coutts and associates' series[69,70] showed a lower pain medication requirement than in the traditionally treated series. The theory commonly employed to explain the surprising tolerance of postoperative patients for passive motion is the "gate" theory of Melzack and Wall.[74] This theory postulates that nonpainful afferent input into spinal cord ganglia can overwhelm pain fiber input, thereby blocking a part of the pain perception otherwise experienced. CPM provides considerable afferent input owing to the effects of motion on proprioceptive receptors. This concept is not universally accepted in postoperative applications of CPM, but at least it seems clear that CPM does not increase pain medication requirements.

Continuous Passive Motion and Wound Healing

No wound disruptions have been reported from application of CPM postoperatively, and, furthermore, postoperative swelling and joint effusions were reduced.[69] The benefits of a relatively brief few days of application of CPM postoperatively appear to significantly outweigh questions of cost or of risk.

Continuous Passive Motion Prophylaxis against Thrombophlebitis

The use of CPM in the various clinical applications described earlier has evoked interest using it in prophylaxis against thrombophlebitis in the postoperative period of high risk.[75] The proposed physiologic basis is the cycling of intramuscular pressure, which occurs during passive motion as the muscles of the limb are lengthened and shortened passively. The passive pressure alteration almost certainly has the same functional effect as active muscle contraction in propelling venous blood back to the heart. Because venous stasis is presumed to be an important factor in venous thrombosis, the use of CPM, which would significantly reduce venous stasis, would be expected to reduce the rate of complications of postoperative thrombophlebitis and pulmonary embolism.

Preliminary results supporting this line of reasoning have been presented by Lynch and coworkers[76] and by Vince and colleagues,[73] but other studies showed no prophylaxis with respect to incidence of deep venous thrombosis as visualized by venogram.[71,72] Several centers have ongoing studies on this problem and will provide considerable information in the near future on the effectiveness of CPM in this application. As is typical of other studies of deep venous thrombosis postoperatively, the size of the clinical series must be very large to be valid statistically.

Other Uses of Continuous Passive Motion

An almost infinite variety of conditions can be treated by CPM. These include elbow contractures after surgical release,[77] hemophiliac joints after synovectomy,[78] and knee contractures after arthroscopy.[79] Recent review articles by Salter and by Mooney highlight other related clinical applications.[40,59] The principles for use of CPM are so fundamental that they are valid for numerous other potential applications, including the spine.

NEW OBSERVATIONS ON MECHANISMS OF THE CELLULAR RESPONSE TO MECHANICAL STIMULI

The tissue adaptation to mechanical forces varies dramatically depending on whether the forces are compressive or tensile. Areas where forces are primarily tensile develop fibrous characteristics, and areas where forces are primarily compressive generally develop cartilaginous characteristics. The obvious example of cartilaginous adaptation is, of course, articular cartilage covering the joint surfaces at the ends of long bones. In other areas where the compressive and tensile forces are mixed, fibrocartilaginous tissue develops; examples include the annulus fibrosus of the intervertebral disc and the meniscus of the knee. These structures share load bearing of longitudinal compressive forces and simultaneously accept considerable tensile load via hoop stresses. The presence of primarily fibrocartilaginous cells in the ACL has been described.[80] Whether this results from stress on the ligament during flexion and extension of the knee or from other causes, such as nutritional factors or meager blood supply, is not clear.

Cartilaginous and fibrocartilaginous tissues lack a significant blood supply, relying on diffusion and convection of fluid, ions, and small molecules for nutrition and homeostasis. Compressive forces undoubtedly force an adaptation toward avascularity because of the tendency of those forces to collapse small vessels and capillaries. However, the adaptation has a large price: the inability of these tissues to achieve intrinsic healing. The lack of vessels and associated primitive perivascular cells eliminates the possibility of scar production after injury. Lack of a healing response of cartilaginous and fibrocartilaginous tissues may affect many structures: intervertebral discs, meniscus and ACL of the knee, the Bankhart lesion of the shoulder, and others.

CELLULAR DIFFERENCES BETWEEN LIGAMENTS

Ultrastructural, histological, biochemical, and biomechanical differences have been described between the ACL and MCL, tissues with strikingly different capacities for healing.[64,80] Light microscopy of the MCL reveals spindle-shaped cells aligned with the long axis of the ligament and interspersed throughout the collagen fiber bundles.[64] The ACL cells are oval and aligned in columns between fiber bundles. Ultrastructurally, MCL collagen fibers are uniformly of large diameter.[80] The fibroblasts have long cellular processes in close apposition to surrounding collagen fibrils. Fibril diameters in the ACL are more heterogeneous. Oval cells are surrounded by an amorphous ground substance and have small microprocesses, which are not in close apposition to collagen fibrils.

A spectrum of fibroblast phenotypes appears to exist, ranging from the spindle-shaped connective tissue fibroblast of dermis, tendon, and fascia to the rounded, nested fibroblast of fibrocartilage. The ACL fibroblast seems to exist near the fibrocartilaginous end of the spectrum in terms of morphologic features. Quite possibly these features are interrelated with cellular function and help determine their response to injury. The form or function suitable for survival in a synovial environment may not be sufficient for mounting and sustaining an effective healing response. The concept that the shape of a cell and its orientation with respect to the surrounding matrix are important factors in modulating its proliferative response to mitogens was proposed by Wessels[81] in studies on skin. These observations were expanded by Gospodarowicz and colleagues.[82]

Fibronectin

Fibronectins are a class of high-molecular-weight glycoproteins proposed as a key element in the structural interrelationship of cells to matrix and to other cells.[83,84] They are associated with an array of cellular functions, including cellular adhesion (both cell-to-cell and cell-to-substratum), intra- and extracellular matrix morphology, cell migration, and reticuloendothelial system function (i.e., phagocytosis and chemotaxis). By having adhesive domains specific to fibrin, actin, hyaluronic acid, collagen, heparin, and cell surface factors, they function to attract and couple key elements in normal, healing, and growing organized tissue. In fact, fibronectins have been shown to facilitate wound healing[85] and to be required for normal collagen organization and deposition by fibroblasts in vitro.[86]

The ACL, MCL, and meniscus have stained positive for fibronectin. The fibronectin is heavily concentrated in the amorphous ground substance surrounding the ACL cells and meniscal cells, whereas in the MCL fibronectin is distributed evenly over the cell membrane, even out along the long cellular processes.

The amount of fibronectin in rabbit periarticular soft tissues has also been quantified.[87] The amounts of total extractable fibronectin found to be present in ACL, PCL, MCL, and pronator teres (PT), respectively, were 2.0, 1.9, 0.8, and 0.7 μg/mg of dry tissue. Although the fibronectin quantities in ACL and PCL were found to be similar, they were over twice as high as the amounts found in either MCL or PT.

Our laboratories have shown that the prolonged disuse of the knee joint in a rabbit model (i.e., 9 and 12 weeks of stress deprivation) resulting in significant alterations in fibronectin concentration in the periarticular connective tissues (ACL, MCL, and PT).

The concentration of fibronectin was measured by competitive enzyme-linked immunosorbent assay (ELISA).[87] Decreases of 54.0 percent and 63.7 percent occurred in the ACL after 9 and 12 weeks. The PT, being tonically stressed by the quadriceps muscles, showed no statistical change. The decreases in total fibronectin concentration observed in this study may reflect increased activity in enzymes that can degrade fibronectin, such as stromelysin. It should also be stated that the decrease in fibronectin occurring after stress deprivation could be explained by the biochemical alterations of the periarticular connective tissues (i.e., ligaments and tendons).

The loss of glycosaminoglycan (GAG)- and collagen-bound fibronectin after stress deprivation also could be related to the degradation of the GAGs and the collogen observed in these periarticular connective tissues.

Although fibronectin levels have been observed to increase in healing tissue,[88-90] it is not known whether differences in the baseline levels of fibronectin affect the healing potential of a tissue such as the cruciate ligament. Baseline levels in the cruciate ligaments are high compared to those in other periarticular tissues, which have a better healing response. Although the importance of fibronectin in various connective tissues is becoming increasingly evident, further studies are required to clarify its role in normal ligament structure and in the ligament healing response.

ADHESIVE PROTEIN RECEPTORS

A new superfamily of adhesion-mediating cell surface glycoproteins (the integrins) has been identified and partially characterized.[91] A major subfamily called the "very late antigens" (VLAs) appears to play a primary role in the adhesion of cells to components of the extracellular matrix, including fibronectin, collagen, and laminin.

The VLAs are transmembrane glycoproteins expressed on a wide variety of cells, including fibroblasts, epithelial cells, and hematopoietic cells. A number of functional roles have been assigned to these adhesive protein receptors, including cell migration, cell-matrix adhesions, wound contraction, and ligament "tensioning."[92]

The adhesive protein receptors of ligament tissue have received little attention to date. Generalizing from other fibroblast-containing structures, it is reasonable to expect that these receptors exist on cells of the cruciate ligaments and other periarticular tissues. Transforming growth factor beta (TGF_β) has been found to regulate the cell surface display of VLAs on a variety of cell types and to modulate the interaction of cells with the extracellular matrix.[93,94] These studies lead us to believe that cell surface receptor distribution and expression may have profound effects on ligament healing capacity. Fundamental studies on these receptors are in progress in several laboratories with respect to distribution in various connective tissue cells and to alteration of expression during the healing process.

CONCLUSIONS

It is abundantly clear by now that rehabilitation and acute therapeutic measures must overlap almost to the point of synonymity. The message of this chapter is one of prevention of the complications of stress deprivation. It is unjustifiable to allow serious and rapidly progressive effects of stress deprivation to occur in disorders or injuries of the musculoskeletal system. In virtually all cases of injury, acceleration of recovery has been demonstrated with the controlled institution of early activity. Education of patients, their families, and medical and paramedical professionals of the importance of this message must be fostered.

This review summarizes the existing knowledge of the roles of stress and motion in synovial joint homeostasis. The deleterious effects of stress deprivation occur rapidly and are profound, influencing joint mechanics, biochemistry, and physiology in fundamental ways. The recovery from this process is not expeditious, requiring many months rather than weeks to re-establish nearly normal values. In fact, composite ligament structures have not regained normal mechanical strength even 12 months after resumption of activity.

The manner in which cells interpret physical signals will be a fundamental topic for investigation in addition to the clinical efforts that will be made in the next decade. Although more and better clinical studies in this field are imperative, exercise as a therapeutic adjunct for rehabilitation of supporting connective tissues will be increasingly employed because of successes already achieved in the several applications described. That repair processes are facilitated by early motion seems an almost universal observation for tendon, ligament, cartilage, and bone. The utility of early motion in treating such widely divergent problems as septic arthritis, hemarthrosis, total joint replacement, and tendon repair indicates the breadth of applications currently employed clinically. Mechanical stimuli appear to be crucial as signals to cell receptors that control synthesis of matrix components and other factors that guide extracellular organization of those components. Clearly, additional efforts are required to clarify the importance and relevance of these principles.

REFERENCES

1. Hemler ME, Huang C, Schwartz L. The VLA protein family. J Biol Chem 262:3300, 1987
2. Akeson WH: An experimental study of joint stiffness. J Bone Joint Surg [Am] 43:1022, 1961
3. Akeson WH, Amiel D, Woo SL-Y: Immobility effects on synovial joints: the pathomechanics of joint contracture. Biorheology 17:95, 1980
4. Woo SL-Y, Kuei SC, Gomez MA et al: Effect of immobilization and exercise on strength characteristics of bone–medial col-

lateral ligament–bone complex. Am Soc Mech Eng Symp 32:62, 1979.

5. Akeson WH, Woo SL-Y, Amiel D, Frank CB: The biology of ligaments. In Hunter L, Funk F (eds): Rehabilitation of the Injured Knee. CV Mosby, St Louis, 1984
6. Frank C, Akeson WH, Woo SL-Y et al: Physiology and therapeutic value of passive joint motion. Clin Orthop Rel Res 185:113, 1984
7. Evans EB, Eggers GWN, Butler JK, Blumel J: Experimental immobilization and remobilization of rat knee joints. J Bone Joint Surg [Am] 42:737, 1960
8. Enneking WF, Horowitz M: The intra articular effects of immobilization on the human knee. J Bone Joint Surg [Am] 54:973, 1972
9. Baker WC, Thomas TG, Kirkaldy-Willis WH: Changes in the cartilage of the posterior intervertebral joints after anterior fusion. J Bone Joint Surg [Br] 51:737, 1969
10. von Reyher C: On the cartilage and synovial membranes of the joints. J Anat Physiol 8:261, 1874
11. Weichselbaum A: Die feineren Veranderungen des gelenk Knorpels bei fungoser Synovitis und Caries der Gelenkenden. Virchows Arch 73:461, 1878
12. Parker F, Keefer CS: Gross and histologic changes in the knee joint in rheumatoid arthritis. Arch Pathol 20:507, 1935
13. Salter RB, Field P: The effects of continuous compression on living articular cartilage. J Bone Joint Surg [Am] 42A:31, 1960
14. Thaxter TH, Mann RA, Anderson CE: Degeneration of immobilized knee joints in rats. J Bone Joint Surg [Am] 47:567, 1965
15. Akeson WH, Woo SL-Y, Amiel D et al: The connective tissue response to immobility: biochemical changes in periarticular connective tissue of the immobilized rabbit knee. Clin Orthop 93:356, 1973
16. Woo SL-Y, Matthews JV, Akeson WH et al: Connective tissue response to immobility. Correlative study of biomechanical and biochemical measurements of normal and immobilized rabbit knees. Arthritis Rheum 18:257, 1975
17. Amiel D, Frey C, Woo SL-Y et al: Value of hyaluronic acid in the prevention of contracture formation. Clin Orthop Rel Res 196:22, 1985
18. Woo SL-Y, Gomez MA, Seguchi Y et al: Measurement of mechanical properties of ligament substance from a bone-ligament-bone preparation. J Orthop Res 1:22, 1983
19. Laros GS, Tipton CM, Cooper RR: Influence of physical activity on ligament insertions in the knees of dogs. J Bone Joint Surg [Am] 53:275, 1971
20. Cooper RR, Misel S: Tendon and ligament insertion. J Bone Joint Surg [Am] 52:1, 1970
21. Tipton CM, Matthes RD, Martin RR: Influence of age and sex on the strength of bone-ligament junctions in knee joints of rats. J Bone Joint Surg [Am] 60:230, 1978
22. Woo SL-Y, Kuei SC, Amiel D et al: The response of cortical long bone secondary to exercise training. Trans 26th Annual Meeting Orthop Res Soc 5:256, 1980
23. Woo SL-Y, Ritter MA, Gomez MA et al: The biomechanical and structural properties of swine digital flexor tendons secondary to running exercise. Orthop Trans 4:165, 1980
24. Woo SL-Y, Gomez MA, Amiel D et al: The biomechanical and biochemical changes of the MCL following immobilization and remobilization. J Bone Joint Surg [Am] 69:1200, 1987
25. Noyes FR, Torvik PJ, Hyde WB, DeLucas JL: Biomechanics of ligament failure. II. An analysis of immobilization, exercise and reconditioning effects in primates. J Bone Joint Surg [Am] 56:1406, 1974
26. Akeson WH, Woo SL-Y, Amiel D et al: The connective tissue response to immobility: biochemical changes in periarticular

27. Swann DA, Radin EL, Nazimiec M: Role of hyaluronic acid in joint lubrication. Ann Rheum Dis 33:318, 1974
28. Akeson WH, Amiel D, LaViolette D: The connective tissue response to immobility. A study of chondroitin 4 and 6 sulfate and dermatan sulfate changes in periarticular connective tissue of control and immobilized knees of dogs. Clin Orthop Rel Res 51:183, 1967
29. Schiller S, Matthews MD, Cifonelli J, Dorfman A: The metabolism of mucopoly-saccharides in animals. Further studies on skin utilizing C14 glucose, C14 acetate, and S35 sodium sulfate. J Biol Chem 218:139, 1956
30. Neuberger A, Slack HGB: The metabolism of collagen from liver, bones, skin and tendon in the normal rat. Biochem J 53:47, 1953
31. Guyton AC, Barber BJ, Moffatt DS: Theory of interstitial pressures. In Hargens A (ed): Tissue Fluid Pressure and Composition. Williams & Wilkins, Baltimore, 1980
32. Brooke JS, Slack HGB: Metabolism of connective tissue in limb atrophy in the rabbit. Ann Rheum 18:129, 1959
33. Peacock EE: Comparison of collagenous tissue surrounding normal and immobilized joints. Surg Forum 14:440, 1963
34. Amiel D, Akeson WH, Harwood FL, Mechanic GL: Effect on nine week immobilization of the types of collagen synthesized in periarticular connective tissue from rabbit knees. Conn Tissue Res 8:27, 1980
35. Klein L, Dawson MH, Heiple KG: Turnover of collagen in the adult rat after denervation. J Bone Joint Surg [Am] 59:1065, 1977
36. Akeson WH, Amiel D, Woo SL-Y, Harwood FL: Mechanical imperatives for synovial joint homeostasis: the present potential for their therapeutic manipulation. p. 47. In Proceedings of the Third International Congress on Biorheology. 1978
37. Akeson WH, Amiel D, Mechanic GL et al: Collagen cross-linking alterations in joint contractures: changes in the reducible cross-links in periarticular connective tissue collagen after nine weeks of immobilization. Conn Tiss Res 5:15, 1977
38. Bailey AJ, Robins SP: Development and maturation of the cross-links in the collagen fibers of skin. Frontiers Matrix Biol 1:130, 1973
39. Jackson DS, Mechanic G: Cross-link patterns of collagens synthesized by cultures of 3T6 and 3T3 fibroblasts and by fibroblasts of various granulation tissues. Biochem Biophys Acta, 000:336, 1974
40. Mooney V, Stills M: Continuous passive motion with joint fractures and infections. Orthop Clin North Am 18:1, 1987
41. Pedowitz RA, Gershuni DH, Crenshaw AG et al: Intraarticular pressure during continuous passive motion of the human knee. J Orthop Res 7:530, 1989
42. Baxendale RH, Ferrell WR, Wood L: Intra-articular pressures during active and passive movement of normal and distended human knee joints. J Physiol 396:179P, 1985
43. Caughey DE, Bywaters EGL: Joint fluid pressure in chronic knee effusions. Ann Rheum Dis 22:106, 1963
44. O'Driscoll SW, Kumar A, Salter RB: The effect of continuous passive motion on the clearance of a hemarthrosis. Clin Orthop 176:336, 1983
45. Danzig LA, Hargens AR, Gershuni DH et al: Increased transsynovial transport with continuous passive motion. J Orthop Res 5:409, 1987
46. Skyhar MJ, Danzig LA, Hargens AR, Akeson WH: Nutrition of the anterior cruciate ligament. Effects of continuous passive motion. Am J Sports Med 13:415, 1985
47. Salter RB, Bell RS, Keeley F: The protective effect of continu-

ous passive motion on living articular cartilage in acute septic arthritis: an experimental investigation in the rabbit. Clin Orthop 159:223, 1981

48. O'Driscoll SW, Salter RB: The induction of neochondrogenesis in free intra-articular periosteal autografts under the influence of continuous passive motion. J Bone Joint Surg [Am] 66:1248, 1984

49. Gelberman RH, Woo SL-Y, Lothringer K et al: Effects of early intermittent passive mobilization on healing canine flexor tendons. J Hand Surg 7:170, 1982

50. Inoue M, Gomez MA, Hollis JM et al: Medial collateral ligament healing: repair vs nonrepair. Trans Orthop Res Soc 11:78, 1986

51. Salter RB, Simmonds DF, Malcolm BW et al: The biological effects of continuous passive motion on the healing of full-thickness defects in articular cartilage: an experimental investigation in the rabbit. J Bone Joint Surg 62:1232, 1980

52. Mooney V, Ferguson AB Jr: The influence of immobilization and motion on the formation of fibrocartilage in the repair granuloma after joint resection in the rabbit. J Bone Joint Surg 48:1145, 1966

53. Hohl M, Luck JV: Fractures of the tibial condyle. J Bone Joint Surg [Am] 38:1001, 1956

54. Convery FR, Akeson WH, Keown GH: The repair of large osteochondral defects. An experimental study in horses. Clin Orthop 82:253 1972

55. Ohlsen L: Cartilage regeneration from perichondrium. Experimental and clinical applications. Plast Reconstr Surg 62:507, 1978

56. Engkvist O: Reconstruction of patellar articular cartilage with free autologous perichondrial grafts. An experimental study in dogs. Scand J Plast Reconstr Surg 13:361, 1979

57. Coutts RD, Amiel D, Woo SL-Y et al: Establishment of an appropriate model for the growth of perichondrium in a rabbit joint milieu. Trans Orthop Res Soc, 8:196, 1983

58. Zarnett R, Salter RB: Periosteal neochondrogenesis for biologically resurfacing joints: its cellular origin. Can J Surg 32:171, 1989

59. Salter RB: The biologic concept of continuous passive motion of synovial joints. Clin Orthop 242:12, 1989

60. O'Driscoll SW, Keeley FW, Salter RB: Durability of regenerated articular cartilage produced by free autogeneous periosteal grafts in major full-thickness defects in joint surfaces under the influence of continuous passive motion. J Bone Joint Surg 70:595, 1988

61. Shimizu T, Videman T, Shimazaki K, Mooney V: Experimental study on the repair of full thickness articular cartilage defects: effects of varying periods of continuous passive motion, cage activity, and immobilization. J Orthop Res 5:187, 1987

62. Engkvist O, Johansson SH: Perichondrial arthroplasty. A clinical study in twenty-six patients. Scand J Plast Reconstr Surg 14:71, 1980

63. Poussa M, Rubak J, Ritsila V: Differentiation of the osteochondrogenic cells of the periosteum in chondrotrophic environment. Acta Orthop Scand 52:235, 1981

64. Amiel D, Frank C, Harwood F et al: Tendons and ligaments: a morphological and biochemical comparison. J Orthop Res 1:257, 1984

65. Burks R, Daniel D, Losse G: The effect of continuous passive motion on anterior cruciate ligament reconstruction stability. Am J Sports Med 12:323, 1984

66. Noyes FR, Mangine RE, Barber S: Early knee motion after open and arthroscopic anterior cruciate ligament reconstruction. Am J Sports Med 15:149, 1987

67. Amiel D, Kleiner J, Akeson WH: The natural history of the anterior cruciate ligament autograft of patellar tendon origin. Am J Sports Med 14:449, 1986

68. Fronek J, Frank C, Amiel D et al: The effect of intermittent passive motion (IPM) on the healing of the medial collateral ligament. Trans Orthop Res Soc 8:31, 1983

69. Coutts RD, Toth C, Kaita J: The role of continuous passive motion in the rehabilitation of the total knee patient. p 000. In Hungerford D (ed): Total Knee arthroplasty — A Comprehensive Approach. Williams & Wilkins, Baltimore, 1983

70. Coutts RD, Kaita J, Barr R et al: The role of continuous passive motion in the postoperative rehabilitation of the total knee patient. Orthop Trans 6:277, 1982

71. Romness DW, Rand JA: The role of continuous passive motion following total knee arthroplasty. Clin Orthop 226:34, 1988

72. Lynch AF, Bourne RB, Rorabeck CH et al: Deep-vein thrombosis and continuous passive motion after total knee arthroplasty. J Bone Joint Surg 70:11, 1988

73. Vince KG, Kelly MA, Beck J, Insall JN: Continuous passive motion after total knee arthroplasty. J Arthroplasty 2:281, 1987

74. Melzack R, Wall PD: Psychophysiology of pain. Evolution of pain theories. Int Anesthesiol Clin 8:3, 1970

75. Fisher RL, Kloter K, Bzdyra B, Cooper JA: Continuous passive motion (CPM) following total knee replacement. Conn Med 49:498, 1985

76. Lynch JA, Baker PL, Polly RE et al: Continuous passive motion: a prophylaxis for deep venous thrombosis following total knee replacement. Am Acad Orthop Surg 1984

77. Breen TF, Gelberman RH, Ackerman GN: Elbow flexion contractures: treatment by anterior release and continuous passive motion. J Hand Surg 13:286, 1988

78. Limbird RJ, Dennis SC: Synovectomy and continuous passive motion (CPM) in hemophiliac-patients. Arthroscopy (J Arthrosc Rel Surg) 3:74, 1987

79. Parisien JS: The role of arthroscopy in the treatment of postoperative fibroarthrosis of the knee joint. Clin Orthop 299:185, 1988

80. Lyon RM, Billings E Jr, Woo SL-Y et al: The ACL: a fibrocartilaginous structure. Trans Orthop Res Soc 14:189, 1989

81. Wessels NK: Tissue Interactions and Development. p. 213. Benjamin-Cummings, Menlo Park, CA, 1977

82. Gospodarowicz D, Neufeld G, Schweigerer L: Cellular shape is determined by the extracellular matrix and is responsible for the control of cellular growth and function. Mol Cell Endocrinol 46:187, 1986

83. Ruoslahti E, Pierschbacher, MD. Arg-Gly-Asp: a versatile cell recognition site. Cell 44:517, 1986

84. Ruoslahti E, Pierschbacher MD: New perspectives in cell adhesion: RGD and integrins. Science 238:491, 1987

85. Nagelschmidt M, Becker D, Bonninghoff N, Engelhardt GH: Effect of fibronectin therapy and fibronectin deficiency on wound healing: a study in rats. J Trauma 27:1267, 1987

86. McDonald JA, Kelley DG, Broekelmann TJ: Role of fibronectin in collagen deposition: Fab' to the gelatin-binding domain of fibronectin inhibits both fibronectin and collagen organization in fibroblast extracellular matrix. J Cell Biol 92:485, 1982

87. Amiel D, Foulk RA, Harwood FL, Akeson WH: Quantitative assessment by competitive ELISA of fibronectin (fn) in tendons and ligaments. Matrix 9:421, 1990

88. Kurkinen M, Vaheri AV, Roberts PJ, Stenman S: Sequential appearance of fibronectin and collagen in experimental granulation tissue. Lab Invest 43:47, 1980

89. Lehto M, Duance VC, Restall D: Collagen and fibronectin in a healing skeletal muscle injury. J Bone Joint Surg [Br] 67:820, 1985

90. Williams IF, McCullagh KG, Silver IA: The distribution of types I and III collagen and fibronectin in the healing equine tendon. Conn Tiss Res 12:211, 1984

91. Dahners LE: Ligament contraction—a correlation with cellularity and actin staining. Trans Orthop Res Soc 11:56, 1986

92. Roberts CJ, Birkenmeier TM, McQuillan JJ et al: Transforming growth factor β stimulates the expression of fibronectin and of both subunits of the human fibronectin receptor by cultured human lung fibroblasts. J Biol Chem 263:4586, 1988

93. Ignotz RA, Massague J: Cell adhesion protein receptors as targets for transforming growth factor-β action. Cell 51:189 1987

26 Muscle Spasticity

SUE C. BODINE-FOWLER
MICHAEL J. BOTTE

Disruption of motor pathways owing to stroke, brain trauma, or spinal cord injury leads to a variety of motor dysfunctions. The *upper motoneuron syndrome* is a common term used to describe the clinical features in patients with abnormal motor functions as the result of lesions to descending pathways at the level of the cortex, internal capsule, brain stem, or spinal cord. Patients with upper motoneuron syndrome suffer from both "negative" symptoms (performance deficits) and "positive" symptoms (abnormal behaviors).[1-5] Negative symptoms include weakness and/or paresis, loss of dexterity (especially of fine manual manipulations of the digits), and fatigability. Positive symptoms include abnormal posture, exaggeration of proprioceptive reflexes, producing "spasticity," and exaggeration of cutaneous reflexes, producing flexion withdrawal spasms, extensor spasms, and the Babinski response. Positive symptoms can be caused by the increased excitability of a specific part of the neural circuit or by the release of one part of the neural circuit from the inhibitory control of another part of the neural circuit.

Spasticity is a common component of the upper motoneuron syndrome and is the result of changes in spinal proprioceptive reflexes. The severity of spasticity and its time course depend largely on the location of the lesion or lesions and the central nervous system pathways involved. The term *spasticity* has an abundance of definitions and meanings.[1,6] For the clinician, the term is often used to describe various phenomena such as (1) increased tendon reflexes; (2) increased resistance to passive movement of the limb; (3) flexor spasms associated with paraplegia; (4) motor dysfunctions, including decreased strength, speed, and range of voluntary movement; and (5) dystonia and rigidity. A widely accepted definition of spasticity is that it is "a motor disorder characterized by a velocity-dependent increase in tonic stretch reflexes (muscle tone) with exaggerated tendon jerks, resulting from hyperexcitability of the stretch reflex, as one component of the upper motoneuron syndrome."[7] Excitability of the stretch reflex is controlled by many different spinal cord circuits, and consequently a change in any one of the components of the circuit could produce a modification in the stretch reflex.

Diagnosis of movement disorders requires an understanding of both the organization of neural networks and pathways that mediate movement, and the integration of the motor system with the sensory system. This chapter reviews the salient neuroanatomic pathways and neurophysiologic mechanisms involved in the production of movement and discusses how alterations in these pathways can lead to the movement disorders characteristic of the upper motoneuron syndrome.

INTEGRATION OF THE MOTOR AND SENSORY SYSTEMS

The motor system is organized hierarchically and consists of four major divisions, each of which contains separate neural circuits that are linked to each of the other regions. The four major divisions are (1) the spinal cord, (2) the brain stem and reticular formation, (3) the motor cortex, and (4) the premotor cortical areas, which include the basal ganglia and cerebellum. The most automatic motor responses are organized at the level of the spinal cord, whereas the least automatic behaviors are controlled by the higher centers.

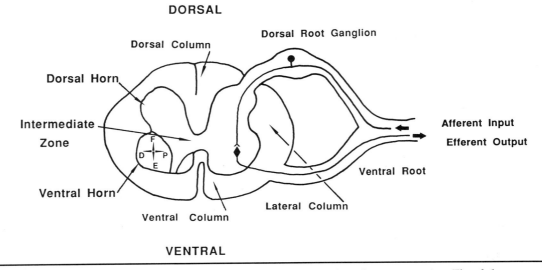

Fig. 26-1. Major subdivisions of white and gray matter of the spinal cord in cross section. The alpha motoneurons in the lateral pool of the ventral horn are grouped according to whether they innervate proximal (P) or distal (D) and flexor (F) or extensor (E) muscles of the limbs.

Spinal Cord

The spinal cord contains both the neural circuitry that is responsible for segmental and proprioceptive reflexes and the circuitry responsible for the reciprocal activation of flexor and extensor muscles during locomotion. Neurons in the spinal cord mediate reflexes and control motor output by processing information from the periphery, other spinal cord neurons, and descending pathways. They also send ascending projections to higher centers.[8]

Spinal Cord Anatomy

In the adult human, the spinal cord extends from the foramen magnum to the lower border of the first lumbar vertebra. Axons enter and exit the spinal cord via the spinal nerves, of which there are 31 pairs: 8 cervical, 12 thoracic, 5 lumbar, 5 sacral, and 1 coccygeal. Each spinal nerve consists of a ventral or efferent root and a dorsal or afferent root (Fig. 26-1). The ventral roots carry output from the myelinated axons of the alpha and gamma motoneurons in the gray matter of the ventral horn to the striated muscles. The dorsal roots carry sensory input from myelinated and unmyelinated axons originating from sensory receptors in the periphery. The cell bodies of the afferent fibers are located in the dorsal root ganglia.

The spinal cord is composed of white and gray matter.[9] The white matter is divided into columns of ascending and descending fiber tracts, which contain myelinated and unmyelinated nerve axons. The gray matter consists of longitudinally arranged neuronal cell bodies, dendrites, glial cells, and myelinated and unmyelinated axons. The gray matter is partitioned into the dorsal horn, intermediate zone, and ventral horn. Three types of neurons are present in the spinal gray matter: (1) neurons that send axonal projections out of the central nervous system via the ventral roots (i.e., alpha and gamma motoneurons), (2) neurons with axonal projections that remain in the spinal cord (i.e., interneurons), and (3) neurons that send ascending axonal projections to supraspinal centers (i.e., tract cells). The spinal gray matter is divided histologically by cell types into nine different regions or laminae[10] (Fig. 26-2). Each lamina contains a specific type of neuron and receives projections from specific sensory axons and descending pathways[9] (Fig. 26-2).

Lower Motoneurons

Gross body movement is generated by the activation of striated skeletal muscles. Skeletal muscles are innervated by lower motoneurons located in the ven-

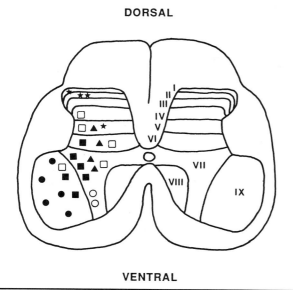

DORSAL

VENTRAL

Fig. 26-2. Location of Rexed's laminae within the ventral horn of the spinal cord. The symbols represent the location of specific cells types within the ventral and dorsal horn: (●) alpha motoneurons, (○) Renshaw cells, (■) projection of type Ia afferents, (□) projection of type II afferents, (▲) projection of type Ib afferents, and (★) nociceptors.

tral gray matter of the spinal cord. Motoneurons are arranged in columns that extend through several spinal segments. The alpha motoneurons are relatively large cells with soma sizes that range from 30 to 70 μm[11] and motor axons that innervate the extrafusal muscle fibers in striated muscles. The gamma motoneurons are smaller than the alpha motoneurons and innervate the intrafusal fibers in the muscle spindles. Within the ventral horn the motoneurons are located in nonoverlapping areas: axial muscles are innervated by medially located motoneurons (lamina VIII) and limb muscles are innervated by more laterally located motoneurons (lamina IX). Within the lateral group of motoneurons (lamina IX), the most medial motoneurons tend to innervate the proximal muscles (i.e., muscles of the shoulder and hip), whereas the more lateral motoneurons tend to innervate the distal muscles (i.e., the muscles of the extremities and digits). Further organization occurs in that the motoneurons innervating the extensor muscles tend to be located ventral to those innervating flexor motoneurons (Fig. 26-2).

The basic functional unit of a muscle is the *motor unit*, which consists of an alpha motoneuron, its motor axon, and all the muscle fibers it innervates.[11] Generally, a motoneuron innervates muscle fibers contained in only one muscle. Sherrington[12] called the motor unit the "final common pathway" because all information, whether direct or indirect, must be processed by the alpha motoneuron for muscle contraction to occur. The alpha motoneuron receives input from three major sources: (1) the sensory system, (2) the pyramidal pathways, and (3) the extrapyramidal pathways. Although the motoneuron receives direct inputs from these systems, the coordination of activity in neural circuits is achieved primarily by interneurons.[8] The interneurons function as a link between the peripheral nervous system, the descending pathways from the cortex and brain stem, and local spinal neurons and motoneurons.

Spinal Cord Reflexes

The simplest level of motor control is a reflex, which can be defined as a stereotyped response to a specific sensory stimulus.[12] A reflex pathway consists of the receptor (i.e., the sensory organ), the effector (i.e., the motoneuron), and the interconnecting neural elements (i.e., the interneurons). Reflexes may be monosynaptic, involving only one synapse between the receptor and the effector, or polysynaptic involving one or more interneurons between the receptor and the effector. Most synapses are polysynaptic. Spinal reflex pathways can be modulated by supraspinal pathways either directly through a mechanism known as presynaptic inhibition or indirectly through interneurons (Fig. 26-3).

Spinal cord reflexes involve the so-called final common pathway and are an integral part of the neural circuitry involved in the maintenance of posture and the production of movement. This section reviews several spinal reflexes: the stretch reflex (myotatic reflex), the clasp-knife response, autogenic inhibition (inverse myotatic reflex), recurrent inhibition, and the flexion withdrawal reflex.

Stretch Reflex (or Myotatic Reflex)

The stretch reflex is a monosynaptic reflex initiated by an afferent discharge from the muscle spindles, which excite the alpha motoneurons, innervating the

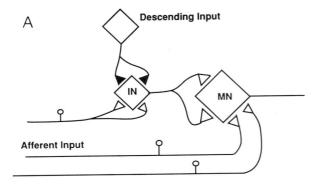

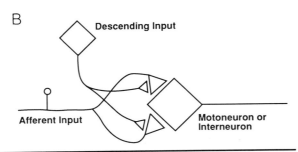

Fig. 26-3. Modulation of afferent input by **(A)** interneurons and **(B)** presynaptic inhibition. **(A)** Interneurons (IN) can enhance or suppress the effect of afferent input. For example, if an interneuron is inhibited by another input (i.e., descending pathways), the excitatory signal from the afferent fiber will have less influence on the alpha motoneurons (MN). **(B)** Additionally, afferent input can be modulated through a mechanism referred to as presynaptic inhibition. An axon (i.e., descending fiber) that synapses with the presynaptic terminal of an afferent fiber will depolarize the terminal, resulting in a reduction in the amount of transmitter released by the afferent fiber. This, in turn, will result in a decrease in the amount of excitatory input transmitted to the alpha motoneuron by the afferent fiber.

muscle from which the afferent discharge originated and synergistic muscles to produce a brisk, transient contraction of the muscle. The stretch reflex can be produced in both flexor and extensor muscles, but it is generally strongest in muscles that function as physiologic extensors, (i.e., those muscles that oppose gravity, which in humans are the flexors of the upper extremity and the extensors of the lower extremity).

Muscle spindles are specialized receptors that are distributed throughout the belly of the muscle and are arranged in parallel to the extrafusal muscle fibers in striated muscles. Each spindle consists of an en-

capsulated group of specialized muscle fibers called intrafusal fibers (Fig. 26-4).[13] The intrafusal fibers are of two types: nuclear bag fibers and nuclear chain fibers, which differ both morphologically and physiologically. The nuclear bag fibers are larger than the nuclear chain fibers, are fast contracting, and have clustered nuclei. The nuclear chain fibers, in contrast, have nuclei that are arranged in a single row and are slow contracting.

Each intrafusal fiber within the spindle is innervated by a gamma motoneuron (Fig. 26-4). Activation of the gamma motoneurons results in contraction of the ends or poles of the intrafusal fiber, causing the noncontractile equatorial region to stretch. When a muscle is shortened, the intrafusal fibers become slack or unloaded and are unable to monitor changes in length. Gamma activation provides a means of controlling both the length of the intrafusal fibers and the ability of the muscle spindle to detect changes in muscle length. Gamma motoneurons generally are coactivated with alpha motoneurons.[8]

Two types of afferent endings are found in muscle spindles: primary and secondary.[13] All intrafusal fibers in the spindle have a primary ending located in the center or equatorial region of the fiber. The primary ending gives rise to a large-diameter, fast-conducting afferent fiber called a *type Ia fiber* (Fig. 26-4). The primary endings are most sensitive to a sudden change in the length of the muscle and are responsible for the phasic component of the stretch reflex. The secondary endings are located primarily on the nuclear chain fibers and give rise to small-diameter, slow-conducting afferent fibers called *type II fibers* (Fig. 26-4). The secondary endings are most sensitive to a steady change in muscle length and are responsible for the tonic component of the stretch reflex.

The phasic stretch reflex is elicited by muscle stretch sufficient to excite the primary afferent (Ia) fibers. Clinically, the stretch reflex is most commonly elicited by tapping on a tendon to produce stretch of the extrafusal muscle fibers, which is detected by the muscle spindle and transmitted to the central nervous system via the Ia afferent fibers.

The Ia afferent fibers project through the dorsal roots and make the following connections in the spinal cord (Fig. 26-5):

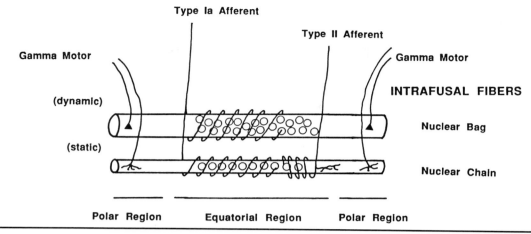

Type Ia Afferent

Type II Afferent

Gamma Motor

Gamma Motor

(dynamic)

INTRAFUSAL FIBERS

Nuclear Bag

(static)

Nuclear Chain

Polar Region   Equatorial Region   Polar Region

Fig. 26-4. Schematic diagram of the intrafusal fibers and their motor (gamma) and sensory (type Ia and type II) innervation.

1. The Ia fiber makes a *monosynaptic excitatory* connection with alpha motoneurons that innervate the same muscle from which it originated (homonymous motoneurons).
2. The Ia fiber also makes a monosynaptic, excitatory connection with alpha motoneurons that innervate synergistic muscles (heteronymous motoneurons).
3. The Ia fibers provide a monosynaptic connection to an inhibitory interneuron referred to as the *Ia inhibitory interneuron*.

The Ia inhibitory interneuron, in turn, projects directly to the alpha motoneurons that are antagonistic to the muscle from which that Ia afferent originated and provides an inhibitory potential to those motoneurons. Consequently, when a muscle is stretched the motoneurons innervating the muscle to which the stretch is imposed and its synergists are excited, whereas the motoneurons innervating the antagonist muscles are inhibited. This pattern of simultaneous inhibition of antagonists and excitation of the homonymous and synergistic motoneurons is referred to as *reciprocal inhibition*.

The type II afferents from the secondary endings have connections similar to those of the type Ia afferents. In addition, the type II afferent fibers make widespread polysynaptic connections in the spinal cord and are thought to play a role in the flexion reflex.[3] The type II afferent fibers are also thought to participate in the *clasp-knife response*, because they produce a length-dependent inhibition of the stretch reflex. The clasp-knife response is characterized by an initial resistance (increase in muscle tone) at the beginning of the stretch, which is followed by a sudden loss of resistance (decrease in muscle tone) once the muscle has been stretched past a certain point.[2,3]

Autogenic Inhibition (or Inverse Myotatic Reflex)

Golgi tendon organs are encapsulated sensory organs located primarily near the myotendinosus junction in muscle. Each Golgi tendon organ is in series with approximately 15 to 20 extrafusal muscle fibers and is innervated by an afferent fiber known as *Ib afferent fiber*. When a muscle contracts, the Ib afferent fiber is compressed and activated. The Golgi tendon organ is most sensitive to active muscle contraction and measures muscle tension.[14]

Activation of Ib afferent fibers results in (1) inhibition of the muscle from which they originated and of synergistic muscles and (2) excitation of antagonistic muscles. This response is opposite to the stretch reflex, which is why it is often referred to as the inverse myotatic reflex. This response is also referred to as *autogenic inhibition*. The Ib afferent fibers make a disynaptic, inhibitory connection to the motoneurons from the homonymous and synergistic muscles, and a disynaptic, excitatory connection to the motoneurons of the antagonistic muscles (Fig. 26-6). The central connections of the Ib afferent fibers have three

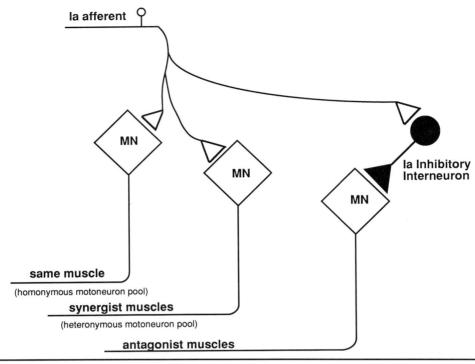

la afferent

MN

MN

la Inhibitory Interneuron

MN

same muscle
(homonymous motoneuron pool)

synergist muscles
(heteronymous motoneuron pool)

antagonist muscles

Fig. 26-5. Diagram of the projections of the type Ia afferent fibers from the muscle spindle to alpha motoneurons (MN) and interneurons within the spinal cord. The type Ia afferent inhibits the motoneurons innervating antagonistic muscles through an inhibitory interneuron (black) known as the Ia inhibitory interneuron.

main features: (1) all connections to motoneurons are through interneurons, (2) Ib afferents make weak connections to flexor muscles but strong connections to extensor muscles, and (3) the central connections of the Ib afferent fibers are more extensive than those of the Ia afferent fibers.[8,14]

Recurrent Inhibition (Renshaw Cell)

Another important inhibitory spinal interneuron is the Renshaw cell.[8] Alpha motoneurons give off a collateral that makes a direct, excitatory connection to the Renshaw cell. The Renshaw cell is an interneuron that projects back to the same motoneuron in addition to sending collaterals to synergistic motoneurons (Fig. 26-7). The Renshaw cell projection to alpha motoneurons is inhibitory. This process is called *recurrent inhibition.* Recurrent inhibition functions to regulate the activation of a particular motor pool.

The Renshaw cell also projects to the Ia inhibitory interneuron (Fig. 26-7). This pathway results in the release of inhibition (or disinhibition) of the antagonist motoneurons by inhibition of the Ia inhibitory interneuron. The Renshaw cell – Ia inhibitory interneuron pathway may function to limit the duration and magnitude of the Ia afferent – mediated reflex response.

Flexion Reflexes

The flexion reflex, also referred to as the withdrawal reflex, the cutaneous reflex, and the nociceptive reflex, is a polysynaptic reflex mediated by myelinated group II and unmyelinated group IV afferent fibers.[8] Generally these afferent fibers carry information from nociceptors, touch and pressure receptors, joint receptors, and also muscle receptors. These afferent fibers, which produce flexion responses, are collectively called *flexor reflex afferents* (FRA).

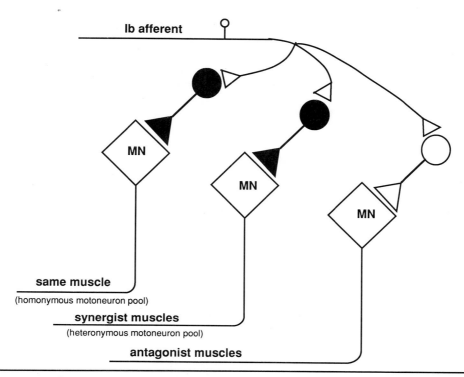

Ib afferent

MN

MN

MN

same muscle
(homonymous motoneuron pool)

synergist muscles
(heteronymous motoneuron pool)

antagonist muscles

Fig. 26-6. Diagram of the projections of the type Ib afferent fibers to neurons within the spinal cord. All projections from type Ib afferents to alpha motoneurons (MN) are through interneurons. The type Ib afferent inhibits the muscle from which it came and the synergistic muscles through an inhibitory (black) interneuron.

The general response to activation of flexor reflex afferents is excitation of the flexor motoneurons and inhibition of the extensor motoneurons on the ipsilateral side, and inhibition of the flexor motoneurons and excitation of the extensor motoneurons on the contralateral side. Contralateral excitation of the extensor motoneurons (also known as the *crossed extension reflex*) serves to stabilize the body as the ipsilateral limb is flexed. The basic circuitry for the flexion reflex is diagrammed in Figure 26-8.

Upper Motoneurons and the Descending Pathways

The descending pathways originate from upper motoneurons in the cerebral cortex and brain stem. These pathways often are divided into pyramidal or corticospinal tract and extrapyramidal tracts. The pyramidal tract originates from neurons in the motor cortex, premotor cortex, and parietal lobe. The extrapyramidal tracts arise from cells in the red nucleus, reticular formation, and vestibular nucleus of the brain stem and give rise to the rubrospinal, reticulospinal, and vestibulospinal tracts, respectively.

Pyramidal or Corticospinal Tract

In humans, the pyramidal tract functions primarily to produce fine, precise movements of the wrist and digits. The upper motoneurons that give rise to corticospinal fibers are distributed as follows: 30 percent are from the motor cortex (Brodmann's area 4), 30 percent are from the premotor cortex (Area 6), and the remaining 40 percent are from the parietal lobe (areas 3, 1 and 2).[15] The axons from these motoneurons course through the internal capsule to the ventral portion of the midbrain. At this level, some axons synapse with cells in the brain stem motor nuclei,

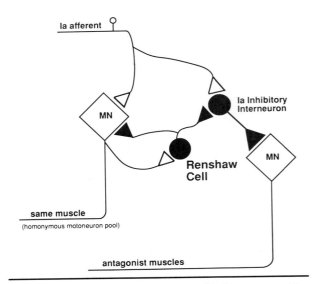

Fig. 26-7. Diagram of the circuit involved in recurrent inhibition. The Renshaw cell is an inhibitory cell (black) that is excited by an alpha motoneuron (MN) and, in turn, inhibits the same motoneuron and the type Ia inhibitory interneuron.

and, therefore, are referred to as *corticobulbar fibers.* At the level of the ventral medulla, the corticospinal axons congregate to form the medullary pyramids. At the junction of the medulla and the spinal cord, 80 percent of the fibers decussate and descend in the dorsal part of the lateral columns (dorsolateral columns) of the spinal cord and form the *lateral corticospinal tract.* The remaining, uncrossed fibers descend in the ventral column of the spinal cord and form the *ventral corticospinal tract* (Fig. 26-9).

In humans, the lateral corticospinal tract projects to (1) sensory neurons in the dorsal horn, (2) interneurons in the intermediate zone, and (3) motoneurons innervating distal limb muscles (Fig. 26-9). It has been shown in primates that motoneurons innervating the distal forelimb receive the highest density of monosynaptic corticospinal projections. The ventral corticospinal tract projects bilaterally to motoneurons located in the ventromedial region of the ventral horn, innervating axial and proximal muscles, and to cells in the intermediate zone (Fig. 26-9A).

The corticospinal pathway appears first in mammals. In the most primitive mammals, the axons connect exclusively to sensory regions of the brain stem and

spinal cord. In higher mammals, there is a gradual increase in the number of corticospinal fibers and an increase in the number of direct connections with alpha motoneurons. In humans, lesions restricted to the corticospinal tract result in the inability to move individual fingers independently and weakness and/or paresis, especially of distal muscles.[3,15,16] Impairment is greatest for fine movements and skilled movements. Generally no atrophy occurs and reflexes are preserved, although they may be mildly reduced. Another indication of a corticospinal lesion is the presence of the Babinski sign, characterized as extension of the big toe and spreading of the other toes in response to stroking the lateral aspect of the plantar surface of the foot.

Extrapyramidal Tracts

The brain stem contains several groups of neurons or nuclei that send direct projections to the spinal cord.[15,16] The three primary descending pathways are the rubrospinal, reticulospinal, and vestibulospinal tracts. These pathways are often referred to as extrapyramidal because they do not pass through the medullary pyramids. These pathways are extremely important in the maintenance of posture and muscle tone and in the modulation of spinal cord reflexes. Descending pathways from the brain stem can be divided into two subgroups according to the location of their descending fibers in the spinal cord. In general, the *ventromedial tracts* project primarily to proximal muscles in the limbs and provide excitation to extensor muscles and inhibition to flexor muscles. In contrast, the *dorsolateral tracts* project primarily to distal muscles, especially of the upper extremity, and provide excitation to flexor muscles and inhibition to extensor muscles.

Rubrospinal Tract

The rubrospinal tract originates in the red nucleus in the midbrain and decussates immediately to descend on the contralateral side in the dorsolateral funiculus of the spinal cord. The rubrospinal tract descends in the same region of the spinal cord as the lateral corticospinal tract and makes connections similar to those made by the corticospinal tract (Fig. 26-9B).[15,16] The major input to the red nucleus comes from the cerebellum and the cerebral cortex, which can modify the descending input from the red nucleus.

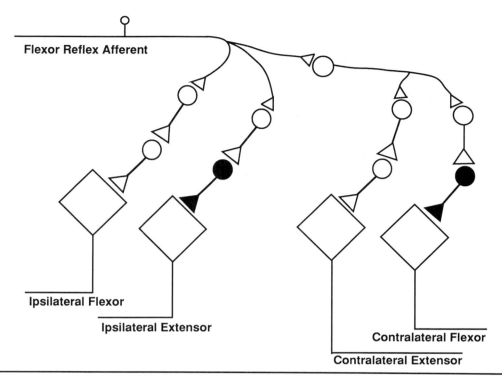

Fig. 26-8. Diagram of the flexion reflex pathway. Through a series of excitatory and inhibitory (black) interneurons, a noxious stimulus can produce ipsilateral flexion and contralateral extension (crossed extension reflex).

The majority of the terminations from the rubrospinal tract are to the interneurons in the intermediate zone of the spinal cord. The rubrospinal tract has been shown to facilitate transmission through the Ia and Ib inhibitory interneurons. The primary influence of the rubrospinal tract to motoneurons is excitation of flexors and inhibition of extensors. The major projections are to the motoneurons innervating distal flexor muscles of the upper extremity.

Reticulospinal Tract

The reticular formation is found in the medulla, pons, and midbrain; however, reticulospinal fibers originate principally from cells in the pons and medulla. Pontine reticulospinal fibers originate from cells in the *dorsolateral reticular formation* and descend uncrossed in the ventromedial funiculus of the spinal cord. These fibers terminate primarily in the ventral medial region of the ventral horn of the spinal cord (Fig. 26-9C). In general, activation of this pathway

results in excitation of extensor motoneurons and inhibition of flexor motoneurons.[15,16] Medullary reticulospinal fibers originate from cells in the *ventromedial reticular formation* and descend in the ventrolateral funiculus of the spinal cord. Fibers from the medullary reticulospinal tract can be crossed and uncrossed. These fibers terminate primarily in the dorsolateral part of the ventral horn of the spinal cord, in the same areas where corticospinal tract fibers terminate (Fig. 26-9C). In general, activation of this pathway produces inhibition of extensor motoneurons and excitation of flexor motoneurons.[15,16]

Vestibulospinal Tract

The major source of the vestibular projections to the spinal neurons is from the lateral vestibular nucleus. The vestibulospinal tract descends, mostly uncrossed, in the ventromedial funiculus of the spinal cord and makes terminations similar to those of the pontine reticulospinal tract (Fig. 26-9D).[15,16] Activa-

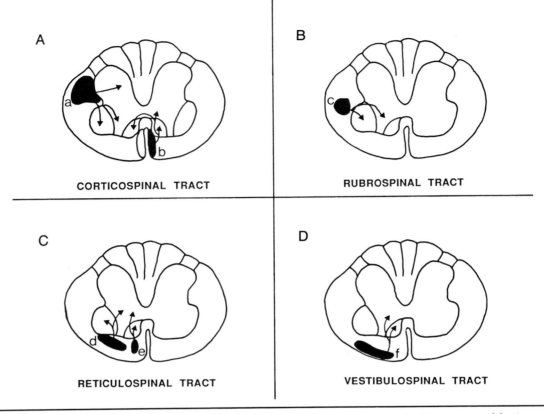

Fig. 26-9. Location of axons from tracts originating from upper motoneurons in the cortex and brain stem. **(A)** Corticospinal tract. **(B)** Rubrospinal tract. **(C)** Reticulospinal tract. **(D)** Vestibulospinal tract. The projection of the lateral corticospinal tract (a), ventral corticospinal tract (b), rubrospinal tract (c), medullary reticulospinal tract (d), pontine reticulospinal tract (e), and vestibulospinal tract (f) to the ventral and dorsal horns of the spinal cord are shown by the arrows.

tion of cells in the lateral vestibular nucleus produces excitation of extensor motoneurons and inhibition of flexor motoneurons.

UPPER MOTONEURON SYNDROME

Lesions of the descending pathways from the cerebral cortex and brain stem occur as the result of spinal cord injury, stroke, or brain trauma and are referred to as *upper motoneuron lesions.* Because of the intermingling of fibers from the cerebral cortex and brain stem, damage is rarely restricted to a single descending pathway. Selective damage of the corticospinal tract at the level of the medullary pyramids or cerebral peduncles produces only minor movement deficits. In general, the only permanent functional defect is the loss of independent control of the digits of the affected upper extremity. Damage to the extrapyramidal fibers or brain stem pathways generally is associated with the appearance of spasticity.

Spasticity is clinically manifested as tendon jerk hyperreflexia and an increase in muscle tone that is usually much greater in antigravity muscles and is highly velocity dependent. Patients with upper motoneuron syndrome rarely exhibit only spastic hypertonia. The upper motoneuron syndrome is characterized by both positive symptoms (abnormal movements) and negative symptoms (performance deficits), and its clinical manifestations depend on the site of the lesion and the pathways affected. Table

Table 26-1. Positive (Abnormal Behaviors) and Negative (Performance Deficits) Symptoms Observed in Upper Motoneuron Lesions at Various Levels

Damaged Pathway	Level of Damage		
	Spinal	Brain Stem Caudal to Red Nucleus	Brain Stem Rostral to Red Nucleus
Pyramidal tract (corticospinal tract)	Weakness, loss of abdominal reflex, and Babinski's sign	Weakness, loss of abdominal reflex, Babinski's sign, hyporeflexia, and hypotonia	Weakness, loss of abdominal reflex, Babinski's sign, seizure, apraxia, hyporeflexia, and hypotonia
Extrapyramidal tract (rubrospinal, reticulospinal and vestibulospinal tracts)	Hyperreflexia, clonus spasticity, and clasp-knife reflex	Hyperreflexia, clonus, spasticity, clasp-knife reflex, and decerebrate posture	Hyperreflexia, clonus, spasticity, clasp-knife reflex, apraxia, and decorticate posture

26-1 lists some of the positive and negative symptoms exhibited with various lesions.

Negative Symptoms

Negative symptoms are generally observed in hemiparetic patients who are suffering from cerebrovascular accidents or traumatic brain injury. Negative symptoms include paralysis, weakness, excess fatigability, and loss of dexterity. In hemiparetic patients, movement deficits may be attributed to the following observations: (1) fewer motor units are activated during a task than would normally be recruited, (2) those units that are recruited are activated at lower than normal frequencies, (3) motor units cannot be driven to discharge at high rates, and (4) it is difficult for a motor unit to sustain discharge once recruited.[17] The loss of recruitment and rate modulation of motoneurons within a given motor pool leads to inefficient muscle activation. Disturbances in the pattern of activation of motor units coupled with co-contraction of agonist and antagonist muscles leads to severe movement disorders.[17,18] Although positive symptoms such as spasticity are more obvious, the major deficits in function generally are the result of negative symptoms.[1-6]

Positive Symptoms

The hemiplegic posture is characterized by flexed and adducted upper limbs and extended lower limbs. This posture results from increased motoneuron activity in the antigravity muscles (i.e., the flexors of the upper limb and the extensors of the lower limb). This posture is often considered to be "spastic"; however,

by strict definition it is not, because (1) the activity in the muscles is continuous even in the absence of movement, and (2) the posture does not result from overactivity in spinal reflex circuits, because interruption of the reflex arc by sectioning the dorsal roots does not abolish the overactivity in the muscles.[19] Consequently, the hemiplegic posture more closely resembles rigidity as opposed to spasticity because movement is necessary to demonstrate a spastic increase in muscle tone. In general, the disabilities in the hemiplegic patient result primarily from weakness and loss of dexterity, not the dystonia or spasticity that may or may not be present.

Alterations of Proprioceptive Reflexes

Lesions to upper motoneuron pathways often result in alterations in the responsiveness of many segmental reflexes. In "spastic" muscles, the resistance to passive stretch (i.e., muscle tone) increases (as measured by electromyographic activity or torque) in proportion to the velocity of the stretch.[1-5,20-22] In a resting state or in a stretched position, so-called spastic muscles are flaccid. The receptor for detecting the imposed stretch is the primary ending of the muscle spindle. Activation of the Ia afferent fibers results in excitation of the homonymous and synergist motoneurons, causing a reflex contraction that opposes the stretch. The increase in muscle tone or resistance to stretch seems to be largely attributable to a reduction in the reflex threshold.[3,4]

Another characteristic feature of spasticity is the clasp-knife phenomenon, which produces "catch" and "give" sensations.[2,3] Rapid passive stretch of a

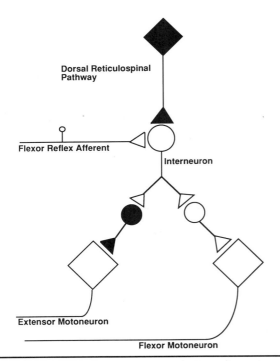

Fig. 26-10. Control of the flexor reflex pathways by the dorsal reticulospinal pathway. The flexor reflex involves a polysynaptic pathway that contains at least two interneurons, which results in excitation of flexor motoneurons and inhibition of extensor motoneurons on the ipsilateral side. This pathway can be modulated by descending input from the dorsal reticulospinal pathway, which can inhibit the first-order interneuron, thereby decreasing the effect of the flexor reflex afferents.

muscle results in a reflex contraction, which opposes the stretch, (i.e., a "catch" sensation). Further stretch, however, results in a decrease in resistance or muscle tone (i.e., the "give" sensation). The receptors thought to be responsible for this phenomenon are the secondary spindle endings and flexor reflex afferents. The flexor reflex pathway is subject to supraspinal control, particularly by fibers from the pontomedullary reticular formation (dorsal reticulospinal tract). This descending pathway inhibits the first-order interneuron in the flexor reflex pathway (Fig. 26-10). Disinhibition of the interneurons in the flexor reflex pathway is a result of lesions of upper motoneuron pathways is thought to be responsible for the clasp-knife phenomenon. Other features often present in spastic patients include an exaggerated tendon jerk and clonus. Clonus is described as a cyclic

hyperactivity of antagonistic muscles in response to stretch.

Alteration of Cutaneous Reflexes

The flexion withdrawal response is mediated by the flexor reflex afferents (FRA), which activate a reflex pathway that produces excitation of flexor motoneurons and inhibition of extensor motoneurons. This pathway is influenced by descending pathways; in particular, the reticulospinal pathways suppress transmission, whereas the corticospinal and rubrospinal pathways facilitate transmission in the FRA circuit.[8,16] The release of reflexes from descending inhibitory control (i.e., disinhibition) often results in flexor or adductor spasms.

BASIS OF THE HYPERTONIA AND HYPERREFLEXIA OF SPASTICITY

Muscle tone may be described as "the sensation of resistance felt as one manipulates a joint through a range of motion."[23] The amount of resistance to passive movement is dependent on both neural and non-neural factors. There is some evidence to suggest that hypertonia is in part related to a decrease in the compliance or an increase in the stiffness of the muscle.[20,24] Although structural changes to the muscle fibers or connective tissue may be occurring, a large component of the increased resistance to stretch is related to a disturbance of reflex pathways resulting in hyperreflexia.

Spinal Mechanisms Underlying Spasticity

Spasticity is the result of changes in segmental spinal circuits, in particular the stretch reflex arc.[3-5] An enhanced reflex response to muscle stretch could occur as the result of (1) an increase in the excitability of the alpha motoneuron or (2) an increase in the amount of excitatory input elicited by muscle stretch, or (3) an increase in both of these. A motoneuron is said to be hyperexcitable if it takes less than normal amounts of excitatory input to recruit the motoneuron or alter its discharge frequency. Stated in another way, the same amount of input generates a greater response. A motoneuron would be at a state of increased excitability if it were constantly depolarized (i.e., if the membrane potential were closer to the threshold for action potential generation). A depolarized state could occur as the result of a change in the balance of excitatory and inhibitory input to the motoneuron. It has been postulated that lesions to upper motoneurons result in a reduction in the amount of inhibitory input to the motoneuron. This could occur owing to a reduction in the input from inhibitory interneurons such as the Renshaw cell, the Ia interneuron, or the Ib interneuron. A motoneuron could also exhibit increased excitability by altering its intrinsic electrical properties such that a given synaptic current generates a larger than normal voltage change in the neuron.

Another possible explanation for the increased response to stretch is that the imposed stretch on the muscle generates more excitatory input to the motoneuron than normal. An increased synaptic current caused by the same amount of stretch could arise if (1) the Ia afferent fiber showed an enhanced response to stretch (i.e., greater rate of firing) because of increased fusimotor bias, or (2) the excitatory interneurons within the neural circuit were more responsive to muscle afferent input. This second alternative could occur owing to (1) collateral sprouting, which would lead to an increase in the number of excitatory synapses, (2) denervation supersensitivity, or (3) a reduction in presynaptic inhibition of the muscle afferent, resulting in greater transmission of the excitatory signal.

Of the mechanisms just mentioned, there is no evidence in support of increased fusimotor activity leading to excessive muscle spindle activity, decreased group II inhibition, or decreased recurrent inhibition.[3,21,22] Evidence does exist, however, to support decreased presynaptic inhibition of Ia afferent fibers, decreased inhibition of antagonists through reciprocal inhibition, and increased motoneuronal excitability.[3,21,22] Experimental evidence in chronically spinally transected cats suggests that motoneuron hyperexcitability is not due to a significant change in the intrinsic properties of the motoneuron.[25,26] Therefore, the changes must occur as the result of alterations in the amount of excitatory or inhibitory input to the cell.

In summary, patients with upper motoneuron lesions demonstrate varying degrees of spastic hypertonia, in addition to paresis and loss of dexterity, flexor spasm, clasp-knife response, and co-contraction of agonist and antagonist muscles. Changes in reflex responses can, in part, be related to a loss of inhibitory control of segmental reflex circuits by supraspinal pathways. In addition, local biochemical or morphologic changes, or both, may occur at the spinal cord level. These local changes could include collateral sprouting of intact dorsal root afferents, shortening of motoneuron dendrites, or denervation supersensitivity.[3,4,21]

REFERENCES

1. Landau WM: Spasticity: the fable of a neurological demon and the emperors of new therapy. Arch Neurol 31:217, 1974
2. Lance JW: The control of muscle tone, reflexes, and movement. Neurology 30:1303, 1980
3. Burke D: Spasticity as an adaptation to pyramidal tract injury. Adv Neurol 47:410, 1988
4. Katz RT, Rymer WZ: Spastic hypertonia: mechanisms and measurement. Arch Phys Med Rehabil 70:144, 1989
5. Young RR: The physiology of spasticity and its response to therapy. Ann NY Acad Sci 531:146, 1988
6. Rushworth G: Some pathophysiological aspects of spasticity and the search for rational and successful therapy. Int Rehabil Med 2:23, 1980
7. Lance JW: Symposium synopsis. p. 485. In Feldman RG, Young RR, Koella WP (eds): Spasticity: Disordered Motor Control. Year Book Medical Publishers, Chicago, 1980
8. Baldissera F, Hultborn H, Illert M: Integration in spinal neuronal systems. p. 509. In Brooks VB (ed): Handbook of Physiology. Section I. The Nervous System. Vol. II. Motor Control, Part I. American Physiological Society, Bethesda, MD, 1981
9. Brown AG: Organization in the Spinal Cord. Springer-Verlag, Berlin, 1981
10. Romanes GJ: The motor cell columns of the lumbosacral spinal cord of the cat. J Comp Neurol 94:313, 1951
11. Burke RE: Motor units: anatomy, physiology and functional organization. p. 345. In Brooks VB (ed): Handbook of Physiology. Section I. The Nervous System. Vol. II. Motor Control, Part I. American Physiological Society, Bethesda, MD, 1981
12. Sherrington CS: The Integrative Action of the Nervous System. Yale University Press, New Haven, CT, 1906
13. Matthews PBC: Muscle spindles: their messages and their fusimotor supply. p. 189. In Brooks VB (ed): Handbook of Physiology. Section I. The Nervous System. Vol. II. Motor Control, Part I. American Physiological Society, Bethesda, MD, 1981
14. Matthews PBC: Proprioceptors and the regulation of movement. p. 93. In Towe AL, Luschei ES (eds): Handbook of Behavioral Neurophysiology. Vol. 5. Motor Coordination. Plenum Press, New York, 1981
15. Kuypers HGJM: Anatomy of the descending pathways. p. 597. In Brooks VB (ed): Handbook of Physiology. Section I. The Nervous System. Vol. II. Motor Control, Part I. American Physiological Society, Bethesda, MD, 1981
16. Schwindt PC: Control of motoneuron output by pathways descending from the brainstem. p. 139. In Towe AL, Luschei ES (eds): Handbook of Behavioral Neurophysiology. Vol. 5. Motor Coordination. Plenum Press, New York, 1981
17. Young RR, Wierzbicka MM: Behavior of single motor units in normal subjects and in patients with spastic paresis. p. 27. In

Delwaide PJ, Young RR (eds): Clinical Neurophysiology in Spasticity. Elsevier, Amsterdam, 1985

18. Knutsson E: Studies of gait control in patients with spastic paresis. p. 175. In Delwaide PJ, Young RR (eds): Clinical Neurophysiology in Spasticity. Elsevier, Amsterdam, 1985

19. Denny-Brown DB: The Cerebral Control of Movement. Liverpool University Press, Liverpool, England, 1966

20. Powers RK, Marder-Meyer J, Rymer WZ: Quantitative relations between hypertonia and stretch reflex threshold in spastic hemiparesis. Ann Neurol 23:115, 1988

21. Pierrot-Deseilligny E, Mazieres L: Spinal mechanisms underlying spasticity. p. 63. In Delwaide PJ, Young RR (eds): Clinical Neurophysiology in Spasticity. Elsevier, Amsterdam, 1985

22. Delwaide PJ: Electrophysiological testing of spastic patients: its potential usefulness and limitations. p. 185. In Delwaide PJ, Young RR (eds): Clinical Neurophysiology in Spasticity. Elsevier, Amsterdam, 1985

23. Lance JW, McLeod JG: A Physiological Approach to Clinical Neurology. 3rd Ed. Butterworth, Boston, 1981

24. Lehmann JF, Price R, deLateur BJ et al: Spasticity: quantitative measurements as a basis for assessing effectiveness of therapeutic intervention. Arch Phys Med Rehabil 70:6, 1989

25. Cope TC, Bodine SC, Fournier M, Edgerton VR: Soleus motor units in chronic spinal transected cats: physiological and morphological alterations. J Neurophysiol 55:1202, 1986

26. Hochman S, McCrea DA: Effect of chronic spinal transection on homonymous Ia EPSP rise time in triceps surae motoneurons in cats. Soc Neurosci Abstr 186:12, 1987

27 Rehabilitation of Neuromuscular Disorders

DAVID B. SIMON
STEVEN P. RINGEL

Disorders affecting the neuromuscular system can impair vital functions, including voluntary movement, speaking, swallowing, and breathing. Whether these conditions develop acutely or progress slowly over time, the disability incurred has a significant impact on functional independence, so that major therapeutic intervention is necessary for maximal rehabilitation.

In this chapter, we first outline the anatomy and physiology of the neuromuscular system. Muscle and nerve biopsies and electrodiagnostic studies — procedures that are valuable in the diagnosis and treatment of neuromuscular disorders — are then reviewed. Specific neuromuscular diseases are described to illustrate problems affecting various levels of the neuromuscular unit. The role of rehabilitative techniques in these conditions is emphasized. Finally, the treatment of functional problems common to a variety of neuromuscular conditions is described in greater detail.

PHYSIOLOGY AND ANATOMY OF THE NEUROMUSCULAR SYSTEM

Cortical control of voluntary muscle function is vested in neurons descending through the white matter of the cerbral hemispheres, brain stem, and spinal cord to synapse directly or indirectly on lower motoneurons in the anterior gray matter of the spinal cord. Afferent sensory fibers provide sensory information to the central nervous system and also convey information from muscle spindles to the lower motoneuron regarding the length and tension of the muscle. A continuous feedback mechanism exists between the mointoring receptors of the muscle fiber and the anterior horn cell to maintain the appropriate degree of muscle tone. The deep tendon or stretch reflex tests the integrity of this circuit.

The anterior horn cell, its axon, and all the muscle fibers innervated by that axon constitute the functional unit (motor unit) of the peripheral nervous system (Fig. 27-1). In general, the finer the control over a particular movement the smaller the number of fibers innervated by an anterior horn cell. For example, for fine hand movements the innervation ratio of muscle fibers per motor unit may be as low as 100; in contrast, the large muscles of the calf may have as many as 2,000 muscle fibers per motor unit.[1]

Efferent axons from motoneurons combine with afferent axons from sensory receptors to form peripheral sensorimotor nerves. These mixed nerves contain fibers of various diameters and conduction velocities. Large myelinated fibers, which include motor axons and sensory fibers mediating position, touch, muscle length, and tension, are the fastest conductors. Medium-sized myelinated fibers carrying information from muscle spindles and vibratory and pressure receptors have intermediate velocities, and small, lightly myelinated and unmyelinated

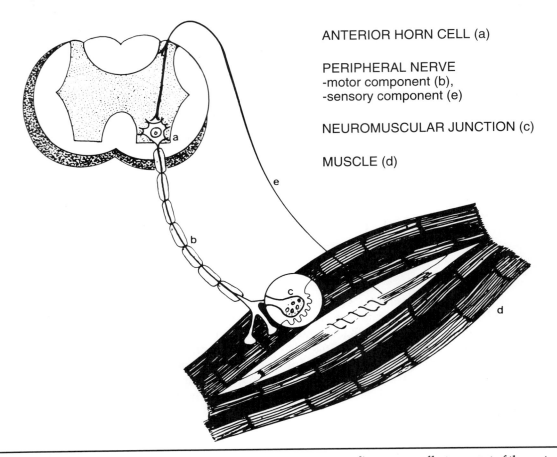

ANTERIOR HORN CELL (a)

PERIPHERAL NERVE
-motor component (b),
-sensory component (e)

NEUROMUSCULAR JUNCTION (c)

MUSCLE (d)

Fig. 27-1. Anatomy of the neuromuscular system. Lower motor neuron diseases can affect any part of the motor unit, which consists of an anterior horn cell **(A)**, axon **(B)**, neuromuscular junction **(C)**, and numerous muscle fibers **(D)**. Afferent fibers arising from the muscle spindle **(E)** provide a feedback loop for monitoring muscle tension and length. (From Simon DB, Ringel SP, Lacey JR: Neuromuscular emergencies. p. 221. In Ernest MP [ed]: Neurologic Emergencies. Churchill Livingstone, New York, 1983)

fibers subserving temperature, pain, and autonomic information transmit most slowly.

The trophic influence of a nerve on the muscle fibers supplied is most easily noted when the nerve supply is damaged, and the muscle atrophies despite the presence of an adequate blood supply. If reinnervation occurs from a nearby nerve branch, the muscle fiber may regain its normal size.

At the neuromuscular junction (the synapse between the nerve and muscle) the neurotransmitter acetylcholine is released; it diffuses across the synaptic cleft and stimulates receptors on the postsynaptic membrane of the muscle fiber. Binding of the neurotransmitter produces changes in the permeability of the endplate region of the muscle membrane, leading to fluxes in sodium and potassium across the muscle fiber that result in depolarization and contraction.

The force of muscle contraction is produced by the contractile proteins actin and myosin. The process of muscular contraction is a complex one, which begins with the release of calcium from the sarcoplasmic reticulum. This calcium is bound by several regulatory proteins, which allow cross-bridges to form between the actin and myosin protein filaments. The resulting muscle fiber shortening requires large amounts of energy, which is produced from the metabolism of glycogen and lipids stored in the muscle as high-energy phosphate bonds.

Muscle fibers are composed of two major types relatively evenly distributed throughout the muscles. The type I fibers (aerobic, slow twitch), which are rich in oxidative enzymes, utilize oxygen through the Krebs cycle. The type II fibers (anaerobic, fast twitch), which are rich in glycogen, are larger and more powerful but fatigue more quickly. Because type II fibers utilize anaerobic metabolism, lactic acid accumulates more readily. All muscle fibers innervated by a motoneuron are of the same type, but a fiber may convert from one fiber type to another if it is denervated from one motoneuron and reinnervated by another.

ELECTRODIAGNOSTIC STUDIES FOR THE EVALUATION OF NEUROMUSCULAR DISORDERS

Assessment of the neurophysiologic integrity of nerve and muscle function can be made through the use of electrodiagnostic studies. A routine electrodiagnostic study consists of nerve conduction velocity (NCV) assessment and electromyography (EMG). NCVs are determined by applying an electrical stimulus to a sensory or motor nerve and recording the generated action potential at a site distant from the stimulation point. Sensory responses are often recorded by stimulating the digits with ringed electrodes and recording the response more proximally. Motor responses are usually determined with recording electrodes placed over isolated motor endpoints and stimulation along a motor nerve at proximal and distal sites. Information that can be obtained includes the latency, which defines the time between the stimulus and the response; the amplitude of the response; and a calculated conduction velocity. Conduction velocity along a nerve segment can be derived by dividing the distance between the stimulation sites by the difference in the latencies (Fig. 27-2).

Slowing of nerve conduction and reduction in amplitude may be due to a variety of disease processes affecting the nerve. Local compression, diseases of myelination and disorders affecting the axon itself may all produce slowing. Disorders affecting primarily myelin generally produce marked slowing (less than 60 percent) of the normal velocity, whereas axonal injury produces minimal slowing. Compressive neuropathies (e.g., carpal tunnel syndrome, tardy ulnar palsy) will usually produce a significant decrement in the velocity across the site of compression or a delay in the motor latency.

In the EMG evaluation, a fine needle is inserted into a muscle and electrical activity is recorded at rest, with minimal muscle contraction, and with full muscular effort. The electrical activity of the muscle can be viewed on an oscilloscope screen and detected audibly. A normal muscle is electrically silent at rest. Abnormal spontaneous activity in the form of fibrillations or positive waves is seen with neuropathic denervation as well as with some primary muscle disorders. During minimal muscle contraction, individual motor unit potentials can be assessed for their configuration, amplitude, and duration.

In primary muscle diseases, the activity of motor units appears as brief-duration, small-amplitude peaks with multiple phases. In primary neuropathic disorders, large-amplitude, long-duration polyphasic peaks may be seen. With maximal contraction diseases of muscle generally produce an early complete interference pattern, whereas in motoneuron or neuropathic disorders usually a reduction in the interference pattern occurs with full effort (Fig. 27-3).

The neuromuscular junction may be assessed by repetitive stimulation studies in which the nerve action potential is recorded while the nerve is excited at rates of 2 to 50 times per second. When transmission across the neuromuscular junction is normal, no decrease or increase in the amplitude of the consecutive evoked muscle action potential is seen. In myasthenia gravis, a decrease of 10 percent or more in the amplitude is characteristic (Fig. 27-3D). In the Eaton-Lambert syndrome, the initial amplitude of the motor response is reduced, but it increases with repetitive stimulation.

BIOPSIES OF MUSCLE AND NERVES

Histochemical analysis of muscle biopsies has greatly aided the specific diagnosis of nerve and muscle diseases. Under local anesthesia, a small piece of muscle about the size of a pencil eraser is excised surgically, quickly frozen, and processed with histochemical stains, which help to distinguish between type I and type II muscle fibers. Neuropathic disorders frequently result in small atrophic fibers with grouping of fiber types. Myopathies produce variable degener-

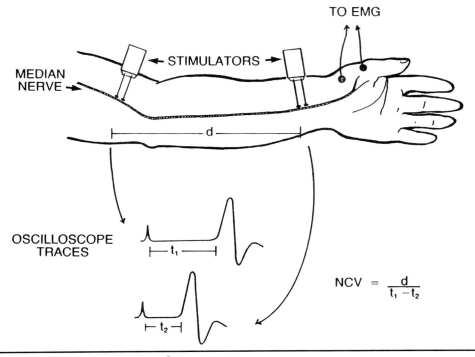

Fig. 27-2. Nerve conduction velocity determination. A peripheral nerve is stimulated proximally and distally and a muscle action potential is recorded. The distance between stimulation points divided by the difference in latencies provides the conduction velocity. (From Simon DB, Ringel SP, Lacey JR: Neuromuscular emergencies. p. 223. In Ernest MP [ed]: Neurologic Emergencies. Churchill Livingstone, New York, 1983.)

ation, necrosis, and alterations in fiber size without regard to fiber type. Characteristic changes are seen in inflammatory disorder, inherited degenerative muscle disorders, and metabolic myopathies.

Biopsy of the sural nerve behind the lateral malleolus can sometimes provide a specific diagnosis of a hypertrophic or inflammatory neuropathy or amyloidosis. Frequently, the nerve biopsy is not diagnostic, although it distinguishes axonal or myelin loss. Therefore, it is not recommended for routine use in patients with peripheral neuropathy.

DISEASES OF THE NEUROMUSCULAR SYSTEM

Although symptoms and signs of diseases affecting different levels of the neuromuscular unit often overlap, characteristic patterns of dysfunction allow an accurate diagnosis to be made. Examples of diseases affecting the motor neuron, peripheral nerve, neuromuscular junction, and muscle are reviewed in this section, with an emphasis on both clinical disability and rehabilitation needs.

Lower Motoneuron Diseases

Diseases affecting the lower motoneurons include the inherited spinal muscular atrophies, polimyelitis, and amyotrophic lateral sclerosis (ALS) (Table 27-1).

Spinal Muscular Atrophies

The spinal muscular atrophies are a clinically heterogeneous group of inherited disorders, characterized by weakness and muscular wasting. Degeneration of the anterior horn cells of the spinal cord and cranial nerve motor nuclei is seen pathologically. These disorders are usually inherited in an autosomal-recessive pattern, although occasionally x-linked recessive or dominant transmission is found.

The spinal muscular atrophies are classified according to the age of onset and severity of involvement. In the most severe infantile form *(Werdnig-Hoffmann*

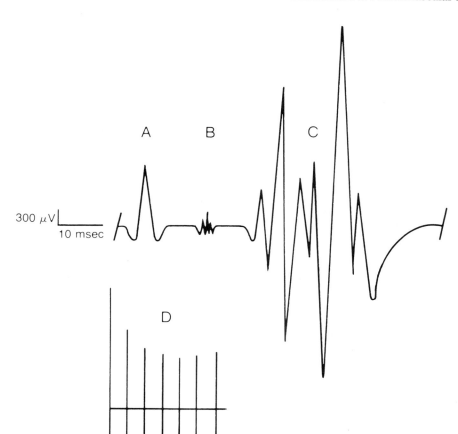

Fig. 27-3. EMG motor unit action potentials. Single motor unit potentials (MUP) in normal muscle **(A)**, myopathy **(B)**, and motor neuron disease **(C)**. Note the striking difference between the small-amplitude, brief duration polyphasic myopathic MUP **(B)** and the large-amplitude, broad polyphasic neuropathic potential **(C)**. A 2/second repetitive stimulation of a motor nerve in a patient with myasthenia gravis produces a normal amplitude first response, but a decremental response in subsequent motor unit action potentials **(D)**. (From Simon DB, Ringel SP, Lacey JR: Neuromuscular emergencies. p. 224. In Ernest MP [ed]: Neurologic Emergencies. Churchill Livingstone, New York, 1983.)

disease), babies are weak and hypotonic at birth, or quickly become weak within the first few months of life. They usually have a weak cry, poor respiratory effort, and difficulty feeding, with frequent aspiration. Because the eye movements are unaffected, the infants usually have alert expressions. This inherited disorder must be differentiated from hypotonic cerebral palsy and a host of uncommon congenital myopathies.

The *intermediate form* of spinal muscular atrophy is seen in children who fail to attain normal motor milestones. They may achieve the ability to sit unsupported and occasionally can stand, but very rarely can they walk. Contractures and kyphoscoliosis are the major complications. Rehabilitation efforts must be directed toward proper wheelchair positioning and the use of body jackets. In carefully selected cases, spinal fusion to delay progressive scoliosis and spinal collapse is performed. Although death in both the infantile and the intermediate forms of spinal muscular atrophy is usually due to respiratory insufficiency, aggressive respiratory therapy may improve survival into the second and third decades.

The juvenile form of spinal muscular atrophy *(Kugelberg-Welander disease)* typically is noted between the ages of 5 and 15 years, when walking becomes in-

Table 27-1. Diseases of the Lower
Motoneuron

I. Spinal muscular atrophies
Infantile (Werdnig-Hoffman)
Intermediate
Juvenile (Kugelberg-Welander)
II. Amyotrophic lateral sclerosis (motoneuron disease)
Progressive bulbar atrophy
Progressive muscular atrophy
Primary lateral sclerosis
III. Poliomyelitis

(From Simon DB, Ringel SP, Lacey JR: Neuromuscular emergencies. p. 226. In Ernest MP (ed): Neurologic Emergencies. Churchill Livingstone, New York, 1983.)

creasingly difficult. Most patients require a wheelchair within 5 to 10 years after the onset of symptoms. Aggressive physical therapy to reduce contractures will often prolong ambulation. Again, aggressive management of kyphoscoliosis and respiratory infections will allow for a more functional life into and often beyond the third decade.

Poliomyelitis

Fortunately, poliomyelitis has become a rare disease in the United States since the introduction of the Salk and Sabin vaccines. However, this reduced incidence has promoted a more casual attitude toward immunization and increases the likelihood of sporadic outbreaks. In any case of a rapid bulbar and spinal paralysis, the diagnosis of poliomyelitis should be considered. The diagnosis can be made with a lumbar puncture, which will demonstrate a marked cerebrospinal fluid pleocytosis.

In recent years, increasing attention has been directed toward progressive weakness that begins many years after an initial episode of poliomyelitis. There is no evidence of viral reactivation in this progressive postpoliomyelitis syndrome. Because it is most apparent in very severely affected patients, it probably represents superimposed loss of anterior horn cells from aging.

Amyotrophic Lateral Sclerosis

Progressive degeneration of the motoneurons in the brain stem and spinal cord results in progressive weakness and wasting of bulbar and extremity mus-

culature. Degeneration of corticospinal tracts leads to spasticity and hyperreflexia. The majority of patients with ALS die within 4 to 5 years, although up to 20 percent of patients have a milder or more localized illness and are alive at 10 years.

Subgroups of ALS have been described, including patients in whom the disease affects primarily the bulbar musculature (*progressive bulbar palsy*), others in whom the primary feature is that of progressive muscular atrophy, and occasionally patients who have primarily long tract findings with a predominance of spasticity (*primary lateral sclerosis*). However, in most cases, as the disease progresses some involvement of bulbar and of lower and upper motoneurons is seen, justifying the inclusive term *amyotrophic lateral sclerosis*.

This sporadic disease may begin any time during adulthood, but it is most commonly seen in men in later years. A few cases (7 percent) are autosomal dominant. Weakness and clumsiness of a limb are the most common early complaints, although speaking and swallowing problems may first bring the patient to a physician's attention. Cognitive function, bowel and bladder control, and ocular motility are spared, as is sensation. Impairment in corticobulbar function may produce a pseudobulbar syndrome, including hyperactive cough reflex, spastic dysphagia, or inappropriate outbursts of laughing or crying.

Examination of the patient with ALS will usually demonstrate both upper and lower motoneuron dysfunction. Weakness, atrophy, and fasciculations may be associated with hypo- and hyperreflexia. Most chemistry studies yield normal results, although serum creatine phosphokinase (CPK) levels may be elevated. Electrodiagnostic studies are usually helpful in demonstrating neuropathic features, including fibrillations, fasciculations, and large motor units with a reduced interference pattern.

As the disease progresses, rehabilitation efforts should attempt to maintain the patient's highest quality of life. Careful monitoring of swallowing function may help to reduce the risk of aspiration. As dysphagia progresses, a decision must be made with the family regarding the use of a feeding tube. Surgical techniques, including sectioning of the nerves to the major salivary glands on one side, can reduce saliva production without causing sedation. Injection of Gelfoam or Teflon into a vocal cord may help to reduce the risk of aspiration. Amitriptyline lessens pseudobulbar symptoms and reduces salivary flow.

Maintaining range of motion of paretic limbs and providing assistive ambulatory devices to maximize independence will help key the patient's quality of life as high as possible. Increasingly, patients with respiratory failure are choosing ventilatory assistance. Considerations regarding home ventilation are reviewed later in this chapter.

Disease of the Peripheral Nerves

Peripheral nerve dysfunction may be due to a wide variety of systemic medical illnesses as well as to specific focal or generalized neuropathic conditions. Mononeuropathies, plexopathies, and polyneuropathies are the most common syndromes of peripheral nerve dysfunction.

Mononeuropathies

Mononeuropathies describe damage to a single peripheral nerve, most commonly as a result of local compression or traction. The *carpal tunnel syndrome* is probably the most frequently seen mononeuropathy; it involves compression of the median nerve as it transits the carpal tunnel in the wrist. Numbness of the first three fingers, pain radiating into the hand or forearm, and occasional weakness in the hand are the most common presenting symptoms. Pain often awakens the patient from sleep. Carpal tunnel syndrome commonly responds to simple maneuvers such as neutral wrist splinting or steriod injections; rarely, surgical decompression is necessary if clinical signs, symptoms, and electrodiagnostic studies point to progressive nerve impairment.[2]

An *ulnar neuropathy* due to injury or compression of the ulnar nerve in the groove at the elbow results in numbness over the fourth and fifth fingers of the hand with weakness and atrophy of the intrinsic hand muscles. In the early stages, attention to preventing further injury and padding the elbow is usually succesful in relieving symptoms. In more chronic or progressive cases, surgical decompression or transposition may be indicated.[2]

Peroneal nerve palsy owing to compression of the peroneal nerve as it crosses the fibular head in the leg will result in weakness of ankle dorsiflexion and impaired sensation over the dorsum of the foot. Prevention of further injury and, at times, an ankle-foot orthosis (AFO) to prevent further ankle damage owing to the foot-drop will eventually result in recovery of function.

Plexopathy

Plexopathy refers to injury of the brachial or lumbosacral plexus, usually resulting from trauma, infection, or invasion by tumor. In *idiopathic brachial neuritis,* a patient initially experiences severe pain in the shoulder, followed by weakness and atrophy of the upper arm. Prior history of trauma, infection, or immunization can sometimes be obtained. The weakness and atrophy usually recover over 1 to 3 years as the damaged nerves regenerate. Support of the paralyzed limb with a sling and physical therapy to maintain range of motion and maximize function allow the most complete level of recovery.

Lumbosacral plexopathy may occur in diabetes when small vessel infarction involves multiple nerves in the plexus rather than limitation to a single nerve. The patient may initially experience severe pain in the upper leg followed by weakness and atrophy. As in the upper extremity plexopathy, there is often nearly complete recovery of the weakness and atrophy over months to years.

Polyneuropathy

Polyneuropathies are seen in a variety of systemic medical disorders in which progressive sensory loss and weakness develop in the extremities in a symmetric pattern. Most commonly the distal portions are affected earliest and most severely, with proximal involvement occurring subsequently over time. Polyneuropathies are usually divided into axonal and demyelinating patterns. In an *axonal neuropathy* the nerve fiber itself (axon) is damaged, whereas in demyelinating neuropathies the insulating myelin is stripped away. The most common causes of axonal neuropathies encountered in general medical practices are those associated with diabetes and alcohol abuse. Such neuropathies can also be seen after exposure to a variety of toxic agents, in heavy metal

Table 27-2. Peripheral Neuropathies

I. Axonal neuropathies
  A. Diabetes
  B. Alcohol related
  C. Uremia
  D. Hypothyroidism
  E. Sarcoidosis
  F. Collagen vascular diseases
    1. Systemic lupus erythematosus
    2. Rheumatoid arthritis
    3. Wegener's granulomatosis
  G. Paraproteinemias
  H. Drugs
    1. Isoniazid
    2. Hydralazine
    3. Nitrofurantoin
    4. Vincristine
  I. Heavy metals
    1. Lead
    2. Arsenic
    3. Mercury
    4. Thallium
  J. Industrial toxins
    1. n-Hexane
    2. n-Butyltketone
    3. Acrylamide
    4. Organophosphate
  K. Amyloidosis
  L. Carcinoma (remote effect)
  M. Tick paralysis
II. Demyelinating neuropathies
  A. Guillain-Barré syndrome
  B. Diphtheria
  C. Porphyria

(From Simon DB, Ringel SP, Lacey JR: Neuromuscular emergencies. p. 231. In Ernest MP (ed): Neurologic Emergencies. Churchill Livingstone, New York, 1983.)

poisoning, and in metabolic or endocrine disorders (Table 27-2).

Identification of any possibly reversible causes and removal of offending toxic agents are the most important therapeutic interventions. Treatment of neuropathic pain with simple analgesics or tricyclic antidepressant agents may be of value. The use of capsaicin-containing agents (Zostrix) may help to relieve painful paresthesias, but this method has not yet been studied systematically. Occasionally, there is weakness in the distal extremities that is significant enough to justify splinting.

In contrast to axonal polyneuropathies, *demyelinating neuropathies* tend to be more rapidly progressive and to involve motor function to a greater degree than sensory function. The most frequently seen disorder, the Guillain-Barré syndrome, is immunologically mediated and often develops after infection, immunization, surgery, or trauma. The syndrome usually begins with paresthesias of the extremity followed by rapidly ascending weakness and areflexia. The weakness may involve respiratory muscles, and respiratory assistance is necessary in 20 to 30 percent of cases. Autonomic dysfunction, including transient hypertension and hypotension as well as cardiac arrhythmias, may occur. Cranial neuropathies are also common and may result in facial weakness and dysphagia. Laboratory studies demonstrate markedly slow NCVs and elevated cerebrospinal fluid protein, with few or no cells.

The treatment of Guillain-Barré syndrome is primarily supportive, with careful monitoring and, if necessary, assistance in respiratory functioning. Corticosteroids have not been shown to be of benefit, but plasmapheresis has been advocated in rapidly progressive conditions. Ninety percent of patients eventually recover after many months, without significant residual disability. Rehabilitation during the acute and recovery phases is important to prevent contractures and aspiration.[3]

Inherited sensorimotor neuropathies progress slowly, resulting in weakness, wasting, and deformity. The most common disorder in this group is Charcot-Marie-Tooth disease. Both axonal (neuronal) and demyelinating (hypertrophic) varieties can occur. The clinical expression is variable, with some affected members showing only pes cavus and loss of reflexes. More severely affected patients will often have severe atrophy of the leg musculature with footdrop requiring (AFOs).

Diseases of the Neuromuscular Junction

Diseases of the neuromuscular junction can interfere with the release of acetylcholine, disrupt the postsynaptic membrane, or interfere with inactivation of acetylocholine (Table 27-3).

Table 27-3. Neuromuscular Junction Disorders

Myasthenia gravis
Botulism
Eaton-Lambert syndrome
Pseudocholinesterase deficiency
Organophosphate intoxication

(From Simon DB, Ringel SP, Lacey JR: Neuromuscular emergencies. p. 235. In Ernest MP (ed): Neurologic Emergencies. Churchill Livingstone, New York, 1983.)

Myasthenia Gravis

The most common disorder affecting the neuromuscular junction is myasthenia gravis, an autoimmune disorder in which acetylcholine receptor antibodies bind to the postsynaptic membrane, interfering with neuromuscular transmission. Approximately 15 percent of patients with myasthenia gravis have evidence of a concomitant autoimmune disorder, such as rheumatoid arthritis, lupus erythematosus, or thyroid disease. The disorder most commonly is first manifested between the ages of 20 and 30 years and is seen in women more often than in men. Typical symptoms include ptosis, diplopia, nasal or slurred speech, and difficulty with chewing and swallowing. The extremities may be affected, but usually to a lesser degree. The diagnosis can usually be confirmed by the use of the edrophonium (Tensilon) test, repetitive nerve stimulation studies, and detection of acetylcholine receptor antibodies in the serum.

Treatment of myasthenia gravis over the years has shifted from symptomatic efforts utilizing cholinesterase inhibitors to focusing on the autoimmune nature of the disease. Corticosteroids, other immunosuppressive agents, and plasmapheresis have all been utilized with good results, although patients may become transiently weaker during the initial administration of steroids. Although the exact role of the thymus gland in myasthenia gravis remains uncertain, thymectomy has been shown to clinically enhance the chance for complete remission in selected patients.

Eaton-Lambert Syndrome

The Eaton-Lambert syndrome occurs owing to the formation of an antibody that binds to the presynaptic membrane and prevents the release of acetylcho-

Table 27-4. Diseases of Muscles

I. Muscular dystrophies
  A. X-linked (Duchenne, Becker)
  B. Facioscapulohumeral (FSH)
  C. Scapuloperoneal
  D. Limb girdle
  E. Progressive external ophthalmoplegias
  F. Myotonic
II. Inflammatory myopathies
  A. Infectious (viral, bacterial, parasitic)
  B. Immune mediated
    1. Polymyositis
    2. Dermatomyositis
    3. Myositis associated with other connective tissue disorders (systemic lupus erythematosus, polyarteritis nodosa, Sjogren's syndrome, rheumatoid arthritis, scleroderma)
III. Endocrine or metabolic myopathies
  A. Hyper- or hypothyroidism
  B. Hyper- or hypocalcemia
  C. Hyper- or hypoadrenalism
IV. Toxic myopathies
  A. Alcohol
  B. Amphotericin B
  C. Vincristine
  D. Chloroquine
V. Inherited metabolic myopathies
  A. Glycogen storage disorders (McArdle's syndrome, phosphofructokinase and acid maltase deficiency)
  B. Lipid myopathies (carnitine and carnitine palmityl transferase deficiency)
  C. Periodic paralyses (hypo-, hyper-, or normokalemic)
  D. Malignant hyperthermia

(From Simon DB, Ringel SP, Lacey JR: Neuromuscular emergencies. p. 239. In Ernest MP (ed): Neurologic Emergencies. Churchill Livingstone, New York, 1983.)

line. It most commonly develops in patients with underlying carcinoma, usually oat cell carcinoma of the lung. Mild weakness of the arms and legs with reduced deep tendon reflexes is the common presenting picture. Identification and treatment of the primary carcinoma may result in improvement in the neuromuscular symptoms, and some patients improve after treatment with corticosteroids.

Diseases of Muscle

A diverse array of disorders may affect the voluntary skeletal muscles, including the dystrophies, inflammatory myopathies, metabolic, toxic, and endocrine myopathies, and several nonprogressive congenital myopathies (Table 27-4). This section focuses primarily on the dystrophies and the inflamatory my-opathies.

The Dystrophies

A variety of inherited muscular dystrophy syndromes have been characterized. New findings have demonstrated specific genetic defects accounting for faulty muscle proteins.[4]

Duchenne muscular dystrophy is an X-linked recessive disorder that is characterized by progressive weakness, elevated serum CPK levels, and the presence of a characteristic myopathic, fibrotic muscle in biopsy specimens. The onset of symptoms is usually insidious, but generally the child's walk is noted to be clumsy by age 4 to 5 years. Pseudohypertrophy of the calf muscles and a tendency toward toe walking as heel cords shorten are characteristic. As the disease progresses, the child loses strength in the hip girdle muscles and resorts to using arm muscles when rising from the floor or from a chair. Most boys require a wheelchair by the age of 10 years, and survival beyond 20 years is uncommon unless ventilatory assistance is provided.[5] Progressive decompensation in respiratory function due to respiratory muscle weakness and scoliosis predisposes the patient to pulmonary failure and infection. Cardiac enlargement, congestive heart failure, and cardiac dysrhythmias may arise in the advanced stages of the disease.

Becker's dystrophy is another X-linked disorder that resembles Duchenne dystrophy, but it is milder and progresses more slowly.[6] Mean age of onset is 11 years, with loss of ambulation occurring by the patient's 20s.

Myotonic muscular dystrophy is a multisystem disorder with an autosomal-dominant inheritance. Muscle weakness, wasting, and myotonia are usually mild, so that many patients remain ambulatory throughout life. Early cataracts, endocrine dysfunction, intellectual deficits, and gastrointestinal complaints are common. Cardiac conduction defects and hypoventilation may produce life-threatening complications.

Facioscapulohumeral (FSH) *and scapuloperoneal* (SP) *dystrophies* are slowly progressive, dominantly inherited diseases that predominantly involve muscles that control shoulder movement. Facial (in FSH) and leg (in SP) weakness may be present to a variable degree. In most patients, the shoulders sag and rotate anteriorly, resulting in protruding clavicles. Inability to elevate the arms over the head and scapular winging are consistent features. Although surgical fixation of the scapula to the chest wall has been attempted, success is often limited. Fortunately, owing to the localizing nature of these dystrophies, life span is usually not shortened.

In limb girdle dystrophy, patients develop slowly progressive weakness in their shoulders and hips. Impaired ambulation and respiratory insufficiency may develop gradually over 5 to 20 years. A variety of toxic, endocrine, metabolic, or inflammatory conditions may result in a limb girdle pattern of weakness, which must be distinguished from the relatively rare recessively inherited limb girdle muscular dystrophy.

In all the muscular dystrophies, the proper use of physical therapy, bracing, and, when necessary, surgery can greatly enhance a person's adjustment to the physical disabilities. Stretching of heel cords and tight hip muscles, regular exercise programs, and appropriate short or long leg bracing can help to prolong the patient's ambulatory phase. Proper wheelchair positioning and the use of body jackets can help to delay progressive deformity and maximize respiratory function.[7] Surgical procedures to lengthen contracted muscle tendons[8] and correct progressive scoliosis in selective patients may help to reduce discomfort, improve motility, and maximize lung expansion.

Inflammatory Myopathies

Muscle may be the site of infectious or immunologically mediated inflammatory reactions. In immunologic disorders of muscle, the weakness usually progresses over weeks to months, although rarely it may be more rapidly progressive. An aching, deep pain is described in about half of the patients with myositis. An elevated serum CPK level is usually present, and EMG will usually show typical myopathic potentials with fibrillations and brief polyphasic potentials. A muscle biopsy usually is diagnostic, demonstrating inflammatory cell infiltrates. Inflammatory myopathies may be associated with a characteristic skin rash (dermatomyositis) or with other connective tissue disorders, including rheumatoid arthritis, lupus erythematosus, polyarteritis nodosa, Sjögren's syndrome, and scleroderma. Patients over the age of 50 years who develop polymyositis or dermatomyositis have a significant risk of an occult malignancy (10 to 20 percent). The use of anti-inflammatory, immunosuppressive agents (corticosteroids, azathioprine, or methotrexate) helps to slow or reverse deterioration from the inflammatory myopathies.

REHABILITATION THERAPY FOR NEUROMUSCULAR DISORDERS

Although the neuromuscular system can be impaired from a variety of disorders at all levels from anterior horn cell to muscle fiber, the ultimate result is the development of weakness, wasting, and decreased range of motion of voluntary muscles. The appropriate use of physical therapy, bracing, and surgery can greatly improve a person's adjustment. The goal of therapy is to maximize existing capabilities and prevent further loss of motion that may develop from contractures of joints and deformity. The initial concern is to maximize ambulation. When the patient is no longer able to walk, the therapeutic emphasis shifts to maintaining proper positioning and functioning in a wheelchair. In children who develop progressive curvature of the spine, surgery may be necessary to avoid spinal collapse and restricted breathing.

Patterns of weakness are manifested in characteristic ways and require specific intervention.

Hip Weakness

Patients with progressive weakness of the legs develop characteristic ways of compensating. Boys with Duchenne muscular dystrophy will attempt to compensate for weakness of the hips by moving the shoulders back, protruding the abdomen, and tilting the pelvis forward. Progressive shortening or muscle fibers and tendons results in contractures that impair the ability to compensate for the hip weakness. From an early age, physical therapy should focus on maintaining stretch of hips, knees, and heel cords (Figs. 27-4 through 27-6). This needs to be part of a daily

routine, with an effort made to stretch the affected limb at least twice per day.

Bracing and Surgery

With progressive neuromuscular disorders, the patient will have an increasingly difficult time with walking despite a vigorous stretching and exercise program. Children may benefit from polypropylene knee-ankle-foot orthoses (KAFOs) with movable locks at the knee (Fig. 27-7A). If there is too much deformity to use braces, surgery may be necessary to release contractures of the heel cords, the hips, and occasionally the knees. Long leg casts are usually applied postoperatively. The child is encouraged to walk as soon as possible after surgery.

In patients with primarily distal weakness resulting in footdrop, an AFO can usually be worn within the patient's shoe (Fig. 27-7B). This can prevent ankle turning and toe drag during the swing phase of walking. Molded AFO braces will usually be more comfortable, although they are somewhat more expensive than the prefabricated braces that are available.

Scoliosis is a problem that is seen more commonly in children than in adults. In children with progressive muscular dystrophies, proper wheelchair positioning can significantly influence the quality and length of life. Use of scoliosis pads and seat inserts is critical. Younger children may benefit from a molded, lightweight plastic body jacket.

Scoliosis Surgery

If, despite the proper wheelchair positioning and use of body jackets, progressive deformity develops to a point where the curve reaches 35° to 40° and appears to be progressing, surgery is usually recommended. The best candidates for surgery are children who have at least 50 percent of their breathing capacity. Potential risks and benefits must be carefully discussed with the family, and the overall life expectancy must be carefully weighed. The patients who are considered for spinal deformity surgery usually have more severe breathing difficulties and therefore have a higher operative mortality. A practical consideration is that the child will no longer be able to bend over to write or eat after spinal fusion. Consequently, the working surface must be raised and mobile arm

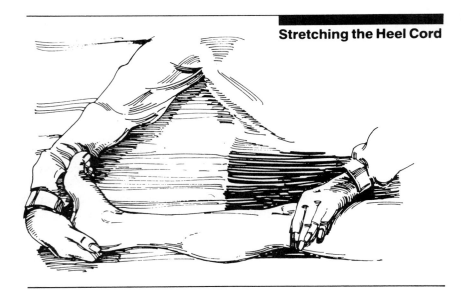

Stretching the Heel Cord

Fig. 27-4. Stretching the heel cord. Cup the heel and pull it down with one hand while the other hand keeps the knee straight. Added leverage is possible by resting the sole of the foot against the forearm to bend the ankle up. Flexing the knee relieves tension but prevents maximal stretching. (From Ringel SP: Neuromuscular Disorders—A Guide for Patient and Family. p. 55. Raven Press, New York, 1987.)

supports provided to compensate for limited arm abduction.

Arm Weakness

If a neuromuscular disorder results in wheelchair dependency, an emphasis should be made on maximizing arm range of motion and strength. Whenever possible the patient should be encouraged to use a manual wheelchair, but a motorized power wheelchair should be considered when it will assist the patient's overall functional independence.

In patients with hand weakness, a variety of adaptive devices are available to make it easier to eat, write, reach, and grasp (Fig. 27-8). Night splints may be

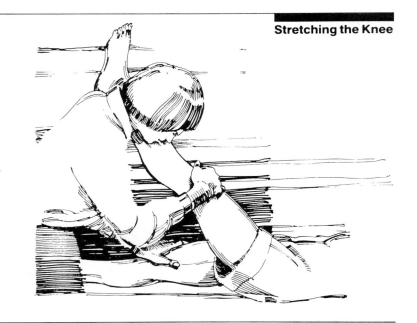

Stretching the Knee

Fig. 27-5. Stretching the knee. The knee is held straight (extended) with one hand while the leg, which rests on the shoulder, is raised to bend the hip. The therapist's other hand stabilizes the other leg to prevent movement. (From Ringel SP: Neuromuscular Disorders—A Guide for Patient and Family. p. 57. Raven Press, New York, 1987.)

Fig. 27-6. Stretching the hip. First the knee is elevated off the table, and the leg is moved out as far as possible. Then the leg is moved in all the way while the knee is still elevated maximally. Pressure is applied with the therapist's other hand over the buttocks to stabilize the pelvis. (From Ringel SP: Neuromuscular Disorders — A Guide for Patient and Family. p. 56. Raven Press, New York, 1987.)

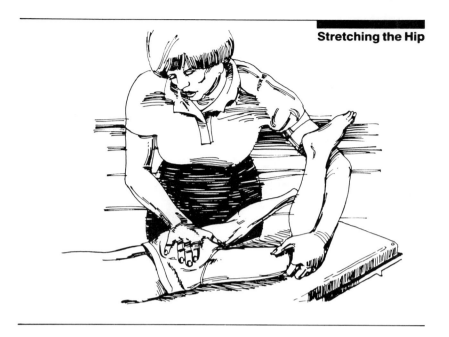

Stretching the Hip

recommended for patients with hand weakness to prevent wrist and finger deformities and preserve hand function. In patients with nonprogressive weakness, tendon transfers occasionally will improve hand dexterity.

For patients with neck weakness, a variety of neck collars may help to provide head support and reduce the pain that results from uncontrollable movements of the head. A styrofoam Philadelphia collar can usually be worn comfortably, although it can be

Fig. 27-7. Long leg brace. This knee-ankle-foot orthosis (KAFO) is lightweight and fits into any shoe. A lock at the knee keeps the leg stiff, when standing, but it can be released to bend the knee when sitting. **(B)** Short leg brace. This AFO positions the foot and ankle and prevents toe drag. It is molded to the contour of the leg and fits into any shoe. Shoe heel height is not varied once the brace is fitted. (From Ringel SP: Neuromuscular Disorders — A Guide for Patient and Family. p. 59. Raven Press, New York, 1987.)

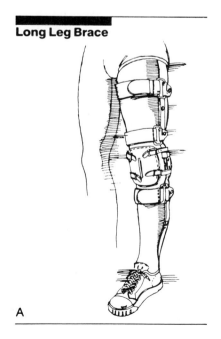

Long Leg Brace

A

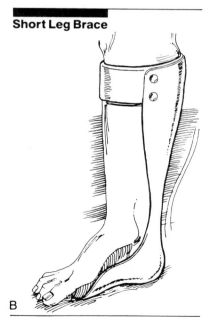

Short Leg Brace

B

Utensil Holders

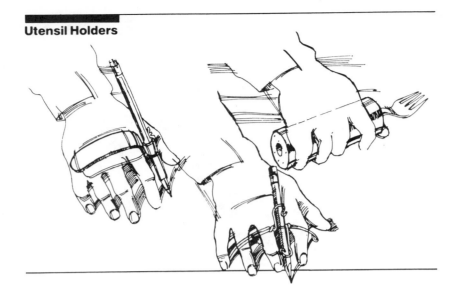

Fig. 27-8. For patients with inadequate strength to grasp, this apparatus can hold a pencil or eating utensil so that it is possible to write and eat independently. (From Ringel SP: Neuromuscular Disorders—A Guide for Patient and Family. p. 70. Raven Press, New York, 1987.)

bulky and hot during the summer months. A thinner, lightweight, rubber-coated metal frame (Hallmark collar) is cooler, although it may not provide as much support.

Dropping of the eyelids may be corrected surgically or mechanically using tape or eyelid crutches (wire loops that attach to the eyeglass frame and hold up the lids). These procedures may result in dry eyes, and appropriate lubricating drops must be used.

Aids to Daily Living

Assistive devices are designed to maximize function and significantly improve a patient's independence and self-esteem. A variety of commonly prescribed devices are available to assist the patient in such activities as dressing, eating, bathing and toileting, and mobility, as well as in maintaining respiratory function.

Dressing

Patients with progressive neuromuscular disorders often solve their dressing problems by modifying the type and style of clothing they wear and by learning easier dressing techniques. Avoiding garments with tiny buttons or zippers in the back, and substituting slacks with elastic waistbands are examples of adaptations. A zipper pull, button hook, sock aid, and long-handled shoehorn can help to reduce the frus-

tration associated with dressing. Velcro fasteners are easier to use than buttons. Many patients find that simple jogging suits are easy to don and are suitable for many activities. Well-fitting shoes that can accommodate an orthotic device are suggested. Many patients prefer lightweight tennis or running shoes, which are comfortable but provide minimal support.

Eating

The ability to eat independently and inconspicuously is extremely important to self-esteem. Simple adjustments such as correct positioning and table height can facilitate independent eating. If the patient rests the elbows on the table, more motion at the elbow, wrist, and hand is possible because the patient does not have to work against gravity. If utensils are difficult to hold, adaptive handles can be added to allow for better gripping surface. The universal cuff wrist strap can hold eating utensils as well as writing implements. For a patient with prominent shoulder weakness, a mobile arm support permanently attached to a wheelchair may allow for independent feeding.

Bathing and Toileting

The bathroom is potentially the most dangerous room in the house, particularly for someone with a neuromuscular disability. Often the room is small, making access with a wheelchair, braces, or crutches

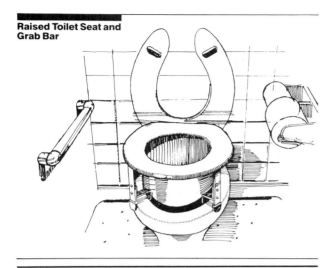

Raised Toilet Seat and Grab Bar

Fig. 27-9. Raised toilet seat, This seat, portable for travel, helps the person with hip muscle weakness come to a standing position more easily. The securely fastened grab bar (left), rather than the toilet paper dispenser (right), is used to support weight. (From Ringel SP: Neuromuscular Disorders—A Guide for Patient and Family. p. 68. Raven Press, New York, 1987.)

difficult; in addition, movement onto the toilet and into the tub or shower may be hazardous.

Even for patients with mild weakness, grab bars should be installed on the inside and outside of the shower to provide for support. A tall shower chair with a back support provides additional steadiness. A long-handled brush or sponge can help a person improve independence in bathing. A patient with moderate weakness can benefit from a bathtub shower seat, a flexible shower hose, and a bath transfer bench, which allows for independent access. As weakness increases, the patient can take a bath using a water-powered bathlift with a seat that extends over the bathtub edge.

Patients with prominent hip weakness may avoid the frustration of getting on and off the toilet by utilizing a 6-inch to 8-inch raised lightweight portable toilet seat (Fig. 27-9). If the bathroom is inaccessible because of size, a portable commode may be the safest device.

Mobility

For patients who have difficulty getting out of low seats, simply raising the seat on wooden blocks makes it much easier to come to a standing position. Easy-lift power chairs are available for patients who cannot get out of a sitting position. Patients who are fearful of walking because they have fallen would benefit from a straight cane, a quad-cane, or a walker.

With progressive neuromuscular disorders, the point is usually reached at which the patient is no longer

Fig. 27-10. Manual wheelchair. Several of the many options available for a wheelchair are illustrated, including (1) removable or solid back, (2) removable desk arm rests, (3) seat and cushion, (4) swing-away foot rests, (5) wheel locks, (6) solid or air-filled rubber tires, (7) hand rim, and (8) seat belt. (From Ringel SP: Neuromuscular Disorders—A Guide for Patient and Family. p. 71. Raven Press, New York, 1987.)

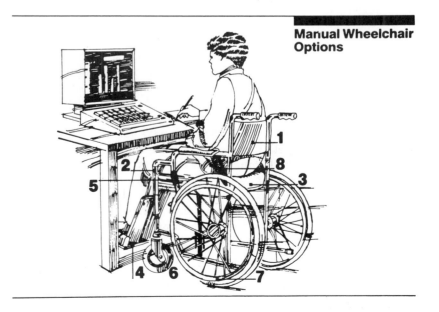

Manual Wheelchair Options

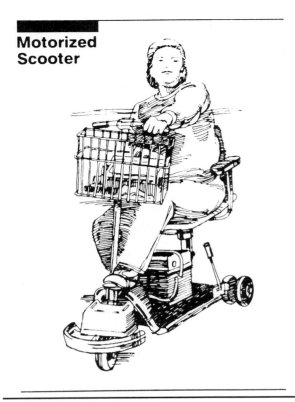

Motorized Scooter

Fig. 27-11. Motorized scooter. These scooters have manual or power adjustments for seat height. Many have interchangeable seats that provide greater trunk support. Some collapse into several components for easy transport in an automobile. (From Ringel SP: Neuromuscular Disorders — A Guide for Patient and Family. p. 73. Raven Press, New York, 1987.)

able to ambulate safely, and a wheelchair must be considered. Attention to the proper fitting of a wheelchair, including appropriate cushions, armrests, foot supports, and easily activated brakes will ensure the maximum benefit from the wheelchair (Fig. 27-10). When a patient does not have adequate strength to propel a manual wheelchair, a motorized chair can provide much-needed access and independence. The major disadvantage of power chairs is their weight and lack of portability. The house must have a ramp for entry, and a van or bus requires a lift if a person wishes to be transported from place to place.

As an alternative to a motorized wheelchair, lighter weight, more portable scooters are available (Fig.

27-11). These tend to provide less support and cannot be used by people with severe weakness of the upper body and poor trunk support.

For patients with advanced weakness, moving in and out of bed may not be possible without assistance. An alternating air mattress or water bed can add comfort and prevent total dependency. Prevention of pressure sores in the later stages of neuromuscular illness is an important priority.

Respiratory Dysfunction

Patients with neuromuscular disease are at risk for respiratory decompensation because of a number of factors. Weakness and incoordination of muscles involved in chewing and swallowing may result in aspiration of liquids and solids. Weakness of respiratory muscles results in impaired air exchange: pulmonary function tests often reveal reduced inspiratory and expiratory pressures, as well as decreases in forced vital capacity. A weak cough impairs a patient's ability to adequately clear the airway, increasing the risk of aspiration pneumonia. Some neuromuscular disorders (acid maltase deficiency, myotonic dystrophy) may have a diminished ventilatory response to falling oxygen or rising carbon dioxide tensions.

Efforts at optimizing respiratory function in patients with neuromuscular disorders must be maintained at all stages of the illness. Inspiratory muscle training, in which the patient inhales against progressively harder inspiratory resistors, may be efficacious in strengthening respiratory muscles. Postural drainage techniques with chest percussion can aid in clearing airway obstruction and preventing microatelectasis. Family members should be instructed in the Heimlich maneuver in case acute airway blockage develops that cannot be cleared by the patient's weakened cough.

The issue of mechanical ventilatory support is a difficult one to address, but it must be considered in patients with progressive neuromuscular diseases. A variety of support systems are available, including gravity units, negative pressure ventilators, and positive pressure ventilators. A *gravity unit*, such as a rocking bed, will assist nocturnal respiration in patients with mild respiratory weakness by causing abdominal contents to be pulled away from and pushed toward the diaphragm. This device is not forceful enough to provide adequate air exchange in patients with advanced respiratory compromise.

Negative pressure ventilators, including a chest cuirass and pneumowraps, work well for nocturnal assistance as long as a good seal is maintained between the chest wall and the thoracic shell. They are not adequate for advanced respiratory insufficiency. *Positive pressure ventilators* traditionally require a tracheostomy, although recent reports have demonstrated that some patients may tolerate custom-fitted oral or nasal interface devices.[9] A physician needs to carefully discuss the ramifications of mechanical ventilatory asistance with the patient and family before recommending these devices. Important issues include third party payment, family and community support systems, vendor contracts, and education of the family and patient.

SUMMARY

Diseases that affect the neuromuscular system produce a wide range of disabilities. Early diagnosis, characterization of individual problems, and attention to maximizing independent functioning can add significantly to the quality of life. Until such time when specific intervention to treat or cure the underlying neuromuscular disease is available, physicians can help these patients by addressing such basic needs as eating, dressing, toileting, and moving with the highest level of independence possible.

REFERENCES

1. Feinstein B, Lindegard B, Nyman E, Wohlfort B: Morphologic studies of motor units in normal human muscles. Acta Anat (Basel) 23:127, 1955
2. Berger AR, Schaumberg HH: Rehabilitation of focal nerve injuries. J Neurol Rehabil 2:65, 1988
3. Berger AR, Schaumberg HH: Rehabilitation of peripheral neuropathies. J Neurol Rehabil 2:23, 1988
4. Gutmann DH, Fischbeck KH: Molecular biology of Duchenne and Becker muscular dystrophy: clinical applications. Annals Neurol 26:189, 1989
5. Brooke MH, Fenichel GR, Griggs RC et al: Duchenne muscular dystrophy: patterns of clinical progression and effects of supportive therapy. Neurology 39:475, 1989
6. Hoffman EP, Kunkel LM Angelini C et al: Improved diagnosis of Becker muscular dystrophy by dystrophia testing. Neurology 39:1011, 1989
7. Ringel SP, Neville HE: The rehabilitation of muscular disorders. J Neurol Rehabil 1:149, 1987
8. Siegel IM, Glantz RH: Orthopedic rehabilitation for stand and walking in selected neuromuscular diseases. J Neurol Rehabil 2:131, 1988
9. McDermott I, Bach JR, Parker C, Sortor S: Custom-fabricated interfaces for intermittent positive pressure ventilation. Int J Prosthodont 2:224, 1989

SUGGESTED READINGS

Brooke MH: A Clinician's View of Neuromuscular Disorders. 2nd Edit Williams & Wilkins, Baltimore, 1986

Dawson DM, Hallet M, Millender LH: Entrapment Neuropathies. Little, Brown Boston, 1983

Mulder DW (ed): The Diagnosis and Treatment of Amyotrophic Lateral Sclerosis. Houghton Mifflin, Boston, 1980

Ringel SP: Neuromuscular disorders — A Guide for Patient and Family. Raven Press, New York, 1987

Section IV

GENERALIZED DISORDERS

28 Cerebral Palsy

M. MARK HOFFER
MARTIN KOFFMAN

HISTORY AND DEFINITIONS

Cerebral palsy is a nonprogressive, nonhereditary disease with many neurologic manifestations. The onset is prenatal and its cause is poorly understood. Little[1] was the first to describe cerebral palsy, and his work was popularized and amplified by Osler and by Freud.[2] Classifications of cerebral palsy have been developed by Balf and Ingram,[3] Minear,[4] Pearlstein,[5] and Phelps.[6] More than 500,000 Americans have cerebral palsy. According to Phelps,[6] one-third of this population has severe involvement and one-sixth has very mild involvement. It is difficult to formulate treatment plans for cerebral palsy patients because of the diffuse manifestations of the disease, but a simple classification scheme has been accepted that is useful in making goals and plans.[7]

There are three general descriptive types of cerebral palsy: spastic, dyskinetic, and mixed. The spastic patient has hyperactive reflexes and clonus. The clonus increases with stretch. The orthopaedic surgeon has most to offer this group of patients. Cerebral palsy patients with motion disorders have extremely complicated conditions that are more difficult to define and treat. Precise definitions have been advanced for spastic motion disorders, such as "athetosis," "chorea," "dyskinesia," and "ataxia." These terms each have different meanings neurologically, but ultimately the differences are not important, because specific measures for managing any of these problems are not yet available. We like to distinguish between those persons who have problems with control of the limb in the pathway of their motion and those who have problems in the endpoint of that motion. Some patients exhibit a mixed picture of spasticity and motion disorder.

Cerebral palsy patients present a continuum of types of severity of bodily involvement. The extent of involvement is another important factor in evaluating cerebral palsy. The person with hemiplegia suffers mainly from involvement of one side. Barring the presence of other preventive conditions, people with hemiplegia will always be able to walk, and they rarely need any therapy to alow them to speak. Their greatest problems seem to be sensory deprivation in the upper extremity and equinovarus deformity in the lower extremity. Commonly hemiplegic patients have involvement of the opposite leg to a lesser degree. Single limb involvement also occurs but it is rare.

In patients with diplegia, the lower extremities are more involved than the upper extremities, yet the upper extremities are almost always involved to some extent. Patients with diplegia often have esotropia as well. The involvement for diplegic persons usually is more severe in the hips and less so in the feet. They tend to have anteverted, adducted hips, valgus, externally rotated knees, and equinovalgus deformity of the feet. The designation of paraplegia is probably not correct for these patients, because that term more clearly defines the person with spinal cord injury.

The patient with total involvement has problems in all four extremities; in addition, speech, swallowing, and cognition are often critically deficient. Again, the word "quadriplegia" is not used because this term is better restricted to a patient with a spinal cord injury. It is the totally involved individual — that is, the cerebral palsy patient — who has the most difficulty in ambulating. Ambulation, in fact, is not usually the goal for these persons. Patients may require surgery and orthoses to aid them in sitting. Scoliosis and dislocated hips do affect the eventual ability of these children to sit and so they may need surgery for the hip and spine.

It is very important to test the reflex levels of these patients because they reveal if the patient is developing balance. Children who have not achieved the balance reaction as demonstrated by parachute reflex, and who have persistent obligatory tonic neck reflexes, by the age of 3 years should not be considered candidates for functional ambulation because of their lack of trunk balance. Furthermore, if they do not develop these reactions by the time they are 6 years old, they will have difficulty with sitting independently.

When studying individual limbs, two general factors must be determined. The sensibility of the limb should be studied by two-point discrimination, graphesthesia, or object identification. The motor control of the limb should be studied for its dependence on or independence of patterns of motion involving other limbs. Muscle testing for grades is an excellent way of testing muscles for selective control. However, most cerebral palsied muscles do not have selective control and thus these tests are not valid.

Finally, the most important abilities of human beings involve their cognition and communication. It is difficult to test intelligence unless the person can communicate. Thus these two crucial factors are interrelated. Nonverbal speech programs may aid these patients.

CLASSIFICATIONS OF MOBILITY

We like to think of three types of sitting: propped, self-propped, and independent. A propped sitter is one who has a straight back and loose hips, and who can be propped up in a wheelchair. These patients have no balance reactions and often require a loose cerebral palsy bracing as a propped device. Ankle and knee orthoses are not necessary in these sitters, nor are operations on the foot and knee, which are performed for ambulatory patients. Hip releases and surgical stabilization of the spine may be more effective operations. Self-propped sitters may need some support, but they can maintain themselves at balance

temporarily. These patients may need modifications of their wheelchairs. Patients who sit independently have balance and support reactions. Attention should be paid to modifying their wheelchairs to make sure that they are permitted the ability to transfer. In addition, some of these patients are able to propel the wheelchair backward and it may be necessary to add equipment for foot control.

There are four types of ambulation or nonambulation used by disabled persons: community, household, physiologic, and nonambulation. In community ambulation, patients walk both indoors and outdoors during most of their activities and may need orthoses for these activities. These patients require wheelchairs only for long trips out of the community. Household ambulation implies that a patient only walks indoors with the support of some type of apparatus. Household ambulators get in and out of chairs and beds with little, if any, assistance and may need a wheelchair only for some indoor activities away from the home. Physiologic or nonfunctional ambulation is used primarily in a therapy session and persons in this classification use wheelchairs for their functional needs. Nonambulatory patients may stand and transfer but they are truly sitters because they cannot maintain the balance necessary for forward progression. All hemiplegics can achieve functional ambulation, diplegics who develop balance reactions by age 3 years and have stable hips will walk functionally, and few totally involved patients will achieve functional ambulation.

SURGICAL PLANNING AND OPERATING PROCEDURES

Lower Extremities

Fortunately, pain is a relatively infrequent indication for surgery in the cerebral palsy patient. Similarly, operations are not often performed for cosmetic purposes alone. By far the most frequent justification for surgical intervention is the expected improvement of function. The deformities and abnormal postures displayed by the cerebral palsy patient from muscle imbalance and imperfect motor control invite a variety of interventions. Unfortunately, surgical correction of a deformity does not always result in improved function. Even so, sometimes it is desirable to advocate prophylactic surgery to prevent progression of a deformity that would otherwise result in loss of function already present. For example, by correcting the progressive subluxation of the hip, loss of ambulation is averted. Nevertheless, a blend of art and science occurs in decision-making when predicting the results of an operation on the peripheral musculoskeletal apparatus in the patient with a central nervous system lesion.

To improve our accuracy in predicting the results of surgery, we rely on classifications, prognostic indicators, the experience of others, and information gained by electromyographic (EMG) studies of the timing of "firing" of individual muscles and muscle groups during the performance of certain functional activities.[7-9] These tools may be augmented in the future with more kinesiologic data and energy cost-of-work studies.

Hemiplegia

All hemiplegic persons will be independently ambulatory. Equinus deformities frequently can be controlled at an early age by combinations of casting, bracing, and night splints. An Achilles tendon lengthening and split anterior tibial tendon transfer (SPLATT) can be performed for equinovarus attitude of the foot present during the entire gait cycle. Posterior tibialis tendon lengthening may need to accompany the SPLATT procedure if there is fixed varus deformity under anesthesia. The Achilles tendon lengthening must accompany the SPLATT procedure if there is fixed equinus deformity under anesthesia.

If the EMG shows posterior tibialis muscle activity during the swing phase but not during the stance phase, transfer of the posterior tibialis tendon through the interosseous membrane to the dorsum of the foot may be a more logical procedure than the SPLATT. To transfer the posterior tibialis tendon through the interosseous membrane when it is active through all phases of the gait cycle by EMG is to establish a tenodesis, which initially results in limited ankle motion but will later subside as the tendon becomes stretched out.

Transferring the posterior tibialis tendon to the lateral side of the foot is never indicated.

An equinus foot deformity is rarely solely responsible for a patient's failure to walk. The deformity can usually be controlled early with braces and splints until the patient is able to walk; then an operation can be performed. In the foot not previously operated upon, a three-level, Hoke-type tenotomy of the Achilles tendon that brings the ankle perpendicular to the tibia while the patient is under anesthesia and then casts the ankle in 5° of plantar flexion is the preferred technique. A short leg, weight-bearing cast is applied postoperatively and worn for 6 weeks.

The technique of advancing the Achilles tendon anteriorly on the os calcis is being evaluated in the treatment of the equinus ankle. Although it is too early to make any definite statements about results, the procedure has its primary application in ankles with adequate motion but in which there is excessive plantar flexion tone and an equinus gait. We have no experience with os calcis osteotomies in correcting the varus foot deformity in this group of patients.

The hip is rarely a clinical problem in early life for hemiplegic persons. Occasionally the excessive internal rotation and adduction during gait will require adductor release and a medial hamstring release or a lateral transfer in a child younger than the age of 6 years who has a passive external rotation range of 20° to 30° at rest. The medial hamstring (semitendinosus) transfer will be most effective if the gait EMG shows it to be active only during the end of swing phase and into early stance phase, as in the patient without neurologic involvement.

More often the adduction and internal rotation attitude during gait will need to be corrected by adductor release. A derotation osteotomy also will be required to correct the anteversion of the femur. Frequently the internal rotation attitude and anteversion are not accompanied by radiographic evidence of hip subluxation, and in these patients the derotation osteotomy can be performed in the distal femur.

The supracondylar approach to the osteotomy has the advantages of permitting early weight-bearing and not requiring hardware to be in the body for an extended period of time.

Diplegia

Diplegic patients who develop some trunk balance will become ambulatory. Some will be grossly restricted to household ambulation with a pick-up walker, whereas others will be independent community ambulators. Therefore, the focus in these patients' lower extremities is at the hips. The hip action brace can be a useful training adjunct to physical therapy when the patient is learning to walk, but if the hip abduction range begins to shrink, adductor releases are indicated.[10] Adductor transfer posteriorly to the ischium has not proved to be superior to adductor release alone. The adductor releases must be performed bilaterally in these patients.

If hip subluxation occurs at any age, derotation-varus osteotomy will be necessary in addition to adductor releases. We tend to use crossed pins to hold the osteotomy in young patients and a small ankle orthosis (AO) plate or the Coventry screw in the older patients. In either instance, a spica cast is always used in the early postoperative period. The gracilis, adductor longus, and adductor brevis muscles are released without performing an obturator neurectomy in these potentially ambulatory children. A crouch gait with excessive lumbar lordosis during gait often calls attention to the presence of hip flexion deformities. If the hip flexion together with the adduction and internal rotation is judged to be contributing to the subluxation of the hip, other muscles in addition to the adductors will need to be released surgically.

If the patient's ambulation has reached a plateau or is deteriorating over a period of several months while under the supervision of a therapist and the patient is younger than 10 years old, surgical correction of the crouch gait associated with excessive lumbar lordosis can be considered. The EMG helps in selecting whether the iliopsoas or the rectus femoris is to be released, and it may also aid in analyzing the gracilis or medial hamstring muscles.

Successive or concomitant corrections of the knee flexion deformity by selective distal hamstring lengthenings and tenotomies are indicated is some patients with a crouch gait. A knee flexion deformity should never be approached surgically without proper attention being given to the hip flexion deformity. Attention must also be paid to the possible un-

deractivity of the triceps surae muscle as at least a contributing factor to some of the patient's crouch posture during gait.

Indications for surgery are clinical[11-13] and not based on the EMG findings. Once the decision to operate has been made on clinical grounds, the gait EMG may aid in selecting the most appropriate muscle among a group on which to operate. The EMG reveals which muscle or muscles are deviating most from their normal phasic pattern of activity during the gait cycle. Surprisingly, several muscles in the lower extremity of diplegic persons will be firing in a normal manner during walking. Also surprisingly, patients exhibiting the same posture during gait may show different variations from the normal EMG patterns to account for these same postures. For example, the hip flexion attitude may be caused by an abnormal iliopsoas muscle in one patient but by an abnormal rectus femoris muscle in another. Alternatively, the internal rotation attitude may be due to an abnormal iliopsoas in one patient and to an abnormal medial hamstring in another.

Rehabilitation professionals are less concerned about postures and attitudes—the cosmesis of gait—than about the cost—that is, the energy expenditure—of walking. Measuring oxygen consumption, either directly or indirectly by monitoring heart rates, to determine efficiency of gait and endurance will become more popular in assessing postoperative results.

We are less concerned about the ankles and feet in diplegic persons than previously.[14] Equinus deformity, although commonly present, is rarely the limiting factor in the patient's ability to walk. Positions at the feet sometimes change in response to hip and knee operations. For that reason, an operation on the feet and ankles is often deferred unless the patient has a significant fixed (not dynamic) deformity, in which case an Achilles tendon lengthening is performed.

Valgus foot deformities are common but are rarely reponsible for a patient's failure to progress in ambulation. Orthotic devices are of limited usefulness and results of peroneal tendon transfers to the medial side of the foot are unpredictable. We find our indications for the Grice procedure to be diminishing with time.

In many cases we would prefer to wait until the patient is at least 12 years old and then perform a triple arthrodesis if the patient is still a functional ambulator.

However, if the valgus deformities are becoming progressively more fixed and skin changes are taking place at sites of excessive pressure in the shoes, Grice procedures are required. Proper attention is given to correcting excessive anteversion before the Grice procedures are performed.

Totally Involved Spasticity

The totally involved spastic patient is not and will not be a functional ambulator. Many of these patients have some combination of spasticity and dyskinesia. Those patients with almost pure dyskinesia frequently do walk, and the following discussion is not meant to apply to them.

Being able to transfer, assisted or unassisted, is the highest functional level that the totally involved spastic patient performs with the use of the lower extremities. These patients will spend most of their waking hours sitting in a chair. This group of patients will include several who appear to resemble diplegic persons but who have more severe involvement of the upper extremities than usual, or who may resemble those with hemiplegia with more severe involvement of the unaffected side.

For the first 8 to 10 years of their lives, patients with total involvement should have aggressive surgical treatment of any subluxation or dislocation of the hip. This treatment encompasses the combinations of soft tissue releases and osteotomies as indicated by static examinations. EMG is of no value in preoperative planning for this group of patients, and tendon transfers have never been shown to offer any advantages over releases. Postoperative splinting or bracing for 12 hours a day is often useful. In this age group the hips rarely are painful. We are less aggressive in operating on deformities about the knees and ankles in these patients, particularly if they are not going to be able to transfer because of the severity of the neurologic involvement, which affect their balance and use of their upper extremities.

The totally involved patient who has reached adolescence or adulthood needs 90° of painless hip flexion range and balanced spinal curvatures to be able to sit propped upright. The adult patient's hip may become painful irrespective of whether it is dislocated. An adult's case is best managed by paying more attention to the clinical status instead of trying to set up criteria for interventions based solely on the radiographic appearance of the hips.

Proximal hamstring-origin releases from the ischium may be useful to gain a range of hip flexion for ease of sitting.

A patient who did not have preoperative pain may develop it postoperatively. If soft tissue releases alone are not sufficient to gain adequate range of hip motion for sitting, femoral osteotomy with skeletal shortening would seem to be preferable to the proximal femoral resection in a painless hip.

Occasionally a quadriceps tendon release may be indicated to gain range of knee flexion for sitting.

Spinal stabilization to the sacrum is sometimes helpful in controlling the increasing spinal deformity and pelvic obliquity that interferes with sitting. Fusions should include posterior procedures to the sacrum when pelvic obliquity is noted. The addition of anterior thoracolumbar fusions is currently advocated to reduce the pseudarthrosis rate.

The problem of the painful hip in the cerebral palsied patient has not yet been solved. The results of proximal femoral resection with or without insertion of a constrained implant have been disappointing to date. Although initially they may be improved, many of these patients have recurrence of their pain 1 to 2 years postoperatively. This disturbance is frequently associated with excessive amounts of heterotopic bone formation and a decrease in the range of motion that developed shortly after surgery.

Upper Extremities

Four factors are to be considered in planning care for the upper limb in cerebral palsy[15]: cognition, sensibility, placement, and control of the muscles of the hand. The problems in assessing cognition and sensibility have already been mentioned.

Placement of the cerebral palsied hand is a combined problem of body, shoulder, and elbow motion. The range of motion is limited by contracture or spasticity of these parts. The speed of placement is limited by the motion disorders that force the arm to make complicated pathways to an object. The precision of placement is limited by those motion disorders affecting the endpoint of such placement activity. It is convenient to document the speed and precision of placement of a hand on the opposite knee and on the top of the head.

The muscle control of the upper extremity in cerebral palsy depends on the degree of spasticity. Minor degrees of spasticity may exist in limbs with good function, but severe spasticity leads to fixed contractures of muscle-tendon units and joints. These fixed contractures rarely develop in sophisticated upper limbs, and when such deformities are seen, function is surely affected.

The retained perinatal reflexes can influence the posture of the whole upper limb in developing mass flexion-extension patterns. Hands that are forcibly constrained by these primitive mass reflexes also have poor potential for rehabilitation.

Realistic goals for hand use are based on the aforementioned four factors. In a patient who has poor cognition, poor sensibility,[16] poor hand placement, and no selective control, a posture that permits hygiene only is a realistic goal. Yet a patient in whom cognition, sensibility, hand placement, and selective control are all good will have no real need for surgical intervention. Thus, any individual for whom a functional goal exists will have to sacrifice some disability, and it is hoped that this would be in the motor area, where an operation has some effect.

The hygiene and cosmetic operations in patients with poor performance in all four factors in upper extremity mobility consist mainly of correcting wrist flexion, thumb-in-palm, and finger flexion contractures. These patients respond inconsistently to muscle transfers or lengthening procedures. Our general policy is to perform radial-to-metacarpal wrist fusions with iliac bone grafts and pin fixation. At the same time the muscle tendon units are lengthened by sublimis-to-profundis transfer and some releases are performed.

Functional procedures are performed in those persons with good cognition, sensibility, and placement, but who have difficulty with muscle control. The problems in muscle control seem to revolve around the three main areas of pinch, grasp, and release. When the thumb-in-palm deformity exists, thumb web releases by Z-plasty and release of the adducted first dorsal interosseous muscle from the thumb metacarpal allow opening of the thumb from the palm.[17] In addition, it may be necessary to augment the thumb extensor muscle by a tendon transfer.[18] Sometimes the thumb metacarpal joint is hyperextended, and for such loose joints, capsulodesis with temporary pin fixation is helpful.

Patients with grasp problems are obliged to use their wrist flexors at the time of finger flexion. This discoordinate action of wrist flexors and finger flexor weakens the effective power of the fingers. In such cases a transfer of the wrist flexor to the wrist extensor will allow the patient to flex the fingers in vigorous grasp while the wrist is extended.[19-21] Before performing such a procedure, it must be ascertained that when the wrist is held in a neutral position the fingers can be actively extended. If they cannot, it is possible that the problem with which the surgeon is faced is one of release.

The patients with problems in releasing find it difficult to open their fingers when the wrist is extended; they are obliged to flex the wrist to open their fingers. In these children there is often synergy between the finger extensors and the wrist flexors. This synergy resembles the tenodesis action seen in paralytics, but in most cerebral palsy patients there is no fixed contracture, the movements being a matter of synergistic activity in release rather than tenodesis. The EMG may help to separate the problems with grasp from those of release, and we tend to obtain electromyograms routinely before an operation. When the flexed wrist release combination is seen, transfer of the wrist flexors to the finger extensors may be helpful.

Numerous other procedures have been introduced for the care of the more functionally capable cerebral palsied hands.[22-24] These include sublimis tenodesis for a hyperextended proximal interphalangeal joint, the use of the flexor carpi radial is muscles, elbow flexor releases, and wrist and finger flexor tendon lengthenings. Flexor slides should not be performed in these more highly functional hands for fear they will lose significant strength. Wrist fusions are poorly tolerated in functional cerebral palsied hands.

When making surgical plans for the cerebral palsy patient's upper extremity, it should be remembered that each child presents different and unique problems. Current experiments with functional orthoses and needle electromyograms may eventually provide more accurate preoperative judgments in these complex problems.

REFERENCES

1. Little WJ: On the influence of abnormal parturition on the child. Trans Obstet Soc Lond 3:293, 1862
2. Freud S: Infantile Cerebral Paralysis (L. Russin, transl). University of Miami Press, Miami, 1978
3. Balf CL, Ingram O: Problems in classification of cerebral palsy in childhood. Br Med J 2:163, 1955
4. Minear WL: A classification of cerebral palsy. Pediatrics 18:841, 1956
5. Pearlstein MA: Infantile cerebral palsy: classification and clinical correlation. JAMA 145:30, 1952
6. Phelps WM: Etiology and diagnostic classification in cerebral palsy. In Proceedings of Cerebral Palsy Meeting. New York Association to Aid Crippled Children, New York, 1950
7. Hoffer MM: Basic considerations and classifications of cerebral palsy. Instr Course Lect 25:96, 1976
8. Perry J, Hoffer MM, Giovan P, et al: Gait analysis of the triceps surae in cerebral palsy. J Bone Joint Surg [AM] 56:511, 1974
9. Perry J, Hoffer MM, Antonelli D, et al: Electromyography before and after surgery for hip deformity in children with cerebral palsy. J Bone Joint Surg [AM] 58:201, 1976
10. Hoffer MM, Garrett A, Koffman M, et al: New concepts in orthotics for cerebral palsy. Clin Orthop 102:100, 1974
11. Bleck EE: Hip deformities in cerebral palsy. Instr Course Lect 20:54, 1971
12. Bleck EE: Locomotor prognosis in cerebral palsy. Dev Med Child Neurol 17:18, 1975
13. Goldner JL: General principles in cerebral palsy. Instr Course Lect 20:20, 1971
14. Bassett FH: Deformities of the feet due to cerebral palsy. Instr Course Lect 20:35, 1971
15. Hoffer MM: The upper extremity in cerebral palsy. Symp Neurol Aspects Plastic Surg 17:133, 1978
16. Tachdjian MO, Minear WL: Sensory disturbances in the hands of children with cerebral palsy. J Bone Joint Surg [AM] 40:85, 1958
17. Matev IB: Surgical treatment of flexion adduction contractures of the thumbs in cerebral palsy. Acta Orthop Scand 41:439, 1970
18. Goldner JL: Reconstructive surgery in the hand in cerebral palsy. J Bone Joint Surg [AM] 37:1141, 1955
19. Green WT, Banks HH: Flexor carpi ulnaris transplant and its use in cerebral palsy. J Bone Joint Surg [AM] 44:1343, 1962
20. Samilson RL: Principles of assessment of upper limbs in cerebral palsy. Clin Orthop 47:105, 1966
21. Samilson RL, Morris JM: Surgical improvement of the cerebral-palsied upper limb. J Bone Joint Surg [AM] 46:1203, 1964
22. Goldner JL: The upper extremity in cerebral palsy. p. 221. In Samilson R (ed): Orthopedic Aspects of Cerebral Palsy. JB Lippincott, Philadelphia, 1975
23. Swanson AB: Surgery of the hand in cerebral palsy and the swan-neck deformity. J Bone Joint Surg [AM] 42:951, 1960
24. Swanson AB: Surgery of the hand in cerebral palsy and muscle origin release procedures. Surg Clin North Am 48:1129, 1968

29 Stroke

MICHAEL J. BOTTE
MARY ANN E. KEENAN
CHRISTOPHER JORDAN

Deficits in cognition and limb function often develop after a cerebrovascular accident. Disruption of upper motoneuron inhibitory pathways leads to muscle spasticity. Spasticity, with its increased muscle tone, results in muscle imbalance, causing limb deformity and posturing. Limb posturing, if prolonged or neglected, will lead to fixed contractures. Fixed contractures inhibit further recovery of function, cause hygiene and dressing problems, can lead to decubitus ulcers, and can contribute to development of peripheral neuropathy. In addition, poor limb sensibility and extremity pain are other problems the stroke patient often faces. The management of patients with who have sustained a stroke is reviewed here, with emphasis on extremity problems and associated treatment.

INCIDENCE

Stroke is the third leading cause of death in the United States. The incidence of stroke is 1 per 1,000 population annually, with 190,000 to 250,000 patients surviving and 200,000 dying per year.[1,2] Stroke is currently the leading cause of acquired hemiplegia in the adult, and over 2 million people have permanent neurologic deficits. The average patient who survives a stroke beyond the first few months has a life expectancy of greater than 5 years.[3,4]

Despite the severe deficits sustained, many stroke patients survive long enough and achieve adequate function to justify aggressive rehabilitation and surgical reconstruction.[3-10] Functional prognosis of survivors is outlined in Table 29-1.[4]

PATHOPHYSIOLOGY

Cerebral function is dependent on a continuous supply of oxygen. An interruption of oxygenation during a cerebrovascular accident (from thrombosis, hemorrhage, or emboli) results in neuron death and subsequent deficits in cognition and sensory and motor function.[1,3,11,12]

Cerebral thrombosis, the most common cause of stroke, accounts for nearly three-fourths of all cerebrovascular accidents. Arteriosclerosis is the most significant predisposing factor.[1,3,12,13] Spontaneous intracerebral or subarachnoid hemorrhage is the second most common cause of stroke, accounting for approximately one-sixth of all cerebrovascular accidents. Hypertension is a predisposing factor in these patients.[3,12] Isolated cerebral emboli account for less than one-tenth of cerebrovascular accidents. Pre-existing extracranial pathology, including carotid arterial atherosclerosis, cardiac valve pathology, or cardiac arrhythmias, is usually present.[14]

Other predisposing factors to cerebrovascular accidents include increased age, genetic predisposition, hyperlipidemia, hypercholesterolemia, obesity, cardiac anomalies (arrhythmias, myocardial infarction, hypotension, mural thrombosis), diabetes mellitus, collagen vascular disease (vasculitis, polyarteritis), hyperviscosity states (sickle cell disease, polycythemia), oral contraceptive use, tobacco smoking, severe cerebrovascular spasm secondary to migraine headaches, and septic vasculitis (tuberculosis, syphilis, and mucormycosis).[1,3,12,14]

Table 29-1. Prognosis after Cerebrovascular Accidents (CVAs)

	Total Number of CVAs (%)	Survival Rate After			Functional Prognosis of Survivors (%)	
		30 Days (%)	5 Years (%)	10 Years (%)		
All CVAs		62			29	Normal
					33	Able to work
					3	Total care
Thrombosis	71	90	43	22	27	Normal
					34	Able to work
					2	Total care
Emboli	8	75	30	15	27	Normal
					34	Able to work
					2	Total care
Hemorrhage, overall	16				49	Normal
					14	Able to work
					49	Total care
Intracerebral bleeding		22	7	0		
Subarachnoid bleeding		55	37	30		

(Modified from Matsumoto et al,[4] with permission.)

ANATOMIC CORRELATIONS

Clinical syndromes often arise from insults to specific areas of the cerebral cortex.[1,9,15] Motor and sensory function of the trunk, upper extremity, and face, in addition to the functions of speech, is controlled chiefly by the cerebral cortex (Fig. 29-1A). The main arterial supply to this area of the brain is the middle cerebral artery (Fig. 29-1B). A stroke involving the middle cerebral artery (the most common type of stroke) produces a typical hemiplegic picture with greater involvement of the upper extremity, face, and speech than of the lower extremity.

Motor and sensory functions of the lower extremity are controlled chiefly by the midcortex in the sagittal plane of the brain (Fig. 29-1A). This area of the brain is supplied by the anterior cerebral artery (Fig. 29-1B). A stroke involving the anterior cerebral artery usually results in hemiplegia with sensory and motor deficits involving chiefly the lower extremity.

Visual functions are controlled by the visual cortex in the occipital region. This area of the brain is supplied by the posterior cerebral artery. Common impairments caused by injury to this artery or to the occipi-

tal lobes or optic tracts by cerebrovascular accidents (Fig. 29-1B)[9,15] include hemianopia (blindness in half of the visual field), loss of depth perception, poor perceptual organization, loss of geometric sense, inability to copy figures, and failure at tasks involving spatial analysis.

Bilateral cortical involvement, especially in the frontal lobes, can lead to severe cognitive deficits, resulting in loss of memory, poor attention span, lack of motivation, and inability to learn.

Injury to the parietal lobe of the nondominant hemisphere may result in a lack of awareness of the involved side of the body, known as *body neglect*. This failure to recognize and use the involved side occurs despite minimal motor involvement.

Cerebrovascular accidents in the vertebrobasilar system are uncommon. When they do occur, deficits in balance and coordination arise from interruption of afferent and efferent pathways between the brain and spinal cord. These deficits make rehabilitation especially difficult.

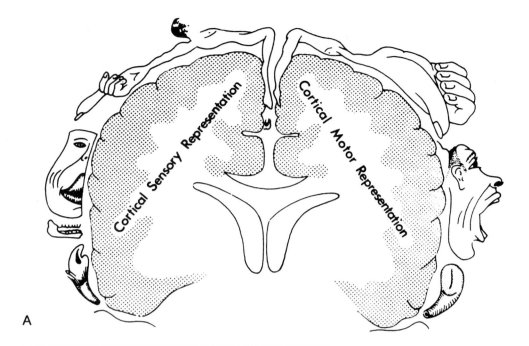

A

Fig. 29-1. Diagrams of the cerebral cortex demonstrating areas that control various functions **(A)** and their corresponding arterial blood supply **(B)**. Note the large area of cortex that is dedicated to controlling the hand and face. The upper extremity and speech are impaired most often when the lateral cortex is injured from middle cerebral artery thrombosis or hemorrhage (thus producing the common hemiplegic pattern, with greater involvement of the upper extremity and speech compared to involvement of the lower extremity). The midportion of the brain in the sagittal plane controls lower extremity function. These functions are impaired from thrombosis or hemorrhage of the anterior cerebral artery.

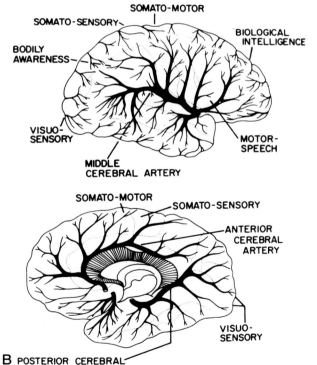

EVALUATION OF THE STROKE PATIENT

Three major areas of impairment in the stroke patient include cognition, sensibility, and motor function.[21]

Cognition

Cognition (i.e., thought processes, mental perception, and memory) can be evaluated by appropriateness of response to questions, ability to follow commands, psychological testing, and direct testing of learning ability in a rehabilitation setting.[1,9,15,16] Decreased ability to learn and loss of short-term memory may become apparent only with specific testing. Cognitive deficits may be severe in patients with frontal lobe impairment, who otherwise have minimal motor or sensibility loss. These patients show clinical features similar to senility, with lack of attention span and little motivation for recovery.

Loss of ability to communicate or understand speech, writing, or signs is known as *aphasia*. Aphasia can be expressive or receptive and commonly occurs with lesions of the left hemisphere, usually without regard to hand dominance. Receptive aphasia has a poor prognosis for rehabilitation because the patient cannot understand instructions. An expressive aphasia, however, may be compatible with rehabilitation if the patient is able comprehend instructions.[9,15,16]

Apraxia is the impairment of execution of a learned purposeful movement in the absence of motor dysfunction. It is characterized an inability to perform routine tasks, such as tying shoelaces or shaking hands. Apraxia occurs more often with right hemispheric involvement. When apraxia is severe, the prognosis usually is poor.[9,15]

Behavioral and psychological aberrations are common. These include hostility, resentment, depression, withdrawal, or emotional lability. The behavior often is a reflection of premorbid personality traits, and therefore, an understanding of premorbid states helps in coping with the difficult patient and establishing a functional prognosis from a psychological standpoint. Psychiatric consultation assists evaluation.

Extremity Sensibility

Sensibility is evaluated by touch, pinprick, two-point discrimination, monofilament testing, proprioception, testing for ability to discriminate size, shape, texture, or point localization, or the evaluation of astereognosis. Consultation and evaluation with occupational or physical therapists specialized in hand therapy is invaluable. Sensibility evaluation often is difficult in the stroke patient with cognitive deficits who is unable to cooperate fully.[17]

A common sensory aberration in the stroke patients is persistent extremity pain, often without an obvious cause. Extremity pain can be severe and can impede rehabilitation efforts. Pain of central origin (i.e., referred pain in the extremities originating in the brain) is characterized by head, arm, and leg pain on the affected side. Other causes of limb pain include reflex sympathetic dystrophy, pain from constant muscle tension or chronic joint position secondary to spasticity or contracture, pain from joint subluxation secondary to muscle imbalance, heterotopic ossification (rare in stroke), and peripheral neuropathy. The shoulder is often afflicted with additional inflammatory conditions such as subdeltoid bursitis and bicipital tendinitis. Flaccidity of the shoulder musculature can lead to painful subluxation of the shoulder and/or traction on the brachial plexus. Pain in an extremity should be evaluated with appropriate physical examination and standard roentgenograms. Specific testing for sympathetic nerve dysfunction is often indicated when reflex sympathetic dystrophy is suspected.

Heterotopic ossification, although rare in the stroke patient, may occur and can be further evaluated with determination of serum alkaline phosphatase levels and technetium bone scans.[18-27] Heterotopic ossification is discussed in Chapter 35.

Body neglect is the failure to recognize or use the involved side. It is evaluated by examination of the patient during standing or attempted ambulation.[16,28] Ambulation is difficult for patients who do not make accommodation for the weight of the unrecognized side. Patients often fail to look across their own midline toward the affected side, and tendency to lean or fall toward that side will be present. Self-drawings sketched by the patients will usually show omissions of extremities on the neglected side.

Visual impairment is best evaluated by appropriate consultation. These tests should be obtained early, because of the prognostic value of these examinations.

Motor Function

Motor evaluation includes assessment of muscle tone, presence of patterned reflexes or volitional control, presence of rigidity or clonus, degree of phasic activity and dexterity, motor strength, activity of stretch reflexes, and presence of fixed joint contractures. In the upper limb, specific testing is performed for selective control in grasp, release, and the ability to position the hand in space. Presence of body neglect (refusal to use the hand despite adequate motor strength) is noted. In the lower limb, the patient is specifically evaluated for presence of body neglect (falling toward the affected side), limb stability and strength for standing, and adequate balance.

An appreciation of the dynamic nature (i.e., changing with time) of motor impairment in stroke is required to understand and evaluate motor function appropriately. After the initial cerebrovascular insult, a transient period of flaccid paralysis or paresis usually occurs, with hypotonia and depression of stretch reflexes. This period of flaccidity or hypotonia, which lasts from several hours to several weeks, then gives way to a period of increasing muscle tone. Stretch reflexes return and there is a progression to hyperactive reflexes that culminates in spasticity. Characteristics of spasticity include increased muscle tone, hyperreflexia, and possible clonus or rigidity.[29-34] Weakness and loss of dexterity are often present concomitantly.[35] Muscle tone and hyperreflexia reach a peak within a few days or weeks. There then follows a long period of spontaneous neurology recovery during which spasticity improves and the muscles return to a more normal, less hypertonic state. Strength, coordination, volitional control, and sensory and cognitive function all improve. In the stroke patient, variable degrees of recovery usually occur over the first 6 months. At the end of this period, little

improvement in motor function, sensibility, or cognition usually occurs. Appreciation of this period of spontaneous neurologic recovery is important both from the standpoint of prognosis (for patient and family education) and for the timing of surgical limb reconstruction (because irreversible surgical procedures usually should be delayed until a patient has reached the end of this recovery period and is no longer making progress in a comprehensive therapy program).

Early in the period of spontaneous recovery, voluntary movement usually returns first in the most proximal muscle groups of the limbs and continues in a proximal-to-distal direction. Voluntary shoulder and hip motor function should be sought and assessed early in the recovery period, when flaccidity or hypotonia are present.

Two types of voluntary motion are evaluated as the patient recovers: pattern movement and selective movement. *Pattern movement,* usually the first to appear, consists of a mass flexor or extensor muscle contraction that is initiated voluntarily by the patient. (For example, mass lower extremity extensor muscle contraction, may be self-initiated by the patient's stroking the thigh. The hip extensors, the knee extensors, and the ankle plantar flexors may all contract simultaneously.) This phenomenon of pattern movement may be somewhat useful in the lower extremity, in which a voluntarily initiated mass contraction of the extensor muscles of the hip and knee can stabilize the lower extremity for support during wheelchair transfers. In the upper extremity, however, pattern movement is usually undesirable and prevents accurate hand positioning. *Selective movement* returns later and consists of precise control of individual muscles. Spastic patients often show coexistance of minimal selective movement in an extremity that has predominantly pattern movement.

Later in the period of spontaneous neurologic recovery, it becomes important to determine when this recovery has ceased and little further improvement of spasticity is likely. As recovery slows, it may be difficult to detect subtle improvements. Team evaluation, with quantitative methods for motor and sensory examinations, is necessary for assessment.

Use of Dynamic Electromyography in Muscle Evaluation

Muscle that contracts at the proper time during a sequence of limb movement is considered *phasic*. Muscle that contracts continuously or is inappropriately overactive is *spastic*. Muscle that shows no activity or minimal activity is *paralytic* (paralysis), or *paretic* (paresis), respectively. Dynamic electromyography (EMG) is helpful in the evaluation of the phasic activity of muscles and will demonstrate muscle that is phasic, spastic, paralytic, or paretic.[28,36-38] During dynamic EMG, electrical activity of the muscle is recorded as the patient performs a specific task (Fig. 29-2). Dynamic EMG is useful when muscle evaluation (during activity) of a deeply situated muscle is difficult to perform by palpation or by physical examination alone. Dynamic EMG is also especially useful in the determination of which specific muscles contribute to a deformity when multiple muscles are involved (such as in elbow flexion deformity and thumb-in-palm deformity).[17,36] When more than one muscle is involved, it often becomes difficult to distinguish which ones are causing the problem by physical examination alone.

Evaluation of Fixed Soft Tissue Contracture

If a spastic limb is not mobilized for a prolonged period, fixed soft tissue contractures (Fig. 29-3) occur. Molecular cross-bridging of the collagen (soft tissue protein) results in stiffness of the soft tissue that prevents the joint from moving. Soft tissues involved in the formation of a contracture can include ligaments, joint capsule, muscle-tendon units, neurovascular bundles, and skin. A soft tissue contracture will persist even after spasticity resolves. Thus, an important aspect of spasticity management is mobilization to prevent contractures.

Limb deformity caused by soft tissue contracture, as opposed to that caused by severe spasticity, can be evaluated with diagnostic motor nerve block to the involved muscles using 1 percent lidocaine hydrochloride. After the nerve block, deformity caused by spasticity will improve, because the nerve impulses causing the muscle to contract will be blocked. However, deformity caused by soft tissue contracture will not change, because the nerve block will have no effect on the fixed stiffness of the ligaments, joint capsule, or myotendinous units. Common sites for nerve blocks include the musculocutaneous nerve for elbow flexion deformity, median nerve in the proximal forearm for wrist and digital flexion, recurrent motor branch of the median nerve for thumb-in-palm deformity, femoral nerve for hip flexion, obturator nerve for hip adduction, and posterior tibial nerve at the level of the knee for equinovarus and toe flexion[1,5,16,33] (Fig. 29-4). These blocks are performed with the aid of an insulated needle with the tip exposed and the hub attached to a nerve stimulator (Fig. 29-5).[1,5,12] The nerve stimulator attached to the insulated needle will indicate proper needle tip position when the noninsulated tip of the needle is in the immediate vicinity of the motor nerve (as will be noted by muscle contractions), thus aiding in the accurate injection of the lidocaine hydrocloride (Fig. 29-5).

A joint held in a fixed position may also be stiff from the formation of neurogenic heterotopic ossification.[19-22,27] Standard roentgenograms usually demonstrate the presence of this abnormality, and technetium bone scans and serum alkaline phosphatase levels help evaluate its degree of activity. Heterotopic ossification is much less common in the stroke patient than in the patient with traumatic brain injury or spinal cord injury.

Potential for Ambulation

The potential of the hemiplegic patient to ambulate is evaluated by assessment of motor function, balance, and joint stability. Requirements for ambulation in the adult with acquired hemiplegia include (1) voluntary hip flexion, (2) adequate standing balance, and (3) limb stability.[1,28,38-41] Active hip flexion to 30° is usually required for limb advancement.[16,28] Occasionally, adductors can substitute for weak hip flexors to assist limb advancement[28] (an important consideration prior to the release of the adductor muscles for adduction deformity).

Adequate balance for sitting and independent standing are prerequisites for ambulation. Patients often lean to the unaffected side to support the body with a cane held in the unaffected hand. Because of upper extremity involvement in hemiplegia, a walker usually is not feasible. The double-limb support standing

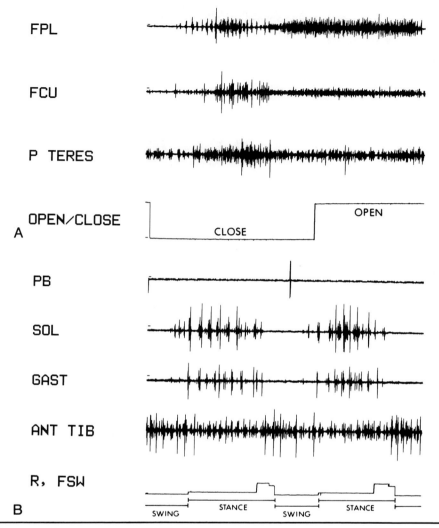

Fig. 29-2. Dynamic electromyograms (EMG) demonstrating continuous (spastic) muscle activity. The patient had spastic hemiplegia. Selected muscles of the upper extremity **(A)** and of the lower extremity **(B)** were evaluated. Muscles tested in the upper extremity **(A)** included the flexor pollicis longus (FPL), the flexor carpi ulnaris (FCU), and the pronator teres (P TERES). The patient attempted to open and close the fist (noted as "open" and "close"). Continuous activity of the muscles is noted on the tracing, indicating spasticity. The FPL should show no activity when the fist is open, because it should relax to allow extension of the thumb. The patient's clinical deformity included a spastic pronated forearm, flexed wrist, and thumb-in-palm deformity. Muscles tested in the lower extremity **(B)** include the peroneus brevis (PB), the soleus (SOL), the gastrocnemius (GAST), and the tibilis anterior (ANT TIB). The phase of gait (i.e., stance or swing phase) is demonstrated from data obtained from a foot switch located inside the shoe (R, FSW = right foot switch). Note the minimal (paretic) activity of the PB and the continuous activity of the ANT TIB. The patient's clinical deformity included equinovarus deformity of the foot. The varus component was secondary to overactivity of the TIB ANT and concomitant weakness of the PB.

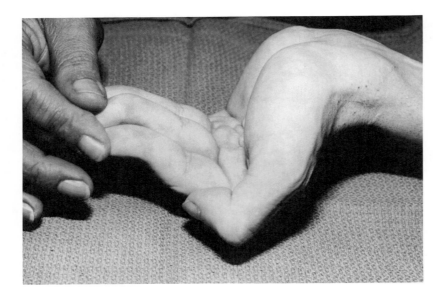

Fig. 29-3. Fixed flexion contracture of the metacarpophalangeal joints of the digits and of the interphalangeal joint of the thumb. These contractures developed from spasticity that was neglected and failure to mobilize the limb. (From Botte MJ et al,[29] with permission.)

test popularized by Perry assesses balance by noting alignment of the trunk and the amount of spontaneous support given by the hemiplegic limb as the patient stands with the aid of a cane.[16,28] Even with profound hemiparesis, a patient should be able to stand by shifting the body weight over to the unaffected side. Falling toward the hemiparetic side suggests body neglect rather than limb disability.[16,28,38,41]

The third requirement for ambulation is limb stability. The hip, knee, and ankle must be stable enough to support body weight during the stance phase. Single-limb stance on the hemiparetic limb is tested. Forward lean of the trunk implies weakness of the hip extensors. Flexion of the knee with ankle dorsiflexion may indicate soleus weakness. Stance with the knee flexed demonstrates adequate quadriceps strength, because the quadriceps muscle is able to support the body weight on the flexed knee. Hyperextension of the knee may indicate weakness of the quadriceps or soleus, or it may be secondary to an ankle plantar flexion contracture. Extensor patterning can aid in stance stability, often useful for wheelchair transfers in the nonambulator.

Evaluation for Peripheral Neuropathy

Peripheral neuropathy can occur in the stroke patient secondary to prolonged limb positioning or posturing. Ulnar neuropathy at the elbow can develop from chronic spastic elbow flexion. The elbow flexion may cause prolonged traction on the ulnar nerve (which passes posterior to the axis of the elbow joint). In addition, ulnar neuropathy at the elbow can be caused by chronic pressure on the nerve if the elbow continually rests on the wheelchair armrest.[34,42,43]

Median neuropathy at the wrist (carpal tunnel syndrome) can occur from chronic spastic wrist flexion. Flexion of the wrist can either contribute to increased pressure within the tunnel or cause compression or ischemia of the contents of the carpal tunnel.

Peripheral neuropathy may be difficult to detect in the stroke patient, because symptoms may be minimal (especially if overlying cognitive, sensory, and motor deficits are present). A patient with intrinsic minus deformity (hyperextension at the metacarpophalangeal joints and flexion at the proximal interphalangeal joints—i.e., claw hand) with concomitant intrinsic muscle wasting needs careful motor and sensory evaluation (if cognition and cooperation will allow testing) and tests of nerve conduction velocity and EMGs to rule out ulnar neuropathy. Likewise, a patient with wrist flexion patterning or contracture and thenar muscle atrophy should undergo evaluation for median neuropathy.

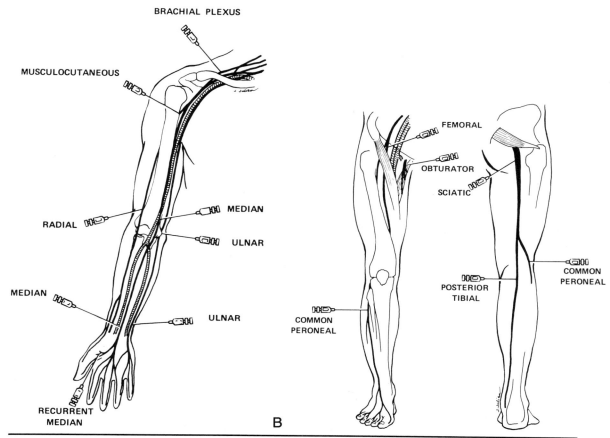

Fig. 29-4. Peripheral nerves commonly blocked to determine whether a deformity is caused by spasticity or by a fixed myostatic or ligamentous contracture. **(A)** Upper extremity; **(B)** lower extremity. One percent lidocaine hydrochloride without epinephrine is injected with the guidance of an insulated needle attached to a nerve stimulator. Deformity caused by spasticity usually will improve after nerve block; deformity caused by fixed contracture will not. Nerves that carry predominantly motor fibers, such as the recurrent motor branch of the median nerve, musculocutaneous nerve, and obturator nerve, can be blocked with phenol, 5 percent aqueous, in a similar closed manner. Blocks with phenol usually last from 6 to 12 weeks. (From Keenan MAE,[33] with permission.)

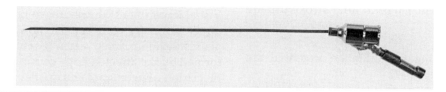

Fig. 29-5. Insulated needle to assist accurate needle positioning and lidocaine infiltration for nerve blocks. The shaft of the needle is coated with Teflon, but the tip is exposed. The hub is connected to a nerve stimulator and the needle is advanced toward the nerve. When the uninsulated exposed tip of the needle is in the immediate vicinity of the nerve, the corresponding innervated muscles will contract from nerve stimulation. Accurate placement of the needle tip adjacent to the nerve is thus assisted.

POTENTIAL FOR STROKE REHABILITATION

Triage in Rehabilitation

A patient's functional potential must be assessed prior to initiating treatment, to strategically select those who will likely make the best rehabilitation candidates and to identify those who would be poor candidates. Because rehabilitation resources usually are limited, they are not optimally spent on attempts at rehabilitation of patients who are not proper candidates. Once a patient is identified as a suitable candidate for rehabilitation, the potential benefits, goals, patient placement, and a family teaching program should be defined by the rehabilitation team *before* therapy begins.

Prognosis for Rehabilitation

Certain specific deficits usually indicate a patient's poor likelihood to benefit from a comprehensive rehabilitation program. These include severe cognitive impairment, receptive aphasia, severe visual impairment (especially in perception), body neglect, prolonged flaccidity (longer than 6 weeks), and rigidity from bilateral cortical involvement. In the upper extremity, loss of sensibility indicates a poor chance for hand rehabilitation.[9,16]

Significant medical problems are also poor prognostic signs for rehabilitation. Poor activity tolerance from cardiopulmonary or metabolic causes or obesity will inhibit successful rehabilitation.

Bowel and bladder incontinence, although not contraindications for rehabilitation, tend to prevent satisfactory home placement. Few bowel-incontinent patients are able to return home. Incontinence present for more than 1 month after stroke usually does not improve.

The factors inhibiting rehabilitation potential are summarized in Table 29-2.

Upper Extremity Functional Potential

Prognosis for recovery of normal upper limb function in the adult with acquired hemiplegia generally is poor. Only two-thirds of stroke patients recover

Table 29-2. Inhibitors of Rehabilitation Potential

Severe inhibitors
  Severely impaired cognition and learning ability
  Decreased activity tolerance secondary to severe medical problems
Relative inhibitors
  Bilateral cerebral damage
  Obesity
  Contralateral extremity problems
  Body neglect
  Impaired balance
  Marked sensory impairment
  Prolonged flaccidity
  Placement in a nursing home

enough partial use of the limb for it to function as an assist to the normal side, and nearly one-third will have a permanently nonfunctional limb.[1,44] This poor outlook is due to the complex nature of upper limb function and to the greater dependence of the upper limbs on normal sensibility and perceptual function.

The requirements for satisfactory upper extremity function include proximal joint stability, adequate motor function and coordination to place the hand in space, ability to grasp and release, intact sensibility, and adequate cognition to recall and carry out learned actions.

Loss or severe impairment of sensibility has a devastating effect on hand function. Loss of proprioception and two-point discrimination will usually prevent spontaneous hand use, despite intact pain and touch sensibility and adequate motor ability.

Body neglect and apraxia are poor indicators for recovery of upper extremity function. Patients cannot remember to use the extremity unless given constant verbal cues.

Visual impairment contributes to poor prognosis for upper extremity recovery. Homonymous hemianopia results in impaired visual feedback for tasks performed by the affected limb, causing difficulty in appreciation of geometric and spatial relationships.

Lower Extremity Functional Potential

Body neglect causes problems with ambulation and also carries a poor prognosis. Loss of proprioception at the hip or knee may prevent ambulation. Poor balance will often prohibit safe ambulation. After a stroke, 20 to 30 percent of patients will regain normal ambulation, and 75 percent will return to some level of ambulation.[38,41]

PRINCIPLES AND METHODS OF MANAGEMENT

Among the most common and challenging extremity problems in the stroke patient are spasticity, contracture, and extremity pain, and the loss of function that is associated with these problems.[1,7–10,12,13,15,16,18,20,28,30,32–35,37,41,45]

Throughout the period of spontaneous neurologic recovery, efforts are directed toward maintaining joint motion to prevent fixed soft tissue contractures. Severe spasticity and contractures interfere with function, passive positioning, hygiene, dressing, balance, and comfort; in addition, they can lead to secondary problems of decubitus ulcers and peripheral neuropathy.[42,43] Treatment of contractures is by prevention through mobilization of joints of the spastic limb. *A joint moved once a day through its full range of motion should not develop a contracture.* Once a contracture is allowed to form, however, its management is time consuming, is uncomfortable to the patient, exhausts considerable rehabilitation resources, and may require operative procedures. Prevention of contractures is achieved through limb mobilization using passive stretching, static splinting or serial casting to reach or maintain corrective positions, strengthening of weak antagonistic muscles, and medication to aid spastic muscle relaxation. Adjunctive therapy includes electrical muscle stimulation of antagonist muscles (which assists limb mobilization and may strengthen the antagonists), serial lidocaine motor nerve blocks (to help temporarily relieve spasticity and allow mobilization), and open or closed phenol motor nerve injections (for longer lasting but temporary relief of muscle spasticity).[9,15,33,34,46–52]

Once a fixed contracture develops from refractory or neglected spasticity, manual joint mobilization and serial casting are utilized to stretch the soft tissues and allow joint motion. When these nonsurgical efforts are not successful in the prevention or resolution of contractures and the patient is beyond the period of neurologic recovery, surgical release or lengthening is usually indicated.[12,13,53–68]

Mobilization and Splinting

Mobilization is the pine qua non for prevention of soft tissue contractures. A joint that is passively mobilized through a full range of motion daily cannot develop a fixed soft tissue deformity. Between therapy sessions, joints are maintained in proper position with well-padded bivalved casts, splints, or static orthoses. Splints decrease muscle tone by decreasing motion, which lessens stimulation to the stretch reflex to decrease spasticity. Dynamic splints (i.e., those employing constant force through spring-loaded or elastic devices) or traction devices are avoided in the spastic limb because the continuous stretch may provide stimulation that increases spasticity or perpetuates clonus. (Serial casting, however, with constant but gentle stretch usually is tolerated satisfactorily without causing clonus. Serial casting is discussed later.)

Lidocaine Nerve Blocks

Local anesthetic nerve blocks are used either therapeutically, to eliminate spasticity temporarily prior to mobilization or serial casting, or diagnostically, to differentiate joint deformity caused by true soft tissue contracture versus that caused by spasticity. Lidocaine hydrochloride, 1 percent, without epinephrine is placed accurately with the aid of a nerve stimulator attached to the hypodermic needle during injection (Figs. 29-4 and 29-5). Serial nerve blocks have been found helpful to decrease spasticity or unwanted patterned contractions permanently.[7,33]

Phenol Nerve Blocks

Motor nerve blocks using phenol provide muscle relaxation for up to 6 months. Nerve injection of a 3 to 5 percent solution mixed in glycerine (for open direct nerve injection)[52] or 5 percent aqueous (for percutaneous injection) denatures the protein in the peripheral nerve, causing axonal degeneration that leads to a chemical axonotmesis. Because the continuity of the nerve sheath is not disrupted, the axons subsequently regenerate and recovery occurs. The duration of the block depends on the time required for axon regeneration.[46–49,51]

Phenol blocks for spasticity are optimally given during the period of neurologic recovery (within 6 months from stroke episode). Because of the relatively short period of recovery in the stroke patient, phenol blocks are given much less frequently than in the patient with traumatic brain injury or spinal cord injury, for which the recovery period is much longer). Thus, phenol nerve blocks are discussed in more detail in Chapter 30. In the stroke patient who is beyond the period of spontaneous recovery and in whom spasticity continues to be a problem, definitive measures such as surgical lengthening or recession are usually considered.

The use of multiple undirected intramuscular phenol blocks to weaken spastic muscles is not advised. Intrathecal phenol blocks also are avoided in the management of these patients, because the intrathecal injection may cause a lower motor nerve lesion, resulting in motor paralysis. The consequent gluteal atrophy can lead to decubitus ulcers. In addition, a spastic but continent bowel and bladder may be converted a flaccid, incontinent bowel and bladder (from the lower motoneuron lesion), resulting in obvious additional problems of hygiene and patient care.[1]

A preparation containing botulinum toxin injected intramuscularly is currently under investigation and shows promise in the management of spasticity.

Oral Muscle Relaxants

Oral antispasmotic medications such as baclofen and dantrolene may help decrease spasticity and provide a valuable adjunct to passive joint mobilization. Diazepam has potent muscle relaxant properties; however, side effects of lethargy and somnolence and the potential addictiveness may make its use less optimal in many patients.

Electrical Stimulation

Electrical stimulation of the weak antagonist muscle to the spastic muscles assists in mobilization of the joints, helps maintain antagonist strength, may inhibit the spastic agonist, and, when strategically timed or controlled, (functional electrical stimulation) can improve limb function.[16,34,38,44,69] Sensorimotor reeducation may be accelerated by increasing the patient's awareness of the sensations of contraction of these weak antagonists.

Serial Casting

Once a soft tissue contracture has formed, serial casting can be an effective means of treatment by slowly stretching soft tissue. The limb is placed in the position of maximum correction and a well-padded cast is applied. Each week, the cast is removed, the patient undergoes passive limb mobilization, and a new cast is applied with any additional correction as needed. Over a 6- to 8-week period, many contractures can be improved significantly. A lidocaine nerve block to the involved spastic muscles prior to cast application may assist in gaining maximal correction. Because patients may have common sensory and cognitive deficits, the casts must be well padded and the skin checked routinely.[1,7,9,12,13,15,28,34,36,39,44,56]

PRINCIPLES OF SURGICAL RECONSTRUCTION

Common limb deformities of the upper extremity in the hemiplegic adult include internal rotation and adduction of the shoulder, flexion of the elbow, pronation of the forearm, flexion of the wrist and digits, and thumb-in-palm deformity (Fig. 29-6).[1,5,7,9,13,16,32,33,44,55,59] Common deformities of the lower extremity include flexion-adduction of the hip, flexion of the knee, equinovarus of the ankle and hindfoot, and flexion of the toes (Fig. 29-7).[7,9,15,28,30,37,70] These deformities are usually a result of overactivity of the spastic flexor-adductor muscle groups combined with relative weakness of the opposing extensor-abductor groups. Limb deformity causes obvious functional deficits, which impair or obliterate volitional control of the limb. Problems with hygiene and skin maceration can arise between the toes and in the axilla, antecubital region, palm of the hand, groin, and popliteal fossa (Fig. 29-8). The skin is at risk for decubitus ulcers at the elbow, as the olecranon of the flexed elbow presses against the bed sheets or wheelchair armrest. The skin in the palm of the hand is liable to break down with a clenched-fist deformity, in which the fingernails may dig into the skin. Over the lateral hip, pressure from the greater trochanter is accentuated with hip flexion deformity,

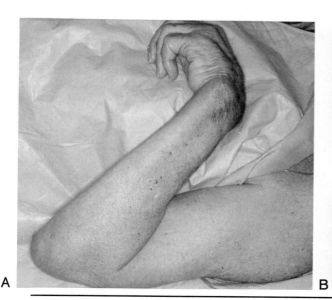 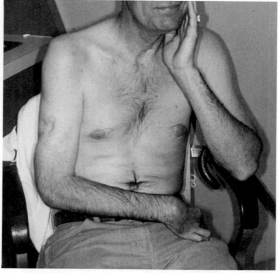

A B

Fig. 29-6. (A & B) Photographs of upper extremities of patients with hemiplegia secondary to stroke. Common upper limb deformity includes internal rotation and adduction of the shoulder, flexion of the elbow, pronation of the forearm, flexion of the wrist and digits, and a thumb-in-palm deformity.

placing the hip and gluteal region at risk. Flexion of the knee may result in pressure against the heels. Positioning and dressing the patient are difficult. Pain often accompanies these deformities, both from the continuous muscle activity and from passive stretch against soft tissue contractures when a limb is used to lift or position these patients.[9,14,33]

Operative management of a spastic limb deformity in the adult with acquired spasticity is indicated when there are correctable deformities that interfere with function, hygiene, or dressing, which have not responded to a comprehensive therapy program. If a patient is still in the recovery period, during which spontaneous improvement still can be expected, open or closed phenol blocks can be considered. If a patient is beyond the recovery period and no further spontaneous limb recovery is expected, operative correction with tendon lengthening, muscles recession, or release is indicated. Reconstructive surgery should not, in general, be performed on patients who are still in the recovery phase or who continue to show improvement in a therapy program.[1,7,13] Occasionally, a patient will develop troublesome refractory fixed myostatic contractures prior to the end of

spontaneous recovery; surgical release can be considered in these patients. Disfigurement alone usually is not an indication for surgical intervention; function, hygiene, positioning, or other aspects of patient care must be impaired as well.

Goals of surgery include prevention of decubitus ulcers and improvement of function, hygiene, positioning, and dressing.[9,13,31,41,44,55] Pain can often also be relieved with the relaxation of spastic muscles by phenol injection, lengthening, or release.[55] Phenol injections are used as a temporizing procedure to augment conventional therapy.

The operative procedures are selected depending on the deformity present and the specific goals intended (functional improvement or facilitation of hygiene). To preserve or improve function and correct deformity, lengthening or recession of the involved muscle or tendon is performed. (Recession of a muscle involves release of its origin while preserving the motor innervation. The limb position is corrected, and the muscle origin is allowed to slide distally to heal and reattach at a new site.)

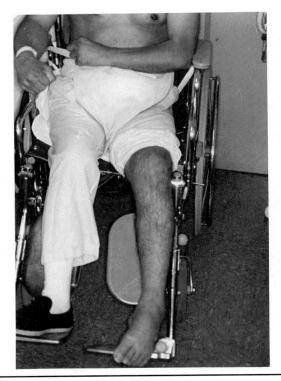

Fig. 29-7. Photograph of relatively young stroke patient with hemiplegia. Lower extremity deformity includes hip and knee flexion and equinovarus deformity of the foot.

If the limb is functionless and the goals of treatment are to facilitate hygiene or help correct positioning problems, release of the involved muscle, tendon, or joint capsule can be performed. Additionally, muscle or tendon lengthening can be considered in these patients to prevent overcorrection, which may occur after complete muscle release.

Upper Extremity

Shoulder

The most common deformity of the shoulder is internal rotation and adduction (Fig. 29-6). The muscles usually responsible for this deformity are the pectoralis major, subscapularis, latissimus dorsi, and teres major. Depending on the activity of the deltoids and patterning of the extremity, abduction of the shoulder may occur. Subluxation of the shoulder rarely occurs as a result of flaccid masculature. To deter-

mine which muscles contribute to the deformity, the arm is abducted and rotated externally. All shoulder muscles but the subscapularis are palpable clinically. If the humerus resists external rotation with the arm at the side, the subscapularis muscle is usually spastic as well.[44] Dynamic EMG also is helpful in distinguishing which muscles are spastic. Spasticity is initially treated with an aggressive mobilization program. Phenol nerve block to the pectoralis major muscle is useful to decrease muscle tone if the patient is within the period of spontaneous neurologic recovery.[46] Although this type of closed phenol block addresses only one of the four muscles possibly responsible for the adduction and internal rotation deformity, it may still significantly improve shoulder mobilization. The pectoralis motor block can be repeated in 2 months as necessary.

If spasticity persists and myostatic contracture of the shoulder develops, hygiene problems in the axilla and difficulty in patient dressing arise. Chronic shoulder pain is common. In these patients, especially in those who are beyond the period of expected spontaneous recovery, surgical release can be considered. The insertions of the pectoralis major and subscapularis are released, as described by Braun and colleagues.[55] If deformity persists from remaining myostatic contracture of the latissimus dorsi and teres major muscles, these muscles are subsequently released as described by Waters and others.[5,8,34,44] An aggressive mobilization program is reinstituted as soon as wound healing and patient comfort permit.

Subluxation of the shoulder occurs rarely and is caused by persistent flaccid musculature. The entire limb is usually functionless because motor function return occurs in a proximal-to-distal direction. The subluxation leads to pain and possible secondary bursitis or tendinitis, resulting in further decreased range of motion. Management includes mobilization, anti-inflammatory medication, and shoulder support by a sling. There is no reliable operative procedure to treat the flaccid shoulder with subluxation. Tendinitis or bursitis may respond to steroid and lidocaine hydrochloride injection.

Elbow

The most common deformity of the elbow is flexion deformity, usually associated with forearm pronation (Fig. 29-6). Flexion posturing is caused by spasticity

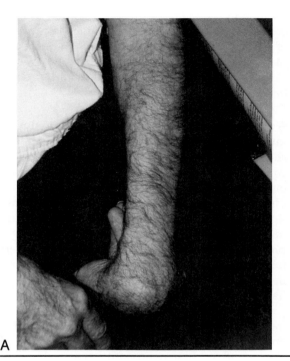

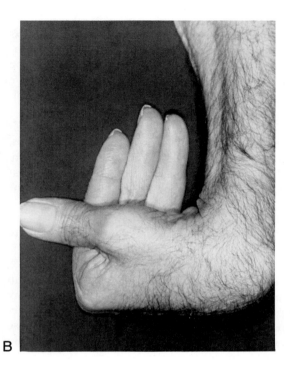

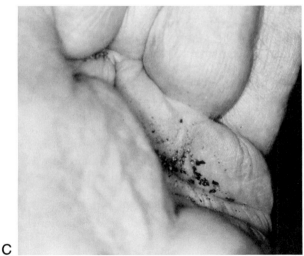

Fig. 29-8. (A & B) Photographs of the hand of a stroke patient with severe wrist and digit flexion deformity. **(C)** Hygiene problem in the palm that developed as a result of the spasticity causing chronic digital and wrist flexion. Note skin maceration, debris, and breakdown within palm.

of the biceps, brachialis, and brachioradialis muscles. Forearm pronation (discussed later) is usually due to spasticity of the pronator teres muscle. Functional difficulty, inadequate hygiene in the antecubital fossa, risk of decubitus ulcers over the olecranon, and problems with positioning and dressing arise. The patient is also at risk for ulnar neuropathy at the elbow from chronic elbow flexion. Initial manage-

ment consists of passive mobilization, splinting, and oral muscle relaxants. If a patient is within the period of neurologic recovery, a phenol nerve block can be given to the musculocutaneous nerve or motor branches to the brachioradialis muscle.[34,47]

Closed phenol blocks usually afford less than 2 months of muscle relaxation. These procedure can be repeated once as needed. Alternatively, an open phenol block (in which the nerve is surgically exposed) can be given. An open block will ensure accurate instillation of the phenol and usually gives a more complete block that lasts longer (up to 6 months). Open blocks can be used primarily or chosen if a closed block proves inadequate.

If fixed myostatic contracture of the elbow develops, serial casting may be successful in regaining motion. Fixed contracture is differentiated from severe spasticity with lidocaine block to the musculocutaneous nerve. When a patient is beyond the recovery phase, definitive procedures such as lengthening release of the elbow flexors or musculocutaneous neurectomy are performed.

In the spastic, nonfunctional elbow with less than 90° of deformity, a musculocutaneous neurectomy can performed.[9,32,34,44,71] Garland and colleagues recommended concomitant elbow flexor release in those with deformity of 75° or more.[71] Residual deformity is corrected by dropout or serial casting. If the brachioradialis muscle has volitional control or spasticity, this radial nerve–innervated muscle will preserve some elbow flexion and prevent a flail or hyperextended (overcorrected) elbow.

In a nonfunctional elbow with a greater than 75° to 90° of contracture, a surgical release is performed as described by Garland and associates[71] and by Waters.[44] Release of the biceps, brachialis, and brachioradialis muscles is usually required. Capsular release usually is unnecessary. Approximately 40° of correction may be obtained. Further elbow extension is usually limited by contracture of the neurovascular structures. Thus, although residual flexion may exist after surgical release of elbow flexors, hygiene and patient care are facilitated.

In the patient with a functional elbow and hand, selective release or lengthening of only the responsible or most involved spastic or contracted elbow flexors is indicated. Preoperative dynamic EMG may identify specific flexors that are most responsible for the deformity. Motor neurectomy, surgical release, or lengthening is restricted to this muscle (or muscles). Preoperative lidocaine nerve block to the musculocutaneous nerve or the radial nerve will enable the surgeon to evaluate the effects of deletion of tone in corresponding muscles prior to surgery. If spasticity of the brachioradialis is found to be selectively at fault for the deformity or impairs active elbow extension, motor neurectomy restricted to this muscle can be performed.[50]

A patient with chronic elbow flexion who develops intrinsic minus (claw hand) deformity of the hand should be suspected of having ulnar neuropathy. The continuous elbow flexion can place chronic tension on the ulnar nerve, thus producing neuropathy. The ulnar nerve supplies motor innervation to the intrinsic muscles of the hand, which provide flexion at the metacarpophalangeal joints and extension at the proximal interphalangeal joints. Loss of this innervation from ulnar neuropathy will result in muscle imbalance, producing intrinsic minus deformity, typified by extension of the metacarpophalangeal joints and flexion at the proximal interphalangeal joints. Patient evaluation includes motor and sensibility examination, nerve conduction velocities, and EMG. Treatment of ulnar neuropathy at the elbow from flexion deformity includes surgical correction of the elbow flexion and anterior transposition of the ulnar nerve.

Forearm and Hand

Deformities of the wrist and hand usually consist of wrist and digital flexion resulting from spasticity of forearm flexors and the intrinsic muscles of the hand (Figs. 29-6 and 29-8). A tightly clenched fist, with the wrist in flexion and a thumb-in-palm deformity is common. This deformity results in loss of selective grasp and release and often causes hygiene problems. Skin breakdown may result from fingernails pressing into the palm. When myostatic contractures are present, attempts to open the hand are painful for the patient.

The wrist flexors commonly develop severe spasticity (Fig. 29-6). Selective finger control may exist despite wrist flexor spasticity. However, grasp will be weak if the wrist is flexed, because the finger flexors will not be at optimum resting length. Although orthoses should be used initially to prevent wrist contractures, they usually interfere with hand function and are cumbersome for long-term use.

In a patient who is within the period of neurologic recovery, a closed phenol block to the motor branches of the wrist and digital flexors can be effective in alleviating flexion deformity. This is performed with a nerve stimulator to accurately place an insulated needle prior to phenol injection. A mean correction of 25° in wrist resting angle for a duration of up to 2 months has been achieved; the technique has been described in detail by Garland and colleagues.[71]

Although there have been no serious complications reported with closed phenol blocks of the forearm, an open phenol block to the motor branches of the median nerve will minimize the theoretical risk of injury to the neighboring brachial, ulnar, and radial arteries, especially when multiple injections are given. Besides the theoretical advantage of safety, open blocks to these motor branches provide a more complete and longer lasting effect. The obvious disadvantage of the open block is the operative nerve exposure and requirement for anesthesia.

Indications for operative release or lengthening in cases of wrist flexor deformity include refractory flexion that interferes with function, hygiene, or dressing in a patient whose spasticity is no longer improving or who has a fixed myostatic contracture. Complete release of the wrist flexors may be considered if digital flexors are intact and can substitute for wrist flexion. A complete release of both wrist and digital flexors should be avoided because this may unmask occult extensor spasticity and result in an overcorrection deformity.

Prior to lengthening or release of wrist flexor tendons, it is desirable to determine whether extrinsic myostatic shortening of the digital flexors will prevent digital extension once the wrist flexion deformity is corrected. Preoperatively, the wrist is held manually in a corrected position while the digits are evaluated simultaneously for adequate active and passive extension. If the digital flexors are contracted as well, lengthening of these muscles at the time of wrist flexor lengthening should be considered.

Identification of specific flexors that contribute to deformity is assessed with palpation of each muscle during attempted wrist and digital extension. Lido-

caine nerve block to the ulnar nerve at the cubital tunnel will eliminate contribution of the flexor carpi ulnaris muscle. If adequate wrist extension occurs after ulnar nerve block, only the flexor carpi ulnaris may need to be addressed operatively. Dynamic EMGs of both the wrist and digital flexors also will help elucidate which muscles are contributing to the wrist flexion.

It has usually not been necessary or advisable to transfer the wrist flexor tendons to the wrist extensors in stroke patients. The degree of spasticity, limited excursion, and pattern of muscular activity are too variable to ensure predictable results. Fortunately, as noted by Waters, most patients with selective finger extension have sufficient strength to extend the wrist after wrist flexor lengthening.[44]

Spasticity of the extrinsic digital flexors (flexor digitorum superficialis and flexor digitorum profundus) that interferes with function or hygiene can be treated operatively. Surgery should only be done when spasticity is no longer improving. Identification of contributing muscles is made by physical examination and dynamic electromyograms. Procedures used to treat spastic extrinsic digital flexors include closed or open phenol block to the forearm flexor muscles (as described earlier), the flexor pronator slide procedure, fractional lengthening, and superficialis-to-profundus transfer.

The flexor pronator slide procedure, as described by Page,[62] and popularized by Braun and colleagues[54] and by Ingles and Cooper[57] is performed by release of the origin of the flexor-pronator muscles mass in the forearm, allowing the muscle bellies to slide distally and reattach by healing in a new, distal position. By allowing these muscles to slide distally, wrist and digital flexion deformity are alleviated. This also helps correct pronation deformity of the forearm caused by the pronator teres muscle.[54,57,62] Advantages of this procedure are the amount of correction it can provide (up to 4 to 5 cm), the possible correction of pronation, and preservation of function. Disadvantages include the possible supination deformity created when the pronator muscle is released (overcorrection) and the resulting weakness soemtimes encountered after origin release.

Because of the disadvantages of the flexor-pronator slide procedure, fractional lengthening (for the functional extremity) or superficialis-to-profundus transfer (for the nonfunctional extremity) have become popular.[5,55,59,60,72] In performing fractional lengthening, some residual finger flexion should be left to avoid overlengthening and grip strength loss. Excursion does not usually improve. Z-lengthening can be done if only one or two fingers are involved; Z-lengthening of multiple tendons in the forearm is not desirable because of adhesion formation. Digital flexor lengthening in the forearm is usually combined with wrist flexor lengthening or release.

In the nonfunctional spastic or contracted, clenched fist, which is associated with hygiene problems, the superficialis-to-profundus transfer usually achieves adequate correction.[56,59,72] This transfer provides a large amount of extrinsic digital flexor lengthening while restricting finger hyperextension and preventing possible overcorrection. The procedure works well with the tightly clenched fist deformity, in which adequate correction is not obtainable with fractional or Z-lengthening. The procedure does not usually improve function, especially if performed on a nonfunctional hand.

Spasticity or contracture of the intrinsic muscles (i.e., lumbricalis and interosseous muscles) of the hand often exists concomitantly with extrinsic finger flexor deformity. The spasticity or contracture, however, may not be apparent because of the overwhelming extrinsic muscle deformity that masks the intrinsic muscle tightness (because the hand is pulled into a clenched fist deformity). Spasticity or myostatic contracture of the interosseous and lumbricalis muscles is addressed at the time of extrinsic flexor phenol block, lengthening, or transfer. In the patient who is within the period of spontaneous neurologic recovery and who has noxious intrinsic spasticity or spasticity unmasked after phenol block to the extrinsic flexors, phenol block to the deep (motor) branch of the ulnar nerve will alleviate spasticity of the interosseous muscles and of the two ulnar lumbricales. If the patient is beyond the recovery period, a more definitive procedure is indicated (such as neurectomy or lengthening of the intrinsic muscles, depending on functional status). A closed phenol block to the motor branch of the ulnar nerve is not advised because of

risk of phenol injury to the neighboring ulnar artery or superficial (sensory) branch of the ulnar nerve. In a nonfunctional hand in the patient who is beyond the period of neurologic recovery, extrinsic release of the flexor muscles should be followed by the intrinsic muscle tightness test as described by Smith.[65] This is accomplished by passively extending the metacarpophalangeal (MCP) joints and testing for tightness during passive flexion at the proximal interphalangeal (PIP) joints (after first confirming adequate passive PIP joint motion with the MCP joints flexed.)[65] If the intrinsic muscles of the hand are tight, the PIP joints will not easily flex passively. If tightness of the intrinsic muscles is not addressed, an intrinsic plus deformity (flexion at the MCP joints with extension at the PIP joints) will usually occur postoperatively. Tightness of the intrinsic muscles can be addressed with either motor neurectomy or muscle release or lengthening.

In the nonfunctional hand with intrinsic muscle tightness, neurectomy of the deep (motor) branch of the ulnar nerve is performed at the time of extrinsic flexor lengthening. Hygiene and cosmetic appearance will be improved. Concomitant adductor pollicis spasticity will be relieved as well. Neurectomy, however, only addresses spasticity, and is less optimal if fixed myostatic contracture exists.

Fixed myostatic contracture of the intrinsic muscles is treated with surgical release or lengthening. Lengthening is performed at the lateral bands of the extensor hood mechanism at the level of the proximal phalanx. A release of the intrinsic muscles may be performed either through the tendinous portion at the level of the MCP joints or at their origin from the metacarpal shafts.[65,73]

Thumb-in-Palm Deformity

Spasticity of the thumb extrinsic flexors and intrinsic muscles (thenar muscles) often leads to thumb adduction and flexion, resulting in the thumb-in-palm deformity. Muscles that can contribute to this deformity include the flexor pollicis longus, flexor pollicis brevis, abductor pollicis brevis, opponens pollicis, adductor pollicis, and first dorsal interosseous muscles. The first four of these are innervated by the median nerve and the last two by the ulnar nerve. In the stroke patient, any or all of these muscles can be spastic or can develop myostatic contractures, resulting in varying degrees of deformity. When the thumb is pulled into the palm, its function as an opposing force is obliterated. Hand grasp and pinch are severely impaired. Hygiene problems in the thenar crease arise. The thumb-in-palm deformity often coexists with a clenched fist deformity, thus compounding functional deficits and hygiene problems.

Initial management includes passive mobilization and splinting. However, the adducted, flexed thumb is difficult to splint into a corrected position. Joint instability and hyperextension at the MCP joint may result from attempts to abduct and extend the thumb when the metacarpal is tightly adducted.[5]

Surgical treatment must be planned carefully because of the many muscles that can be involved and their variable degree of contribution. Preoperative evaluation includes physical examination, diagnostic lidocaine nerve blocks, and dynamic EMGs. A deformity resulting from spasticity of the thenar muscles is exemplified by flexion at the thumb MCP joint with a supple, or extended, interphalangeal joint. A deformity resulting from spasticity of the flexor pollicis longus muscle is evident by predominant flexion at the interphalangeal joint with variable flexion at the MCP joint. Involvement of the adductor pollicis muscle causes flexion at the MCP joint and adduction of the metacarpal bone toward the midpalm. Involvement of the first dorsal interosseous or the opponens pollicis muscle is evident by an adducted position of the metacarpal in the plane of the palm, resulting in tightness of the thumb web space.[5,17]

The specific muscles responsible cannot always be identified easily by physical examination alone, especially when multiple muscles are involved. Sequential diagnostic lidocaine nerve blocks to the median and ulnar nerves at the wrist will help differentiate the contributions from the intrinsic muscles innervated by the median and ulnar nerves. Additional lidocaine block to the median nerve proximal to the elbow will establish involvement of the flexor pollicis longus muscle. Fixed contracture (as opposed to spasticity) of the myotendinous units or joints capsule can be identified by persisting deformity following nerve blocks. Dynamic EMG is used to further identify or confirm involvement of specific muscles.

In the patient within the recovery period of spasticity who has a deformity caused by the thenar muscles, a closed phenol injection can be given to the recurrent motor branch of the median nerve.[49] Definitive surgical procedures, directed only toward those muscles contributing to the deformity, are performed in the patient who is beyond the period of spontaneous recovery.

When the flexor pollicis brevis, abductor pollicis brevis, and opponens pollicis are involved, recession of their origin is performed (thenar origin recession). If needed, the adductor pollicis muscle is released at this time. This procedure allows the muscles to reattach with the thumb in a corrected position. Function is preserved and overcorrection avoided.[17] Release of the origin of the adductor pollicis has the advantage of preserving function (since the muscle will reattach as it heals). Release at the insertion, although technically easier, will obliterate the muscle's function.

When fixed flexion deformity exist at the interphalangeal joint of the thumb, arthrodesis provides a satisfactory means of correction. It is also useful if joint instability is present. If secondary web space contracture has developed, the web space is surgically deepened with a two- or four-quadrant Z-plasty.

In patients with a combination of upper extremity deformities, multiple procedures can be performed at the same time.

Lower Extremity

Hip

The major problems associated with the hip in the stroke patient are adductor and flexor spasticity and their associated myostatic contractures. Muscles that contribute to hip flexion are the rectus femoris, the iliopsoas, the tensor fascia lata, and the sartorius. Muscles that contribute to adduction deformity are the adductor longus, adductor brevis, pectineus, gracilis, and adductor magnus. There is no orthosis that is feasible for treating these deformities. Mobilization and intermittent positioning in a prone position can be instituted initially for hip flexion. Serial obturator bupivacaine (marcaine) nerve blocks or a closed phenol nerve block may help alleviate adductor spasticity and allow stretching exercises while the patient is in the period of neurologic recovery.[13] Adductor spasticity in a hemiplegic person rarely causes problems with hygiene if it is unilateral and adequate motion of the contralateral hip allows for skin care. Scissoring, however, may impede ambulation of affect balance during wheelchair transfers. Definitive procedures such as partial adductor release (leaving the adductor magnus muscle intact to prevent overcorrection) or anterior obturator neurectomy are then indicated if the patient is beyond the period of neurologic recovery and is no longer making progress in a conventional therapy program. Care must be taken to avoid adductor release or neurectomy in a patient whose adductor muscles are the sole means of limb advancement. Such patients walk with the lower extremity externally rotated. Preoperative lidocaine hydrochloride nerve block to the obturator nerve will simulate neurectomy and allow evaluation of ambulation prior to performing a definitive neurectomy. Dynamic EMG also is helpful in these instances.

Flexion deformity or contractures of the hip are initially treated with passive mobilization and prone positioning. If these fail, and persistent spasticity or contracture results in a flexed attitude during ambulation, surgical release is indicated. Muscles addressed include the iliopsoas, the rectus femoris, the tensor fasciae latae, and the sartorius. In a nonambulator, release will assist in hygiene, positioning and dressing the patient. Ipsilateral hip and knee flexion deformity should be released simultaneously to prevent recurrence. If a patient has a functional extremity, Z-lengthening of the iliopsoas (instead of complete release) can be performed to preserve some hip flexor function.

Knee

Two common problems associated with the knee in the stroke patient are inadequate knee flexion and flexion contracture.[16,28] Inadequate knee flexion is a dynamic problem during gait and is caused by inappropriate quadriceps activity. The quadriceps contracts during the terminal stance phase and early swing phase to prevent knee flexion, causing a stiff-legged gait.[31,38,67] The patient must hike the pelvis and circumduct the limb so the foot clears the floor. There is no effective nonoperative treatment for this deformity. EMG studies have shown that the abnormal activity may be restricted to the rectus femoris and vastus intermedius. Waters and coworkers have shown that release of these isolated portions of the quadriceps will allow knee flexion and good results in 88 percent of the patients.[38,67]

If all four heads of the quadriceps are overactive, release of the rectus femoris and vastus intermedius will usually not be sufficient. Release of all four heads is not indicated because some extensor function must be preserved to stabilize the knee. These patients often are not surgical candidates.[38,67]

Knee flexion contractures cause two major problems. In the nonambulatory patient, decubitus ulcers often develop on the heels or sacrum. In the ambulatory patient, increased quadriceps demand is required to stabilize the knee in the flexed position during stance. Energy consumption is greatly increased. Increased hip extensor demand is also required to stabilize the hip. Stretching exercises, splinting, or serial casting is instituted initially. If these fail, surgery is indicated. In the nonambulatory patient, treatment consists of distal release of the hamstring mucles.[74] Residual capsular contracture can be treated with serial casting after hamstring release. In the ambulatory or potentially ambulatory patient, selective release or fractional lengthening is performed on the basis of EMG studies. If concomitant hip flexion attitude is present, it is desirable to preserve the hip extensor function of the hamstrings. This can be performed with distal transfer of the hamstrings from the proximal tibia to the distal femur.[75]

Selective release or lengthening of specific offending muscles can be performed, depending on dynamic EMG studies. If muscle lengthening is performed, the knee is immobilized for 3 to 4 weeks.

Ankle and Foot

Deformities of the hindfoot and ankle include equinus, equinovarus, varus, and planovalgus. Equinovarus is the most common. Equinus is caused by

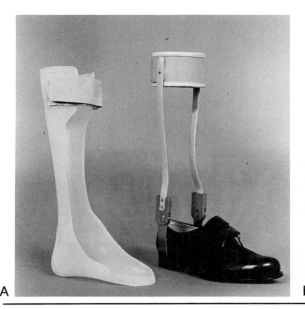

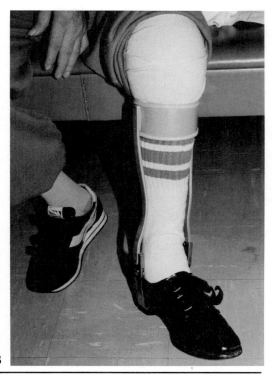

Fig. 29-9. Ankle-foot orthoses (AFO). **(A)** Polypropylene on left and double upright on the right. Both of these orthoses are commonly used to help control equinus and varus (or valgus) deformity. The double upright orthosis can be spring-loaded or locked into one position. It can control or prevent both plantar and dorsiflexion. It is strong and can control moderately severe deformities. Among its disadvantages are the facts that it is heavier, that it can only be used in one pair of shoes to which it is installed, and that it is more obvious. The polypropylene orthosis is of lighter weight, can incorporate a hinge or stop, can be used interchangeably with many types of shoes, and fits within the shoe under the pants and is thus less noticeable. It is form fitted, can be easily modified, and can disperse forces over a wider area. An arch support, metatarsal bar, or other modifications can be incorporated. It is, however, less sturdy than the double-upright and will not afford quite the same amount of control. **(B)** Double upright in place, adequately controlling equinovarus deformity.

overactivity of the gastrocnemius and soleus muscles with lesser contributions from the flexor hallucis longus, flexor digitorum longus, and tibialis posterior. The varus component is due to overactivity of the tibialis anterior, flexor digitorum longus, and flexor hallucis longus, with variable contributions from the tibialis posterior. Paralysis or weakness of the peroneus longus and peroneus brevis (which both help evert the foot) add to the varus deformity (Figs. 29-2B and 29-7). Initial management consists of correction by a locked ankle-foot orthosis (AFO), bivalved casts, or intermittent casting combined with passive mobilization, if feasible (Fig. 29-9). If bracing alone cannot control deformity, and a patient is in the recovery phase of spasticity, phenol motor nerve blocks to the gastrocnemius-soleus, tibialis posterior, flexor hallucis longus, and flexor digitorum longus muscles are indicated.

Definitive surgical reconstruction is delayed until the patient is beyond the period of neurologic recovery. Surgical indications for reconstruction include a deformity that is so severe that an AFO cannot be fitted (Fig. 29-10), residual deformity that interferes with ambulation despite use of an AFO, or a deformity that is correctable with an AFO in a patient who may become brace free after the reconstruction. Surgical reconstruction should also be considered in a wheel-

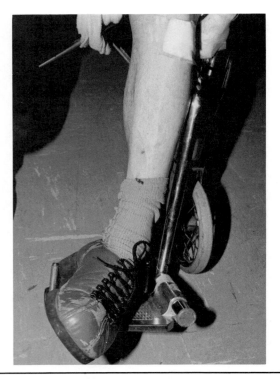

Fig. 29-10. Equinovarus deformity in stroke patient. Note the bandage over the area of skin breakdown, caused by pressure from the orthosis. This patient, whose deformity cannot be treated adequately with an orthosis, is a reasonable candidate for surgical reconstruction.

chair-bound patient in whom there is no hope for ambulation, but in whom a correction may produce a plantigrade foot that can be placed more comfortably on the wheelchair platform and allow dressing and shoes or footwear to keep the feet warm when the patient is taken outdoors.

Surgical correction of the equinus component is accomplished with tendo Achillis lengthening (TAL). Many methods for this procedure have been described and include open Z-lengthening, fractional lengthening, and percutaneous triple hemisection tenotomy.[33,38,63,64,66,68] If only the gastrocnemius muscle is spastic, selective fractional lengthening of this muscle can be performed. In the patient who has had a previous tendo Achillis lengthening and has a recurrent deformity, open lengthening is indicated because previous lengthening usually produces adhe-

sions that interfere with percutaneous lengthening. An open procedure in these patients allows precise control of lengthening. Whether only the gastrocnemius is involved can be determined by noting the disappearance of the equinus configuration when the gastrocnemius is relaxed by flexing the knee.

Ankle varus deviation may be caused by spasticity of the tibialis anterior, flexor hallucis longus, flexor digitorum longus, soleus, and, less commonly, the tibialis posterior muscles.[62,71] Pain and eventually decubitus ulcers may develop on the lateral aspect of the foot. Treatment consists of correction by a locked ankle orthosis. Surgical correction for varus deformity is indicated either for inadequate correction with an orthosis or to allow a patient to walk without an orthosis. Proprioception and adequate calf strength are required for brace-free ambulation. Preoperative EMG helps determine specific muscles responsible for the varus deformity. In stroke and brain injury, the tibialis anterior is often involved. The split anterior tibialis tendon transfer (SPLATT) is used to correct the varus component. The procedure consists of transfer of the lateral two-thirds of the tibialis anterior to the cuboid or third cuneiform bone, thus converting the deforming force to a corrective force. Overcorrection is prevented by the remaining nontransferred portion of the tendon. It is usually combined with a TAL to correct an equinovarus deformity[38,51] and with toe flexor release to avoid toe flexion deformity from tight extrinsic toe flexors, which are unmasked when the foot is corrected to a plantigrade position.[61]

CONCLUSION

With an aging population and improved methods of emergency transport, the number of stroke patients will continue to increase. Aggressive rehabilitation of appropriate candidates is justified. In the period of spontaneous recovery, efforts are made to prevent fixed contractures utilizing passive mobilization, splinting, nerve blocks, oral muscle relaxants, and electrical stimulation. If deformity persists and the patient is no longer recovering, surgical intervention can help alleviate the functional and hygiene problems associated with these limb deformities.

REFERENCES

1. Jordan C, Waters RL: Stroke. p. 277. In Nickel VL (ed): Orthopaedic Rehabilitation. Churchill Livingstone, New York, 1982
2. Waters RL, Botte MJ, Jordan C et al: Symposium: Rehabilitation of stroke patients—the role of the orthopaedic surgeon. Contemp Orthop 20:311, 1990
3. Bloch R, Bayer N: Prognosis in stroke. Clin Orthop 131:10, 1978
4. Matsumoto N, Whisnant JP, Kurland LT. Natural history of stroke in Rochester, Minnesota, 1955 to 1969. Stroke 4:20, 1973
5. Botte MJ, Keenan MAE: Reconstructive surgery of the upper extremity in the patient with head trauma. J Head Trauma Rehabil 2:34, 1987
6. Garland DE, Capen D, Waters RL: Surgical morbidity in patients with neurologic dysfunction. Clin Orthop; 45:189, 1979
7. Garland DE, Keenan MAE: Orthopedic strategies in the management of the adult head-injured patient. J Am Phys Ther Assoc 63:2004, 1983
8. Keenan MAE: Surgical decision making for residual limb deformities following traumatic brain injury. Orthop Rev 17:1185, 1988
9. McCollough NC III: Orthopaedic evaluation and treatment of the stroke patient. Instr Course Lect. 24:29, 1975
10. Rhoades ME, Garland DE: Orthopedic prognosis of brain-injured adults. Part I. Clin Orthop 131:104, 1978
11. Baker CC, Oppenheimer L, Stephens B et al: Epidemiology of trauma deaths. Am J Surg 140:144, 1980
12. Botte MJ, Waters RL, Keenan MAE et al: Orthopaedic management of the stroke patient. Part I. Pathophysiology, limb deformity, and patient evaluation. Orthop Rev 17:637, 1988
13. Botte MJ, Waters RL, Keenan MAE et al: Orthopaedic management of the stroke patient. Part II. Treating deformities of the upper and lower extremities. Orthop Rev 17:891, 1988
14. Lubic LG, Palkovity HP: Stroke. Medical Examination Publishing Company, Hyde Park, 1983
15. MaCollough NC III: Orthopaedic management in adult hemiplegia. Clin Orthop 131:38, 1978
16. Perry J, Waters RL: Orthopedic evaluation and treatment of the stroke patient, Instr Course Lect. 24:40, 1975
17. Botte MJ, Keenan MA, Gellman H et al: Surgical management of spastic thumb-in-palm deformity in adults with brain injury. J Hand Surg [Am] 14:174, 1989
18. Couvee LMJ: Heterotopic ossification in the surgical treatment of serious contractures. Paraplegia 19:89, 1981
19. Garland DE, Blum CE, Waters RL: Periarticular heterotopic ossification in head injured adults: incidence and location. J Bone Joint Surg [Am] 62:1143, 1980
20. Garland DE, Hanscom DA, Keenan MAE et al: Resection of heterotopic ossification in the adult with head trauma. J Bone Joint Surg [Am] 67:1261, 1985
21. Garland DE: Clinical observations on fractures and heterotopic ossification in the spinal cord and traumatic brain injured populations. Clin Orthop 233:86, 1988
22. Garland DE, Razza BE, Waters RL: Forceful joint manipulation in head-injured adults with heterotopic ossification. Clin Orthop 169:133, 1982
23. Garland DE, Alday B, Venos KG, Vogt JC: Diphosphonate treatment for heterotopic ossification in spinal cord injury patients. Clin Orthop 176:197, 1983
24. Mendelson L, Grosswasser Z, Najenson T et al: Periarticular new bone formation in patients suffering from severe head injuries. Scand J Rehabil Med 7:141, 1975
25. Meilants H, Vanhove E, Deneels J, Beys E: Clinical survey of and pathogenic approach to para-articular ossification in long-term coma. Acta Orthop Scand 46:190, 1975
26. Orzel JA, Rudd TG: Heterotopic bone formation: clinical, laboratory, and imaging correlation. J Nucl Med 26:125, 1985
27. Wharton GW: Heterotopic ossification. Clin Orthop 112:142, 1975
28. Perry J: Lower extremity management in stroke. Examination: A neurologic basis for treatment. Instr Course Lect. 24:26, 1975
29. Botte MJ, Nickel VL, Akeson WH: Spasticity and contracture: physiologic aspects of formation. Clin Orthop 233:7, 1988
30. Braun RM: Spasticity in the upper extremity. Clin Orthop 104:80, 1974
31. Garland DE, Rhoades ME: Orthopedic management of brain-injured adults. Part II. Clin Orthop 131:111, 1978
32. Garland DE: Head injuries in adults. p. 257. In Nickel VL (ed): Orthopaedic Rehabilitation. Churchill Livingstone, New York, 1982
33. Keenan MAE: The orthopaedic management of spasticity. J Head Trauma Rehabil 2:62, 1987
34. Keenan MAE: Management of the spastic upper extremity in the neurologically impaired adult. Clin Orthop 233:116, 1988
35. Young RR, Wiegner AW: Spasticity. Clin Orthop 219:50, 1982
36. Keenan MAE, Romanelli RR, Lunsford BR: The use of dynamic electromyography to evaluate motor control in the hands of adults who have spasticity caused by brain injury. J Bone Joint Surg [Am] 71:120, 1989
37. Perry J, Waters RL, Perrin T: Electromyographic analysis of equinovarus following stroke. Clin Orthop 131:47, 1978
38. Waters RL, Perry P, Garland DE: Surgical correction of gait abnormalities following stroke. Clin Orthop 131:54, 1978
39. Jordan C: Current status of functional lower extremity surgery in adult spastic patients. Clin Orthop 233:102, 1988
40. Keenan MAE, Perry J, Jordan C: Factors affecting balance and ambulation following stroke. Clin Orthop 182:165, 1984
41. Waters RL, Montgomery J: Lower extremity management of hemiparesis. Clin Orthop 102:133, 1974
42. Keenan MAE, Kauffman DL, Garland DE, Smith CW: Late ulnar neuropathy in the brain-injured adult. J Hand Surg [Am] 13:120, 1988
43. Stone L, Keenan MAE: Peripheral nerve injuries in the adult with traumatic brain injury. Clin Orthop 233:136, 1988
44. Waters RL: Upper extremity surgery in stroke patients, Clin Orthop 131:30, 1978
45. Botte MJ, Moore TJ: The orthopaedic management of extremity injuries in head trauma. J Head Trauma Rehabil 2:13, 1987
46. Botte MJ, Keenan MAE: Percutaneous phenol blocks of the pectoralis major muscle to treat spastic deformities. J Hand Surg [Am] 13:147, 1988
47. Braun RM, Hoffer MM, Mooney V: Phenol nerve block in the treatment of acquired spastic hemiplegia in the upper limb. J Bone Joint Surg [Am] 55:580, 1973
48. Garland DE, Lilling M, Keenan MAE: Percutaneous phenol blocks to motor points of spastic forearm muscles in head-injured populations. Arch Phys Med Rehabil 65:243, 1984
49. Keenan MAE, Botte MJ: Technique of percutaneous phenol block of the recurrent motor branch of the median nerve. J Hand Surg [Am] 12:806, 1987
50. Meals RA: Denervation for the treatment of acquired spasticity of the brachioradialis. J Bone Joint Surg [Am] 70:1081, 1988
51. Mooney V, Frykman G, McLamb J: Current status of intraneural phenol injections. Clin Orthop 63:132, 1969

52. Wood KM: The use of phenol as a neurolytic agent: a review. Pain 5:205, 1978
53. Baker LD: A rational approach to the surgical needs of the cerebral palsy patient. J Bone Joint Surg [Am] 38:313, 1956
54. Braun RM, Mooney V, Nickel VL: Flexor origin release for pronation-flexion deformity of the forearm and hand in the stroke patient. An evaluation of the early results in eighteen patients. J Bone Joint Surg [Am] 52:907, 1970
55. Braun RM, West F, Mooney V: Surgical treatment of the painful shoulder contracture in the stroke patient. J Bone Joint Surg [Am] 53:1307, 1971
56. Braun RM, Vise GT, Roper B: Preliminary experience with superficialis to profundus tendon transfer in the hemiplegic upper extremity. J Bone Joint Surg [Am] 56:466, 1974
57. Inglis AE, Cooper W: Release of the flexor-pronator origin for flexion deformities of the hand and wrist in spastic paralysis. A study of eighteen cases. J Bone Joint Surg [Am] 48:847, 1966
58. Keenan MAE, Todderud EP, Henderson R, Botte MJ: Management of intrinsic spasticity in the hand with phenol injection or neurectomy of the motor branch of the ulnar nerve. J Hand Surg [Am] 12:734, 1987
59. Keenan MAE, Korchek JI, Botte MJ et al: Results of transfer of the flexor digitorum superficialis tendons to the flexor digitorum profundus tendons in adults with acquired spasticity of the hand. J Bone Joint Surg [Am] 69:1127, 1987
60. Keenan MAE, Abrams RA, Garland DE, Waters RL: Results of fractional lengthening of the finger flexors in adults with upper extremity spasticity. J Hand Surg [Am] 12:575, 1987
61. Keenan MAE, Gorai AP, Smith CW, Garland DE: Intrinsic toe flexion deformity following correction of spastic equinovarus deformity in adults. Foot Ankle 7:333, 1987
62. Page CM: An operation for the relief of flexion contraction of the forearm. J Bone Joint Surg 5:233, 1923
63. Silfverskiold N: Reduction of the uncrossed two-joint muscles of the legs to one-joint muscles in spastic conditions. Acta Chir Scand 56:315, 1924
64. Silver CM, Simons SD: Gastrocnemius muscle recession (Silfverskiold operation) for spastic equinus deformity in cerebral palsy. J Bone Joint Surg [Am] 41:1021, 1959
65. Smith RJ: Intrinsic muscles of the fingers: function, dysfunction and surgical reconstruction. Instr Course Lect. 24:200, 1975
66. Strayer LM Jr: Recession of the gastrocnemius. J Bone Joint Surg [Am] 32:671, 1950
67. Waters RL, Garland DE, Perry J et al: Stiff-legged gait in hemiplegia: surgical correction. J Bone Joint Surg [Am] 61:927, 1979
68. White JW: Torsion of the Achilles tendon: its surgical significance. Arch Surg 46:784, 1943
69. Botte MJ, Nakai RJ, Waters RL et al: Motor point delineation of the gluteus medius muscle for functional electrical stimulation: an in vivo anatomic study. Arch Phys Med Rehabil 72:112, 1991
70. Perry J, Giovan P, Harris L et al: The determinants of muscle action in the hemiparetic lower extremity. Clin Orthop 131:71, 1978
71. Garland DE, Thompson R, Waters RL: Musculocutaneous neurectomy for spastic elbow flexion in nonfunctional upper extremities in adults. J Bone Joint Surg [Am] 62:108, 1980
72. Botte MJ, Keenan MAE, Korchek JI, Waters RL: Modified technique for the superficialis-to-profundus transfer in the treatment of adults with spastic clenched fist deformity. J Hand Surg [Am] 12:639, 1987
73. Harris C Jr, Riordan DC: Intrinsic contracture in the hand and its surgical treatment. J Bone Joint Surg [Am] 36:10, 1954
74. Keenan MAE, Ure K, Smith CW, Jordan C: Hamstring release for knee flexion contractures in spastic adults. Clin Orthop 236:221, 1988
75. Eggers GWN: Transplantation of hamstring tendons to femoral condyles in order to improve hip extension and decrease knee flexion in cerebral spastic paralysis. J Bone Joint Surg [Am] 34:827, 1952

30 Traumatic Brain Injury

MARY ANN E. KEENAN
MICHAEL J. BOTTE

Injury to the brain is a leading cause of death and disability in the United States and most developed countries.[1-7] An epidemiologic study of traumatic brain injuries occurring in San Diego County, California, in 1981 revealed an annual incidence of 180 per 100,000 population.[8] Extrapolating this rate to the 1980 United States population census would yield an estimate of 410,000 new cases of traumatic brain injury each year. Eleven percent of these patients will die shortly after the injury. Approximately 80 percent of the survivors will have a good or moderate neurologic recovery. Most traumatic injuries to the brain occur in persons who are less than 45 years old, and those who survive have a normal life span despite the injury.

PATHOPHYSIOLOGY OF BRAIN INJURY

Brain injuries can be broadly classified as either open or closed wounds. Open wounds generally are penetrating injuries such as gunshot wounds. Closed or nonpenetrating wounds generally have a combination of both compression and acceleration-deceleration injuries.

Pure compression injuries to the brain are infrequent and result primarily in focal brain damage. More destructive are the shearing forces of acceleration-deceleration, which cause widespread damage to the brain. Blunt trauma causes a combination of minor focal damage from the compression aspect of the injury but also more widespread damage from the acceleration-deceleration forces. Rotational forces to the head cause shearing injuries with tears of the white matter (long tracts), cranial nerves, and vessels. The severity of brain injury depends on the extent rather than the location of the injury.

Trauma to the head commonly causes contusion and lacerations located on the temporal lobes and inferior surfaces of the frontal lobes as a result of impingement on the bony ridges in the base of the skull. These temporal and frontal lobe injuries are usually bilateral. Bilateral temporal lobe injuries result in memory impairment. Prefrontal lesions result in personality changes. Loss of consciousness occurring after a head injury results from the shearing forces on nerve fibers, especially those of the reticular activating system, located in the brain stem. If an injury to the posterior cerebral artery occurs with occipital infarction, visual field deficits can result. Spasticity and weakness are caused by shearing of the pyramidal nerve fibers. Rigidity can be seen as a result of damage to the basal ganglia. Ataxia is caused when there is damage to the cerebellar pathways.

A subdural or intradural hematoma will increase the risk of residual hemiparesis. An increased incidence of epilepsy is seen after an open injury to the brain, a depressed skull fracture, an intradural hemorrhage, or the occurrence of early seizures. Computed tomographic (CT) scanning of the brain is relatively insensitive to contusions and shear injuries, although hematomas are well visualized. Magnetic resonance (MA) imaging scans of the brain more clearly delineate damage to the white matter.

361

Table 30-1. Glasgow Coma Scale

Eye opening	Spontaneous	4
	Speech	3
	Pain	2
	None	1
Motor response	Obeys	6
	Localizes	5
	Withdrawal	4
	Abnormal flexion	3
	Extensioin	2
	None	1
Verbal response	Oriented	5
	Confused	4
	Inappropriate	3
	Incomprehensible	2
	None	1

PROGNOSIS

Prognosis after traumatic brain injury has commonly been predicted on the basis of the Glasgow Coma Scale (Table 30-1),[5-7] which evaluates a patient's responses to eye opening, motor responses, and verbal responses. The Glasgow Outcome Scale is frequently used to determine outcome after brain injury (Table 30-2). When the results of the Glasgow Coma Scale score obtained within 24 hours of the patient's admission to the hospital are used, a coma score of 11 or greater is associated with an 82 percent probability of moderate or good neurologic recovery. A coma score of 8 to 10 results in a 68 percent probability of a moderate or good recovery. Coma scores of 5 to 7 indicate severe injuries and result in only a 34 percent incidence of moderate or good neurologic recovery. Scores lower than 5 have a significantly higher incidence of severe sequelae.

Age has an important effect on outcome after brain injury regardless of the severity of injury. Sixty-two percent of patients under the age of 20 years at the time of brain injury can expect a moderate or good neurologic recovery. Forty-six percent of patients between the ages of 20 and 30 will experience a moderate or good neurologic recovery. In a series of pediatric patients with brain injury, 90 percent achieved a moderate or good neurologic recovery and only 8 percent died or remained in a persistent vegetative state. Young children with a Glasgow Coma Scale score of 5 or better have a good prognosis for recovery.

The duration of coma is another indicator of prognosis. If emergence from coma occurs within the first 2 weeks of brain injury, 70 percent of patients can be expected to achieve a good recovery. If the coma persists beyond 4 weeks, the chance of good recovery is much diminished. Brain stem involvement, as indicated by the presence of decerebrate or decorticate posturing, has a poor prognosis for outcome. If decerebrate posturing occurs and resolves within the first week after injury, 40 percent of patients will attain a good neurologic recovery. If decerebrate posturing persists beyond the first week, only 9 percent of patients will achieve a good neurologic recovery.

Similarly, the duration of posttraumatic confusion can also be an indicator of prognosis. If the confusion persists for more than 4 weeks, one-third of the patients will have a poor neurologic outcome. It should be remembered, however, that prognosis is a probability statement and, although various factors can be used as guidelines, none is an absolute indicator in the individual patient.

REHABILITATION GOALS FOR THE BRAIN-INJURED PATIENT

The primary question that arises after brain injury is whether or not the person is a candidate for a comprehensive rehabilitation program. In general, rehabilitation goals are dictated by the patient's age, the current level of function and potential for further neurologic recovery, and the placement of the patient after the discharge from the rehabilitation facility. Three primary questions must be asked: What is the current level of function? What is the prognosis for further neurologic recovery? Based on this information, what can the rehabilitation team do for this person? Specific areas of function to be considered are communication, cognition, feeding, respiration, positioning, mobility, bladder and bowel control, activities of daily living, and hygiene and grooming.

Table 30-2. Glasgow Outcome Scale

Dead
Persistive vegetative state
Severely disabled
Moderately disabled
Good recovery

Communication and Cognition

The first rule is to establish communication with the patient. In a nonverbal patient, it is important to have a buzzer available at the bedside so that nursing staff can be alerted to a patient's needs. Simple "yes" and "no" signals can be established depending on the patient's physical abilities. An alphabet or picture board is an uncomplicated means for the patient to spell out a message or point to a desired object (Fig. 30-1). More sophisticated electronic communicators also are available.

When evaluating oral communication skills, factors such as cognition, linguistic skills, speech production ability, and auditory acuity must all be considered.[9] As patients emerge from coma after a closed brain injury, they can be expected to follow a predictable pathway as described by the Rancho Levels of Cog-

Table 30-3. Rancho Levels of Cognitive Functioning

I	No response
II	Generalized response
III	Localized response
IV	Confused—Agitated
V	Confused—inappropriate, nonagitated
VI	Confused—appropriate
VII	Automatic—appropriate
VIII	Purposeful—appropriate

nitive Function (Table 30-3).[10] The approach to the patient with low cognitive levels, such as Rancho Cognitive Level II or III with decreased response, is an organized program of stimulation (Table 30-4). Random stimulation, such as television or radio playing, has no therapeutic benefit. For a Rancho Cognitive Level IV with a confused and agitated patient or a level V patient who is no longer agitated but remains confused, the therapeutic approach is a great deal of external structure and a daily routine. When patients achieve a higher level of cognitive functioning with automatic or purposeful responses, such as Cognitive Levels VII and VIII, community reintegration training proceeds.

Feeding

Feeding is a basic necessity in considering function in the brain-injured patient. Adequate nutrition is critical to the prevention of unnecessary complications. If the patient is unable to swallow, a nasogastric tube should be inserted. This tube should be changed on a weekly basis, alternating nostrils to prevent irritation and skin breakdown. In addition, adhesive tape should be avoided to protect the skin of the nose. The tube can be positioned with twill tape wrapped around the tube and then tied around the head. The services of the dietitian should be obtained to calculate the patient's nutritional needs and plan an adequate diet. If it is necessary for the patient to have

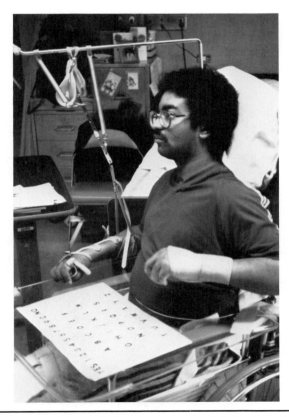

Fig. 30-1. A nonverbal patient uses an alphabet board to communicate.

Table 30-4. Therapeutic Strategies Based on Cognition

Cognitive Level	Recovery Phase	Therapeutic Approach
II, III	Decreased response	Stimulation
IV	Agitated response	External structure
V, VI	Confused response	External structure
VII, VIII	Automatic response	Community activities

tube feeding for a prolonged period of time, gastrostomy or jejunostomy tube insertion should be considered. With the advent of the percutaneous endoscopic technique of gastrostomy (PEG), the morbidity of this procedure has been greatly reduced.

If the patient has adequate control of the intraoral muscles to begin a feeding program, several factors should be considered. First, it is necessary that the patient be placed in a seated upright position for a proper alignment of the swallowing structures to help prevent aspiration. Second, the use of thickened foods or liquids will greatly facilitate the patient's swallowing response, especially in view of the delayed motor responses. Pureed foods and gelatin not only help to stimulate the swallowing response but also will move more slowly in the oral pharynx, allowing the patient more time to respond and helping to prevent aspiration.

Tracheostomies

When a tracheostomy is necessary, the dressings around the tracheostomy tubes should be removed as soon as the surgical wound is healed. Leaving dressings in place causes them to serve as a sponge to absorb secretions and promotes infection. The tube should be changed to an uncuffed tracheostomy tube as soon as possible to help prevent tracheal stenosis. When the patient is medically stable and no longer requires respiratory support, attempts at plugging the tracheostomy tube can be started. The time interval for plugging the tracheostomy tube is gradually increased as patient tolerance allows. Usually when the patient is able to tolerate 3 consecutive days of having the tracheostomy tube plugged, it can be removed safely.

Positioning

It is necessary to evaluate the patient for adequate positioning in the bed, in a wheelchair, with orthotic devices, or for shoewear. Improving the ability to position a patient often requires the treatment of spasticity and contractures. Frequent nursing checks of agitated patients are needed to be certain that they are in a safe position in the bed. When a patient is able to begin sitting, adequate support in the chair is necessary. Frequently lap belts and head control devices are needed. A soft roll between the knees or a firm pillow is useful if hip adductor spasticity is present. If the patient has difficulty with upright sitting balance, a lap board applied to the wheelchair (available in varying thicknesses) may help the patient maintain an upright posture without unduly restricting motion.

Mobility

Early mobilization is a goal in all patients. Patients should be evaluated for their ability to move safely and adequately to reposition themselves in the bed. If the patient is unable to bear weight or has inadequate balance for ambulation training, wheelchair mobility is considered. This may involve the use of a manual wheelchair, a chair that can be propelled with the use of one upper extremity, or an electric wheelchair. When the patient is ready to begin ambulation training the need for orthotic support and upper extremity assistive devices is considered (Fig. 30-2).

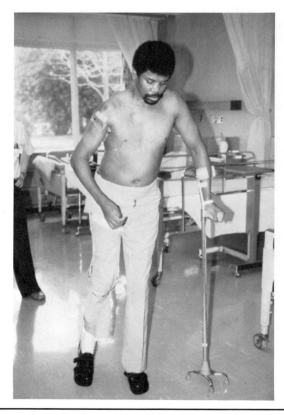

Fig. 30-2. A hemiplegic patient uses a knee-ankle-foot orthosis (KAFO) and a quad cane during gait training.

Bladder and Bowel Control

In general all tubes—including Foley catheters—should be removed as soon as possible because they are potential sources of infection. Incontinence is not an indication for an indwelling Foley catheter. As soon as the patient's condition is medically stable the indwelling catheter should be removed and urinary incontinence managed with the use of an external catheter or diapers.

In the brain-injured patient, bladder and bowel continence is generally a function of the patient cognitive abilities rather than physiologic control of the bladder and bowel. If an indwelling Foley catheter has been used for an extended period of time, an intermittent catheterization program may be necessary to re-establish bladder tone and control. Because the patients generally are confused, daily regimentation of bladder and bowel habits will be helpful in retraining the patient to regain continence.

Activities of Daily Living

The nursing staff and the physical and occupational therapists are actively involved with patients in assessing their abilities to perform personal hygiene, grooming, and dressing tasks. In the brain-injured patient, once again cognition is the major limiting factor. Spasticity, loss of motor control, and the presence of early contractures also may interfere with the use of the extremities in performing daily tasks. This requires a complex program of cooperation between the nursing, therapist, and physician staff.

ORTHOPAEDIC MANAGEMENT OF BRAIN INJURY

Acute Phase

The orthopaedic management of brain injury can be divided into three distinct time periods.[11,12] The initial phase of management occurs immediately after the injury in the acute care hospital. More than 50 percent of traumatic brain injuries are the result of a motor vehicle accident, and therefore multiple trauma is common. Because the injuries usually are multiple, the orthopaedic surgeon is commonly a consultant, but one with a critical role. It is imperative

to be aggressive in the treatment of orthopaedic injuries at an early stage.

The first rule of orthopaedic care is to make the diagnosis. Because of the turmoil of a multiple trauma situation, with many life-threatening injuries being present and resuscitation efforts taking place, missed injuries such as fractures or major peripheral nerve injuries are not uncommon. In a review of patients admitted to the Adult Brain Injury Service at Rancho Los Amigos Medical Center, 10 percent of the patients were noted to have contractures and 34 percent were noted to have previously undiagnosed peripheral nerve injuries.[13-16] In the comatose patient radiographs of all major joints and any other areas suspected of being injured should be obtained on a routine basis. It is also important to avoid assuming that all neurologic deficits present are from the central nervous system injury. Especially in the presence of a limb fracture, a peripheral nerve injury may have also occurred.

The second rule in orthopaedic care is to assume that the patient will make a good neurologic recovery. Therefore, all orthopaedic injuries should be treated appropriately (Fig. 30-3).[17,18]

The third rule is to expect lack of patient cooperation. As patients emerge from coma they may be expected to go through a period of agitation and confusion. Fracture care should be made as fail safe as possible because patient cooperation cannot be expected. Therefore, traction and external fixators for treatment of extremity fractures should be avoided where possible. Fractures should be fixed stably internally whenever this is feasible.

Subacute Phase

After traumatic brain injury, spontaneous neurologic recovery can occur over a prolonged period of time. The general rule of thumb is that improvement can be made for up to 18 months. In general, the majority of improvement in motor control occurs within the first 6 months after injury. However, after 18 months the patient can be assumed to have achieved maximum spontaneous improvement in motor control. Cognitive changes are also being made most rapidly in the early phases after brain injury, but these can continue for a very long period of time.

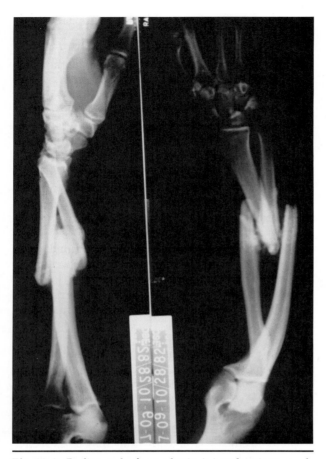

Fig. 30-3. Radiographs from a brain-injured patient on admission to the rehabilitation hospital reveal a forearm fracture, which was allowed to heal in a shortened, rotated, and angulated position. This was the patient's only functional upper extremity and surgical correction of the malunion was necessary.

It is during the subacute phase that the patient is generally in a rehabilitation facility. Serious head injury requiring a period of rehabilitation is frequently complicated by spasticity.[19-26] This spasticity often is severe and prevents adequate range-of-motion therapy for the joints. It also interferes with the maintenance of limb position despite the most conscientious and aggressive treatment attempts by family members, nursing staff, and therapists. Even in those situations in which joint motion can be maintained by a knowledgeable therapist, this commonly requires much force, which is painful for the patient, potentially harmful, and very time consuming. Lesser degrees of spasticity can also impede a patient's function or require the use of positioning devices that interfere with the use of an extremity.

There are many complications of spasticity. These include the formation of contractures. Limited positioning and myotatic contractures combined with the patient's diminished nutritional status can result in decubitus ulcers or hygiene problems (Fig. 30-4). When fractures are present, fracture malunion can occur if there is uncontrolled spasticity. Joint subluxation also can develop from prolonged spasticity or from attempts to range a joint in cases of severe spasticity. This is most commonly seen at the knee joint with posterior subluxation of the tibia. Spasticity also appears to be one of several etiologic factors in the formation of heterotopic periarticular bone (Fig. 30-5). A final complication of spasticity is acquired peripheral neuropathy, most commonly ulnar neuropathy at the elbow from severe flexion and continuous pressure on the ulnar nerve; carpal tunnel syndrome secondary to severe wrist flexion and pressure of the median nerve against the leading edge of the transverse carpal ligament (Fig. 30-6); or common peroneal nerve palsy associated with hip flexor spasticity and limited positioning, resulting in pressure on the nerve at the head of the fibula.

Evaluation of Limb Deformity

The period of potential possible neurologic recovery after head injury is prolonged, definitive surgical procedures should be avoided during this transitional stage. In a brain-injured patient, it is frequently difficult to distinguish among multiple possible causes of decreased range of motion in a joint. These possibilities include increase muscle tone, a myotatic contracture, the presence of periarticular heterotopic ossification, an undetected fracture or dislocation, pain, or the lack of patient cooperation secondary to diminished cognition. Bony deformities such as a fracture or dislocation may not be manifested by an obvious clinical deformity but can be ruled out by radiography. Heterotopic ossification is manifested clinically by an intense inflammatory reaction about the joint with redness, warmth, severe pain, and rapidly decreasing range of motion.[27] Heterotopic ossification becomes obvious at approximately 2 months after the traumatic brain injury, and generally a radiograph will show evidence of the heterotopic bone.

Fig. 30-4. A spastic quadriplegic patient with rigid hip and knee flexion contractures had very limited positioning in bed. This commonly results in the development of trochanteric and sacral decubitus ulcers.

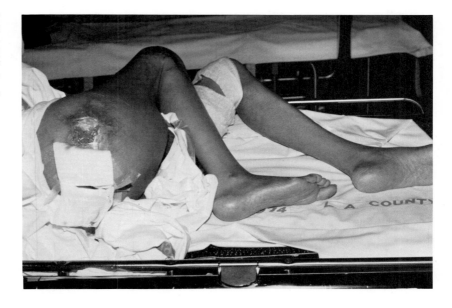

Diagnostic (Anesthetic) Nerve Blocks

Differentiating between the relative contributions of pain, increased muscle tone, and contracture can be difficult. Anesthetic nerve blocks are extremely useful in assessing a patient's joint range of motion. The blocks can be performed at the bedside or in the clinic without the use of special devices (Figs. 30-7 and 30-8). By temporarily eliminating the pain and muscle tone, patient cooperation is gained and the amount of fixed joint contracture can be determined. Through use of local anesthetic blocks the strength and motor control of the antagonistic muscle group can also be evaluated.

Fig. 30-5. Radiograph shows a bridge of periarticular heterotopic bone anterior to the elbow joint of a patient with marked elbow flexor spasticity.

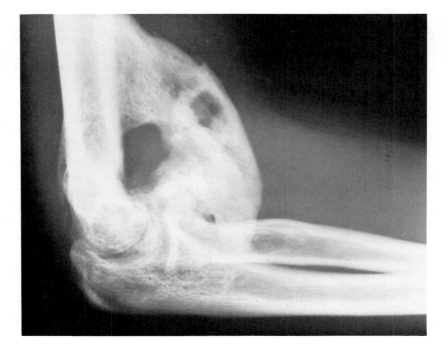

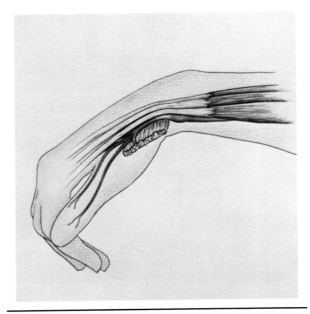

Fig. 30-6. A wrist flexion deformity in a spastic patient causes the median nerve to be compressed against the proximal edge of the transverse carpal ligament. Pressure from the taut finger flexor tendons results in a chronic "active" Phalen's maneuver.

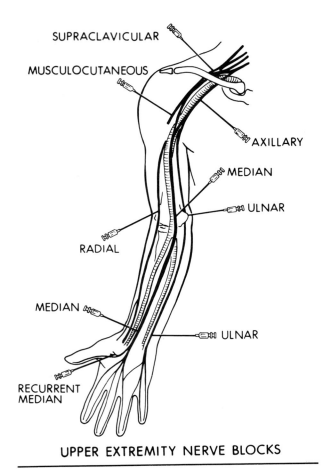

UPPER EXTREMITY NERVE BLOCKS

Fig. 30-7. Common sites of anesthetic nerve blocks used in the upper extremity to differentiate between dynamic deformities caused by spasticity and fixed myostatic contractures. (From Keenan,[26] with permission.)

Temporary Control of Spasticity

The treatment of spasticity depends on the time since injury and the prognosis for further recovery. Several choices are available for treatment. Drugs have been used in the treatment of spasticity; however, most cause unwanted drowsiness, which can seriously hamper the progress of the patient. Other serious side effects, such as hepatotoxicity, can occur. In our experience these drugs have been of limited effectiveness in the treatment of severe spasticity in the brain-injured patient. We therefore prefer to use techniques directed at specific muscles or joints.

A combination of peripheral nerve blocks and casting or splinting techniques is commonly used to give temporary relief of spasticity. Casting maintains muscle fiber length and diminishes muscle tone by decreasing sensory input. Local anesthetic nerve blocks are very helpful when done prior to cast application, because relieving the spasticity allows for easier limb positioning. Casts are used primarily for the correction of contractural deformities; for this pur-

pose a cast is applied on a weekly basis. If a patient is in an upright position, a dropout cast for an elbow flexion contracture is very helpful (Fig. 30-9). Serial casting is most successful when a contracture has been present for less than 6 months. Although some carryover effect can be seen in diminishing spasticity with casting, this generally is not a practical treatment modality.

Repeated anesthetic nerve blocks also will give some carryover effect in relieving spasticity and maintaining joint range of motion. Repeating lidocaine blocks on a daily basis, however, generally is not practical. In this situation, a longer acting agent, such as phenol

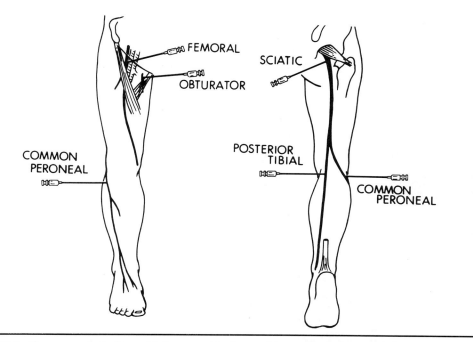

Fig. 30-8. Common sites of anesthetic nerve blocks used to evaluate the spastic lower extremity. (From Keenan,[26] with permission.)

or alcohol, is used to block nerve function.[20,23–26,28–34] Phenol denatures the protein in the peripheral nerve, causing axonal degeneration. The axons then regenerate because the continuity of the nerve sheath has been maintained. The average duration of a phenol block is therefore approximately 6 months. The action of phenol is nonspecific and phenol affects all nerve fibers alike.

Techniques of Phenol Blocks

Phenol blocks are used to decrease spasticity only during the period of potential neurologic recovery. It is hoped that by the time the nerve has regenerated the patient will have recovered more control of the affected muscle. If excessive spasticity occurs and the patient still has potential for further spontaneous recovery, the phenol nerve blocks can be repeated. Several techniques of phenol blocks are used, depending on the anatomic accessibility of the nerve and its composition. The direct injection of a peripheral nerve gives the most complete and longest lasting block; however, when a peripheral nerve has a large sensory component, direct injection is not recommended because loss of sensation is undesirable

and some patients may develop painful hyperesthesia. In some cases it is necessary to surgically dissect the individual motor branches of a nerve to a muscle and inject each separately. Another approach is to localize the motor points of the muscles using a needle electrode and nerve stimulator. Motor point injections do not completely relieve spasticity but can be helpful in reducing tone. The duration of motor point blocks is approximately 2 months; these blocks can be repeated as necessary.

Phenol Blocks for Common Types of Spasticity

Shoulder Adduction. Shoulder adduction and internal rotation spasticity are common in the upper extremity. This deformity interferes with hygiene and upper body dressing. Phenol motor point blocks of the pectoralis major muscle are effective in reducing tone and improving shoulder adduction (Fig. 30-10).[35] In addition, blocks of the thoracodorsal nerve can also be performed.

The Flexed Elbow Deformity. When spasticity of the biceps and brachialis muscles interferes with

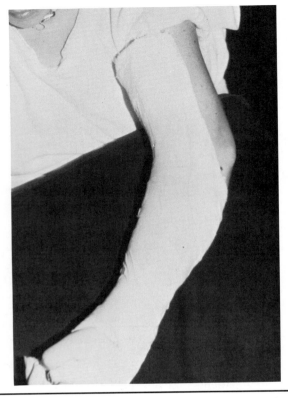

Fig. 30-9. An elbow dropout cast is useful to correct a flexion contracture in a patient who can be upright. The weight of the cast applies an extension force to the elbow. The anterior portion of the cast prevents elbow flexion.

elbow extension, a phenol block of the musculocutaneous nerve can provide temporary relief (Fig. 30-11).[23,36] The block is most commonly performed percutaneously at the bedside. Because the musculocutaneous nerve has a minimal sensory component and minimal corticosensory representation, percutaneous phenol injection will not interfere with sensation in the upper extremity. The advantages of performing the musculocutaneous nerve blocks percutaneously are that it is more readily done, does not require general anesthesia, and provides only a partial blockade of the action of the biceps and brachialis muscles. The partial block preserves the potential for upper extremity fractional training.

The brachioradialis muscle has been shown by dynamic electromyographic studies to be the most spastic of the elbow flexor muscles. Because this muscle is innervated by the radial nerve, it is commonly necessary to also perform a motor point block of the brachioradialis muscle (Fig. 30-12). The motor points are first localized on the surface of the brachioradialis muscle using a surface stimulator. An insulated teflon-coated needle is then used in conjunction with a nerve stimulator to localize more accurately to the motor points. Approximately 1 ml of a 5 percent solution of phenol in saline is then injected at each of two points. The ensuing block of the brachioradialis muscle takes effect over the following 24

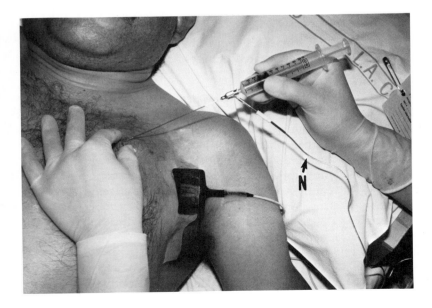

Fig. 30-10. A spinal needle electrode insulated with Teflon is connected to a nerve stimulator (N) and used to identify the motor points within the pectoralis major muscle. One milliliter of 5 percent phenol is injected at each motor point to diminish spasticity in the pectoralis major muscle.

Fig. 30-11. The musculocutaneous nerve is identified beneath the biceps muscle percutaneously using a needle electrode and a nerve stimulator. Three milliliters of 5 percent phenol are then injected into the nerve to diminish spasticity in the biceps and brachialis muscles. (From Keenan, 42, with permission.)

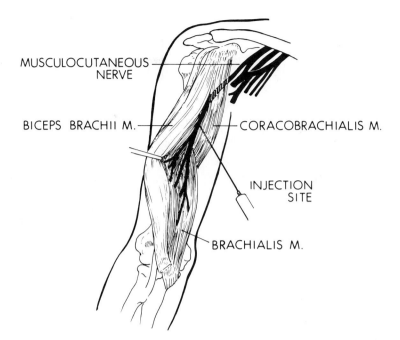

hours. If a myotatic contracture of the elbow is also present, an elbow dropout cast or serial casting is used to correct the contractural deformity.

Wrist and Finger Flexor Spasticity. Spastic forearm flexor muscles causing wrist and finger flexion deformities can be treated by phenol motor point blocks.[24] Because of the large sensory components of both the median and ulnar nerves at the forearm

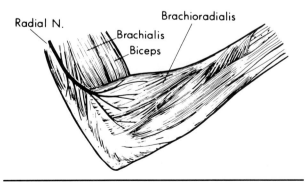

Fig. 30-12. The brachioradialis muscle is the most spastic of the elbow flexors. The motor points of the brachioradialis are located using an insulated needle and nerve stimulator for injection of phenol. (From Keenan et al,[36] with permission.)

level, an injection of the nerve proper is undesirable. Surgical dissection of the motor branches of these nerves would be extensive and would cause excessive scarring for only temporary relief of spasticity. For these reasons, an attempt is made to localize the point of entry of the motor branches into the muscles using surface electrical stimulation. The points of maximal responses are marked. Then, additional stimulation is applied using a needle electrode to further define the motor points of the muscles (Fig. 30-13). When the motor points have been localized, 1 ml of 5 percent phenol solution is injected at each point.

Intrinsic Spasticity in the Hand. Spasticity involving the intrinsic muscles of the hand is common but may be masked by spastic deformities in the extrinsic finger flexors. An adducted thumb, limited extension of the metacarpophalangeal joints, or swan-neck positioning of the fingers should alert the physician to the possibility of underlying intrinsic spasticity. A permanent deformity can be avoided by performing phenol block of the two motor branches of the ulnar nerve in Guyon's canal after surgical exposure (Fig. 30-14).[37]

Thumb-in-Palm Deformity. The thumb-in-palm deformity is heterogeneous in appearance and may

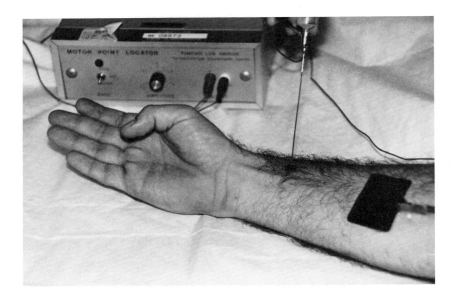

Fig. 30-13. A motor point block using phenol will temporarily reduce spasticity of the forearm flexor muscles, such as the flexor pollicis longus.

be secondary to spasticity of multiple muscles. If flexion of the interphalangeal joint of the thumb is present, a motor point block of the flexor pollicis longus is performed (Fig. 30-13).[24] When the thumb is in a severely adducted position, a surgical block of

the motor branches of the ulnar nerve using phenol is performed (Fig. 30-14).[37] When the adduction deformity of the thumb is also secondary to spasticity of the median nerve–innervated muscles of the thenar eminence, a phenol block of the recurrent motor

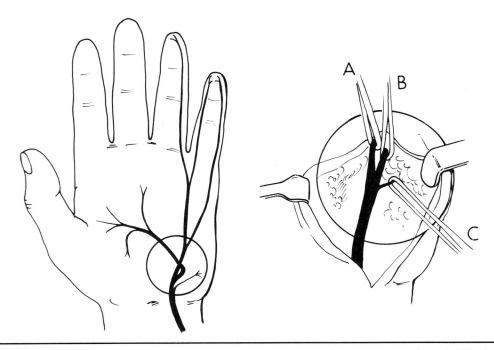

Fig. 30-14. The motor branches of the ulnar nerve **(B and C)** are isolated from the sensory branch **(A).** The motor nerves are then injected with phenol to eliminate intrinsic spasticity.

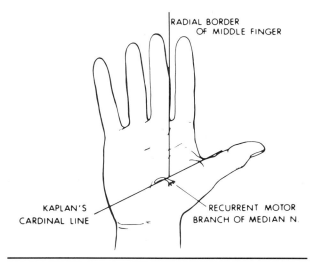

RADIAL BORDER
OF MIDDLE FINGER

KAPLAN'S
CARDINAL LINE

RECURRENT MOTOR
BRANCH OF MEDIAN N.

Fig. 30-15. The recurrent motor branch of the median nerve can be located at the intersection of Kaplan's cardinal line and a line drawn along the radial border of the long finger. Injection of the recurrent median nerve with phenol is useful in diminishing spasticity in the thenar muscles. (From Keenan and Botte,[38] with permission.)

branch of the median nerve can be done (Fig. 30-15).[38] The block can be performed percutaneously using an electrode needle and nerve stimulator. The recurrent motor branch of the median nerve enters the thenar mass at the junction between Kaplan's cardinal line and a line drawn along the radial border of the long finger. Kaplan's line is drawn parallel to the proximal palmar crease beginning at the apex of the first web space.

Hip Adductor Spasticity. Severe spasticity of the hip adductor muscles results in multiple problems, including poor hygiene, limited position of the patient in the bed or chair, and decubitus ulcers. In patients with greater function, the increase in tone causes scissoring of the legs when the patient is upright, which interferes with balance, transfers, and ambulation. A phenol block of the obturator nerve can be performed percutaneously to provide relief of the increased tone. It is advisable to do an anesthetic nerve block first to rule out a myotatic contracture. The obturator nerve is injected as it emerges from the obturator canal.

Hip Flexor Spasticity. Severe spasticity of the hip flexor muscles not only causes hip flexion contrac-

tures but may also contribute to knee flexion deformities. When hip flexor spasticity cannot be controlled by the use of a long leg cast or by proning or positioning devices, percutaneous paraspinal blocks of the upper lumbar nerve roots can be performed to diminish hip flexor spasticity.

Knee Flexor Spasticity. When severe hamstring spasticity is present, knee flexor contractures develop very rapidly. Because of the large sensory component of the sciatic nerve, direct injection with phenol is undesirable. The dissection required to identify the multiple motor branches of the hamstring muscles is extensive and often impractical. Attempts at motor point injections of the hamstring muscles have been made but generally were not effective. Prevention of knee flexion contractures is done by performing repeated anesthetic nerve blocks of the sciatic nerve and casting the limb in extension. An anesthetic block of the sciatic nerve will also temporarily eliminate calf spasticity and allow for serial casting of an equinus contracture of the foot if present (Fig. 30-8).

When serial casting and sciatic nerve blocks fail to correct a knee flexion deformity or when posterior subluxation of the tibia occurs secondary to the hamstring tightness, a lengthening of the hamstring muscles can be performed even in the early stages after injury. The biceps femoris, gracilis, and semimembranosus muscles have myotendinous junctions that permit a fractional lengthening. The semitendinosus muscle is either divided or lengthened by Z-shaped incision (Z-lengthening). Casting is still commonly needed after a hamstring lengthening to correct the residual flexion deformity.

The Equinus Foot Posturing. Excessive spasticity of the gastrocnemius and soleus muscles causing equinus posturing of the foot is very common. When the spasticity is mild, it can generally be contained and an equinus contracture prevented by the use of an ankle-foot orthosis. At times the muscle tone is too severe to be adequately controlled by a brace. The patient may exhibit ankle clonus while in the upright position, causing the foot to piston up and down in the brace.

A phenol block of the posterior tibial nerve is performed as a surgical procedure to preserve sensation to the plantar aspect of the foot (Fig. 30-16).[23] An

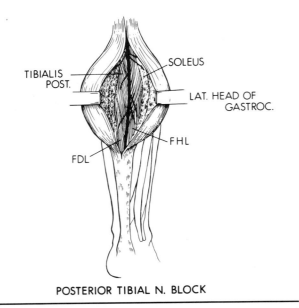

POSTERIOR TIBIAL N. BLOCK

Fig. 30-16. Phenol injection of the surgically exposed motor branches of the posterior tibial nerve is an effective means of controlling spasticity of the calf muscles. FDL, flexor digitorum longus; FHL, flexor hallucis longus.

incision is made on the posterior aspect of the calf at the midline beginning just distal to the popliteal crease. The posterior tibial nerve is identified by dissecting between the heads of the gastrocnemius muscle and is traced distally. A nerve stimulator is used to identify the motor branches. When all of the motor branches to the gastrocnemius, soleus, posterior tibialis, flexor hallucis longus, and flexor digitorum muscles have been identified, each is protected from the surrounding tissue by a moistened gauze sponge. The motor branches are then injected with a 5 percent phenol solution in glycerin. Postoperatively the patient must be protected with an ankle-foot orthosis to maintain the ankle in a neutral position to protect the calf muscles while the block is in effect. The duration of the surgically performed block of the posterior tibial nerve is generally 6 months.

Knee Extension Deformity. Severe spasticity of the quadriceps muscles may be seen in brain stem injuries or anoxic brain damage. When knee range of motion cannot be maintained because of the quadriceps tone, a percutaneous phenol block of the femoral nerve can be performed. This block, in combina-

tion with the use of a continuous passive motion machine, is then use to regain and maintain adequte knee range of motion. Even in a severely injured patient, knee and hip flexion range should be preserved to allow adequate sitting in a chair.

Hip Extension Deformity. Severe spasticity of the hip extensor muscles can occur with brain stem or anoxic injuries. Percutaneous phenol injection of the inferior gluteal nerve as it enters the belly of the gluteus maximus muscle is an effective technique in reducing hip extensor tone and maintaining the ability to flex the hip. The inferior gluteal nerve enters the gluteus maximus muscle at the center of the muscle belly just proximal to the midportion of the piriformis tendon. The nerve is carefully localized with an electrode needle and a nerve stimulator prior to injection.

Residual Phase

When spontaneous neurologic recovery has ceased to occur, the brain-injured patient is commonly left with residual limb deformities from spasticity, contractures, and muscle imbalance. It is at this time that definitive orthopaedic surgical procedures are performed to rebalance the muscle forces and correct the residual deformities.

Upper Extremity Surgery

Preoperative Evaluation

Assessment of Cognition and Communication. Upper extremity function requires complex and highly sophisticated mechanisms working together in unison. Improving the functional use of a hand and arm requires careful systematic evaluation. The goals must be practical and clearly understood by the patients and their family members. General principles of patient assessment include an evaluation of cognition and communication skills.[39-42] This is done during the physical examination. Patients should be capable of following simple commands and also should be able to cooperate with a postoperative therapy program. In addition, they should have sufficient cognition to incorporate the improved motor function into their use of the extremity. Adequate memory is needed to retain what is taught during the postoperative therapy.

Sensory Evaluation. Intact sensation is essential to the functional use of the hand.[40,42] The basic modalities of pain, light touch, and temperature must be present. Two-point discrimination is a useful predictive test, because a patient will rarely use the hand for functional activities if the distance for discrimination is greater than 10 mm. Proprioception and kinesthetic awareness of the limb in space are important. Kinesthetic awareness is tested in a hemiplegic person by placing the spastic limb in a position and asking the patient to duplicate this position with the sound limb while keeping the eyes closed. Stereognosis is not a practical test in spastic patients, who lack the fine motor control necessary to manipulate an object in the hand.

It is helpful to observe the patient's spontaneous use of the hand. A patient with impaired sensation may use a hand on request, relying on visual feedback, but may not necessarily use the extremity in activities of daily living even as a functional assist. Visual perceptual deficits add increased problems involving motion of the limb and even awareness of the limb itself.

Detecting Fixed Deformities. The presence of fixed deformities such as myotatic contractures, bony deformities, and heterotopic ossification must be determined. Anesthetic nerve blocks are used to differentiate between contractures and severe spasticity limiting joint motion.[26] Radiographs are obtained to detect bony deformities, such as occult fractures, and heterotopic ossification.

Evaluation of Motor Control. The evaluation of motor control is complex because spasticity will often mask underlying control. In the upper extremity, the most common pattern of spasticity is one of flexion. Unmasking of primitive patterning reflexes further contributes to the motor impairment. Spasticity (hyperactive response to quick stretch), rigidity (resistance to slow movement), or movement dystonias may be present.[43] Judgment of motor control based on the position a limb assumes at rest or during an activity can be misleading. Position is often the result of multiple muscle forces. By selectively eliminating or reducing specific muscle forces using anesthetic nerve blocks, a more accurate assessment can be obtained of control and the extent of contractures (Figs. 30-7 and 30-8).

The patient should first be observed clinically in a variety of functional tasks. If there is doubt as to the action of specific muscle groups, more sophisticated laboratory assessment is needed. Dynamic, multichannel electromyography (EMG) has been shown to be a useful supplement to clinical examination when evaluating muscle function in both normal and spastic persons.[44-51] It is important, however, to differentiate between cause and effect with prudence when evaluating muscle activity patterns on EMG.

Definitive Surgical Procedures to Improve Function

Functional Elbow Release. Hand placement depends on both shoulder and elbow motor control. Flexion of the shoulder generally is not a problem in the upper extremity with potential for function. Smooth control of elbow flexion and extension is commonly impaired and limits the patient's ability to perform activities of daily living even when good hand control is present.

The clinical picture is one of cogwheel motion on attempted extension of the elbow with a very prolonged period of extension and often incomplete range of motion. Dynamic electromyography shows that the most common pattern seen is that all three heads of the triceps muscle are operating in a normal phasic pattern, and the brachioradialis muscle shows severe spasticity with continuous activity during both flexion and extension. Both heads of the biceps muscle are moderately spastic, with activity continuing during elbow extension. A lesser degree of spasticity is observed in the brachialis muscle.[41,51]

To correct this problem, a proximal release of the brachioradialis muscle by myotomy is performed using electrocautery and is combined with Z-lengthening of the biceps tendon and fractional lengthening of the brachialis tendon through a curved incision on the anterior aspect of the elbow (Fig. 30-17). Postoperatively the patient is placed in a cast with the elbow in 45° of flexion for 4 weeks, after which a program of active therapy is begun.[42] This procedure has significantly enhanced the fluid control of elbow motion and improved hand placement in properly selected patients.

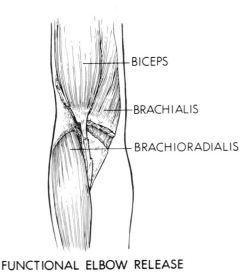

FUNCTIONAL ELBOW RELEASE

Fig. 30-17. Elbow motion is improved in the spastic patient by proximal release of the brachioradialis muscle and lengthening of the biceps and brachialis muscles.

Wrist and Finger Flexor Lengthening. The fingers are held in a clenched-fist position. This may be accomplished by wrist flexion as well. The degree of motor control may be masked by the severe amount of tone present in the finger flexors. Passive range of motion should be established first. After this, the patient is asked to open and close the fingers and to flex and extend the wrist. If no active wrist or finger extension is seen, it is still important to determine whether the patient appears to have active control of finger flexion. In the continuum of neurologic impairment and recovery, control of wrist and finger flexion is seen prior to active control of extension.[44] A finger is placed in the patient's palm and the patient is asked to grasp it. Often an increase in the pressure of grasp can be felt, indicating underlying muscle control.

Next, an anesthetic block of the median and ulnar nerves is performed at the elbow to temporarily eliminate flexor tone. With the flexor muscles relaxed, the activity of the extensor muscles can be evaluated more accurately. When extensor control returns, it is generally seen in the extensor indicis proprius muscle first.[44] If any uncertainty remains concerning the pattern of muscle control, dynamic electromyographic studies can be utilized to further elucidate the situation.

Although active wrist and finger extension is desirable for good hand function, a review of fractional lengthening of the finger flexors in the spastic upper extremity showed that control of grasp was more important to hand function than active finger extension.[52]

The surgery is performed through an incision on the volar surface of the forearm. The palmaris longus tendon is divided, and the flexor carpi radialis and flexor carpi ulnaris tendons are transected for Z-lengthening if a wrist flexion deformity is present. Median neuropathy is common in the presence of a wrist flexion deformity, and it is advisable to perform a carpal tunnel release (Fig. 30-6).[16] The lengthening of the flexor digitorum superficialis and flexor digitorum profundus tendons is performed by incising the flexor tendon with a Z cut at the musculotendinous junction and then passively extending the digit, allowing the tendon to slide distally (Fig. 30-18). To prevent further lengthening of the muscle-tendon unit, the tendon is sutured in the lengthened position. The flexor pollicis longus tendon is lengthened in an identical manner. The amount of lengthening is determined prior to cutting the flexor tendons of the digits by placing the wrist and digits in the position of maximum active extension seen preoperatively. The wrist and fingers are then passively extended and the amount of excursion measured. The tendons are lengthened by half the measured excursion. If a Z-lengthening of the wrist flexors is performed, the tendons are repaired with the wrist in a neutral position using a nonabsorbable suture.

Postoperatively the wrist and hand are immobilized for 3 weeks in a plaster cast. The wrist is held in 20° of extension and the fingers are immobilized with the metacarpophalangeal joints in 60° of flexion and the interphalangeal joints extended. The patient is begun on a program of active exercise when the cast is removed. Resting splints are worn at night for an additional 3 weeks to protect the tendons from inadvertent stretching.

Intrinsic Muscle Spasticity. When spasticity of the extrinsic flexors is present, intrinsic muscle spasticity

Fig. 30-18. The flexor tendons in the forearm are lengthened by making a Z-shaped cut in the tendon over the muscle belly and passively extending the finger to achieve the desired amount of correction. The tendon is then sutured in this position. The technique is technically simple and maintains the blood supply to the tendon.

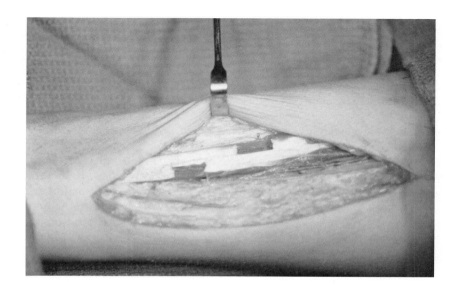

should be expected also.[37,53,54] Extension of the fingers at the metacarpophalangeal joints may be blocked by spasticity of the interosseus and lumbrical muscles of the hand. Another manifestation of intrinsic muscle spasticity is the tendency toward swan-neck positioning of the fingers.

The degree of tension caused by the intrinsic muscles can be demonstrated by comparing the amount of proximal interphalangeal joint flexion obtained with the metacarpophalangeal joints both flexed and extended. If there is less proximal interphalangeal joint flexion with metacarpophalangeal joint extension, the intrinsic tendons are tight. This test should be performed both before and after a lidocaine block of the ulnar nerve at the wrist to distinguish between intrinsic tone and contracture.

Two techniques for controlling intrinsic muscle spasticity are used (Fig. 30-14).[37] The first technique is a phenol block of the motor branch of the ulnar nerve in Guyon's canal. This provides temporary relief of the spasticity. The second technique is a neurectomy of the motor branch of the ulnar nerve to provide permanent ablation of intrinsic muscle function.

If contracture of the intrinsic muscles is already present, release of the tendons is needed. Release is performed on the lateral bands of the extensor hood

mechanism at the level of the proximal phalanx (Fig. 30-19). A neurectomy of the motor branches of the ulnar nerve is done simultaneously to prevent recurrence of the intrinsic muscle spasticity plus deformity from spasticity of the interosseous muscles. Postoperatively the patient's hands are immobilized in splints for 3 weeks, after which a therapy program is begun.

Thumb-in-Palm Deformity. A thumb-in-palm deformity is frequently seen secondary to spasticity in

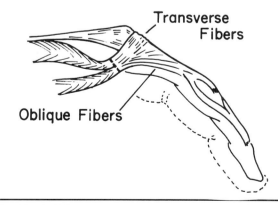

Fig. 30-19. When an intrinsic contracture is present, a release of the lateral bands is performed in conjunction with a neurectomy of the motor branches of the ulnar nerve in the hand.

the flexor pollicis longus muscle as well as the median and ulnar nerve–innervated thenar muscles. A flexion deformity of the interphalangeal joint of the thumb indicates spasticity of the flexor pollicis longus muscle. Surgical lengthening of the tendon will improve thumb extension. Arthrodesis of the interphalangeal joint is usually performed with a Moberg screw for added stability during lateral pinch.

Generally all of the thenar muscles are spastic or contracted, and a proximal myotomy is required to reposition the thumb and decrease the underlying tone to improve pinch function (Fig. 30-20).[55–57] Distal releases are to be avoided because these result in a hyperextension deformity of the metacarpophalangeal joint of the thumb.

An incision is made along the thenar crease on the palm. The neurovascular structures and flexor tendons are retracted ulnarly. The adductor pollicis, flexor pollicis brevis, opponens pollicis, and abductor pollicis muscles are detached from their origins and allowed to slide distally. If the first dorsal interosseus muscle is to be released, an incision is made on the dorsum of the thumb metacarpal. By releasing these muscles from their origins, they are allowed to retract radially and reattach in an improved position, preserving function and preventing a hyperextension

deformity of the metacarpophalangeal joint. Postoperatively the patient's thumb is immobilized in a thumb spica cast for 4 weeks.

Contracture Releases in the Nonfunctional Arm

Shoulder Release. An adducted and internally rotated shoulder causes problems with hygiene, difficulty in dressing and positioning, and sometimes pain. Release of the pectoralis major, latissimus dorsi, teres major, and subscapularis muscles is required to relieve the deformity.[39,40,42,58] Postoperatively, careful positioning of the arm is important to prevent recurrence.

Elbow Release. Flexion contractures of the elbow result in skin maceration and breakdown.[39,40,42,58] They also are frequently associated with a compression neuropathy of the ulnar nerve.[14,15] The release is performed through a longitudinal incision on the lateral side of the elbow. It is necessary to transect the brachioradialis muscle and biceps tendon. When the deformity is not severe, the brachialis muscle is lengthened at its myotendinous junction but left to counterbalance any pull by the triceps muscles. When the elbow flexion contracture is severe and has been present for many years, it may be necessary to

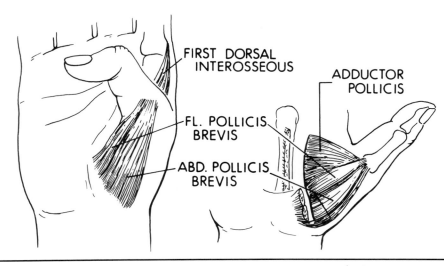

Fig. 30-20. A proximal release of the spastic and contracted thenar muscles is performed to correct a thumb-in-palm deformity. The flexor pollicis longus is also lengthened and the interphalangeal joint of the thumb is fused to provide a stable lateral pinch.

completely release the brachialis muscle. Approximately 50 percent correction of the deformity can be expected at surgery without causing excessive tension on the contracted neurovascular structures. Serial casting or dropout casts can be used to obtain further correction over the ensuing weeks.

Wrist and Finger Flexor Release. In the hand with no active motor control and poor sensibility, flexion deformities of the wrist and fingers can be obtained by release of the palmaris longus, flexor carpi ulnaris, and flexor carpi radialis tendons. The flexor pollicis longus tendon is lengthened and the interphalangeal joint of the thumb is stabilized with a Moberg screw. The finger flexors are lengthened using the superficialis-to-profundus tendon transfer (Fig. 30-21).

In the superficialis-to-profundus tendon transfer, the four superficialis tendons are first sutured together distally and then transected.[53,54] The profundus tendons are sutured together proximally and then cut. The fingers are extended, and the distal ends of the superficialis tendons are then sutured en masse to the proximal ends of the profundus tendons. This procedure allows for extensive lengthening of the spastic flexor tendons while still maintaining a passive tether should any extensor tone develop.

Several other surgical procedures are routinely done in combination with the superficialis-to-profundus tendon transfer. A neurectomy of the motor branch of the ulnar nerve is needed to prevent an intrinsic plus interosseous muscle deformity from developing.[54] A carpal tunnel release is done to decompress the median nerve. To prevent a recurrent wrist flexion deformity from occurring as a consequence of passive wrist flexion, the wrist must be stabilized. Wrist extensor tenodesis has been attempted but often the tendon will stretch out with time. A cock-up wrist splint can be worn, but patient compliance is poor. A fusion of the wrist in 15° of extension provides the most reliable means of maintaining hand position. A proximal release of the thenar muscles is often needed as well to correct a thumb-in-palm deformity.

Surgical Procedures for the Lower Extremity

The goals of rehabilitation must be established prior to performing any surgical procedures. The common goal is to prevent or correct spastic or contractural deformities in nonfunctioning limbs that could interfere with hygiene and nursing care.[59-61] Achieving the goal commonly requires surgical release of con-

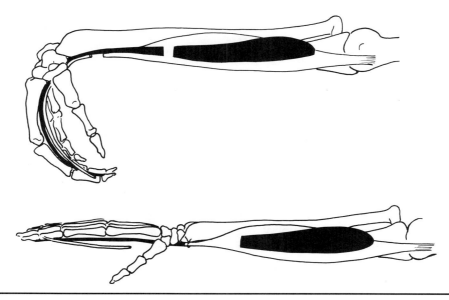

Fig. 30-21. The superficialis (white)–to–profundus (black) tendon transfer provides maximal lengthening for correction of a severely spastic wrist and finger flexion contracture in a nonfunctional hand.

tractures or neurectomy for relief of spastic muscles. In the patient with the potential for function, the rehabilitation program should stimulate the patient to use other neurologic pathways during therapeutic activities.

In the lower extremity, standing balance, limb advancement, and limb stability are needed for independent ambulation. Standing balance is the result of spontaneous neurologic recovery facilitated by therapeutic exercise. It correlates very closely with ambulation potential and is dependent on adequate motor control in the limb as well as intact proprioception.[62] Limb advancement requires functioning trunk muscles and hip flexor muscles. These are the minimal muscles required for walking. Limb stability is required during the stance phase to keep the leg from collapsing. The stability normally is provided by the hip extensors, quadriceps, gastrocnemius, and soleus muscles. Static positioning can provide stability as long as the patient can maintain the center of gravity posterior to the axis of rotation of the hip and anterior to the knee. Ankle stability can be provided by an ankle-foot orthosis.

The surgical indications in the nonambulatory patient who might be considered to have functional potential are those that improve positioning in a wheelchair and allow shoewear. Contracture releases may be valuable to ease nursing care of the patient.

Preoperative Evaluation

A careful and thorough preoperative evaluation is necessary for predictable surgical results. Clinical examination should include an assessment of balance, sensation, and the quality of muscle control in the extremity. Strength testing done by manual muscle testing is not appropriate in a spastic patient because of motor control difficulties. Local anesthetic nerve blocks that temporarily eliminate spasticity can be useful in previewing the results of the surgery and also can serve to identify which muscles are causing the major deformities.[26]

The most useful preoperative test is a dynamic electromyogram done with wire electrodes implanted in each of the muscles potentially causing deformity (Fig. 30-22).[41,61,63,64] The muscle data recorded during walking provide a complete picture of what each muscle is doing during each phase of the gait cycle. Armed with these data, the surgeon can plan the appropriate tendon transfers.

Definitive Surgical Procedures

Equinus Foot Deformity. Equinus is the most common spastic deformity causing gait difficulty (Fig. 30-23).[59,60,64,65] It results from the overactivity or premature activity of the gastrocnemius and soleus muscles. Surgical lengthening of the Achilles tendon is indicated when the patient's foot and ankle position is not adequately controlled by an orthosis or when attempting to make the patient brace-free. Adequate lengthening of the Achilles tendon can be performed using the Hoke triple hemisection technique percutaneously. Postoperative management requires 6 weeks in a short leg walking cast following by use of an ankle-foot orthosis for an additional $4\frac{1}{2}$ months.

Toe Clawing. Toe clawing, or toe curling, is a common accompaniment of overactivity of the gastrocnemius muscle. Toe curling is also caused by overactivity of the flexor hallucis longus and flexor

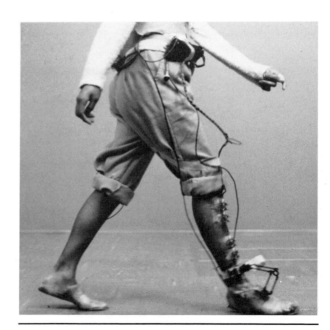

Fig. 30-22. Dynamic electromyography using wire electrodes during gait accurately identifies muscle action and aids in preoperative planning of tendon transfers.

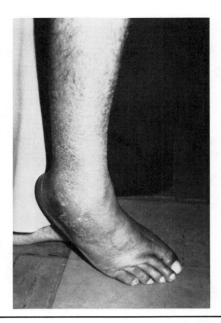

Fig. 30-23. A spastic equinovarus deformity is the most common condition causing gait problems in the brain-injured patient. The equinus deformity is caused by overactivity in the gastrocnemius and soleus muscles. The varus deformity results from spasticity of the tibialis anterior muscle.

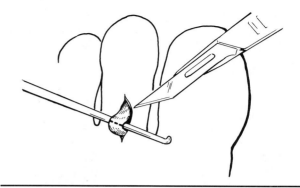

Fig. 30-24. The long and short toe flexor tendons are transected through small incisions at the base of each toe to prevent or correct spastic toe clawing deformities.

In approximately 10 percent of brain-injured patients the tibialis posterior muscle is also spastic and can contribute to the varus deformity. Clinically this is evidenced by the increased heel varus in addition to the forefoot varus caused by the tibialis anterior

digitorum muscles as well as the short toe flexor and occasionally the intrinsic muscles of the foot. The condition can be corrected by releasing the toe flexor tendons and intrinsic tendons through individual longitudinal incisions on the plantar base of each toe (Fig. 30-24).[66] Postoperative management consists of a soft dressing and immediate ambulation. This procedure is commonly done in combination with an Achilles tendon lengthening because bringing the foot into a plantargrade position will worsen the toe curling.

Varus Foot Deformity. Varus deformities occur as the result of overactivity of the tibialis interior muscle (Fig. 30-23). This deformity is corrected by a split anterior tibial tendon transfer (SPLATT), in which the lateral half of the tibialis anterior tendon is transferred to the lateral side of the foot and passed through a tunnel in the cuboid bone (Fig. 30-25).[59,60,64,65] The tendon is drawn through the bone channel and sutured to itself, holding the foot in a corrected position.

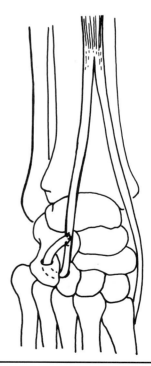

Fig. 30-25. The split anterior tibialis tendon transfer (SPLATT) is performed by transferring the lateral half of the anterior tibialis tendon through a passage in the cuboid bone to correct a spastic varus deformity.

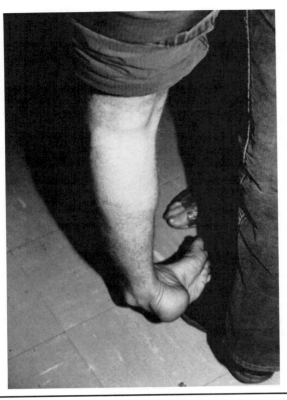

Fig. 30-26. When excessive heel inversion is seen in addition to the forefoot varus deformity, spasticity of the tibialis posterior muscle should be suspected. Lengthening of the tibialis posterior tendon should be done in combination with the SPLATT.

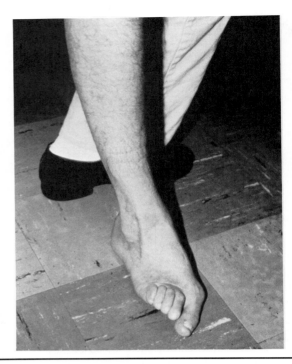

Fig. 30-27. Overactivity of the peroneus longus muscle can cause a spastic valgus deformity of the foot.

muscle (Fig. 30-26). When spasticity of the tibialis posterior muscle is present, a myotendinous lengthening of the tendon is performed posterior and slightly proximal to the medial malleolus. Complete release of the tibialis posterior tendon is not recommended because a planovalgus deformity may occur secondarily. Postoperatively the patient is placed in a short leg walking cast for 6 weeks, followed by an ankle-foot orthosis for an additional 4½ months. Most commonly the SPLATT is performed in conjunction with the Hoke lengthening of the Achilles tendon and a toe flexor release.

Valgus Foot Deformity. A spastic valgus deformity may be seen from overactivity of the peroneus longus muscle (Fig. 30-27). This can occur as an isolated deformity but more commonly is seen in combination with spastic equinovarus. In the "spastic combination foot" deformity, equinovarus is observed during the swing phase from premature and prolonged firing of the tibialis anterior and gastrocnemius-soleus muscles (Fig. 30-28A). The planovalgus deformity occurs during stance from the inappropriate activity of the peroneus longus muscle (Fig. 30-28B). The pronation deformity may be accentuated by a premorbid tendency to flatfoot or by the presence of an equinus contracture.

When spastic valgus deformity occurs in isolation, release of the distal insertion of the peroneus longus tendon is performed. When a combined deformity is present, a SPLATT is performed along with a tendo Achillis lengthening and toe flexor release to correct the swing phase abnormalities. The peroneus longus is released distally to eliminate the valgus force during stance phase. The peroneus longus tendon can then be transferred subcutaneously across the dorsum of the foot to the tarsal navicular bone to support the longitudinal arch of the foot during stance.

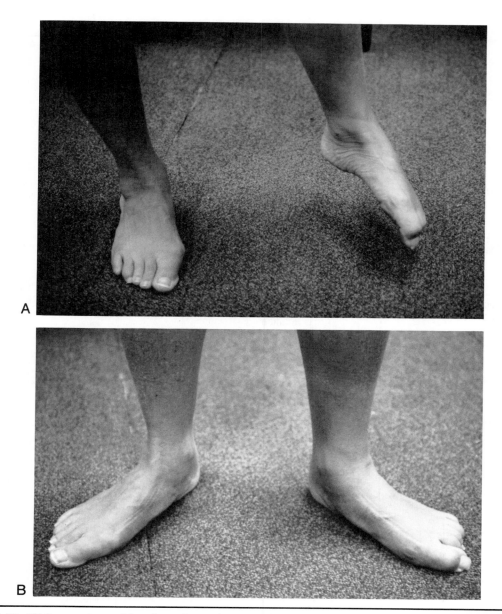

Fig. 30-28. (A) In a patient with a "spastic combination foot" deformity, an equinovarus deformity is seen during swing phase. This is caused by spasticity of the gastrocnemius, soleus, and tibialis anterior muscles. **(B)** In the same patient, a spastic planovalgus deformity is seen during stance phase from overactivity of the peroneus longus muscle. The planovalgus deformity may be further accentuated by the presence of an equinus contracture.

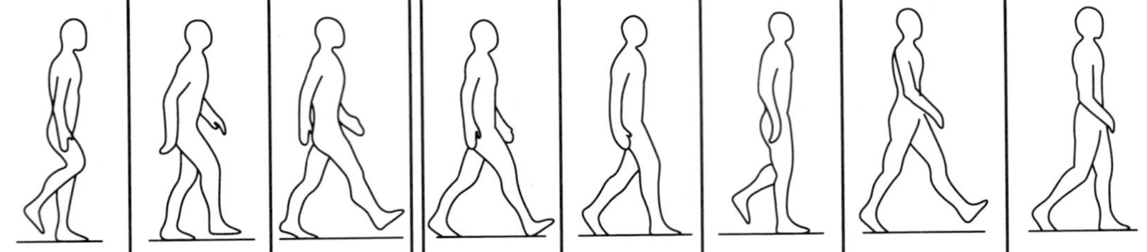

	Swing 40%			Stance 60%				
	Initial Swing	Mid-Swing	Terminal Swing	Initial Contact	Loading Response	Mid-Stance	Terminal Stance	Pre-Swing
Trunk	Erect Neutral	Erect Neutral	Erect Neutral	Erect Neutral	Erect Neutral	Erect Neutral	Erect Neutral	Erect Neutral
Pelvis	Level: Backward Rotation 5°	Level: Neutral Rotation	Level: Forward Rotation 5°	Level: Maintains Forward Rotation	Level: Less Forward Rotation	Level: Neutral Rotation	Level: Backward Rotation 5°	Level: Backward Rotation 5°
Hip	Flexion 20° Neutral Rotation Abduction Adduction	Flexion 20° to 30° Neutral Rotation Abduction Adduction	Flexion 30° Neutral Rotation Abduction Adduction	Flexion 30° Neutral Rotation Abduction Adduction	Flexion 30° Neutral Rotation Abduction Adduction	Extending to Neutral Neutral Rotation Abduction Adduction	Apparent Hyperext 10° Neutral Rotation Abduction Adduction	Neutral Extension Neutral Rotation Abduction Adduction
Knee	Flexion 60°	From 60° to 30° Flexion	Extension to 0°	Full Extension	Flexion 15°	Extending to Neutral	Full Extension	Flexion 35°
Ankle	Plantar Flexion 10°	Neutral	Neutral	Neutral Heel First	Plantar Flexion 15°	From Plantar Flexion to 10° Dorsiflexion	Neutral With Tibia Stable and Heel Off Prior to Initial Contact Opposite Foot	Plantar Flexion 20°
Toes	Neutral	Neutral	Neutral	Neutral	Neutral	Neutral	Neutral IP Extended MP	Neutral IP Extended MP

Fig. 30-29. In normal gait, the quadriceps muscles are inactive during the preswing period (initial contact of the opposite limb), allowing the knee to flex with the forward momentum of the body. (From Orthopaedic Knowledge Update-I. Neuromuscular Disorders and Gait Section. p. 74. American Academy of Orthopaedic Surgeons Publication.)

After surgery the foot is immobilized in a short leg walking cast for 6 weeks followed by an ankle-foot orthosis with an arch support for an additional $4\frac{1}{2}$ months.

Stiff-Legged Gait. A stiff-legged gait is defined as inadequate knee flexion during the swing phase of gait and results from overactivity of the quadriceps muscle.[41,67] Normally the quadriceps muscle is active in midswing and through the early stance phase (Fig. 30-29). In some patients the quadriceps is active during terminal stance and the early swing phase, which prevents the knee from bending. When knee flexion is blocked by this inappropriate quadriceps activity, the patient compensates by hip hiking and circumducting the leg, both of which are very energy-consuming gait deviations. Approximately 24 percent of patients will have a dynamic electromyographic pattern that shows inappropriate firing limited to the rectus femoris muscle. Another 16 percent will show inappropriate firing of both the rectus femoris and vastus intermedius muscles. In the remaining patients, all four muscles of the quadriceps complex are firing inappropriately.

When the premature activity is limited to the rectus femoris or vastus intermedius muscle, selective release of these muscles just proximal to the knee will improve knee flexion during swing while maintaining sufficient quadriceps strength for limb stability during stance (Fig. 30-30). A dynamic electromyogram is necessary to determine whether a patient is a candidate for surgery.

Knee Flexion Contracture. A knee flexion contracture is caused by overactivity of the hamstring muscles.[68] With severe spasticity of the hamstring muscles or a knee flexion contracture of greater than $60°$, attempts to correct the knee position with casting or bracing may result in posterior subluxation of the tibia. Distal release of the hamstring tendons does not prevent a patient from becoming ambulatory.

In a nonambulatory patient with a marked increase in muscle tone, hip flexor spasticity is frequently present also. If the hip flexion contracture or spasticity is not corrected at the same time as the hamstring release, a recurrent knee flexion contracture is likely

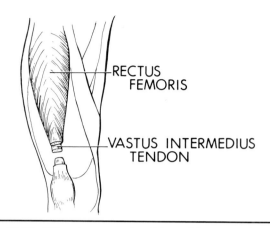

Fig. 30-30. When inappropriate firing of the rectus femoris or vastus intermedius muscle during the preswing period blocks knee flexion, release of these tendons above the knee will improve knee flexion while maintaining limb stability.

to develop, which is very resistant to surgical correction.

With the patient in the supine position, a longitudinal incision of approximately 8 cm is made on the lateral aspect of the distal thigh just proximal to the knee joint (Fig. 30-31A). The peroneal nerve is isolated and protected and the biceps femoris tendon is divided just proximal to its insertion using the electrocautery. The portion of the iliotibial band that is posterior to the axis of knee flexion is also divided transversely. A longitudinal incision is then made on the medial aspect of the knee and the tendons of the gracilis, semimembranosus, and semitendinosus muscles are isolated and divided (Fig. 30-31B).

Use of electrocautery allows the procedure to be performed easily without a tourniquet, which facilitates localization and protection of the posterior tibial artery, vein, and nerve. Following localization of the neurovascular bundle, any remaining restricting bands are divided as required. The posterior fascia at the knee is often thickened, limiting extension, and may require release. The posterior joint capsule is not released.

After surgery, the extremity is immobilized in a long leg cast. Approximately 50 percent correction of the

386 / Orthopaedic Rehabilitation

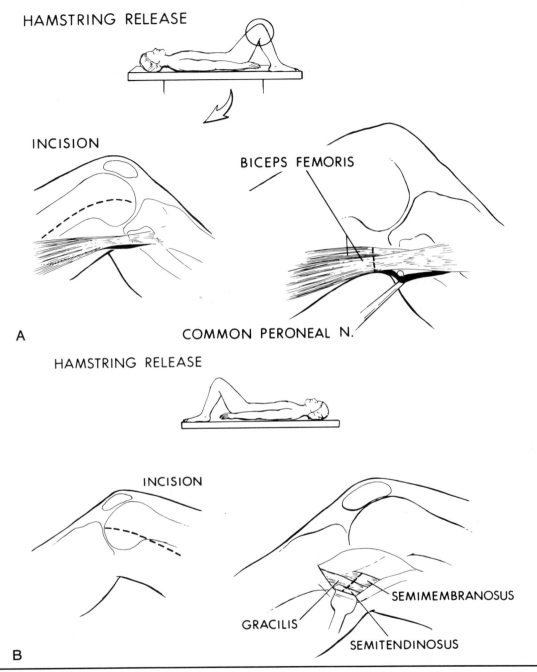

Fig. 30-31. (A) Using a lateral aspect incision, the biceps femoris tendon and iliotibial band are released to correct a knee flexion contracture. **(B)** The semimembranosus, gracilis, and semitendinosus tendons are released through a medial aspect incision on the contracted knee.

knee flexion deformity can be expected at the time of surgery. Further correction is limited owing to tethering of the neurovascular structures. The extremity is casted in the position of knee extension it assumes while being supported under the heel, without attempting forced extension. Forced knee extension can result in limb ischemia. The long leg cast is changed weekly until full knee extension has been obtained. Splints are used at night for an additional 4 weeks to maintain correction.

When a lesser degree of hamstring spasticity is present, a partial release or lengthening can be performed. The indications for hamstring lengthening are (1) overactivity of the hamstring muscles causing a dynamic flexion deformity of the knee or (2) a flexion contracture of 45° or less in a patient with volitional motor control in the leg. The procedure can be performed through medial and lateral incisions on the knee with the patient in the supine position as described for a distal hamstring release. Alternately, a single posterior incision can be utilized with the patient in the prone position.

The iliotibial band is released if tight. The tendon of the biceps femoris muscle is sharply transected over the muscle belly and allowed to slide distally to provide a myotendinous lengthening. In a similar manner, on the medial side the semimembranosus tendon is fractionally lengthened. The semitendinosus and gracilis tendons are transected or Z-lengthened.

A long leg cast is placed after surgery with the leg in maximal extension without force. The cast is changed weekly until full knee extension has been obtained. A night splint is used for an additional 4 weeks. Gait and transfer training can be started as soon as it is tolerated by the patient.

Hip Flexion Contracture. A hip flexion contracture or severe spasticity in a nonambulatory patient causing poor hygiene or decubitus ulcers that cannot heal because of limited positioning of the patient requires surgical release (Fig. 30-4).[58] An adduction contracture of the hip and a flexion deformity of the knee are commonly associated with a hip flexion contracture in the severely spastic patient. These deformities are common in patients with traumatic brain injury, stroke, cerebral anoxia, and multiple sclerosis. As

with any contracture, preoperative radiographs should be obtained prior to performing soft tissue releases to rule out the presence of heterotopic ossification or an underlying bony deformity that would prevent correction.

When a severe adduction contracture of the hip is present, it may be necessary to perform a percutaneous release of the adductor longus tendon in the groin to allow for adequate positioning of the patient and preparation for further surgery.

With the patient in the supine position, an anterior incision is made beginning 2.5 cm distal to the anterior superior iliac spine and is carried distally following the course of the sartorius muscle for a short distance (Fig. 30-32). The incision should not extend over the iliac crest because the patient will be expected to lie in the prone position postoperatively to gain further correction of the deformity. The lateral femoral cutaneous nerve is identified as it passes distal to the anterior superior iliac spine and protected. The sartorius muscle is detached from its origin on the anterior superior iliac spine. The rectus femoris muscle is released from its origin on the anterior inferior spine of the pelvic bone. The femoral nerve and vessels are gently retracted medially to expose the

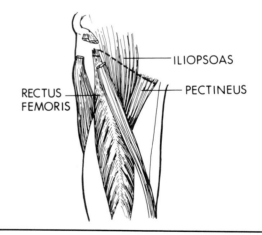

Fig. 30-32. A release of a severe hip flexion contracture is performed by transecting the rectus femoris and sartorius muscles at their origins on the ilium. The iliopsoas and pectineus muscles are transected over the pelvic brim to prevent reattachment and recurrence of the flexion deformity.

iliopsoas muscle on the anterior aspect of the hip. The iliopsoas and pectineus muscles are carefully divided over the pelvic brim using electrocautery to diminish postoperative bleeding. Because the iliopsoas muscle has capsular insertions, release of the iliopsoas tendon from the lesser trochanter of the femur does not provide a complete release. The tensor fasciae latae and the anterior portion of the gluteus medius muscle and gluteal aponeurosis may be released from the iliac crest if necessary. The hip joint capsule is not released.

In a patient severe with contraction, care must be taken to identify all structures prior to release because the anatomy is frequently distorted by the long-standing deformity. A large dead space is left after releasing the hip flexor muscles, and a drain should be used. Careful wound closure and a compressive dressing are helpful in preventing postoperative infection.

As with release of other contracted joints, approximately 50 percent of the deformity will be corrected at the time of surgery. Daily wound care will help prevent infection in this area, where bacterial contamination is likely and the large dead space increases the potential. Placing the patient in a prone position three times a day for increasing periods and gentle stretching exercises will assist in correcting any residual hip flexion deformity. When a release of a knee flexion contracture has been performed simultaneously, the weight of the long leg cast will also provide a correcting force. Sitting in a wheelchair is allowed for short periods.

Hip Adduction Deformity. A hip adduction contracture that interferes with nursing care and hygiene in a nonambulatory patient or causes excessive limb scissoring during attempted transfers and ambulation in a patient with active function requires surgical release.[58,59] In a severely spastic patient, flexion contractures of the hip and knee commonly occur in conjunction with an adduction contracture. As with any contracture, radiographs should be obtained prior to performing soft tissue releases to rule out the presence of heterotopic ossification or an underlying bony deformity that would prevent correction.

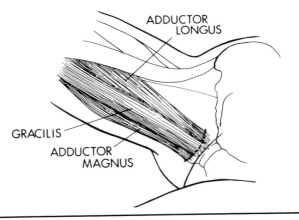

Fig. 30-33. A hip adduction contracture is released by transecting the origins of the adductor longus, adductor brevis, gracilis, and adductor magnus (anterior portion) muscles.

With the patient in the supine position, a longitudinal incision is made along the inferior border of the adductor longus muscle distal to the groin crease (to place the incision in a more hygienic location). A longitudinal incision is used to decrease tension on the wound edges as the leg is brought into a corrected position after surgery. The anterior branch of the obturator nerve is identified and transected. The adductor longus, gracilis, and adductor brevis muscles are released close to their pelvic origin using electrocautery to diminish postoperative bleeding (Fig. 30-33). The wound is closed over a drain.

Daily wound care is essential to prevent infection in this potentially contaminated area. The hips should be kept in abduction for 4 weeks using casts or an abduction pillow splint to prevent recurrence of the deformity during wound healing.

REFERENCES

1. Anderson DH, McLaurin RL: The national head and spinal cord injury survey. J Neurosurg 53:S1-S43, 1980
2. Baker CC, Oppenheimer L, Stephens B et al: Epidemiology of trauma deaths. Am J Surg 140:144, 1980
3. Heiden JS, Small R, Caton W et al: Severe head injury and outcome: a prospective study. p. 181. In Popp AJ (ed): Neural Trauma. Raven Press, New York, 1979
4. Jane JA, Rimel RW et al: Outcome and pathology of head injury. In: Proceedings of the Fourth Chicago Conference on

Neural Trauma: Seminars in Neurological Surgery, Chicago, 1980

5. Jennett B, Teasdale G, Galbraith S et al: Severe head injuries in three countries. J Neurol Neurosurg Psychiatry 40:291, 1977
6. Jennett B, Teasdale G, Braakman R et al: Prognosis of patients with severe head injury. Neurosurgery 4:283, 1979
7. Jennett B, Teasdale G: Management of Head Injuries. FA Davis, Philadelphia, 1981
8. Kraus JF, Black MA, Hessol M et al: The incidence of acute brain injury in a defined population. Am J Epidemiol 119:186, 1984
9. Groher M: Language and memory disorder following closed head injury. Speech Hearing Res 20:212, 1977
10. Hagen C, Malkmus D, Durham P: Levels of cognitive functioning. p. 87. In Rehabilitation of the Head Injured Adult: Comprehensive Physical Management. Professional Staff Association of Rancho Los Amigos Hospital, Downey, CA, 1979
11. Garland DE, Rhoades M: Orthopedic management of brain-injured adults. Clin Orthop 131:111, 1978
12. Garland DE, Keenan MAE: Orthopedic strategies in the management of the adult head-injured patient. Phys Ther 63:2004, 1983
13. Garland DE, Bailey S: Undetected injuries in head-injured adults. Clin Orthop 155:162, 1981
14. Stone L, Keenan MAE: Peripheral nerve injuries in the adult with traumatic brain injury. Clin Orthop 233:136, 1988
15. Keenan MAE, Kauffman DL, Garland DE, Smith C: Late ulnar neuropathy in the brain-injured adult. J Hand Surg [Am] 13:120, 1988
16. Orcutt SA, Kramer WG, Howard MW et al: Carpal tunnel syndrome in patients with spastic wrist flexion deformity. J Hand Surg 15A:940, 1990
17. Garland DE, Waters RL: Extremity fractures in head injured adults. p. 134. In Meyer MH (ed): The Multiply Injured Patient with Complex Fractures. Lea & Febiger, Philadelphia, 1984
18. Botte MJ, Moore TJ: The orthopedic management of extremity injuries in head trauma. J Head Trauma Rehabil 2:13, 1987
19. Booth BJ, Doyle M, Montgomery J: Serial casting for the management of spasticity in the head-injured adult. Phys Ther 63:1960, 1983
20. Braun RM, Hoffer MM, Mooney V, et al: Phenol nerve block in treatment of acquired spastic hemiplegia in the upper limb. J Bone Joint Surg [Am] 55:580, 1973
21. Caldwell CB, Braun RM: Spasticity in the upper extremity. Clin Orthop 104:80, 1974
22. Garland DE, Thompson R, Waters RL: Musculocutaneous neurectomy for spastic elbow flexion in non-functional upper extremities in adults. J Bone Joint Surg [Am] 62:108, 1980
23. Garland DE, Lucie RS, Waters RL: Current uses of open phenol nerve block for adult acquired spasticity. Clin Orthop 165:217, 1982
24. Garland DE, Lilling M, Keenan MA: Phenol blocks to motor points of spastic forearm muscles in head-injured adults. Arch Phys Med Rehabil 65:243, 1984
25. Katz J, Knott LW, Feldman DJ: Peripheral nerve injections with phenol in management of spastic patients. Arch Phys Med Rehabil 48:97, 1967
26. Keenan MAE: The orthopaedic management of spasticity. J Head Trauma Rehabil 2:62, 1987
27. Garland DE, Blum C, Waters RL: Periarticular heterotopic ossification in head-injured adults. Incidence and location. J Bone Joint Surg [Am] 62:1143, 1980
28. Copp EP, Keenan J: Phenol nerve and motor point block in spasticity. Rheumatol Phys Med 11:287, 1972
29. Khalili AA, Betts HB: Peripheral nerve block with phenol in the management of spasticity: indications and complications. JAMA 200:1155, 1967
30. Khalili AA, Harmel MH, Forster S, Benton JG: Management of spasticity by selective peripheral nerve block with dilute phenol solutions in clinical rehabilitation. Arch Phys Med Rehabil 45:513, 1964
31. Mooney V, Frykman G, McLamb J: Current status of intra-neural phenol injections. Clin Orthop 63:132, 1969
32. Moritz U: Phenol block of peripheral nerves. Scand J Rehabil Med 5:160, 1973
33. Wainapel SF, Haigney D, Labib K: Spastic hemiplegia in a quadriplegic patient: treatment with phenol nerve block. Arch Phys Med Rehabil 65:786, 1984
34. Wood KM: The use of phenol as a neurolytic agent: a review. Pain 5:205, 1978
35. Botte MJ, Keenan MAE: Percutaneous phenol blocks of the pectoralis major muscle to treat spastic deformities. J Hand Surg [Am] 13:147, 1988
36. Keenan MAE, Tomas E, Stone L, Gersten LM: Percutaneous phenol block of the musculocutaneous nerve to control elbow flexor spasticity. J Hand Surg [Am] 15:340, 1990
37. Keenan MAE, Todderud EP, Henderson R, Botte MJ: Management of intrinsic spasticity in the hand with phenol injection or neurectomy of the motor branch of the ulnar nerve. J Hand Surg [Am] 12:734, 1987
38. Keenan MAE, Botte MJ: Technique of percutaneous phenol block of the recurrent motor branch of the median nerve. J Hand Surg [Am] 12:806, 1987
39. Botte MJ, Keenan MAE: Reconstructive surgery of the upper extremity in the patient with head trauma. J Head Trauma Rehabil 2:34, 1987
40. Waters RL, Keenan MA: Surgical treatment of the upper extremity after stroke. p. 1449. In Chapman M (ed): Operative Orthopaedics. JB Lippincott, Philadelphia, 1988
41. Keenan MAE: Surgical decision making for residual limb deformities following traumatic brain injury. Orthop Rev 27:1185, 1988
42. Keenan MAE: Management of the spastic upper extremity in the neurologically impaired adult. Clin Orthop 233:116, 1988
43. Botte MJ, Nickel VL, Akeson WH: Spasticity and contracture: physiologic aspects of formation. Clin Orthop 233:7, 1988
44. Keenan MAE, Romanelli RR, Lunsford BR: The use of dynamic electromyography to evaluate motor control in the hands of adults who have spasticity caused by brain injury. J Bone Joint Surg [Am] 71:120, 1989
45. Boivin G, Wadsworth GE, Landsmeer JMF, Long C: Electromyographic kinesiology of the hand: muscles driving the index finger. Arch Phys Med Rehabil 50:17, 1969
46. Close JR, Todd FN: The phasic activity of the muscles of the lower extremity and the effect of tendon transfer. J Bone Joint Surg [Am] 41:189, 1959
47. Hoffer MM, Perry J, Melkonian DVM: Dynamic electromyography and decision-making for surgery in the upper extremity of patients with cerebral palsy. J Hand Surg 4:424, 1979
48. Long C: Intrinsic-extrinsic muscle control of the fingers. Electromyographic studies. J Bone Joint Surg [Am] 50:973, 1968
49. McFarland GB, Weathersby HT: Kinesiology of selected muscles acting on the wrist: electromyographic study. Arch Phys Med Rehabil 43:165, 1962
50. Samilson RL, Morris JW: Surgical improvement of the cerebral palsied upper limb. Electromyographic studies and results of 128 operations. J Bone Joint Surg 45:1203, 1964

51. Keenan MAE, Haider TT, Stone LR: Dynamic electromyography to assess elbow flexor spasticity. J Hand Surg 15:607, 1990
52. Keenan MAE, Abrams RA, Garland DE, Waters RL: Results of fractional lengthening of the finger flexors in adults with upper extremity spasticity. J Hand Surg [Am] 12:575, 1987
53. Braun RM, Vise GT, Roper B: Preliminary experience with superficialis to profundus tendon transfer in the hemiparetic upper extremity. J Bone Joint Surg [Am] 56:466, 1974
54. Keenan MAE, Korchek JI, Botte MJ, Garland DE: Results of transfer of the flexor digitorum superficialis tendons to flexor digitorum profundus tendons in adults with acquired spasticity of the hand. J Bone Joint Surg [Am] 69:1127, 1987
55. House JH, Gwanthmey FW, Fidler MO: A dynamic approach to the thumb-in-palm deformity. J Bone Joint Surg [Am] 63:216, 1981
56. Matev I: Surgical treatment of spastic "thumb-in-palm" deformity. J Bone Joint Surg [Br] 45:703, 1963
57. Botte MJ, Keenan MA, Gellman H et al: Surgical management of spastic thumb-in-palm deformity in adults with brain injury. J Hand Surg [Am] 14:174, 1989
58. Ough JL, Garland DE, Jordan C, Waters RL: Treatment of spastic joint contractures in mentally disabled adults. Orthop Clin North Am 12:143, 1981
59. Jordan C: Current status of functional lower extremity surgery in adult spastic patients. Clin Orthop 233:102, 1988
60. Smith CW, Leventhal L: Surgical management of lower extremity deformities in adult head injured patients. J Head Trauma Rehabil 2:53, 1987
61. Waters RL, Perry J, Garland DE: Surgical correction of gait abnormalities following stroke. Clin Orthop 131:54, 1978
62. Keenan MAE, Perry J, Jordan C: Factors affecting balance and ambulation following stroke. Clin Orthop 182:165, 1984
63. Waters RL, Frazier J, Garland D et al: Electromyographic gait analysis before and after treatment for hemiplegic equinus and equinovarus deformity. J Bone Joint Surg [Am] 64:284, 1982
64. Keenan MA, Creighton J, Garland DE, Moore T: Surgical correction of spastic equinovarus deformity in the adult head trauma patient. Foot Ankle 5:35, 1984
65. Roper BA, Williams A, King JB: The surgical treatment of equinovarus deformity in adults with spasticity. J Bone Joint Surg [Br] 60:533, 1978
66. Keenan MAE, Gorai AP, Smith CW, Garland DE: Intrinsic toe flexion deformity following correction of spastic equinovarus deformity in adults. Foot Ankle 7:333, 1987
67. Waters RL, Garland DE, Perry J et al: Stiff-legged gait in hemiplegia: surgical correction. J Bone Joint Surg [Am] 61:927, 1979
68. Keenan MAE, Ure K, Smith CW, Jordan C: Hamstring release for knee flexion contractures in spastic adults. Clin Orthop 236:221, 1988

31 Anoxic Brain Injury

REID ABRAMS
SARA WELLS-RAWSON

EPIDEMIOLOGY AND FUNCTIONAL OUTCOME

Although there are various causes of acquired anoxic encephalopathy in the child (e.g., asphyxiation, severe anemia, cardiac failure, carbon monoxide poisoning), this chapter discusses orthopaedic rehabilitation of the child with anoxic encephalopathy resulting from near drowning, because our experience with pediatric anoxia is primarily in nearly drowned children.

In a Los Angeles Children's Hospital study involving 94 patients, almost 90 percent of drownings occurred in children less than 5 years old. The overall incidence of drowning in the general population is 3.2 to 5.6 per 100,000 population, and it has been estimated the risk of drowning or near drowning is ten times higher in children 1 to 2 years old.[2,3] Consequently, this chapter focuses on the orthopaedic consequences of anoxic encephalopathy acquired at what is generally the toddler age.

Near drowning is defined as underwater submersion of sufficient gravity to warrant hospitalization that does not result in death within 24 hours. If the patient dies within the first 24 hours after the accident, this is termed *drowning*. This definition is sufficiently loose to account for the vast differences in prognosis seen in the literature.[1,2,5-8] Nevertheless, between 5 and 20 percent of nearly drowned children sustain severe anoxic encephalopathy (SAE). Although few long-term follow-up studies exist dealing with prognostic indicators and functional outcome in patients who sustain anoxic brain injury from near drowning, those that do exist show that functional outcome can range from no apparent neurologic deficit to subtle cognitive deficits to vegetative state.[8-10] Factors that correlate with severity of involvement are cold versus warm water immersion, length of submersion, whether the patient required cardiopulmonary resuscitation on arrival at the emergency room, initial arterial pH, Glasgow Coma Scale Score and brain stem auditory evoked potentials.[1,2,4-6,11]

Our long-term follow-up study from Children's Hospital and Health Center in San Diego is the only one of which we are aware that discusses the frequency of different functional levels of involvement in a defined population after long-term follow-up[8] (Fig. 31-1). Of those admitted with altered mental status or respiratory or cardiac arrest, 34 percent were discharged neurologically normal, 30 percent had SAE, and 36 percent died in the days after injury.[8] Among those who were neurologically normal, some have subsequently been found to have subtle cognitive deficits such as learning disabilities.[9] Of the patients with SAE, approximately 30 percent became ambulatory. All patients who sat independently by discharge (and a few patients who could not sit independently by discharge) eventually became ambulators. Ambulation occurred a median of 4 months after injury. All of the ambulators ate independently except one patient, who did not have the cognitive ability to do so.

The remainder of the encephalopathic patients were nonambulatory quadriplegics. Most of them were dependent sitters, with 20 percent able to feed themselves. Those who could not feed themselves required oral or gastrostomy feedings by a care provider. About half of the quadriplegic patients were vegetative (or responsive only to pain) and half had increased but variable degrees of responsiveness to their environment. It is of note that about half of the patients who were vegetative (or responsive only to pain) at discharge had improved their functioning by the time of average follow-up of 4 years. This improvement ranged from developing indications of

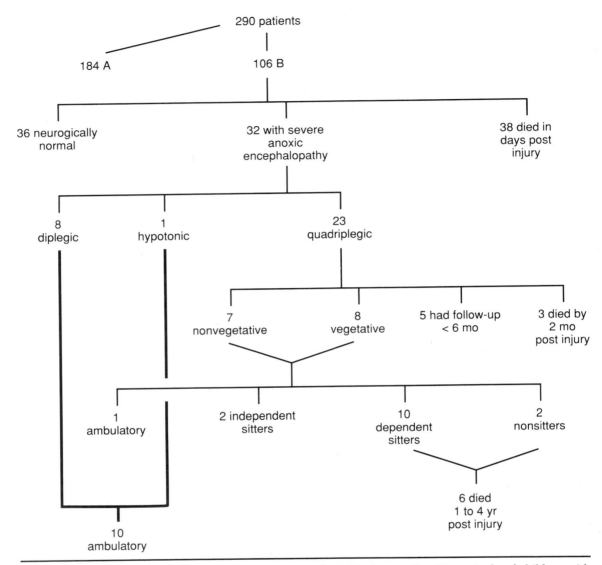

Fig. 31-1. Outcome summary of Children's Hospital and Health Center–San Diego study of children with acquired anoxic brain injury from near drowning. Group A: neurologically normal at discharge, 24 to 48 hours after injury or died within 24 hours; Group B: history of altered neurologic status, respiratory or cardiac arrest. (From Abrams and Mubarak,[8] with permission.)

awareness of surroundings (i.e., social smile) to the ability to feed themselves, drive an electric wheelchair, and use a computer communication device.

ORTHOPAEDIC PROBLEMS

The orthopaedic problems in pediatric anoxia are essentially the same as those seen in other pediatric spastic disorders, such as cerebral palsy and trau-

matic brain injury. These include soft tissue spasticity and contracture, hip subluxation and dislocation, spastic dislocation of joints other than the hips (such as radiocapitellar and shoulder joints), scoliosis, and fractures due to disuse osteoporosis. Heterotopic ossification has been conspicuously absent in nearly drowned encephalopathic patients in our experience. *The unique aspect of the pediatric patient with anoxic encephalopathy is the malignancy of the spasticity,* with

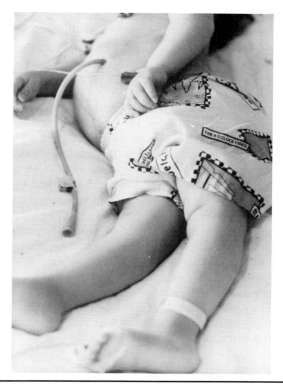

Fig. 31-2. Typical posturing pattern of a patient with acquired anoxic encephalopathy.

early opisthotonus and almost constant or frequent decerebrate or decorticate posturing (Fig. 31-2).

Treatment of a patient with acquired anoxic encephalopathy must deal with the acute, subacute, and chronic periods. The acute period occurs during the initial hospitalization, during which time medical stabilization takes place. The subacute period is the time during which neurologic recovery occurs. The chronic period is when the neurologic status and, more specifically, spasticity has somewhat stabilized. With some exceptions to be discussed later, irreversible surgery prior to neurologic stabilization is inappropriate. It is unclear when neurologic improvement plateaus, but this probably takes place about 1 to 2 years after injury. Some parents and care providers, however, have noted functional improvement up to 10 years after the injury. We are uncertain whether this represents actual neurologic improvement or a capacity for learning that results in increasing adaptation, or both.

When considering intervention in the pediatric patient with anoxic encephalopathy, especially one in whom the neurologic status has stabilized, the physician must individualize functional goals and care. Important considerations are: How cognitively intact is the patient? How is the patient's balance? Cognition and balance are major determinants for ambulation. Patients who do not at least have independent sitting or, more importantly, kneeling balance will be unlikely to walk. If the patient will not be able to walk, will dependent or independent sitting be possible? When sitting, can the hands be free for tasks other than maintaining upright posture?

In general, ambulatory patients have not had markedly disabling cognitive deficits, although exceptions have been seen. Upper extremity function has been good and has not required any operative intervention. In some patients, lower extremity function has been improved by operative intervention similar to that employed (with similar indications) for spastic diplegia from cerebral palsy. Significant hip dysplasia or scoliosis was not seen in the ambulatory patients we reviewed.

Extensive surgical intervention for the bedridden noninteractive patient must be considered cautiously. Goals should be realistic and are aimed primarily at enhancing custodial care and hygiene. This could also include facilitation of dependent sitting. In patients who have pain, this may entail maintaining reduced hips. However, extensive risky surgical procedures in the lower extremities and spine may not be appropriate in some of these children. For example, a recent study in scoliotic children with severe cerebral palsy showed minimal difference in respiratory status between operated and unoperated children. This suggests that factors other than theoretical risk of respiratory compromise must be considered in the decision to perform risky spinal surgery in these severely involved children.[12]

Quadriplegic patients who are more cognitively intact but have poor balance are candidates for dependent sitting. A dependent sitter will require wheelchair modifications and possibly surgical interventions to enhance positioning, decrease scoliosis, and maintain reduced hips. Sitting will make these patients easier to manage and feed and will enhance their disposition.[13] Some children with bet-

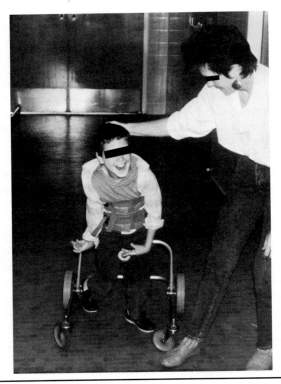

Fig. 31-3. A patient using a Mulholland walker who has balance problems and problems with selective control over his lower extremities, but who has good cognition and control over mass patterned movement.

ter balance can sit independently, although some require maintaining upright posture with their upper extremities. Again, wheelchair modifications can often free up the upper extremities for other activities. Some nonverbal patients with adequate cognitive function have used communication devices with their upper extremities.

In our experience, with quadriplegic patients, selective control of the upper extremities has not been sufficient to justify surgery to improve function and, in general, hygiene problems in the upper extremities also have not been significant enough to require surgical intervention. This must be individualized and, if the surgeon believes that upper extremity surgery may be of benefit, indications and procedures similar to those used in cerebral palsy would be recommended. Some quadriplegic patients have control over mass patterned motion of the lower extremities but still have poor balance. These patients can sometimes ambulate with a Mulholland walker (Fig. 31-3).

Ambulation occasionally can be optimized with surgical intervention, usually after neurologic status has plateaued.

MANAGEMENT OF SPASTICITY

It is usually spasticity that precipitates consultation of the orthopaedist during the acute hospital phase. Generally the patient is in the intensive care unit, only a few days after injury. If barbiturate-induced coma was used, spasticity begins shortly after the medication is discontinued and increases within several days (Fig. 31-2). The most common posturing places the shoulders in internal rotation and adduction, elbows in full extension or flexion, forearms in pronation, and wrists and fingers flexed. Hips are usually held in adduction and extension (or flexion), knees are usually extended, and feet are in equinus. Patients are frequently opisthotonic. Sometimes spasticity has been difficult to distinguish from contracture early on, because the tone can be so extreme that it often cannot be overcome.

Our approach to the management of spasticity has been to start with range-of-motion exercises with the notion that if the affected joint can be put through a full range several times daily, it will rarely develop a contracture. The most successful short-term reduction in spasticity and posturing has been observed with the techniques of proximal proprioceptive input at the shoulders and hips followed by truncal rotation. Some success has been seen with promotion of motion in a side-lying position. Slow movements or rocking in a dark and quiet room frequently reduces agitation and tone and promotes more success with range-of-motion exercises. However, in no other pediatric spastic disorder are physical and occupational therapists so frustrated, because, despite timely vigilant range-of-motion techniques, motion is almost invariably lost.

Serial casting is next in our armamentarium. This diminishes spaxticity by decreasing stimulation of the stretch reflex.[14] We have not, in general, used phenol nerve blocks in this population, but this may be a consideration in certain cases.[15-17] These blocks should not be used in mixed motor and sensory nerves owing to problems with dysesthesia.[15] Finally, surgical lengthening is used in patients with refractory spasticity or fixed contracture. In general, sur-

Fig. 31-4. The most common sites of soft tissue tightness seen at some time in the postinjury course in nearly drowned encephalopathic children.[2] (From Abrams and Mubarak,[8] with permission.)

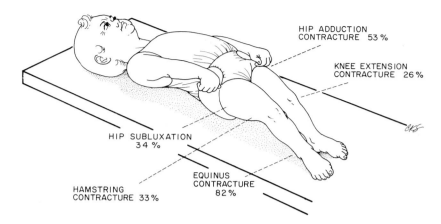

HIP ADDUCTION CONTRACTURE 53%

KNEE EXTENSION CONTRACTURE 26%

EQUINUS CONTRACTURE 82%

HAMSTRING CONTRACTURE 33%

HIP SUBLUXATION 34%

gery is reserved for the chronic period, although there are important exceptions.

Lower Extremity Spasticity

The most troublesome spasticity is in the lower extremities, equinus deformity being the most common (Fig. 31-4). Although serial casting is useful, up to 50 percent of patients have had skin breakdown.[8] Because timely tendo Achillis lengthening (TAL) has been a simple solution and has not been complicated by overlengthening in the population we studied, it has been difficult to justify open phenol nerve blocks to the gastrocnemius-soleus. The latter requires meticulous dissection of the motor branches to the gastrocnemius-soleus and is usually used as a temporary treatment until neurologic improvement plateaus. Tendo Achillis lengthening should probably not be done in a child before 1 year post injury. This is especially important in the ambulatory child. If the TAL is performed prior to the reduction in spasticity brought about by spontaneous neurologic improvement, excessive lengthening of the heel cord may occur, resulting in a crouched gait.

Other common areas of lower extremity spasticity are the hip adductors, the quadriceps, and the hamstrings (Fig. 30-4). Again, in cases of severe spasticity range-of-motion exercises have been unsuccessful, and in the face of quadriceps and hamstring spasticity these exercises have been complicated with femur fracture. Dropout casting has not been used owing to the cumbersome casts that would be required for the frequently simultaneous hamstring and quadriceps (and tendo Achillis) tightness. Abduction casting and

pillows have also been unsuccessful in the management of hip adductor spasticity. We have not tried obturator nerve block, and it may be a rational consideration because it has been useful in decreasing adductor spasticity in adults with stroke and traumatic brain injury.[16,17] In patients with less severe spasticity who are destined to become ambulators, conservative measures have been more successful and severe contractures have not developed. Frequently, with the aid of gait analysis, timely surgical procedures can be done to enhance ambulation after neurologic improvement plateaus. These usually entail TAL and distal hamstring lengthening, or occasionally tendon transfers about the foot (i.e., anterior or posterior tibial tendons).

Management of spasticity in the lower extremities in the nonambulatory child is aimed at preventing hip subluxation and enhancing sitting ability. We believe that hip adductor spasticity is an exception to the rule of performing lengthenings only after neurologic improvement plateaus. If the hips cannot be abducted to 45°, especially if there are signs of subluxation on radiographs, surgical lengthening is required because of the propensity for rapid hip subluxation in the patient with severe hip adductor spasticity (see later discussion). Hamstring lengthening in the patient able to sit is done proximally and can be performed through a groin incision usually at the time adductor lengthening is done. Psoas lengthening is also sometimes necessary. Caution is necessary because we have found a high rate of infection in these groin wounds. Proper postoperative dressings that protect against soilage are imperative. Quadriceps lengthenings distally have occasionally been necessary to improve sitting ability.

Upper Extremity Spasticity

Our approach for upper extremity spasticity has started with passive range-of-motion exercises. Usually casts or splints are necessary to maintain range-of-motion in the wrist and digits. We have not uniformly employed motor point phenol blocks to diminish spasticity (as is done in adult acquired spasticity) because theoretically its use in small extremities (in children 1 to 3 years old) may lead to significant muscle necrosis (i.e., in the case of motor point blocks in the volar forearm and pectoralis muscle).[18,19] Musculocutaneous nerve blocks could be a consideration, although significant elbow flexion spasticity has been rare. Among our patients, who ranged from very functional ambulators to the most severe quadriplegics, the number of patients requiring upper extremity procedures for spasticity at long-term follow-up has not been significant. No hygiene problems or problems with function amenable to surgical intervention were seen. Should such a case arise, our approach would be similar to that used for cerebral palsy. In the patient with a potentially functional spastic upper extremity, consideration must be given to aptitude, proximal positioning, sensibility, and selective motion.

Hip Subluxation

A more rapid hip subluxation and a higher incidence of subluxation are seen in children who have nearly drowned than in children with other spastic disorders[8,20] as a result of two factors: (1) the almost constant severe hip adductor spasticity in almost every patient, but especially those destined to remain quadriplegic, and (2) the time at which most near drownings occur, the toddler age, when the hip is easily influenced. We found subluxation or dislocation in 48 percent of our quadriplegic patients and in none of our ambulatory patients. Hip subluxation has been seen as early as 1 month and at a median of 10 months after injury in nearly drowned children[8] (Fig. 31-5). Hip subluxation is usually seen later in cerebral palsy by an average age of 7 years and, in traumatic brain injury, not before 1 year post injury (with a mean of 31 months).[8,20-23] Hip subluxation or dislo-

cation in encephalopathic nearly drowned children frequently occurs before the bony dysplastic changes usually seen concomitantly with subluxation in cerebral palsy.[8,24]

Because hip subluxation can be painful in the spastic patient and can lead to or exacerbate pelvic obliquity and paralytic scoliosis, and consequently hamper seating, we have been aggressive in management of spasticity about the hip (especially hip adductor spasticity). An anteroposterior pelvic radiograph is recommended 1 month after injury and every month thereafter during the acutely spastic period. Forty-five degrees of hip abduction is maintained. Soft tissue release is performed at the first signs of subluxation when severe spasticity or contractures occur. Varus derotational osteotomy (VDRO) is added for increasing subluxation. With dislocation, closed or open reduction and capsulorrhaphy are performed with VDRO and soft tissue release. If the acetabulum is deficient, acetabuloplasty is added[25] (Fig. 31-5). On occasion, in addition to hip adductor release, proximal hamstring and psoas muscle releases are indicated.

Scoliosis

In our follow-up study of the orthopaedic consequences of pediatric near drowning, scoliosis was seen in 18 percent of the patients.[8] This incidence is higher than that seen in pediatric traumatic brain injury,[20,22,26] and is also the same as or slightly higher than that seen in cerebral palsy.[27] Scoliosis develops more slowly than the problems seen in the hips. It is usually amenable to bracing, but posterior spinal fusion may be necessary about the time of the growth spurt, when curves have been noted to progress. Segmental instrumentation from the T2 vertebral level to the sacrum is recommended. Interestingly, during the early opisthotonic period, scoliosis was not seen. Opisthotonus may be protective owing to locking of the posterior facets. This has also been seen in children with muscular dystrophy who maintain a lordotic posture.[28] Radiographic follow-up on a yearly basis is appropriate until the growth spurt, when radiographs may be indicated every 4 to 6 months depending on the rate of progression. Clinical parameters are also useful in judging when radiographs are

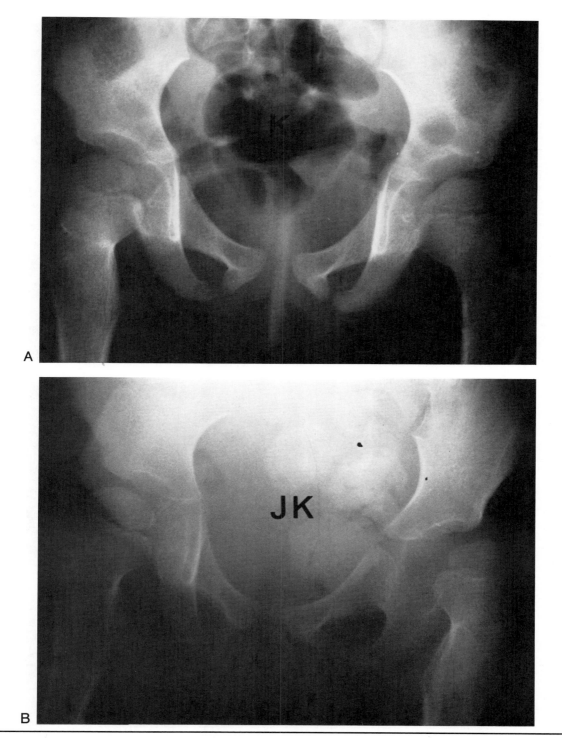

Fig. 31-5. An example of bilateral hip subluxation in a severely encephalopathic quadriplegic girl secondary to near drowning. **(A)** Pelvic radiograph made 2 weeks after near drowning (child is $3\frac{1}{2}$ years old). **(B)** Radiograph made 6 months after near drowning showing bilateral hip subluxation. *(Figure continues.)*

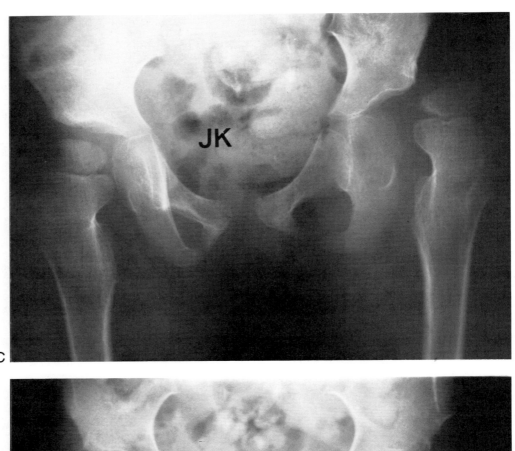

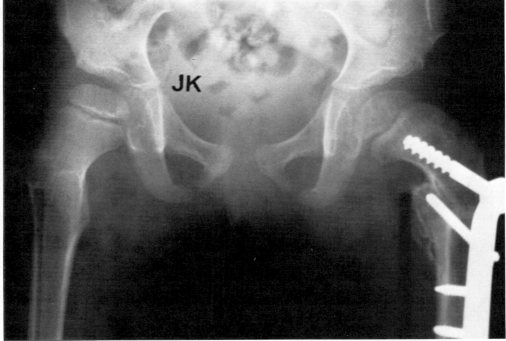

Fig. 31-5 *(Continued)*. **(C)** Radiograph made 9 months after near drowning showing right hip subluxation and left hip dislocation (preoperative). **(D)** Radiograph made 6 months postoperatively; bilateral hip adductor and psoas lengthening, left varus derotation osteotomy, open reduction, and capsulorrhaphy were performed. Earlier soft tissue releases would have eliminated the need for osteotomy and open reduction. *(Figure continues.)*

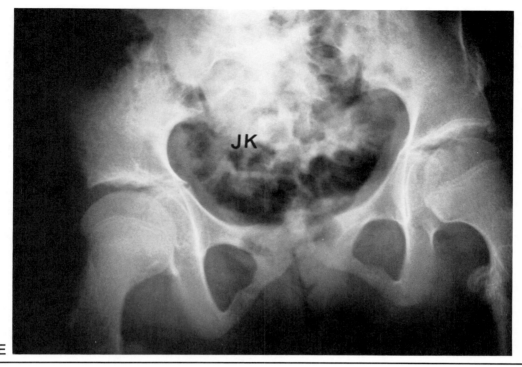

Fig. 31-5 *(Continued).* **(E)** Radiograph made 8 years after operation demonstrating hips concentrically reduced with normal acetabular development. (From Abrams and Mubarak,[8] with permission.)

indicated. Sitting or standing anteroposterior thoracolumbar spine radiographs are the most informative.

SUMMARY

Our experience with acquired pediatric anoxic encephalopathy from near drowning shows that approximately 30 percent of patients ambulate a median of 4 months from injury and the rest are quadriplegic. Independent sitting or better function by discharge from the hospital (usually 1 to 3 months after injury) indicates a good prognosis for ambulation. Of the quadriplegic children, about 66 percent were dependent sitters, and around 50 percent of them showed some awareness of or interactiveness with their environment.

Children with acquired anoxic encephalopathy (from near drowning) have a uniquely malignant type of spasticity. This form is characterized by frequent or constant decerebrate or decorticate posturing and opisthotonus during the acute period, which may or may not resolve as neurologic recovery plateaus (depending on the severity of the insult to the central nervous system).

The most significant orthopaedic problems include functionally disabling spasticity and contractures, hip subluxation and dislocation, and scoliosis. The rapidity of hip subluxation distinguishes these patients from those with other pediatric spastic disorders. Hip subluxation was present in 34 percent of nearly drowned encephalopathic children and in 48 percent of those who were quadriplegic with onset as early as 1 month (with a median of 10 months) after injury. This justifies an aggressive approach with maintenance of hip abduction, close radiographic observation, and early soft tissue release (even before neurologic recovery plateaus, if necessary). Spasticity and soft tissue contrature (other than of the hip adductor) are treated with range-of-motion exercises and serial casting, but often these are refractory, especially in the lower extremities, and frequently require surgical lengthening. The most common functionally disabling spasticity or contractures are in the lower extremities involving the heel cords, hip adductors, hamstrings, and quadriceps. Scoliosis has been seen in 18 percent of patients and is amendable to bracing but is progressive, especially at the growth spurt, and sometimes requires surgery.

REFERENCES

1. Dean JM, Kaufman ND: Prognostic indicators in pediatric near drowning: the Glascow Coma Scale. Crit Care Med 9:536, 1981
2. Rogers M (ed): Textbook of Pediatric Intensive Care. p. 721. Williams & Wilkins, Baltimore, 1987
3. O'Carrol PW, Alkon E, Weiss B: Drowning mortality in Los Angeles County, 1976 to 1984. JAMA 260:380, 1988
4. Allman FD, Nelson WB, Pacentine GA, McComb G: Outcome following cardiopulmonary resuscitation in severe pediatric near drowning. Am J Dis Child 140:571, 1986
5. Kruus J, Bergstrom L, Suutarinen T, Hyvonen R: The prognosis of near-drowned children. Acta Paediatr Scand 68:315, 1979
6. Peterson B: Morbidity of childhood near drowning. Pediatrics 59:364, 1977
7. Pearn JH, Bart RD, Yomaoka R: Neurologic sequelae after childhood near drowning: a total population study from Hawaii. Pediatrics 64:187, 1979
8. Abrams RA, Mubarak S: Musculoskeletal consequences of near drowning in children. J Pediatr Orthop (in press)
9. Children's Hospital and Health Center–San Diego long term functional outcome study (unpublished data)
10. Kalichman MA: The variability of "severe" deficits—functional outcome of survivors of near drowning. Orthop Trans, 10:149, 1986
11. Fisher B, Peterson B: Determination of neurologic recovery by brain stem auditory evoked responses after near drowning in children. Presented at the Society for Critical Care Management, New Orleans, June 4, 1989.
12. Kalen V, Conklin M: The effects of untreated scoliosis in severely involved patients with cerebral palsy. Dev Med Child Neurol 31(suppl 59):12, 1989
13. Rang M, Douglas G, Bennet G, Koreska J: Seating for children with cerebral palsy. J Pediatr Orthop 1:279, 1981
14. Zablotny C, Andric M, Gowland C: Serial casting: clinical applications for the adult head-injured patient. J Head Trauma Rehabil 2:46, 1987
15. Khalili A, Betts H: Peripheral nerve block with phenol in the management of spasticity. JAMA 200:1155, 1967
16. Keenan MA: The orthopedic management of spasticity. J Head Trauma Rehabil 2:62, 1987
17. Botte M, Waters R, Keenan M et al: Orthopedic management of the stroke patient. Part II: treating deformities of the upper and lower extremities. Orthop Rev 27:891, 1988
18. Casey J, Moore M, Nickel V: Spasticity: what to do when it becomes harmful. J Musculoskel Med 2:29, 1985
19. Keenan M: Management of the spastic upper extremity in the neurologically impaired adult. Clin Orthop Rel Res 233:116, 1988
20. Hoffer M, Garret A, Brink J et al: The orthopaedic management of brain injured children. J Bone Joint Surg [Am] 53:567, 1971
21. Samilson RL, Tsou P, Aamotg G et al: Dislocation and subluxation of the hip in cerebral palsy. J Bone Joint Surg [Am] 54:863, 1972
22. Hoffer M, Brink J: Orthopedic management of acquired cerebrospasticity in childhood. Clin Orthop Rel Res 110:244, 1975
23. Blasier D, Lets M: The orthopedic manifestations of head injury in children. Orthop Trans 11:43, 1987
24. Huang S, Eilert R: Important radiographic signs for decision making in surgery of the hip in cerebral palsy. Orthop Trans 9:87, 1985
25. Mubarak S, Mortonson W, Katz M, Wenger D: One stage surgical correction of the spastic dislocated hip: value of pericapsular acetabuloplasty to improve coverage. Submitted to JBJS Nov. 1989
26. Gillogly SD: Orthopaedic problems in head injured children and adolescents. Orthop Trans 11:43, 1987
27. Bonnett C, Brown J, Grow T: Thoracolumbar scoliosis in cerebral palsy. J Bone Joint Surg [Am] 58:328, 1976
28. Cambridge W, Drennan J: Scoliosis associated with Duchenne muscular dystrophy. J Pediatr Orthop 7:436, 1987

32 Extremity Fractures in the Brain-Injured Patient

SERENA YOUNG
MARY ANN E. KEENAN

Management of acute fractures in a patient who has sustained a brain injury can present a challenging problem for the orthopaedic surgeon. Initial resuscitation efforts can interfere with early diagnosis and treatment of extremity fractures. Diagnosis is further delayed if the patient is comatose or confused and agitated because the patient is unable to direct the physician's attention to a painful extremity or cooperate during a thorough physical and sensory examination. Once the injury is diagnosed, the appropriate treatment can remain uncertain because of poor understanding of the extent of brain injury and the prognosis. Inadequately treated fractures can present special problems, especially in the presence of spastic muscles. Spasticity can cause displacement of fractures that are treated with immobilization or skeletal traction.

GENERAL PRINCIPLES

Five basic concepts have emerged from several studies involving the management of adult brain-injured patients with fractures[1-3]: (1) anticipate the diagnosis, (2) expect good neurologic recovery, (3) anticipate uncontrolled limb motion, (4) avoid casting in a flexed position, and (5) avoid traction method.

Anticipate the Diagnosis

The prevalence of missed musculoskeletal injuries in the brain-injured patient is 10 percent.[4] Missed peripheral nerve injuries are found in as many as 34 percent of these patients.[5] A patient who has decreased cognition from a brain injury may be unable to direct the physician's attention to the injured extremity. Because delay in diagnosis can lead to suboptimal management of the fracture or nerve injury, initial radiographs should include anteroposterior (AP) and lateral views of the cervical spine and AP views of the pelvis, hips, and knees. Anteroposterior radiographs of the entire extremities in the comatose patient may screen for more discrete fractures. A high index of suspicion is needed for the diagnosis of peripheral nerve injuries. A common error is for the physician to assume that all neurologic deficits are the result of the central nervous system injury. Serial examinations as well as evaluation with electromyography can help with the diagnosis.

Expect Good Neurologic Recovery

Treatment should be based on the assumption that the patient who survives a brain injury will make a good neurologic recovery. The overall fatality rate for patients who sustain brain injury is 17 percent. Among these hospitalized, the fatality rate is 6 percent, but for those with severe brain injury it is 58 percent. Of the survivors, nearly 90 percent have a good recovery on discharge from hospital, almost 4 percent have moderate or severe outcome, and 0.5 percent remain in a persistent vegetative state.[6] Inadequately treated fractures may lead to long-term disability. An insignificant musculoskeletal disability for the neurologically normal person often is catastrophic to someone with permanent neurologic impairment, who may not be able to compensate.

Anticipate Uncontrolled Limb Motion

Closed treatment of fractures with slings, splints, casts, and braces may be difficult in a patient who is confused and agitated. Frequent appliance adjustments are required, as are checks for skin irritation and neurovascular compromise. Because of the difficulty of immobilizing the limb in a patient with agitation, stable internal fixation of the fracture is usually justified.

Avoid Casting Joints in a Flexed Position

Spasticity occurring after brain injury can cause joints to assume a flexed position. Although immobilizing joints in flexion can help align the fracture, this can result in a flexion contracture in the presence of spasticity. Open reduction internal fixation of a fracture should be seriously entertained if muscle spasticity is present. This would also allow for early mobilization and avoidance of prolonged bed rest.

Avoid Traction Methods

The use of skeletal or skin traction in confused and agitated patients may add to the difficulty of providing nursing care, may cause patients to injure themselves from poorly padded slings or malaligned ropes and weights, and will prolong immobilization. Traction is useful in the initial management of fractures by providing temporary reduction while the patient's condition is being stabilized for surgical clearance. Early stable internal or external fixation of fractures in the brain trauma patient can facilitate overall care.

ANESTHESIA

The risks of complications from general anesthesia in a patient who has sustained a recent brain injury are high. Monitoring the neurologic status in a patient who is comatose is difficult. Uncal herniation or decreased cerebral perfusion resulting in cortical ischemia can occur from hypercarbia or anesthetic agents that increase intracranial pressure during intubation.[3] Most neurosurgeons recommend that general anesthesia be delayed until neurologic status is stable or has not worsened over a 24-hour period. Cerebral

edema appears within 24 hours of injury. Maximal edema is reached 3 to 5 days after injury and usually subsides in 7 to 10 days. Most elective orthopaedic procedures may be undertaken safely at 10 to 14 days.

Major fractures should be treated with stable internal fixation as soon as the patient's medical condition will permit. Open fractures in a medically unstable patient should be treated with as much adequate débridement and irrigation as the patient's condition will allow. Further débridement and definitive fracture stabilization should be deferred until the patient's medical status stabilizes.

FRACTURE HEALING

Although brain-injured patients have a tendency to develop neurogenic heterotopic ossification, the overall rate of fracture healing is essentially the same as in the general population. Exuberant callus may occasionally occur from increased motion at the fracture site in an agitated patient who is thrashing about or in a fracture in which rigid internal fixation was not achieved.[7]

FRACTURE CARE

Upper Extremity Fractures

Upper extremity injuries are not as common as lower extremity injuries in the brain-injured population. The most commonly missed fractures are those about the shoulder girdle and the minimally displaced distal radius fracture.[3]

Shoulder Girdle

The most common injuries in the upper extremity are fractures about the clavicle and scapula and separation of the acromioclavicular joint. Standard orthopaedic care can be applied here because these injuries do not usually pose any significant problems. A high index of suspicion is needed to recognize an associated peripheral nerve injury. An underlying brachial plexus injury should be assumed until proved otherwise in a brain-injured patient with a flail upper extremity.

Humerus

Treatment of humeral fractures relies on gravity to hold the reduction. However, in a confused and uncooperative patient who is bedridden, the use of a hanging cast or coaptation splint may result in malalignment of the fracture. Skeletal traction can cause further damage to soft tissue and prolong bed rest in the uncooperative patient. Internal fixation either with a compression plate or with an intramedullary rod for humeral shaft fractures can facilitate early mobilization of the patient and prevent contractures. Open reduction can provide the opportunity for exploration of the radial nerve if injury is suspected.

Elbow

Three major problems result from injuries about the spastic elbow. These are (1) heterotopic bone formation; (2) ulnar nerve neuropathy; and (3) flexion contracture. If the elbow injury is treated with closed methods, the elbow should be casted in 45° of flexion. This position will help in preventing a flexion contracture if spasticity is present. Open reduction internal fixation is the recommended treatment, especially if the fracture is displaced or if there is intra-articular involvement. This will allow early mobilization as well as facilitate muscle strengthening and re-education.

Heterotopic bone in fractures and dislocations about the elbow (Fig. 32-1) is evident more frequently in neurologically impaired patients than in the general population and occurs in up to 90 percent of all injuries.[3,4] Early passive and active range-of-motion exercises for the elbow may minimize the formation of heterotopic bone.

Ulnar nerve entrapment in the cubital canal occurs frequently in the brain trauma patient. Nerve compression can be caused by heterotopic bone formation within the ulnar groove or by compression or stretch spasticity causing sustained hyperflexion of the elbow. Recognition of ulnar nerve neuropathy is usually delayed in this population because of impaired cognition and failure to call the physician's attention to the neuropathy. Clinical findings often include intrinsic wasting and clawing of the fingers. Electromyography and nerve conduction studies will confirm the diagnosis. Anterior transposition of the ulnar nerve is the treatment of choice. Resection of heterotopic bone often is required, even if it is immature, so that the nerve can be freed.

Forearm

The management of forearm fractures in the brain trauma patient can pose several problems, including difficulty in maintaining reduction, loss of supination and pronation, and missed or delayed diagnosis of compartment syndrome. Although nondisplaced fractures of the radius or ulna can be treated by closed methods, maintenance of the reduction may be difficult in the presence of spastic muscles or in an agitated patient. Open reduction internal fixation is the optimal method of treatment.

The prevalence of synostosis in the general population ranges from less than 1 percent to 8 percent, whereas in the brain-injured patient, the frequency is reported to be as high as 33 percent.[8] The cause of synostosis is multifactorial. The intersseous membrane appears to have intrinsic potential to ossify after central neurologic insult. Initial malreduction of the forearm fracture and delay in surgical intervention may result in callus formation across the membrane. Extensive soft tissue dissection during internal fixation may further potentiate ossification of the membrane. Minimal surgical dissection during operative reduction is highly recommended. Stable internal fixation not only allows for anatomic alignment but also enhances early mobilization, thereby minimizing soft tissue contracture and loss of range of motion.

Resection of the ankylosis is recommended only if neurologic recovery has returned enough so that some voluntary control is present in the involved extremity and the deformity is unacceptable. Otherwise, a large gain in motion is highly unlikely. Aggressive physical therapy and administration of indocin and diphosphonates are employed postoperatively.

A high index of suspicion is required for the diagnosis of compartment syndrome in the brain-injured patient. Frequent monitoring of muscle tenseness by physical examination and compartment pressure measurements will facilitate its diagnosis.

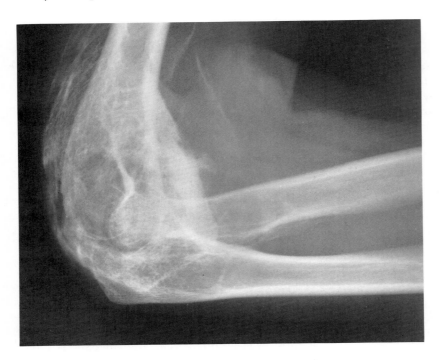

Fig. 32-1. Formation of heterotopic bone after a posterior elbow dislocation.

Distal Radius

Distal radius fractures are one of the most commonly missed fractures in the brain-injured patient, especially if there is minimal displacement. Problems resulting from this injury include malunion, limited supination and pronation, and median nerve neuropathy. Closed reduction and immobilization with a sugar tong splint or a cast that has been bivalved is recommended if acceptable anatomic alignment can be achieved. Special attention should be given to swelling and edema, which can cause constriction of the median nerve or compartment syndrome.

Median nerve neuropathy can be confirmed with electromyography and nerve conduction studies, because many of these patients may not be cognitively able to complain about dysesthesia or cooperate during a good physical examination. Release of the carpal tunnel and correction of the malunion with removal of any loose bony fragments that may be impinging on the nerve should alleviate the problem.

Associated distal radioulnar disruption (Fig. 32-2A) can result in limited range of motion and should be ruled out with adequate initial x-ray examination.

The treatment of choice would include open reduction internal fixation of the distal radius and reduction of the distal radioulnar joint (Fig. 32-2B). Resection of the distal ulna is indicated if the radial deformity is severe and pronation and supination are limited.

Lower Extremity Injuries

Pelvis

Fractures of the pelvis occur in as many as 50 percent of surviving pedestrians who are struck by motor vehicles.[9,10] These injuries can be serious, leading to uncontrolled blood loss. Associated injuries to the bladder or urethra can be evaluated with urinalysis and retrograde urethrogram. Sling or skeletal traction is not well tolerated in an agitated patient, and unstable fractures should be reduced with either internal or external fixation. This will allow early mobilization and facilitate nursing care. Stable pelvic fractures usually heal uneventfully.

Acetabulum and Hip

Hip dislocations and acetabular fractures in brain-injured patients pose several dilemmas for the orthopaedic surgeon. Approximately 10 percent of these

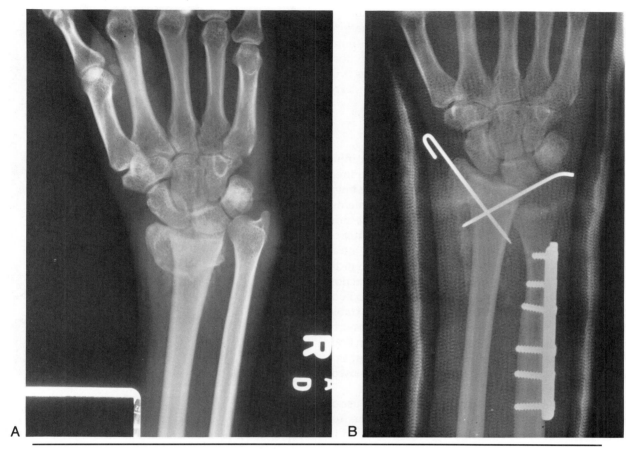

Fig. 32-2. (A) A missed distal radius fracture with disruption of the distal radioulnar joint. **(B)** Open reduction of the distal radius and fixation with K-wires was performed. Shortening of the ulna with plate fixation was required to prevent an ulnar plus deformity.

injuries go undetected.[10] The prevalence of heterotopic bone formation is high. Many of these fractures require traction, which prolongs bed rest and is not well tolerated in an incoherent patient. If open reduction internal fixation is performed, surgical dissection should be kept to a minimum because myositis ossificans is likely to occur. Whether open or closed methods are elected, early motion should be initiated to minimize the development of heterotopic bone. If the patient does not have voluntary control of the involved hip, indocin and diphosphonates should be employed, even if ossification has not appeared on the radiographs yet. Patients with selective control of the hip and without radiographic evidence of heterotopic bone should be followed closely. Patients who develop spasticity should be watched for

hip redislocation. Associated sciatic nerve injury should be suspected in a flail lower extremity.

Reflex sympathetic dystrophy can occasionally result from formation of heterotopic bone around the sciatic notch, causing mechanical compression of the sciatic nerve. If the ossification has not matured, as documented by decreased activity on bone scan and a nearly normal alkaline phosphatase level, a Bier block with lidocaine and steroid can be placed in the lower extremity. Other modalities such as transcutaneous electrical nerve stimulation (TENS) and aggressive physical therapy also should be employed. Lumbar sympathetic blocks can be used if the patient can cooperate.

Femoral neck and intertrochanteric fractures should be treated with open reduction internal fixation. Subtrochanteric fractures should be treated with intramedullary rods and locked proximally when possible. Stable internal fixation of these injuries will avoid prolonged traction and facilitate nursing care as well as early mobilization.[11,12]

Femur

Femoral fractures are the most common major injuries of the lower extremity. Stable fixation is required to control the fracture in the presence of spastic muscles that tend to rotate or angulate the fragments. Open reduction with extensive soft tissue dissection is discouraged because of the increased prevalence of myositis ossificans. The closed technique using intramedullary rods with interlocking screws when indicated is the treatment of choice. Skeletal traction should be used only as a temporary measure to hold the fracture until the patient is neurologically stable for surgery. Traction prolongs bed rest and is poorly tolerated by the agitated patient, and in addition both femoral shortening and angulation are common as a result of spastic muscles when this procedure is used.

If the patient is not a candidate for surgery, the use of a cast brace is a viable option. External fixators for open fractures should be employed with caution in confused patients because these patients can cause injury to themselves and to the nursing staff.

Knee

Intra-articular fractures in the distal femur and proximal tibia require restoration of the joint surface as in the general population. Internal fixation is the treatment of choice. Postoperatively, the knee should be cast in a neutral position to prevent a flexion contracture. A cast brace can provide protection and allow for early mobilization of the knee if internal fixation has been achieved.

Compartment syndrome can occur after internal fixation of tibial plateau fractures. This diagnosis often is delayed in a patient who is mentally impaired. Close observation with frequent pressure monitoring should be carried out. If extensive soft tissue swelling is present at the time of surgery, an adjunctive fasciotomy is recommended.

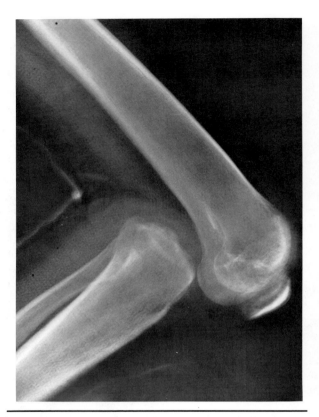

Fig. 32-3. Posterior knee dislocation occurred after the development of hamstring spasticity in a patient who had ruptured her posterior cruciate ligament in a bicycle-auto accident.

Early repair of knee ligament injuries in this population is usually not necessary. Postoperative immobilization requires that the knee be placed in flexion. However, if repair is performed on the spastic hemiplegic side, a flexion contracture can result from this position. Repair in the normal person requires intensive physical therapy and a high level of cooperation postoperatively. In a patient who is mentally impaired and who has difficulty with attention span, the problem is further complicated. Thus, in a brain-injured patient, cast immobilization is usually sufficient. If neurologic recovery occurs to a degree such that the patient is symptomatic, reconstruction surgery can be performed at that time.

Posterior cruciate ligament injuries should be observed closely because dislocation of the knee can occur if hamstring spasticity develops (Fig. 32-3).

Tibia

Tibial fractures are the second most common lower extremity injury in the brain-injured patient. Long leg cast immobilization with the knee and ankle in a neutral position is adequate treatment for fractures with a stable configuration. A patellar tendon bearing cast can be employed when the fracture has achieved partial union and can be adequately controlled. Union rate is 94 percent and occurs at an average of 5.6 months.[13]

Fractures with an unstable configuration are best treated with intramedullary rodding and interlocking screws. This will allow early mobilization of the patient and obviate frequent x-ray evaluation to ensure that displacement of the fracture has not occurred.

Open tibial fractures account for 50 percent of all tibial fractures.[13] External fixators should be used with caution in an agitated patient because these patients can injure both themselves and the nursing staff. A metatarsal pin should be placed in the first metatarsal and connected to the external fixator to hold the ankle in a neutral position. This will prevent equinus contracture.

The indications for early gastrocnemius or soleus muscle flap to provide coverage for exposed bone are essentially the same as for patients in the general population. The use of free muscle flaps with microvascular reconstruction should be delayed until the patient has achieved sufficient neurological recovery to be able to cooperate postoperatively.

The Ilizarov method to treat large bone defects in brain-injured patients should be used only in carefully selected cases. Corticotomy is performed either proximal or distal to the defect. Multiple transfixing wires are placed so that the corticotomized fragments can be slowly drawn away from each other to fill the bone defect (Fig. 32-4). Multiple problems have been encountered with this technique in the brain-injured population.

Spasticity is often present when there is central nervous system injury. Transfixing muscles from the Ilizarov wires can further potentiate the spasticity through a feedback mechanism. Thus, flexion con-

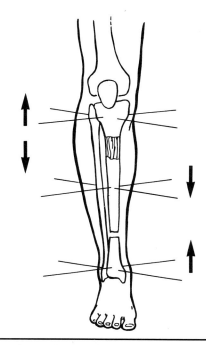

Fig. 32-4. A treatment technique utilizing the Ilizarov method to correct for a large bone defect in the distal tibia. A proximal corticotomy is performed. The tibial fragment is slowly lowered using Ilizarov wires, which are connected to a central ring. Once the gap has been filled, axial compression is applied to stabilize the pseudarthrosis and cause regeneration of bone.

tractures often result in the knee or equinus contractures occur in the ankle. Even with hamstring or tendo Achillis lengthening, these contractures can still recur. Premature ossification takes place in the intercalary segment, making it necessary to bring the patient back to the operating room for repeat corticotomies. The confused patient will often disassemble the external fixator. Thus, the Ilizarov method should be used only in a patient who is functioning at a high cognitive level and who has no spasticity or contractures, and the surgeon should be prepared to take the patient back to the operating room a number of times for repeat corticotomies if premature ossification should occur (S. A. Green, M.D., personal communication).

A high index of suspicion is needed to diagnose a peroneal nerve palsy in the brain-injured patient. The prevalence has been reported to be 17 percent.[7,13]

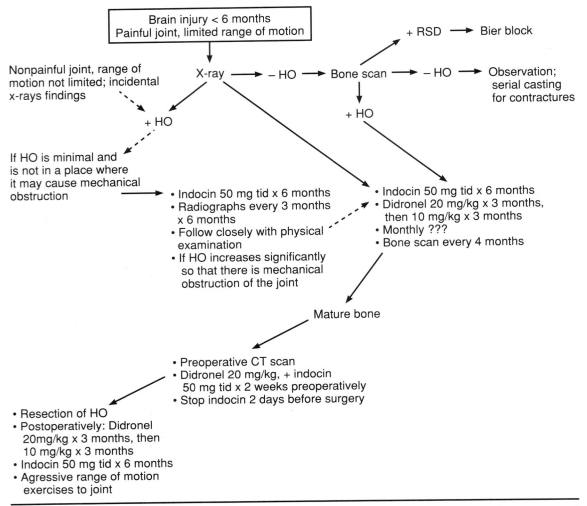

Fig. 32-5. Algorithym for work-up of painful joints or joints with limited range of motion in brain-injured patients. HO, Heterotopic ossification; RSD, reflex sympathetic dystrophy; AP, alkaline phosphatase.

Electrodiagnostic studies are often required to confirm the diagnosis.

Compartment syndromes of the tibia must always be considered, especially in the comatose or mentally impaired patient with a closed tibial fracture. Frequent clinical examination with aggressive compartment pressure measurements should be undertaken.

Ankle and Foot

Displaced or comminuted fractures of the ankle should be treated with stable internal fixation as in the general population to allow for early mobiliza-

tion. Stable fractures that are treated with closed methods should be in well-padded casts with the ankle in a neutral position.

HETEROTOPIC BONE

The prevalence of heterotopic bone formation is increased among brain-injured patients, especially in the presence of fracture dislocation of the elbow, forearm fractures, and acetabular and hip injuries. Heterotopic bone is rarely seen about the knee. When unexplainable pain is present, x-ray evaluation should be performed to rule out a missed fracture or the formation of heterotopic bone. If no fracture or heterotopic bone is seen, the physician should rule out reflex sympathetic dystrophy, which is present in 13 percent of this population, by obtaining a bone scan. Reflex sympathetic dystrophy can be treated with sympathetic nerve blocks or Bier blocks consisting of lidocaine and steroid.

If heterotopic bone is seen on radiographs and the patient is within 6 months of having suffered the brain-injury, a regimen of indocin (50 mg three times a day for 6 months) and diphosphonates (20 mg/kg body weight/day for 3 months and then decreased to 10 mg/kg/day for an additional 3 months) should be instituted. Resection of the heterotopic bone should be performed when it is mature as indicated by radiographs, bone scan, and a nearly normal alkaline phosphatase level. Aggressive physical therapy and the use of indocin and diphosphonates should be employed postoperatively for an additional 6 months (Fig. 32-5).

Because of the high rate of heterotopic bone formation in the presence of acetabular fractures, especially if internal fixation has been performed, patients who have spasticity on the involved side are empirically placed on a regimen of indocin and diphosphonates, even if there is not yet x-ray evidence of bone formation.

REFERENCES

1. Garland DE: Head injuries in adults. p. 257. In Nickel VL (ed): Orthopaedic Rehabilitation. Churchill Livingstone, New York, 1982
2. Garland DE, Rhoades ME: Orthopedic management of brain-injured adults. Part II. Clin Orthop 131:111, 1978
3. Garland DE, Waters RL: Extremity fracture in head injured adults. p. 134. In Meyer MH (ed): The Multiply Injured Patient with Complex Fractures. Lea & Febiger, Philadelphia, 1984
4. Garland DE, O'Hollaren RM: Fractures and dislocations about the elbow in the head-injured adult. Clin Orthop 168:38, 1982
5. Kraus JF, Black MA: The incidence of acute brain injury and serious impairment in a defined population. Am J Epidemiol 119:186, 1984
6. Garland DE, Bailey S: Undetected injuries in head-injured adults. Clin Orthop 155:162, 1981
7. Stone L, Keenan MAE: Peripheral nerve injuries in the adult with traumatic brain injury. Clin Orthop 233:136, 1988
8. Garland DE, Dowling V: Forearm fractures in the head-injured adult. Clin Orthop 175:190, 1983
9. Garland DE, Glogova SV, Waters RL: Orthopedic aspects of pedestrian victims of automobile accidents. Orthopedics 2:242, 1979
10. Garland DE, Miller G: Fractures and dislocations about the hip in head-injured adults. Clin Orthop 186:154, 1984
11. Garland DE, Rothi B, Waters RL: Femoral fractures in head-injured adults. Clin Orthop 166:219, 1982
12. Botte MJ, Moore TJ: The orthopedic management of extremity injuries in head trauma. J Head Trauma Rehab 2:13, 1987
13. Garland DE, Toder L: Fractures of the tibial diaphysis in adults with head injuries. Clin Orthop 153:189, 1980

SUGGESTED READING

Garland DE, Capen D, Waters RL: Surgical morbidity in patients with neurologic dysfunction. Clin Orthop 145:189, 1979

Garland AD, Chick R, Taylor J et al: Treatment of proximal-third femur fractures with pins and thigh plaster. Clin Orthop 180:86, 1981

Garland DE, Blum CE, Waters RL: Periarticular heterotopic ossification in head-injured adults: incidence and location. J Bone Joint Surg [Am] 62:1143, 1980

Green SA, Wall DM: The Ilizarov method transfixion wire technique. Mediguide to Orthopedics 8:1, 1989

Ilizarov GA: The tension-stress effect on the genesis and growth of tissues. Clin Orthop 238:249, 1989

Rhoades ME, Garland DE: Orthopedic prognosis of brain-injured adults. Clin Orthop 131:104, 1978

33 Spinal Cord Injury

DANIEL A. CAPEN
JACK E. ZIGLER

Trauma to the spinal cord results in a very specific set of symptoms and signs that create specialized patient care requirements. Spinal cord injury is the most disabling survivable injury that occurs to humans. It can be defined as a traumatically induced dysfunction of the spinal cord that results in a nonprogressive loss of sensory and motor function distal to the point of injury. This definition excludes paralysis resulting from diseases of the central nervous system, such as degenerative diseases, primary or metastatic neoplasms, or vascular diseases, because these conditions are not traumatic and most often are progressive. However, certain patients with a vascular anomaly, such as arteriovenous malformation, or with vascular accidents, such as a ruptured aorta or degenerative disk disease, may experience a sudden onset of nonprogressive paralysis as the result of the process or its treatment. These patients are treated as if they had a traumatic lesion. There is usually an associated injury to the spine, impairing its structural stability. Loss of spine stability and gunshot injuries are the most common causes of spinal cord injury. Effective management of the injury to the spine and spinal cord in the initial phases must recognize the interrelationship of these structures.

Two broad categories of spinal cord injury are recognized: complete and incomplete. A complete spinal cord injury is one in which there is no detectable sensory or voluntary motor function below the level of injury. The most significant feature of complete injury is irreversible functional loss occurs, except for root recovery. An incomplete injury is one with par-

tial preservation of sensory or motor function below the level of injury. Consequently, persons with incomplete injuries are capable of further functional recovery.

Injury to the spinal cord anywhere from the first cervical segment through the first thoracic segment produces sensory and motor deficits in all four limbs and is referred to as quadriplegia or tetraplegia. Injuries to the second thoracic segment and below spare the upper extremities and result in paraplegia.

PREVALENCE, INCIDENCE, AND CAUSES

Accurate prevalence and incidence figures are difficult to obtain, and published reports are few. To give a rough idea, the 1971 prevalence rate for persons with complete or partial paralysis as the result of injury was 0.8 per 1,000 population or 145,000 to 170,000 persons in the United States.[1]

The annual incidence of spinal cord injury is estimated at 25 to 35 injuries per 1 million population.[1] In one study in northern California, the incidence was 52.4 per million per year.[2] If subjects who were dead on arrival or who died immediately after admission to the hospital were excluded, the incidence rate was 32 per million per year.[2] In the same study, the case fatality rate was 48.3 percent, of which 79 percent of subjects died prior to arrival at the hospital. The case fatality rate for persons admitted to the hospital was 17 percent. In a survival study conducted on Veterans Administration Hospital patients, the 10-year survival for patients who survived the first 3 months was 86 percent for paraplegics and 80 percent for quadriplegics.[3] Studies indicate that survival

Supported in part by the National Institute for Disability and Rehabilitation Research Grant No. G008535134

411

for quadriplegics now approaches 80 percent of actuarial life expectancy and for paraplegics is 90 to 95 percent of actuarial expectancy.

The leading causes of spinal cord injury are motor vehicle accidents, gunshot wounds, falls, sports injuries (particularly diving), and water injuries.[1]

HISTORICAL PERSPECTIVE

Until World War II, little effective rehabilitation was even considered for victims of spinal cord injury, and most persons so injured died within a short time of injury. Dr. Donald Munro, who set up a unit at Boston City Hospital, reported in 1954 on results of 445 patients treated since 1930.[4] He emphasized that comprehensive rehabilitation could allow return of the spinal cord–injured patient to a productive life in the community. During World War II, more patients survived spinal cord injury, and Sir Ludwig Guttmann founded the National Spinal Cord Injury Center at Stokes-Mandeville, England. In large measure based on Guttmann's results, the concept of a comprehensive spinal cord injury center gained worldwide acceptance. In the United States, the Veterans Administration set up similar centers for American veterans with spinal cord injuries. The American system now has grown to 18 centers. With the support of the industrial accident insurance carriers, and more recently the U.S. Department of Health and Human Services and the National Institutes of Health, regional spinal cord injury centers have been established throughout the country. They all follow the principles established by Munro and Guttmann: that the care and rehabilitation of spinal cord–injured patients are best provided in spinal cord injury centers to which the patients are admitted for comprehensive treatment as soon as possible after injury.

Now, many regionalized spinal cord injury units are found throughout the United States. These centers are linked by an information network that facilitates a relatively standardized rehabilitation treatment.

GENERAL PHILOSOPHY OF TREATMENT

The basic treatment goals for spinal cord injury are to minimize functional deficits, prevent complications, and use all remaining function, both voluntary and reflex, to the maximum extent so that the patient can return in as short a time as reasonable to a productive life in society. It must be borne in mind that with modern care the spinal cord–injured person has a nearly normal life expectancy, and this potential should not be compromised to achieve short-term objectives.

The first treatment priority is survival of the patient; therefore, dealing with associated life-threatening injuries and conditions is essential. The second priority is to reverse, if possible, the effects of the injury to the spinal cord by immediate spinal realignment by halo, tongs, or other traction methods. It might be argued that this should be the first priority. However, surgical intervention can be delayed until life-threatening conditions are stabilized. Because there is no pharmacologic treatment that has been shown to be efficacious in reversing the neurologic deficit, appropriate stabilization and decompression of the spine is the only method currently available to facilitate neural recovery. The rehabilitation process starts early after the initial treatment.

The care of the spinal cord–injured person is complex and requires the skill of members from diverse professions. This care is best delivered by the team headed by a single responsible physician who has knowledge of all aspects of the care and rehabilitation of the patient. This essential body of knowledge is of a multidisciplinary nature, and no single specialty can legitimately claim primacy for the direction of the care. The leader of the team must appreciate and understand the roles of all the medical and allied medical specialists involved and treat them as professionals with needed expertise. There is no ideal team makeup, but representatives from at least the areas of general medicine, general surgery, plastic surgery, urology, neurology, neurosurgery, orthopaedics, physical therapy, occupational therapy, social work, psychology, and nursing should be included.

As soon as the extent and nature of the injuries to the spinal cord, spine, and other parts of the body are determined, it should be possible to establish a prognosis for survival and neurologic recovery. On the basis of this knowledge, therapeutic and rehabilitation goals can be established, and an estimate can be made of the time required to meet those goals. It is important to set this timetable as early as possible so that both the patient and the family know what to expect and can begin planning and preparing. These goals may be difficult for the patient and the family to accept initially and may require modification and change, depending on the patient's progress. Early treatment is directed toward preservation of joint range of motion and prevention of atrophy and deformity. Later treatment emphasizes enhancement of function and reeducation to deal with functional losses effectively.

EVALUATION OF THE PATIENT

General Care

The general examination with a complete history and physical examination is as important in the patient with spinal cord injury as it is in any other patient. A point to emphasize is that the neurologic injury may obscure or eliminate important findings usually relied on, such as pain, tenderness, and muscle spasm. The laboratory examination includes complete blood count; determination of blood urea nitrogen, sodium, potassium, chloride, calcium, phosphorus, and alkaline phosphatase levels; and determination of pH, oxygen partial pressure, and carbon dioxide partial pressure of arterial blood. The basic roentgenographic examination should include lateral radiographs of the entire spine, chest radiograph, and anteroposterior views of the injured area of the spine. The need for additional spinal radiographs is determined according to the level involved. In the cervical area in particular, oblique views and an open-mouth anteroposterior view of the C1 level are important for a complete examination of the cervical spine. Radiographs should be taken of an extremity with external evidence of trauma, abnormal or false motion in any of the long bones, or abnormal motion of any joint. If head trauma is also present, some examiners favor a complete skeletal survey by radiographs to avoid missing fractures.

A complete and accurately recorded neurologic examination is the single most important procedure in establishing treatment for the injured spinal cord. It serves as the basis for determining further diagnostic evaluation, treatment, prognosis, and planning of rehabilitation. The sensory examination is best recorded on an outline drawing or, in the emergency phase, directly on the patient. The baseline neuro-

logic examination will be important in formulating surgical planning because neurologic deterioration is an indication for emergency surgery.

Anatomy and Mechanisms of Injury

Figure 33-1 shows the major sensory and motor tracks and blood supply to the spinal cord. The anterior spinal artery supplies the anterior two-thirds of the central gray matter and the white matter anterior to the posterior horn. The paired posterior spinal arteries supply the posterior one-third, and the interconnecting circumferential arteries supply the narrow band in the periphery of the cord. Of particular importance is the fact that the lateral corticospinal tract and the lateral spinothalamic tract not only are in close anatomic relationship but also have a common blood supply. Therefore, sparing of pain and temperature sensation carries a favorable prognosis for further recovery of both sensory and motor function.

In experimental spinal cord injury, the first effects are seen in the gray matter, with decreased blood flow, decreased oxygen content, intra- and extracellular edema, and petechial hemorrhage. This process then evolves, with enlargement and coalescence of the hemorrhagic areas and cellular necrosis, and advances into the white matter. In complete injuries, the process extends to the periphery of the cord, and all neural elements in this area are destroyed. In incomplete injuries the same processes are seen but they are less intense and do not extend to the periphery of the cord. The fibers in the long tracts going to and from the sacral segments are located peripherally, which is believed to be the basis for sacral sparing as possibly the only sign of an incomplete injury. The entire process of hemorrhagic necrosis in experimental models evolves over a 4- to 8-hour period. However, the neurologic deficit is usually instantaneous. The process in the experimental model can be modified and ameliorated by a variety of physical and pharmacologic manipulations, such as cooling, myelotomy, steroids, and sympatholytic drugs. To date, however, none of these manipulations has been shown to work consistently for humans.[5]

Neurologic Examination

The first element of the neurologic examination relevant to the spinal cord injury is the determination of the level of the sensory and motor loss. In determin-

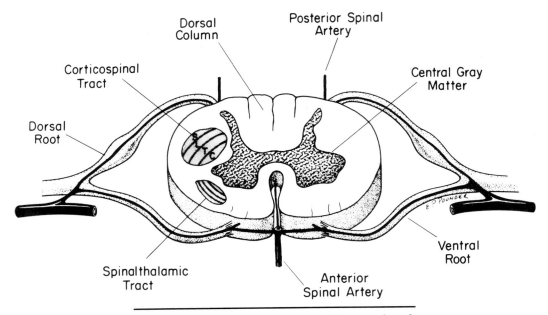

Fig. 33-1. Cross-sectional anatomy of the spinal cord.

ing the neurologic level, it is important to remember that segments C5 through T1 are not represented on the anterior portion of the trunk but are found only on the arms. If the level of injury is determined only by testing the trunk in any cervical trauma, the neurologic level will be found at the junction of the C4 and T2 dermatomes 4 to 5 cm below the clavicle. When doing this part of the examination, it is most convenient to place the patient's arms away from the sides of the body in the palm-up position. The testing is then done in the midaxillary line, moving across the axilla and then down the postaxial border of the arm, across the palm and up the preaxial border of the arm to the shoulder. In this way, each dermatome from T2 to C4 is crossed in succession. The accurate determination of the neurologic level, particularly in the zone between C7 and T3, is especially important because the corresponding segments of the spine are difficult to demonstrate by standard radiographic technique. It is often necessary to use special radiographic techniques, such as swimmer's views, oblique views, computed or plain tomography, and even fluoroscopic examination, to adequately visualize the spine in this area. The authors have seen on several occasions major dislocations in the C7, T1, and T2 areas missed because the neurologic level was not accurately defined and therefore the radiographic examination was not complete.

The next step is to determine if the injury is complete or incomplete. This may be obvious and already determined along with the level; however, particularly in extremely acute injuries, preserved function may be confined to sacral segments (the so-called sacral sparing). Only after careful examination of the perineal and genital regions has been carried out and checks for motion of the toe muscles and sphincter reveal no sparing can the patient be considered to have a complete injury. This examination should be repeated after satisfactory spine alignment has been obtained. The diagnosis of complete spinal cord injury depends on emergence from spinal shock, heralded by return of the bulbocavernosus reflex.

Table 33-1 lists the incomplete spinal cord injury syndromes, their major features, and their prognoses for recovery.[6] Several generalizations can be made. The earlier and more rapidly the recovery occurs the better the end result. Motor sparing carries the best prognosis for major functional improvement, followed by preservation of the pain sensation. It is common for a patient with a definitely incomplete injury to go as long as 3 weeks before the first signs of motor recovery are seen. Stauffer, in discussing prognosis based on neurologic examination, stated that in the presence of complete spinal shock as evidenced by a complete state of areflexia, the absence of sacral

Table 33-1. Incomplete Spinal Cord Injuries and the Prognoses for Recovery

Syndrome	Salient Features	Prognosis
Brown-Séquard syndrome (functional hemi-section)	Motor loss one side, pain and temperature loss opposite side	Good
Central cord syndrome	Usually cervical; all sensory motor functions involved; involvement greatest at level of lesion; greater sparing distally	Variable: spasticity and poor hand function
Anterior cord syndrome	Complete or partial loss of pain, temperature and motor function; touch and position sense spared	Poor for motor recovery unless pain sensation is spared
Posterior cord syndrome	Normal pain; temperature and motor loss; absent touch and position sense	Extremely rare
Concussion	Complete or partial loss momentary with rapid recovery	Normal within 48 hours

(From Bedbrook,[6] with permission.)

sparing may not indicate a complete lesion.[7] The bulbocavernosus reflex (reflex contraction of the anal sphincter on squeezing the glans penis or clitoris or tugging on the catheter) is usually the first reflex to return, often so quickly after injury that it can be questioned whether it was ever lost. Stauffer used the return of this reflex to indicate the end of the spinal shock phase and noted that, at this point, if there is no sacral sparing, the injury can be truly considered to be complete.[7] The experience at other centers may provide rare exceptions to this hypothesis, but we believe that the return of the bulbocavernosus reflex basically permits the examiner to determine that the patient's injury is complete. We have found, however, that some patients have spasticity with hyperactive deep tendon reflexes immediately after injury, and that these patients' injuries become incomplete, as evidenced by the appearance of sensory sparing even though initially there was none. Therefore, although we consider testing for the bulbocavernosus reflex an integral part of the initial complete neurologic examination, we have not been able to relate the presence or absence of this reflex to final neurologic outcome.[7-9]

For prognosis and to enable the rehabilitation team to plan the patient treatment program, we suggest that the functional diagnosis does have value. Although certain injuries are technically incomplete spinal cord injuries, it is clear that functional goals for the individual patient are quite limited. The anterior cord syndromes are associated with some sensory sparing but generally do not, except for root recovery, progress well with a great deal of functional return. In addition conus lesions with only minimal sensory function do not, as a group, have bright prospects for return of function. Although the team never takes

away hope of potential recovery, it is always best to make an optimistic but realistic rehabilitation plan for these patient groups.

Standard Radiographic Examination

The standard radiographic examination of the spine includes anterior, posterior, and lateral views of all spinal segments. All views should be obtained without moving the patient. In addition, oblique views of the cervical spine, which can be obtained without moving the patient by angling the x-ray tube 50°, are vital to determine the presence of unilateral facet dislocations, dislocations in the lower cervical and upper thoracic spine, and fractures of pedicles, facets, and laminae. Oblique views are of little value in the thoracic spine owing to superimposed rib shadow, but they may help to define some injuries in the lumbar spine. The open-mouth view for the odontoid fracture should be included in patients with head trauma or cervical spine injury. Computed tomography (CT) or polytomography aids in defining the skeletal injury, particularly if the standard radiographs are equivocal or if the spine is obscured by superimposed structures. Lateral views in flexion and extension should be obtained when static films fail to show an injury in patients with spine pain or neurologic deficit. These views, however, should be obtained carefully and only by personnel experienced in performing such studies in spine-injured persons, and usually under fluoroscopic control.

Neuroradiologic Examination

Magnetic resonance (MR) imaging is the most recent advance in neuroradiologic technique. This method can provide information concerning bone, disc soft tissue, and hematoma. Actual intrathecal lesions such as hematomyelia, necrosis, and hemorrhage can also be detected. MR imaging with or without computed tomography (CT) scanning is our preferred method of diagnostic study. Combined CT and MR scans have essentially supplanted the previously popular myelographic studies. Myelography in the acute injury is rarely indicated and, in our experience, nearly always reveals a "complete block" owing to posttraumatic edema.

CT of the spine, with or without the addition of water-soluble contrast material, can be helpful, especially in the subacute phase and when MR imaging is unavailable. The enhanced image shows both the spine and spinal cord and demonstrates fractures and other pathologic conditions that cannot be picked up on myelography alone.

The experience with MR imaging and CT technique in spinal cord injury is growing, and their proper role in the evaluation of such injuries is clear. These methods constitute the standard for spinal cord and spinal canal evaluation at present. Other tests that may be used are electromyography and evoked cortical potentials. In general, a careful neurologic examination will yield as much useful clinical information as these electrodiagnostic tests. The diagnostic studies may, however, distinguish between spinal cord and plexus or peripheral nerve injuries. They also have value in the evaluation of patients with altered states of consciousness when the usual neurologic examination gives unreliable information. Gas myelography combined with polytomography can demonstrate soft disc and bone in relation to neural elements but is rarely required.[10]

ACUTE MANAGEMENT

General Care

The general care of the acutely injured patient is directed first toward survival. The standard care applicable to any victim of trauma is given: frequent monitoring of vital signs, urinary output, arterial blood gases, serial hemoglobin and hematocrit, white blood count, and serum electrolyte levels. In our center, steroids are avoided because most studies fail to document beneficial effects. If steroids are employed it is critical to also provide treatment against potential gastrointestinal complications.

The patient must be repositioned every 2 hours to avoid decubitus ulcers. This can be accomplished in a regular hospital bed, even with the patient in traction, by log rolling from side to back to side. Specialized beds and frames may make this safer and simpler and require fewer personnel, but no single such device is universally applicable. Patients with injuries at cervical levels of C4 and above do not tolerate the prone position—because of their decreased ventilation fatal hypoxia can result. The Circoelectric bed in particular is thought not to be appropriate for acutely injured patients. These patients may have severe postural hypotension during turning; the gravitational loading of the spine during turning can cause displacement, and the pressure placed on the heels during rapid turning results in decubitus ulcers of the plantar surface of the heels. No turning device can substitute for good nursing care.

The leading cause of early morbidity and mortality is pulmonary dysfunction. Close monitoring of the pulmonary status by auscultation of the chest, chest radiographs, and arterial blood gas determinations will enable the physician to anticipate problems. Chest physical therapy should be instituted at once, with deep breathing exercises, assisted coughing exercises, and mechanical aids such as the incentive respirometer, intermittent positive-pressure breathing machine, and abdominal binders. In patients unable to mobilize their secretions, nasotracheal suctioning or therapeutic bronchoscopy may be needed. If it is necessary to use a mechanical ventilator, endotracheal intubation by the oral or nasal route is preferable to immediate tracheostomy. If the need for long-term ventilatory support is anticipated, elective tracheostomy can be performed 5 to 10 days after injury.

The prompt restoration of normal spine alignment and mobilization of the injured segments of the spine are the next priorities. For cervical spine injuries, these goals are best accomplished by skeletal traction, using either calvarial tongs or the halo ring. The halo ring has the advantage of being able to be incorporated into an orthotic device or cast. It provides rigid immobilization of the spine and allows early mobilization of the patient. Reduction of cervical dislocation should ideally be accomplished within 4 to 8 hours by increasing weights and close radiographic monitoring. Closed manipulation is not routinely practiced or advocated in the United States, in contrast to Australia and South Africa. If it is done, it should be carried out only by someone experienced in the technique. If reduction cannot be obtained by closed means, emergency open reduction should be performed unless contraindicated by the condition of the patient. If open reduction is performed, it should be accompanied by internal fixation and fusion. There is less unanimity concerning the handling of thoracic and thoracolumbar fracture-dislocation.[3,11-14] The postural reduction techniques advocated by Guttmann[15] have the greatest worldwide acceptance. In the United States, open reduction internal fixation using the Harrington instrumentation system, C-D system, or pedicle screw system is advocated. As an alternative, traction reduction via the pelvic band or the halo femoral traction can be effective.[16,17]

Life-threatening thoracic and abdominal injuries take precedence in the treatment plan, even over emergency spinal surgery. The treatment of associated extremity fractures makes use of the same general therapeutic principles applied to comparable injuries in the patient whose spinal cord is not injured, with two exceptions. Solid circular casts without extra cast padding should never be applied below the level of injury, and traction is difficult to manage, particularly with spasticity and the need for routinely turning the patient. Whenever possible, taking into consideration the type of fracture and condition of the patient, early open reduction and internal fixation will significantly simplify the care of the patient and the fracture. External skeletal fixation may be ideal for spinal cord–injured patients in that the method eliminates the need for casts and immobilization of adjacent joints. Therefore, it allows continual skin inspection and early range of motion of adjacent joints without the need for major surgical procedures.

The total program of rehabilitation begins on the day of injury. This includes accurate recording of muscle strength and joint range of motion, range-of-motion exercises several times per day of all paralyzed joints, and active exercises for the unparalyzed muscles. Resting splints should be fabricated for the hands of all quadriplegic persons, and they must be worn continuously except during exercise periods and inspec-

tion. The patient should be positioned to prevent the development of deformities, in particular equinus deformity of the feet and ankles, adduction and internal rotation deformity of the shoulders, and flexion deformity at the elbows. Whenever and as soon as possible, the patient should begin self-feeding and doing light hygiene activities, even though on bed rest and in traction.

Deep venous thrombosis and thromboembolic disease pose real hazards to the spinal cord–injured patient. The frequency varies widely, in large measure related to the criteria for diagnosis, but it has been reported to be as high as 80 percent. There is no standard accepted means for prevention in the spinal cord–injured patient, as in the rest of orthopaedic practice. The various preventive means advocated as beneficial range from frequent range-of-motion exercises through wearing of stocking and intermittent compression boots to anticoagulation with heparin or warfarin. The lethal potential of this complication is such that some measure should be taken for prevention and early recognition so that a massive, fatal, pulmonary embolus can be avoided. Despite best efforts at prophylaxis, there is still a low but definite incidence of fatal pulmonary embolus.

Early Urologic and Bowel Care

The accepted standard in most spinal cord injury units for bladder management is intermittent catherization. This means emptying the bladder at regular 4- to 8-hour intervals using an aseptic technique of catherization. The intervals of catheterization and the fluid intake must be adjusted so that no more than 500 ml of urine is allowed to accumulate in the bladder between catheterizations. If it is necessary to monitor urinary output closely or to give large amounts of fluids such as blood or plasma, the patient is best put on constant catheter drainage until these needs are past.

Reflex ileus occurs after most spine fractures and spinal cord injuries. The patient should not be given liquids or food orally until coordinated intestinal activity returns, as evidenced by passage of flatus and feces. If there is any tendency to abdominal distention, gastric dilatation, or vomiting, a nasogastric tube should be passed to decompress the stomach until coordinated intestinal function resumes. A daily program of suppository use is started with a small enema every 3 days if there is no result from the suppository, until a pattern of regular fecal elimination is established. This program is usually modified in a few weeks to one bowel movement every other day for both the patient's and the staff's convenience. This establishes a pattern that the patient should retain for life, with minimal risk of "accidents" between periods of bowel evacuation.

Skin Care

Routine pressure relief of insensate skin must occur at least every 2 hours. Nursing care for bed turning and patient education for wheelchair relief by cushion and raises are essential. When skin breakdown occurs, immediate attention must be given.

Consultative services by plastic surgeons who can provide flap coverage are often utilized during early rehabilitation. Also, some chronic care of decubitus ulcer will be needed in the group of patients who have excessive spasticity and contractures and who develop chronic ulcers about the pelvis.

SPINE STABILIZATION

The mechanical function of the spine is to provide a flexible axial support for the body in the upright position, and the goal of treatment is to restore this function. Support is provided by the combined effect of the vertebrae, ligaments, and spinal musculature. The keys are the osseous integrity of the vertebra and the continuity of its ligaments. The structural stability anteriorly is provided by the vertebral bodies, the intervertebral disc, and the anterior and posterior longitudinal ligaments. Posteriorly the facet joints, their capsular ligaments, the interspinous ligaments, the interlaminar ligamentum flavum, and the attached muscles provide the stability. The posterior complex is the key to alignment of the spine, because it is composed of the arthrodial or gliding joints that limit motion by their structure.

The spine when injured heals by three means: healing of the fractured bones, spontaneous fusion between injured vertebrae, and healing of the disrupted ligaments. Spinal fractures heal through the normal processes of fracture healing, which results in solid bony union. The spontaneous fusion between vertebrae occurs most commonly through the formation of new bone anteriorly between injured vertebra or across the disc spaces at the point of dislocation. These two forms of healing bring about the most stable form of union. The healing of torn ligaments is accomplished, however, by the formation of fibrous scar tissue. This fibrous scar often is not as strong as the original ligament and does not prevent abnormal mobility in the area of injury. When the healing process consists of only this type of healing, abnormal mobility or instability is frequently the result.

Late instability after spinal injury can take two forms. The first and most common is the result of a failure of the healing process, leading to persisting abnormal mobility in the area of injury. This is usually the result of inadequate immobilization during the healing phase or inadequate length of time of immobilization to allow adequate healing. The second form of late instability is progressive deformity in the area of injury. This results from healing in a markedly deformed position so that normal gravitational and muscular stresses produce a progressive deformity. Many cervical spinal injuries will heal if the patient is immobilized by bed rest and bracing in an appropriate position, with traction. This process is usually completed within 3 months and only rarely is the degree of damage and deformity so great as to prevent it. The primary exception is the ligamentous injury, is seen in cervical spine dislocations in which the resulting ligamentous scar is insufficient to prevent abnormal mobility. Many injuries are potentially chronically unstable owing to a combination of bony and ligamentous injury.

The current methods of treatment available are bed rest with traction, orthotic support, and surgical stabilization, which is usually accompanied by some form of internal fixation. Bed rest with or without traction results in stable healing in many instances. This, of course, eliminates the risks associated with surgery but, particularly in units not accustomed to dealing with acute injuries, increases the risk of such complications as pneumonia, atelectasis, decubitus ulcers, deep venous thrombosis, and restriction of joint motion. Orthotic support alone can provide immobilization of the injured thoracic or lumbar spine. The halo-vest or halo-brace combinations will immobilize the cervical spine sufficiently in many cases to allow healing without confining the patient to bed. When the skin underneath the orthotic device is anesthetic, there is a risk of pressure necrosis, but in patients with incomplete injuries halo-brace immobilization is an ideal nonoperative means of stabilization that allows early mobilization of the patient. Operative stabilization in properly selected patients will allow early mobilization of the patient, but these procedures should be performed only by surgeons experienced in such operations in spinal cord–injured patients.

Stabilization of Various Segments of the Spine

Cervical spine stabilization is classically obtained by the use of skull traction and bed rest. Turning frames help in maintaining spine alignment, but they are not essential. The traction device most widely used today is the Gardner-Wells tongs, which are easily applied and need no additional equipment beyond the tongs themselves. The halo can be used as a traction device in the same way as the tongs; later it can be attached to an orthotic device if indicated. The traction, in addition to immobilizing the spine, is used to reduce the displacement and deformity. Surgical stabilization can be obtained by anterior or posterior fusion, depending on the nature of the skeletal injury. The anterior approach is primarily reserved for cases in which decompression of the spinal canal is necessary. It usually combines resection of the fractured body and replacement with a fibula or iliac strut graft. If present, facet joint dislocations should be closed prior to anterior fusion, because it is difficult to reduce facet dislocations indirectly from the anterior approach.[18] The interbody types of fusions, such as the Cloward procedure used for cervical disk disease, are not appropriate for this class of injury, because they do not treat instability created by the fractured vertebral body. Posterior fusion is used to treat posterior instability. The posterior wiring and fusion technique is the procedure of choice with facet dislocations, either as part of open reduction of locked facet dislocations or as a stabilizing measure for a previously reduced facet dislocation.

For present purposes, this discussion of the *thoracic spine* is limited to the segments of the thoracic vertebral column. These segments' articulation with ribs attached to the sternum provides stabilization of vertebral segments themselves in addition to the intrinsic spinal structures. Of the three areas of the spine, this region is least frequently associated with spinal cord injury. When injured, it is usually by extreme and often direct force and is associated with injuries to the thorax and intrathoracic structures. The spinal cord injury in this region is usually complete and surgical intervention is indicated only extremely rarely. The bony injury is often complex: typically, it is one of multiple fragments that, despite a tendency toward gross displacement, go on to solid bone union. Therefore, injuries in this region of the spine stabilized by the ribs can be mobilized more quickly and rarely require surgical stabilization. If it is necessary, posterior fusion fixation with Harrington rods is the method of choice. Many injuries to the thoracic spine will achieve stabilization by nonsurgical treatment.

Injuries to the *thoracolumbar spine* — that is, the eleventh thoracic through second lumbar vertebrae — initially are the most unstable encountered. Most of these injuries are caused by a combination of flexion, rotation, and compression forces, resulting in the slice fracture-dislocation or burst fracture.[14] Either of these conditions can seriously disrupt the anterior and posterior bony and ligamentous structures. Prompt closed reduction similar to that used in cervical spine injury is more difficult, but recent experience with traction methods is encouraging.[16,17] The accepted closed method has been "postural" reduction, in which pads or pillows slowly correct the anteroposterior deformity but not the rotary or lateral deformity. Owing to the instability and difficulty in reduction, operative reduction through internal fixation has been advocated by a number of authorities.[6,7,15,19] Currently, the most popular technique is correction and internal fixation using Harrington distraction rods or the C-D system.[20] The rods should extend at least two segments above and below the injured segments, and autogenous bone grafts should be added for fusion. Compression devices are used to prevent overdistraction or for injuries with primary flexion deformity and intact posterior structures.

Surgical Versus Nonsurgical Stabilization

In considering surgical versus nonsurgical stabilization, several points must be weighed. Fractured vertebrae, like other bones, will heal if the fragments are in reasonable approximation and adequately immobilized for a sufficient time. Purely ligamentous injuries heal less well, but in most instances there is sufficient injury to the bone or periosteal tissue to stimulate spontaneous intersegmental fusion. Therefore, at least 80 to 90 percent of spinal injuries will heal within 12 weeks on a program of recumbent immobilization. Most spinal fractures and dislocations can be realigned satisfactorily by closed traction or postural means. The neurologic outcome has not been improved by surgical stabilization. The only clear difference is a shorter period of bed rest in the surgically stabilized group and a slightly shortened initial hospital stay.[20] In each instance, therefore, the physician must weigh the risk of surgery, the type of operation required, and the benefit expected from the reduction of the period of bed rest. Certainly, there is no clear advantage that would allow a statement that surgical stabilization is the preferred method of treatment.

PHYSICAL REHABILITATION

The Rehabilitation Team

The rehabilitation team is the keystone of the basic treatment team. Classically, it is composed of physical and occupational therapists under the direction of a physician who has primary responsibility for overall treatment of the patient so that all aspects of rehabilitation and treatment remain coordinated. Other members of the team are orthotists, driver training instructors, and other specialized types of therapists. The exact composition is determined in large measure by the institution and the individual patient needs.

Other members of the rehabilitation team — in particular, nursing personnel — play a pivotal role, because they have the closest and most frequent contact with the patient and must reinforce the newly learned skills, provide supervision, and, most importantly, insist that the patient use the new skills. Social workers, psychologists, and vocational counselors must be up to date as to the patient's potential and inform the team of specific therapy needs of which they may become aware.

The working relationships between the members of the team depend on the establishment of responsibility for the various aspects of rehabilitation. As in any team, all members must know their responsibilities and assignments. Usually this means assigning specific aspects to specific therapy groups or therapists, such as assigning dressing to occupational therapy and transferring to physical therapy. However, there can be no hard and fast rules in this regard, and much depends on institutional organization, training, and tradition. It matters little who does what so long as each job is done and the entire program is accomplished. Regular team meetings are essential to keep the patient's program coordinated and give everyone the opportunity to contribute expertise.

Rehabilitation Methods and Techniques

The first rehabilitation treatment goal is to maintain a normal range of motion in all joints. This is accomplished by proper positioning and range-of-motion exercises — active assistance for those portions of the body with functioning muscles and passive exercises for paralyzed joints. Therapy is started as soon as the patient is injured. Formal range-of-motion exercises by a therapist should be carried out at least daily, and more frequently if the patient has restricted motion or is developing restriction of motion. This problem is most apt to appear in joints with an unopposed major muscle, such as at the elbow when the biceps is of normal strength yet triceps function is absent. Range-of-motion exercises are supplemented by static positioning orthoses or other devices, such as blocks or pillows. These aids prevent deformity, particularly of the hands and wrists in quadriplegic patients and equinus deformity of the foot and ankle in all patients with paralysis of the legs. The patient is instructed as soon as possible in carrying out range-of-motion and other exercises.

The nursing team participates informally in range of motion by positioning the patient properly to prevent loss of motion and deformity. The patient in the side-back-side turning program should have the lower leg positioned in full extension at the hip and knee, and the upper leg positioned in full flexion at the hip and knee. This means that every time the patient is turned, these joints are carried through a full range of motion. A common deformity, especially in patients in turning frames, is internal rotation and adduction deformity of the shoulder. This can be prevented by positioning the arms in abduction and external rotation through part of the day.

The modalities of heat, cold, ultrasound, and diathermy play a small role in rehabilitating the spinal cord–injured patient. Extreme care must be exercised when these treatment methods are used in areas of reduced sensation so as not to injure the patient. The primary value of these methods is to relieve pain and spasm and to gain the patient's cooperation in the range-of-motion program. No one technique is clearly superior to the others, and different modalities may be effective in different patients with the same problem.

Prescribing appropriate orthotic devices and equipment is one of the most important aspects in rehabilitation of the spinal cord–injured person. The proper equipment can make the patient more independent, make employment possible, and improve the quality of life.

The single most important item for most patients is the wheelchair. The basic objective must be to keep the chair as light and narrow as possible. The back height should be adjusted to align just below the point of the scapula so it will not interfere with pushing. The seat depth is measured to make the front edge 5 cm proximal to the popliteal crease, and the foot rests are adjusted so that the knees are slightly lower than the hips. This increases the weight carried by the thighs, takes weight off the ischial region, and distributes the weight over the greatest possible surface, all of which help decrease the risk of ischial decubitus ulcers. Manual propulsion is feasible for most patients with functional levels below C6, although modifications of the rims may be needed for the quadriplegic patient. High backs and reclining backs are rarely needed, and then only for patients with functional levels at C4 and above.

Motorized wheelchairs are needed for most patients with functional levels of C5 and higher. The best controller is the proportional hand or joystick control. Nonproportional control may be needed in patients with poor arm control, spasticity, or involuntary movements. Chin control would be adequate for the majority of patients unable to use hand controls, but some patients may require other means, such as the tongue switch, puff and sip, or more sophisticated control mechanisms.

A proper cushion is equally vital. No cushion exists that completely prevents decubitus ulcers. The patient or the care providers must periodically relieve the weight on the sitting surfaces or decubitus ulcers will develop. The most satisfactory cushion remains the 7.5- to 10-cm thick, latex, pin core, foam rubber variety. Other cushions of special materials, construction, or configuration may be needed in special circumstances — in particular, for those patients with scars from previous decubitus ulcers or fixed deformities.

Patients with functional levels between C5 and C7 may benefit from a functional hand orthosis. The two most useful such orthoses are the wrist-driven, flexor-hinge hand splint for those with functioning wrist extensors, and the ratchet hand splint for patients without wrist extensor function. The ratchet splint is a modification of the wrist-driven splint, giving passive prehension by means of a one-way ratchet.

Paraplegics with functional levels below L1 and L2 may achieve functional ambulation with the use of lower limb orthoses. For limbs without knee, ankle, or foot control, the long leg brace or a knee-ankle-foot orthosis (KAFO) will be needed. Essential features of this brace are the rigid foot-ankle unit and either a drop lock or bail lock knee unit. The Scott Craig orthosis is one of the most satisfactory forms of KAFO. It is rare for a patient who requires bilateral KAFOs to become functionally ambulatory. For a limb with knee control but with little or no foot or ankle control, a short leg brace or ankle-foot orthosis (AFO) is needed. The molded plastic insert orthoses are very satisfactory in these instances. Patients who require a KAFO on one side and an AFO on the other or bilateral AFOs will frequently become functionally ambulatory.

Table 33-2. Functional Goals of Spinal Cord–Damaged Patients by Level of Injury

Functional Spinal Cord Level	Muscle Function	Functional Goals
C4	Neck control	Manipulate electric wheelchair with devices
	Scapular elevators	Mouth stick (communication)
		Use environmental controls
C5	Partial shoulder control	Independent in light hygiene and feeding activities with devices
	Partial elbow flexion	Propel wheelchair with assistive devices or electric wheelchair
		Swivel bar transfer
		Adapted sports: swimming, archery, bowling
C6	Shoulder control	Independent in dressing activities
	Elbow flexion	Independent in transfer activities, car, and bed
	Wrist extension	Driving with adapted equipment
	Supinators	Adapted sports: track and field, table tennis
C7 and C8	Shoulder depression	Independent in eating without adapted devices
	Elbow extension	Independent in application of condom drainage
	Some hand function	Independent transfers—car, bed, commode chair, or tub stool
		Assisted bowel care
T1–T5	Normal upper extremity muscle function	Total wheelchair independence
		Independent transfers—wheelchair to tub
		Move from wheelchair to floor and back
		Assisted standing activities
		All wheelchair sports
T6–T10	Partial trunk stability	Exercise ambulation with bilateral long leg brace and crutches
T11–L1	Trunk stability	Possible household ambulation
L2	Hip flexors	Household ambulation
L3–L4	Adductors, quadriceps	Community ambulation
L5–S2	Hip extensors, abductors	Community ambulation
	Knee flexors	
	Ankle control	

Patient and family teaching is an essential part of the rehabilitation. Patients should become the experts in their own care. Even if they are unable to carry it out themselves, they should be able to instruct others in their care. Family members should also be instructed in this care, particularly for the more dependent patient. Typical complications, such as decubitus ulcers, contractures, and bowel and bladder problems, can be prevented by a knowledgeable patient and family.

Table 33-2 lists the goals for the average spinal cord–injured patient according to functional level, and the equipment that helps the patient meet and sustain those functional expectations. As soon as the patient's functional level has become stable, the goals should be set and explained to the patient, and a timetable should be established to meet the goals. However, every person is an individual, and the table lists only average expectations. Age-associated problems body size, and development may modify these goals for given patients. The goals are based on the functional level at the time the rehabilitation program is instituted, not on some vague expectation of future recovery. If the functional level improves, the goals can be changed to meet the new conditions.[13]

Bladder Rehabilitation

The goals of bladder rehabilitation are achieving adequate bladder emptying, either reflexively or by external pressure, and avoiding chronic urinary tract infection. The technique that best meets these objectives is bladder retraining by intermittent catheterization. This is started in the acute phase at 4- to 6-hour intervals. When the patient begins to void, the intervals between catheterizations can be increased and the fluid restrictions relaxed. The bladder is considered balanced when the postvoiding residuals are less than 100 to 150 ml and the emptying is achieved without high intravesical pressure. A urologist experienced in the care of the neurogenic bladder is a vital member of the team.

Bowel rehabilitation is started immediately after the injury to establish the regular pattern of bowel evacuation. Suppositories and rectal stimulation are the usual means of achieving evacuation. The best schedule to strive for is bowel evacuation every day or every other day at the same time of day (usually following a meal) to take advantage of normal gastrocolic reflexes. A stool softener or lubricator, such as dioctyl sodium sulfosuccinate (Colace), helps maintain proper consistency and on occasion a mild laxative, such as milk of magnesia or concentrated prune juice, will help facilitate regular evacuation. There is significant individual variation, but once an effective program is established, it should be strictly adhered to.

PSYCHOSOCIAL AND VOCATIONAL REHABILITATION

Effective psychosocial rehabilitation is as essential as aggressive physical rehabilitation for spinal cord – injured patients to retain and maintain their maximum potential. Patients who cannot accept injury and disability and cannot see themselves as valuable members of society and who will not cooperate in the rehabilitation process or take care of themselves will develop a never-ending series of complications. Psychosocial rehabilitation involves close interaction among the patient and all members of the rehabilitation team. Of special importance in this regard are the social workers and psychologists working with the patient and family. At one time it was popular to categorize stages of readjustment to the injury, but with increasing experience psychologists and psychiatrists working with spinal cord – injured patients are discarding such theories. Unquestionably, most if not all patients initially deny the seriousness and permanency of the injury and its functional consequences, but with time the majority come to terms with themselves and their disabilities sufficiently to work toward effective rehabilitation.

Community placement is one of the major goals. Ideally, this means returning patients to their homes. Such structural alterations as ramps, wide doors, and adapted bathrooms may be required. Planning should begin as soon as patients are admitted. Plans must be made for selection and training of an attendant when required, whether it be a family member, friend, or paid attendant. If appropriate living arrangements cannot be identified, some alternative must be found, such as congregate or communal facilities. Institutional placement should be considered a last resort for the spinal cord – injured patient.

Vocational and educational counseling and training are frequently needed. The average patient is in the early 20s and has not made a career choice or completed education. If the reintegration of such patients into society is to be truly complete, they must be trained in an appropriate skill or occupation. With a proper attitude and education, there is no degree of disability that precludes the patient from finding a meaningful vocation. Obviously, however, the choices and opportunities are more limited for the more severely disabled.

SPECIAL PROBLEMS

Heterotopic Ossification

Heterotopic ossification is a condition of unknown cause in which new bone begins forming outside its normal location, in the soft tissues near major joints below the level of injury, most frequently in hip joints. In its most severe form it can lead to bony ankylosis of the joint. Especially when complete ankylosis occurs, the patient will be unable to reach the expected rehabilitation goals and will become completely dependent. In these instances, surgical resection of the ankylosing bar will restore functional range of motion and the functional capability of the patient.[21]

Surgery must not be performed until the process has fully matured or massive recurrence is inevitable. The signs of maturity are smooth cortical outline in the new bone mass, a normal serum alkaline phosphatase level, and, most important, a stable, low uptake ratio on bone scan for at least three consecutive months. This is determined by serial bone scan in which the activity in the highest uptake area of the new bone is compared to the activity in a normal reference bone by using computerized counting.[22] The uptake ratio will reach a maximum when the process is most active and then decrease to a stable lower level. At this point, resection of the ankylosing bar can be performed and major recurrence will not occur.[23] Frequently 2 years are required from the time the process first appears to the time when sufficient maturity for a safe surgical resection has been reached.

Decubitus Ulcers

Decubitus ulcers are the most common avoidable complication of spinal cord injury. They are formed when sustained pressure exceeds capillary filling pressures, which then leads to necrosis of skin and underlying soft tissue. Decubitus ulcers most commonly occur in two distinctly different settings with typical sores unique to each.

The first setting is the sacrum or heel in the newly injured patient. These ulcers result from inadequate turning and positioning during the period of vascular instability in the immediate postinjury period. Prevention requires turning every 2 to 3 hours, plus protecting bony prominences with pillows; in particular, the heels must be kept off the bed. Most heel ulcers are allowed to heal by granulation and re-epithelialization, because this is a difficult area to treat surgically. Sacral ulcers, if small, can heal in a similar way, but large ones may require skin grafting or flaps. What is most distressing about these ulcers is that they may delay rehabilitation by at least 3 to 4 months and leave the patient with permanently scarred skin before rehabilitation even begins.

The second setting is the "sitting ulcer" in the rehabilitation patient. These are most common in the ischial and trochanteric regions, and the most common cause is lack of proper care by the patient. They can be prevented by using a properly fitted wheelchair and having the patient regularly relieve pressure by raising off the cushion. These ulcers frequently require surgical closure.

The sine qua non of decubitus ulcer treatment is to keep the ulcer free of pressure at all times. As Vilan, a French plastic surgeon, has said, "You can put anything but the patient on the sore and it will heal." It is a mistake to make the patient with an ulcer get up even if for only a short time if the objective is to heal the ulcer.

The High Quadriplegic

In the past 10 years, improved emergency treatment and pulmonary therapy have made possible the appearance of the "high quadriplegic," that is, someone with a neurologic level of C4 or higher. These persons have no functional limb musculature, and their diaphragmatic function is compromised or absent.

In the initial phases, artificial ventilation and intensive pulmonary care are the keys to survival. If the patient has a complete injury (having a level of C3-C4, or higher), elective tracheostomy will improve care and make the patient more comfortable. This decision should be made within the first 10 days. When diaphragm function is compromised, weaning is easier with a tracheostomy, and if the diaphragm is completely paralyzed tracheostomy is essential. If the zone of injury includes the region of C3 and C4, the anterior horn motor neurons have been destroyed, meaning that permanent, artificial ventilation by means of a ventilator is required. If the zone of injury is above this level, resulting in diaphragmatic paralysis of the upper motor neurons, ventilation by electrical stimulation of the phrenic nerves is possible through the use of an implanted electrophrenic pacemaker.

High quadriplegics can utilize breath-activated environmental control units. By this means they can operate a number of electrical appliances and components, such as radios, televisions, telephones, tape recorders, alarms, door openers, typewriters, wheelchairs. These units are available commercially. Their use gives the patient a form of independence and in some cases can make possible some type of income-producing occupation.

Reconstructive Hand Surgery

In certain carefully selected quadriplegics, surgery on the hands can bestow improved function. The total patient and the patient's level of function must be taken into consideration, particularly transfer capability and wheelchair propulsion. There are two basic points to keep in mind: (1) never compromise active wrist extension, and (2) do not utilize spastic muscles for transfer. The results are always better in hands with good sensation, specifically those with two-point discrimination.

FUTURE DIRECTIONS

Spinal Cord Regeneration

An increasing amount of basic research is being conducted into the problem of regeneration. It is necessary to gain an understanding of the factors that influence axon growth, myelination, and glial growth within the central nervous system. Peripheral axons attempt to grow into the central nervous system and will grow into connective tissue scar, but they do not seem to be able to grow into regions where glial cells produce myelin and support the axon. If the processes of axonal growth within glial support structures could be understood, it might be possible to accomplish regeneration.

Acute Care and Reversal of Cord Damage

Since the first experiment by Allen,[24] a wide variety of physical and pharmacologic treatments of the experimentally injured spinal cord in laboratory animals have resulted in reversal or lessening of the effect of injury. To date none of these treatments has been shown to produce a similar effect in a clinical series of spinal cord–injured patients. A number of explanations can account for this: species differences, mode of injury, and the time from injury to start of treatment. Emergency medical services are improving rapidly, and now treatment of a variety of conditions is started at the scene of the accident by paramedics. Perhaps other specific therapies can be started within minutes of injury to minimize the extent of cord damage. Newer techniques of diagnosis, in particular, CT scanning, can supply better information more rapidly and further point to specific therapies. Prevention and early reversal are more likely to be effected before restoration of function through regeneration.

Rehabilitation Engineering

The gains in engineering technology in the past two decades have been phenomenal. Humans can control complex machines at the edge of the solar system and purchase at the corner drugstore a pocket computer with a greater capability than the prototype computer, which filled a room. Some of these advances have been used to improve the capabilities and the lives of spinal cord–injured persons, but much of this current knowledge and technology have not as yet been applied to rehabilitation. Increasingly engineers and rehabilitation professionals are working together, and in almost every instance this collaboration has been beneficial to the disabled person. This trend will continue and increase in magnitude, and, if past experience is an indicator, the rewards will be great. Functional electrical stimulation has the possibility of providing useful function in muscles without central nervous system control. Electrophrenic pacemakers can now successfully give a patient diaphragmatic function over prolonged periods of time. Obstacles that sill must be overcome to make functional electrical stimulation practical are the problems of fatigue, synchronization, and recruitment. Implanted stimulators operated by computer are being investigated.

Modern technology is also being applied to mobility aids. Vans have been designed that can be operated safely by quadriplegics who less than 10 years ago were considered practically or legally incapable of driving a vehicle. This technology will be applied to other mobility aids, such as the wheelchair, which has not had a major design modification since it was introduced.

Great strides have been made in the care and rehabilitation of the spinal cord–injured patient. The value of specialized spinal cord injury units has now become well accepted, and nationwide systems of spinal cord injury centers are established. These centers are now functioning within regional trauma systems so that persons with a spinal cord injury are rapidly transferred there for treatment. However, considering the number of patients sustaining spinal cord injury and the number of existing centers, it is obvious that most patients in the United States, still are not receiving this type of care.

With technologic advances comes social and governmental responsibility in dealing with prevention. Speed laws, drunk driving legislation, vehicle safety, and gun control legislation remain a vital part of the preventive aspects of treatment of spinal cord injury. Water safety education also can assist in reducing the incidence of cervical injury. Treatment clearly is a team effort but the preventive medicine aspects of spinal cord injury also require a team effort.

REFERENCES

1. Young JS, Northrup NE: Statistical information pertaining to some of the most commonly asked questions about SCI, Part I. SCI Dig 1:11, 1979
2. Kraus JF, Franti CE, Riggins RS, et al: Incidence of traumatic spinal cord lesions. J Chronic Dis 28:471, 1975
3. Messard L, Carmody A, Mannarino E, Ruge D: Survival after spinal cord trauma. Arch Neurol 35:78, 1978
4. Munro D: Boston City Hospital, Boston, 1954
5. Tator CH: Acute spinal cord injury: a review of recent studies of treatment and pathophysiology. Can Med Assoc J 107:143, 1972
6. Bedbrook GM: Spinal injuries with tetraplegia and paraplegia. J Bone Joint Surg [Br] 61:267, 1979
7. Stauffer ES, Kaufer H: Fractures and dislocations of the spine. p. 817. In Rockwood CA, Green DP (eds): Fractures. JB Lippincott, Philadelphia, 1975
8. Rossier AB, Fam BA, di Benedetto M, Sarakarati M: Urethrovesical function during spinal shock. Urol Res 8:53, 1980
9. Stauffer ES, Niel JL: Biomechanical analysis of structural stability of internal fixation of fractures of the thoracolumbar spine. Clin Orthop 112:159, 1975
10. Rossier AB, Berney J, Rosenbaum AE, Hachen J: Value of gas myelography in early management of acute spinal cord injuries. J Neurosurg 42:330, 1975
11. Akbarnia BA, Fogarty JP, Tayob AA: Contoured Harrington instrumentation in the treatment of unstable spinal fractures. Clin Orthop 189:186, 1984
12. Drummond D, Guadagni J, Keene JS et al: Interspinous process segmental spinal instrumentation. J Pediatr Orthop 4:397, 1984
13. Gertzbein SD, MacMichael D, Tile M: Harrington instrumentation as a method of internal fixation of fractures of the spine: a critical analysis of deficiencies. J Bone Joint Surg [Br] 64:526, 1982
14. Holdsworth FW: Fractures, dislocations and fracture-dislocations. J Bone Joint Surg [Am] 52:1534, 1970
15. Guttmann L: Spinal Cord Injuries: Comprehensive Management and Research. Blackwell Scientific Publications, Oxford, England, 1973
16. Cahal AS: Care of spinal cord injuries in the armed forces of India. Paraplegia 13:25, 1975
17. Wang FJ, Whitehill R, Stamp WG Rosenberger R: The treatment of fracture dislocations of the thoracolumbar spine with halo-femoral traction and Harrington rod instrumentation. Clin Orthop 142:168, 1979
18. Rossier AB, Hussey RW, Kenzora JE: Anterior fibular interbody fusion in the treatment of cervical spinal cord injuries. Surg Neurol 7:55, 1977
19. Burke DC, Murray DD: The management of thoracic and thoracolumbar injuries of the spine with neurological involvement. J Bone Joint Surg [Br] 56:72, 1974
20. Dickson J, Harrington P, Erwin W: Results of reduction and stabilization of the severely fractured thoracic and lumbar spine. J Bone Joint Surg [Am] 69:799, 1978
21. Hussey RW, Stauffer ES: Spinal cord injury: requirements for ambulation. Arch Phys Med Rehabil 54:544, 1973
22. Tanaka T, Rossier AB, Hussey RW et al: Quantitative assessment of para-osteoarthropathy and its maturation on serial radionuclide bone images. Radiology 123:217, 1977
23. Rossier AB, Bussat P, Infante F et al: Current facts on para-osteoarthropathy. Paraplegia 11:38, 1973
24. Allen AR: Surgery of experimental lesion of spinal cord equivalent to crush injury of fracture dislocation of spinal column. JAMA 57:878, 1911

34 Extremity Problems in Spinal Cord Injury

MICHAEL J. BOTTE

The loss of extremity function after acute spinal cord injury is well recognized. However, even beyond the acute effects on the musculoskeletal system, chronic problems and subsequent complications can further impede functional and emotional recovery. Although many of these extremity problems are unavoidable or are the result of the initial spinal cord injury, many complications may be preventable or minimized with a high index of suspicion, prompt diagnosis, and proper management. In this chapter, musculoskeletal complications and problems in the spinal cord injury patient are discussed. These problems include fractures, spasticity and contracture, paralysis, problems associated with upper extremity weight bearing (rotator cuff injury, bursitis, tendinitis, peripheral neuropathy), and miscellaneous complications (skin ulceration, infection, thrombophlebitis, reflex sympathetic dystrophy, and gravitational edema). Heterotopic ossification, an important extremity affliction, and reflex sympathetic dystrophy are discussed separately in other chapters.

EXTREMITY FRACTURES IN SPINAL CORD INJURY

Extremity fractures in the spinal cord–injured patient can be divided into three types: (1) acute fractures sustained in normal bone at the time of spinal cord injury, (2) subsequent pathologic fractures sustained in osteoporotic bone in the patient with a long-standing paretic extremity, and (3) a fracture sustained in a normal limb above the level of paralysis (i.e., in normal bone) in a patient with long-standing spinal cord injury.[1,2] These fractures, especially the first two types, present challenges in both diagnosis and treatment.

Acute Fractures Sustained at the Time of Spinal Cord Injury

Acute fractures sustained at the time of spinal cord injury occur in previously normal bone and usually involve high-speed injuries.[1-3] In configuration and anatomic location these fractures are similar to those in patients without spinal cord injury. The reported prevalence of extremity fractures occurring in the multiple-trauma spinal cord–injured patient is between 9 and 20 percent[1,2,4] with long bone fractures accounting for 26 to 44 percent of these. Eleven to 19 percent of long bone fractures occur in the upper extremity and 19 to 47 percent occur in the lower extremity. Pelvic fractures occur in up to 28 percent of spinal cord–injured patients.[2,3] Malunion and delayed union are common;[1,3] the frequency of reported nonunion varies between 4 and 16 percent.[1]

Clinical diagnosis of fracture in the paretic extremity may not be apparent initially because pain is absent owing to impaired sensibility. Additionally, deformity may not be seen in incomplete fractures or occult fractures that occur in the carpus or tarsus. In the multiple-trauma patient, the examiner is often misdirected toward more obvious injuries. Decreased patient cognition may further obscure the diagnosis. Presence of swelling, ecchymosis, warmth, lacerations, abrasions, and crepitus requires careful further examination and appropriate radiographic evaluation. The multiple-trauma patient deserves routine pelvic and spinal radiographs. Careful examination and a low threshold for radiographic examination will help reveal these difficult to diagnose fractures.

Management of acute fractures in the spinal cord–injured patient is directed toward early fracture stabilization to allow patient mobilization and early rehabilitation, and to minimize complications associated with prolonged bed rest. Operative stabilization and early mobilization have been shown to decrease the frequency of deep venous thromboses and decubitus ulcers.[5] Internal fixation of fractures also obviates casts, splints, and traction, all of which are poorly tolerated in the anesthetic or spastic extremity. Impaired sensibility increases the chances of skin ulceration with cast or splints. In addition, spastic limbs with increased muscle tone or clonus are difficult to manage in traction or with splints. Plaster devices prevent joint mobilization, interfere with self-care, and hinder wheel-chair transfers. Also, the physical weight of these devices can be difficult to manage by the patient with a paretic limb.

If the patient is medically stable and there are no contraindications, open reduction and internal fixation of major long bone fractures is desirable.[2,3] These procedures can often be performed at the time of initial spine stabilization. Most fractures are treated according to standard orthopaedic principles. Some fractures that might otherwise be treated with closed methods (such as those of the clavicle, metacarpals, and metatarsals) may be difficult to manage if spasticity or paralytic muscle imbalance is present and causes unacceptable deformity.[6] Open reduction and internal fixation in these fractures should be considered (Fig. 34-1). Intramedullary nailing of humerus fractures may allow early upper extremity weight bearing for wheelchair transfers. If operative surgery for extremity fractures is contraindicated, the use of well-padded splints or bivalved casts may provide a reasonable alternative,[2] with internal fixation being considered for a later date when the patient's condition becomes medically stable. Any external immobilization devices must be well padded and the extremity checked frequently for evidence of skin irritation or ischemia.

Pathologic Fractures in Long-Standing Spinal Cord Injury

Patients with long-standing spinal cord injury can develop severe osteoporosis from lack of weight bearing on paralytic limbs. These limbs are at risk for

pathologic fractures. Fractures often occur from minimal trauma or low-energy injuries. Falls from wheelchairs or during transfers, careless abrupt positioning in bed, or aggressive manual mobilization of a joint are common modes of injury. Fractures in long bones occur more often in paraplegic than in quadriplegic patients because paraplegic persons are at risk of injury from their increased levels of activity and greater participation in physical activities. Most fractures are sustained in metaphyseal areas of the lower extremity, commonly near the knee. Other common sites for fracture include the distal tibia, intertrochanteric region of the femur, femoral neck, and diaphysis of the femur or tibia.[7] Because of impaired sensibility and the minimal trauma required to fracture an osteoporotic bone, the fracture often goes unrecognized initially. With incomplete fracture or minimal deformity, swelling, ecchymosis, and warmth may be the only physical signs. Fractures occurring near joints can clinically mimic infection, heterotopic ossification, or thrombophlebitis. A high index of suspicion will promote proper examination and radiographic confirmation.

The cause of osteoporosis in the spinal cord–injured patient is stress deprivation in the paralytic limbs, owing to both lack of muscular forces acting on the bone and lack of weight bearing. The loss of bone mass commences after spinal cord injury and is accompanied initially by a negative calcium balance. Although calcium balance usually becomes positive by the sixth month after injury, the degree of osteoporosis may not change significantly if normal muscular forces are not acting on bone.[7] The degree of osteoporosis varies, and in some patients a year may be required before osteoporosis is sufficiently advanced that pathologic fractures will occur.[8]

Management of pathologic fracture in the spinal cord–injured patient depends on the type of fracture and the degree of limb paresis or spasticity. In the paralytic nonfunctional extremity with little or no spasticity, pathologic fractures can usually be managed nonoperatively, utilizing well-padded splints or bivalved casts.[7-9] Operative stabilization is avoided because fixation is often difficult to achieve or easily lost in the osteoporotic bone. There is also an increased frequency of infection owing to the atrophy of the surrounding muscle and skin. Fortunately, most of these pathologic fractures heal without surgery. In the nonambulatory patient, a moderate de-

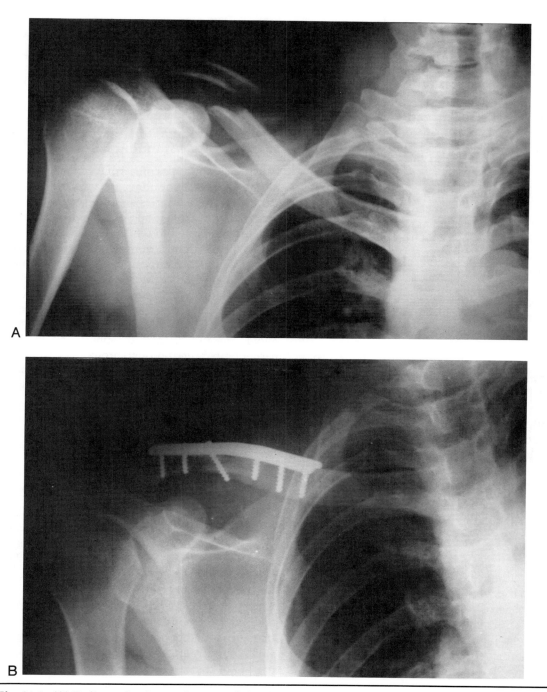

Fig. 34-1. **(A)** Radiograph of acute fracture of the clavicle in a patient with concomitant cervical spinal cord injury. This fracture is usually treated with closed methods (splinting) when it is an isolated injury. However, when it occurs along with spinal cord injury or brain injury, open reduction and internal fixation **(B)** will stabilize a spastic shoulder girdle and allow early motion to facilitate rehabilitation.

gree of fracture deformity may be acceptable, as long as previous function is preserved and fracture deformity or callus does not result in areas of increased pressure on the skin. Ease of positioning, sitting, and transfers must be maintained. Fractures of the femoral neck treated nonoperatively may form a pseudarthrosis. Pseudarthrosis of the femoral neck may cause no additional disability to the nonambulatory patient, provided there are no major rotational deformities. In some patients, pseudarthrosis of the hip may actually allow an increased range of motion.[8] Nonambulatory patients with fractures in paralytic limbs usually have little or no discomfort, so the fracture usually can be easily reduced and maintained in well-padded splints or bivalved casts.[8] Nonunion may occur in severely displaced fractures or in those with soft tissue interposition. Management of these fractures may require operative stabilization.

In the paraparetic patient who has residual function of the lower extremities or who was ambulatory prior to fracture, treatment is directed toward functional restoration. Open reduction and internal fixation of displaced femoral neck fractures minimizes the chances of pseudarthrosis of the neck and avascular necrosis of the femoral head. Open reduction and internal fixation of displaced intertrochanteric or subtrochanteric fractures can prevent shortening or varus malunion. Internal fixation of severely shortened diaphyseal femoral fractures minimizes chances of limb length discrepancy. Displaced intra-articular fractures in the ambulatory patient require operative restoration of the articular surface. In severely displaced fractures or those with soft tissue interposition, surgery may be required to achieve union.

Pathologic fractures can occur in the upper extremity of quadriparetic patients. The goals of fracture management emphasize restoration of pre-existing extremity function. Fractures must be satisfactorily reduced, utilizing internal fixation as necessary. If internal fixation is required in severely osteoporotic bone, addition external immobilization with splints may be necessary. Postoperative therapy for mobilization of the limb is individualized.

When severe extremity spasticity is present, it may be difficult or impossible to manage a fracture with closed methods.[6,10–12] If adequate bone stock exists,

open reduction and internal fixation should be considered. Alternatively, a phenol nerve block to the involved muscles may allow closed treatment of the fracture. The phenol block will decrease spasticity and lasts 3 to 6 months,[13–16] usually enough time to allow fracture healing. Phenol blocks are discussed later in this chapter.

Fracture of a Normal Extremity in Long-Standing Paraplegia

Fractures of this type consist of traumatic injuries that occur in normal bone above the level of longstanding paralysis. These injuries are often high-energy fractures and occur in a group of patients who are vigorous and motivated to remain active[2] (many of these patients drive motor vehicles). In the treatment of these fractures, an effort is made to maintain the patient's independence. Most fractures can be treated in a fashion similar to those in the patient without spinal cord injury, with similar indications for operative stabilization. An aggressive operative approach avoids the use of casts or splints and thus allows earlier limb mobilization to promote rapid rehabilitation. In fractures of the diaphysis of the humerus, intramedullary nailing usually allows earlier weight bearing for wheelchair transfers.

SPASTICITY IN SPINAL CORD INJURY

Correlation between Type of Injury and Clinical Presentation

Injury to the spinal cord can produce different effects on muscle, including paralysis (which denotes no volitional muscle function), paresis (weak muscle function), or spasticity (which includes increased tone, hyperactive reflexes, clonus, and/or rigidity). The effect on muscle depends on the type and level of spinal cord injury, the involvement of nerve roots, and the time elapsed from injury. Immediately after a severe spinal cord injury, flaccid paralysis develops below (distal to) the level of the lesion. Flaccidity usually lasts less than 24 hours and is followed by development of spasticity.[8] Spasticity is manifested as a result of disruption of the upper motoneuron inhibitory pathways from the brain to the anterior horn cells of the spinal cord. Muscle control from the brain is impaired or eliminated. Primitive reflex action predominates from the uninjured spinal cord below the level of injury. Thus, the period of flaccidity is followed by a period of increasing muscle tone, return of stretch reflexes, and a progression to hyperactive reflexes. In addition, sudden muscle contractions or spasms may become frequent and occur with minimal stimulus to the muscle or overlying skin. Clonus, rigidity, and the clasp-knife reflex frequently develop. At this point, with increased tone and hyperactivity, the muscles are considered to be spastic.[17]

Spasticity develops in the muscles distal to the level of cord damage, mediated by primitive reflex activity from the intact spinal cord distal to the injury. However, spasticity does not develop *at* the level of cord injury, because the spinal reflex arc is disrupted at this level. Instead, flaccid paralysis (no function) or paresis (weakness) occurs at the level of injury. Nerve root injury may also contribute to or account for weakness at the level of injury and is discussed further later in this chapter. If spinal cord injury is incomplete, some neurologic recovery may occur. Muscles that are spastic may improve (become less spastic) with time, and the muscles return to a less hyperreflexic state. Gradual recovery of volitional control can occur as well (in the incomplete lesion) and contribute to improved extremity function. This "recovery period" is variable and usually occurs over a 6 to 12-month period after the initial spinal cord injury. Approximately 1 year after injury, most patients with an incomplete spinal cord injury will have reached the end of the recovery period (when spontaneous neurologic recovery usually occurs), after which little or no further neurologic recovery can be expected.

In addition to injury to the spinal cord, nerve roots or anterior horn cells in the vicinity of the cord lesion may be injured. Trauma that injures the cervical cord often injures the neighboring nerve roots, especially roots in the foramen between dislocated or fractured vertebrae. The nerve root may originate from the normal spinal cord proximal to the injured segment and be damaged as it leaves the foramen,[8] thus resulting in some muscle function loss that is above the level of cord injury. When a nerve root is damaged, the injury is a lower motoneuron lesion. Paralysis or weakness (but not spasticity) of the corresponding muscles results. Therefore, in spinal cord injury there may be a group of flaccid or weak muscles (from

nerve root injury) that are proximal to the level of spastic muscles (from cord injury). If the nerve root is only partially injured and remains structurally intact (neurapraxia or axonotmesis), the impaired function of the corresponding muscle may gradually return. This may explain why some patients with a complete spinal cord injury subsequently gain the function of one or two root levels over time. It is actually a peripheral nerve (which is a lower motor nerve lesion) that is recovering, not the spinal cord. If the continuity of the nerve root is disrupted (neurotmesis), function will not recover spontaneously, and the affected muscles will remain weak or flaccid.

To summarize, depending on the type of injury to the spinal cord and neighboring nerve roots, three clinical presentations with different types of muscle impairment may ultimately occur at or below the level of injury: (1) paralysis, (2) paresis, and (3) spasticity. At the level of injury, muscles will be weak or flaccid, either owing to damage to the cord at this level (thus disrupting both volitional control and spinal reflex activity) or owing to nerve root injury (resulting in a peripheral nerve injury and paresis). Below the level of spinal cord injury, the muscles will be paralyzed or paretic (depending on completeness of the cord injury), and spasticity will usually be present, owing to loss of upper motoneuron inhibitory control.

In many complete cervical spinal cord injuries that involve the spinal cord between the C5 and T1 root levels, muscles in the upper extremity are predominantly weak or flaccid, with little or no spasticity. This occurs because the cord or nerve roots have been damaged segmentally over a few levels, and spinal reflex arcs at these levels are disrupted and spasticity cannot occur. Because spasticity occurs only in areas where the spinal reflex is intact, upper extremity spasticity, if present, usually develops at the more distally innervated muscles (innervated by roots C7, C8, or T1), because these levels are more apt to be distal to the injured segment of the spinal cord (and thus the spinal reflex arc is intact). Spasticity does, however, rarely occur in the more proximally innervated muscles in the upper extremity (such as C5 or C4) if the spinal cord lesion is proximal to these levels. Many of these patients, however, do not survive because of paralysis of the diaphragm and resulting respiratory failure. Therefore, in most spinal cord–injured patients, spasticity is seen less often in the upper extremity than in the lower extremity; paralysis and paresis are the predominant upper extremity problems.

Injuries to the lumbar spine can produce either upper motoneuron or lower motoneuron injuries. The cauda equina begins near the L2 level. Injuries proximal to this usually produce upper motoneuron lesions (with varying degrees of lower motoneuron involvement if nerve roots are injured). These injuries usually result in muscle spasticity distal to the injury. Distal to the conus medullaris, lower motoneurons exist, and trauma to these areas produces peripheral nerve injuries manifested by paralysis or paresis without spasticity. In reality, many injuries in the vicinity of L2 injure both the spinal cord above the conus and associated nerve roots or parts of the cauda equina; therefore clinical presentations with both spasticity and flaccidity are possible.

In spinal cord injuries the degree of spasticity is variable. In the incomplete cord lesion, some volitional control may be possible for either spastic or paretic muscles below the level of injury. Volitional control does not return in the true complete spinal cord injury.

Muscle strength in the spinal cord–injured patient should not progressively decrease. Ascending or progressive loss of muscle function is worrisome. In the acute stages of spinal injury this may indicate progressive nerve or spinal cord compression (e.g., from disc protrusion, hematoma, edema, loss of spine reduction). In the later or subacute period of spinal cord injury, progressive loss of muscle function may indicate ascending syrinx formation within the spinal cord or loss of spine stability. Progressive muscle loss in any of these settings requires immediate evaluation.

In the following sections, problems associated with spasticity and paralysis and their management are discussed. Although these two topics are covered separately, it must be kept in mind that they often occur in the same extremity simultaneously (e.g., spastic paralysis).

Weakness is often predominant in the upper extremities and spasticity often predominates in the lower extremities. Management of these problems has evolved so that efforts in the upper extremities are usually directed toward restoring function of weak muscles using reconstructive procedures such as tendon transfers and tenodeses. In the lower extremities, however, efforts are directed more toward the control of noxious spasticity, using muscle or tendon releases or lengthenings.

Patterns of Spasticity in Spinal Cord Injury

Following the initial period of flaccidity that occurs immediately after spinal cord injury, increased muscle tone progressively develops and culminates in spasticity of varying degrees.[18] Spasticity occurs in both complete and incomplete spinal cord injury. In some patients spasticity is mild, and the muscles remain predominantly weak or flaccid. In others spasticity is so severe that it can prohibit joint mobilization or cause sudden violent muscle contractions from minimal muscle stimulation.

The spasticity in the spinal cord–injured patient differs in character from that in the brain–injured, stroke, and cerebral palsy patient. In the last three conditions, chronic increased tone or continuous static muscle contractions are often seen. In the spinal cord–injured patient, however, spasticity is often manifested by periodic distinct sudden muscle contractions triggered by minimal stretch or cutaneous stimulation. Two patterns of muscle contraction often occur: (1) those in which the major limb flexors contract, thus withdrawing the limb toward the body (known as flexor patterning), and (2) those in which the extensor muscles contract, resulting in the limb extending away from the body (known as extensor patterning). Patients often have alternating flexor and extensor patterning. The type of patterning may depend, in part, on the type of stimulation initiating the response or on the position of the limb at the time of stimulation.

Problems Associated with Spasticity

Joint mobilization of a limb can be dificult when spasticity is severe. Passive motion, although a necessary part of management, is often painful, is time consuming, and, if performed too aggressively, can potentially cause injury to the limb. If spasticity prevents or impairs limb mobilization, difficulty with positioning the extremity occurs. It may not be possible to position the feet on the wheelchair platform.

Sitting, transfers, and positioning in bed can be challenging. Dressing the patient also becomes time consuming. Proper hygiene may be prevented, especially in the groin and popliteal fossa. Mobilization of the joint for articular cartilage and soft tissue nutrition is prevented. Spasticity likewise can interfere with joint mobilization carried out in the management of heterotopic ossification. If the joints cannot be mobilized adequately, stiffness of soft tissues can lead to fixed joint contracture.[17,19] Chronic limb deformity or prolonged positioning can lead to unrelieved pressure on the surface and result in skin ulceration.

Occasionally severely spastic muscles will produce sudden violent muscle contractions that are hazardous to the patient. These sudden contractions are able to propel a patient out of a wheelchair or bed and make operation of a car or machinery dangerous. Wheelchair transfers are sometimes prevented. These sudden spasms are often painful when they occur in areas of retained sensibility.

In the patient with an incomplete spinal cord injury, spasticity may be superimposed on a limb with retained motor and sensory function. The spasticity can severely impair what residual function remains. If sensibility is intact, chronic increased muscle tone and sudden muscle contractions can be painful.

Spasticity as an Aid to the Patient

Occasionally, the hyperactive reflexes or increased muscle tone can be of use to the spinal cord–injured patient, and this must be kept in mind prior to the surgical elimination of spasticity. By changing muscle position or by manual stimulation of the overlying skin, some patients are able to trigger an extension spinal reflex of the lower extremity, thereby facilitating limb stability for standing or wheelchair transfers. Pinching the calf of the leg can cause a flexor reflex and thus can help in dressing the lower extremities.[20] Reflex activity can also be used to provoke desired reflexes to assist with functional electrical stimulation during gait.[21]

Evaluation of Spasticity

Assessment of degree of spasticity can be difficult, because concomitant conditions cause stiffness or loss of joint motion. These include fixed soft tissue contracture, heterotopic ossification, undetected fracture or dislocation, and extremity pain from various causes (reflex sympathetic dystrophy, bursitis, tendinitis).[14] Differentiating among the relative contributions of pain, increased muscle tone, and contracture as a cause of decreased joint motion can be difficult. Diagnostic lidocaine nerve blocks can help differentiate the relative contributions to joint immobility by temporarily eliminating pain and muscle tone, thereby allowing the relative contributions of fixed soft tissue contracture to be evaluated. Effective diagnostic nerve blocks have been outlined by Keenan[14] (see Chapter 30), with blocks to the sciatic, femoral, obturator, and posterior tibial nerve being particularly useful in the spinal cord–injured patient. Detection of heterotopic ossification as a cause of joint stiffness can usually be made radiographically (except within the first few months, when ossification may not be adequately mature to appear on radiographs). Heterotopic ossification is usually also accompanied by an inflammatory reaction, increased alkaline phosphatase, concentration, and increased activity on technetium bone scan, all of which are useful from a diagnostic standpoint. Clinically occult fracture or dislocation causing loss of joint motion can often be demonstrated by careful clinical examination or by radiographs.

A relatively sudden increase in spasticity in the limbs may be a signal indicating occurrence of an occult pathologic process, one of which the patient is not aware because of impaired sensibility. Such processes include urinary tract infection, renal calculi, blockage of a catheter, or infected decubitus ulcers.[20] An increase in spasticity should promote evaluation for these possible problems.

Management of Spasticity in Spinal Cord Injury

Goals in the management of spasticity are to decrease muscle tone that interferes with function, retain limb motion to prevent contractures, and relieve the pain that is often associated with spasticity. These are optimally accomplished by a multidisciplinary approach with a well-coordinated rehabilitation team. Management can include manual joint mobilization, limb splinting in a desirable position between therapy sessions, use of a standing frame, electrical stimulation of antagonist muscles to facilitate relaxation of the agonist, oral muscle relaxants, serial lidocaine nerve blocks and phenol nerve blocks, surgical neurectomy, and surgical reconstruction. In the initial 12-month period of neurologic recovery (when spasticity may be decreasing), irreversible procedures such as neurectomy or tendon lengthenings should usually be avoided, because spontaneous recovery may make these procedures unnecessary or result in an "overcorrection" deformity. In this 12-month period, mobilization, splinting, oral medication, and lidocaine or phenol nerve blocks should be utilized to their utmost effectiveness to avoid joint contracture.

Mobilization is performed by passive joint manipulation with proper splinting between mobilization sessions. The multiple benefits of joint mobilization include maintenance of lubrication efficiency of the joint, maintenance of the normal patterns of the soft tissue matrix, assistance of orientation of new collagen fibers according to stresses, and prevention of increased cross-links in the collagen matrix, which cause fixed contractures. Electrical stimulation can be used as an adjunct. Electrical stimulation of an agonist muscle not only provides a method of moving the joint, but also assists in the relaxation of the antagonist and possibly strengthens the agonist.

Oral medication can be used to decrease muscle tone. Systemic agents such as baclofen, diazepam, and dantrolene sodium are useful to help control sudden muscle contractions and to help alleviate increased tone.[6] Baclofen blocks release of excitatory transmitters, thereby decreasing the severity of sudden muscle spasms. Given in divided doses of 10 to 60 mg/day, it is well tolerated, has few side effects, and is less sedative than other medications used to decrease muscle tone. Diazepam enhances presynaptic inhibition, also resulting in reduction of painful spasms. It can be given in divided doses of 4 to 30 mg/day. Major side effects are sedation and tolerance, and this drug is potentially habit forming. Dantrolene sodium exerts an inhibitive effect directly on muscle, acting at sites within the cell membrane, and has no central nervous system depressant effect.[20] Side effects are minimal, and tolerance is not known to occur. Hepatotoxicity is a potential side effect of all of these medications. Drugs under investigation for treatment of spasticity include propranolol, thymoxamine, and Tizanidine.[21]

Lidocaine and bupivacaine nerve blocks are effective temporary methods of decreasing spasticity. Regional lidocaine nerve blocks are helpful diagnostically to distinguish deformity caused by spasticity versus that caused by fixed contracture. Lidocaine nerve blocks can also be accomplished in a serial fashion, prior to mobilization therapy. In some cases, daily nerve blocks will help alleviate spasticity. Lidocaine nerve block prior to serial casting will ease joint mobilization and cast application. Bupivacaine is a longer-acting agent than lidocaine and can be used when a prolonged block is desired.

Phenol nerve blocks have proved to be useful in the management of spasticity.[6,13,15,16,22-25] Phenol denatures the protein in a peripheral nerve, causing axonal degeneration. Because the continuity of the nerve sheath is not disrupted, the axons regenerate and nerve function returns.[14,25] Phenol, therefore, provides a much longer nerve block than lidocaine. A 5 percent solution can be injected in a closed or open (surgical) fashion. Five percent aqueous solutions are used with closed blocks, and 3 to 5 percent solutions in glycerin are used with open blocks. Glycerin helps provide continued slow release of the phenol.[14] Phenol injection into a mixed nerve (containing both motor and sensory components) generally should be avoided in the patient with intact sensibility, because painful paresthesias from the sensory fibers may result. If sensibility is present, the phenol blocks should be reserved for nerves or nerve branches that carry predominantly motor fibers (such as the motor branches of a mixed nerve where they enter the muscle, or the motor points within the muscle). Injection into the motor branches is most accurately and safely performed by open block under direct visualization. When injected in a closed fashion, a Teflon-insulated needle with an exposed tip guided by a nerve stimulator will assist with accurate placement of phenol. Closed phenol nerve blocks often provide relief from spasticity for up to 3 months. Open blocks, using a 5 percent solution in glycerin injected directly into the motor branches of the nerve, will usually provide longer relief, often up to 6 months. It should be mentioned, however, that phenol is not currently approved for this use by the Food and Drug Administration (FDA), and proper patient consent is required. Phenol should not be sterilized with the autoclave, because it can be denatured. Phenol optimally used within the period of neurologic recovery. It is hoped that, as the nerve regenerates from the phenol block, the spasticity will decrease (if spontaneous recovery continues). If excessive spasticity remains when neurologic recovery has reached a plateau, definitive surgery can be planned.[14,22]

Open motor neurectomy can be performed in the patient with persistent noxious spasticity in whom no further neurologic recovery is occurring or expected (i.e., the patient is beyond the 12-month period of spontaneous recovery). Prior to neurectomy, the effects of the neurectomy can be simulated with a lidocaine or phenol block. If the block produces the desired results, neurectomy is considered. It must be realized that neurectomy alone will not correct a fixed contracture; it will only address the spastic component of the muscle (and does not affect fixed ligament or joint capsule contracture). Prior lidocaine block will help differentiate the relative contributions of spasticity and fixed contracture causing the deformity. The spastic component will be obliterated with the block; the fixed contracture will remain. Common motor neurectomies include the musculocutaneous nerve (for elbow flexion), motor branch to the brachioradialis (for elbow flexion), deep motor branch of the ulnar nerve (for intrinsic plus deformity of the hand), superficial branch of the obturator nerve (for adduction deformity of the thighs), motor branches of the femoral nerve (for hip flexor or knee extensor spasticity), motor branches of the sciatic nerve (for knee flexion spasticity), and motor branches of the posterior tibial nerve (for equinovarus deformity). In performing a neurectomy, it is desirable to remove a segment of nerve to prevent spontaneous repair from axonal regeneration.

Intrathecal injections to control noxious spasticity have been reported; however, they are mentioned here only to discourage their use. These injections, using either alcohol or phenol, in general should not be performed; they produce permanent lower motoneuron lesions, which results in a flaccid paralysis. The loss of all spasticity allows severe soft tissue atrophy to occur, placing the lower extremities at higher risk for decubitus ulcers. Any functionally useful extensor patterning is lost, such as that used for wheelchair transfers. The spastic bowel and bladder are converted to a flaccid bowel and bladder, resulting in

loss of reflex evacuation and subsequent incontinence. There should never be a need or indication for intrathecal injection. The peripheral nerves or muscles should be addressed instead of the spinal cord at the level of the intrathecal space. Peripheral phenol nerve blocks, motor neurectomies, or muscle lengthenings or releases are adequate to control even the most noxious spastic muscles.

Severance of part or all of the spinal cord has been performed to disrupt the reflex arc and convert a severely spastic extremity into a flaccid extremity. Similar complications to those just mentioned for intrathecal injection may occur. Therefore, it is my opinion that these procedures are not indicated. Treatment at the level of the peripheral nerve or muscle, as already described, seems preferable.

CONTRACTURE AND DEFORMITY

A fixed joint contracture is a condition of soft tissue "stiffness" that restricts joint motion. Contractures originate from prolonged immobilization (see Chapter 25). Contractures result in loss of passive (or active) joint motion and are one of the most disastrous and often preventable complications of spasticity or paralysis. If a joint is not mobilized, either actively or passively, a soft tissue contracture will develop. Contractures can develop after immobilization from spasticity, paralysis, or heterotopic ossification, or after joint or bone injury. A joint moved once daily through its full range of motion will not develop a contracture. Contractures occur from loss of elasticity, leading to fixed shortening of soft tissues. The tissues involved can include the joint capsule, ligaments, muscle-tendon units, skin, nerves, and vascular structures. A fixed contracture that prevents any joint motion will secondarily cause subsequent irreversible joint changes, such as articular cartilage erosions, fatty infiltration, and formation of intra-articular adhesions.[26-29] Contractures with concomitant limb deformity will interfere with function and hygiene. Joint contractures restrict limb positioning, cause problems with wheelchair transfers, interfere with dressing and sitting, and secondarily increase the potential for decubitus ulcer formation. Proper hygiene may be difficult to maintain, especially in the groin and popliteal fossa. Skin maceration can lead to ulceration and infection. In addition, the contractures themselves are often painful, especially when the limb is forcibly manipulated or used to lift or position the patient. *Therefore, one of the most important goals in the management of spasticity is to maintain range of joint motion to prevent a fixed contracture.*

Management of Contractures in Spinal Cord Injury

Contractures are difficult to treat. They require considerable time, cause discomfort to the patient, and often require surgical intervention. The most important aspect in the treatment of contractures is *prevention.* Joint mobilization and proper splinting should be initiated early after spinal cord injury, commencing when the patient is still in the intensive care unit, as soon as medical stability permits. Once established, treatment of a contracture includes manual mobilization followed by well-padded serial casting as needed. Casts are changed weekly to inspect skin, allow further limb mobilization, and achieve further correction in a new cast. Serial dropout casts are effective in the management of contracture. Dynamic splints may be attempted; however, these will not work if considerable spasticity coexists, especially if clonus is present.

The following paragraphs discuss management of contractures. These contractures are usually caused by spasticity or muscle imbalance. It should be noted, however, that in the upper extremity of the spinal cord–injured patient, paralysis is usually the predominant problem, not spasticity with contracture. However, when spasticity does occur in the upper extremity, fixed contracture can develop. The management of paralysis is discussed later in this chapter.

Specific Contractures or Deformities

Shoulder Contracture

Involvement of the shoulder with spasticity is uncommon in the spinal cord–injured patient, because injuries that occur proximal to the C5 root level result in paralysis of the diaphragm (C4) and often lead to respiratory failure. However, in the survivors of these proximal cervical spinal cord injuries, spasticity can be severe. Extremity function is usually minimal, and reconstruction is difficult because of lack of available donor muscles and presence spasticity throughout the limb. Deformity of the shoulder with spasticity usually is manifested by adduction and internal rotation. Muscles responsible for the deformity include the pectoralis major, subscapularis, teres major, and latissimus dorsi. Problems with hygiene, positioning, and dressing can arise. Rehabilitation efforts are initially directed toward mobilization to prevent contracture. Orthoses are not practical to correct this deformity. Phenol nerve blocks to the pectoralis muscle can be performed if the patient is in the period of neurologic recovery from spasticity.[13] If the patient has reached a plateau in improvement, no further neurologic recovery is expected, surgical release of spastic muscles can be performed to aid positioning and hygiene. Releases of the pectoralis major and subscapularis muscles are performed first, followed by the teres major and latissimus dorsi muscles as needed.[30]

Elbow Contracture

Contracture from spasticity of the elbow is rare, because these muscles are innervated primarily by nerve roots from the C5 level; therefore, for spasticity to occur, the lesion must be proximal to this level. Many patients with more proximal lesions do not survive. If spasticity is present, initial treatment is mobilization to prevent contracture and use of well-padded splints between therapy sessions to maintain correction. During the period of neurologic recovery, closed phenol nerve block to the musculocutaneous nerve can aid mobilization. If spasticity is severe and there is no volitional control in the extremity of a patient who is beyond the period of spontaneous recovery, motor neurectomy or surgical release of the biceps, brachialis, and brachioradialis muscles can be performed. These releases will facilitate hygiene, positioning, and dressing. If volitional control is preserved, selective lengthening of the elbow flexors can be performed to augment function.[31]

Hand and Wrist

Contractures from spasticity of the hands and wrist can occur in the spinal cord–injured patient but are usually associated with proximal spinal cord lesions with spasticity throughout the upper extremity. In the severely affected patients, there is usually flexion deformity at the wrist and the hand (combined with flexor patterning of the upper extremity—i.e., elbow flexion and shoulder adduction and flexion). The hand can assume an "intrinsic plus" position (flexion at the metacarpophalangeal joints with extension at the proximal interphalangeal joints) if the intrinsic muscles are spastic and the extrinsic muscles paretic or paralytic.[15] If contracture develops, fixed shortening of the flexor tendons of the wrist or digits can be treated with mobilization, serial casting, or tendon lengthening as needed. If lengthening is necessary, fractional lengthening is preferred when volitional control is present.[32] Fixed intrinsic contracture can be treated with lengthening of the intrinsic hood.[22,31]

In the more distal cervical cord injuries (e.g., C8/T1 root levels), an "intrinsic minus" hand deformity may develop. This deformity is due to loss of nerve root or cord disruption at the C8 or T1 level, resulting in paralysis of the intrinsic muscles of the hand. If the extrinsic flexors and extensors are intact (because these are innervated by nerves from a more proximal spinal cord level), the imbalance will produce the intrinsic minus or claw hand deformity. This problem is discussed later in this chapter with paralysis of the upper extremity.

Hip

Flexor patterning of the lower extremity results in hip flexion and adduction. Hip flexion is usually caused by spasticity of the rectus femoris and iliopsoas muscles. The anterior portion of the tensor fascia lata may contribute to hip flexion. Hip adduction is usually caused by spasticity of the adductor longus, adductor brevis, adductor magnus, and gracilis muscles. Problems with hygiene in the groin are common. Difficulty in transfers, standing, and dressing also occur. There is no feasible orthosis to treat flexion and adduction deformities of the hip. Mobilization may be initiated and prone positioning attempted to prevent contracture. Serial femoral and obturator lidocaine nerve blocks or closed phenol nerve blocks can be given. Open phenol blocks to the motor branches of the obturator nerve or femoral nerve can be given if closed phenol blocks are not adequate. Nerve blocks to the quadriceps muscles will also decrease knee extension, which may or may not be desirable. It is difficult to block the motor nerve to the iliopsoas muscle. If the patient has reached a plateau in a physical therapy program providing mobilization

and the period of expected neurologic recovery has passed, muscle lengthenings or releases can be considered. If the patient is nonambulatory, adduction deformity can be addressed with tenotomy of the adductor longus, adductor brevis, gracilis, and possibly a portion of the adductor magnus muscles. Alternatively, anterior obturator neurectomy can be performed; however, this may not alleviate a deformity caused by fixed muscle-tendon contracture. If the patient is ambulatory, the adductor magnus muscle should be preserved to provide some adduction of the hip and prevent undesirable overcorrection, manifested by hip abduction. In the nonambulatory patient, chronic refractory hip flexion deformity can be managed with release of the rectus femoris, iliopsoas, sartorius, and anterior portion of the tensor fasciae latae muscles.

When surgical lengthenings or releases are considered, care must be taken in assessing the functional status of the limb. If the patient has functional lower extremities, muscle lengthenings should usually be performed instead of complete muscle releases. At the hip, this can include Z-lengthening of the iliopsoas tendon, fractional lengthening or release of the rectus femoris, and partial release of the adductor muscles (release of the adductor longus, adductor brevis, and gracilis, with preservation of the adductor magnus). Fixed contractures of these muscles can be treated by lengthening or release, depending on functional status. Residual contracture of the joint capsule can usually be corrected with mobilization or prone positioning once the deforming spastic or contracted muscle forces are eliminated.

Knee

Knee flexion deformity is caused either by spasticity of the medial and lateral hamstring muscles or imbalance due to paresis of the quadriceps. This deformity increases the potential for development of decubitus ulcers on the hindfoot, makes transfers difficult, and causes hygiene problems in the popliteal fossa. If sudden muscle spasms occur, the patient can be propelled from the wheelchair. Initial treatment of chronic knee flexion deformity from spasticity includes mobilization to prevent contracture and medications to control spasticity. Serial lidocaine nerve blocks to the sciatic nerve in the proximal thigh may help alleviate hamstring spasticity. Closed phenol nerve block to the sciatic nerve can be performed in the patient without sensibility. The sciatic nerve is blocked in a closed fashion by percutaneous injection at the distal margin of the gluteus maximus, guided with the nerve stimulator and insulated needle. If sensibility is present in the lower extremity, closed phenol block to the sciatic nerve should not be performed because painful paresthesias can occur from the phenol injection into a nerve containing sensory fibers. In these patients, open phenol block to the motor branches of the sciatic nerve can be performed, thus avoiding injection of phenol into sensory fibers. However, this requires a large surgical exposure to adequately identify and inject the motor branches to the hamstrings. It is difficult to inject many of the more distal branches in the thigh. In the ambulatory patient with knee flexor spasticity that interferes with function, and who has reached a plateau in neurologic recovery, surgical lengthening of the hamstring muscles can be performed. In the nonambulatory patient with noxious knee flexor spasticity that interferes with transfers, positioning, or hygiene, and who has reached a plateau in neurologic recovery, release of the distal hamstrings can be performed.

Occasionally, knee extensor spasticity is present. This can be troublesome or beneficial. Sudden muscle spasms can propel the patient from the bed or wheelchair. However, the patient may use knee extensor patterning to stabilize the limb during wheelchair transfers. When knee extensor spasticity is difficult to control or unsafe for the patient, phenol block to the femoral nerve in the proximal thigh will help to control quadriceps spasms temporarily. If the patient is beyond the recovery period (1 year after spinal cord injury), selective release of the distal quadriceps or neurectomy of the motor branches of the femoral nerve may be performed. However, these procedures may accentuate knee flexion spasticity and should be avoided or performed cautiously in the patient who also has alternating knee flexor spasticity or patterning.

Foot and Ankle

Equinus deformity of the foot is common, caused by spasticity of the gastrocnemius and soleus muscles. Severe deformity causes difficulty with standing, transfers, wearing shoes, and placement of the feet on the wheelchair platform. Manual mobilization, splinting, and pharmacologic control of spasticity are initiated first. Serial lidocaine nerve blocks to the posterior tibial nerve in the popliteal fossa can help alleviate spasticity. Serial casting with well-padded casts can be performed for fixed contracture; however, frequent cast replacement is necessary to allow skin inspection. If the patient is no longer improving in a therapy program and is beyond the period of expected neurologic recovery, tendo Achillis lengthening can be performed. If hindfoot varus deformity is present, this can be addressed with lengthening of the tibialis posterior or tibialis anterior tendon. The split tibialis anterior tendon transfer (SPLATT procedure) is only rarely performed in the spinal cord–injured patient, because this procedure does not address the commonly spastic tibialis posterior muscle.[33]

Toes

Clawing of the toes (hyperextension at the metatarsophalangeal joints, flexion at the proximal interphalangeal joints) can cause skin irritation on the dorsum of the toes from pressure against the shoes. Clawing can be caused by intrinsic muscle weakness or imbalance or by spasticity of the extrinsic extensors and flexors. Correction of deformity can be performed with lengthening or release of the extensor tendons (and flexors as necessary). These procedures can be combined with resection arthroplasty or arthrodesis of the proximal interphalangeal joint if fixed joint deformity exists. Phalangectomy should generally be avoided, because the loss of bony and ligamentous stability can result in lateral deviation of the toes if spasticity is present.

Occasionally only flexion deformities will be present, manifested by flexion at the metatarsophalangeal and interphalangeal joints. Painful skin irritation on the distal tip of the toe can result as the toes are flexed into the shoe or floor. Release of the both the long and short flexors can be performed. Release of the toe flexors can be carried out through incisions on the plantar aspect of the toes. Loss of active toe flexion usually is not a problem.[33]

If flexion deformity is present only at the proximal interphalangeal joint, without flexion at the distal phalangeal joint, the short toe flexors may be responsible. Involvement of these muscles can be verified with a posterior tibial nerve block at the ankle. This will selectively block the intrinsic flexors, leaving the extrinsic toe flexors functioning. If the deformity is corrected with this block, it is the short toe flexors that are responsible, and these can be released selectively.[33]

PARALYSIS OF THE UPPER EXTREMITIES

Loss of upper limb function constitutes one of the most severe problems that the quadriplegic patient faces. On a questionnaire survey, many quadriplegic patients indicated they would prefer restoration of hand function over restoration of walking capacity, bladder or bowel function, or sexual function.[34] Orthoses and surgical reconstruction play an important role in the rehabilitation of the upper extremity. New techniques in functional electrical stimulation of the upper extremity have shown promising results in the restoration of function.

Surgical Reconstruction

Principal Functions to Restore

It has been estimated that 70 percent of patients with traumatic tetraplegia can be helped by surgical reconstruction.[35] Two of the most desirable functions to aim to restore are (1) active elbow extension, and (2) single hand grip (usually provided by lateral pinch).[35–38] In addition, reconstruction of finger flexion has been emphasized.[39] Other desirable functions include forearm pronation and intrinsic muscle augmentation (for claw deformity), but these should be considered only after restoration of elbow extension and single hand grip functions, provided that suitable donor muscles are available.

Elbow extension can be reconstructed if a functional deltoid muscle is present, using a deltoid-to-triceps tendon transfer (Fig. 34-2). Restoration of elbow extension allows patients to stabilize themselves in the wheelchair and improves control of self-help devices. Patients may gain the ability to hang up clothes or to take objects down from an overhead shelf. In rare cases patients may gain the ability to move from bed to wheelchair or to pivot without help (even

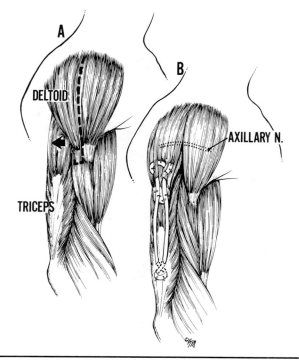

Fig. 34-2. Example of reconstructive procedure used to restore function in the spinal cord–injured patient. The posterior deltoid-to-triceps transfer (Moberg) can provide active elbow extension. **(A)** The posterior border of the muscle belly is isolated, preserving as much of the tendinous insertion as possible. **(B)** An intercalary tendon graft is required, usually obtained from the lower extremity. The posterior portion of the deltoid is then connected to the triceps through the tendon graft, and thus the posterior deltoid functions as an elbow extensor. (From McDowell,[36] with permission.)

though these bed-to-chair functions depend more on muscles that forwardly flex and depress the humerus, such as the pectoralis). These motions allow locking of the elbow in extension, providing adequate elbow stability for transfers.

Single hand grip can be accomplished by different methods: (1) use of a wrist-driven flexor hinge orthosis, powered by volitional wrist extension to provide pinch (Fig. 34-3), (2) tendon transfer (i.e., brachioradialis to extensor carpi radialis brevis) to provide or augment weak wrist extension to power a wrist-driven flexor hinged orthosis and provide pinch, and (3) Moberg tenodesis procedure to provide lateral pinch (Fig. 34-4) plus opponensplasty to provide

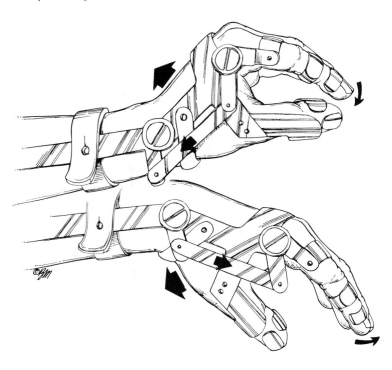

Fig. 34-3 Wrist-driven orthosis. Active wrist extension with the orthosis in place provides a means of single hand grasp. The device is dependent on adequate wrist extensor strength. As the wrist is dorsiflexed, the fingers are flexed to bring them into contact with the thumb, which is stabilized by the orthosis. As the wrist is palmar flexed, the fingers are extended. If wrist extensor strength is not adequate, a tendon transfer to provide extensor strength can be considered (provided an adequate and appropriate donor muscle, such as the brachioradialis, is available). A similar but static ratchet type of orthosis is available that will hold the fingers in pinch position if the wrist is passively extended into a locked mode. (From McDowell,[36] with permission.)

thumb-to-finger pinch.[39] These are discussed later in this chapter.

Patient Selection and Classification

Selection of tetraplegic patients for any type of surgical reconstruction can be difficult because of the complexity of the physical examination, the possibility of changing neurologic status over the first 12 months, and the multiple subjective factors that should be considered (patient's age, occupation, interests, and expectations). Methods of surgical reconstruction of each of the different functional levels are discussed separately. However, general considerations are overviewed first.

Selection for surgical reconstruction depends on existing motor and sensory function. In the past, quadriplegic patients were classified by the cervical spine segment injured, assuming that the level of paralysis and sensory loss coincided with the bone injury (Fig. 34-5).[38] However, this classification was not consistently accurate, because the level of bone injured may not coincide with the actual level of spinal cord injury. In addition, spinal injury may not be symmetrical, and there may be unusual patterns of sparing of

sensory or motor function. Nerve root injury from a higher spinal level may coexist with the spinal cord lesion. Therefore, a more useful classification was developed by McDowell and coworkers and approved by an international group of surgeons working with tetraplegic persons.[40,41] This classification is based on the most distal muscle available for transfer, and patients are assigned to ten groups. The groups are further subdivided according to sensibility (Table 34-1). In group 0 (the most severely affected group) only the deltoid muscle is available for transfer; the rest of the upper extremity is paralytic or paretic. In group 9 (the least involved in this patient classification) the only weak muscles are the hand intrinsic muscles, and numerous muscles are available for transfer. Specific transfers are discussed later.

Sensory Evaluation

Successful surgical reconstruction of the upper limbs depends on the presence of adequate sensibility. Sensory evaluation should include stereognosis and two-point discrimination. In most patients, stereognosis and two-point discrimination of 10 mm or less are required for pinch or grip to be useful.[35,37] If two-point discrimination of 10 mm or less is not present,

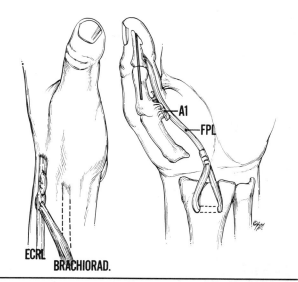

Fig. 34-4. Drawing of Moberg reconstruction to provide key pinch. Strong wrist extension is a prerequisite. If wrist extension is weak, the brachioradialis muscle can be transferred to the extensor carpi radialis brevis to provide wrist extension. Salient features of this reconstruction include: (1) tenodesis of the flexor pollicis longus to the distal palmar radius, to provide thumb flexion and create key pinch when the wrist is actively extended; (2) resection of the proximal annular pulley of the thumb to permit the tendon to bowstring and increase the strength of the key grip; (3) internal fixation of the interphalangeal joint of the thumb to prevent interphalangeal joint flexion and maintain a broad contact surface; and (4) tenodesis of the extensor hood mechanism to the metacarpal of the thumb to prevent hyperflexion of the metacarpophalangeal joint. (From McDowell,[36] with permission.)

grip must be guided or regulated by direct vision. Using direct vision to regulate grip usually means only one hand can be guided at a time.[42] Therefore, a prerequisite for surgical reconstruction of grip is the presence of two-point discrimination and stereognosis in at least one hand.

The motor group classifications are subdivided according to sensibility. When sensibility is adequate to regulate grip, the classification of "Cu" (cutaneous) is given, which indicates cutaneous afferents good enough to lead the grip. If sensibility is not adequate to lead the grip, direct vision is required to regulate grip, and the sensory classification is "O." For example, a patient with the brachioradialis muscle avail-

able for transfer and adequate sensibility in both hands is classified as CuCu 9 (Table 34-1).

Timing of Surgical Reconstruction

Surgical reconstruction in the quadriplegic upper extremity is usually not performed earlier than 1 year after injury. This usually provides adequate time for the neurologic recovery to reach a plateau and allows the patient sufficient time to adjust psychologically to the paralysis and to realize that there will be no further recovery. In addition, recovery from spasticity usually becomes static by 1 year after injury, thus providing a static clinical picture of limb function. If there is any evidence of continuing neurologic recovery or improvement in function in a therapy program, surgical reconstruction should be delayed until there is no longer any motor or sensory improvement.

Basic Principles in Limb Reconstruction

Principles of limb reconstruction have been outlined by many authors.[35–38,43,44] The least affected limb should usually undergo reconstruction first. Surgery should be performed on the dominant extremity first if both are the similarly impaired. If adequate cutaneous sensibility is not present, surgery should be done only on the side with the better residual motor function, using vision to guide the grip in this extremity. Only one surgical procedure should be performed at a time. Restoration of elbow extension should precede other procedures that restore pinch or grasp to the hand. Simplicity in surgery is the safest, utilizing available muscles of the extremity to strive for one or two simple functions. True opposition in pinch usually is not necessary; lateral pinch (key pinch) is more useful. Severe spasticity or fixed contractures must be controlled or corrected prior to tendon transfers.

Surgical Procedures

Surgical procedures are discussed according to motor classification. To reiterate, two-point discrimination of 10 mm or less and intact stereognosis must be present for useful hand function without guidance by direct vision, and a person can visually guide only one hand at a time. Therefore, at least one hand should have adequate cutaneous sensibility; direct vision can guide the other. For further information on reconstruction in patients with tetraplegia, including

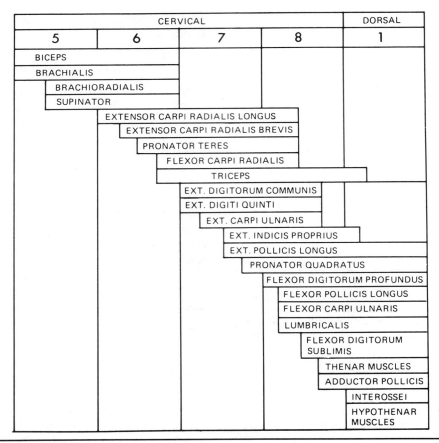

Fig. 34-5. Segmental innervation of muscles of the elbow, forearm, and hand. (From Zancolli,[38] with permission.)

details of surgical procedures, the reader is referred to the excellent discussions and original published works by McDowell,[36] Moberg,[35,37] Freehafer and colleagues,[9,39] House and coworkers,[45-47] Waters and associates,[48] Zancolli,[38,44] Kelly and coworkers,[49] and Lamb and Chan.[50]

Group 0

In general, patients in group 0 have functioning deltoid muscles but no muscle function below the elbow suitable for transfer (Table 34-1). This corresponds roughly to a C5 functional level. If elbow extension itself is lacking, it can be restored provided that the deltoid is functional. The posterior portion of the deltoid is transferred to the triceps, using an intercalary tendon graft harvested from the tensor fascia lata, toe extensor, or tibialis anterior (Fig. 34-2). Patients in

group 0 may be candidates for an externally powered orthosis. Most of these patients can use some assistive devices attached to one hand.

Group 1

Patients in group 1 have a strong brachioradialis muscle but poor muscle function distally, including poor wrist extensors. Transfer of the brachioradialis into the extensor carpi radialis brevis or longus, or to both, can provide sufficient wrist extension to power a wrist-driven flexor hinge orthosis. This can provide a type of single hand grip. In addition, lateral pinch can be augmented or reconstructed as needed with either the Moberg reconstruction for key pinch or the wrist-driven flexor hinge hand described by Nickel and coworkers.[35,37,43] The Moberg reconstruction requires strong wrist extension as a prerequisite. Re-

Table 34-1. International Classification for Surgery of the Hand in Tetraplegia.
Edinburgh 1978 (Modified Giens 1984)

Sensibility O or Cu	Group	Motor Characteristics[a]	Description of Function
	0	No muscle below elbow suitable for transfer	Flexion and supination of the elbow
	1	BR	
	2	ECRL	Extension of the wrist (weak or strong)
	3[b]	ECRB	Extension of the wrist
	4	PT	Extension and pronation of the wrist
	5	FCR	Flexion of the wrist
	6	Finger extensors	Extrinsic extension of the fingers (partial or complete)
	7	Thumb extensor	Extrinsic extension of the thumb
	8	Partial digital flexors	Extrinsic flexion of the fingers (weak)
	9	Lacks only intrinsics	Extrinsic flexion of the fingers
	X	Exceptions	

[a] BR, brachioradialis; ECRL, extensor carpi radialis longus; ECRB, extensor carpi radialis brevis; PT, pronator teres; FCR, flexor carpi radialis.

[b] Caution: It is not possible to determine the strength of the ECRB without surgical exposure.

Notes:

1. This classification does not include the shoulder. It is a guide to the forearm and hand only. Determination of patient suitability for posterior deltoid to triceps transfer or biceps to triceps transfer is considered separately.
2. The need for triceps reconstruction is stated separately. It may be required in order to make brachioradialis transfers function properly (see text).
3. There is a sensory component to the classification. Afferent input is recorded using the method described by Moberg and precedes the motor classification. Both ocular and cutaneous input should be documented. When vision is the only afferent available the designation is "Oculo" (abbreviated O). Assuming there is 10 mm or less two-point discrimination in the thumb and index finger, the correct classification would be Cu, indicating that the patient has adequate cutaneous sensibility. If two-point discrimination is greater than 10 mm (meaning inadequate cutaneous sensibility), the designation O would precede the motor group (example O 2).
4. Motor grouping assumes that all listed muscles are grade 4 Medical Research Council (MRC) or better and a new muscle is added for each group; for example, a Group 3 patient will have BR, ECRL, and ECRB rated at least grade 4 (MRC).

(Modified from McDowell,[36] with permission.)

construction of lateral pinch consists of (1) tenodesis of the flexor pollicis longus to the distal palmar radius, to provide thumb flexion and create lateral pinch when the wrist is actively extended; (2) resection of the proximal annular pulley of the thumb to permit the tendon to bowstring and increase the strength of the key pinch; (3) internal fixation of the interphalangeal joint of the thumb to prevent flexion at the interphalangeal joint and maintain a broad contact surface; and (4) tenodesis of the extensor hood mechanism to the metacarpal of the thumb to prevent hyperflexion of the metacarpophalangeal joint (Fig. 34-4). Many modifications of this procedure have been described.[42,51-53] An alternative reconstruction is the wrist-driven flexor hinge hand described by Nickel and colleagues.[43] This includes stabilization of the thumb and interphalangeal joints of the index and long fingers with arthrodesis, and tenodesis of the profundus tendons of the index and long fingers to the distal radius so that the tips of these two fingers are brought into contact with the thumb during wrist extension.[43] Alternative methods of achieving pinch have been further discussed by other authors,[9,39,45-47,49] and include transfer of the brachioradialis to a rerouted flexor digitorum superficialis muscle (from the ring finger, routed across the palm) to insert into the abductor pollicis tendon or splitting of the rerouted flexor digitorum superficialis and transfer into the dorsum of the thumb over the proximal phalanx.

Group 2

Patients in group 2 have function of the extensor carpi radialis longus muscle. They are able to operate a wrist-driven wrist orthosis for single hand grip and are also candidates for single hand grip or lateral pinch reconstruction, as already described. Because the extensor carpi radialis brevis is such an effective wrist extensor, and because wrist extension is so valuable, this muscle should not be transferred.[9,39] However, the brachioradialis is available for transfer and can be used in different ways (because it is not needed to provide wrist extension, as in group 1 patients). Possible options include transfer of the brachioradialis to the flexor pollicis longus muscle to increase strength of pinch[33,42] or to the extensor pollicis longus, extensor pollicis brevis, or abductor pollicis longus muscle to open the thumb–index finger web space to improve the release phase of the grasp-release sequence. The usefulness of these procedures does not seem to be as promising as had been anticipated, however,[36,37] and transfer of the brachioradialis muscle in group 2 patients is not recommended by McDowell.[36]

Group 3

Patients in group 3 have function of the both the extensor carpi radialis longus and extensor carpi radialis brevis muscles. This group is similar to patients with C6 functional level. Many patients are content with a wrist-driven flexor hinge orthosis to provide pinch. These patients are good candidates for surgical reconstruction for key pinch. In addition, with both wrist extensors functioning, the extensor carpi radialis longus becomes available for transfer (leaving the extensor carpi radialis brevis as the remaining wrist extensor because of its more central insertion). In this group of patients, Zancolli has described a two-stage reconstruction to provide digital release, prevent clawing, and provide digital flexion.[36,38,44] In the first stage, digit and thumb extension tenodeses are performed to provide release during wrist palmar flexion. To prevent or reduce clawing, each flexor digitorum superficialis tendon is joined to itself around the A-1 (first annular pulley), maintaining slight flexion at the metacarpophalangeal joint (lasso procedure). Arthrodesis is performed on the thumb interphalangeal joint to prevent hyperflexion. In the second stage of the reconstruction, digital flexion is established with transfer of the extensor carpi radialis longus muscle to the flexor digitorum profundus, and the brachioradialis is transferred to the flexor pollicis longus.[38,44,48] In many patients in groups 2 and 3, lack of forearm pronation may present an additional problem. These patients have active wrist extension

and utilize the tenodesis effect for grasp and release. If the forearm cannot be pronated, however, gravity cannot be utilized to produce palmar flexion of the wrist and digital extension for release of grasp. In these patients, the biceps tendon can be transferred around the radial side of the radius, transforming it into a forearm pronator.[38,44]

Group 4

In group 4 patients the pronator teres is intact. This muscle provides a useful antagonist to the supination provided by the biceps. Therefore, function of the pronator is valuable, and its use as a donor for transfer is controversial. Zancolli has described its transfer to the flexor carpi radialis to strengthen wrist extension and augment wrist-activated tenodesis reconstructions.[38,44]

Group 5

The flexor carpi radialis is intact in group 5 patients, and these patients have active flexion and extension of the wrist. Patients in this group are similar to those with C7 functional level. Reconstruction efforts are directed toward providing digital flexion and extension. Because wrist flexion is valuable, the flexor carpi radialis usually is not transferred as long as the brachioradialis, extensor carpi radialis longus, and pronator teres are available for transfer. House and colleagues have described a two-stage reconstruction that provides digital flexion and release.[45-47] The first stage (extensor phase) involves either tenodesis of the common extensors and the extensor pollicis longus to the distal radius or a transfer of the brachioradialis to the common extensors and the extensor pollicis longus for digital extension. Stabilization of the thumb is accomplished by carpometacarpal joint arthrodesis or tenodesis of the abductor pollicis longus. In the second stage (flexor phase), the extensor carpi radialis longus is transferred to the profundus tendons to the index, long, ring, and little fingers. The pronator teres is transferred to the flexor pollicis longus. Intrinsic tenodeses as described by Zancolli (group 3) are also performed, because the intrinsic muscles are not functioning.

Group 6

The extensor digitorum communis is strong in group 6 patients; however, the extensor pollicis longus is too weak to extend the thumb out of the palm. The extensor pollicis longus can be sutured to the common extensors so that active extension of the fingers will produce extension of the thumb.[21]

Group 7

In group 7 patients the extensor pollicis longus is strong and need not be augmented. Attention is directed toward reconstruction of weak digital flexion and intrinsic muscle augmentation, using the lasso procedure described by Zancolli.[36,38,44]

Group 8

Patients in group 8 lack strength in extrinsic finger flexion. Occasionally the ulnar flexors have adequate strength, but flexor power to the radial flexors is weak. These can be balanced by suturing all four profundus tendons together.[21] Active flexion to the thumb can be provided with transfer of the brachioradialis to the flexor pollicis longus. Because the intrinsics muscles are also weak, augmentation is usually required, utilizing the lasso procedure as mentioned earlier.

Group 9

Patients in group 9 lack intrinsic muscle strength, and clawing is usually present. Intrinsic muscle augmentation can be performed to eliminate hyperextension deformity at the metacarpophalangeal joints.

Postoperative Care

After most tendon transfers, the transferred tendon is immobilized for approximately 4 weeks or mobilized early in a protected range. A closely supervised hand therapy program follows, in which active and passive motion are initiated.

Functional Electrical Simulation in the Upper Extremity

Electrical stimulation of muscle is a relatively new means of producing contraction of muscle in cases of neuromuscular impairment. Electrical stimulation with muscle contraction can assist mobilization of the joint to prevent contractures, can help relax spastic antagonist muscles, and, if timed or controlled carefully, can augment function of the limb. In addition, there is evidence that electrical stimulation of muscle strengthens the muscle and improves endurance.[54] If the muscle is stimulated to provide a specific movement or function of the extremity (i.e., digital flexion for grasp, ankle dorsiflexion during gait), the stimulation is called functional electrical stimulation. The muscles can be stimulated by surface electrodes placed on the skin or by surgically implanted electrodes placed either on the epimyseal surface of the muscle or near the respective motor nerve.[55-59]

In the tetraplegic upper extremity, functional control by electrical stimulation has been studied by various investigators.[55,57,58] Restoration of key pinch, grasp, and release have been studied using a percutaneous electrode system. Patients have included those in groups 0 and 1 (functional levels C5 or C6), with cutaneous sensibility that was usually intact. At these levels of cord injury few muscles are available for tendon transfer. Prerequisites for successful use of electrodes include control of spasticity, adequate seated balance, and nearly full range of movement of the shoulder, elbow, and fingers. Intact lower motoneurons are required, and the muscle must be electrically excitable by stimulation of its peripheral nerve. The electrodes are strategically placed in the forearm to stimulate the digital and thumb flexors and extensor muscles (Fig. 34-6). The electrodes are connected to a controller, which in turn is connected to a transducer placed on the contralateral shoulder. Firing of the electrodes is controlled volitionally by the patient via contralateral shoulder movements through the transducer. The electrodes usually remain in place over a year. This system requires no voluntary control below the level of the elbow, yet it yields adequate key grip or lateral pinch to handle small objects and palmar prehension to handle large objects.

Many alternative methods of volitional control of muscle excitation have been developed, including potentiometers mounted on a fixed surface and moved by the patient's opposite extremity; potentiometers attached to an orthosis that measures position of the wrist; on/off switches that select a slowly increasing or decreasing command; and voice control.[57,58] Using two grasp patterns, the user can hold objects such as eating utensils and writing implements and position the hand for functions such as the use of a keyboard or control of switches and knobs.[55,58]

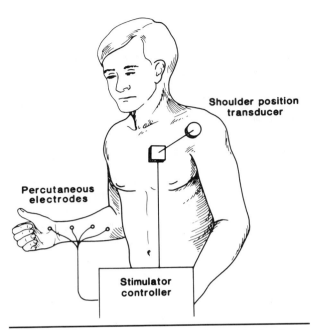

Fig. 34-6. Diagram of percutaneous electrical stimulation system. Percutaneous electrodes are placed in the forearm to stimulate digital and thumb flexor and extensor muscles. Stimulation of these muscles is controlled volitionally by the patient via the transducer placed on the contralateral shoulder. Specific movements of the shoulder are processed by the stimulator controller, and the muscles are stimulated to produce the desired function. (From Keith et al,[55] with permission.)

PARALYSIS OF THE LOWER EXTREMITIES

Patients with spinal cord lesions proximal to the conus have upper motoneuron lesions; therefore, severe spasticity is often present. Severe noxious spasticity is often an overwhelming but treatable condition. In these patients, the problems with spasticity often overshadow problems of weakness or paresis; consequently, reconstructive efforts are directed mostly toward ablation of spastic deformity using tendon lengthenings and releases. Less emphasis is placed on reconstruction to restore strength to weak muscles using tendon transfers, and these transfers are not generally feasible until severe spasticity is controlled and contractures eliminated.

Injuries that occur distal to the level of the second lumbar vertebra injure the cauda equina and produce lower motoneuron lesions that result in lower ex-

tremity weakness. These injuries therefore do not produce spasticity. Injury of varying severity to nerve roots may occur, and incomplete lesions causing different patterns of weakness may result. Hence, clinical presentations of specific root-level injuries are often not seen. The affected muscles become flaccid or paretic. In these patients, reconstructive efforts are directed toward reconstruction of the flaccid or paretic paralytic limb, and many of the concepts of bracing and tendon transfers developed for peripheral nerve injuries or anterior horn cell diseases are feasible. Use of functional electrical stimulation is gaining popularity, and this modality is discussed briefly in the following section.

Reconstructive Procedures

Weakness of the Hip and Knee

Requirements for ambulation include adequate balance, limb stability, and a means of hip advancement. Paraplegic patients with functional levels between T1 and T5 will lack trunk balance and are usually wheelchair dependent. Patients with functional levels between T6 and T10 will have some trunk stability, and exercise ambulation with bilateral long leg braces and crutches or parallel bars may be possible. Stability of the knee can be provided with a knee-ankle-foot orthosis (KAFO). With functional levels between T11 and L1, trunk stability will be present; however, hip advancement is lacking and limited, if any, household ambulation will be possible. In the patient with L2 functional level, some hip flexion will be intact, and household ambulation may be possible. If L3 or L4 levels are intact, the quadriceps and hip adductors will be functioning, and community ambulation will be possible. Ankle stability can be provided with an ankle-foot orthosis (AFO).

Weakness of Ankle Plantar Flexion

Ambulatory patients may have weakness of the gastrocnemius-soleus that allows the ankle to collapse into dorsiflexion during stance. This results in excessive forward advancement of the tibia. Compensatory flexion at the knee occurs, which increases demands on the quadriceps during stance. This can result in loss of stability at both the knee and ankle. Many patients with gastrocnemius-soleus weakness subsequently develop a second gait pattern in which the knee is passively locked in extension at or immediately after floor contact. This prevents knee collapse during stance and avoids the increased demand on the quadriceps if the knee is in flexion during stance. Although this gait pattern increases stability, the chronic hyperextension stresses on the knee can eventually lead to genu recurvatum and knee pain, especially in the active patient. Treatment of the weak gastrocnemius-soleus is aimed at providing ankle stability using a rigid AFO. Double upright orthoses are the most stable and generally the most effective. However, they are heavy and can be difficult to use in the paretic limb. New designs in polypropylene orthoses may provide adequate stability and are much lighter.

Weakness of Ankle Dorsiflexion

Inadequate dorsiflexion with a footdrop is caused by weakness of the tibialis anterior, extensor hallucis longus, and extensor digitorum longus muscles. The patients often drag the toes on the floor during the swing-through phase of gait. Treatment is stabilization with an AFO. A flexible polypropylene orthosis allows a small amount of controlled ankle motion during stance and provides adequate dorsiflexion during swing. If footdrop is the only gait problem, a lightweight flexible polypropylene orthosis with posterior trimlines is sufficient to provide a neutral toe position during swing. Its flexibility allows some ankle motion during stance.

Weakness of Foot Eversion

A varus deformity may result either from spasticity of the inverters of the foot (tibialis posterior or tibialis anterior) or from the weakness of the everters (peroneus longus and peroneus brevis). Deformity caused by weakness of the foot everters can usually be improved with an AFO. Lightweight flexible polypropylene orthoses are usually adequate.

Functional Electrical Stimulation in the Paraparetic Lower Extremity

Function in the lower extremity can be augmented with electrical stimulation. In paraparetic patients (those with preservation of some lower extremity function), functional electrical stimulation is able to improve standing or walking. These systems promise to provide significant gains in function. However, the systems are not always practical. Patients must be carefully selected, goals must be realistic, and obstacles such as adapting to and maintaining equipment need to be overcome.

Kralj and coworkers have developed a successful system to augment standing and walking in the paraparetic patient.[56] In their system, the patient utilizes and incorporates as much preserved function as possible into the restoration of ambulation. Patient capabilities are utilized to the maximal extent, including remaining motor skills and preserved reflexes. A four-channel stimulation unit is utilized. The four-channel gait pattern is controlled by the patient via trigger switches built into the handles of walkers or crutches. Standing is accomplished by stimulation of the quadriceps, enabling the patient to stand with exaggerated lordotic posture. Gravity is used to stabilize the extended hips. Limb advancement is accomplished by stimulating a reflex synergistic flexion in the extremity, combined with the patient's shifting of body weight using the upper extremities and the walker or crutches. In Kralj and coworkers' series, only 15 percent of all admitted patients were selected as candidates. Of those selected, 75 percent of patients with T4-T5 lesions were able to utilize the four-channel walking system. Only 60 percent continued to use the system at home because of time required to apply the equipment.

Although relatively few well-documented studies in functional electrical stimulation (FES) have been performed, investigations by Kralj and others seem to support several conclusions. FES for standing is an important function enabling patients to perform tasks in an upright position. Such standing may extend the transfer capabilities for patients and may be considered a therapeutic modality. FES used to augment walking seems to be able to provide useful but limited household ambulation. Its importance and role in the daily life of spinal cord–injured patients must be determined. For long-term use, the time required for donning and removing the device is an important consideration. In addition, cosmesis and availability of the FES-assisted devices are of prime importance. Surgically implantable systems, although still somewhat experimental, have advantages over the surface-applied systems and may ultimately prove superior for long-term use. Surface systems are useful for short-term use, such as therapeutic, training, and evaluation purposes to prepare and select patients for implantation.[56]

PROBLEMS ASSOCIATED WITH UPPER EXTREMITY WEIGHT BEARING IN PARAPLEGIA

The paraplegic patient relies on the upper extremities for activities of daily living, locomotion, and wheelchair transfers. These activities result in higher stresses on the shoulders, elbows, wrists, and hands, which can precipitate problems associated with overuse. Frequent problems include extremity pain (especially at the shoulder) and peripheral neuropathies.[60–67]

Upper Extremity Pain (Rotator Cuff Tears, Tendinitis, Bursitis)

Studies have shown that a high percentage (51 to 100 percent) of spinal cord–injured patients eventually develop pain in their upper extremities. The pain is usually associated with or aggravated by wheelchair use or crutch walking. The reported incidence of extremity pain increases with time, from 52 percent during the first 5 years to up to 100 percent after 20 years.[62,64,65,67]

The shoulder joint has the highest incidence of pain, with one third to one half of all patients developing shoulder pain during wheelchair transfers within the first 5 years and 70 percent at 10 years. Among the causes implicated in chronic shoulder pain are rotator cuff tears, bicipital tendinitis, and bursitis. Arthrography performed in paraplegic patients with persistent shoulder pain revealed a 45 percent incidence of rotator cuff tears. Intra-articular pressures of the shoulder joint are elevated during active transfers, reaching pressures greater than 250 mm Hg. Although increased stresses and activity at the shoulder seem to contribute to soft tissue injury, degenerative arthritis does not develop universally, even in patients with paraplegia of long duration or in those who have used crutches for swing-through gait for many years. Gait studies in paraplegic crutch-walkers imply occurrence of increased loads through the glenohumeral and acromiohumeral joints during upper extremity weight bearing.[67]

Subdeltoid (subacromial) bursitis of the shoulder is manifested by pain under the acromion. The pain is increased with activity and sometimes increased with abduction (as in rotator cuff injury). Diagnosis of bursitis is usually made by exclusion of other causes. Chronic rotator cuff attritional injuries can be excluded with arthrography or magnetic resonance imaging. Tendinitis of the rotator cuff may be difficult to exclude. Radiographs may show calcifications in the supraspinatus tendon. Bicipital tendinitis causes pain along the biceps tendon in the bicipital groove on the anterior surface of the humeral head. Pain is well localized and increased with elbow flexion against resistance. Bursitis and tendinitis are usually self-limiting and often can be controlled by rest, decreasing activity, and anti-inflammatory medications. Because wheelchair patients require use of the upper extremities for activities of daily living, decreasing activity may cause them difficulty. Occasional and limited lidocaine and steroid injections can be useful in the treatment of bursitis and tendinitis. Treatment of rotator cuff tears depends on the extent of injury and limitations of the patient. Rarely have chronic attritional tears of the cuff been of sufficient magnitude to require surgical repair. In general, indications for surgical repair are the same as for patients in the general population.

Besides the shoulder, the hand also is commonly involved with pain. About 9 percent of patients complain of hand pain, most frequently in the palm. Pain in the palm is usually due to direct soft tissue irritation from repeated trauma during wheelchair propulsion. A second source of hand pain is the development of carpal tunnel syndrome (discussed in the next section). Pain also occurs in the elbow and forearm in approximately 5 percent of patients.[62,64,67] Bone density in the forearm has been noted to be increased in paraparetic patients who rely on swing-through crutch-walking for ambulation.[67]

Carpal Tunnel Syndrome

Carpal tunnel syndrome has been associated with wheelchair use and transfers.[60,62,68] Up to 64 percent of paraplegic patients studied had signs or symptoms consistent with carpal tunnel syndrome, and the prevalence was noted to increase with the length of time from spinal cord injury. This high prevalence has been attributed to both the frequent use of the wrist in an extended position during lifting and transfers and the repetitive trauma sustained to the palmar aspect of the wrist while propelling a wheelchair. Concurrent ulnar neuropathy at the elbow was noted in 40 percent of paraplegic patients with carpal tunnel syndrome.[60]

In the paraplegic patient with symptoms, signs, and electrodiagnostic confirmation of carpal tunnel syndrome, treatment should include standard initial measures of rest, splinting, and anti-inflammatory medications. However, splinting may not be practical in this population and persistent or severe symptoms usually require surgical decompression. Prolonged recovery of grip strength and persistent incisional discomfort are common, probably related to dependence on upper extremity function for activities of daily living.

Cubital Tunnel Syndrome

In addition to carpal tunnel syndrome, an increased frequency of ulnar neuropathy has been associated with upper extremity use in paraplegic patients.[60,66] Of those with carpal tunnel syndrome, concurrent cubital tunnel syndrome was noted in 40 percent.[60] An awareness of this problem and appropriate evaluation of nerve function will allow prompt detection and appropriate management.

MISCELLANEOUS PROBLEMS

Additional problems in the musculoskeletal system faced by the patient with spinal cord injury include reflex sympathetic dystrophy, thrombophlebitis, gravitational edema, and decubitus ulcers.

Reflex Sympathetic Dystrophy

Reflex sympathetic dystrophy is a recognized cause of upper extremity pain in the tetraplegic patient, with reported prevalence in spinal cord injury as high as 10 percent.[64,69-72] Common findings include diffuse hand or extremity pain, swelling, and stiffness. Less frequently, trophic changes of skin and hyper-

hydrosis are present. Radiographs often show macular and periarticular osteopenia. Three-phase radionuclide scintigraphy is a sensitive and specific diagnostic study to confirm the diagnosis. Management of this problem includes mobilization and splinting to prevent contractures, peripheral nerve or stellate ganglion block, systemic medication (sympatholytic medications such as alpha blockers or calcium channel blockers) and surgical sympathectomy. This disorder is discussed in more detail in Chapter 47.

Venous Thrombosis

Venous thrombosis usually occurs within the first 40 days of hospitalization and appears to be more common in spinal cord–injured patients than in other hospitalized patients. Contributing factors include lack of mobilization and the loss of pump action from active muscle contraction. If sensibility is not intact, diagnosis may be difficult. Findings include edema, warmth, and an increase in calf circumference. Minor edema may be the only presenting sign. Differential diagnosis includes heterotopic ossification, infection, tumor, gravitational edema, and pathologic fracture. Venography is usually diagnostic. Treatment is by anticoagulation, usually beginning with intravenous heparin followed by oral long-term anticoagulant drugs such as warfarin sodium. Physical therapy should cease temporarily during the acute stage. Late venous thrombosis also can occur, appearing in the second or third month after injury.

Gravitational Edema

Gravitational edema is caused by extravascular fluid pooling as a result of dependence of the limb and lack of active muscle action. It occurs mostly in the lower extremities. Gravitational edema usually subsides within a few hours after elevation of the extremities. It is mentioned here briefly because it can mimic or mask other, more serious disorders, such as thrombophlebitis, infection, occult fracture, or heterotopic bone formation.

Decubitus Ulcers

Decubitus ulcers are one of the most preventable complications in the spinal cord–injured patient. Although proper care should completely eliminate this

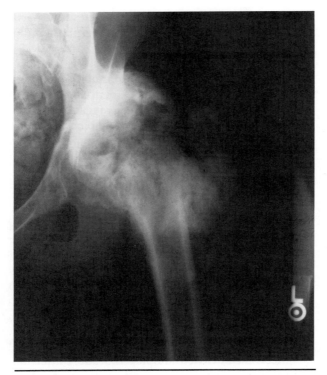

Fig. 34-7. Anteroposterior radiograph of left hip of spinal cord–injured patient with heterotopic ossification. Restricted motion led to difficulty with wheelchair transfers and positioning and ultimately contributed to formation of decubitus ulcers.

problem, these ulcers continue to be a common problem in the spinal cord–injured patient. A single indiscretion in care can lead to persistent, repeated ulceration with resultant hospitalization, loss of independence, and disruption of social adjustment. Areas where subcutaneous tissue is thin and skin overlies a bony prominence are at high risk for ulceration. Common sites include the ischial tuberosities, sacrum, great trochanter, malleoli, and os calcis. Flexion contractures or joint stiffness from spasticity or heterotopic ossification increases the risk owing to limited or prolonged positioning (Fig. 34-7). Continuous pressure leads to ischemia of all tissues between the skin and underlying bone. Lack of sensibility and paralysis do not promote or allow patients to reposition themselves to relieve the ischemic area. Necrosis follows, usually in the subcutaneous fat (which has a lesser blood supply than the dermis). Healing may occur, and the ulcer fills with dense, nonresilient scar tissue covered with thin epithelial tissue. Thick cicatrix covered with thin epithelium has poor resistance to repeated breakdown, and repeated or chronic ulcers may result. Chronic ulcers also are high risk for infection. Osteomyelitis can develop in a bony prominence, such as the greater trochanter, that becomes exposed in the ulcer (Fig. 34-8).

Treatment of decubitus ulcers is prevention. Proper padding, frequent positioning, and constant surveillance for early evidence of skin ischemia must be instituted. Established ulcers require unloading of the pressure, local wound care, control of infection, correction of nutritional deficiencies, correction of contractures or spasticity that may be contributing to pressure areas, and surgical reconstruction if needed.[73] Surgery often involves resection of infected bone, soft tissue débridement, and coverage using skin grafting and local pedicle or distant tissue flaps.

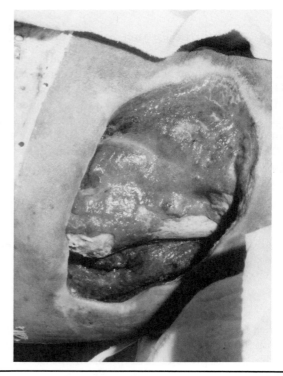

Fig. 34-8. Large decubitus ulcer in hip region with exposed greater trochanter. Osteomyelitis commonly develops when bone is exposed. It must be emphasized that the most important aspect of treatment of such ulcers is prevention.

CONCLUSION

The many possible complications involving the musculoskeletal system in the patient with spinal cord injury have been outlined. The numerous problems possible, and the consequences of delay in diagnosis or improper management, emphasize the need for a constant high index of suspicion for complications and an aggressive treatment approach in the management of these patients. Although some of the problems presented here are unavoidable or are an unchangeable consequence of spinal cord injury, many can be prevented or minimized with an awareness of the potential problems, the use of proper preventive measures, and a thorough evaluation when a problem is suspected.

REFERENCES

1. Comarr AE, Hutchinson RH, Bors E: Extremity fractures of patients with spinal cord injuries. Am J Surg 103:732, 1962
2. McMaster WC, Stauffer ES: The management of long bone fracture in the spinal cord injured patient. Clin Orthop 112:44, 1975
3. Garfin SR, Shackford SR, Marshall LF, Drummond JC: Care of the multiply injured patient with cervical spine injury. Clin Orthop 239:19, 1989
4. Tricot A, Hallot R: Traumatic paraplegia and associated fractures. Paraplegia 5:211, 1968
5. Garland DE: Clinical observations on fractures and heterotopic ossification in the spinal cord and traumatic brain injured populations. Clin Orthop 233:86, 1988
6. Botte MJ, Moore TJ: The orthopaedic management of extremity injuries in head trauma. J Head Trauma Rehab 2:13, 1987
7. Ragnarsson KT, Sell GH: Lower extremity fractures after spinal cord injury: a retrospective study. Arch Phys Med Rehabil 62:418, 1981
8. Stauffer ES: Long-term management of traumatic quadriplegia. In Pierce DS, Nickel VL (eds): The Total Care of Spinal Cord Injuries. Little, Brown and Company, Boston, 1977
9. Freehafer AA: Long-term management of lumbar paraplegia. In Pierce DS, Nickel VL (eds): The Total Care of Spinal Cord Injuries. Little, Brown and Company, Boston, 1977
10. Garland DE, Reiser TVC, Singer DI: Treatment of femoral shaft fractures associated with acute spinal cord injuries. Clin Orthop 197:191, 1985
11. Garland DE, Saucedo T, Reiser TV: The management of tibial fractures in acute spinal cord injury patients. Clin Orthop 213:237, 1986
12. Garland DE, Jones RC, Kuncle RW: Upper extremity fractures in the acute spinal cord injured patient. Clin Orthop 233:110, 1988
13. Botte MJ, Keenan MAE: Percutaneous phenol blocks of the pectoralis major muscle to treat spastic deformities. J Hand Surg [Am] 13:147, 1988
14. Keenan MAE: The orthopaedic management of spasticity. Head Trauma Rehabil 2:62, 1987
15. Keenan MAE, Todderud EP, Henderson R, Botte MJ: Management of intrinsic spasticity in the hand with phenol injection or neurectomy of the motor branch of the ulnar nerve. J Hand Surg [Am] 12:734, 1987
16. Keenan MAE, Botte MJ: Technique of percutaneous phenol block to the recurrent motor branch of the median nerve. J Hand Surg [Am] 12:806, 1987
17. Botte MJ, Nickel VL, Akeson WH: Spasticity and contracture: physiologic aspects of formation. Clin Orthop 233:7, 1988
18. Guttmann L: Spinal shock and reflex behaviour in man. Paraplegia 8:100, 1970
19. Jordan C: Current status of functional lower extremity surgery in adult spastic patients. Clin Orthop 233:102, 1988
20. Davis R: Spasticity following spinal cord injury. Orthop Clin 112:66, 1975
21. Marsolais EB, Kobetic R: Development of a practical electrical stimulation system for restoring gait in the paralyzed patient. Clin Orthop 233:64, 1988
22. Botte MJ, Keenan MAE: Reconstructive surgery of the upper extremity in the patient with head trauma. J Head Trauma Rehabil 2:34, 1987
23. Braun RM, Hoffer MM, Mooney V: Phenol nerve block in the treatment of acquired spastic hemiplegia in the upper limb. J Bone Joint Surg [Am] 55:580, 1973
24. Garland DE, Lilling M, Keenan MA: Percutaneous phenol blocks to motor points of spastic forearm muscles in head-injured adults. Arch Phys Med Rehabil 65:243, 1984
25. Mooney V, Frykman G, McLamb J: Current status of intraneural phenol injections. Clin Orthop 63:132, 1969
26. Akeson WH, Amiel D, Woo SL-Y: Immobility effects on synovial joints: the pathomechanics of joint contracture. Biorheology 17:95, 1980
27. Akeson WH, Amiel D, Abel MF et al: Effects of immobilization on joints. Clin Orthop 219:28, 1987
28. Woo SL-Y, Matthews JV, Akeson WH et al: Connective tissue response to immobility: correlative study of biomechanical measurements of normal and immobilized rabbit knees. Arthritis Rheum 18:257, 1975
29. Woo SL-Y, Gomez MA, Young-Knyn W, Akeson WH: Mechanical properties of tendons and ligaments. II. The relationships of immobilization and exercise on tissue remodeling. Biorheology 19:397, 1982
30. Braun RM, West F, Mooney V: Surgical treatment of the painful shoulder contracture in the stroke patient. J Bone Joint Surg [Am] 53:1307, 1971
31. Keenan MAE: Management of the spastic upper extremity in the neurologically impaired adult. Clin Orthop 233:116, 1988
32. Keenan MAE, Abrams RA, Garland DE, Waters RL: Results of fractional lengthening of the finger flexors in adults with upper extremity spasticity. J Hand Surg [Am] 12:575, 1987
33. Waters RL, Garland DE: Acquired neurologic disorders of the adult foot, p. 332. In Mann RA (ed): Surgery of the Foot. CV Mosby, St. Louis, 1986
34. Hanson RW, Franklin WR: Sexual loss in relation to other functional losses for spinal cord injured males. Arch Phys Med Rehabil 57:291, 1976
35. Moberg EA: Upper limb surgical rehabilitation in tetraplegia. In Evarts CM (ed): Surgery of the Musculoskeletal System. Churchill Livingstone, New York, 1983
36. McDowell CL: Tetraplegia. In Green DP (ed): Operative Hand Surgery. Churchill Livingstone, New York, 1988
37. Moberg E: The Upper Limb in Tetraplegia, George Thieme, Stuttgart, 1978
38. Zancolli EI: Structural and Dynamic Bases of Hand Surgery. p. 231. JB Lippincott, Philadelphia, 1979
39. Freehafer AA, Vonhaam E, Allen V: Tendon transfers to im-

prove grasp after injuries of the cervical spinal cord. J Hand Surg [Am] 56:951, 1974

40. McDowell CL, Moberg EA, Graham-Smith A: International conference on surgical rehabilitation of the upper limb in tetraplegia. J Hand Surg 4:387, 1979

41. McDowell CL, Moberg EA, House JH: The Second International Conference on Surgical Rehabilitation of the Upper Limb in Tetraplegia (quadriplegia). J Hand Surg [Am] 11:604, 1986

42. Smith AG: Early complications of key grip hand surgery for tetraplegia. Paraplegia 19:123, 1981

43. Nickel VL, Perry J, Garrett AL: Development of useful function in the severely paralyzed hand. J Bone Joint Surg [Am] 45:933, 1963

44. Zancolli E: Surgery for the quadriplegic hand with active strong wrist extension preserved. A study of 97 cases. Clin Orthop 112:101, 1975

45. House JH, Gwathmey FW, Lundsgaard DK: Restoration of strong grasp and lateral pinch in tetraplegia due to cervical spinal cord injury. J Hand Surg 1:152, 1976

46. House JH, Shannon MA: Restoration of strong grasp and lateral pinch in tetraplegia: a comparison of two methods of thumb control in each patient. J Hand Surg [Am] 10:22, 1985

47. House JH: Reconstruction of the thumb in tetraplegia following spinal cord injury. Clin Orthop 195:117, 1985

48. Waters RL, Moore KR, Graboff SR, Paris K: Brachioradialis to flexor pollicis longus tendon transfer for active lateral pinch in the tetraplegic. J Hand Surg [Am] 10:385, 1985

49. Kelly CM, Freehafer AA, Peckham PH, Stroh K: Postoperative results of opponensplasty and flexor tendon transfer in patients with spinal cord injuries. J Hand Surg [Am] 10:890, 1985

50. Lamb DW, Chan KM: Surgical reconstruction of the upper limb in traumatic tetraplegia: a review of 41 patients. J Bone Joint Surg [Br] 65:291, 1983

51. Brand PW: Clinical Mechanics of the Hand. CV Mosby, St Louis, 1985

52. Hentz VR, Brown M, Keoshian LA: Upper limb reconstruction in quadriplegia: functional assessment and proposed treatment modifications. J Hand Surg 8:119, 1983

53. Hiersche DL, Waters RL: Interphalangeal fixation of the thumb in Moberg's key grip procedure. J Hand Surg [Am] 10:30, 1985

54. Ragnarsson KT: Physiologic effects of functional electrical stimulation-induced exercises in spinal cord–injured individuals. Clin Orthop 233:53, 1988

55. Keith MW, Peckham PH, Thrope GB et al: Functional neuromuscular stimulation neuroprostheses for the tetraplegic hand. Clin Orthop 233:25, 1988

56. Kralj A, Bajd T, Turk R: Enhancement of gait restoration in spinal injured patients by functional electrical stimulation. Clin Orthop 233:34, 1988

57. Peckham PH: Functional electrical stimulation: current status and future prospects of applications to the neuromuscular system in spinal cord injury. Paraplegia 25:279, 1987

58. Peckham PH, Keith MW, Freehafer AA: Restoration of functional control by electrical stimulation in the upper extremity of the quadriplegic patient. J Bone Joint Surg [Am] 70:144, 1988

59. Waters RL, Campbell JM, Nakai R: Therapeutic electrical stimulation of the lower limb by epimysial electrodes. Clin Orthop 233:44, 1988

60. Aljure J, Eltorai I, Bradley WE et al: Carpal tunnel syndrome in paraplegic patients. Paraplegia 23:182, 1985

61. Bayley JC, Cochran TP, Sledge CB: The weight-bearing shoulder: the impingement syndrome in paraplegics. J Bone Joint Surg [Am] 69:676, 1987

62. Blankstein A, Shmueli R, Weingarten I et al: Hand problems due to prolonged use of crutches and wheelchairs. Ortho Rev 14:29, 1985

63. Davis R: Pain and suffering following spinal cord injury. Orthop Clin 112:76, 1975

64. Gellman H, Sie I, Waters RL: Late complications of the weight-bearing upper extremity in the paraplegic patient. Clin Orthop 233:132, 1988

65. Nichols PJR, Norman PA, Ennis JR: Wheelchair user's shoulder? Shoulder pain in patients with spinal cord injuries. Scand J Rehabil Med 11:29, 1979

66. Stephaniwsky L, Bilowitt DS, Prasad SS: Reduced motor conduction velocity of the ulnar nerve in spinal cord injured patients. Paraplegia 18:21, 1980

67. Wing PC, Tredwell SJ: The weight-bearing shoulder. Paraplegia 21:107, 1983

68. Gellman H, Chandler D, Sie I et al: Carpal tunnel syndrome in paraplegic patients. J Bone Joint Surg [Am] 70:517, 1988

69. Andrews LG, Armitage KJ: Sudeck's atrophy in traumatic quadriplegia. Paraplegia 9:159, 1971

70. Gellman H, Eckert RR, Botte MJ et al: Reflex sympathetic dystrophy in cervical spinal cord injury patients. Clin Orthop 233:126, 1988

71. Ohry A, Brooks ME, Steinbach TV, Rozin R: Shoulder complication as a cause of delay in rehabilitation of spinal cord injured patients. Paraplegia 16:310, 1978

72. Wainapel SR, Freed MM: Reflex sympathetic dystrophy in quadriplegia: case report. Arch Phys Med Rehabil 65:35, 1984

73. Shea JD: Pressure sores: classification and management. Orthop Clin 112:89, 1975

35 Heterotopic Ossification

DOUGLAS E. GARLAND

Abnormal bone formation, often called heterotopic ossification (HO), is the consequence of many diseases and various types of trauma. The primary entities associated with HO that physicians are most likely to encounter are neurologic insults, traumatic brain injury, spinal cord injury, and other types of trauma (violent or surgical). These more common disorders leading to HO have some clinical similarities, such as location in the body (although sites about a joint may vary), natural history, and treatment modalities. Knowledge of the commonalities assists the clinician in evaluating and selecting appropriate treatment plans. These similarities may help the researcher to identify possible systemic and/or local cell regulators and various cell types responsible for HO.

GENETICS AND PATIENT PREDISPOSITION

Strong support for some type of genetic predisposition to HO formation comes from the hereditary disorder fibrodysplasia ossificans progressiva (FOP). FOP is inherited as an autosomal-dominant trait with full penetrance and variable expression; it is a disorder of connective tissue with skeletal malformations and HO.[1] The natural history of HO associated with FOP has similarities to the natural history of HO from other causes, especially neurogenic HO. Although the majority of cases of FOP-associated HO are spontaneous, some cases also occur after trauma. A predilection of HO for certain locations (i.e., the axial musculature and proximal limbs) is documented that is common in both traumatic and neurogenic HO. HO frequently recurs after surgical resection, including not uncommonly after resection of neurogenic HO and occasionally traumatic HO.

Primary osteoma cutis is also a dominantly inherited disease wherein multifocal subcutaneous ossifications occur. The HO may occur around joints, including distal joints, which are rarely involved by HO of traumatic or neurogenic origin.[2]

The association of human leukocyte antigens (HLAs) with neurogenic HO has been documented. An increased prevalence of HLA-B18, HLA-B27, and HLA-DW7 antigens has been reported in patients with HO in comparison to normal subjects.[3,4] However, follow-up studies from other centers have not confirmed these findings,[5] and this system cannot at present predict subjects' susceptibility to HO.

The HO of traumatic brain injury is predictably associated with spasticity, especially if the patient is evaluated early after the neurologic insult.[6] As neurologic recovery occurs, spasticity about a joint with HO may diminish. The persistence of limb spasticity is an excellent predictor of functional outcome and recurrence of HO after its resection.[7] The HO of spinal cord injury also is associated with spasticity, although HO may occur in flaccid limbs. Patients with limb spasticity are at increased risk of developing HO.[8,9] Patients with massive HO have severe spasticity, and it is also in this group that recurrence after resection is the highest.[10] Trauma to a joint or surgical repair (iatrogenic trauma) of a fracture greatly increases the occurrence of HO in the patient with central nervous system disease.[11,12] In addition, decubitus ulcers about a proximal joint increase the risk of HO.[8]

453

Other nongenetic risk factors, especially in patients undergoing total hip replacement, have been associated with HO. The most consistently mentioned and generally accepted risk factors are male sex and presence of osteoarthritis and osteophyte formation. Other risk factors, for which there is no consensus, are surgical approach to treatment, age, other prior surgeries, trochanteric osteotomy, and length of surgery. Likewise, there is no concensus such that HO will develop on the opposite hip after it has formed in a total hip replacement patient.[13,14]

PREVALENCE AND ONSET

Prevalence

The reported prevalence varies for most types of HO, but much of this difference may be the result of methodology and institutional variations. The type of center, (acute care versus rehabilitation) and the type of patient (with hemiplegia, paraplegia, or quadriplegia) influence the results. Methodology also affects study outcomes. Prospective versus retrospective studies, whole-body radiographs versus hip only, and 6-month versus 1-year follow-ups have potential to influence final data.

The prevalence of clinically significant HO—that which limits joint motion—as opposed to HO of purely academic interest or that which is solely a radiographic observation, is similar when studies from similar institutions and methodologies are compared regardless of its cause. The most commonly reported prevalence of clinically significant HO is 10 to 20 percent.[6,9,13-18] Joint ankylosis occurs in less than 10 percent of the lesions. This similar rate of occurrence from the varying causes suggests an underlying patient predetermination.

Onset

The onset of HO regardless of cause ranges from 4 to 12 weeks after the precipitating event, with a peak occurrence at 2 months. Occasionally, HO may be detected prior to 3 weeks and after 3 months.[6,9,13-23]

DIAGNOSIS

Physical Examination

Limited joint motion is the most common physical finding and frequently the earliest sign of HO. Localized swelling is the second most common sign. Joint erythema and warmth occasionally require differentiation from a septic joint, especially after total joint replacement. Lower limb swelling may mimic thrombophlebitis, most notably in the HO of spinal cord injury. The most common symptom of HO is pain. An increase in pain, relative spasticity, or muscle guarding should alert the examiner of the possibility of HO.

Serum Alkaline Phosphatase Determination

Early reports on HO failed to detect elevated serum alkaline phosphatase (SAP) levels. However, follow-up studies have demonstrated that elevated levels of SAP are associated with clinically significant HO.[21,24,25] SAP levels begin to rise, although remaining in the normal range, within 2 weeks of injury. Elevated levels may occur by 3 weeks, and the duration of persistent high levels averages 5 months (Fig. 35-1).[21] The majority of patients who develop so-called clinically significant HO will have an elevated SAP level. SAP concentration does not correlate with inactivity, peak activity, or number of HO lesions. SAP determination is nonspecific and not absolute but it may constitute the earliest and certainly is the most convenient and least expensive laboratory test for early detection of HO. In addition, many neurologic patients are in intensive care units and cannot undergo special studies. SAP level is easy to determine and is an excellent presumptive test for HO. Medicinal treatment may be initiated solely on the basis of SAP elevation if fractures are not present.

Radionuclide Bone Imaging

Radionuclide bone imaging (RNBI) became efficient as a diagnostic tool in the late 1960s and early 1970s. Early bone scan technique employed injection of technetium-99m polyphosphate with follow-up scans obtained approximately 4 to 5 hours after injection. At present, the "three-phase" bone scan is the best method for early detection of HO; this test involves injection of ^{99m}Tc-labeled methylene diphosphonate followed by imaging in three phases:

Phase I—a dynamic blood flow study with frequent photoscans for approximately 1 minute;
Phase II—a static scan for blood pool after the completion of phase I.
Phase III—a 2- to 4-hour bone scan to determine the degree of the labeled radionuclide in bone.

The first two phases are the most sensitive for the earliest detection of HO and may show abnormal

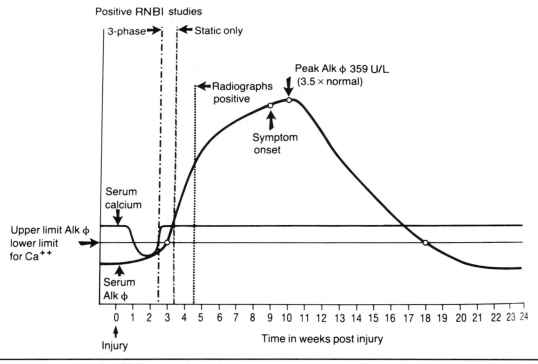

Fig. 35-1. Serum alkaline phosphatase level (Alk 0) and calcium (Ca⁺⁺) behavior in acute heterotopic bone formation and relationship to radionuclide bone imaging (RNBI) studies. (From Orzel and Rudd,[21] with permission.)

results within 2 to 4 weeks after injury even though the osseous tissue uptake may be normal (phase III). This period of positive uptake in phases I and II with a negative phase III may range from 2 to 4 weeks. Likewise, phase III may be positive up to 4 weeks before HO is observed radiographically.[16]

A large definitive prospective or even retrospective study of the RNBI phase III evaluation of HO is not available. Correlation of RNBI and evolution of radiographic features has not been performed. It does appear that the majority of bone scans return to baseline within 7 to 12 months while a slowly downward activity occurs in many of the remainder of the scans. A few scans remain fully active during the first year.[16] The RNBI may become reactivated after a quiescent period.

Quantitative radionuclide bone scans compare the ratio of uptake in normal versus heterotopic bone. Because HO uptake decreases with time, it is assumed that serial decreases or a steady state in the ratio of uptake between normal and heterotopic bone is an indication of HO maturity. It is proposed that the incidence of recurrence of HO is decreased after resection if HO is removed during a radionuclide steady state. Unfortunately, this premise has not been adequately verified in a large homogeneous series. Two large surgical resection series demonstrated that this steady state was not a predictor of recurrence.[7,10] Patients with persistent active scans predictably had recurrence whereas patients with baseline scans not uncommonly had recurrence. Consequently, it seems that neither the natural history of HO nor treatment guidelines based on RNBI activity have been adequately established.

Radiography

Before RNBI became available, radiographs provided confirmatory evidence of HO. Although plain films may detect HO as early as 3 weeks after injury, radiographic detection generally is not confirmatory until 2 months after the stimulus.

Radiographs offer other benefits. They can identify the site of HO at the joint and are an easy, cheap, and reliable method for evaluation of treatment. Radiographs permit evaluation of maturation of HO, especially when coupled with results of SAP determinations and physical examination. Radiographic grading of the amount of HO has some predictive value for recurrence after resection.[10] In addition, radiographic quantitative assessment may eventually allow standard grading, may assist in evaluation of treatment methods, and may predict recurrence after resection.

Computed Tomography

The precise role of computed tomography (CT) scanning as a clinical tool for diagnosis and a measure of maturation of HO is not established. CT may aid in preoperative surgical planning. Involvement of varying sites at a joint may be identified in situations in which standard radiographs do not allow such discrimination (Fig. 35-2). CT scan may more clearly define localization of HO and its relationship to muscle, vessel and nerve.[26]

LOCATION

Heterotopic bone most commonly forms in the proximal joints and limbs. Varying causes produce predictable patterns of formation about a specific joint. Spasticity may partially direct the site specificity in neurogenic HO.[6] The HO associated with trauma may be para-articular or peri-articular in location, whereas neurogenic HO is para-articular.

Shoulder

Traumatic Brain Injury

The frequency of HO of the shoulder is less common than HO at the hip, is similar to the frequency of HO at the elbow, always less frequent than HO of the shoulder joint.[6] A pseudoarthrosis is frequently present. Ankylosis is rare. Internal rotator muscle spasticity is present both early and late if neurologic recovery does not occur.

Spinal Cord Injury

Heterotopic bone is uncommon in the upper extremity and rare in the elbow. The appearance of HO may be nonspecific or similar to the HO observed in the shoulder in traumatic brain injury.

Trauma

HO may occur in any and all planes about the shoulder after trauma. It is also commonly present in the vicinity of the coracoacromial ligament.

Elbow

Trauma

HO may form in all planes in single sites or in various combinations. The most common locations are medial and lateral, and the bone develops adjacent to or may encircle the collateral ligaments (Fig. 35-3).[12] HO in the vicinity of the ulnar collateral ligament is associated with tardy ulnar palsy.[27] The HO lesion may encircle the ulnar nerve. Anterior HO lies beneath the brachialis muscle whereas posterior HO is located beneath the triceps muscle.

Traumatic Brain Injury

The most common site for HO associated with traumatic brain injury is posterior, which is also the most common location for ankylosis in all such cases.[7] Posterior HO is usually associated with extensor rigidity, but with neurologic recovery triceps spasticity subsides. The heterotopic bone usually forms posterolaterally but may be posteromedial or involve the entire posterior surface (Fig. 35-4). Anterior HO is usually associated with flexor spasticity. HO in the vicinity of the collateral ligaments is uncommon and rarely requires resection regardless of the cause. Tardy ulnar palsy occurs in chronic pressure paralysis in the bedridden patient with an enkylosed elbow or from the inflammatory response of HO.[27]

Hip

Trauma

HO associated with trauma may appear hazy and diffuse. The HO lesion may be peri- or para-articular. HO may form in a single posterior site as a consequence of a posterior dislocation. If an open reduction–internal fixation was necessary, HO may occur in the abductor region (Fig. 35-2).[11]

Total Hip Replacement

Two main forms of HO develop after total hip replacement. The more common type occurs laterally in the vicinity of the abductor muscles. This HO appears similar to traumatic HO detected after open reduction–internal fixation of acetabular-peritro-

Fig. 35-2. (A) Anteroposterior (AP) radiograph of the hip. The patient had concomitant traumatic brain injury and dislocation of the hip. An open reduction was required. Neurogenic HO formed anteriorly (a), traumatic (or surgical) HO formed posteriorly (b), and surgical HO formed in the abductor region (c). **(B)** Computed tomography (CT) scan of the hip. Note the space between the neurogenic HO (a) and the posterior HO (b) and the hip capsule. Neurogenic HO does not involve the joint capsule. A posterior approach was employed to remove the posterior and abductor (c) HO. One week later, an anterior approach was utilized to remove the anterior HO.

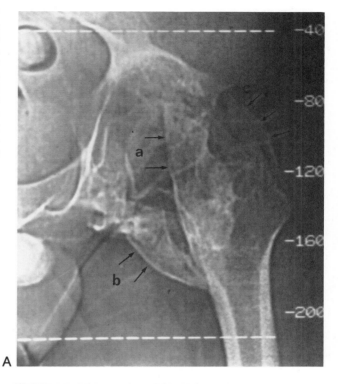

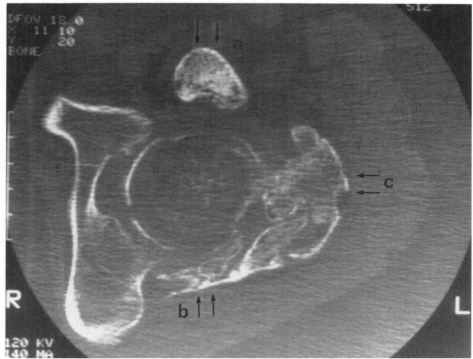

chanteric fractures. The other type occurs about the femoral neck. In the mild form the HO lesion has the appearance of traumatic HO. However, as the ossific deposit progresses in size the radiographic appearance is quite distinct and predictable when adjacent to the femoral neck medially, laterally, or both.

Spinal Cord Injury

The HO of spinal cord injury is most commonly located aneriorly and may have varying appearances, but it generally forms within a plane from the anterior superior iliac spine toward the lesser trochanter (Fig. 35-5).[18] This HO forms proximally above the joint, distally about the lesser trochanter, or between the two. The hip is in flexion and adduction. If a decubitus ulcer is present about the greater trochanter, the lesion may form in this vicinity. HO may occur in the abductor region or at a posterior site, although this type is less common.

Traumatic Brain Injury

Three main forms of HO associated with traumatic brain injury develop and are the most distinctive of the hip patterns.[7] Anterior HO lies in a plane from the anterior superior iliac spine to the greater trochanter, in contradistinction to HO of spinal cord injury, in which the bone is directed toward the lesser trochanter. The hip posture is slight flexion and external rotation. Inferomedial HO is found distal to the hip joint and medial to the femoral shaft. This variety of HO is associated with adductor muscle spasticity. Posterior HO lies immediately posterior to the femoral head and neck and is often accompanied by a mild flexion contracture. Occasionally, combined patterns or even an abductor muscle location may occur (Fig. 35-2).

Femur and Knee

No site specificity is apparent in the femur or knee. Quadriceps HO occurs in various locations, predictably at the site of blunt trauma. Quadriceps HO is also observed distally after spinal cord injury and occasionally after traumatic brain injury (Fig. 35-6). HO about the knee itself is the second most common location of the HO of spinal cord injury,[18] although it is rarely seen in HO of traumatic brain injury. The most common site is medial and the radiographic appearance often is similar to that of Pellegrini-Stieda disease. Posterior and lateral sites of ossification occur. HO in these locations responds to symptomatic treatment and range-of-motor exercises; surgical excision is seldom necessary.

NATURAL HISTORY

The natural history of HO is defined mainly through radiographs and is infrequently emphasized. The natural radiographic history is similar and predictable in the majority of patients regardless of the precipitating cause. It also closely parallels the elevation of SAP level (Fig. 35-1). Some minor variations occur among the different entities associated with HO and within similar patient populations, but these usually affect only a small percentage of a given population. However, these variations cause continuing confusion. The lack of awareness and emphasis on the natural history combined with these minor variations gives rise to many of the conflicting reports concerning interpretation of laboratory data as well as treatment outcomes.

Total Hip Replacement

A noteworthy study concerning the natural radiographic evolution of the HO of total hip replacement involved a double-blind study of placebo versus etidronate disodium treatment to prevent HO after total hip replacement.[15] Sequential radiographic evaluation of 124 untreated total hip replacement patients demonstrated that the majority of HO occurred within 15 weeks of surgery. Clinically significant HO was noted in 19 percent of the hips. The aggregate of HO lesions plateaued at 4.5 to 6 months after surgery (Fig. 35-7).

Spinal Cord Injury

In a prospective study, clinically significant HO occurred in 18.5 percent (14 of 75) of patients with spinal cord injury, with an average time to diagnosis of 62 days (range, 32 to 156 days).[17] Nine patients were treated with etidronate disodium at 10 mg/kg of body weight and followed radiographically for an average of 14 months. The average radiographic progression occurred over 5.3 months. In two patients

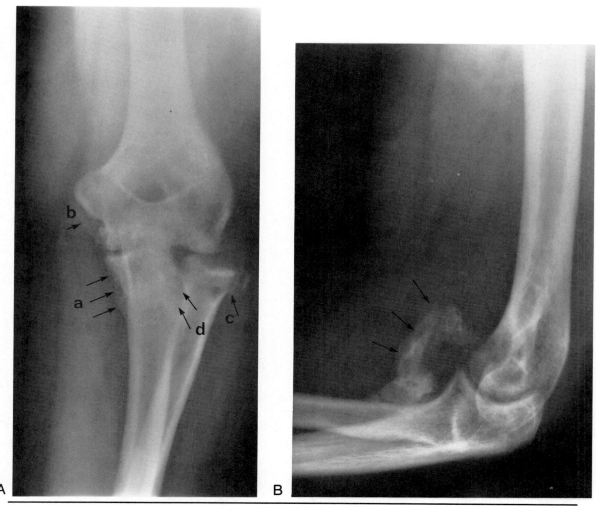

Fig. 35-3. AP **(A)** and lateral **(B)** radiographs of the elbow. The patient sustained a traumatic brain injury and a dislocation of the elbow. HO is located anteriorly (a), at the medial collateral ligament (b), at the lateral collateral ligament (c), and in the interosseous membrane (d). An ulnar neuropathy was present. A transfer of the ulnar nerve was performed through a medial approach and an anterolateral approach was employed to remove the anterior HO. The medial and lateral HO lesions were not excised. Excision of the interosseous heterotopic bone can be accomplished with the anterolateral approach or a separate posterolateral approach.

the HO progression continued after 1 year. Range of hip flexion averaged 90°.

A review of radiographs in a retrospective study of 19 patients who underwent resection of HO over a 15-year span demonstrated a greater than 6-month radiographic progression of HO in each instance.[10] Patients had moderate or larger amounts of HO. In some instances significant RNBI activity persisted for years. Approximately 3,000 patients underwent re-

habilitation during this period and did not either develop or require resection of HO. Consequently, this HO lesion involves only a small percentage of the spinal cord injury population.

In the study already cited,[15] 104 placebo-treated spinal cord–injured patients were studied radiographically. Over 80 percent developed HO within 150 days of injury, and clinically significant HO occurred in 16 percent. Patients were treated with either eti-

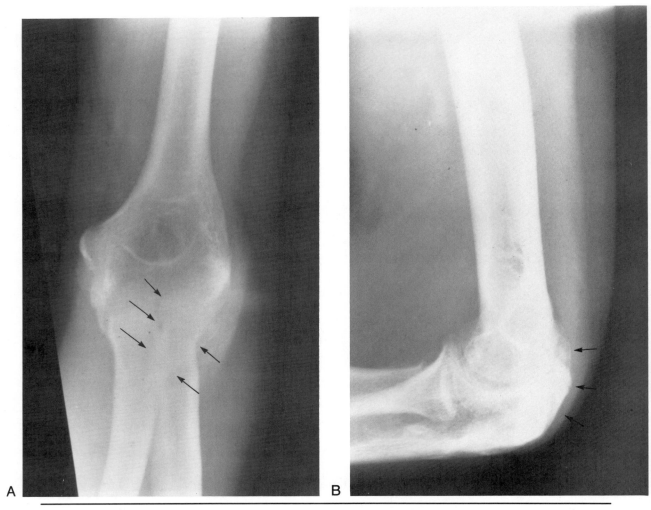

Fig. 35-4. AP **(A)** and lateral **(B)** radiographs of the elbow. This posterolateral site (arrows) is the most common location for HO in traumatic brain injury at the elbow and the most commonly involved by ankylosis. A simple posterolateral approach allows removal.

dronate disodium at 10 mg/kg of body weight or a placebo for 3 months after diagnosis of HO. Ten percent of etidronate disodium–treated patients versus 30 percent of the placebo-treated patients developed clinically significant lesions at the 9-month follow-up after cessation of treatment.

Based on these studies, some inferences can be made. The majority of cases of HO associated with spinal cord injury occur between 2 and 3 months after injury. Radiographic evolution of HO occurs over a 6-month span. A small percentage of the spinal cord injury population with HO—10 to 20 percent—have a greater than 6-month radiographic progression of HO. It is in these joints that bony ankylosis occurs, as does increased RNBI activity lasting for years (Fig. 35-8).[28]

Traumatic Brain Injury

In a retrospective review of 23 traumatic brain-injured patients who underwent resection of HO at an average of 28 months after injury,[7] patients were

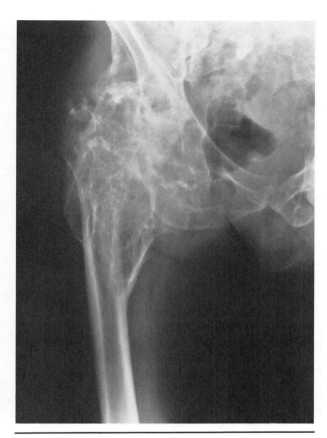

Fig. 35-5. Typical HO of spinal cord injury in an antero-medial plane at the hip. This patient had had two previous HO resections with recurrence. The hip has dislocated. Recurrence, fracture of the femoral neck, and dislocation are common in the class II spinal cord injury.

classified as belonging to classes I to V according to their neurologic recovery. Class I patients had near-normal neurologic recovery, whereas class V patients had severe cognitive deficits and spasticity. Class I patients rarely had recurrence after resection; in contrast, every class V patient had recurrence regardless of the site of every HO. Radiographic progression subsided by 6 months, and SAP levels and RNBI activity were normal or significantly decreasing in patients who were making an early normal neurologic recovery. Patients with severe motor compromise had larger amounts of ossific bone, which progressed in some instances for more than 1 year; elevated SAP levels for 2 years or longer; and occasionally persistent activity on RNBI (Fig. 35-9)

TREATMENT

HO runs a gamut from being undetected (and therefore untreated) to having a poor response to all treatment methods. Some patients with minimal HO require no treatment, whereas others may require physical therapy, medicine, manipulation, surgical excision, or all of these. The majority of patients with HO maintain functional joint motion with standard physical therapies, medicines, and occasionally forceful manipulations. A small group require surgery, with some developing recurrence of HO.

Medical Treatment

Medical treatment including radiation, is used prophylactically in two general situations: (1) to prevent HO formation after the primary insult and (2) to prevent recurrence of HO after its surgical resection.

Ethylhydroxydiphosphonate (Etidronate Disodium)

In the early 1960s, research with polyphosphates and their inhibitory activity on calcium phosphate precipitation led to evaluation of diphosphonates, most specifically ethylhydroxydiphosphonate (EHDP), for similar effects. Definitive studies demonstrated that diphosphonates inhibited the precipitation of calcium phosphate from clear solutions, delayed aggregation of apatite crystals into layer clusters, blocked the transformation of amorphous calcium phosphate into hydroxyapatite, and delayed dissolution of crystals. All effects seemed related to their affinity for hydroxyapatite. The ability of EHDP to inhibit experimental soft tissue ossification as well as normal mineralization of bone led to the clinical use of EHDP to prevent HO.[29,30]

Clinical research has not irrefutably proved or disproved the effectiveness of EHDP in prevention of clinical HO.[15-17,23,31,32] Some authors have supported its effectiveness, but none has been able to prove absolute arrest of HO when the studies are subjected to strict scientific scrutiny. Other authors have stated that EDHP is not effective in preventing HO.[33]

The desired response to EHDP dictates the proper dosage and duration of treatment. Simplistically speaking, EHDP prevents conversion of the amor-

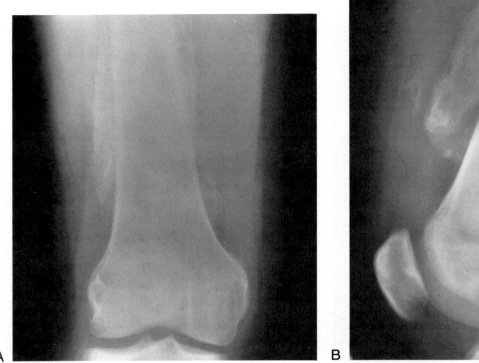
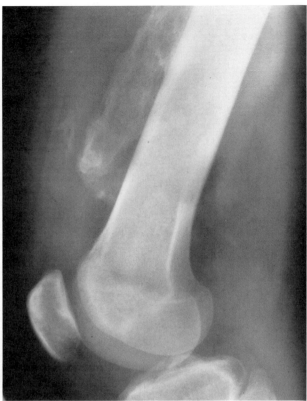

A   B

Fig. 35-6. AP **(A)** and lateral **(B)** radiographs of the distal part of the femur with neurogenic HO in a traumatic brain-injured patient. This locaiton is more common for HO in spinal cord–injured patients. The ability of the knee to move responds to standard therapy techniques, and the HO seldom requires resection.

phous calcium phosphate compounds into hydroxy-apatite crystals, which is one of the final steps of bone formation. Because the majority of HO evolves radiographically over a period of 6 months, it is concluded that EHDP should generally be taken for this 6-month span. Lower EHDP doses are adequate to inhibit crystal resorption, but they are less effective in inhibiting crystal growth. Therefore, the 20-mg/kg dosage is necessary to prevent HO formation. It is anticipated that treatment for this duration and at this dosage should prevent HO lesions in the majority of patients and also decrease the incidence of the so-called recovery phase of "rebound" calcification. A small group, approximately 10 to 20 percent, continues to exhibit formation of HO after 6 months, and the incidence of "rebound" should be expected to remain in this range in any study. Prolonged treatment at high doses of EHDP produces undesirable

side effects, such as long bone fractures, in dogs.[34] Therefore, dosages of 20 mg/kg for longer than 6 months' duration may not be warranted, and continued treatment may be deleterious. EHDP will not be effective for the massive heterotopic bone–forming patient regardless of dosage and duration of treatment.

Quantitative histomorphometry demonstrates an increased number of osteoclasts, as well as osteoblasts, in the HO lesion compared to normal bone.[35] EHDP at a much lower dosage than that necessary for the inhibition of ossification interrupts osteoclastic function but does not destroy the osteoclasts. They eventually recover full function but over a prolonged period. This effect, although somewhat overlooked in the treatment of HO by EHDP, is extremely undesirable because resorption is an important aspect in HO

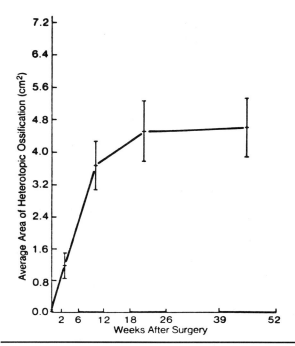

Fig. 35-7. Severity of HO as a function of time after hip replacement. Forty-five untreated patients without HO prior to the hip surgery, but in whom heterotopic bone formed after surgery, were evaluated. Patients included in this analysis had radiographs available for observation at the following times after surgery: at 2 or 6 weeks; at 12 weeks or at 18 or 26 weeks; and at 39 or 52 weeks. The diagnosis of HO was based on average area measurements of HO obtained by two independent radiologists working without knowledge of the patient's clinical course. Bars denote ±1 standard error. (From Finerman and Stover,[15] with permission.)

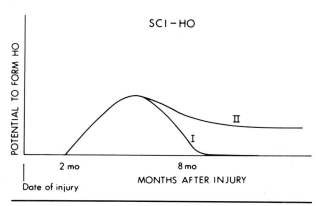

Fig. 35-8. The two main clinical responses of HO in spinal cord injury. Class I patients have roentgenographic progression and SAP activity for 5 to 6 months. Thereafter, the HO becomes relatively inert, and the bone scan returns to normal. Class II patients have persistent potential to form HO, although after a 6-month period the potential diminishes with regard to the amount of HO produced when stimulated. The bone scan often remains active in these patients. Traumatic HO appears to occur in these two classes of patients. Also, this model is similar to the antigen-antibody response: the antigen is introduced (date of injury) and a delay occurs (2 months). The immunoglobulin M antibody is produced for a short period of time (class I), and the immunoglobulin G antibody is produced for years (class II). (From Garland,[28] with permission.)

maturation, which involves partial or even complete resorption of the HO lesion. With cessation of treatment, the osteoid may ossify immediately, while the resorptive capability remains impaired until osteoclastic function returns. This may influence the rebound phenomenon as well as resorption. The effect of EHDP on osteoclasts, the recovery or rebound phase, the length of treatment, patient compliance, and the cost of the medication may eventually contribute to the selection of another drug for treatment of HO.

Indomethacin

Dahl is generally credited with demonstrating the prophylactic effects of indomethacin on HO formation after total hip replacement.[36] Other studies have verified its effectiveness, including one double-blind study.[37,38] The ability of indomethacin to inhibit prostaglandin synthetase is proposed as the primary mechanism for HO prevention, although many effects on bone formation are known. Prostaglandins are mediators of inflammation, and part of indomethacin's effect is due to inhibition of the inflammatory response or supression of mesenchymal cell proliferation. Indomethacin dosage is 25 mg three times a day for 6 weeks after total hip replacement. Ibuprofen and aspirin may also be effective when used in a similar fashion. The effectiveness of nonsteroidal anti-inflammatory drugs (NSAIDs) to prevent HO in the neurologic patient has not been established.

Radiation

The ability of radiation to inhibit bone growth has been known by radiotherapists for years. Irradiation prevents conversion of precursor cells to bone-forming cells. Early reports of irradiation in the treatment of myositis ossificans were often anecdotal. Now it

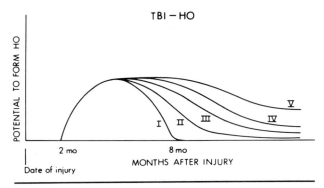

Fig. 35-9. The clinical responses of HO in traumatic brain injury. Although in spinal cord injury genetic programming may dictate HO patterns, this is overridden by neurologic outcome in the HO of traumatic brain injury. Class I patients recover early from their injury and HO runs a short course. Class V patients remain neurologically compromised and the potential to form HO may persist indefinitely. (From Garland,[28] with permission.)

apears that 1,000 rad at 200 rad/day immediately after total hip replacement is effective in preventing HO.[39,40] The location of HO formation in the neurologic patient cannot be predicted. Because radiation is relatively ineffective once HO is detected, its use in prevention of initial neurognic HO may be limited.

Manipulation

Using manipulation as a method of treatment is controversial. Some authors state that benign neglect is more desirable than continuing range of motion, claiming that moving joints through their range increases the inflammatory response, which in turn increases the HO mass. Supporters claim that experimental HO can be caused by forceful manipulation of rabbit quadriceps,[41] but in actuality this model represents traumatic HO. Consequently, this comparison is not necessarily justified because modification of the neurogenic HO pathway through manipulation has not been demonstrated.

Observations appears to show that moving joints through their range of motion does not accelerate HO formation and maintains or increases joint mobility.[9,18,42] To abstain from such exercises in the event of an inflammatory response allows fibrous ankylosis to occur even in the absence of HO formation or with mild HO. In certain instances and especially in the traumatic brain injury population, manipulation under general anesthesia is the most beneficial means to maintain range of motion (Fig. 35-10). Manipulations every 1 to 2 months may be necessary to achieve the desired results while neurologic recovery ensues. More than three manipulations generally is unwarranted.

Surgery

Surgery is indicated for joint mobility, limb positioning, or sitting. Various operative procedures have been described. Precise timing for surgery is infrequently mentioned with respect to the quiescent state, indicated by normal SAP levels, mature radiographic appearance, and baseline RNBI. The natural history of HO is seldom mentioned from a surgical vantage point. Postoperative complications are common, especially in comparison to standard orthopaedic procedures.

Trauma and Total Hip Replacement

A precise time for surgical excision is mentioned infrequently in cases of HO associated with trauma or total hip replacement. An appropriate interval may be selected on the basis of natural history and physical examination with support from the laboratory findings. The HO should not be resected earlier than 6 months after onset. No joint pain or swelling should be present. Radiographic progression should have stabilized and some HO involution may be evident. SAP levels should have returned to baseline, and RNBI will be declining. If the laboratory results remain abnormal or if the patient had ineffective prophylactic treatment, a further delay of up to 6 months may be warranted. Medical prophylaxis after surgery is desirable. Indomethacin and radiation, as outlined previously, are beneficial. EHDP, if used, should be given at 20 mg/kg for a minimum of 3 months. If any clinical or laboratory parameters are abnormal, treatment should continue for three additional months.

Spinal Cord Injury

A definitive surgical date for HO associated with spinal cord injury is seldom outlined. Consideration for HO excision should be planned at approximately 1 year after injury in the majority of patients. Surgery should be delayed to between 1½ and 2 years in the

Fig. 35-10. **(A)** Radiograph of inferomedial or adductor HO in a traumatic brain injury patient. **(B)** Limb posture at bed rest. The patient would not allow passive range of motion of the hip or the knee. (*Figure continues.*)

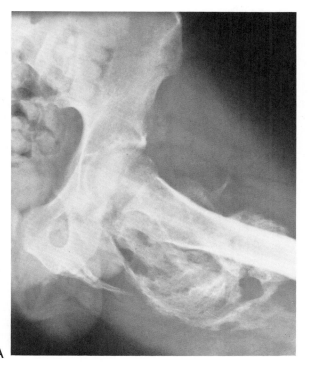

A

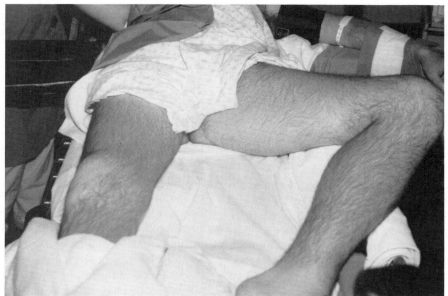

B

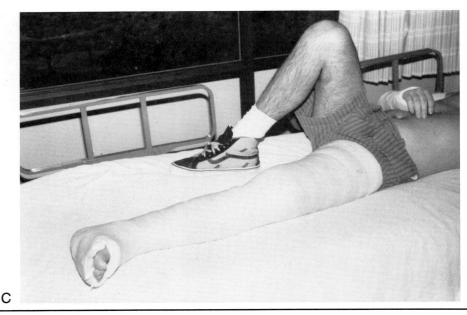

Fig. 35-10 *(Continued)* **(C)** Position of the limb after manipulation under general anesthesia. The hip will become ankylosed in a neutral position, and the hamstrings cannot develop a contracture. Therapy to include transfers and standing may proceed.

young male patient with an ankylosis or near-ankylosis of the hip, radiographic progression of HO for longer than 6 months, more than moderate amounts of HO radiographically, severe spasticity, persistent elevation of SAP, continued uptake in RNBI, and poor response to prophylactic medications. Procrastination longer than 2 years may permit development of possible complications, such as intra-articular joint ankylosis and fractures in the osteoporotic bone with initiation of joint motion after resection.[10]

EHDP has been evaluated, with mixed reviews, for its effectiveness in postoperative prevention of HO recurrence.[32] Because EHDP affects the final phase of ossification, it does not seem necessary to begin medication prior to surgery. Three months of treatment is usually adequate in the majority of patients if treatment proves effective. A full 6-month course of EHDP is necessary in the small group of patients who form massive amounts of HO because the propensity to form HO remains high. Physical therapy must continue during this 3- to 6-month period. The natural tendency is to lose joint motion while HO is forming.[10] The efficacy of irradiation and indomethacin

prophylaxis in preventing postoperative HO in spinal cord injury has not been demonstrated.

Traumatic Brain Injury

The natural history of neurologic recovery is the best indicator for surgical excision, recurrence, and functional outcome.[7] The majority of motor recovery occurs by 1½ years. Excision in the patient with a rapid neurologic recovery may be undertaken when guidelines similar to those for excision of HO associated with trauma, total hip replacement, and the majority of spinal cord injury cases are met. Surgery should be delayed longer than 1½ years if the motor recovery is prolonged. Recurrence is common in the presence of normal or abnormal laboratory values in the neurologically compromised patient, and delaying excision because of abnormal laboratory values is not warranted. Surgery is indicated for limb positioning in the neurologically compromised patient.

No studies currently available have defined the role of medical prophylaxis after resection. The stimulus to form HO has subsided in the normal recovery group and medical prophylaxis may not be necessary for these patients. Because the neurologically compromised patient continues to form HO after resection, present prophylaxis methods may be inadequate for this group. A mildly to moderately neurologically compromised patient should respond to prophylaxis after resection.

SUMMARY

In rare instances HO is genetically transmitted. An innate predisposition to HO is suspected and realized as a consequence of the primary disease. Varying amounts of HO may be attributable to variable genetic expression or penetrance and the influence of various risk factors. These risk factors are probably additive, as is illustrated in a patient who sustains a concomitant traumatic brain injury and a proximal joint injury; such a patient has a greatly increased incidence of traumatic HO over that of the general population. The occurrence of HO is predictably increased even further if surgery is required for open reduction and internal fixation of the joint. Spinal cord–injured patients with decubitus ulcers about the hip have an increased frequency of HO about the hip than do such patients with intact skin.

Clinically significant HO develops in 10 to 20 percent of predisposed patients. The average onset is 2 months after insult. Decreased motion and pain are commonly the first evidence of HO. A rise in SAP level in the absence of fractures should alert the physician that clinically significant HO is imminent. Early confirmation is best established by triple-phase RNBI. Site-specific location, grading, and response to treatment are accomplished with standard radiographs. Quantitative RNBI as an indicator for the appropriate time to resect HO has not been reliably verified. CT may aid the surgeon in preoperative planning and surgical approach.

The common entities associated wth HO are all characterized by development of bone at the proximal limbs and joints. However, the specific sites about these joints that are involved vary, tending to be very specific to the underlying cause. The radiographic appearance of HO at the hip often permits reliable prediction of the underlying disease.

The natural history of HO is similar with respect to SAP level and radiographic evolution regardless of its cause. The heterotopic bone formation probably begins soon after the insult but is not detected radiographically for 2 months. In 80 percent or more of cases of HO, the disorder runs a relatively benign course. The patient experiences pain, swelling, and some decrease in joint motion. Radiographically HO evolves for a period of 6 months, with a return of SAP level to baseline by that time and RNBI thereafter. Another, smaller group of patients undergo a different clinical and laboratory course. These patients experience a significant loss of joint motion. Radiographic evolution continues for more than 6 months and large amounts of bone are formed. Elevated SAP levels may persist for 1 to 2 years, and RNBI may be persistently active. The identity of this latter group maybe summarized as follows: large amounts of heterotopic bone by 6 months; continued radiographic progression while undergoing medical treatment or more than 6 months after insult; persistently elevated SAP level; prolonged RNBI activity; and severe spasticity. Identification of this group is important for decisions about outcome of both ongoing and future treatment, such as surgical resection.

Various forms of treatment are available. The only drug studied extensively in neurologic prophylaxis is EHDP, and its efficacy has not been definitively determined. The dosage should be 20 mg/kg body weight for 6 months based on the natural radiographic history. In a small number of spinal cord–injured patients the HO will continue to progress after cessation of treatment, and this group can be predicted as described previously. A traumatic brain-injured patient with persistent spasticity at 6 months will have progression of HO after cessation of the EHDP, but continued use may not be warranted owing to harmful side effects or persistent neurologic compromise. The role of NSAIDs and irradiation has not been defined in this population.

The timing of surgical intervention is based on the natural history of the underlying disease and on both clinical signs and symptoms and laboratory evaluation. Resection of traumatic HO may be considered at 6 months in the general population. Because the stimulus for HO seems to persist slightly longer in the spinal cord–injured patient, resection is considered at 1 year after HO initiation. Finally, because traumatic brain-injured patients improve neurologically for a prolonged period, surgical excision is considered at neurologic stability or at approximately $1\frac{1}{2}$ years.

Treatment with irradiation and indomethacin after HO resection to prevent recurrence has proved effective in HO developing after trauma or total hip replacement. The effectiveness of these modalities in neurologic patients has yet to be determined. EHDP therapy after resection has met with varying results in the total hip replacement population and has not been thoroughly evaluated in the population with neurogenic disorders.

REFERENCES

1. Connor JM, Evans DAP: Fibroplasia ossificans progressiva. The clinical features and natural history of 34 patients. J Bone Joint Surg [Br] 64:76, 1982
2. Fawcett HA, Marsden RA: Hereditary osteoma cutis. J Soc Med 76:697, 1983
3. Larson JM, Michalski JP, Collacott EA et al: Increased prevalence of HLA-B27 in patients with ectopic ossification following traumatic spinal cord injury. Rheumatol Rehabil 20:193, 1981
4. Minare P, Betuel H, Girad R, Pilonchery G: Neurologic injuries, paraosteoarthropathies, and human leukocyte antigens. Arch Phys Med Rehabil 61:214, 1980
5. Garland DE, Alday B, Venos KG: Heterotopic ossification and HLA antigens. Arch Phys Med Rehabil 65:531, 1984
6. Garland DE, Blum CE, Waters RL: Periarticular heterotopic ossification in head injured adults: incidence and location. J Bone Joint Surg [Am] 62:1143, 1980
7. Garland DE, Hanscom DA, Keenan MA et al: Resection of heterotopic ossification in the adult with head trauma. J Bone Joint Surg [Am] 67:1261, 1985
8. Lal S, Hamilton B, Heinemann A, Betts HB: Risk factors for heterotopic ossification in spinal cord injury. Arch Phys Med Rehabil 70:387, 1989
9. Wharton GW, Morgan TH: Ankylosis in the paralyzed patient. J Bone Joint Surg [Am] 52:105, 1970
10. Garland DE, Orwin JF: Resection of heterotopic ossification in patients with spinal cord injuries. Clin Orthop 242:169, 1989
11. Garland DE, Miller G: Fractures and dislocations about the hip in head-injured adults. Clin Orthop 186:154, 1984
12. Garland DE, O'Hollaren RM: Fractures and dislocations about the elbow in the head-injured adult. Clin Orthop 168:38, 1982
13. Brooker AF, Bowerman JW, Robinson RA, Riley LH: Ectopic ossification following total hip replacement. J Bone Joint Surg [Am] 55:1629, 1973
14. DeLee AF, Charnley J: Ectopic bone formation following low friction arthroplasty of the hip. Clin Orthop 121:53, 1976
15. Finerman GAM, Stover SL: Heterotopic ossification following hip replacement or spinal cord injury. Two clinical studies with EHDP. Metab Bone Dis Rel Res 3:337, 1981
16. Freed JH, Hahn H, Menter MD, Dillion T: The use of the three-phase bone scan in the early diagnosis of heterotopic ossification (HO) and in the evaluation of Didronel therapy. Paraplegia 20:208, 1982
17. Garland DE, Alday B, Venos KG, Vogt JC: Diphosponate treatment for heterotopic ossification in spinal cord injury patients. Clin Orthop 176:197, 1983
18. Stover L, Hataway CG, Zieger HE: Heterotopic ossification in spinal cord injured patients. Arch Phys Med Rehabil 56:199, 1975
19. Mendelson L, Grosswasser Z, Najenson T et al: Periarticular new bone formation in patients suffering from severe head injuries. Scand J Rehabil Med 7:141, 1975
20. Mielants H, Vanhove E, de Neels J, Veys E: Clinical survey of and pathogenic approach to para-articular ossifications in long-term coma. Acta Orthop Scand 46:190, 1975
21. Orzel JA, Rudd TG: Heterotopic bone formation: clinical, laboratory, and imaging correlation. J Nucl Med 26:125, 1985
22. Sazbon L, Najenson T, Tartakovsky M et al: Wide-spread periarticular new bone formation in long-term comatose patients. J Bone Joint Surg [Br] 63:120, 1981
23. Stover L, Hahn HR, Miller JM: Disodium etidronate in the prevention of heterotopic ossification following spinal cord injury. Paraplegia 14:146, 1976
24. Furman R, Nicholas JJ, Jivoff L: Elevation of the serum alkaline phosphatase coincident with ectopic bone formation in paraplegic patients. J Bone Joint Surg [Am] 52:1131, 1970
25. Kjaersaard-Anderson P, Peidersen P, Kristensen SS et al: Serum alkaline phosphatase as an indicator of heterotopic bone formation following the total hip arthroplasty. Clin Orthop 234:102, 1988
26. Bressler EL, Marn CS, Gore RM, Hendrix RW: Evaluation of ectopic bone by CT. AJR 148:931, 1987
27. Keenan MAE, Kauffman DL, Garland DE, Smith C: Late ulnar neuropathy in the brain injured adult. J Hand Surg [Am] 13:120, 1988
28. Garland DE: Clinical observations on fractures and heterotopic ossification in the spinal cord and traumatic brain injured populations. Clin Orthop 233:86, 1988.
29. Fleisch H: Diphosphonates: history and mechanisms of action. Metab Bone Dis Rel Res 3:279, 1981
30. Russell RGG, Smith R: Diphosphonates—experimental and clinical aspects. J Bone Joint Surg [Br] 55:66, 1973
31. Spielman G, Gennarelli TA, Rogers CR: Disodium etidronate: its role in preventing heterotopic ossification in severe head injury. Arch Phys Med Rehabil 64:539, 1983
32. Stover SL, Nieman KM, Miller JM: Disodium etidronate in the prevention of postoperative recurrence of heterotopic ossification in spinal cord injury patients. J Bone Joint Surg [Am] 58:683, 1976
33. Thomas BJ, Amstutz HC: Results of administration of diophosphonate for prevention of heterotopic ossification after total hip arthroplasty. J Bone Joint Surg [Am] 67:400, 1985
34. Flora L, Hassing GS, Cloyd GG et al: The long-term skeletal effects of EHDP in dogs. Metab Bone Dis Rel Res 3:289, 1981
35. Puzas JE, Miller MD, Rosier RN: Pathologic bone formation. Clin Orthop 245:269, 1989
36. Dahl HK: Kliniske Observasjoner. In Symposium about Hip Arthrosis. MSD, Blindern, Norway, 1974
37. Ritter MA, Sieber JM: Prophylactic indomethacin for the prevention of heterotopic bone formation following total hip arthroplasty. Clin Orthop 196:217, 1985
38. Schmidt SA, Kjaersgaard-Anderson P, Pederson NW et al: The use of indomethacin to prevent the formation of heterotopic bone after total hip replacement. J Bone Joint Surg [Am] 70:834, 1988

39. Ayers DG, Evarts C, McC, Parkinson JR: The prevention of heterotopic ossification in high-risk patients by low-dose radiation therapy after total hip arthroplasty. J Bone Joint Surg [Am] 68:1423, 1986

40. Coventry MB, Scanton PW: Use of radiation to discourage ectopic bone. J Bone Joint Surg [Am] 63:201, 1982

41. Michelsson J, Granroth G, Anderson JC: Myositis ossificans following forcible manipulation of the leg. J Bone Joint Surg [Am] 62:811, 1980

42. Garland DE, Razza BE, Waters RL: Forceful joint manipulation in head-injured adults with heterotopic ossification. Clin Orthop 169:133, 1982

36 Peripheral Nerve Injury

ROBERT M. SZABO
BRUCE FOERSTER

The intricacy of orchestrated movements in executing hand function becomes apparent when viewing a patient who has had a peripheral nerve injury of the upper extremity. The important balance of muscular actions of the hand is dramatically disrupted with the loss of a single nerve. The loss of tactile skin sensibility, concomitantly with the deeper sensory fibers responsible for proprioception and muscle tension afferents, results in a significant alteration in hand function. Loss of sudomotor function further compromises the hand, causing dry, atrophic skin and its sequelae. Although similarities among them exist, specific nerve injuries are greatly affected by patient factors, including age, occupation, patient adaptability and education, and anatomic variations. A team approach is necessary when considering the many facets of the patient's clinical problem. In addition to the hand surgeon, an experienced electrophysiologist, an upper extremity rehabilitation expert, an occupational therapist, and an orthotist are essential in maximizing outcome of treatment.

The common goal is to restore function for the patient, at the same time avoiding tunnel vision and not focusing on the hand alone. Simpler is better for some patients. Always enlist the patient's help in decision making.

HISTORICAL PERSPECTIVES

Clinicians, neuroanatomists, and neurophysiologists have contributed to our knowledge of peripheral nerve injury and its treatment. In 1838, Schwann described the sheath surrounding the cylindrical peripheral nerve. Waller, in 1850, demonstrated on the hypoglossal and glossopharyngeal nerves in frogs that when a nerve is severed, its distal portion undergoes degeneration while the proximal segment remains viable. This basic concept has become known as *wallerian degeneration.* In 1878, Ranvier identified the nodal pattern found in peripheral axons. During this period, Nissl studied the intracellular structures of the anterior horn cell, which participate in peripheral nerve regeneration.

Clinical understanding of nerve injuries is largely derived from wartime experience. Tinel, in France, and Hoffman, in Germany, studied recovering nerve injuries in World War I soldiers. Tinel's classic paper on the "tingling sign" observed in patients with regenerating axons after nerve injury was published in 1915.[17] Seddon's valuable contributions during and after World War II included classifying the physiologic responses to traumatic nerve lesions and monitoring their rate of recovery.[1] With detailed studies on the internal neuroanatomy of peripheral nerves, Sunderland further classified the stages of nerve injury.[2-4]

Nevertheless, the surgeon's ability to influence nerve regeneration is impaired by the inability to reunite peripheral receptors and motor units with their original cortical representations.

ANATOMY, PHYSIOLOGY, AND FUNCTION

A peripheral nerve is formed from motor, sensory, and sympathetic fibers with accompanying connective tissue. The ultimate function of a peripheral nerve is to conduct both afferent and efferent impulses to and from the central nervous system for processing and execution. The axon is the fundamental unit of conduction and may be myelinated or unmyelinated, motor or sensory. Sympathetic fibers are unmyelinated. In both myelinated and unmyelinated nerve fibers, a number of Schwann cells in sequence are associated with the axons. However, in the unmyelinated nerve, one Schwann cell may surround many axons, whereas in a myelinated nerve an axon has only one associated Schwann cell at a given level. The Schwann cell membrane repeatedly spirals around the axon, forming a layered myelin sheath. Nodes of Ranvier define the intervals between one Schwann cell and the next along a myelinated fiber. Myelination is a property that determines conduction velocity and susceptibility to and recovery from injury; thus, it is an important characteristic of axons.

Myelinated nerve fibers, or axons, their Schwann cells and myelin sheath, and groups of unmyelinated axons are surrounded by a connective tissue stroma called endoneurium. This endoneurial tube serves as a supporting structure for a group of axons, providing a homeostatic barrier and resisting stretch of its nerve fibers.

Groups of nerve fibers are organized into bundles called fascicles (Fig. 36-1). A fascicle is surrounded by a sheath of connective tissue, the perineurium. The perineurium is extremely important to the normal function of its fascicles. It not only protects the nerve fibers within it but also serves as a diffusion barrier and helps to maintain intrafascicular pressure, thereby assisting with axonal transport. Injury to the perineurium will therefore cause nerve dysfunction.

The epineurium is the loosely arranged connective tissue that encircles and separates fascicle bundles. External epineurium is the circumferential sheath around a peripheral nerve; internal epineurium is the collagenous tissue separating nerve fascicles within the nerve.

Sunderland has shown that these connective tissue structures contribute from 25 to 75 percent of a normal nerve's cross-sectional area, depending on the nerve and the particular location along that nerve.[3] For instance, as nerves cross joints the percentage of connective tissue is relatively increased, which serves as a protective mechanism and enhances excursion of the nerve with joint motion.[5] Additionally, the connective tissue components proliferate in response to injury.

The natural undulating pattern or waviness of both the conductive and connective tissues of a peripheral nerve is described by Sunderland.[2] This pattern provides elasticity for a physiologic range of stretch to assist in the nerve's longitudinal excursion, which is necessary as it crosses joints.[6] As longitudinal tension is applied across a nerve, initially the epineurium (the loosest of layers) will stretch. Next fascicular bundles followed by their individual axonal fibers will stretch and will straighten their undulating patterns. The perineurium is the strongest of the layers and most resistant to stretch; it protects the neural tissues it surrounds. In general, a nerve can sustain about 20 percent elongation before losing continuity.

Nerve function is critically tied to the vascularity of the nerve. Perfusion studies have shown a rich intraneural vasculature present as plexuses in the epineurium, perineurium, and endoneurium.[7,8] Numerous anastomotic linkages are found between these three vascular supplies. After a nerve injury, both the status of the internal vasculature and the vascularity of the surrounding soft tissues in the zone of injury play a crucial role in recovery of nerve function. The nerve's intrinsic blood supply is sensitive to both increased tension and pressure. Compromise of blood flow is known to affect nerve function.

NATURAL HISTORY OF NERVE INJURY

The mechanism of nerve injury may be laceration, compression, contusion, traction, or thermal injury. The outcome depends more on the severity of the

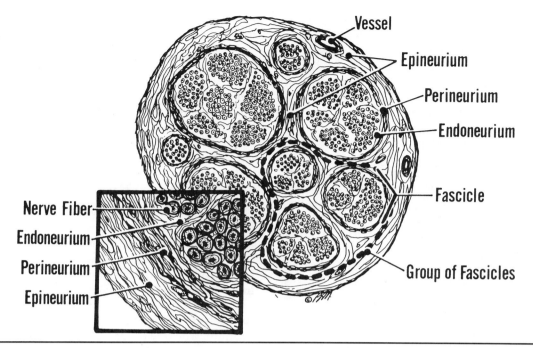

Fig. 36-1. Cross-sectional anatomy of a peripheral nerve. (From Wilgis EFS: Nerve repair and grafting. p. 1375. In Green's Operative Hand Surgery. 2nd ed. Vol. 2. Churchill Livingstone, New York, 1987, with permission. Copyright Elizabeth Roselius.)

injury than on the mechanism. Seddon described three basic degrees of nerve injury: neurapraxia, axonotmesis, and neurotmesis.[1,9]

In neurapraxia axonal continuity is maintained but the myelin sheath is damaged, which adversely affects conduction. Recovery of nerve function usually occurs in minutes to weeks. Typical examples of neurapraxia are tourniquet paralysis, radial nerve palsy after humeral shaft fracture, and Saturday night palsy. Because no degeneration of the neural elements distal to the site of injury occurs in neurapraxia, recovery is dependent not on regenerating axons but rather on an adjustment to their normal biologic milieu.

Axonotmesis is an injury to the nerve in which the epineurium, perineurium, and endoneurium remain intact but axonal continuity is interrupted. Wallerian degeneration occurs, with proliferation of Schwann cells distal to the site of injury and accumulation of macrophages. With relative preservation of the

nerve's connective tissue supporting structures, a more organized axonal regenerative process is expected. At the time of injury, patients show both motor and sensory loss. Recovery depends on the time required for regenerating proximal axons to penetrate their endoneurial tubes distally and then elongate to the peripheral target. The less scarring that is present at the injury site the greater the percentage of functional recovery that will occur. Once axonal regeneration has crossed the site of nerve injury, it progresses distally within the endoneurial tubes at an approximate rate of 1 mm/day. This may be observed in patients after a nerve injury or repair by monitoring the rate of the advancing Tinel's sign.

Neurotmesis refers to complete severance of a nerve. This may be secondary to direct laceration, avulsion, or blast injury. The continuity of neural elements and accompanying connective tissue is completely disrupted, with concomitant injury to the surrounding tissues further complicating the lesion. All nerve function distally is lost acutely, and the prognosis for recovery is poor. The proximal nerve stump forms a neuroma with whorls of disorganized axonal sprouts, Schwann cells, and connective tissue. The distal stump forms a glioma with proliferation of Schwann cells and connective tissue. The neural elements undergo Wallerian degeneration distally, and macrophages assist in their resorption.

Peripheral targets and the proximal nerve cell show significant changes with axonal injury. The neuron cell body (located in the anterior horn of the spinal cord for motor neurons and in the dorsal root ganglia for sensory neurons) swells, producing subsequent nuclear enlargement and eccentricity. Chromatolysis (dissolution of the Nissl bodies or rough endoplasmic reticulum), increased RNA synthesis, and increased lipid and protein synthesis all occur as the nerve cell ''gears up'' for the regenerative process and increasing axonal transport. The normal bidirectional axonal transport is interrupted at the site of injury, and the neuron responds to this change in retrograde transport.

Distal to the neuromuscular junction, the muscle cells atrophy with loss of cross-striations and increasing deformity of muscle fibers. Muscle enzyme concentrations decrease, metabolic activity slows, and membrane potentials drop secondary to loss of neurotropic signals from the motor endplate. The proportion of connective tissue elements increases within the muscle, and in the absence of regeneration this eventually leads to fibrosis. Intermittent electrical stimulation and range-of-motion exercises cannot prevent the metabolic aberrations from occurring, but they may succeed in diminishing contracture of the muscle as fibrosis progresses over time. Denervated muscle changes worsen with time, and therefore restoration of nerve function will yield greater functional recovery of muscle action the sooner it occurs.

The sensory target organs, whether they are mechanoreceptors, thermoreceptors, proprioceptors, or nociceptors, however, show no microscopic or macroscopic degenerative processes after denervation. Yet, recovery of normal sensory function after nerve injury is rare because sensation is a cortical perception of a composite response of many axons firing simultaneously, but in a specific pattern. The probability of restoring the anatomic cortical representation is very low.

PATIENT EVALUATION

Functional recovery after peripheral nerve injury requires a coordinated program of evaluation, surgery, therapy, and re-education. It is important to elicit and record both historical and objective information on initial contact with the patient.

History

Historical factors affecting the end result include the patient's age, handedness, occupation, motivational factors (self-employed versus worker's compensation, anger, potential financial reward, poor self-image), previous upper extremity injuries, the type of injury, and additional medical problems. With regard to age, authors have noted better recovery of nerve function after repair in children and adolescents than in adults. The rate of return is more rapid in children owing to a greater rate of regeneration of axons. The central nervous system of children is more plastic, as it adapts more readily to changes in cortical input.

The overall health of a patient is important in determining treatment and prognosis. Patients with serious systemic illnesses or debilitating medical conditions must be approached cautiously when considering neurorrhaphy or a long course of reconstructive procedures.

Motivation has a truly beneficial effect. The best results for functional recovery after nerve injury are found in patients who are self-employed, bear no anger or resentment regarding the cause of the injury, have no potential financial rewards that are proportional to their resulting disability, and possess the personality to persist with postinjury rehabilitation.

The type of injury will dictate the pathophysiology at the injury site and effect treatment and prognosis. For example, a low-velocity civilian gunshot wound will produce less extensive tissue damage than a high-velocity military weapon injury, although neurotmesis may exist in both situations. Laceration of a nerve with a sharp kitchen knife will likely result in better return of function than a high-voltage electrical burn to the same nerve if all other variables are similar. The length of time since injury also is important to establish.

Objective Physical Findings

Additional objective findings on physical examination that are important to assess are the level of injury, presence of associated injuries, condition of the wound, presence of infection, presence of a partial or complete lesion, and presence of anatomic pathway variations. Distal injuries generally yield better results than proximal ones, and pure motor or pure sensory nerves have better prognoses for recovery than mixed nerves.

The initial evaluation of a patient with a nerve injury requires accurate testing of motor function and sensibility. Voluntary motor testing establishes the level of the lesion on the basis of presence or absence of motor activity. Muscle strength testing is recorded using the British Medical Research Council's scale from 0 (total paralysis) to 5 (normal) as an estimate of motor activity.

"Trick Movements"

"Trick movements" are learned attempts to replace active function that is no longer possible because of paralysis from nerve injury. These are usually a sign of a highly motivated patient who wants to maximize the function of the hand by substituting for motor deficits. These substitute movements should not necessarily be discouraged, but they should be controlled. However, if strong habits develop, the muscles may be more difficult to retrain after later reconstructive procedures and secondary deformities may occur across abnormally motored joints. For instance, in low ulnar and median nerve palsy, some patients utilize simultaneous contraction of the long thumb flexor and extensor to obtain a lateral squeeze pinch. If this activity persists, flexion deformities may occur at the interphalangeal and metacarpophalangeal joints with extension at the carpometacarpal joint. Any results of reconstructive tendon transfers are compromised because this habit is resistant to retraining.

Sensibility Testing

Sensibility tests evaluate the acceptance of a stimulus, the subsequent afferent impulse, and the cortical interpretation of that stimulus. There are no true objective physical tests of sensibility. Testing sensation with a piece of cotton for soft touch, a pin for pain, and a cool or warm test tube for temperature sensation have shown no correlation with estimation of sensory functional loss.

Numerous tests of sensibility have been described (Table 36-1), but we have found that the most valuable information is obtained by testing moving touch, two-point discrimination, and localization of light pressure using the Von Frey test.[10,11] The *Von Frey test* is performed using Semmes-Weinstein monofilaments (Fig. 36-2). Each monofilament is applied perpendicular to the skin, and pressure is gradually increased until the monofilament bends. The patient is then asked to localize the point or area of application. The pressure required to bend the monofilament depends on its diameter. The Von Frey test is a threshold test, and because it is very sensitive, it is best suited for more subtle nerve injuries, such as in nerve compression syndromes.[12]

Two-point discrimination represents an innervation density test in which the patient must distinguish between being touched with one and with two points. The normal minimum distance at which discrimination between two points occurs is 6 mm on the fingertips (Fig. 36-3). *Moving touch* is tested by gently stroking the area of skin to be examined with a blunt object. The patient is asked to identify the area with eyes closed. The patient also may be asked to compare the quality of sensations from one area to another as being greater or less. The examiner can use the opposite extremity, or an area innervated by a different nerve on the same extremity, for comparison.

The sympathetic nerves are affected in sensory nerve injury. Loss of sweating indicates compromised sudomotor function. In a chronic lesion, the skin may appear atrophic and dry, and occasionally it has desquamated areas consistent with the distribution of the injured nerve. The *ninhydrin test* provides a quantitative estimate of sympathetic innervation by staining for the amino acids found in sweat. A dense

Table 36-1. Tests of Peripheral Nerve Function

Test	Effect of Neurotmesis	Comment
1. Sudomotor activity	Loss of sweating in affected distribution	Test by starch-iodine, ninhydrin, or palpatioin; correlates loosely with sensory loss
2. Wrinkle test	Deinnervated skin immersed in warm water for 30 minutes will not wrinkle	
3. Volitional muscle action	Lost distal to lesion	Palpate the muscle belly rather than simply looking at distal motion. Test all muscles (distal to proximal) to localize lesion. Nerve block of parallel nerves may be useful
4. Electromyography	Fibrillation action potentials in deinnervated muscle	Seen several weeks after neurotmesis
5. Nerve conduction velocity	Response to stimulus distal to lesion is not seen proximally, or velocity is reduced in partial lesion	A true sensory test, unlike nos. 6–8, which are sensibility tests depending on cortical integration
6. Static and moving two-point discrimination	Lost; recovery shows increasing acuity	May be confused by overlapping receptive fields; difficult to adminsiter consistently
7. Semmes-Weinstein monofilaments	Lost; recovery shows increasing acuity	Nos. 7 and 8 are threshold tests, best suited to follow nerve status after compression injury when nerve is intact
8. Tuning fork or vibrometer	Lost; recovery shows increasing acuity	
9. Tinel's sign	In recovery, percussion over regenerating front produces tingling in area of distribution	Failure to progress distally is indication for surgery
10. Pick-up test	Lost; with recovery, speed and accuracy improve	Reflects functionality of the repair (combined sensory, motor, and cortical function)

(From Szabo and Madison,[26] with permission.)

grouping of dots after "fingerprinting" represents a functioning sweat gland orifice on the pulp of the digit. An iodine-starch technique also is available and gives similar results. An advantage of these tests is that neither requires any subjective interpretation by the patient. Therefore, a patient who might not have the ability to cooperate, or one who is deliberately uncooperative, may be assessed objectively with these techniques.

Another objective test utilizes the observation that the skin of denervated digits does not wrinkle when immersed in warm water. The *wrinkle test* is performed by immersing the hand into a warm water bath at 40°C for 20 to 30 minutes. Smooth skin after 20 to 30 minutes would signify denervation.

Functional Testing

Functional tests assess the patient's ability to perform certain activities requiring multiple actions in concert. The activities represent composites of the actions of many muscle-tendon units, and such tests can provide quantitative information for both the evaluator and the patient. *Moberg's pick-up test* involves gathering several small objects from a tabletop, identifying them, and then placing them in a small container.[13] Seddon described a coin identification test.[9] Additional evaluations may involve writing numbers or letters on the digits and asking the patient to identify them.

A quantitative measure of grip strength uses the *dynamometer*, which is adjustable to fit the span of the patient's palm and fingers. A normal grip strength for a male adult averages 90 to 125 pounds of force. The uninjured contralateral hand is used as a control, and the differential between the nondominant and the dominant hand is usually 5 to 15 pounds. The power grasp requires a composite of functioning anatomy, such as normal skin; adequate sensation, innervation, power, and excursion of the digital flexor and hand intrinsic muscles; supple joints; and active wrist extension for mechanically advantageous positioning of the hand in space. A weakened grip strength must be interpreted with these factors in mind.

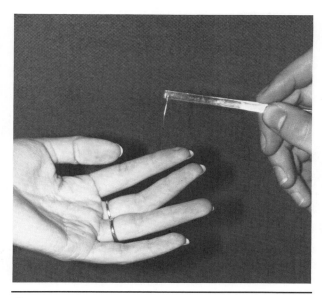

Fig. 36-2. Von Frey test using Semmes-Weinstein monofilaments (see text).

Swanson and coworkers have described, for the significantly weakened hand, a more sensitive evaluation of grip strength.[14] They used a rolled, partially inflated blood pressure cuff that comfortably fits in the patient's palm and measures the increase in pressure with grasp in millimeters of mercury.

Finger pinch, both tip to tip (Fig. 36-4) and lateral (Fig. 36-5), are measured using a *pinch gauge.* Lateral key pinch usually measures 13 to 20 pounds, with fingertip pinch averaging approximately one-half of that value.

Anatomic Variations

The "classic" pattern of anatomic innervation of the muscles of the upper extremity is found in less than half of the population. For example, the flexor digitorum profundus (FDP) muscle is supplied by both the median and the ulnar nerves. Classically, the median nerve, through its anterior interosseous branch, innervates the FDP to the index and long fingers, whereas the ulnar nerve innervates the FDP muscles to the ring and little fingers. However, variations include the ulnar nerve supplying the entire muscle, the median nerve supplying it, or complete dual innervation by both nerves.[15]

The Martin-Gruber anomaly is a neural communication whereby motor fibers from the median nerve or its anterior interosseous branch are carried through the ulnar nerve to supply many intrinsic muscles of the hand. This connection occurs in the proximal part of the forearm and has been found in up to 15 percent of the population.

Fig. 36-3. Two-point discrimination test. Pressure is applied in the longitudinal axis of the digit just enough to blanche the skin. The patient is asked to distinguish between being touched with one or two points while the eyes are closed.

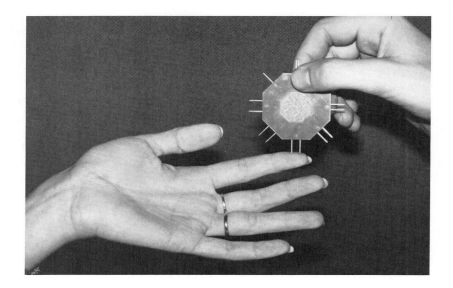

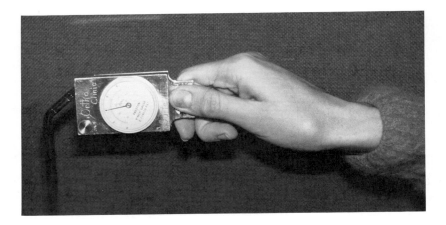

Fig. 36-4. Tip pinch measured using a pinch gauge.

Riche and Cannieu[16a,16b] have described another neural communication between the recurrent branch of the median nerve and the deep branch of the ulnar nerve. This connection should be considered when a patient has a complete low ulnar nerve lesion but without the classic clawing of the little and ring fingers. Another anatomic variation that may explain this clinical picture occurs when the median nerve supplies all four lumbrical muscles without the presence of an ulnar–median nerve connection.[17]

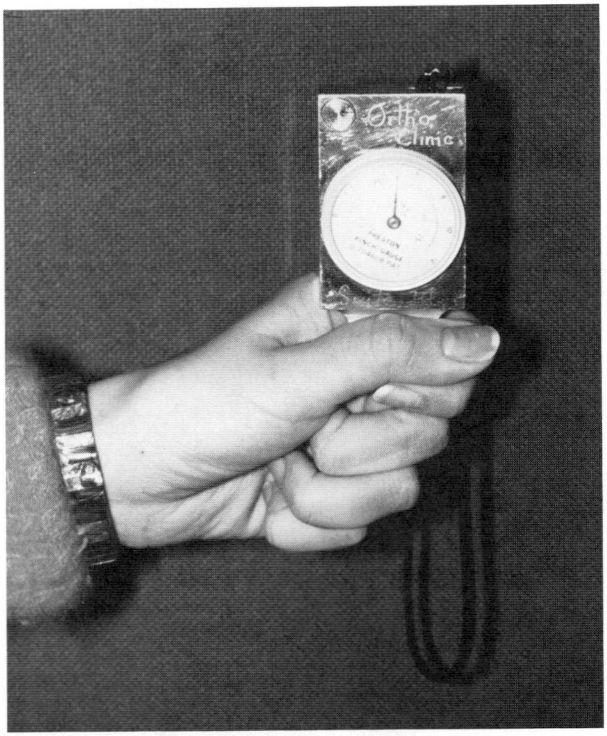

Use of Nerve Blocks

A detailed, complete physical examination of all motor units and sensory distributions cannot be replaced with a quick survey of function when evaluating patients with peripheral nerve injuries. A valuable clinical test that may be incorporated into the evaluation of a patient with an atypical deficit is a nerve block. A regional block of a functioning nerve will provide additional information and clarify the extent of a particular nerve palsy. For instance, a patient with a suspected high ulnar nerve lesion with absent sensation in the little finger but good intrinsic function would benefit from a median nerve block at the elbow to delineate innervation of the intrinsic muscles by a Martin-Gruber connection.

Electrical Diagnostic Studies

Electromyography is an integral part of the evaluation of patients with peripheral nerve injuries. Normally, a resting muscle is electrically silent. With voluntary contractions, motor unit action potentials are recorded. After denervation, the resting muscle produces denervation or fibrillation potentials, which appear as low-voltage, short-duration, monophasic or diphasic spikes. With attempted voluntary contraction, there is no change. Two to 3 weeks may elapse after denervation before this electromyographic pattern becomes evident. Wallerian degeneration may not be complete until approximately 2 to 3

Fig. 36-5. Lateral key pinch measured using a pinch gauge.

weeks after division of a nerve; therefore, in the first 3 weeks after a peripheral nerve injury, electromyograms (EMGs) may be falsely negative.

Nerve conduction studies are also helpful and may localize a peripheral nerve lesion. Decreased velocities and increased motor or sensory latencies are valuable measurements, and a contralateral normal nerve provides the best control.

RESTORATION OF UPPER EXTREMITY FUNCTION AFTER PERIPHERAL NERVE INJURY

The upper extremity surgeon selects from various treatment options, including observation, neurolysis, nerve repair, nerve grafting, and secondary reconstructive procedures such as tendon transfers, tenodeses, joint arthrodeses, or amputation. Not every patient will require surgery, but each patient should be enrolled in a rehabilitation program. Joints must be kept supple in anticipation of the return of motor function. Insensate hands must be protected from injury. Reeducation is initiated to help compensate for a permanent deficit.

Observation

Initial treatment of a peripheral nerve injury depends on the nature of the injury. In closed injuries due to traction or contusion, in which neurapraxia or axonotmesis is expected, initial observation is warranted. After evaluation of the initial deficit, a therapy program is started to maintain supple joints and soft tissues, including splinting to prevent secondary soft tissue deformities. The patient is re-examined monthly and the changing status of the injured nerve is charted. Early on, evaluation may rely on the presence or absence of an advancing Tinel's sign distal to the site of nerve injury, signifying the progression of regenerating axons along the distal nerve segment. Later, the presence of returning distal motor or sensory function will precede the process of functional recovery.

For example, 90 percent of patients with a high radial nerve palsy occurring after a humeral shaft fracture show spontaneous recovery within 1 to 4 months.[18]

Initially, we give our patients a wrist extension splint, or sometimes a low-profile long metacarpophalangeal (MCP) dynamic extension splint, and instruct them in a daily regimen of passive extension exercises to prevent stiffness or contractures. If, after 1 month, the patient shows no sign of nerve function recovery, a baseline EMG is obtained.

Periodic clinical re-evaluation is performed every 4 to 6 weeks to monitor the progression of recovery. When no motor or sensory recovery is demonstrated distal to the site of injury after 4 to 6 months, the patient has a stationary Tinel's sign, and repeat electrodiagnostic studies confirm lack of reinnervation, nerve exploration is considered. Neurolysis, nerve repair, or nerve grafting is performed, depending on the findings at exploration.

Neurosurgical Procedures

Neurolysis

In the event that a neuroma-in-continuity is identified at surgery, the surgeon must decide between neurolysis or resection of the neuroma with repair or grafting. The neuroma is exposed from the normal portions of the nerve proximally and distally toward the lesion. The epineurium is incised and released around the neuroma. All scar tissue from the neuroma is excised. Using the operating microscope, the fascicular continuity is evaluated. Intraoperative nerve stimulation or evoked potentials are often helpful to provide additional information regarding axonal continuity.[19,20] If exploration of the neuroma after neurolysis reveals fascicular continuity or if electrical activity is evident across the lesion, neurolysis without resection should lead to improved functional recovery. Postoperatively, the patient is followed with periodic evaluations to monitor recovery of nerve function.

Nerve Repair

In open injuries, lacerations, or penetrating injuries with or without associated fractures, any nerve that is injured is explored acutely during the initial wound irrigation and débridement. The lesion is usually a neurotmesis, and repair is indicated. Contraindications for acute repair include heavily contaminated or infected wounds and uncertainty of the extent of damage in the transected ends of the nerve. High-velocity gunshot wounds, farm machinery injuries, high-energy crush injuries, and high-voltage electrical burns are situations in which nerve repair is best delayed.

The technique for nerve repair is the only prognostic factor under control of the surgeon. Controversies exist regarding which technical aspects of nerve repair make a difference.[21-26] The goal in peripheral nerve repair is to join the two nerve ends in such a manner that a primary union of the connective tissue elements occurs. This will allow reconstitution of the future regenerating axons across the repair site to their distal endoneurial tubes. Efforts to minimize scar formation at the repair site will aid regeneration.

Magnification is necessary to identify anatomic landmarks so that nerve ends may be oriented in their proper relationship. The fascicle pattern and surface blood vessels on either side of the interrupted nerve are observed for proper rotational alignment.[27,28] Prior to repair, the traumatized nerve ends are sharply cut to facilitate fascicular mapping and remove roughened edges. Epineural repair is performed using fine interrupted simple sutures. During coaptation of the nerve ends, efforts to minimize scar formation at the repair site are taken. The nerve ends are handled atraumatically with jeweler's forceps to grasp only the epineurium. No pressure or traction is applied to the fascicles. Using mobilization techniques, nerve transposition, and joint positioning, the surgeon may suture the nerve ends without tension. However, excessive mobilization destroys collateral blood supply to the nerve and increases scar formation.

Fascicular repair utilizes perineurial sutures to reapproximate fascicles directly. There is no convincing evidence that either epineural or fascicular repair is superior. In selected situations, a combined fascicular and epineural repair may be employed. For instance, repair of a median nerve laceration at the wrist is usually accomplished by a fascicular repair of the motor bundle and epineural repair of the sensory components. The choice of technique is based on the level of injury and the internal topography of the nerve.

Nerve Grafting

If a peripheral nerve repair cannot be accomplished without tension after mobilization, rerouting, or joint positioning, autologous nerve grafting is utilized. Nerve graft segments are interposed between the dissected fascicular bundles of each nerve end, and interfascicular or grouped fascicular suturing is employed. Necessary prerequisites for nerve grafting include a mature, viable, well-vascularized soft tissue bed. Interposition nerve grafts require knowledge of interneural topography to restore continuity between corresponding sectors or quadrants of nerve across the gap.[29-32]

Choice of donor nerve graft is made with respect to donor deficity and donor site morbidity. The sural nerve from the posterolateral aspect of the leg has minimal donor site deficit with loss of sensation over the lateral aspect of the foot and ankle. It is easily harvested using multiple small incisions starting just posterior and distal to the lateral malleolus and moving proximally (Fig. 36-6). A tendon stripper can also be used to harvest the sural nerve from one incision at the ankle. The sural nerve provides excellent diameter and length; up to 35 cm may be obtained from each leg. The graft is then sutured without tension, spanning the nerve gap (Fig. 36-7).

Postoperative care after nerve repairs or grafting is designed to protect the suture junctions. Initially the extremity is immobilized in a plaster-reinforced bulky compressive dressing for 10 days. Once wound sutures are removed, the patient is placed in a cast with joints comfortably positioned to prevent tension or motion at the coaptation sites for a total of 6 weeks. At 4 weeks the patient's cast is changed to add some gradual joint mobilization for the remaining 2 weeks. Therapy and splinting are employed during the recovery period to prevent secondary deformities or contractures, to improve range of motion, and eventually to begin strengthening exercises.

Tendon Transfers

Tendon transfers may be performed in combination with efforts to restore neural continuity, or alone if the nerve injury is irreparable or unreconstructable. Tendon transfers restore motor balance to an extrem-

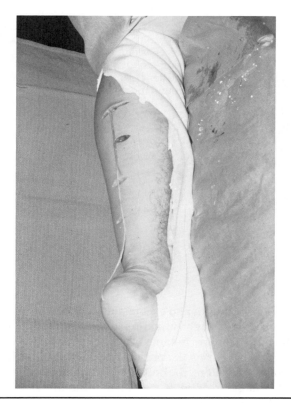

Fig. 36-6. Harvesting the entire sural nerve for nerve grafting. At times multiple incisions can be avoided with the use of a tendon stripper.

ity adversely affected by loss of muscle-tendon action by redistributing motor assets to maximize function. Muscle tension and excursion are important factors when considering moving a muscle-tendon unit.[33,34] A given transfer must provide enough tension to restore motor balance while also allowing the necessary range of motion of the joints that it is crossing.

One grade of strength on the Medical Research Council scale can be expected to be lost after tendon transfer. Brand has shown that the efficiency of the transferred muscle is changed by modifying the length-tension relationship of that particular muscle.[35] Normally, the elastic properties of the connective tissues in and around a muscle do not compromise the length-tension relationship of a muscle because these tissues are very compliant and stretch easily. However, when a muscle is moved to another

location, it can become surrounded by scar tissue. The muscle then must expend a greater portion of its generated tension in attempting to stretch scar tissue, and therefore it has decreased strength.

An important principle in tendon transfers is thus minimizing scar formation and passing the transferred tendon through compliant tissue. Small transverse skin incisions are favored to harvest the tendon and reroute it atraumatically through viable, unscarred, compliant soft tissues by tunneling with a blunt-nosed tendon passer. Any evidence of a continuing inflammatory process, persistent swelling, or significant joint stiffness in the hand or forearm should warn the physician against performing a tendon transfer at that time. Delaying tendon transfers until tissue homeostasis has been achieved will yield better results.

Before considering specific tendon transfers for a patient, all muscles of the upper extremity should be examined and graded individually. Functional deficits should be identified; available muscles for transfer are considered both for the tension they can generate and for their potential excursion. The moment arm of the transferred tendon is carefully considered. The efficiency of a muscle in achieving desired joint motion depends on the torque applied to that joint. Torque is a product of force (or tension) and moment arm (or distance from the tendon to the joint axis). A greater moment arm produces greater torque and a stronger, more competent muscle transfer. Increasing the moment arm will decrease the effective excursion of the transferred muscle, however, leading to a decreased range of motion.

Timing of the Transfer

Timing of tendon transfers for a peripheral nerve palsy is debated.[36-40] Initial efforts focus on treating the nerve injury directly, with neurolysis, nerve repair, or grafting. If this is accomplished, or if the nerve injury is irreparable, the patient starts an outpatient occupational therapy regimen, including splinting. This period of treatment and therapy serves several purposes. It allows the patient time to understand his or her functional deficits. When tendon transfer becomes necessary, the patient will be a

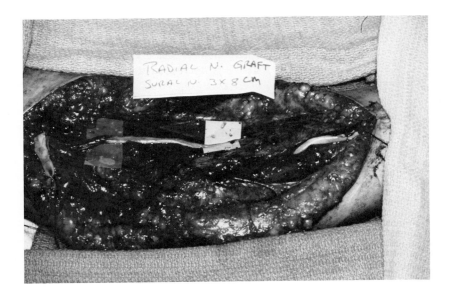

Fig. 36-7. Sural nerve was used to bridge an 8-cm gap in this radial nerve lesion. The graft was sutured using grouped fascicular repair. The junctions lie underneath the background material.

more active and informed participant. The surgeon also has time to assess the patient's motivation, cooperation, and compliance. During this observation period, nerve regeneration is monitored, and prognosis for recovery is more predictable. Time is allowed for tissue homeostasis with resolution of inflammation, swelling, and stiffness. Finally, direct attention is given, through splinting and therapy, to preventing the secondary deformities and contractures seen in the motor muscle–unbalanced upper extremity.

In time, however, a palsied hand tends to develop secondary deformities because the soft tissues on the paralyzed side of a joint stretch as a result of the unbalanced pull of the unaffected antagonist muscles. The antagonist muscles begin to shorten, losing sarcomeres, and decrease their resting length to return to their normal resting tension. The soft tissues on the paralyzed side undergo stress relaxation, and eventually they stretch out sufficiently to allow joint deformities. The hyperextension of the MCP joints and flexion of the proximal interphalangeal (PIP) joints with incompetent, over-stretched palmar plates and central slips seen in the long-standing claw hand deformity of an ulnar nerve palsy is a classic example. Therefore, tendon transfers are performed before secondary deformities develop.

The surgeon can also take advantage of the property of soft tissue viscoelasticity. Frequently, a surgeon must transfer a tendon with adequate tension but diminished length and excursion. Muscle fibers react to a constant slightly increased resting tension by adding sarcomeres in series. This increases the resting length and returns the muscle to the original resting tension. Therefore, the only way to lengthen a muscle is to maintain it in a stretched position while at rest.[34,35] To gain some excursion during a tendon transfer, the tendon is attached under slight tension and the joint it crosses is immobilized postoperatively so that the tension is relieved during the healing period. Once the splint is removed, the joint returns to the normal position, and the transferred muscle will gradually add sarcomeres in response to its increased resting tension.

Tendon Transfers for Specific Nerve Palsies

Radial Nerve Palsy

The major functional deficit with radial nerve injury above the elbow involves a weakened grasp and inability to release. Radial nerve function is essential in two of the three phases of grasp described by Riordan.[41] Phase I involves opening the hand and requires extrinsic extensor function of all digits in addition to function of the intrinsic muscles. In phase 2 the fingers surround the object, which requires function of the extrinsic flexor and the intrinsic muscles and is the only phase of grasp *not* affected by radial nerve injury. Phase 3 involves gripping the object between the fingers and palm or thumb, with wrist stabilization by the wrist extensors required to prevent the powerful finger flexors from pulling the wrist into flexion. Finally, release requires extrinsic extensor function.

Tendon transfers to restore these functions of grasp and release are relatively dependable and reproducible.[18,42,43] The "standard" procedure involves transferring the pronator teres insertion into the extensor carpi radialis brevis for wrist extension. The flexor carpi ulnaris (FCU) is transferred to the extensor digitorum communis, and the palmaris longus tendon to the rerouted extensor pollicis longus. This set of transfers requires little retraining, yields predictable results, and is our recommended transfer in older patients and in patients who require less independent digital control. However, the FCU has inadequate excursion to allow active digital extension with simultaneous wrist extension.

In manual laborers, the importance of a functioning FCU as a wrist stabilizer and ulnar deviator should be considered. Brand has shown that sacrifice of this mucle has a detrimental effect on activities such as hammering, drilling, and other actions requiring power.[33,35] In patients who wish to return to heavy labor, transfer of the flexor carpi radialis (FCR) for digital extension is more advantageous. In addition to maintaining the FCU as an ulnar wrist flexor, this transfer provides 25 percent more excursion because the mean resting fiber length of the FCR is longer. This yields improved, but not complete, digital extension with the wrist extended (Fig. 36-8).

Another option that is best utilized in younger patients who might require independent finger extension is a modification of the Boyes transfer.[42,43] The pronator teres is again used for wrist extension, with the flexor digitorum superficialis of the ring and long fingers providing extension of the digits.[44] The FCR is transferred to the first dorsal extensor compartment to provide thumb abduction. An out-of-phase digital flexor used to restore extension generally is not a problem to retrain in younger, well-motivated patients.

In patients with injury to the posterior interosseous nerve at the elbow or below, wrist extension will be intact when there is at least one unaffected radial wrist extensor. Because of the dominance of radially directed forces, the FCU should *not* be sacrificed for transfer to restore digital extension. Thumb and finger extension is best accomplished using one of the other transfers described earlier.

Our postoperative regimen is similar for these transfers. Initially, a bulky, plaster-reinforced, long arm compression dressing is applied with the elbow at 90°, the forearm in neutral rotation, the wrist in 45° of dorsiflexion, the MCP and all IP joints of the hand in 0° of extension, and the thumb in full extension and radial abduction. At 10 days, this dressing is removed for suture removal, and a long arm cast is applied without changing the position. At 4 weeks postoperatively, the patient is given a removable short arm splint with the wrist in 45° of dorsiflexion and the MCP joints in 20° of flexion. The IP joints are then left free. Occupational therapy is begun at this stage to start retraining the transfers. The splint is usually discontinued after 8 weeks postoperatively or when no further extensor lag is noted at the MCP joints. A gradual program of strengthening and resistive exercises is started after 8 weeks only if no extensor lag exists.

Median Nerve Palsy

Restoration of apposition is a priority in patients with a median nerve deficit. Apposition is a composite motion requiring palmar abduction of the thumb and pronation so that the pulp surfaces of the thumb and fingers face each other.[45] Classically, the median nerve–innervated thumb intrinsic muscles are the abductor pollicis brevis, opponens pollicis, and superficial head of the flexor pollicis brevis. Anatomic variations in innervation are common, and each patient's functional deficit is assessed carefully.

The muscle to be transferred should closely match the normal force and excursion of thumb apposition in addition to its direction of pull and insertion. The transfer must pull from the direction of the pisiform bone, thereby paralleling the fibers of the abductor pollicis brevis. The tendon transfer must substitute for several weakened thumb intrinsic muscles with

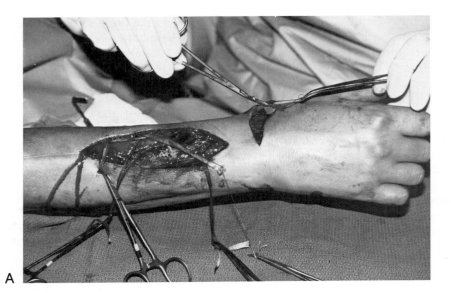

A

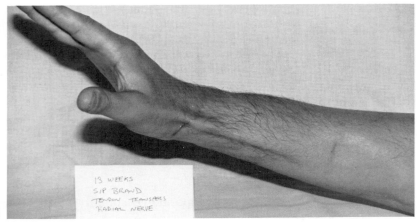

B

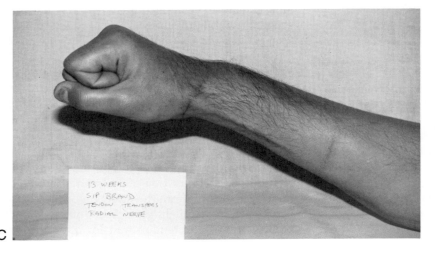

C

Fig. 36-8. Brand radial nerve tendon transfers. **(A)** Intraoperative view showing transfer of palmaris longus to rerouted extensor pollicis longus. The flexor carpi radialis tendon is tagged with a suture and will be weaved into the extensor digitorum communis. A hemostat tags the pronator teres, which lastly will be weaved into the extensor carpi radialis brevis. **(B)** Thirteen weeks postoperatively the patient demonstrates ability to extend his wrist, thumb, and fingers. **(C)** Uncompromised finger flexion is shown.

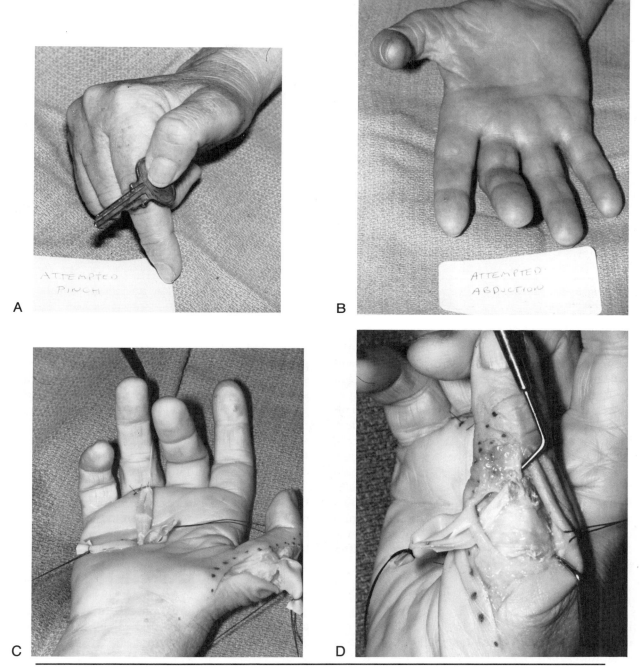

Fig. 36-9. Sixty year old woman with Charcot-Marie-Tooth disease who has severe weakness of thumb intrinsic muscle function as a result of low median and ulnar nerve involvement. **(A)** Patient demonstrates Froment's sign when attempting key pinch. Notice the substitution of flexor pollicis longus for adductor pollicis brevis function. **(B)** The patient is unable to abduct her thumb from the palm. **(C)** A ring finger superficialis tendon was used to restore a combination of abduction and adduction (Royle-Thompson opponensplasty). **(D)** In this case the insertion was made into the tendon of the abductor pollicis brevis on the ulnar base of the proximal phalanx and the extensor pollicis longus to restore balance to the thumb. *(Figure continues.)*

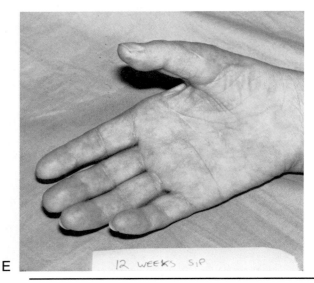 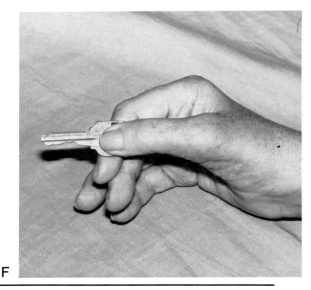

E 12 WEEKS S/P

F

Fig. 36-9 *(Continued).* **(E)** Twelve weeks postoperatively, abduction is improved. **(F)** Key pinch in the patient is also stronger.

one motor unit[45-47] (Fig. 36-9). Insertion is made into the tendon of the abductor pollicis brevis and the ulnar base of the proximal phalanx. The most common motor nerves utilized are either a flexor digitorum superficialis or the extensor indicis proprius; however, the extensor digiti quinti, extensor carpi ulnaris, palmaris longus, and abductor digiti quinti muscles have all been utilized successfully in special situations. Regardless of the motor muscle selected, the postoperative care is similar. The thumb should be immobilized in full palmar abduction for 4 weeks. Recovery of mobility is then initiated by utilizing a removable thumb abduction splint, and the patient is instructed to touch the tips of each finger with the thumb. Strengthening exercises are then begun after 8 weeks.

High Median Nerve Palsy

In high median nerve palsy, the patient exhibits paralysis of the flexor pollicis longus (FPL), the flexor digitorum superficialis (FDS), the pronator teres, the pronator quadratus, and usually the flexor digitorum profundus of the index and long fingers; in addition, there is weakness of the intrinsic muscles of the thumb. Weakness of the FPL is most reliably treated

by thumb interphalangeal fusion in 20° of flexion. The brachioradialis may be transferred to the FPL in patients who require active thumb IP flexion. To restore flexion to the index and long fingers, the extensor carpi radialis brevis may be transferred through a generous window in the interosseous membrane to the index and long finger profundus muscles. This will provide sufficient power for grip, but the finger will be somewhat limited in excursion so that full digital flexion should not be expected.

With palsy of the anterior interosseous branch of the median nerve, weakness is seen in the FPL, median nerve–innervated flexor profundus, and the pronator quadratus. The lack of active distal interphalangeal (DIP) flexion of the index and long fingers may be managed with fusions of these joints because the superficial flexors are intact. If DIP mobility is required, the profundus muscles of the index and long fingers may be sutured to the ulnar nerve–innervated profundus muscles. This allows the weakness to be shared among all the profundus muscles. Alternatively, independent thumb flexion can be maintained by transferring a ring superficialis tendon to the FPL. Grip strength will remain unchanged, but DIP mobility is obtained.

Ulnar Nerve Palsy

Damage to the ulnar nerve results in several motor deficiencies, including loss of key pinch, loss of independent flexion at the MCP joints, and loss of IP extension of all fingers. This is the basis for the claw hand deformity. The patient's sequence of flexion of the digits in grasp changes to flexion at the DIP joints initially rather than flexion of the MCP joints; therefore, the patient cannot place the hand around the object. The lumbrical and interosseous muscles pass palmar to the axes of the MCP joints and dorsal to the IP joints to the lateral bands of the fingers. Therefore, tendon transfers to correct the loss of the intrinsic muscles must duplicate these moment arms. Many authors have described the use of several motor muscles to accomplish these functions.[41,46,48-50] The extensor carpi radialis longus or brevis, the combined extensor indicis proprius and the extensor digiti minimi, and a FDS have all been utilized. It is best to use one of these as a replacement for the intrinsic muscles to all fingers, prolonging the tendon transfer with a four-stranded tendon graft (four-tailed graft) (Fig. 36–10). Static intrinsic procedures directed at limiting MCP hyperextension are reserved for the patients with combined nerve palsy.

Other deficits noted in patients with ulnar nerve lesions include loss of flexion and ulnar deviation of the wrist, weakening of flexion of the ring and little fingers, and loss of abduction-adduction of all fingers. With loss of the FCU, the patient experiences a generalized weakness in a variety of wrist actions but no total loss of any action, nor any resulting deformity. Manual laborers may note this deficit more significantly. It may be useful in selected cases for transfer of the FCR to the ulnar side of the wrist to provide flexion and ulnar deviation.

To replace adduction and abduction of the fingers, eight separate motor muscles would be necessary. This is neither practical nor beneficial. Weakened flexion of the ring and little fingers causes no deformity because the functioning superficialis tendons provide some extrinsic flexor power and motion. However, the manual laborer again might notice a significant deficit because of weakened ulnar-sided

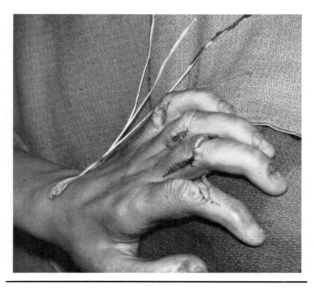

Fig. 36-10. Extensor carpi radialis longus prolonged with a four-tailed plantaris tendon for the reconstruction of intrinsic muscle function in an ulnar nerve palsy. Each tendon slip is sutured to the radial lateral band except on the index finger, where it is attached to the ulnar lateral band. It is important that each tendon slip course palmar to the transverse intermetacarpal ligament before its insertion.

grip. The use of a hammer will demonstrate this gross disability in workers with ulnar nerve palsy through a decrease in the hand's effective width in power grasp. Methods to reduce this deficit include side-to-side suturing of ring and little finger flexor digitorium profundus (FDP) tendons to the FDP of the long finger. This does not strengthen grasp, but it allows the weakness to be shared more evenly in the hand. In patients who wish to return to heavy labor, transfer of the extensor carpi radialis longus to the ring and little finger FDP has also been successful.

The weakness of key pinch in ulnar nerve palsy is demonstrated by the appearance of Froment's sign with IP flexion and MCP hyperextension as the patient attempts a lateral pinch (see Fig. 36–9A). If this pattern persists, a tendon transfer utilizing the long finger FDS or extensor carpi radialis longus around a pulley created by palmar fascia can be performed to restore pinch. Frequently, the longitudinal column of the thumb articulations is unstable, and a MCP arthrodesis is performed to stabilize the thumb in key pinch. The thumb MCP is positioned in 15° of flexion with slight abduction and pronation to improve function.

Postoperative immobilization after transfer for intrinsic muscle function should be prolonged to prevent the increased tendency of these transfers to stretch out. An intrinsic plus position is utilized for 4 weeks in a cast with MCP joints flexed to 90° and IP joints in extension. The patient is begun in the re-education phase by concentrating first on MCP flexion and then on IP extension. An intrinsic plus splint is used for an additional 8 to 12 weeks following cast removal.

Combined Nerve Palsies

The importance of direct nerve repair in patients with multiple peripheral nerve injuries must be emphasized. The greater loss of muscle-tendon function severely limits the available motors for transfer. In addition, the sensory loss is more significant and may be the major disability in these patients. The use of reconstructive procedures such as tendon transfers in conjunction with joint fusions, tenodeses, and capsulodeses will provide stability and improve function. The reader is referred to sources on the treatment of the severely paralyzed hand for discussion of tendon transfers in these patients.[51]

REHABILITATION OF THE NERVE-INJURED PATIENT

Therapy and splinting are crucial to the rehabilitation process of a patient who has sustained a peripheral nerve injury. Occupational therapists provide regular monitoring of the patient's motion and sensibility status, vocational information and retraining, and intervention to improve or maintain range of motion, correct existing soft tissue contractures or joint deformities, and diminish the detrimental effects of abnormal, compensatory movement patterns.

Because of the prolonged recovery time while a patient is awaiting nerve function restoration, it is beneficial to include activities of daily living assessment and training. Work tolerance evaluations also will provide useful information on the patient's functional deficits.[52] Sensory re-education techniques have been described that are supposed to help patients recognize new sensory patterns from their reinnervated digits.[53] Although we have attempted to use these techniques over the years, we have been unable to demonstrate any significant improvement in sensory perceptions.

Splinting, always combined with motion exercises, may utilize two approaches. Corrective splinting with therapy is necessary if joint deformities or contractures are present (Fig. 36-11). Once these static deformities are overcome and joint motion is passively supple, substitution splinting may be incorporated. Substitution splinting diminishes complications in the palsied upper extremity by positioning the joints so that the soft tissues on the paralyzed side of the joint will not stretch beyond their elastic limits and the soft tissues on the antagonist side will not contract to reduce motion and excursion. The second important benefit of substitution splinting is that it positions the hand to allow improved function.

In radial nerve palsy, the emphasis in a splinting program is to position and stabilize the wrist in dorsiflexion to improve grasp. Motion exercises are then included to protect the extensor mechanism of all digits to prevent stretching of these dorsal soft tissues. In some patients who require an improved arc of finger extension, a low-profile, dynamic MCP extension splint may be used (Fig. 36-12). Most patients, however, find the wrist extension splint satisfactory and are not significantly limited with the lack of MCP extension.

In patients with a median nerve injury, usually the loss of sensation in the thumb, index finger, and long finger is more disabling than the actual motor loss. The patient must adapt either through direct visual observation to assist with prehension or use of an ulnar nerve–based pinch, which is very awkward. Splinting in low median nerve injuries utilizes an opponens splint or simple thumb web spacer to maintain carpometacarpal stability and motion. In high median nerve palsies, splinting is specifically individualized but will focus on assisting finger flexion dynamically with thumb opposition.

Fig. 36-11. A dynamic splint used in a patient with ulnar nerve palsy, thumb web, and PIP flexion contractures.

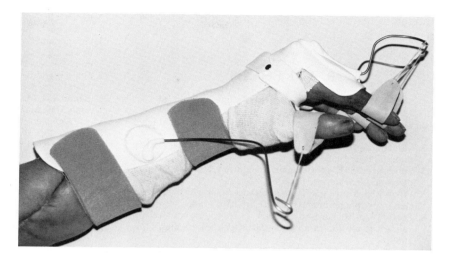

In patients with ulnar nerve lesions, the most common deformity to avoid is clawing. In a supple hand, the tendency toward clawing may be blocked using a static lumbrical bar or dynamic watchband splint. Both prevent MCP hyperextension by maintaining these joints in flexion and allow the patient's extrinsic extensors to actively extend the IP joints.

In combined nerve injuries of the upper extremity, the deficits become more profound and disabling. The available options for reconstructive procedures diminish, and rehabilitation efforts must be aggressive and long-term. Functional orthoses such as a wrist- or shoulder-driven flexor hinge orthosis may be necessary to provide grasp and release in the absence of suitable muscles for transfer or reconstruction.

Remembering that maximal rehabilitation can take years, one must avoid tunnel vision in dealing with the nerve-injured patient. The patient needs emotional and social support. Although the physician and therapist may focus on hand function, the patient's greatest concern may be earning enough

Fig. 36-12. A dynamic radial nerve palsy splint provides wrist, finger, and thumb extension.

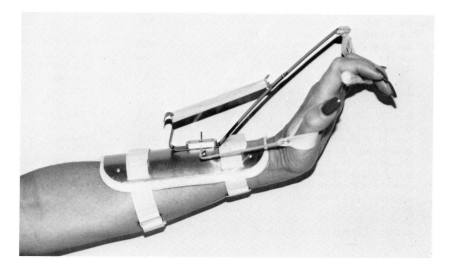

money to feed a family. Never lose sight of the patient's *needs*.

REFERENCES

1. Seddon HJ: Three types of nerve injury. Brain 66:237, 1943
2. Sunderland S: Nerves and Nerve Injuries. 2nd Ed. Churchill Livingstone, Edinburgh, 1978
3. Sunderland S: The connective tissues of peripheral nerves. Brain 88:841, 1965
4. Sunderland S: The intraneural topography of the radial, median and ulnar nerves. Brain 68:243, 1945
5. Wilgis EFS, Murphy R: The significance of longitudinal excursion in peripheral nerves. Hand Clin 2:761, 1986
6. Bora FW Jr, Richardson S, Black J: The biomechanical responses to tension in a peripheral nerve. J Hand Surg 5:21, 1980
7. Lundborg G: Structure and function of the intraneural microvessels as related to trauma, edema formation, and nerve function. J Bone Joint Surg [Am] 57:938, 1975
8. Lundborg G: The intrinsic vascularization of human peripheral nerves: structural and functional aspects. J Hand Surg 4:34, 1979
9. Seddon HJ: Surgical Disorders of the Peripheral Nerves. 2nd Ed. Churchill Livingstone, Edinburgh, 1975
10. Gelberman RA, Szabo RM, Williamson RV, Dimick MP: Sensibility testing in peripheral-nerve compression syndromes. An experimental study in humans. J Bone Joint Surg [Am] 65:632, 1983
11. Szabo RM, Gelberman RH, Dimick MP: Sensibility testing in patients with carpal tunnel syndrome. J Bone Joint Surg [Am] 66:60, 1984
12. Szabo RM: Nerve Compression Syndromes—Diagnosis and Treatment. Slack Inc, Thorofare, NJ, 1989
13. Moberg E: Evaluation and management of nerve injuries in the hand. Surg Clin North Am 44:1019, 1964
14. Swanson AB, Mays JD, Yamauchi Y: A rheumatoid arthritis evaluation record for the upper extremity. Surg Clin North Am 48:1003, 1968
15. Kaplan EB: Functional and Surgical Anatomy of the Hand. 2nd Ed. JB Lippincott, Philadelphia, 1961
16a. Richie P: Le Nerf Cubital et les Muscles de l'Eminence Thenar. Bull Mem Soc Anat. Paris, 5:251, 1897
16b. Cannieu JMA: Recherches sur une Anastomose Entre la Branche Profunde du Cubitale et Le Médian. Bull Soc d'Anat Physiol. Bordeaux, 18:339, 1897
17. Spinner M: Injuries to the Major Branches of Peripheral Nerves of the Forearm. WB Saunders, Philadelphia, 1972
18. Chidgey LK, Szabo RM: Radial nerve palsy. p. 1379. In Chapman MW, Madison M (eds): Operative Orthopaedics. Vol. 2. JB Lippincott, Philadelphia, 1988
19. Gaul JS Jr: Electrical fascicle identificaton as an adjunct to nerve repair. J Hand Surg 8:289, 1983
20. Jabaley ME: Electrical nerve stimulation in the awake patient. Bull Hosp Joint Dis 44:248, 1984
21. Bora FW Jr, Pleasure DE, Didizian NA: A study of nerve regeneration and neuroma formation after nerve stuture by various techniques. J Hand Surg 1:138, 1976
22. Omer GE: Evaluation of the extremity with peripheral nerve injury and timing for nerve suture. Instr Course Lect 33:463, 1984
23. Omer GE, Spinner M: Peripheral nerve testing and suture techniques. Instr Course Lect 24:122, 1975
24. Sunderland S: The anatomical basis of nerve repair. p. 14. In Jewett DL, McCarroll HR Jr (eds): Nerve Repair and Regeneration. CV Mosby, St. Louis, 1980
25. Sunderland S: The pros and cons of funicular nerve repair. J Hand Surg 4:201, 1979
26. Szabo RM, Madison M: Principles of Nerve Repair. In Chapman MW, Madison M (eds): Operative Orthopaedics. Vol. 2. JB Lippincott, Philadelphia, 1988
27. Jabaley ME, Wallace WH, Heckler FR: Internal topography of major nerves of the forearm and hand. J Hand Surg 5:1, 1980
28. Williams HB, Jabaley ME: The importance of internal anatomy of the peripheral nerves to nerve repair in the forearm and hand. Hand Clin 2:689, 1986
29. Millesi H: Interfascicular nerve grafting. Orthop Clin North Am 12:287, 1981
30. Millesi H, Meissl G, Berger A: The interfascicular nerve-grafting of the median and ulnar nerves. J Bone Joint Surg [Am] 54:727, 1972
31. Millesi H, Meissl G, Berger A: Further experience with interfascicular grafting of the median, ulnar, and radial nerves. J Bone Joint Surg [Am] 58:209, 1976
32. Seddon HJ: Nerve grafting. J Bone Joint Surg [Br] 45:447, 1963
33. Brand PW: Clinical Mechanics of the Hand. CV Mosby, St. Louis, 1985
34. Brand PW, Beach RB, Thompson DE: Relative tension and potential excursion of muscles in the forearm and hand. J Hand Surg 6:209, 1981
35. Brand PW: Biomechanics of tendon transfer. Orthop Clin North Am 5:205, 1974
36. Brand PW: General principles for restoration of muscle balance following paralysis in forearm and hand. p. 1401. In Chapman MW, Madison M (eds): Operative Orthopaedics. Vol. 2. JB Lippincott, Philadelphia, 1988
37. Burkhalter WE: Early tendon transfer in upper extremity peripheral nerve injury. Clin Orthop 104:68, 1974
38. Omer GE: The technique and timing of tendon transfers. Orthop Clin North Am 5:243, 1974
39. Omer GE: Timing of tendon transfers in peripheral nerve injury. Hand Clin 4:317, 1988
40. Omer GE, Spinner M (eds): Management of Peripheral Nerve Problems. WB Saunders, Philadelphia, 1980
41. Riordan DC: Tendon transfers in hand surgery. J Hand Surg 8:748, 1983
42. Boyes JH: Tendon transfers for radial nerve palsy. Bull Hosp Joint Dis 21:97, 1960
43. Chuinard RG, Boyes JH, Stark HH, Ashworth CR: Tendon transfers for radial nerve palsy: use of superficialis tendons for digital extension. J Hand Surg 3:560, 1978
44. North ER, Littler JW: Transferring the flexor superficialis tendon: technical considerations in the prevention of proximal interphalangeal joint disability. J Hand Surg 5:498, 1980
45. Cooney WP, Linscheid RL, Kai-Nan AN: Opposition of the thumb: an anatomic and biomechanical study of tendon transfers. J Hand Surg [Am] 9:777, 1984
46. Brand PW: Tendon transfers for median and ulnar nerve paralysis. Orthop Clin North Am 1:447, 1970
47. Burkhalter WE: Tendon transfers in median nerve paralysis. Orthop Clin North Am 5:271, 1974
48. Brand PW: Tendon grafting illustrated by a new operation for

intrinsic paralysis of the fingers. J Bone Joint Surg [Br] 43:444, 1961

49. Omer GE Jr: Reconstructive procedures for extremities with peripheral nerve defects. Clin Orthop 163:80, 1982

50. Zancolli EA: Structural and Dynamic Bases of Hand Surgery. 2nd Ed. JB Lippincott, Philadelphia, 1979

51. Eversmann WW: Tendon transfers for combined nerve injuries. Hand Clin 4:187, 1988

52. Fess EE: Rehabilitation of the patient with peripheral nerve injury. Hand Clin 2:207, 1986

53. Dellon AL, Curtis RM, Edgerton MT: Reeducation of sensation in the hand after nerve injury and repair. Plast Reconstr Surg 53:297, 1974

37 Poliomyelitis

JACQUELIN PERRY

Prior to 1955 poliomyelitis was an active paralyzing disease in the United States, with the severity of the epidemics increasing each decade. Introduction of the Salk vaccine abruptly reversed this course. Subsequent use of the Sabin vaccine (introduced in 1963) virtually eliminated acute poliomyelitis in the Western world (Fig. 37-1).

Recently a late form of postpoliomyelitis disability has emerged. Patients with an initial good recovery 30 or more years ago (ranging from 20 to 60 years) now are experiencing new muscle weakness, fatigue, and pain.[1,2] The ages of these patients range from 35 to 85 years. The impairment is sufficient to deprive some of them of the ability to work, whereas others are having difficulty with community mobility and self-care. This disability had been termed postpolio muscular atrophy (PPMA),[3] the *postpolio syndrome*,[4] or the late effects of poliomyelitis.[1]

Although the present situation has evolved over the past 10 years, it is not a new phenomenon. Charcot published the first report more than 100 years ago,[5] and sporadic articles have appeared in the worldwide literature since then.[6,7] The number of persons estimated to be susceptible to the postpolio syndrome has increased from 125,000[6] to 300,000[8] and most recently 1,600,000 (combined paralytic and nonparalytic cases, National Center for Health Statistics, unpublished data) as awareness of this problem has grown. The large potential population relates to the high incidence of poliomyelitis in the 1935 to 1955 era.[8] Hence, the late effects of poliomyelitis represent a clinical entity necessitating an organized mode of management.

The acute and late forms of poliomyelitis have very different rehabilitation needs. Each is reviewed in this chapter.

ACUTE POLIOMYELITIS

The rarity of acute poliomyelitis in the United States today has made this an almost unrecognized disease. Acute viral invasion of the anterior horn cells in the spinal cord causes pain, stiffness, fever, and paralysis. Poliomyelitis is abrupt in onset and often is confused with influenza.[9] Acute inflammatory cells in the spinal fluid are the most positive sign other than viral isolation; but the number of cells may be small.[9] Another identifying characteristic is the variation in muscle involvement. Although severe paralysis has an anatomic pattern, the degree of partial paresis can differ markedly in adjacent muscles. Involvement may vary from a brief weakness in one limb to total body dysfunction.

Poliomyelitis is a purely motor cell impairment; sensation and central control are normal. The rare patient with an otherwise typical "polio paralysis" pattern will have involvement of sensation, but this is too infrequent to consider except by extensive exclusion.

Acute Care

Treatment of the acute inflammatory state is limited to making the patient comfortable, because there is no known cure. The basic measures are bed rest, general support, and analgesia.[9,10] Hot packs are the most effective means of relieving the very intense muscle pain.[9] Designed by Sister Kenny, these packs are pieces of wool blanket soaked in boiling water, rapidly wrung out, quickly wrapped around the limbs and the trunk, and covered with a matching dry blanket section (Fig. 37-2). Triangles best fit the shoulder and hips, whereas rectangles are used to cover the limb and trunk muscles.[11] The joints are left uncovered to allow motion. When moving the pa-

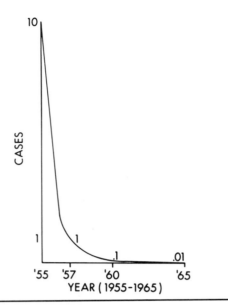

Fig. 37-1. Rate of decline of acute poliomyelitis after introduction of the Salk vaccine (incidence per 100,000 cases).

tient to apply the pack, grasping the joints rather than squeezing the tender muscle bellies also avoids unnecessary pain.[9,11,12] The packs are applied for several hours each day. These are supplemented by gentle range of motion exercises and positioning, which prevents deformity. There should be no rush to strengthen the muscles.

Rehabilitation

Prevention of Contractures

The first concern is prevention of contractures, because spontaneous activity is inhibited by muscle "spasm" as well as by muscle weakness. The intramuscular inflammation makes the tissues very sensitive to motion, causing the pain threshold to be reached long before tissue tension is felt by the therapist. Ranging, thus, is done slowly, with constant observation for signs of pain. Gentle teasing at the end of the arc helps to gain greater mobility. Forcing the tissues only leads to rapid loss of both mobility and patient cooperation. Positioning and protective splints also are indicated to preserve neutral ankle dorsiflexion, full knee extension, and complete hip extension.[9,13] Similar efforts in the upper extremity

are directed to maintaining complete (140°) elbow flexion, full hand opening and grasp, wrists at neutral, and free shoulder rotation in all planes. When there is a likelihood that muscle recovery may be poor, selective functional contracture also should be maintained.[14] The critical positions are neutral ankle and wrist positions and a straight spine. Light plaster body jackets are an effective means of protecting the spine during upright activities.

Recovery of muscle strength follows three paths. The partially injured anterior horn cells heal.[15] Axon sprouting by adjacent neurons allows adoption of some of the muscle fibers orphaned through the destruction of their motoneurons (see Fig. 37-5).[16-19] Muscle hypertrophy is gained through exercise. The final result depends on the extent of the initial anterior horn cell damage.

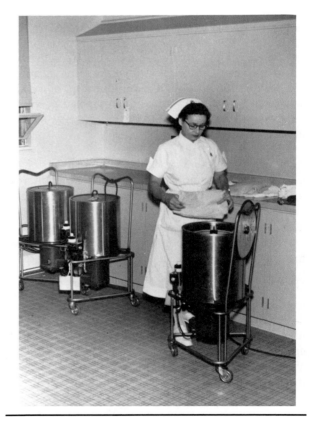

Fig. 37-2. Nurse packing a hot pack steam machine for bedside application.

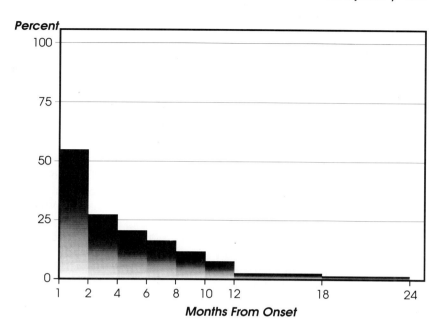

Fig. 37-3. Rate of recovery of strength after acute poliomyelitis. Percentage of cases showing a one-grade gain. (Adapted from Sharrad,[21] with permission.)

Exercise

Exercise begins after comfort has been reestablished. How vigorous it should be, however, has been debated throughout the history of poliomyelitis. Experience has taught the need to progress slowly[9,20]; strength can be lost by overly aggressive exercise. Assistive techniques precede active exercise. Resistance is added only as the muscles respond with increased strength. Exercise increments should be gradual because the paretic muscles are highly sensitive to overuse. There are no clinical signs by which the weakness of disuse atrophy can be differentiated from that of muscle fiber loss. Repetitive high demand can damage the muscle fibers. Thus, the rehabilitation program should induce fatigue of only moderate and short duration. The patient's course should be one of gradual progress. Loss of strength with exercise is the sign of overdemand. With early protection, the overuse injury can be reversed. Continuing the strain on the assumption that exercise is the only "cure" can lead to permanent loss of function.

Sharrard, in a study of 3,000 muscles, found the rate of recovery was greatest in the first month of convalescence, with 55 percent gaining one grade (Fig. 37-3).[21] With each subsequent month the recovery rate declined. By the end of 1 year, only 5 percent of the muscles registered a gain of one grade. Thirty-one percent of the muscles studied made no recovery.

Orthoses

Orthoses and crutches, while enabling patients to be ambulatory, also protect the weak muscles from overuse and deleterious stretch. Very commonly these devices will have served their purpose within a year or two.[11,22]

With the infrequent occurrence of acute poliomyelitis today, appropriate bracing must be obtained through other programs. For the lower extremity, the knee-ankle-foot (KAFO) and ankle-foot (AFO) orthoses used in management of the late effects of poliomyelitis are also appropriate for acute rehabilitation.[23-25] The hand, elbow, and shoulder impairments stemming from poliomyelitis can be met by the orthoses now used for the upper extremity sequelae of spinal cord injury or hand trauma.[26]

Reconstructive Surgery

Another means of improving function involves reconstructive surgery.[22] Soft tissue releases and osteotomies are used to correct fixed deformities.[27] Tendon transfers and selective joint fusion are means of eliminating the need for bracing and also help provide for a general gain in function. Because the post-polio syndrome rather than the acute disease is the more common situation today, most of the surgical procedures are described in the section dealing with that entity.

Spine

Deformity in any direction (scoliosis, lordosis, or kyphosis) and gross postural collapsing can follow paralysis of the spinal muscles. During the growing years prophylactic body jackets can delay the rate of progression.[12] Although it would be best to avoid operating when continuing growth is anticipated, excessive progression of the deformity should not be accepted. Surgery is indicated when forced-bend radiographs show the residual deformity is nearing the limits of acceptability. If spinal growth is still present, the subsequent changes induced by a unilateral rigid bony bar (the fusion) must be considered. In particular, a lordotic posture should be avoided with a posterior fusion. Stabilization of a collapsing spine can markedly improve the patient's level of function and endurance.[12]

Hip

Hip surgery most commonly consists of flexion contracture releases. This procedure can be avoided by early corrective positioning and lower extremity bracing, which encourages standing in hip hyperextension. Joint fusion to provide indirect knee stability and brace-free ambulation is an old practice, but there will be increased strain at both the back and the knee several years later, and then there is no recourse. Transfer of the iliopsoas muscle,[28] iliotibial band,[29] or lateral trunk muscles[30,31] is a means of replacing an incompetent gluteus medius muscle. Early results were good, but there are no long-term reports on follow-up. The traditional technique of iliotibial band sectioning should be replaced with Z-lengthening to preserve passive control at both the hip and the knee.

Knee

Epiphysiodesis in the proximal tibia or distal femur offers a means of equalizing leg length during the growing years.[32,33] The appropriate timing is calculated from predictive charts, of which Green's is the traditional standard.[34] The best program consists of annual leg length radiographs (scanograms) beginning with the child's first visit so the rate of unequal growth can be determined. Surgical timing should be based on bone age determined from reference charts, not chronological age.[35]

Ankle/Foot

Fusion of the subtalar joint is a common means of correcting deformity and stabilizing the paralytic foot.[22] When neutral alignment sagittally and transversely was attained, the long-term results of a triple arthrodesis were good. Residual varus (and less frequently valgus) deformity is a too-frequent outcome. Debilitating arthrotic changes at the ankle are likely to occur about 30 years later. Pantalar arthrodeses also are a means of gaining stability for brace removal. Late changes in the knee and the remaining foot joints cause significant disability. Tendons of muscles working in stance rather than swing (out of phase) that were transferred to restore ankle dorsiflexion do not appear to have survived for even a short time.

Upper Extremity

Phasic transfer of muscles with at least good strength has proved to be a reliable means of restoring thumb opposition. Out-of-phase muscle transfers, however, have not been effective. A shoulder fusion is an excellent means of gaining functional arm stability. The optimum position is approximately 30° abduction, 20° flexion and 15° of internal rotation. This provides useful arm elevation while avoiding scapular winging when the arm is at the side of the body. A valuable technique is to make the protective cast before surgery with the patient standing so a good body fit is obtained. In addition, internal fixation should be planned.

LATE EFFECTS OF POLIOMYELITIS

Disability related to the late effects of poliomyelitis is of two types. Orthopaedic impairment such as contractures, stretched ligaments, or intercurrent injuries are readily recognized and accepted by the medical community.[22,36] More subtle and poorly understood is the loss of muscle function.[36,37]

Late Loss of Muscle Function

Of primary concern has been the cause of this "new" muscle dysfunction. Several causes have been proposed. The possibility of poliovirus reactivation appears to be unlikely on the basis of Bodian's anterior horn cell data, which showed disappearance of the virus within 3 weeks.[15] Amyotrophic lateral sclerosis (ALS) was also considered but the patient's course of disease differs.[4,38] Late failure of the secondary axonal sprouts is the most persistent hypothesis.[3,5] This diagnosis is based on characteristic abnormalities in single motor unit electromyographic (EMG) studies.[3,38–42] However, more recent testing of "old" poliomyelitis patients with and without new loss of function showed similar EMG findings in the two groups.[8,43–45] These authors concluded that the EMG changes represented old motor unit loss rather than new axonal sprout failure.[3,42,44,46] Occasionally the patient experiences a very rapid loss of strength, and this is accompanied by EMG signs of acute denervation.

Muscle damage from chronic overuse may be a more likely cause for the late loss of strength.[47] Dynamic EMG recordings during walking have demonstrated increased intensity as the weakened muscles attempted to meet the force demands (Fig. 37-4).[36,48] The symptomatic muscles also exhibited longer than normal periods of activity as they substituted for less able muscles at adjacent joints.[36] Experimental overexercise of partially denervated muscles resulted in fiber damage and corresponding loss of strength.[49,50] Studies of exhaustive exercise in elite athletes also have demonstrated inflammatory reactions, enzyme changes, and muscle fiber damage.[51] Two characteristics of the acute poliomyelitis course make the patients sensitive to muscle overuse: (1) anterior horn cell destruction reduces the number of motor units within the muscle[15] (Fig. 37-5), and (2) the phenomenon of axon sprouting, by adopting orphaned muscle fibers, clusters them and creates overly large motor units (Fig. 37-5).[19] This exaggerated grouping of the muscle fibers would decrease the opportunity for trade-off to allow rest and recovery. Hence, the post-polio muscles, being smaller than normal and less efficient, are subject to overuse strain.

Several authors have correlated patients' late loss of strength with aggressive activity.[7,52–54] Bennett termed this "overwork weakness."[53] A significant weight gain also has been related to the late-onset weakness.[52] Chronic strain is implied by the patients' reports that they had learned to accept low-grade pain and periodic acute exacerbation as the price of having had poliomyelitis.[55] They routinely "pushed through it" to accomplish their vocational and family demands.

The unique characteristic of poliomyelitis is its random pattern of muscle weakness. This paralytic picture is consistent with the 95 percent anterior horn cell invasion described by Bodian and a recovery varying between 12 and 91 percent.[15] Hence, the areas of residual damage occur by chance. Muscles with similar nerve root innervation can vary markedly in strength. For example, the gluteus maximus may be strong and the gastrocnemius without any function. Both are supplied by the first sacral root.

Intact sensation, depressed reflexes, and normal neural control combined with a history of poliomyelitis and a typical therapeutic program are other supportive findings. Significant deformity is infrequent. Atrophy, an expected sign of flaccid paralysis, has been obscured by two intramuscular physiologic reactions. Muscular stretch from eccentric demands has stimulated the addition of sarcomeres to lengthen the contracting chain.[50] This preserves muscle bulk but does not improve muscle strength because the number of fibers was not increased. The natural muscle contours also have been maintained by body fat occupying the space of the lost fibers.

Rehabilitation

To minimize the late effects of poliomyelitis, the primary therapeutic focus is the elimination of deleterious strain on the muscles, ligaments, and joint surfaces. The rehabilitation plan is designed to match functional demand with physical ability using five programs: (1) life-style modification, (2) exercise, (3) anti-inflammatory medication, (4) functional devices (including orthoses), and (5) reconstructive surgery.

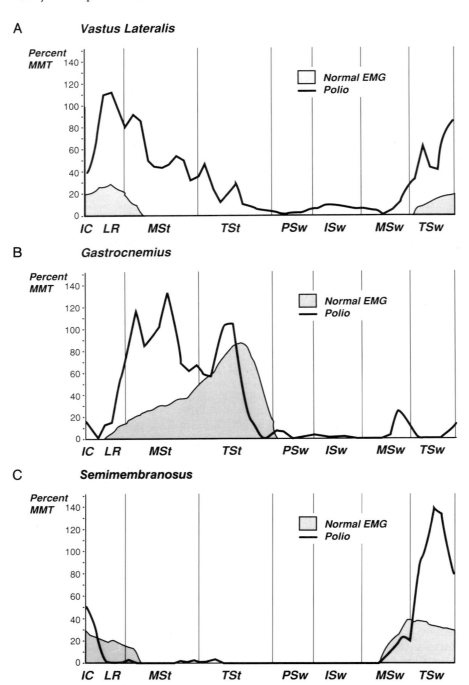

Fig. 37-4. Postpolio muscle function during walking compared to normal. EMG records identify timing and intensity of individual case examples. **(A)** Vastus lateralis (grade 4) muscle shows excessive intensity and duration, evidence of overuse. **(B)** Gastrocnemius (grade 4−) shows premature high intensity and normal duration, indicating overuse. **(C)** Semimembranosus (grade 4) shows high intensity in swing and curtailed stance action; overuse is avoided. Heavy line represents muscle affected by poliomyelitis. Shaded area represents normal function ($n = 25$ each). Percent MMT, percentage of maximum manual strength test. Gait phases identified are as follows: IC, initial contact; LR, loading response; MSt, midstance; TSt, terminal stance; PSw, preswing; ISw, initial swing; MSw, midswing; TSw, terminal swing.

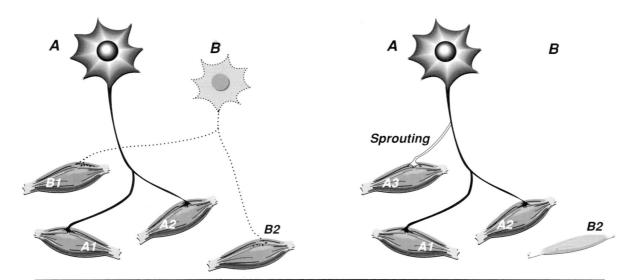

Fig. 37-5. Axon sprouting diagram showing partial adoption of orphaned muscle fibers with corresponding preservation of function. The interaction is displayed by two motor units. Each includes a motor cell, its axon, and branches to two muscle fibers. **(Left)** Motor unit A is healthy and innervates its two muscle fibers (A1, A2). Motor unit B (light shading) has been killed by poliovirus. Its axon and branches have atrophied. Muscle fibers B1 and B2 have lost their innervation. **(Right)** Motor unit A has formed a new axon branch (sprout) to adopt one of the orphaned muscle fibers (B1, now A3). Muscle fiber B2, which has no nerve supply, will die.

Life-Style Management

Life-style modification is the basic program. Prolonged or repetitive high-demand tasks (such as heavy housework or volunteering for every chore at work) either are eliminated or are reduced to the patient's tolerance. Tasks are broken to provide short intervals of activity followed by significant periods of rest. An essential first step in life-style modification is having the patients understand the panthomechanics of their disability and the activity/rest (A/R) ratio guidelines. Psychologically, cutting back on their activities is very difficult to accept because the patients were trained to push despite discomfort and pain.

The physiologic balance between activity and rest has been demonstrated by research with elite athletes for repetitive exercise at their maximum capacity. Duchateau and Hainaut found a rapid decline in strength after 30 seconds, and exhaustion occurred within 1 minute when the activity interval was twice as long as the rest period (A/R = 2:1).[56] Reversing the ratio so that the rest interval was twice as long as the activity segment (A/R = 1:2) resulted in good endurance (i.e., fatigue was avoided). Monad reported a quadratic rather than a linear relationship between activity and rest during repetitive function.[57] The duration of activity that was tolerated deteriorated at an accelerated rate as the intensity (percentage of maximum strength) increased. For example, at a 22 percent effort level the activity could be continued for 80 percent of the cycle (i.e., an A/R ratio of 4:1). In contrast, a 60 percent effort could be tolerated for only 30 percent of the interval, making the acceptable duration ratio (A/R) equal to 1:2.[57] Hence, educating patients to a basic 1:2 activity-rest ratio and increasing their awareness that more intense efforts shorten the nonstressful period is very significant in promoting improvement.

Exercise

Exercise falls into two major classifications, aerobics and strengthening. Each has specific objectives and specific effects on the extremity muscles.

Aerobic exercises are popular today as a means of improving cardiopulmonary health to meet the stresses of an active life-style. Such programs, however, use the arm and leg muscles over an extended period of time to train the heart and lungs. The possibility of causing extremity muscle strain is not usually given much consideration, but in the postpolio patient this becomes an issue. Although some patients benefit from these exercises, in others the postpolio symptoms become accentuated. Only if there are major muscle groups that can accept the challenge without experiencing increased fatigue, weakness, or pain are aerobics appropriate. The usual walking, running or jumping, and twisting in an aerobics class, however, should be replaced with bicycling, swimming, and arm aerobics, which are good substitutions because they can be moderated more easily. When widespread weakness is present, the musculature is not sufficient to significantly challenge the heart when exercised. Recent clinical trials of multiple repetitions of brief (2 to 4 minutes) low-resistance exercise interrupted by 1-minute rest periods has proved to be a means of developing some aerobic gains in persons with limited strength.[58]

Strengthening exercise has a selective role in the late postpolio state.[59,60] Muscle pain is a contraindication because this is a sign that damage already has occurred and is continuing. An exercise trial, however, is justified when the complaints are limited to weakness or fatigue, because there are no clinical indicators to differentiate underuse from overuse. Muscle strain is minimized by a nonfatiguing program. The exercises are of short duration (five to 10 repetitions) with moderate resistance (50 percent of maximum strength). These can be done as a home program, although the discipline and equipment of formal physical therapy appears more effective. The patients are advised to continue their program only if they feel good. If their symptoms increase, reducing the resistance by half is tried. With continuing symptoms the exercise is discontinued. Exercise intolerance signifies there is no disuse to be strengthened.

Among 77 patients in this type of a strengthening exercise program, improved function was experienced by 39 percent.[61] These patients could resume some of their previous activities or had more endurance for the same routine. Only nine of these patients, however, registered a strength increase of at least one-half manual grade. No gain was achieved by 34 percent, and the others suffered further fatigue or pain prior to stopping their program. None experienced any permanent deterioration.[62] The ability to make a functional gain through exercise was greater in the muscles of the lower extremities than in those of the arms.[62] A secondary value to using an exercise trial was the demonstration of the patient's functional limits. This helped them accept the need for life-style modifications. Even 91 percent of the patients who benefitted from their exercise needed to reduce the intensity of their lifestyles.

Anti-inflammatory Medication

Edema and the other inflammatory reactions to overuse muscle damage can be reduced by the use of nonsteroidal anti-inflammatory drugs (NSAIDs). The choice among medications appears to depend on gastric tolerance. The relative effectiveness of the NSAIDs in relieving symptoms is similar. Analgesics and transcutaneous electrical nerve stimulation (TENS) units have limited indications because they merely mask the damage and, thus, can encourage the patients to continue their overuse habits.

Functional Devices

The various devices available today to augment or replace lost function fall into four major categories: orthoses, walking aids, wheelchairs and carts, and upper extremity equipment. Although there are more opportunities to compensate for lower extremity dysfunction than upper extremity impairment, the needs are proportional. Among 442 postpolio patients studied, 56 percent had solely lower extremity symptoms, both upper and lower limbs were involved in 33 percent, and just 11 percent had only upper extremity complaints.

Lower Extremity Management

When lower extremity function becomes unavoidably painful or ineffective, walking aids, orthoses, and wheeled devices are the options for preserving the patient's locomotor capability. The choice often represents a balance between functional need and the patient's cosmetic concerns. Most commonly an orthosis is the first approach, although a few patients will desire to start with a cane. Electric carts often are preferred over wheelchairs as the means of reducing the distances walked.

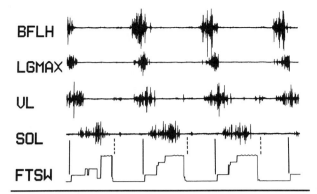

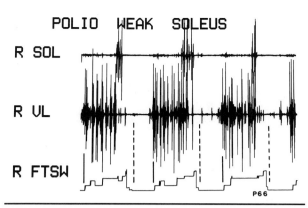

Fig. 37-6. The normal sequence of lower extremity extensor muscle action during walking displayed by dynamic electromyography. BFLH (biceps femoris long head, LGMAX (lower gluteus maximus), VL (vastus lateralis), SOL (soleus), FTSW (footswitch, baseline is swing and staircase is stance indicating progression from heel to flat foot to forefoot support.

Fig. 37-7. EMG recording of prolonged postpolio quadriceps muscle (R VL) action to substitute for a weak soleus (R SOL). High-amplitude bursts are characteristic of enlarged motor units that are reduced in number. R FTSW, Right foot switch. Baseline is swing. Elevated trace shows an irregular progression from heel to foot flat. Heel-off is the abnormally brief high burst at the end of stance. This indicates soleus inadequacy.

Normal extensor control of the limb begins with the hamstrings, proceeds to the gluteus maximus and quadriceps, and then extends to the triceps surae (Fig. 37-6).[63] For the hip extensors and quadriceps, the period of activity is relative short (20 percent of the gait cycle) and the intensity moderate (25 percent of maximum by manual testing). Greater strain is normally placed on the soleus muscle because it serves to stabilize the tibia so body momentum can replace the quadriceps as a knee extensor. The common activity pattern includes a rise in intensity to 80 percent of the normal maximum heel rise capability and duration over 40 percent of the gait cycle.

The weakness and pain of the postpolio syndrome most often are displayed by the triceps surae and quadriceps muscles. Both of these muscle groups are intimately involved in knee stability during stance[64] and, thus, are readily subjected to overuse. With triceps surae muscle weakness, quadriceps activity is increased both in intensity and duration (Fig. 37-7). Conversely, the presence of a weak quadriceps necessitates a much stronger soleus effort (Fig. 37-8). Participation by the hamstrings and gluteus maximus also is increased (Fig. 37-9).

Orthoses. Orthoses offer the advantage of localized control at the knee, ankle, or foot. The reason for choosing this device may be protection of overused muscles, relief of joint pain, or replacement of lost

weight-bearing stability.[23] Modern plastic materials allow better joint control, significantly reduce the weight of the devices, and improve cosmesis. Orthoses still, however, carry the disadvantage of being a visible sign of disability. Also, for many poliomyelitis survivors, returning to the need for an orthosis is extremely difficult psychologically, because one of their early successes was getting rid of the brace during the initial recovery period.

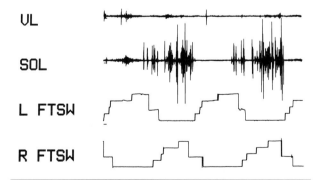

Fig. 37-8. EMG recording (right limb) of premature postpolio soleus (SOL) muscle action substituting for a very weak quadriceps (VL). Muscle timing is demonstrated by the left and right footswitch recordings (FTSW). Soleus onset is in swing (R FTSW at baseline) and then continues with high-amplitude spikes through stance (elevated trace) until the end of single limb support, when the other foot starts its stance (elevated trace in L FTSW).

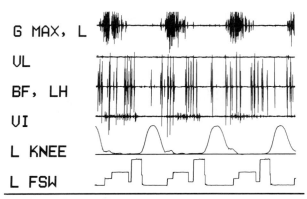

Fig. 37-9. EMG recording of prolonged muscle action of the gluteus maximus (G Max, L), with a good motor unit supply (dense EMG) and the long head of the biceps femoris (BF, LH) with sparse, enlarged motor units substituting for very weak quadriceps (VL, VI) function. Knee goniometer record (L KNEE) shows brief flexion at the onset of stance (elevated L FSW trace) and then rapid full extension. The high arc of flexion in swing (baseline L FSW) is normal in timing and amplitude.

The functional interdependence between the triceps surae and quadriceps muscle groups is very significant in determining orthotic needs.

Quadriceps Weakness. Not all situations require an orthosis. There are two very effective substitutions. Patients with normal triceps surae strength, grade 4 hip extensors, and no knee flexion contracture have good stability and endurance. They use premature activation of the soleus muscle to remove the heel rocker that normally induces knee flexion as the limb is loaded. Prolonged gluteus maximus action assists in maintaining a fully extended knee. Knee hyperextension is a second substitution. This allows the body vector to stabilize the knee. As a result, much less hip and calf muscle strength is needed.

Orthotic assistance is needed when these substitutions are lacking or painful. There are two basic designs based on knee joint mobility, free or locked orthoses.

Free knee orthoses are indicated when there is painful hyperextension (Fig. 37-10A).[23] This may develop as the ligaments fail under continued strain and the knee posture becomes excessive. The pain may either be posterior, in the stretched capsule, or anterior,

where the joint margins of the femur and tibia impact. A knee orthosis with an offset, free-range joint is the device of choice (Fig. 37-10B). It is set to reduce the hyperextension to 10 to 15°. This arc preserves passive stance stability. Unloading the limb for swing allows the patient free knee flexion (Fig. 37-10C). When the deformity is mild and the limb slender, a custom-molded knee orthosis may suffice (Fig. 37-11). Most patients, however, require the full KAFO because the contour of the limb does not allow adequate stabilization without excessive pressure. The minimum foot attachment may be a simple heel cup with a narrow posterior leaf, which allows prompt ankle plantar flexion on heel contact. A hinged ankle joint with appropriate dorsiflexion or plantar flexion controls is added as needed.

Locked knee orthoses are necessary when there is weakness of all the extensor muscles (grade 3 or less) in a knee that lacks a stabilizing hyperextension range or has any flexion contracture. In this case the KAFO must provide both femoral and tibial control to ensure optimum weight-bearing stability of the limb (Fig. 37-12). Thigh control is gained with a well-contoured posterior cuff (or shell) with its proximal edge 2 cm below the ischium (1½ fingerbreadths). This captures as much femoral length as possible while allowing a small arc of pelvic motion to lock the hip by postural hyperextension. The proximal cuff also must be contoured to provide medial groin relief while giving high lateral stability. In addition, its mediolateral dimension should be as narrow as possible to provide coronal plane stability. The modern narrow mediolateral contoured plastic shell design adds further stability. With a well-designed thigh segment (metal or plastic), no pelvic band is needed. A short thigh segment, however, fails to control femoral alignment and knee flexion occurs within the KAFO.

The knee is maximally stable in full extension, so this should be the position of the orthotic knee joint. Aligning the knee joint slightly anterior to the anatomic axis adds further stability. Commercial orthotic knee joints built in full extension require the least modification by the orthotist. If the patient has a flexion contracture, the knee should be extended within 5° of its stretch range to gain all possible postural stability.

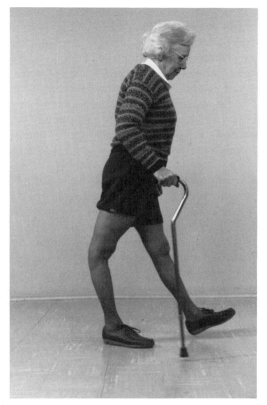

A

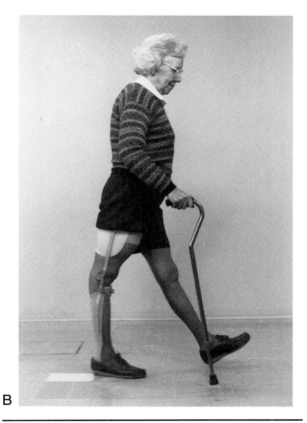

B

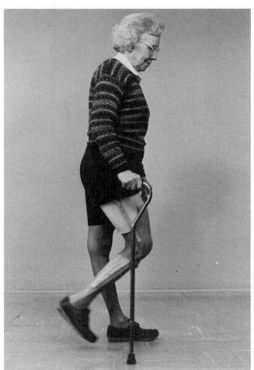

C

Fig. 37-10. Excessive knee hyperextension occurring after years of substitution for a weak quadriceps. **(A)** Maximum strain in terminal stance when body weight is ahead of foot. **(B)** Knee-ankle-foot orthosis (KAFO) with limited hyperextension to remove knee joint strain yet preserve postural substitution for the weak quadriceps. **(C)** Free orthotic knee joint allows voluntary flexion in swing.

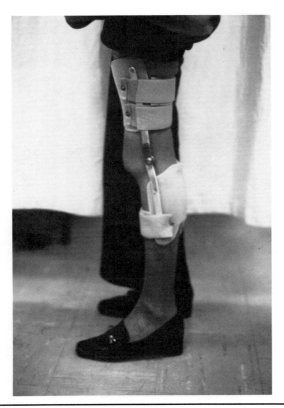

Fig. 37-11. An orthosis limited to the knee (KO) is sufficient if the hyperextension is mild and the limb is well contoured.

Tibial control with a pretibial cuff (or a high tibial band) provides better knee stability than the customary four-buckle knee cage. Further stability is gained with a dorsiflexion stop at the ankle (5° of dorsiflexion). The usual free ankle allows a longer step but offers no stance stability. If the limbs are of equal length, a ½-inch lift to the other foot is needed for toe clearance at initial swing. Otherwise, destructive back strain is introduced as circumduction, hip hiking, or lateral lean is used to lift the foot. Many patients also need a cane or crutch to assist their balance during the swing phase.

Quadriceps Fatigue. Painful overuse of a grade 4+ quadriceps also can result from the increased demands imposed by weakness of the calf muscles. The appropriate device is a hinged AFO with a dorsiflexion stop to replace the lost soleus function. An essential quality is free ankle plantar flexion during the loading response. Otherwise, the demand on the quadriceps has been increased.

Soleus Weakness. The soleus muscle is commonly involved in the postpolio syndrome. Signs of an incompetent soleus are muscle fatigue or pain, lack of a heel rise during the second phase of single-limb support (terminal stance), a flexed knee despite a full passive range, and a short contralateral step (Fig. 37-13A).[65] Late heel rise after the other foot has contacted the floor does not indicate a competent soleus, because body weight is rapidly being transferred to the contralateral limb.

Soleus weakness is confirmed by the standing heel rise strength test.[66] A normal, healthy person can do 20 full-range, single-limb heel rises before tiring.[62] Patients with gait signs of soleus weakness do fewer rises, wobble, or substitute with knee flexion. Soleus strength tested manually with the patient supine will be greatly overestimated because the average force the examiner can exert is only 30 percent of body weight (i.e., one-third of that needed for the first heel lift).[67] Because the primary role of the soleus is tibial stabilization, good function also can be gained from a

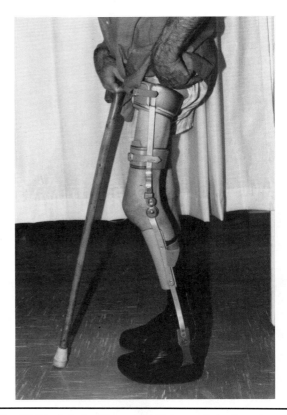

Fig. 37-12. A locked knee KAFO is needed when there is both a weak quadriceps and a flexion contracture.

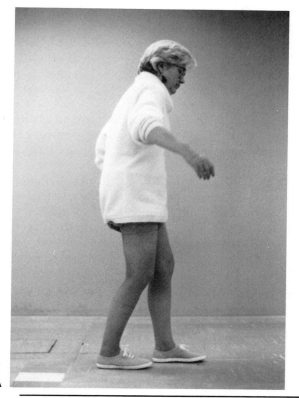
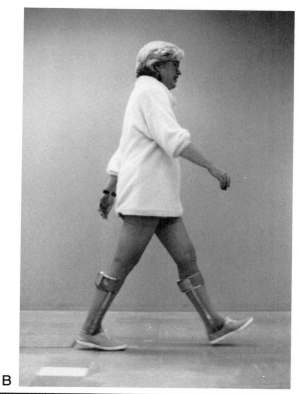

A   B

Fig. 37-13. Midstance limb control with a weak soleus. **(A)** The knee is flexed because the inadequate soleus allowed the tibia to fall into excessive dorsiflexion (trailing limb). Step length was shortened by the resulting instability. **(B)** Ankle-foot orthosis (AFO) with a dorsiflexion stop provides tibial stability to supplement the weak soleus. Not shown is the free plantar flexion allowed during loading response to avoid the knee flexion thrust of a heel rocker. Although metal uprights are shown here, a hinged plastic orthosis can provide similar mechanics.

moderate plantar flexion contracture, which limits the ankle to neutral dorsiflexion on weight bearing.

A *dorsiflexion stop orthosis,* which restricts ankle dorsiflexion, is the appropriate assistance for a weak soleus. Generally, 5° dorsiflexion is allowed so body weight can be rolled onto the forefoot while the tibia keeps its relatively posterior alignment. The basic orthosis has a hinge that allows rapid ankle plantar flexion after floor contact by the heel (Fig. 37-13B). To this is added a dorsiflexion stop. The polypropylene design with a posterior strap is good for lighter patients (under 160 pounds) (Fig. 37-14). Otherwise the double adjustable metal ankle joint is needed. The anterior channels contain stops that limit forward ankle motion to 0° to 5° dorsiflexion while the posterior channel is open to allow free plantar flexion. If dorsiflexion assistance also is needed, a very

light spring can be placed in the posterior channels, but this still must preserve easy plantar flexion.

The use of a solid posterior polypropylene shell as the dorsiflexion stop orthosis rarely is indicated. Patients tolerate this design only if the quadriceps is truly normal. A rigid AFO accentuates the heel rocker, causing the tibia to advance as rapidly as the forefoot drops to the floor. This both accelerates and increases the range of knee flexion as the limb is loaded, creating an added demand on the quadriceps. Positioning the shell in 10° or 15° of plantar flexion to reduce the heel rocker is a tolerable alternative only if the knee has significant hyperextension to allow limb advancement in mid stance and terminal stance.

Tibialis Anterior Paralysis. In cases of tibialis anterior paralysis, an orthosis seldom is indicated unless the patient has difficulty accommodating because of

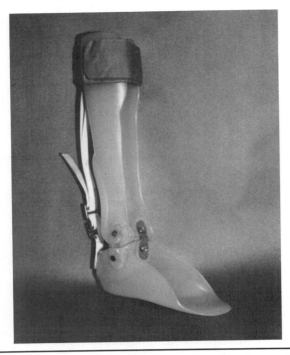

Fig. 37-14. Hinged polypropylene ankle-foot orthosis with a posterior strap to limit dorsiflexion and free plantar flexion (DF-stop-AFO) is a lighter aid for soleus muscle weakness.

flexion after floor contact by the heel. Any orthosis that inhibits this ankle freedom causes the tibia to move forward at the same rate as the foot falls. Knee flexion is accelerated and the arc doubled (30°). A quadriceps with a manual grade less than normal strength will fatigue rapidly with such a demand.

Foot Deformities. Contoured and padded inserts are useful in relieving areas of localized pressure. Their effectiveness, however, hinges on an accurate diagnosis of the cause. Excessive valgus deformity is a common substitution for ankle equinus alignment. Normal subtalar eversion includes a dorsiflexion component. In addition, it unlocks the midfoot. With ankle equinus deformity body weight stretches both ranges. The functional diagnosis is excessive valgus deformity but a corrective insert will not be effective unless the ankle equinus deformity also is accommodated by a heel lift or surgery.

Overuse of the perimalleolar muscles as a substitution for soleus weakness also can cause foot dysfunction. Inversion by the posterior tibialis, first metatarsal head pressure by the peroneus longus muscle, and toe clawing from the long toe flexors are common complications. A dorsiflexion stop AFO is indicated in these circumstances.

Hip Pain. Although there are no effective orthoses for the paralytic hip, function can be improved by attention to knee and ankle stability. Weak abductor muscles most commonly are protected from strain by a lateral trunk lean to the weak side (Trendelenburg limp).[68] Patients with ankle or knee instability or ankle muscle weakness may not be able to adopt this substitution, particularly if the two limbs are of equal length. Consequently, in the management of a painful hip, consider abductor muscle overuse. One therapeutic approach is to make the knee and ankle stable with an appropriate orthosis.

Walking Aids. Walking aids transfer a portion of the weight-bearing load to the arms. The primary indication for a cane or crutch is to substitute for weak hip muscles because there is no effective orthosis. A second strong indication is partial unloading of a painful lumbosacral spine. Persons with moderate weakness at other joints occasionally prefer a cane to a knee or ankle orthosis.

limited hip flexor capability. Extreme passive plantar flexion would be a second indication. The customary answer is a thin polypropylene posterior shell orthosis that fits within the shoe. This is light and has good cosmesis. If the patient has a subnormal quadriceps (grade 4+ or less) the orthosis should have a narrow (¾-inch) distal, posterior shank to preserve free ankle plantar flexion while providing the desired foot pickup in swing. Breakage is not a common problem, but the patient should be alerted to look for margin cracks. If the shank wraps around the heelcord at all, it will obstruct the ankle plantar flexion, increase the heel rocker, and secondarily accelerate knee flexion.

Varus or Valgus Deformities. Rigid AFOs commonly are prescribed for subtalar malalignment.[24] When these are being prescribed for a poliomyelitis survivor, it is essential that the strength of the quadriceps also be considered. The problem is the ease with which the knee flexion of limb loading can be exaggerated by the loss of the normal controlled plantar

Because walking aids always transform the arms into weight-bearing structures, it is necessary to consider the load-carrying capacity of the arms. If there is any local muscular weakness, an intolerable load may be imposed on the shoulder, elbow, wrist, or thumb. The shoulder is particularly vulnerable because upward displacement of the humerus has the potential for rotator cuff impingement unless there is dynamic protection. Safe crutch walking requires normal strength in the rotator cuff muscles as well as the scapular depressors (pectoralis major and latissimus dorsi muscles).

Canes are cosmetically more acceptable, but the small force they accept makes forearm crutches more appropriate for the postpolio patient. If the added trunk stability of axillary crutches is needed, the potential for brachial plexus compression by weight bearing on the axilla must be avoided by fitting them 3 inches below the axilla and using appropriate padding. Impressing the patient with the danger of hand and wrist paralysis is critical.

Wheelchairs and Carts. With the addition of electric carts as an alternative to walking, patients have three choices: manual wheelchair, motorized wheelchair, and electric cart.

Manual Wheelchair. The shoulders, as the primary mover, experience most of the stress from manual wheelchair propulsion. Secondary degeneration and muscle weakness in long-term manual wheelchair users are common findings today (Fig. 37-15). Consequently, the transition of the poliomyelitis survivor from crutches to a manual wheelchair may be a limited solution.

Motorized Wheelchairs. When the shoulders lack the ability to propel a chair, battery power must be substituted. This is a major decision because it markedly challenges the patient's opportunity to drive an automobile unless the limited power of a removable motor is adequate. The weight and bulk of a (noncollapsible) permanent-motor wheelchair make it impractical for use with an automobile; generally a van and motorized lift are required. This is a major expense, which only a few patients can manage. The alternative solution is two wheelchairs, manual for

automobile travel and powered for home or office use.

Electric Carts. These trim, versatile units have become an attractive and practical means of eliminating long-distance ambulation for persons who still have sufficient walking ability for home (or office) independence (Fig. 37-16). They are less suggestive of disability than a motorized wheelchair. Several styles can be broken down for storage in an automobile trunk. Others can be supported by a rack fastened to the back of the car.

Management of the Spine

Back pain is a frequent complaint among postpolio patients. Chronic strain from postural substitutions for lower extremity weakness and the loss of the normal shock absorption by the knee and ankle is common. Excessive lumbosacral loading accompanies the posterior and lateral trunk sway used to substitute for hip extensor or abductor weakness (Fig. 37-17). The impact of abrupt ground contact with locked knees and the unequal limb lengths add further stress to lumbar facet joints. Relief from strain requires improving lower limb efficiency as well as modifying the ways the back is used.

The most effective back support is a Hoke lumbosacral corset (Fig. 37-18). This should have firm paraspinal stays and a good grasp about the pelvis. A good compromise between hip flexion freedom for sitting and an adequate pelvic grasp is provided by an elastic wedge over the thigh with a $\frac{1}{2}$-inch tape sewn across the base for a continuous fixation band (Fig. 37-18). The combination of lateral laces and anterior Velcro straps provides good adaptability for comfort and stability. Diaphragm freedom for persons with limited breathing capacity is gained by not tightening the upper one or two straps.

For collapsing scoliosis, a light polyethylene jacket is a more effective source of trunk support, but it must be prescribed with caution. The rigidity provided often interferes with transferring. Hip flexion is partially restricted, and the trunk has been made longer.

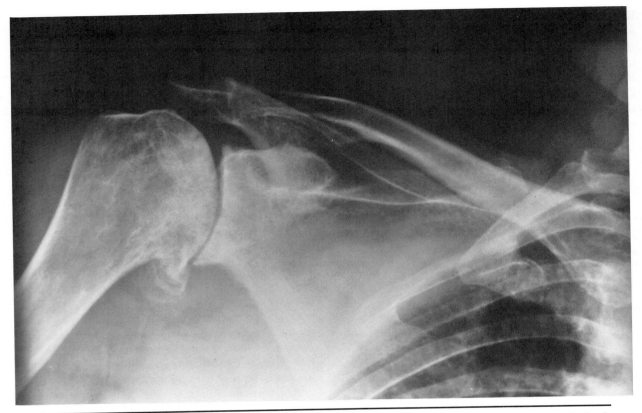

Fig. 37-15. Shoulder joint degeneration occurring after years of crutch walking and subsequent manual wheelchair propulsion.

Both of these devices, however, interfere with walking if trunk sway is used for hip stability. Crutches often are the preferred answer because they reduce the load on the spine. A wheelchair often is the best answer for the spine in late poliomyelitis.

Upper Extremity Management

Shoulder impairment is a common late effect of poliomyelitis. Approximately one-third of the patients studied reported some acute upper extremity involvement initially. During routine function the shoulder muscles lift the weight of the whole arm as well as of any object being lifted.[69] Use of the arms to assist in rising from chairs and other transfer actions is a source of strain.

Control of the highly mobile shoulder depends on a complex interplay between the deltoid and rotator cuff.[69,70] The scapular muscles have the dual role of expanding arm range and stabilizing the arm on the trunk. Both areas are subject to strain.

These muscles are relieved of overuse by modifying the way tasks are performed and by providing substitutive devices. Because self-care, home chores, and work involve such a variety of shoulder functions, the design of an adequate therapeutic program and selection of the appropriate protective equipment requires detailed analysis of the person's activities. Home or office visits often are indicated. Creativity by the occupational therapist is an essential ingredient to reducing upper extremity strain.

There are three basic functions of the shoulder: arm suspension, reaching, and lifting.[71] Although they are functionally integrated, these three activities should be individualized for therapeutic planning.

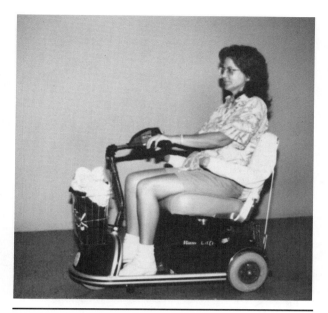

Fig. 37-16. An electric cart is an excellent means of preserving community mobility while reducing shoulder and lower extremity strain.

Passive Suspension. Passive suspension of the arm on the trunk by the clavicular system is possible only if the person sits or stands in a fully erect or slightly reclined posture. The customary forward lean used for most tasks relies on dynamic support by the pos-

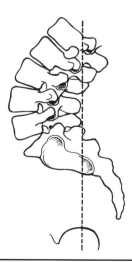

Fig. 37-17. Weight bearing on a lordotic lumbar spine transfers body weight posteriorly and loads the facet joints excessively.

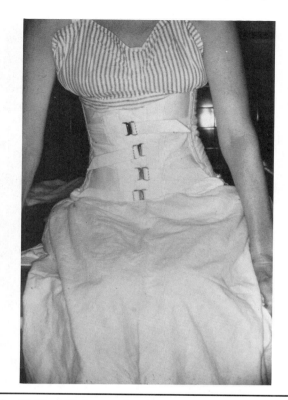

Fig. 37-18. A Hoke-type lumbosacral corset is an effective means of providing trunk support and relieving low back pain.

terior scapular musculature (levator scapulae, trapezius, and rhomboid muscles). In addition, the neck muscles must support the forward head. Overuse of these muscles has become a common industrial complaint. Postpolio sequelae add further susceptibility. Modification of the work area to eliminate forward trunk lean is needed to reduce the muscular demands. Effective approaches include a tilted tabletop, lapboard, and other aids that allow the patient to lean back about 10° from the vertical while still working at a desk or table (Fig. 37-19).

Glenohumeral suspension by the supraspinatus muscles and capsular ligaments is a source of shoulder joint stress. Relief in such cases depends on various commercial or custom-designed arm supports.[72] Overhead activities are particularly demanding on the supraspinatus muscle. Frequent rest intervals constitute the first means of reducing the strain. Otherwise, self-care and work habits must be modi-

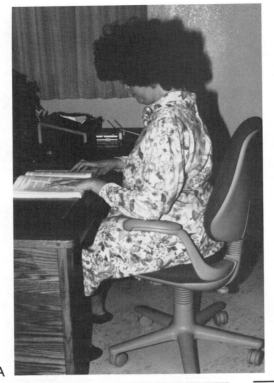

A

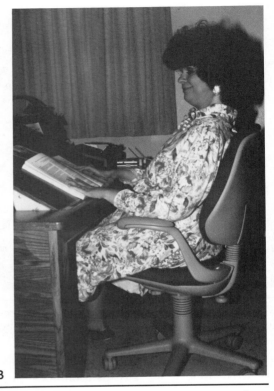

B

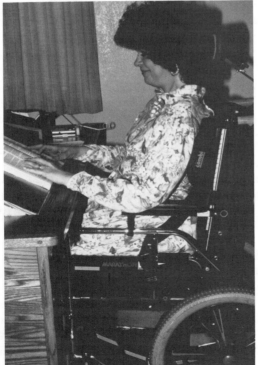

C

Fig. 37-19. Use of a tilted desktop and chair to relieve shoulder and neck pain. **(A)** The problem is the forward lean needed with a flat desktop. **(B)** Secretarial chair with a backward tilt (a bit too much for this patient). **(C)** Tilted wheelchair seat and head rest (better alignment for this patient).

fied to use alternative arm postures or arm supports (Fig. 37-20).

Reaching Devices. Reaching devices offer a means of recovering objects from overhead (Fig. 37-21). They provide an extension for the arm but require a good hand to operate the grasping end. Rearranging the work area and the addition of "Lazy Susan" rotating storage units are ways of bringing needed objects only a forearm's length away.

A mobile arm support (MAS), now classified as a balanced forearm orthosis (BFO), takes the load off the muscles while restoring moderate reaching abil-

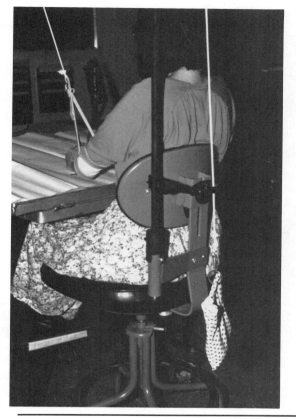

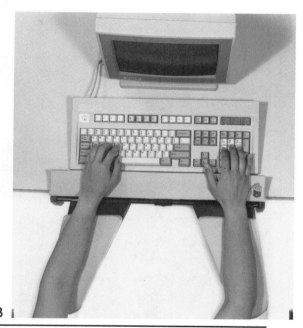

A

B

Fig. 37-20. (A) A counterbalance to suspend the arm and remove the weight-bearing demands on the shoulder. Horizontal mobility is preserved. This patient was an architect with need to compose large drawings at a drafting table. **(B)** Recently a new type of arm support to relieve strain in the wrists, elbows, and shoulders of computer operators has become available. (Courtesy of LMB Hand Rehab Products, San Luis Obispo, CA.)

ity.[26] Because the device is aligned to use gravity as the source of added mobility, the MAS requires a fixed base. For the ambulatory patient, the MAS is attached to a particular table, desk, or other structure. This limits the person to a single work area. Wheelchair-dependent persons carry their MAS with them (Fig. 37-22). In this situation the radial arm design is preferable because it does not interfere with doorways.

Lifting Devices. Lifting and carrying are relieved by the use of wheeled carts and job redesign. Home chores can sometimes be reassigned to other household members or provided through arrangements for outside help. The heaviest object many persons lift is their body during crutch walking. This demand also

must be considered in planning a shoulder protection program.

Reconstructive Surgery

Some of the old poliomyelitis operations are being revived. Tendon releases and osteotomies are used to correct old deformities that require excessive substitutive posturing or cause local joint strain. Transferring of tendons is indicated either to supplement muscle weakness or to remove a deforming force. The much greater age of the poliomyelitis survivors than the young patient with acute poliomyelitis introduces a greater tendency for contracture formation during periods of immobilization. Also, substitutions necessary to perform routine tasks during the healing period are more difficult to accomplish.

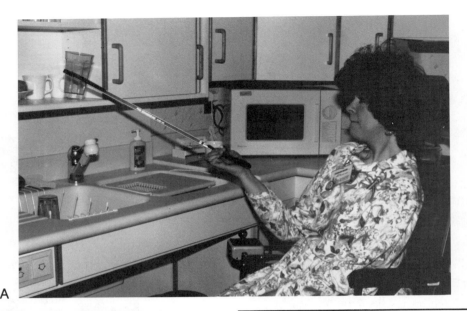

A

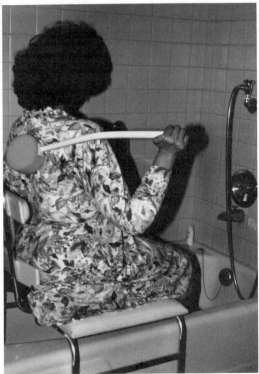

B

Fig. 37-21. Reaching devices help to protect the shoulder from overhead strain. **(A)** Assistance in getting objects from a high shelf. **(B)** Curved bath brush for the back.

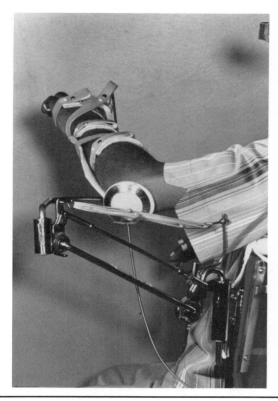

Fig. 37-22. A linear mobile arm support assumes the weight of the arm while allowing horizontal reaching. The design illustrated here also provides limited upward reach.

Hence, the postoperative program must include plans for prevention of deformity and a means of self-care at home.

Ankle and Foot

The ankle and foot have proved to be the areas of greatest need for surgical correction. The problems are equinus deformity, soleus weakness, varus and valgus deformities and claw toe deformities.

Equinus Deformity. Equinus contractures can be at the ankle or within the foot. The two are differentiated by a lateral weight-bearing radiograph that includes the distal tibia (8 inches) as well as the entire foot (Fig. 37-23). Only if there is an area of uncovered talar dome will a tendo Achillis lengthening (TAL) improve foot alignments (Fig. 37-23). The frequently occurring rigid forefoot equinus deformity requires a midfoot osteotomy to re-establish good weight-bear-

ing alignment (Fig. 37-24).[27] Generally, it is an equinovarus deformity that develops. This requires internal rotation at the osteotomy site to lift the lateral side of the foot, as well as a dorsal wedge resection. Primary healing follows the normal time frame, but maturation is slow. As a result, the site should be protected with a functional orthosis for several months.

Correcting the drop-foot with a tendon transfer depends on the presence of a viable substitutive motor muscle. Dynamic electromyographic testing has revealed that long-term substitutions occasionally resulted in a useful phase change of the tibialis posterior, one of the peroneal muscles, or to a lesser extent the lateral gastrocnemius. Successful tendon transfers require two findings in a muscle: at least grade 4 strength and activity during the swing phase as determined by preoperative dynamic EMG. If a muscle is not available for transfer, bracing is continued. Rarely is an ankle fusion appropriate, because the knee flexion thrust will be increased with a correspondingly greater demand on the quadriceps.

Soleus Weakness. Many patients have retained useful strength in the peroneal muscles, tibialis posterior, and/or toe flexors despite major paralysis of the soleus and gastrocnemius. The early concept of transferring the available muscles to the os calcis to supplement calf strength has proved of value in late postpolio disability.[73] To lessen postoperative morbidity from the pressure of a tendon fixation button in the arch, the tendon is made to exit from the os calcis through a medial or lateral hole in the os calcis and sewn to itself with the entry site remaining posterior. Care is taken to preserve maximum bony leverage. All available motor muscles are used. The final distribution of the tendons is determined by an accompanying need for an added eversion or inversion force as well as plantar flexion. During the 6 weeks of cast immobilization prior to returning to the orthosis, great care must be taken to prevent knee and hip flexion contractures.

Valgus and Varus Deformities. Seldom are orthoses or shoe inserts effective in the presence of marked imbalance of the subtalar muscles. Consequently, appropriate tendon transfers are indicated to restore dynamic balance between the inverting and

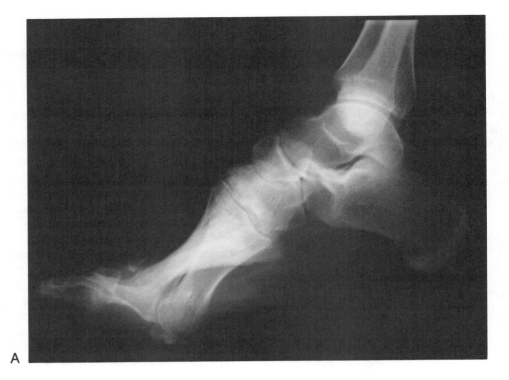

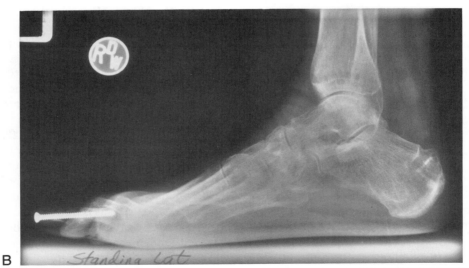

Fig. 37-23. Equinus angulation with the primary deformity in the foot, not at the ankle. **(A)** The close proximity of the anterior margin of the tibia to the anterior limit of the dome of the talus indicates that little of the deformity is at the ankle. Within the foot there is marked forefoot (tarsal and metatarsal) plantar flexion. In addition, there is further depression of the first metatarsal. The indicated treatment is two dorsiflexing osteotomies (midfoot and first metatarsal). **(B)** Postoperative result in a patient with a similar tarsal equinus deformity. Forefoot alignment was corrected by cuneiform-cuboid (healed) osteotomy. Note ankle at maximum dorsiflexion (demonstrated by the slight forward tilt of tibia on talus). The screw is stabilizing an interphalangeal fusion for hammer toe.

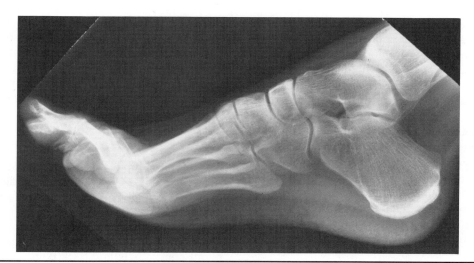

Fig. 37-24. Equinus deformity at the ankle. The anterior margin of the tibia is well posterior to the anterior edge of the dome of the talus. The foot contour is relatively normal. Lengthening of the tendo Achillis is indicated.

everting muscles. Most commonly the transfers are inserted into the heel. Occasionally the muscle is used as a dorsiflexor.

Only when there is no means of restoring dynamic balance is a triple arthrodesis recommended. The long-term follow-ups seen in my postpolio clinic have emphasized the need to align the foot with the ankle and not the knee. External tibial torsion is a common consequence of distal paralysis. Because this causes outward rotation of the ankle, the foot also must be placed in that plane; otherwise the arthrodesis results in an inverted foot.

Claw Toes. Claw toe deformity often is a sign of long toe flexor substitution for a weak soleus. Consequently, these muscles are transferred to the os calcis to enhance this function, rather than merely being released. Management of the toe deformities, per se, follows the routine techniques.

Knees

The knee problems that may be improved surgically include quadriceps paralysis, medial or lateral angulation, and a flexion contracture. Osteotomies and tendon transfers are the procedures of choice.

Quadriceps Paralysis. Quadriceps paralysis is best treated by anterior transfer of the hamstrings if the patient does not have a hyperextension range for knee stability.[74,75] Follow-up of acute poliomyelitis results has shown that the outcome can be excellent but also that the operator may be ineffective, leading to patellar subluxation or excessive genu recurvatum. The ideal candidate has equally strong medial and lateral hamstrings (grade 4) and a mild flexion contracture (5° to 10°). Patients with less favorable muscle patterns also can gain knee extensor stability under particular circumstances. Experience indicates an isolated transfer of the biceps is unlikely to create lateral patellar displacement if the difference in the anatomy and function of the two heads of the biceps is respected. The long head of the biceps, arising from the ischium, is the desired muscle for transfer. It is active in stance and, when transferred, follows a longitudinal course to the patella. In contrast, the short head of the biceps, which inserts into the same tendon, arises from the femoral shaft. This presents a fairly transverse course to the patella that could easily lead to subluxation. In addition, the short head of the biceps is active in swing, a time when the substitute knee extensor should be relaxed. Hence, the biceps tendon should be split and only the long head transferred to the patella.

A second potential problem is variability in medial hamstring activity. Dynamic EMG has shown that the semimembranosus and semitendinosus muscles may function individually. Also, only one or the other may have remained functional after poliomyelitis. In cross section, the semimembranosus is three times larger than the semitendinosus. Hence, it is important to know accurately the relative activity of these two muscles. The third surgical pitfall is the inability to isolate the hamstring muscle during manual muscle test. Their hamstring's combined action of hip extension and knee flexion can be reproduced by gluteus maximus action at the hip and either biceps short head or gastrocnemius pull at the knee. Consequently, the patient may pass the clinical test with hamstrings that are inadequate for surgical transfer. This complexity in the diagnosis of hamstring function implies that an accurate surgical plan requires preoperative dynamic EMG analysis.

Flexion Contracture. The underlying cause of a postpolio flexion contracture is quadriceps paralysis, which thereby limits the opportunities for surgical correction. Permanent loss of knee motion is the likely outcome of either soft tissue sectioning or osteotomy because the patient lacks the motor muscles to provide the intrinsic motion needed to prevent adhesions. Supracondylar osteotomies present a higher risk than those performed in the tibia because of the relative proximity to the knee joint. A high tibial osteotomy, therefore, is preferable. The optimum program includes internal fixation of the osteotomy, external protection with a well-fitted KAFO, and immediate continuous passive motion, which is continued at home for 6 weeks.

Varus and Valgus Angulation. Varus and valgus deformities often require a corrective tibial osteotomy to permit effective bracing in addition to relieving knee pain (Fig. 37-25). Sectioning the fibula should be included, because this is a sturdy bone. In addition, considerable angular correction generally is needed. Early mobilization to preserve knee mobility as outlined earlier, also is required. In planning the osteotomy it must be recognized that much of the deformity may lie within the knee joint.

Excessive Hyperextension. Excessive hyperextension is difficult to restrain by surgical means in mature adults. The previously described triple tenodesis depends on the vigor of youthful tissues and residual limb growth for success.[76] A new combination of a total patellar tendon allograft and capsular reefing

has had promising results. The problem is the need to retain 10° to 15° of hyperextension because the patient still must substitute for quadriceps weakness. Consequently, the surgical reconstruction is protected for a full year by a free knee, offset joint orthosis that allows slightly less hyperextension than the graft.

Hip

Although the hip is the area least likely to gain from surgery, there are some specific indications. These include iliotibial band contracture, joint dysplasia, and degenerative arthritis.

Iliotibial Band Contracture. The presenting complaint generally is low back pain. Clinically the patient displays significant lordosis during standing without a fixed spine deformity or abdominal muscle weakness. Testing the hip demonstrates an apparent flexion contracture with the limb in neutral alignment that is relieved when the hip is abducted. The diagnosis is a contracted iliotibial band (ITB). Release of the tensor fascia lata muscle from the iliac crest corrects the flexor component of the contracture. A Z-plasty lengthening of the central ITB component restores neutral abduction. The tenotomy site is reinforced with the freed tensor muscle. Reconstruction rather than simple release of the tight ITB preserves both passive hip abduction stability and knee extension by the gluteus maximus through its ITB insertions as a substitute to compensate for quadriceps weakness.

Joint Dysplasia. Painful instability of a dysplastic joint may develop spontaneously or follow acute trauma, such as a fall. The patient's precarious soft tissue balance has been destabilized. When nonoperative measures fail, a corrective osteotomy is indicated. A Chiari operator has proved effective in one patient, although restoration of a functional sitting and walking range was slow. A second indication would be to realign a dysplastic hip to create weight-bearing capability. When additional leg length is desired, I have used a Salter rotational acetabular osteotomy.[77]

Degenerative Arthritis. Degenerative arthritis combined with hip abductor weakness is a third postpolio problem. The wisdom of doing a total joint

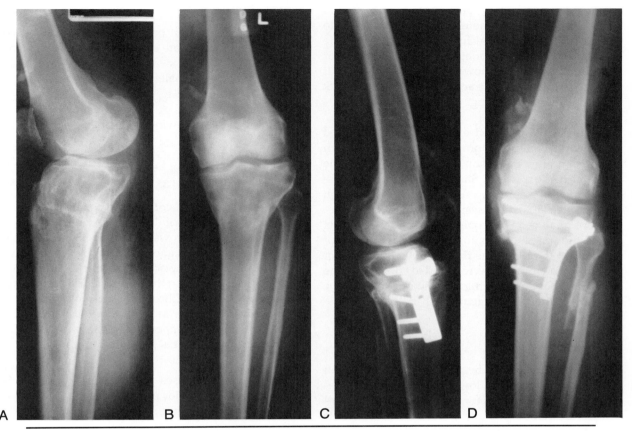

Fig. 37-25. (A & B) A knee with recurvatum **(A)** and varus **(B)** deformities from years of strenuous substitution for quadriceps weakness. **(C & D)** Postoperative tibial osteotomy with internal fixation for early joint mobilization. **(C)** Anterior. **(D)** Lateral.

replacement rests on the presence of adequate abductor muscle strength to prevent postoperative dislocation. At present there are no firm rules, but muscle strength of 3+ or better has proved to be adequate. This is comparable to the strength of patients disabled by rheumatoid arthritis. The strength of both the hip extensors and abductors should be assessed.

Spine and Trunk

The indications for surgery of the spine and trunk tend to involve failure of orthotic management. Both instability and pain are surgical indicators.

Abdominal Fascial Transplant. Experience with one patient demonstrated that adults with late dysfunction can gain significant trunk stability from a

Lowman criss-cross abdominal fascial transplant.[78] If the patient also has considerable back weakness (as was present in my case), the fascial insertion on the ribs should be at the midaxillary line to avoid an excessive flexion force. With strong back muscles the fascia are attached to the ribs just lateral to the nipple line. After 2 weeks of bed rest, a Hoke corset provided postoperative protection for 3 months. In the preoperative evaluation it also should be determined that ITB tension is not needed for knee extensor stabilization in walking (normal quadriceps or dependent on KAFOs).

Spine Fusion. A complete spine fusion to stabilize the paralytic spine for head positioning and effective bulbar muscle function was introduced over 30 years ago.[79] Progressive weakening of paretic muscles is creating the need for this operation in a few postpolio survivors. Recent treatment of one patient by halo fixation and total cervical fusion confirmed that the technique still is appropriate. Head positioning for good bulbar function, however, was more difficult because pharyngeal contractures from chronic neck flexion were more limiting.

Spine fusion is indicated even in the middle-aged patient with a painful or progressive deformity. Both scoliosis and low back pain can be a problem in the adult postpolio patient. Stabilization of a progressively collapsing spine is a feasible undertaking with today's internal fixation systems. The lack of protective musculature may require a light external jacket during the year-long healing phase. Stabilization of the lumbar spine reduces the patient's potential for walking if pelvic motion is required to take a step. The indications for surgery in low back pain tend to be failure of orthotic management of the patient's disability.

Upper Extremity

There have been few indications for late surgery on the upper extremity. Follow-up studies of well-designed opponensplasties for the thumb show continued good function in some patients. Other patients display effective means of substitution, and seldom is there a good motor muscle available. A flexorplasty, which included the flexor ulnaris as well as the other epicondylar muscle mass, has been effective in restoring independent elbow function. Mayer and Green's midshaft placement of the bony button avoided excessive forearm pronation.[80] Demands on the patient's limited strength (3+) were lessened when a deliberate 35° flexion contracture was induced. Rehabilitation was facilitated with a postoperative spring-assist, hinged orthosis until antigravity strength was developed.

Other Vital Functions

Respiratory System

Previously impaired respiratory muscles experience the same pattern of overuse deterioration as do the extremities. Generalized fatigue, dyspnea, and sleep apnea are the complaints.[81,82] Mechanical ventilation and medicinal aids increase endurance.

Bulbar Muscles

A small percentage of patients had bulbar involvement during their acute episode. Late developments include difficulty in swallowing. Eating habits are modified by using smaller bites, softer food, and positioning of the head to preserve optimum pharyngeal muscle length. A cervical pillow facilitates breathing and swallowing, particularly when reclining.[79,83]

SUMMARY

Invasion of the spinal cord by the poliomyelitis virus can cause two forms of disability. Acute paralysis of varying severity follows the initial infection, and most patients make a good, often apparently normal recovery from this episode. Experience during the past decade has shown that a secondary loss of function also can occur. Chronic overuse of a muscle or muscles made smaller and less efficient than normal by the poliomyelitis appears to be the cause. A different form of treatment is therefore indicated.

Strengthening exercises and encouragement to be fully active were major elements in the recovery of optimum function after the acute infection. For patients of today with the postpolio syndrome, however, exercise must be used cautiously. Instead, the major treatment program focuses on ways to reduce the demands on the muscles without inducing disuse atrophy. Orthoses and selected reconstructive surgery are effective means of increasing function in both forms of poliomyelitis.

REFERENCES

1. Halstead LS, Rossi CD: Post-polio syndrome: clinical experience with 132 consecutive outpatients. Birth Defects 23:13, 1987
2. Perry J: Orthopedic management of post-polio sequelae, p. 193. In Halstead LS, Wiechers DO (eds): Late Effects of Poliomyelitis. Symposia Foundation, Miami, 1985
3. Dalakas MC, Sever JL, Madden DL et al: Late postpoliomyelitis muscular atrophy: clinical, virologic, immunologic studies. Rev Infect Dis 6(Supp 2):562, 1984
4. Brown S, Patten BM: Post-polio syndrome and amyotrophic lateral sclerosis: a relationship more apparent than real. Birth Defects 23:83, 1987
5. Wiechers DO: Late effects of polio: historical perspectives. Birth Defects 23:1, 1987
6. Codd MB, Kurland LT: Polio's late effects. In 1986 Medical

and Health Annual, Infectious Diseases. p. 249 Encyclopedia Britannia, Chicago, 1985

7. Hayward M, Setton D: Late sequelae of paralytic poliomyelitis: a clinical and electromyographic study. J Neurol Neurosurg Psychiatry 42:117, 1979

8. Windebank AJ, Daube JR, Litchy WJ et al: Late sequelae of paralytic poliomyelitis in Olmstead County, Minnesota. Birth Defects 23:27, 1987

9. Spencer WA: The Treatment of Acute Poliomyelitis. p. 103. Charles C Thomas, Springfield, IL, 1954

10. Stokes J Jr: Poliomyelitis. p. 479. In Nelson WE (ed): Mitchell-Nelson Textbook of Pediatrics. WB Saunders, Philadelphia, 1945

11. Krusen FH: Mechanotherapy: Exercise. p. 595. In Physical Medicine, The Employment of Physical Agents for Diagnosis and Therapy. WB Saunders, Philadelphia, 1941

12. Garrett AL: Poliomyelitis. p. 449. In Nickel VL (ed): Orthopedic Rehabilitation. Churchill Livingstone, New York, 1982

13. Mercer W: Orthopaedic Surgery. Williams & Wilkins, Baltimore, 1991

14. Adkins HV, Robbins V, Eckland F et al: Selective stretching for the paralytic patient. Phys Ther 40:644, 1960

15. Bodian D: Motoneuron disease and recovery in experimental poliomyelitis. p. 45. In Halstead LS, Weichers DO (eds): Late Effects of Poliomyelitis. Symposia Foundation, Miami, 1985

16. Hoffman H: Local re-innervation in partially denevated muscle: a histo-physiological study. Austr J Exp Biol Med Sci 28:383, 1990

17. Thompson W, Jansen JKS: Extent of sprouting of remaining motor units in partially denervated immature and adult rat soleus muscle. Neuroscience 2:523, 1977

18. Weiss P, Edds MV: Spontaneous recovery of muscle following partial denervation. Am J Physiol 145:587, 1946

19. Wohlfart G: Collateral regeneration in partially denervated muscles. Neurology 8:175, 1958

20. Pohl JF, Kenny E: The Kenny Concept of Infantile Paralysis and its Treatment. p. 173. Bruce Publishing, Minneapolis, 1949

21. Sharrad WJ: Muscle recovery in poliomyelitis. J Bone Joint Surg [Br] 37:63, 1955

22. Ingram AJ: Anterior poliomyelitis. p. 1418. In Edmonson AS, Crenshaw AH (eds): Campbell's Operative Orthopaedics. CV Mosby, St. Louis, 1980

23. Clark DR, Perry J, Lunsford TR: Case studies — orthotic management of the adult postpolio patient. Orthot Prosthet 40(1):43, 1986

24. Fishman S, Berger N, Edlestein JE et al: Lower limb orthoses. p. 204. In American Academy of Orthopedic Surgeons: Atlas of Orthotics. CV Mosby, St. Louis, 1985

25. Perry J: Kinesiology of lower extremity bracing. Clin Orthop 102:18, 1974

26. Fishman S, Berger N, Edelstein JE et al: Upper-limb orthoses. p. 195. In American Academy of Orthopedic Surgeons: Atlas of Orthotics. CV Mosby, St. Louis, 1985

27. Smith H: Ankylosis and deformity. p. 1146. In Edmonson AS, Crenshaw AH (eds): Campbell's Operative Orthopaedics. CV Mosby, St. Louis, 1980

28. Mustard WT: Iliopsoas transfer for weakness of the hip abductors. Preliminary report. J Bone Joint Surg [Am] 34:647, 1952

29. Legg AT: Tensor fasciae femoris transfer in cases of weakened gluteus medius. N Engl J Med 209:61, 1933

30. Ober FR: An operation for relief of paralysis of the gluteus maximus muscle. JAMA 88:1063, 1927

31. Thomas LI, Thompson TC, Straub LR: Transplantation of the external oblique muscle for abductor paralysis. J Bone Joint Surg [Am] 32:207, 1950

32. Blount WP, Clarke GR: Control of bone growth by epiphyseal stapling. J Bone Joint Surg [Am] 31:464, 1949

33. Phemister DB: Operative arrestment of longitudinal growth of bones in the treatment of deformities. J Bone Joint Surg [Am] 15:1, 1933

34. Anderson M, Green WT, Messner MB: Growth and prediction of growth in the lower extremities. J Bone Joint Surg [Am] 45:1, 1963

35. Greulich WW, Pyle SI: Radiographic Atlas of Skeletal Development of the Hand and Wrist. Stanford University Press, Palo Alto, CA, 1950

36. Perry J, Barnes G, Gronley J: Post-polio muscle function. Birth Defects 23:315, 1987

37. Beasley WC: Quantitative muscle testing: principles and applications to research and clinical services. Arch Phys Med Rehabil 42:398, 1961

38. Dalakas MC: Amyotrophic lateral sclerosis and post-polio: differences and similarities. Birth Defects 3:63, 1987

39. Cruz Martinez A, Ferrer MT, Perez Conde MC: Electrophysiological features in patients with non-progressive and late progressive weakness after paralytic poliomyelitis. Electromyogr Clin Neurophysiol 24:469, 1984

40. Cruz Martinez A, Perez Conde MC, Ferrer MT: Chronic partial denervation is more widespread than is suspected clinically in paralytic poliomyelitis. Eur Neurol 22:314, 1983

41. Fetwell MR, Smallberg G, Lewis LD et al: A benign motor neuron disorder: delayed cramps and fasciculation after poliomyelitis or myelitis. Ann Neurol 11:423, 1982

42. Wiechers DO: Pathophysiology and late changes of the motor unit after poliomyelitis. p. 91. In Halstead LS, Wiechers DO (eds): Late Effects of Poliomyelitis. Symposia Foundation, Miami, 1985

43. Borg K, Borg J: Conduction velocity and refractory period of single motor nerve fibres in antecedent poliomyelitis. J Neurol Neurosurg Psychiatry 50:443, 1987

44. Jubelt B, Cashman N: Neurological manifestations of the postpolio syndrome. Crit Rev Biomed Eng 3:199, 1987

45. Ravits J, Hallett M, Baker M et al: Clinical and electromyographic studies of postpoliomyelitis muscular atrophy. Muscle Nerve 13:667, 1990

46. Cashman NR, Siegel IM, Antel JP: Post-polio syndrome: an overview. Clin Prosthet Orthot 11:74, 1987

47. Dawson MJ, Gadian DG, Wilkie DR: Contraction and recovery of living muscles studied by Q31WP nuclear magnetic resonance. J Physiol 267:703, 1977

48. Perry J, Barnes G, Gronley JK: The postpolio syndrome: an overuse phenomenon. Clin Orthop 223:145, 1988

49. Herbison GJ, Jaweed MM, Ditunno JF: Exercise therapies in peripheral neuropathies. Arch Phys Med Rehabil 64:201, 1983

50. Kinney CL, Jaweed MM, Herbison GJ, Ditunno JF: Overwork effect on partially denervated rat soleus muscle. Arch Phys Med Rehabil 67:286, 1986

51. Vihko V, Rantamaki J, Salminen A: Exhaustive physical exercise and acid hydrolase activity in mouse skeletal muscle. Histochemistry 57:237, 1978

52. Anderson AD, Levine SA, Gellert H: Loss of ambulatory ability in patients with old anterior poliomyelitis. Lancet 2:1061, 1972

53. Bennett RL, Knowlton GC: Overwork weakness in partially denervated skeletal muscle. Clin Orthop 12:22, 1958

54. Herbison GJ, Jaweed MM, Ditunno JF Jr: Clinical management of partially innervated muscle. p. 163. In Halstead LS,

Wiechers DO (eds): Late Effects of Poliomyelitis. Symposia Foundation, Miami, 1985

55. Lee FS: Fatigue. Harvey Lect 1:169, 1906
56. Duchateau J, Hainaut K: Isometric or dynamic training: differential effects on mechanical properties of a human muscle. J Appl Physiol 56:296, 1984
57. Monad H: Contractility of muscle during prolonged static and repetitive dynamic activity. Ergonomics 28(1):81, 1985
58. Jones DR, Speier J, Canine K et al: Cardiorespiratory responses to aerobic training by patients with postpoliomyelitis sequelae. JAMA 261:3255, 1989
59. Feldman RM: The use of strengthening exercises in post-polio syndrome. Orthopedics 8:889, 1985
60. Perry J, Young S, Landel RS: The use of strengthening exercises in post-polio patients, abstracted. Arch Phys Med Rehabil 68:660, 1987
61. Perry J, Mulroy SJ, Gronley JK: Etiology and secondary complications of the late effects of poliomyelitis: Final report for NIDRR. Grant no. G008635206, 1989
62. Perry J, Mulroy SJ, Renwick S: The relationship between lower extremity strength and stride characteristics in patients with post-polio syndrome. Arch Phys Med Rehabil 71:805, 1990
63. Perry J, Gronley JK, Bontrager EL: The sequence of extensor muscle control in walking. Trans Orthop Res Soc 15:556, 1990
64. Pathokinesiology Department, Physical Therapy Department: Observational Gait Analysis Handbook. The Professional Staff Association of Rancho Los Amigos Medical Center, Downey, CA, 1989
65. Perry J: Normal and pathologic gait. p. 76. In American Academy of Orthopaedic Surgeons (ed): Atlas of Orthotics. Biomechanical Principles and Applications. CV Mosby, St. Louis, 1985
66. Kendall FP, McCreary EK: Muscles Testing and Function. Williams & Wilkins, Baltimore, 1983
67. Mulroy SJ, Perry J, Gronley JK: A comparison of testing techniques for ankle plantar flexion strength. p. 24. Unpublished Master's Thesis, University of Southern California, Los Angeles, 1990
68. Inman VT: Functional aspects of the abductor muscles of the hip. J Bone Joint Surg 29:607, 1947
69. Perry J: Muscle control of the shoulder. p. 17. In Rowe CR (ed): The Shoulder. Churchill Livingstone, New York, 1988
70. Inman VT, Saunders DM, Abbot LC: Observations on the function of the shoulder joint. J Bone Joint Surg 26:1, 1944
71. Perry J: Normal upper extremity kinesiology. Phys Ther 58:265, 1978
72. Perry J, Hsu JD, Barber L, Hoffer MM: The use of orthoses in patients with brachial plexus injuries. Arch Phys Med Rehabil 55:134, 1974
73. Green WT, Grice DS: The management of calcaneous deformity. Amer Acad Ortho Surg Instr Case Lecture 13:135, 1956
74. Schwartzman JR, Crego CH: Hamstring-tendon transplantation for the relief of quadriceps femoris paralysis in residual poliomyelitis. J Bone Joint Surg [Am] 30:541, 1948
75. Sutherland DH, Bost FC, Schottsteadt ER: Electromyographic study of transplanted muscles about the knee in poliomyelitic patients. J Bone Joint Surg [Am] 42:919, 1960
76. Perry J, O'Brien JP, Hodgson AR: Triple tenodesis of the knee. A soft-tissue operation for correction of paralytic genu recurvatum. J Bone Joint Surg [Am] 58:978, 1976
77. Salter RB: Innominate osteotomy in the treatment of congenital dislocation and subluxation of the hip. J Bone Joint Surg [Br] 43:518, 1961
78. Lowman CL: Abdominal Fascial Transplant. Privately published, Los Angeles, 1954
79. Perry J, Nickel VL: Total cervical-spine fusion for neck paralysis. J Bone Joint Surg [Am] 41:37, 1959
80. Mayer L, Green W: Experience with the Steindler flexor plasty at the elbow. J Bone Joint Surg [Am] 36:775, 1954
81. Fisher DA: Poliomyelitis: late pulmonary complication and management. p. 192. In Halstead LS, Wiechers DO (eds): Late Effects of Poliomyelitis. Symposia Foundation, 1985
82. Fisher DA: Sleep-disordered breathing as a late effect of poliomyelitis. Birth Defects 23:115, 1987
83. Robins V, Adkins HV, Linquist J et al: Physical therapy techniques for bulbar poliomyelitis. Phys Ther Rev 38:523, 1958
84. Perry J: Etiology and Secondary Complications of the Late Effects of Poliomyelitis, Final Report. p. 8. NIDDR Grant #G008635206, 1989

38 Brachial Plexus Injury

RICHARD M. BRAUN

Brachial plexus injuries involve the spinal roots, trunk, cords, and nerve elements, which all form a complex system of innervation of the upper limb. These brachial plexus elements emanate from the fifth cervical vertebral level and continue through the first thoracic root. They are responsible for all motor function and sensibility in the arm, forearm, and hand.

Brachial plexus palsy in adults may originate from a full spectrum of injuries. The vast majority of the patients have a history of high-speed motorcycle or automobile accidents, with occasional injuries caused by industrial trauma, direct penetrating injuries, and falls from substantial heights. Iatrogenic injuries from surgery or radiation therapy are rare. Special consideration is given to birth injuries in the department of pediatric orthopaedics. Injuries associated with brachial plexus palsies may include head trauma with associated upper motorneuron disease, cervical spinal cord injuries, spinal and extremity fractures, burns or areas of skin loss, and frequent instances of combined neurologic and vascular injury. The importance of these associated injuries cannot be overestimated in discussing rehabilitation planning.

NEED FOR EARLY REHABILITATION PLANNING

It is common for the acute-care facility's personnel to devote their entire efforts toward the patient's survival or restoration of limb viability, only to ignore areas of potential function that will be essential to the long-range rehabilitation of the patient. I have seen patients arrive after 3 months of excellent, intensive, acute care who nevertheless have joint contractures,

limb edema, poorly united fractures, open wounds or decubitus ulcers, and even unstable cervical spine injuries. The early evaluation of the entire problem is essential in the care of these complex injuries, but this is not always possible when a rehabilitation program begins only after an acute-care program is completed. Rehabilitation must begin *early* for optimal results to be attained in a seriously injured patient, who will usually have significant residual physical impairment despite any treatment program now available. Two typical examples illustrate this situation.

Case Example A

An adolescent boy sustained a transection of his brachial plexus by crashing through a glass door while skateboarding. He was seen by an orthopaedic surgeon in a nearby hospital emergency room. The patient was in deep shock because the axillary vessels were severed. Resuscitation with 4 liters of lactated Ringer's solution, emergency vessel ligation, packed cell transfusion, and antibiotic prophylaxis were started immediately. A vascular surgeon was called. The patient was ready for a general anesthetic within an hour and a repair of the artery and vein was performed successfully. Another surgeon was called to repair the brachial plexus. All the major nerve divisions were repaired in optimal fashion with the aid of optical magnification (Fig. 38-1) and modern suture technique. The wound was closed over suction drains and primary uncomplicated healing occurred. The patient's mother noted major swelling in the forearm 3 days after surgery: however, the patient had no pain and the vascular surgeon who had repaired the nerves did not see the patient at that time, because the results of nerve repair would require months or even

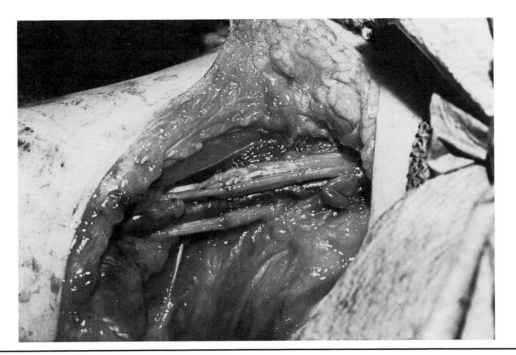

Fig. 38-1. A transection of the brachial plexus has been repaired operatively. Reconstitution of the brachial artery and the major peripheral nerves is seen at the level of the axilla in a patient who sustained an injury by crashing through a glass door while skateboarding.

years of follow-up. The orthopaedic surgeon who saw the boy initially also reassured the parent that the patient would be started on a rehabilitation program as soon as possible.

The patient was seen "for splinting and rehabilitation" about 8 weeks after the accident. His discharge had been approved by the vascular surgeon, who considered the case to be a successful major vessel repair. Figure 38-2 illustrates the Volkmann's contracture the patient sustained. He had no complaint of pain because his nerve injury had destroyed his protective sensibility. His forearm and hand were completely anesthetic. Ischemic fibrosis and contracture of muscle had already resulted in a wrist flexion contracture and compensatory contractures in the fingers in the pernicious claw position. The limb was edematous and the joints were stiff. The rehabilitation program required total limb evaluation, surgery, dynamic and static splinting, elevation with intermittent compression splinting to reduce edema,[1] and an education program for appropriate instruction in this schedule for the patient and parent as well as instruc-

tion for one-handed activities. Tendon transfer surgery and therapy were later required to restore grasp function.

The patient's life had been saved but his rehabilitation was delayed for months by acute-phase factors that increased his final functional deficits.

Case Example B

A middle-aged, healthy, oil field worker caught his hand in a drilling rig. His arm was pulled upward with great violence. Examination in the emergency room showed that the patient was in deep shock. A large hematoma was present in the periclavicular area, the hand was partially degloved, and the humerus had a displaced fracture of the midshaft. Resuscitation commenced with fluid replacement, and a skilled vascular team performed an emergency subclavian-to-brachial artery graft.

The patient was seen 2 months later for rehabilitation. Initial examination at the Rancho Los Amigos Hospital was performed in consultation with a dis-

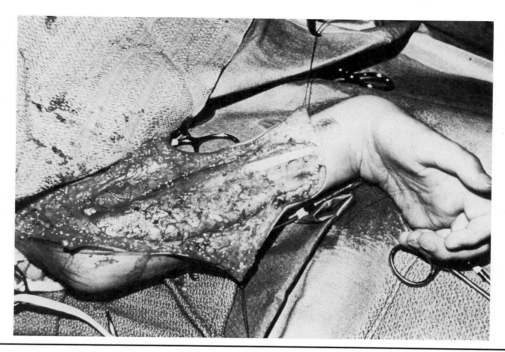

Fig. 38-2. A Volkmann's contracture with ischemic muscle in the volar compartment of the forearm is seen 8 weeks after the initial injury noted in the patient in Figure 38-1. The patient had lost protective sensibility and was unable to complain of pain because of the nerve severance in his axilla. Necrotic muscle is noted in the forearm; it is associated with contracture in the wrist and fingers.

tinguished visiting professor of orthopaedic upper limb surgery who had more than four decades of experience with trauma of this type. His comment was appropriate: "It's too bad that so much has been done to save so little." The patient had a cool but viable limb with a barely palpable radial pulse. The limb was anesthetic, completely paralyzed, painful, and swollen, with open hand wounds and a displaced, angulated, ununited fracture of the humerus. Amputation through the humerus fracture site was advised with difficulty—the patient had already tolerated 2 months of pointless heroics. A postoperative program was designed to restore lost shoulder motion and begin prosthetic training.

DIAGNOSIS AND REHABILITATION PROGNOSIS

In ideal cases, an appropriate diagnosis and a reasonable prognosis can be made at an early stage, and the rehabilitation effort can begin as soon as possible. If the diagnosis is in doubt, or if the condition is changing, the program should be designed to anticipate these changes and assist recovery in every possible way.

An exact diagnosis of brachial plexus injury is often difficult to make when the patient is first seen. The usual mechanism of injury is a stretching type of trauma that injures the complex nerve cables in an irregular manner so that a distinct single level of injury is often not seen. A complete transection may be present in some nerve fibers, whereas in another area of the same nerve or feeding tributary, there is only a neurapraxis owing to a mild stretching force. The area of mild or moderate stretching will recover if further injury is prevented. The area of complete transection will not recover unless nerve ends are approximated by chance or by an operation. The reader is referred to descriptions of the technology of brachial plexus nerve repair and the relative indications for surgery[2-4]

The general areas of injury, however, do play an important role in the rehabilitation program and should be familiar to all physicians treating these patients. Injuries to the cephalad routes of C5 and C6 (+C7), which spare the distal routes of C8 and T1, result in loss of shoulder and elbow control. Some of these patients may also lose portions of limb extension control in areas supplied by the radial nerve. Flexion and pronation of the forearm and hand and the function of the intrinsic hand muscles remain intact. Injuries to lower routes of C8 (±C7) and T1 result in preservation of shoulder and elbow flexion but loss of forearm and hand flexion, as well as loss of intrinsic muscle function. Loss of sensibility usually follows a familiar pattern, with C5 and C6 representing the thumb and index fingers, C7 the long finger, and C8 and T1 the ulnar fingers and forearm. An injury to the entire plexus results in an entirely anesthetic and paralyzed limb. However, an injury that appears complete at an early stage may show some spontaneous return of function at a later time.

Factors with a poor prognosis for recovery include fractures of the cervical spine in the area of the cord, foramen, root egress area, or transverse processes. A Horner's sign (Fig. 38-3) or obvious atrophy in the thoracoscapular muscles or paralysis of the diaphragm also carries a poor prognosis, because these are the hallmarks of a proximal injury that cannot improve spontaneously. In my experience at Rancho Los Amigos Hospital, a functional diagnosis is quite adequate for rehabilitation purposes. Exact nerve testing may not be required for the patient's basic evaluation and treatment program.

The initial history of injury and primary treatment is obtained by the occupational therapist, who can easily learn the technical aspects of taking a basic and accurate medical history. The therapist then performs a sensory and muscle examination of the upper limb and records the findings on the chart along with the elapsed time since the initial injury. The therapist also palpates the area for the presence of point tenderness or a Tinel's sign and records other findings that may be significant, such as a Horner's sign indicating a stellate ganglion–level injury or the presence of severe pain in the limb, shoulder, or neck. The relationship between counterbalancing or elevating the arm and change in the pain pattern is noted, along

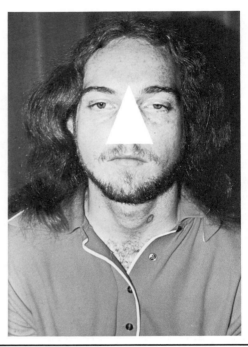

Fig. 38-3. A Horner's sign is demonstrated with ptosis of the eyelid, construction of the pupil, and dryness of the face. A circle marked on the patient's neck indicates the approximate level of the stellate ganglion, which lies adjacent to the vertebral bodies. This sign carried a poor prognosis when associted with brachial plexus injury, because it defines a proximal nerve lesion in the region of the spinal cord and nerve root egress area.

with the presence of contracture in the joints and skin condition. A well-motivated therapist can gain enough experience in this work to take a history, perform a regional physical examination, and make a major contribution to the rehabilitation plan for the patient.

The physician may augment this evaluation with additional testing. After discussion with the therapist, the physician may elect to request a myelogram or electromyogram. These tests do not replace the basic examination; rather, they may add an important depth of information. The presence of a meningocele seen on the cervical myelogram (Fig. 38-4) does not absolutely prove an irreparable nerve avulsion, because dural sleeve tears occasionally spare nerve elements, yet the presence of two or more meningoceles carried a very poor prognosis when combined with a

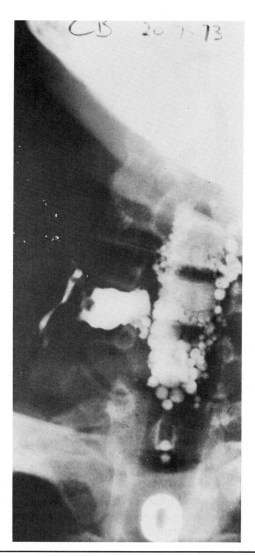

Fig. 38-4. A cervical myelogram demonstrates the presence of a large meningocele in the cervical area by the dye tracking into the region of a root avulsion. This usually carries a grim prognosis of irreparable nerve injury, but it does not always mean that the nerve root in this area has sustained avulsion.

history of major trauma and any findings of marked paralysis in the arm. Fasciculations on electromyograms may indicate areas of complete denervation. Sometimes electromyographic evidence may point out early electrical recovery that may even precede clinical evidence of returning muscle function. In these cases, continued splinting and exercises for preservation of joint range of motion plus the rest of the rehabilitation program must be continued under proper professional supervision.

REHABILITATION PLANNING

The basis of all rehabilitation is to allow the patient to attain maximal function with the residual permanent impairment. At Rancho Los Amigos Hospital, we attempt to minimize the effects of the injury and maximize the function remaining in the injured area and the untapped potential function in the remaining areas of normality. Neither of these objectives can be reached if the patient has a problem with residual pain in the area of injury. A painful limb will not be used or exercised. Contractures of joints and muscles compound the problem. Medications are frequently abused or overused. Vocational training and functional use of the injured limb are rarely accomplished. Psychological regression, dependence, and depression appear, and all chance for rehabilitation is dissolveed in a sea of pills and pity.

We use four methods for dealing with the persistent pain problems seen in about 25 percent of our patients with brachial plexus injury. Three of these methods have given good results on occasion and may be used in conjunction with each other. The fourth, the use of analgesic medication, is considered a necessary evil to be avoided whenever possible. When drugs are given, they are only used in moderation. Medication has never removed pain in a completely satisfactory manner in any patient we have treated. The long-term use of any narcotics or similar medication is obviously to be avoided.

Splinting

Pain can occasionally be controlled by correct splinting. Splinting seems to work because it removes the traction effect of a paralyzed limb, which weighs about 9 kg and hangs without functional muscle counterbalance on the stretched nerves of the brachial plexus. This weight distracts those affected nerves that have already been stretched to the point of injury, which naturally results in pain. Several patients have gained early, satisfactory, and apparently permanent pain relief when the weight of the arm has been transferred directly onto the pelvis with a mo-

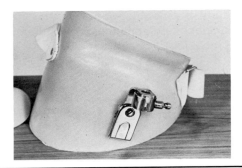

Fig. 38-5. A molded plastic pelvic support is used to transfer the weight of the arm directly onto the pelvis. Fabrication of this orthotic device is simple and relatively inexpensive. The contour of the pelvic portion allows for weight-bearing transfer onto the iliac crest.

bile forearm support splint with pelvic brim purchase that our group has designed (Figs. 38-5 through 38-8). This device may be fabricated rapidly to allow the weight of the arm to be transferred away from the shoulder-plexus-neck area and permit direct loading of the weight onto the pelvic brim.[5]

Hikers have traditionally made use of this principle to carry heavy loads without tranferring the weight of the pack to their shoulders, secured to the skeleton only by the thin strut of the clavicle and the thoracic muscles. If the shoulder straps sag, the hiker may experience brachial plexus injury as the clavicle is

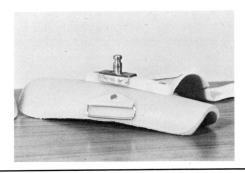

Fig. 38-6. The forearm support of the orthotic device is seen in the inverted position. The metal peg fits into the socket on the pelvic portion. The forearm rests in the trough, as seen in Figure 38-7. The metal pin is adjusted along the length of the trough to provide for appropriate balance in the forearm. Most patients prefer this pin in the center of the forearm to allow for elevation of the hand and wrist by depression of the elbow and shoulder. This position is adjustable.

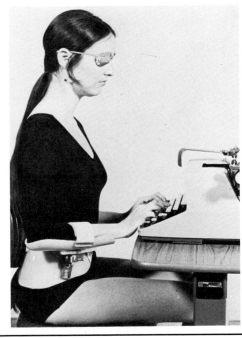

Fig. 38-7. The orthotic device is seen assembled. It is worn in the functional position. In this case, the patient wearing the device is able to function as a typist and secretary while using the device. Two years after her injury, enough strength had returned to her upper limb to warrant discontinuing the device, which remained functional for 2 years.

forced down onto the first rib by the weight of the pack. Relief of pain has been seen in several patients with such an injury within days of splint fitting. The pelvic girdle of molded plastic has been used for backpack type support if heavy loads are carried (Fig. 38-9). It can be modified easily to allow the patient both a backpack and a forearm support splint. In most cases we attempt to fit the patient with this type of support shortly after injury; however, in one case a patient was fitted with the device 2 years after the injury. His pain subsided within a month and, although his injured arm remained completely flail, his pain relief was extremely satisfying both to him and to the members of the rehabilitation team, who are now able to teach him one-handed activities, retrain him for gainful employment, and gradually wean him from the medications that impaired his level of awareness. This orthotic device is now routinely used on brachial plexus palsy patients with a painful upper

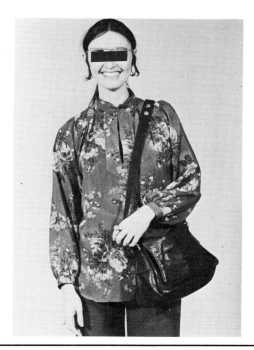

Fig. 38-8. The orthotic device is cosmetically concealed by the use of a slit in the patient's blouse, through which the metal prong protrudes. Another small slit in the undersurface of the sleeve allows for coupling to the forearm trough support. The fact that the device is not readily apparent improves the probability that will be worn at work or in social situations. In the case shown, an ocular prosthesis was later applied to improve the appearance of this woman even further.

limb after trauma or other injuries that have led to a neuritis in the brachial plexus.

Surgery

Surgery may be effective in some cases requiring pain control. Our operative procedures have included those for extraneural decompression, intraneural decompression, and sensory ablation. The decompression procedures may be quite effective in those cases with partial injury from such causes as impingement between the clavicle and the first rib[6] or compartment syndromes in the upper arm in the arterial sheath area of the brachial plexus[7] Orthopaedic surgical evaluation should be obtained in brachial plexus injuries to rule out possibilities that may yield to surgical intervention in the arm, in the thoracic outlet, or even in the area of the cervical spine. It is common for cervical disc disease to commence with the same in-

jury that directly injures the plexus. An acute, soft disc rupture proximal to the area of plexus injury may produce severe pain yet not result in diagnostic unilateral reflex loss or motor deprivation because the effect of more distal peripheral nerve injuries is masked. Special cervical radiographs may show reduced cervical motion, narrowed disc spaces, arthrosis, or fracture in the area of injury. Myelography or computed tomography may define a disc or cord lesion amenable to surgery.

Intraneural neurolysis may be effective in pain management. Multiple branching within proximal nerve elements makes this procedure complex and not

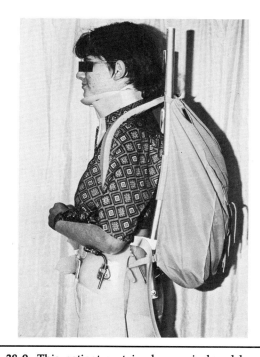

Fig. 38-9. This patient sustained a cervical and brachial plexus injury. Appropriate surgery stabilized the patient's neck. Spontaneous recovery was anticipated in the brachial plexus if further traction on the arm could be avoided. Because the patient wished to attend college, an orthotic device was fabricated allowing her to take all of the weight off her injured arm and transfer it to the pelvis through the mobile arm support. Her college books were carried in a backpack without any transfer of weight onto the cervical spine, the clavicle, or the upper limb. The patient experienced no discomfort in her arm while carrying weights up to 30 pounds and she was able to continue attending college while she recovered motor power in her arm spontaneously.

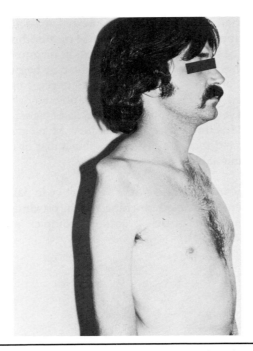

Fig. 38-10. This patient sustained a complete brachial plexus avulsion injury. Exploration of the plexus in the cervical area indicated an irreparable situation. The patient became addicted to narcotic medications because of his constant sever pain. His education level and rehabilitation level were good and it was decided to perform cervical laminectomy for coagulation of the dorsal root entry zone in the cervical area. The patient achieved virtually complete pain relief, discontinued medication, and has been restored to a useful life as a one-handed individual.

without risks. Nevertheless, a patient with a persistent, exquisitely tender mass in the neck who has not shown improvement over a period of several months may deserve exploration, internal neurolysis, and removal of scar and epineurium. The scarring will certainly recur, but it is reasonable to assume the scalpel is less traumatic than the original stretching injury, and diminished pain has been reported by several patients who have undergone this procedure. Good operative technique requires the knowledge of difficult anatomy, delicate microsurgical instruments, excellent illumination, and some type of suitable optical magnification.

Neurosurgical procedures designed to control pain, such as sensory rhizotomy and cordotomy, have usually yielded disappointing results. However, these procedures on the cord itself can be helpful in some carefully selected cases (Fig. 38-10). A neuro-surgical consultant who is interested in this type of work is a valuable asset in such cases. Encouraging early postoperative results have been seen in patients with intractable pain from root avulsion injury. A surgical procedure using a controlled radiofrequency to coagulate areas of the dorsal root entry zone has been described by Nashold and Ostdahl.[8] The procedure has been extremely helpful to several of patients who received no significant benefit from stellate ganglion block, transcutaneous stimulation, narcotic medications, appropriate splinting, or a behavior modification program. Patient selection is not easy. The operations are difficult and carry substantial risk, which the patient must understand.

Pain Programs

Frequently the patient with a painful brachial plexus injury will need to attend "pain clinic." These clinics use behavior modification in helping the patient cope with pain. The use of these clinics is not without risk. The referring physician may send a patient to the clinic simply because the patient has pain, takes excessive medication, and is difficult to deal with. One risk is that an area of potential intervention may have been missed because the evaluation was not thorough enough, leading to an error of omission. The risk may be compounded in the pain clinic, where it may be assumed that the patient would not be there if any chance of an organic cause for the pain had been found. Therefore the patient is started on a psychologically oriented program without a basic medical evaluation and to the error of omission is added on error of commission.

The occupational therapist is ideally suited to keep communications open between the organically oriented physician directing the physical program and the representative of the pain program. The therapist may also act in a medically, psychologically, and socially supporting role to the patient, who has sustained major functional loss and has debilitating symptoms. The therapist also is the ideal person to work with the patient in the use of a cutaneous nerve stimulator for pain relief. The patient and the therapist form their own team to determine those anatomic areas, patterns of stimulation, and techniques that may prove useful in helping the patient to reduce medications, cope with painful stimuli, and continue to function in the re-education program.

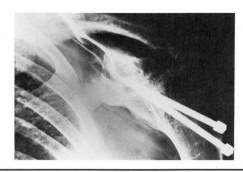

Fig. 38-11. Arthrodesis of the shoulder may prove helpful in cases with permanent paralysis of the deltoid and rotator cuff musculature. This stable platform allows the periscapular muscles to elevate the upper limb. Inta-articular and extra-articular bony arthrodeses are seen on this radiograph.

ROLE OF ORTHOPAEDIC SURGERY

Surgical treatment of the residual muscle weakness of brachial plexus palsy is oriented toward direct nerve repair or compensatory substitutions of unaffected muscle-tendon units for paralytic ones. The loss of deltoid and supraspinatus function is usully considered irreparable, and glenohumeral arthrodesis may provide a shoulder that is stable and pain-free (Figs. 38-11 and 38-12). Mobility due to pericapsular musculature will usually allow a patient to raise the arm to almost 90° from the rest position at the side. Shoulder fusion should be the last step in upper limb reconstruction. It is extremely difficult to carry out effective forearm or chest-arm muscle transfers when the proximal shoulder joint is stiff and cannot be appropriately positioned to facilitate exposure of forearm muscle or the inner aspect of the upper arm in the area of the axilla. In addition, positioning the patient on the operating table when an arthrodesis is present in the shoulder may put excessive stress on the fused area. Fracture of the arthrodesis or the humerus may occur. Arthrodesis position is also dependent on the ability of the patient to flex the elbow and should therefore be determined after all attempts at elbow flexorplasty have been completed and the final range of elbow function is determined. In general, more shoulder abduction is required in cases of weak elbow flexion.

High lesions of C5-C6 routes frequently spare pectoral or forearm motor groups, yet they result in losses of elbow flexion. Transfer of the pectoral mus-

cles and flexorplasty using forearm musculature are reliable procedures for restoring usable elbow flexion. Certain modifications of pectoral transfer for elbow flexion may obviate shoulder arthrodesis if the tendon of the pectoral muscle is inserted on the scapular acromion. We prefer not to build motor power out beyond areas of good sensibility. In general, but not always, distal extremities with major sensory deprivation are not used for function even after motor power has been restored.

Surgical technology is beyond the scope of this chapter, and complete descriptions of the numerous practicable operations cannot be furnished here. Nevertheless, the basic goal of surgery and its place in the rehabilitation program should be understood. An experienced therapist is frequently the best-qualified team member to request a surgical evaluation. Competent therapists usually have a good relationship with the patient, know the patient's goals and potential function, and are aware of the motor power available for transfer to an adjacent area of function with reasonable sensibility. Patients must understand what an operation has to offer and what they may risk in time, functional deficit, and emotional disappointment if the procedure fails to deliver the expected functional return. They must be willing to participate in a preoperative and a postoperative training program for muscle strengthening in functional use of the operated area. The new function must improve their activities of daily living and leave them with no additional functional loss.

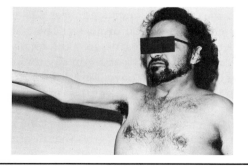

Fig. 38-12. This patient has good scapular musculature with paralysis of the deltoid and rotator cuff. Shoulder arthrodesis enables him to elevate his arm to 90° of abduction or forward flexion.

As an example of a failure of preoperative evaluation, a personal experience is cited here. A girl who had lost her elbow flexion was operated on with transfer of the triceps anteriorly. She obtained an active range of elbow flexion from 30° to 95°. I was pleased until the patient told me that she could no longer lift her arm out of the water during swimming, her favorite sport. The operation was a technical success and a functional failure. It is important not to simply perform "operative procedures" on patients who are already seriously disabled. A thorough understanding of the patient's activities and daily living patterns is the most important aspect of choosing the most appropriate surgical procedure. Patients with a low lesion may not be a candidate for any surgery owing to impaired sensibility in the hand; nevertheless, if their job or activities they enjoy call for a helper hand function and they are intelligent and able to use some eye control, they may well derive real functional benefit from a procedure that restores function (Figs. 38-13 through 38-16). Our clinic's policy involves the patient, the family, and the therapist in this final aspect of surgical planning. All of these persons have spent many long hours wrestling with the patient's vocational and family situation, whereas the surgeon usually has not been so closely involved.

VOCATIONAL REHABILITATION

The real measure of a rehabilitation program is the number of patients who return to society as integrated, related, and, ideally, employed persons. It is obvious not all injured persons can return to a competitive labor market; nor can a sociopath be expected to return to productive society. Despite this, even socially, psychologically, and intellectually deprived patients may become motivated after sustaining a serious, chronic, physical disability. This shift may occur because these persons are now totally separated from their former peer group environments or because they suddenly have a great deal of time to consider their values and their future in society. During these initial months, patients rely heavily on the therapist as a friend, someone who cares and is interested in them when their peer group has disappeared. The physician is too far removed, too powerful an authority figure, and unfortunately "too busy" to form a basic supportive relationship with patients, who definitely do need help from someone in whom

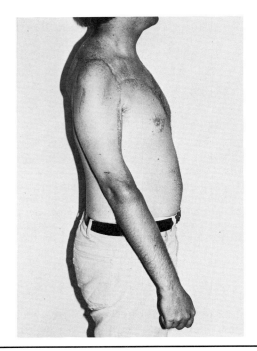

Fig. 38-13. This patient sustained a brachial plexus injury resulting in permanent loss of elbow flexion and shoulder abduction. Good sensibility and reasonably good motor power were present in the forearm and hand. He realized that a return to competitive motorcycle racing was unrealistic, but he had a great desire to return to riding a motorcycle and working in a motorcycle parts and repair factory. He is intelligent and well motivated. Surgical reconstruction of the upper limb was undertaken and the patient was enrolled in a training program to become a motorcycle mechanic.

they can confide. Vocational rehabilitation plays an important role in this phase of treatment, which requires restoration of self-esteem. Appropriate testing may uncover a previously unrecognized skill or talent. Educational training programs may not only allow patients to become employable but also allow them to regain some faith in themselves as persons. No rehabilitation program can succeed without restoration of patient motivation. Some patients can spur themselves on with minimal assistance and others require great strength, persistence, and reasonable prodding by all team members.

One anecdote may illustrate this situation. Gary, a 25-year-old patient, wandered phlegmatically around Rancho Los Amigos Hospital for 2 years. A

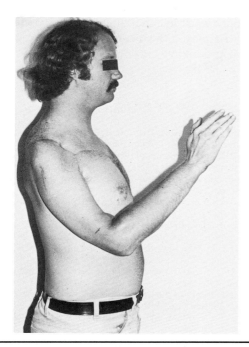

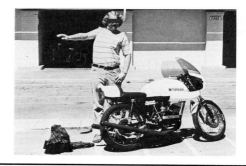

Fig. 38-16. The patient returned to his desired activity of riding motorcycles. His arm was functionally adequate to perform this activity. He completed a satisfactory training program in a junior college and now owns a shop for motorcycle repair.

Fig. 38-14. Reconstruction of strong elbow flexion is accomplished by transfer of the pectoral muscle from the chest wall onto the arm and by proximal migration of the flexor carpi ulnaris to the distal aspect of the medial-surface of the humerus. This patient required both pectoral and forearm flexorplasty. Good range of strong motion in flexion against gravity is demonstrated.

vocational rehabilitation evalution showed that he had a real talent for art and painting. His therapist believed he would benefit from elbow surgery, and a flexorplasty was successful in restoring elbow flexion. Yet Gary did nothing. He had no motivation, but

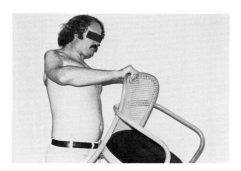

Fig. 38-15. Good strength in the remaining forearm muscles of the other limb, restoration of elbow flexion, and shoulder fusion stability resulted in the restoration of function with good strength.

he continued attending the clinic every month without making up his mind about any future plans. All attempts at support and suggestion failed, so the rehabilitation team attempted a radical approach. At a formal conference in the clinic, he was told that the State of California had given him all that it could. He knew his exercise program and our recommendations and he also knew that he had done nothing about any of them. He was discharged from the clinic and given a dime for a telephone call. He was explicitly instructed that he could use that dime at any time to call vocational counseling at the hospital to request completion of his commercial art training and job placement. He was informed that the choice was his —he could either step forward and accept responsibility or remain "on the dole." He was told not to return unless he wished to help himself. A few days later the telephone rang. Gary is now gainfully employed as a commercial artist and paints for a hobby.

Vocational rehabilitation counselors have assisted in training one-handed typists who have passed civil service employment examinations, discovered talent in art and planning required for training in interior design, helped construction laborers become construction draftsmen, funded educational programs for a warehouseman to become a commercial property and real estate assessor, found baby tending and child care services to allow a disabled mother to return to finish her college education, and helped an injured motorcycle racer gain the training to open his own motorcycle parts shop. The vocational counselor participates in the clinic and functions as a vital team member to prevent the patient from dropping out of a productive life during the initial peirod of disability.

SUMMARY

Rehabilitation of the brachial plexus palsy patient requires a combined effort of a team dedicated to helping the patient to return to society with as much function as possible. An appropriate diagnosis of functional impairment is the initial requirement. Therapy to prevent contractures, assist in strengthening, and document returning functional areas continues throughout the program. Surgical intervention may help the patient recover some nerve function or replace lost functional areas with transferred motor power. Pain control may be initiated through splinting or bracing methods, electrical cutaneous stimulation, or occasionally surgical procedures. Prolonged narcotic medication should be avoided. Behavior modification programs have been beneficial to some patients but must be used judiciously.

The major factor in rehabilitating these patients is their own ability to become motivated to return to society as productive citizens.

REFERENCES

1. Greenberg S, Braun RM: Therapeutic use of the air bag splint for the injured hand. Am J Occup Ther 31:318, 1977
2. Leffert RD: Reconstruction of the shoulder and elbow following brachial plexus injury. p. 805. In Omer G Spinner M, (eds): Management of Peripheral Nerve Problems. WB Saunders, Philadlphia, 1980
3. Millesi H: Surgical management of brachial plexus injuries. J Hand Surg 2:367, 1977
4. Narakas A: Plexo braquial. Rev Ortop, Traum 16:855, 1972
5. Perry J: Orthotic components and systems prescription principles. p. 81. In Atlas of Orthotics, Biomechanical Principles, and Application. CV Mosby, St. Louis, 1975
6. Braun RM: Iatrogenic compression of the thoracic outlet. Johns Hopkins Med J 145:74
7. Braun RM: Injury to the brachial plexus during brachial arteriography. J Hand Surg 3:90
8. Nashold BS, Ostdahl, RH: Dorsal root entry zone lesions for pain relief. J Neurosurg 51:59, 1979

39 Muscular Dystrophy and Neurogenic Atrophy

JOHN D. HSU
IRENE S. GILGOFF

Muscular dystrophy and neurogenic atrophy are neuromuscular disorders that are manifested by weakness. The loss of muscle strength and muscle tissue can be localized or generalized. The muscle weakness may follow a specific pattern — for instance, being proximal or distal. It may progress, either slowly or rapidly, and affect other areas of the body. The weakness may or may not result in loss of function, because frequently the body can adapt either by strengthening another area or by the use of substitution, which can mask the muscle weakness for a long time. Knowledge and recognition of the problem and its underlying cause is of the upmost importance in the care of patients suffering from neuromuscular disorders.[1-3] The purposes of this chapter are the following:

1. To help the reader identify these conditions.
2. To bring forward current knowledge on the care of patients with neuromuscular disorders and to recommend treatment programs.
3. To identify secondary problems and possible complications.

DIAGNOSIS

The identification of the underlying muscle disease is very important in planning overall care and in discussing the prognosis with the patient and the family. This is especially true in a child with young parents who may desire to have more children, because many neuromuscular disorders are transmitted genetically.

History

Knowledge of the onset of muscle weakness, whether related to another condition, a febrile episode, an accident, or an injury, is important. Has the weakness progressed rapidly, been slowly progressive, or remained unchanged? Are any specific areas affected? Are certain activities becoming more difficult to do? Has there been any change in daily habits? Is there any discomfort or pain, at rest or with activity? Is there any cramping of the muscles? Does the person have difficulty releasing a grip on an object? Is fever present? Is there a specific time of day when the symptoms occur? Have measures been taken to help the condition? Is there a change in the patient's work or work capacity? Have recreational activities been modified or abandoned? The history should also include a detailed family history to see if similar problems have occurred within the family in question. In a child it is also important to obtain details of the birth and to see what the child's developmental milestones have been.

Physical Examination and Functional Evaluation

In addition to the general physical examination, special attention needs to be given to the physical characteristics of the body of the patient. Is there adequate head control or trunk control? What is the posture? How does the patient move about? Is the patient able to transfer from standing to seated and from seated to lying? Can he or she get up from a lying position, from an examination table, from a chair, or from the floor? Did these movements evoke Gower's maneuver?

A detailed and specific manual muscle testing of each muscle is probably not necessary during the preliminary examination, but knowledge of how muscle groups function and an understanding of areas of weakness may help identify the condition. Is the weakness proximal? Are the shoulder girdle and hip girdle involved? Is there weakness only in the hands and feet? Is the weakness symmetrical? Is there any localized weakness? Does a repetitive movement become easier or more and more difficult?

A functional evaluation is an integral part of the clinical evaluation and is frequently made through the efforts of the physical therapist or occupational therapist. A home visit may be necessary so that the patient can be seen in the natural environment.

Laboratory Studies

Complete blood count, urinalysis, electrolyte determination, and biochemical studies are useful preliminary screening tests. At present, the most reliable test to determine whether muscle tissue breakdown is present is the creatine phosphokinase (CPK) determination. Specific laboratory tests are being developed for the analysis for muscular dystrophy, including the Dystrophin test.

Electrodiagnostic Studies

Electromyography (EMG) and nerve conduction studies continue to be used to aid in the diagnosis of neuromuscular disorders. Specific electrical patterns are identified with myopathic and neuropathic disorders and with myotonia. Nerve involvement and nerve degeneration or damage can be confirmed via nerve conduction studies.

Children may not be able to tolerate a detailed electrodiagnostic study because they may be quite uncomfortable. In this event, single-muscle EMG should be considered.

Ultrasound Studies

At present there is evidence that certain neuromuscular conditions can be identified by ultrasound, a noninvasive study.

Muscle Biopsy

The muscle biopsy is useful in determining the exact nature of the muscle changes that occur when histochemical and ultrastructural properties are involved. Information that can be gained from interpreting muscle may include the following.

Extent of Muscle Involvement

Are the muscle changes generalized or are only specific parts of the muscle affected? Are there any focal changes? Does the actual muscle biopsy involvement mirror the clinical changes and does it support the clinical picture? Muscle biopsy findings relating to an inflammatory condition may be seen throughout the muscle when they are in the acute or subacute stage; however, in the chronic stage, secondary changes may become prevalent and may be misleading. In contrast, if the physician or technician is looking for a focal change (e.g., the presence of echinococcal cysts) or for the granulomas seen in sarcoidosis, these changes may not be visible if there is insufficient material sample or if the area of the muscle biopsied happens not to be involved.

Myopathic or Neuropathic Pattern

As in EMG interpretations, certain patterns may exist and allow the interpreter to come to a reasonable conclusion as to whether the disease process is primary to the anterior horn cell or nerve or primary to the muscle.

Other Information

Congenital disorders may be identifiable when special ultrastructural studies are made.

Extent of Muscle Involvement Versus Clinical Picture

If the muscle biopsy shows end-stage disease, identification of the exact problem, whether it is myopathic or neuropathic, may not be possible. The results may,

Table 39-1. Differentiation of Neuromuscular Disease

Disease	Etiology	Course	Pattern of Weakness	CPK[a]	Other Signs and Symptoms	Anatomic Site of Disease
Myopathic						
Duchenne muscular dystrophy	Sex linked	Progressive	Proximal	Marked increase	Pseudohypertrophy; learning problems	Muscle
Fascioscapulohumeral muscular dystropy	Autosomal dominant	Slowly progressive	Proximal	Normal to slight increase	Facial weakness	Muscle
Limb girdle dystrophy	Autosomal recessive; sometimes dominant	Slowly progressive	Proximal	Normal to slight increase	Syndrome of many diseases	Muscle
Myotonic dystrophy	Autosomal dominant	Slowly progressive	Distal	Usually normal	Myotonic reflex, ptosis, cataracts, baldness, facial weakness; EMG[b] may be diagnostic	Muscle
Congenital myopathics	Usually sporadic; sometimes inherited	Usually static; occasionally progressive	Variable	Usually normal	Biopsy or electron microscopic diagnosis	Muscle
Polymyositis	Acquired autoimmunity	Acute relapsing; treat with steroids	Variable	Elevated	Painful	Muscle
Neuropathic						
Spinal muscular atrophy	Autosomal recessive	Slowly progressive or static	Proximal	Normal	Fasciculations; minior polymyoclonus	Anterior horn cell
Amyotrophic lateral sclerosis	Usually sporadic; rare cases familial	Progressive	Asymmetric	Mild to moderate increase	Fasciculations; hyperreflexia	Multiple areas affected: motor cortex, cranial nerves, brain stem, spinal cord, peripheral nerves
Charcot-Marie-Tooth disease	Autosomal dominant (some recessive)	Slowly progressive	Distal	Normal	Nerve conduction studies may be diagnostic	Peripheral nerves
Guillain-Barré syndrome	Acquired: ?autoimmune; postviral	Acute paralysis with variable recovery	Distal	Normal	Abnormal lumbar puncture	Peripheral nerves
Virus: poliomyelitis, echovirus, coxsackievirus	Acquired: viral	Acute paralysis with variable recovery	Asymmetric	Normal	Pain in acute stage	Anterior horn cell

[a] CPK, creatine phosphokinase.
[b] EMG, electromyogram.

however, confirm the clinician's suspicion of severe muscle weakness and allow for the future treatment planning, including recommending supportive equipment.

CLASSIFICATION

Table 39-1 lists the clinical characteristics, etiology, and laboratory findings of the major neuromuscular disorders for which patients may be referred for entry into a rehabilitation program. Figure 39-1 shows the muscle biopsy findings. Patients with severe muscle weakness are most likely to require a multidisciplinary approach. Confirmation of the diagnosis would be valuable because team members could then evaluate the patient's needs so that self-care functions can be maximized and appropriate equipment prescribed. In most instances continued medical treatment is necessary.

Knowledge of the prognosis is important. Is the neuromuscular disease a stable one? Will changes need to be made in the house or is it necessary to re-equip the room to accommodate the patient with the disability? For patients whose disorders nad weaknesses have not changed significantly for a period of time—for instance, the adult with spinal muscular atrophy who may be working in the community—certain transportation adaptations or car modifications may be all the equipment that is needed. For the patient with Charcot-Marie-Tooth disease, ankle weakness can be helped by the use of high-topped shoes or boots or by the prescription of an ankle-foot orthosis (AFO). On the other hand, patients with disorders that progress quite rapidly—for instance, amyotrophic lateral sclerosis (ALS)—may need suctioning or ventilatory assistive equipment in the earlier stages of their disorder. Sometimes the progression may be more predictable, such as in Duchenne's pseudohypertrophic muscular dystrophy. Progressive weakness in the second decade of life makes children with this disorder wheelchair dependent.

Functional Evaluation

The patient's functional status can be classified as follows:

1. Community ambulation.
2. Limited or assisted community ambulation.
3. Physiologic ambulation.
4. Wheelchair dependency with activities of daily living (ADL) function.
5. Wheelchair dependency requiring assistance.
6. Totally dependent.

The goal is to achieve the highest level possible, and this may depend on (1) available muscle strength; (2) the ability of the patient to cooperate (e.g., the mental status); (3) the presence or absence of fixed contractures; and (4) the use of assistive devices. After a complete evaluation, equipment may need to be prescribed and fitted individually.

Mental retardation, the environment, and the availability of family or community assistance may play a large role and become major factors in the success or failure of a planned rehabilitation program for patients with neuromuscular disorders.[4]

REGIONAL PROBLEMS AND CONSIDERATIONS

Head, Trunk, and Body Control

Weakness of the paraspinal and trunk supporting muscles may be due to the underlying neuromuscular disorder. When there is inadequate trunk and head control, independent sitting and ambulation may not be possible. In the seated patient with spinal collapse, if the trunk is unsupported, the body weight will need to be borne by the forearms and elbows on the wheelchair rests. This will limit function and can cause decubitus ulcers.[5] The trunk can be supported either internally or externally, and if a body jacket or custom-molded seating device is used, attachments such as a cloverleaf for the occiput can help support the head, thus maintaining an upright posture (Fig. 39-2). It is important to position the head properly so that eye level can be horizontal. When the primary disease process or spinal fusion has resulted in a residual lordotic position, unless the head can be flexed significantly to correct the lordotic attitude of the cervical spine, looking forward can become a problem. Special prismatic glasses may need to be used for straight-ahead vision.

Shoulder

Mild shoulder weakness generally does not present a problem because substitute movements will allow the patient to reach forward, to groom, and to put

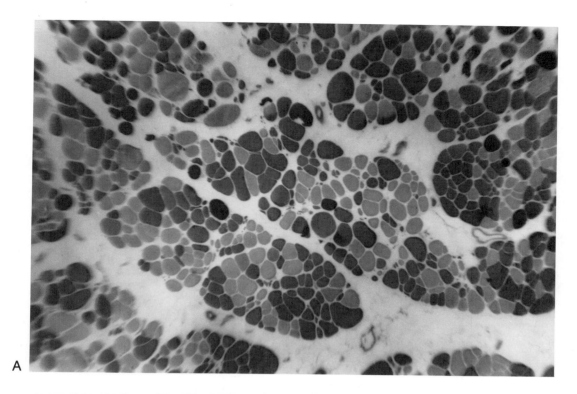

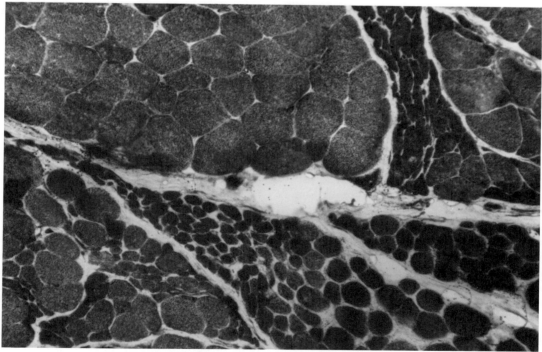

Fig. 39-1. (A) Muscle biopsy (frozen section, ATPase 9.4 stain) from patient with Duchenne muscular dystrophy. Both type I and type II fibers are affected. Some fatty infiltration is also seen. **(B)** Muscle biopsy (frozen section, DPNH stain) from a patient with Charcot-Marie-Tooth disease. Type grouping and group atrophy is seen.

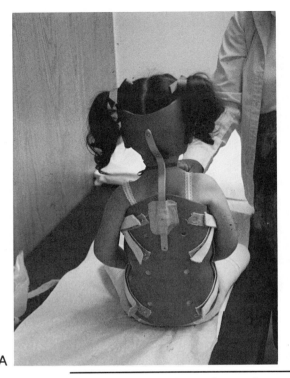 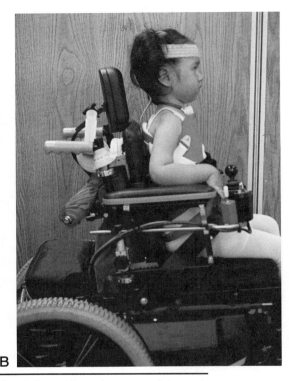

Fig. 39-2. Child with spinal muscular atrophy sitting with equipment and support.

glasses on and off. This is frequently seen in the early stages of a person with facioscapulohumeral (FSH) muscular dystrophy. Persistent and extreme weakness can limit the use of the hands to tabletop or chest-level activities. With marked proximal weakness and good distal function, fixing the scapulae surgically and stabilizing them to the spinal processes or to the rib cage may eliminate some of the wasted motion and allow for the maintenance of some shoulder-level function. Shoulder contractures are frequently present in the patient with a neuromuscular disorder with upper extremity weakness. As a result of limitation caused by the contracture and the osteoporotic nature of the bony structure, fracture at the upper humerus can occur with forcible stretching and with transfers.

Elbow

Elbow contractures should be prevented or limited. When elbow function is limited, feeding and self-care activities may be compromised. Elbow contractures limiting extension require repositioning of wheel-

chair rests, tabletop equipment, and electronic supplies. When seen early, elbow contractures can be treated by serial casting. After improvement of the position, dropout casts can be made so that motion can be maintained either passively or actively. Heterotopic ossification generally is not seen in the patient with muscle disease. Surgical release of elbow contracture does not give satisfying or good long-term results.

Wrist, Hand, and Fingers

In disorders in which there is distal weakness, the hands and fingers may be affected sufficiently that function is impaired. Minor amounts of weakness can affect penmanship and the ability to hold light objects, and adaptive equipment may be required to perform simple tasks. Wheelchair controls may need to be positioned so that they be used efficiently and safely. Unfortunately, when one particular task requiring grasping is performed constantly, such as the need to control a knob or switch to drive an electric wheelchair, fixed flexion contractures of the fingers can form, as frequently occurs in electric wheelchair drivers.[6] When muscle imbalance exists, especially in disorders in which the intrinsic muscles of the hand may be affected, splinting or surgical correction may be recommended, especially when the underlying neuromuscular disease is a mildly progressive or nonprogressive one.

Spine

In spinal involvement, lordosis is seen in the standing and walking patient because of muscle imbalance and adaptation. Proximal muscle weakness involving the hip musculature, anterior abdominal muscles, and quadriceps contributes to the lordotic posture so that balance can be maintained with a widened base. Any changes to this very delicate balance may cause instability. In the standing or ambulatory patient, a body jacket to reduce lordosis encumbers the spine and may cause inability to walk. Therefore, the standing and walking patient should not be fitted with a body jacket.

In the wheelchair-dependent patient, the spine needs to be examined periodically and, if there is doubt whether or not a spinal curve is present, radiographic examination should be made in the seated position. If the radiographic examination shows a curve of the spine, it is generally a neuromuscular curve or a long C-shaped curve. This is due to paraspinal muscle weakness. If the curve progresses, the spine needs to be supported. In cases in which the progression is rapid, surgical intervention is indicated. Spinal fusion is an excellent way to control a spinal curvature and, in the mature spine, is an excellent method to stabilize the spine (Fig. 39-3). Long, multiple-segment fusions are made, generally from the upper thoracic spine to the sacrum.[7] Evaluation of the breathing capacity, whether or not a functional cough is present, and the need to prepare for the blood loss are extremely important factors that need to be taken into account preoperatively. Postoperative care may include ventilatory assistance and this should be anticipated. In the immature spine, provisions must be made for future growth and the posterior spinal elements must be preserved. Temporary control of scoliosis can be made by internal splinting without fusion.

Hip

Hip contractures occur with muscle imbalance and also can develop in patients who spend most of their time upright in a seated position. Generally 30° of hip flexion contracture can be acceptable and does not interfere with function. Early fixed hip contractures, as seen in the patient with congenital myopathy, congenital muscular dystrophy, or spinal muscular atrophy, may cause a delayed or a compromised development of the hip joint. Muscle weakness can also allow the femoral head to become subluxated or dislocated (Fig. 39-4). Unfortunately, these cases cannot be treated by standard orthopaedic methods that were developed for the treatment of congenital dislocated or subluxated hip. In this instance, when spasticity is not present, neither adductor release nor open reduction is indicated. The hips can easily be relocated by adduction of the legs and maintained by the use of multiple diapers or an adduction pillow. The Pavlik harness is not effective. Frequent checks by clinical evaluation and occasional radiographic confirmation should be made. In the wheelchair-dependent patient, generally bilaterally subluxated or dislocated hips do not present a problem for seating, but a unilaterally dislocated hip is undesirable. The "windblown" attitude with pelvic obliquity leads to scoliosis and difficulty in providing the patient with a comfortable seating system.

Unless contractures also exist and interfere with function, hip releases generally are not recommended. In the case of resultant pelvic obliquity, the side on which the hip is adducted is most likely to become dislocated and would be the side that required initial correction. In abduction contracture, which is frequently seen in patients with poliomyelitis residuals, lateral release including fascia lata release may need to be considered. Pelvic osteotomy may be required for the correction of pelvic obliquity.

Osteoporosis is frequently present and associated with fixed contractures. Precautions need to be taken in stretching and with transfers to avoid fractures.

Knee

Knee flexion contractures need to be prevented so that standing and walking can continue. Mild contractures of less than 15° can be tolerated; however,

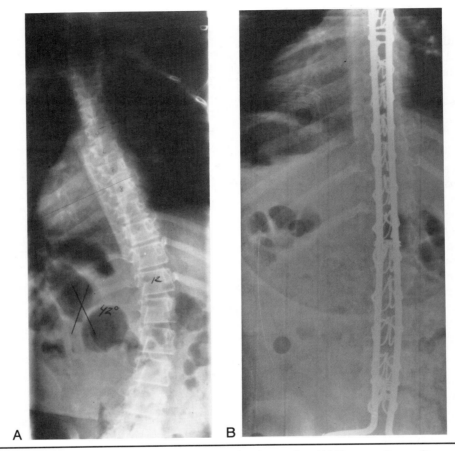

Fig. 39-3. Fifteen-year-old boy with Duchenne muscular dystrophy. **(A)** Preoperative radiograph showing spinal collapse. **(B and C)** Radiographs after fusion with correction. *(Figure continues.)*

more severe contractures will require a shift of the body weight for a person to continue standing, and this generally is poorly tolerated by the ambulatory patient with a neuromuscular disorder, whose balance is already precarious. Some of the patients will become wheelchair dependent because of increasing knee flexion contractures. If there is good musculature proximally so that hip control is not compromised significantly and if the quadriceps muscles activity is fair or better, the likelihood of the patient's being able to continue to stand and walk is good and knee releases should be made. A lateral release of the iliotibial band may be sufficient to correct 15° to 20° of a recent-onset knee flexion contracture; however, fractional lengthening of the hamstrings posteriorly is indicated if the contracture cannot be fully corrected. Capsular release is seldom necessary at the

posterior aspect of the knee and may be difficult. After knee release, postsurgical casting is necessary. When long leg casts are used, the patient should be allowed to ambulate as soon as possible to prevent further muscle deterioration. A lightweight brace (knee-ankle-foot orthosis) using carbon strip reinforcement can be used to support the limb and maintain correction (Fig. 39-5).

In the seated patient, up to 90° of fixed knee flexion contracture is acceptable, although not desirable. This does not appear to interfere with function. However, it also does not allow patients to lie comfortably on their backs or abdomens unless the legs are properly supported. Fixed knee flexion contractures of over 90° can occur when the wheelchair-seated patient does not use foot rests, places the feet

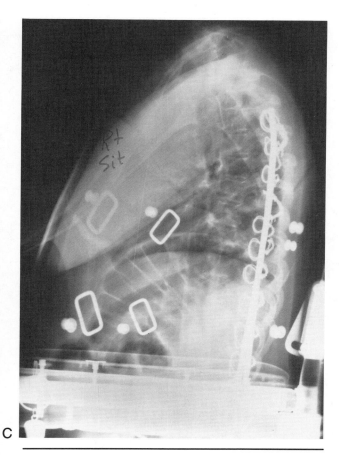

C

Fig. 39-3 *(Continued).*

the legs to prevent this from occurring in the wheel-chair-dependent sitter.

Ankle and Foot

In the ambulatory patient, ankle and foot deformities can lead to lower extremity instability. The development of callosities on the ankles and feet may lead to pain and difficulty in fitting footwear. The nature of the muscle imbalance must be assessed so that improvements can be made. If weakness is the sole problem and there are no dynamic or fixed contractures, the use of appropriate supportive devices may be helpful. A lightweight AFO made of polypropylene material with or without reinforcement with carbon fiber may be used for the person with a weak, collapsing ankle. Shoes need to be lightweight and modified to allow for the incorporation of the orthosis. When dynamic contractures are present, muscle testing would determine the nature of this problem and correction can be effected by the use of appropriate muscle balancing techniques. For instance, the posterior tibial tendon can be transferred anteriorly through the interosseous membrane to correct pes cavus or pes equinovarus deformity[8] seen in the child with Duchenne muscular dystrophy or in the patient with Charcot-Marie-Tooth disease[9] and to correct a varus foot, which can be seen in the patient with myotonic dystrophy.[10] After correction, reassessment of the muscle strength should be made and bracing prescribed if needed.

on the wheelchair seat, or uses a poorly designed or poorly fitted wheelchair. An increase of the flexion contracture can lead to anterior knee pain and difficulty in putting on clothing. It can also allow moisture to collect in the posterior aspect of the knee, causing decubitus ulcers and skin breakdown. Treatment at this stage can be very difficult; stretching is no longer effective and surgical releases—even with the severance of the tight hamstring tendons and capsulotomy—give very little correction. Forceful correction leads to tibiofemoral joint subluxation. Pain and paresthesias occur when the fixed knee contracture becomes stretched out past the limit of endurance of the neurovascular structures. The best method of treatment is awareness of the problems that can be encountered with marked knee flexion contractures and adaptation of methods to support

For feet with fixed deformities, knowledge of the underlying problem as well as an assessment of muscle strength of the anterior tibial, posterior tibial, peroneal, gastrocnemius-soleus, toe flexors, and extensors is necessary. Bony deformities need to be assessed radiographically. Coalitions may exist, which may be better delineated with computed tomography (CT). Bony deformities and fixed soft tissue contractures are correctable by releasing the contractures surgically and by osteotomy. When the corrected foot and ankle have consolidated sufficiently postsurgically, muscle testing needs to be repeated to see if there is a need for dynamic correction using tendon transfer. AFOs are frequently used to maintain correction.[11]

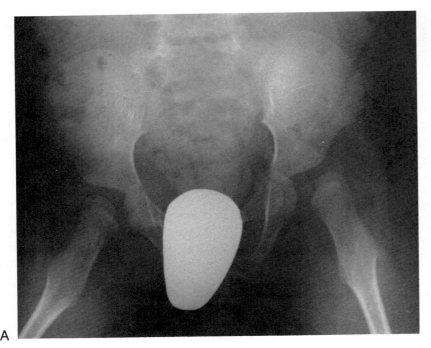

A

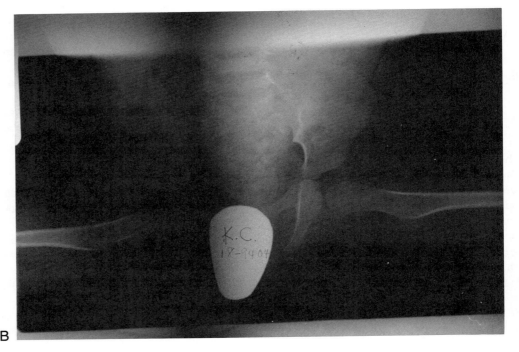

B

Fig. 39-4. Child with congenital myopathy. **(A)** Left hip showing subluxation. **(B)** The subluxation is reduced by wide abduction. *(Figure continues.)*

Fig. 39-4 *(Continued).* **(C)** Positioning of patient using an abduction pillow to maintain corrected position of hip.

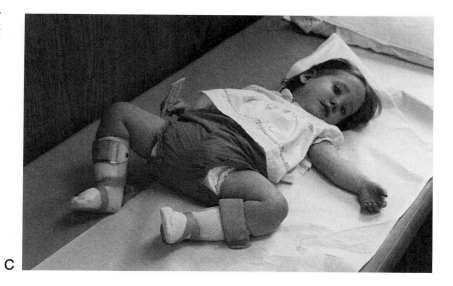

C

Cardiopulmonary Aspects

Respiratory failure is the leading cause of death in patients with neuromuscular disease.[12] Muscular disease affects more than the extremities and the spinal supportive muscles; it also extends its devastation to the muscles of respiration. Although respiratory failure can occur acutely, it usually develops slowly as the respiratory muscles gradually weaken. The onset is insidious. Ironically, in the patient with neuromuscular disease, respiratory death occurs with the lung parenchyma remaining intact and healthy, yet useless because of mechanical failure of the respiratory pump.

The treatment of respiratory failure in the patient with neuromuscular disease requires an understanding of the underlying disease process. In diseases in which progression of muscle weakness is expected to occur, anticipation of problems is possible and early intervention becomes a key aspect of the care plan. Just as it is possible to anticipate the need for a powered wheelchair to assist in mobility, so too it is possible to anticipate the need for aggressive pulmonary intervention. The criteria for establishing a diagnosis of impending respiratory failure must be lenient to allow for early intervention. When progressive weakness of the respiratory muscles can be expected to produce an increasing stress on the respiratory system, identifying impending respiratory failure

early allows the physician to address the problem before emergency intervention becomes necessary. Because the respiratory muscles in the patient with neuromuscular disease are working at an optimal level, any sign of hypoxia (pO_2 less than 60 mm Hg) or hypercapnia (pCO_2 greater than 50 mm Hg) with the patient at rest is ominous.[13] Abnormalities such as these indicate that a compensatory response is no longer possible during times of stress, such as pneumonia.

The presentation of respiratory failure differs from disease to disease. Age at onset varies in disorders of differing severity of muscle involvement. In some of the congenital myopathies, respiratory failure may occur shortly after birth, and in Werdnig-Hoffmann disease, the severe form of spinal muscular atrophy (SMA), it occurs within the first year of life. Rare reports also document the occurrence of respiratory failure during the first 5 years of life in childhood peripheral neuropathy.[14] In Duchenne's muscular dystrophy (DMD), however, respiratory failure classically does not occur until the late teens or early twenties, and in ALS it occurs in late adulthood.

The pattern of respiratory failure is also variable. Much of this has to do with the age at which respiratory muscle failure occurs. Patients with severe weakness of the intercostal muscles during the early developmental years do not develop a stable chest

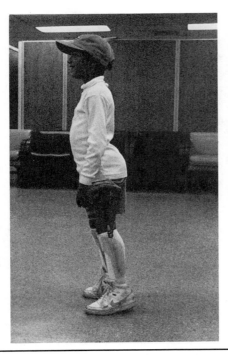

Fig. 39-5. Nine-year-old boy with Duchenne muscular dystrophy. The leg is supported by a knee-ankle-foot orthosis (KAFO) using lightweight components.

wall. This is typical of the classic patient with severe SMA. In these patients, lack of integrity of the chest wall causes paradoxical breathing and actually encourages lung collapse and atelectasis.[15] The tendency of the chest wall to collapse on deep inspiration makes it necessary for patients with severe weakness of the intercostal muscles to breathe with rapid, shallow respirations. In turn, the rapid respiratory rate required to maintain adequate ventilation during times of health leaves little reserve available at times of respiratory illnesses, such as upper respiratory infections or pneumonia. Hypoxia is often the presenting sign of respiratory failure.[13]

In patients in whom respiratory failure does not occur until later in life, such as the teenage patient with DMD and the ALS patient, development of the chest wall has already occurred. The intercostal muscles have successfully elevated the rib cage into a normal position prior to the onset of significant muscle weakness. The chest wall maintains its integrity even as the diaphragm begins to fail; consequently lung collapse is rare in DMD patients. Respiratory failure, unless complicated by an acute pneumonia, is a gradual and insidious process, which often is manifested first during sleep with hypercapnea rather than hypoxia.[16]

Other associated muscle groups directly influence the respiratory system and consequently contribute to the onset of respiratory failure. Severe weakness of the bulbar muscles interferes with coordinated swallowing and increases the risk of aspiration and pneumonia. Some congenital myopathies, such as nemaline rod myopathy, are associated with severe bulbar muscle involvement. Weakness of the abdominal muscles limits the effectiveness of a patient's cough and may prohibit adequate clearance of secretions from the upper airway, again increasing the risk of infection in the lower respiratory tract.[17] SMA is a good example of this. Clearance of secretions from the respiratory tract is often the most serious initial complication related to the respiratory system in children with this disorder.

Because respiratory failure is known to be the overwhelming cause of death in the patient with neuromuscular disease, the key to effective care is early prediction. Education of the family and patient (if old enough) and a coordinated and well-planned course of intervention are mandatory.

Intervention occurs at varying levels. First, aggressive management of all respiratory infections is essential, as are preventive measures, such as annual influenza vaccination and prophylaxis with the pneumococcal vaccine. However, even with the best and most rapid treatment of acute lung infections, the underlying respiratory muscle weakness remains and eventually these muscles fail.

Failure of the respiratory muscles is basically a mechanical problem and definitive treatment eventually also involves mechanical means in the form of a respirator. Respirator support is becoming a more commonly used treatment option in this patient population. Just as treatment in the early stages of each neuromuscular disease requires an understanding of the disease process, this is no less important as the end stage of the disease approaches. Treatment options continue to exist late in the course. Respirators

Muscular Dystrophy and Neurogenic Atrophy / 545

vary from negative-pressure devices[18] such as the iron lung and the cuirass respirators to positive-pressure devices. Positive pressure may now be delivered through nasal[19] or mouth[20] masks or through the tracheostomy.[16,20] Other disease-related options include use of the respirator either for nighttime only or for full-time assistance.[21]

In SMA, respiratory failure appears to evolve in stages. Just as plateaus in strength of the muscles of the extremities are well documented,[22] similar plateaus in the strength of the respiratory muscles may occur. Fatigue of these muscles plays a significant role because the patients maintain a rapid respiratory rate throughout their lives. Resting of these fatigued muscles at night through the use of nighttime ventilator assistance may offer the patient many years of freedom from full-time ventilator use.

The plateaus in muscle strength that occur in SMA make early prediction of respiratory failure difficult. Intervention is usually reserved for patients with recurrent pneumonia. Prediction of ensuing problems may also be made in patients with severe involvement of the bulbar muscles or in patients with a nonfunctional cough secondary to severe abdominal muscle weakness. In these patients a tracheostomy for clearance of secretions may be necessary, eliminating the possibility of other modes of respirator support that are useful in other patients with neuromuscular disease.

In contrast to SMA, patients with DMD do not experience plateaus in muscle strength. Instead, gradual and continual weakening occurs just as predictably in the respiratory muscles as in the muscles of the extremities. Forced vital capacity (FVC) values show reliable increases through the early years of growth, followed by predictable decline during adolescence.[23] Once the FVC reaches 500 cubic centimeters, respiratory failure usually develops within 6 months to 1 year.[16] Respirator options have varied in different medical centers with successful use of both positive and negative pressure systems.

Cardiomyopathy is a feature in several of the neuromuscular diseases, with DMD being a classic example.[24] Respiratory assistance in patients with cardiomyopathy must take into account the cardiac condition. Early respiratory support, however, may prevent worsening of the cardiomyopathy through prevention of cor pulmonale.

Although significant disease-specific variability exists in the course of respiratory failure in the neuromuscular diseases, some aspects of care are universal. Regardless of the disease, individual patients continue to demonstrate numerous possibilities for a fulfilling life on a respirator. The portability of modern machines allows them to fit easily beneath a patient's wheelchair. Children on respirators attend regular school and are now participating fully in many of life's "normal" activities — including recreational pursuits and social activities. Patients have found employment, have married, and have had children. Although cures for most of the neuromuscular diseases of childhood have not as yet been found, respirator assistance now allows the patient and family options, whereas previously death was the only possibility.

Acknowledgment. The authors would like to thank Mrs. Mary Schindler for typing the manuscript.

REFERENCES

1. Walton J (ed): Disorders of Voluntary Muscle. 4th Ed. Churchill Livingstone, Edinburgh, 1981
2. Dubowitz V: Color Atlas of Muscle Disorders in Childhood. Year Book Medical Publishers, Chicago, 1989
3. Drennan JC: Orthopaedic Management of Neuromuscular Disorders. JB Lippincott, Philadelphia, 1983
4. Hsu JD, Lewis JE: Challenges in the care of the retarded child with Duchenne muscular dystrophy. Orthop Clin North Am 12:73, 1981
5. Lehman M, Hsu AM, Hsu JD: Spinal curvature, hand dominance, and prolonged upper extremity use of the wheelchair-dependent DMD patient. Dev Med Child Neurol 28:628, 1986
6. Hsu JD, Taylor D: Upper extremity deformities in Duchenne muscular dystrophy patients. p. 150. In Fredricks S, Brody GS (eds): Symposium on the Neurologic Aspects of Plastic Surgery. CV Mosby, St. Louis, 1978
7. Hsu JD: Spine care of the patient with Duchenne muscular dystrophy. Spine: State Art Review. 4:161, 1990
8. Hsu JD: Management of foot deformity in Duchenne's pseudohypertrophic muscular dystrophy. Orthop Clin North Am 7:979, 1976
9. Hsu JD: Orthopaedic care for children and adolescents with Charcot-Marie-Tooth disease. p. 409. In Lovelace RE, Shapiro HK (eds): Charcot-Marie-Tooth Disorders: Pathophysiology, Molecular Genetics, and Therapy. Wiley-Liss, New York, 1990
10. Ray S, Bowen JR Marks HG: Foot deformity in myotonic dystrophy. Foot Ankle 5:125, 1985
11. Hsu JD, Jackson RB: Treatment of symptomatic foot and ankle

deformities in the nonambulatory neuromuscular patient. Foot Ankle 5:238, 1985

12. Brooke MH: A Clinician's View of Neuromuscular Diseases. Williams & Wilkins, Baltimore, 1986

13. Gilgoff IS, Kahlstrom E, MacLaughlin E, Keens TG: Long-term ventilatory support in spinal muscular atrophy. J Pediatr 115:904, 1989

14. Iannaccone ST, Guilfoile T: Long-term mechanical ventilation in infants with neuromuscular disease. J Child Neurol 3:30, 1988

15. DeTroyer A, Heilporn A: Respiratory mechanics in quadriplegia. The respiratory function of the intercostal muscles. Am Rev Respir Dis 122:591, 1980

16. Gilgoff I, Prentice W, Baydur A: Patient and family participation in the management of respiratory failure in Duchenne's muscular dystrophy. Chest 95:519, 1989

17. Siebens A, Kirby NA, Poulos DA: Cough following transection of spinal cord at C-6. Arch Phys Med Rehabil 45:1, 1964

18. Curran FJ: Night ventilation by body respirators for patients in chronic respiratory failure due to late stage Duchenne muscular dystrophy. Arch Phys Med Rehabil 62:270, 1981

19. Kerby GR, Mayer LS, Pingleton SK: Nocturnal positive pressure ventilation via nasal mask. Am Rev Respir Dis 135:738, 1987

20. Bach JR, O'Brien J, Krotenberg R, Alba AS: Management of end stage respiratory failure in Duchenne muscular dystrophy. Muscle Nerve 10:177, 1987

21. Heckmatt JZ, Loh L, Dubowitz V: Nocturnal hypoventilation in children with nonprogressive neuromuscular disease. Pediatrics 83:250, 1989

22. Dubowitz V: Infantile muscular atrophy a prospective study with particular reference to a slowly progressive variety. Brain 87:707, 1964

23. Rideau Y, Jankowski LW, Grellet J: Respiratory function in the muscular dystrophies. Muscle Nerve 4:155, 1981

24. Stewart GA, Gilgoff I, Baydur A, et al: Gated radionuclide ventriculography in the evaluation of cardiac function in Duchenne's muscular dystrophy. Chest 94:1245, 1988

40 Myelomeningocele

REID ABRAMS
DENNIS R. WENGER

Closure of the embryonal neural tube normally occurs between the third and fourth weeks of gestation, with incomplete closure resulting in spinal dysraphism. Because neural tube closure begins centrally and progresses both cranially and caudally, abnormalities in this process may result in coexisting defects in the thoracic or lumbar region and in the cephalic region (Chiari malformations).

The continuum of abnormalities represented by the term *spinal dysraphism* ranges from spina bifida occulta (lack of fusion of the vertebral arches) to myelomeningocele. Meningocele is the condition in which there is a vertebral defect with a meningeal sac protruding through it. In myelomeningocele, the sac contains abnormal neural elements with a neurologic deficit caudal to the lesion. The skin over the sac is nearly always incomplete.

Genetic, environmental, and nutritional factors have all been suggested as etiologic factors in myelomeningocele. The incidence varies from 1 to 2 cases per 1,000, in the general population throughout the world, and is slightly higher in females. The risk of occurrence in subsequent siblings of an index case increases from 0.1 to 5 percent.[1]

Serum and amniotic fluid α-fetoprotein determinations allow antenatal diagnosis. α-Fetoprotein is normally present in fetal tissues and can be found in amniotic fluid and maternal serum until the fetal abdominal wall and neural tube close by 3 to 4 weeks of gestation. If α-fetoprotein is found in maternal serum thereafter, it is abnormal, and confirmatory amniocentesis should be performed. Diagnosis of neural tube defects can be made in 80 to 90 percent of cases.[1] Thus, depending on the wishes of the parents, termination of the pregnancy or early planning for management can be selected.

GENERAL NONORTHOPAEDIC CONSIDERATIONS

Allowing severely deformed infants to die in infancy has become increasingly more controversial in an era of expanded neonatal technology and capability. The issue of selection is difficult to address, there being many moral, ethical, philosophical, and legal considerations. No absolute criteria noted at birth can specifically determine which, if any, child with severe myelomeningocele (and associated disorders) should be allowed to die in infancy.[1,2] However, early examination of the neonate with myelomeningocele by a neurosurgeon (and an orthopaedist) should help the parents in understanding the prognosis. With parental informed consent, early aggressive care includes emergent neurosurgical closure of the myelomeningocele as a first step. Delay increases the risk of central nervous system sepsis. Thus, a neurosurgeon is an essential component of a multidisciplinary team that cares for a child with myelomeningocele.

Hydrocephalus

Approximately 90 percent of patients have hydrocephalus.[2] Therefore, early decompression by shunting may be necessary depending on the adequacy of cerebrospinal fluid circulation. During subsequent growth, head circumference should be measured at regular intervals. Shunting may become indicated later in childhood. Neurologic deterioration may indicate worsening hydrocephalus in patients without shunts or shunt failure or infection in those with shunts.

547

It was initially thought that the intelligence quotient (IQ) was significantly diminished in those children whose hydrocephalus was severe enough to need shunting.[3] However, subsequent studies have shown that the mean IQs of children with and without shunts were normal when those who had developed shunt infections were selected out. In other words, it is probably not the shunt or the presence of hydrocephalus severe enough to require the shunt that explains the reduction in IQ, which instead is the result of central nervous system infection.

Urologic Considerations

Because 30 percent of children with myelomeningocele have associated congenital anomalies, 13 percent of which are urologic,[4] early work-up with renal ultrasound and intravenous pyelogram are recommended.[1] Thus, the urologist becomes a part of the multidisciplinary team.

Multidisciplinary Care

During infancy and in later periods of growth and development, the child with myelomeningocele is confronted with many difficulties, including neurologic, urologic, and orthopaedic problems, requiring the ongoing consultation of these specialists. In addition, problems with skin ulceration may require a plastic surgeon. Approximately 17 percent of adults with myelomeningocele have problems with non-healing decubitus ulcers.[2] Ongoing physical therapy is usually needed, and orthoses are nearly routinely required. A social worker and psychologist may aid in the inevitable emotional difficulties encountered by the patient and parents. A special educator and vocational counselor may further assist in assimilation of the patient into the community. (Only 30 percent of all adults with myelomeningocele are employed full- or part-time.[2]) The most successful care of the child or adult with myelomeningocele occurs in facilities with a multidisciplinary approach with easy availability of the above-mentioned specialists. Ideally all of these consultants can all be present in a single clinic where they can discuss realistic goals and communicate with the patient and parents (Fig. 40-1). Unfortunately, institutionally based multidisciplinary clinics can sometimes become so complex and confusing that some families dislike them. Certain families may choose to see the required subspecialty consultants independently and individually.

Psychosocial Development

Psychosocially the child with myelomeningocele is fragile. Specialists caring for these children must anticipate and promote as normal as possible progression through developmental milestones while caring for the patients' physical disabilities.

Birth marks the beginning of the sensorimotor stage of development as described by Piaget.[5] This is the stage during which the child is exposed to, actively participates in, and experiences a stimulating environment. Hindrance of this important experiential period of learning, even in the absence of organic intracranial pathology, can lead to developmental delay. Studies have suggested that healthy psychosocial development starts immediately after birth with bonding.[6] Children with myelomeningocele are already off to a suboptimal start because frequently they are in the intensive care unit, isolated from their mothers and from the usual neonatal stimuli. In addition, maternal bonding with the child is hampered by the child's abnormality. Counseling and spina bifida support groups should be made available to inevitably troubled parents.

During the first 6 months, when the child is observing the environment, learning head control and how to smile,[6] orthopaedic interventions such as serial casting of equinovarus feet or the closed treatment of dislocated hips will not interfere. By 6 months, the child should have good head control and begin independent sitting, thus freeing the hands for manipulation. A child with myelomeningocele may have considerable difficulty with sitting if there is a marked kyphosis. In this instance a body jacket may be indicated to promote hand-free sitting and thus more normal development. Conversely, interventions that maintain the patient supine may impede sensorimotor development.

At about 1 year of age, the able-bodied child's world expands with ambulation, experience and parental interaction increase, and the child begins to learn speech. Again, the child with myelomeningocele is

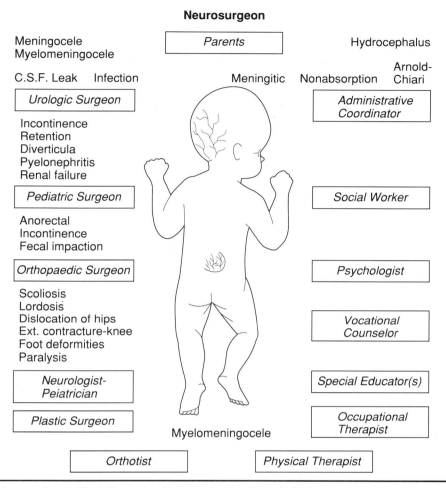

Neurosurgeon

Meningocele
Myelomeningocele

Parents

Hydrocephalus

Arnold-
Chiari

C.S.F. Leak   Infection

Meningitic   Nonabsorption

Urologic Surgeon

*Administrative
Coordinator*

Incontinence
Retention
Diverticula
Pyelonephritis
Renal failure

Pediatric Surgeon

Social Worker

Anorectal
Incontinence
Fecal impaction

Orthopaedic Surgeon

Psychologist

Scoliosis
Lordosis
Dislocation of hips
Ext. contracture-knee
Foot deformities
Paralysis

*Vocational
Counselor*

*Neurologist-
Peiatrician*

Special Educator(s)

Plastic Surgeon

*Occupational
Therapist*

Myelomeningocele

Orthotist

Physical Therapist

Fig. 40-1. Schema of multidisciplinary involvement in the care of children with myelomeningocoele. (From Tachdjian,[1] with permission.)

disadvantaged. Promotion of upright posture and mobility can optimize this stage of development. Goals must be realistic and individualized.

By about 2 years of age, the next stage of cognitive development is reached, heralded by the ability to remember (object constancy).[5] Sensorimotor exploration and mobility are less important as the child develops operational thinking. During this stage, orthopaedic interventions that may limit mobility are less detrimental.

The self-concept of the child with myelomeningocele has thus far been influenced by feedback from adults. Peer input begins when school starts, and this may

adversely affect the child's self-image. Adolescents are preoccupied with their bodies and for teenagers with myelomeningocele, not only is their disability disturbing to them but also their body image is further jeopardized by deterioration (with the possible onset of worsening scoliosis, obesity, loss of ambulation, and confinement to a wheelchair). Peer input reflects more intensely than ever on self-image during adolescence, especially the opinions of members of the opposite sex. Another adolescent task hampered by disability is the development of independence. Appropriate extraparental adult attentions by the medical team can aid in the development of a healthy self-image, and appropriate orthopaedic intervention and orthoses can enhance autonomy. Wheelchair sports programs and other special athletic programs such as handicapped skiing are excellent builders of self-esteem.

AMBULATION

Determinants of Ambulation

Most medical literature dealing with orthopaedic problems defines function according to "level" of involvement. For example, an "L4-level" myelomeningocele patient has no neurologic function distal to the L4 nerve root. Adults with myelomeningocele with an L2 level or higher uniformly use a wheelchair. Of those persons with lesions at the L3, L4, or L5 levels, 78 percent use a wheelchair at least part of the time. In general, if a child with myelomeningocele who has had appropriate treatment cannot stand independently by 6 years of age, that child will be unlikely to walk; the pattern developed by age 10 years will most likely persist into adulthood.[2]

The determinants of ambulation in the patient with myelomeningocele have been discussed by many authors.[7-10] The most significant factor is neurologic level, with the L4 level being the cutoff above which community ambulation into adulthood is unlikely. More specifically, good quadriceps strength and at least antigravity hamstring power is necessary.[7] Consequently, ascending neurologic level is one cause of loss of ambulation (as can be seen with a tethered cord, diasteatomyelia, or hydromyelia.)[1,2,11]

Hip Stability and Prognosis for Ambulation

Lindseth noted hip subluxation to be associated with a decreased likelihood of ambulation in the L4- and L5-level patients,[10] and L3-level patients 8 years of age or more were noted by Asher and Olsen to be less likely to be walking in the presence of hip deformity (i.e., contracture and subluxation or dislocation, or both).[7] Ambulatory capacity in those patients with involvement of levels above L3 does not appear to be influenced by hip abnormalities. Other determinants are musculoskeletal deformity, obesity, and motivation. Age appears to play a role, but this is probably related to increasing weight associated with increased stature.[1,7] By and large, transitions in ambu-

latory status are downward, related to many of the aforementioned factors. Generally, when walking demands too much energy, patients are relieved to use a wheelchair.[7]

Clearly, the goal of severely handicapped children (including those with myelomeningocele, cerebral palsy, and similar diseases) is mobility. Mobility often is achieved more readily and speedily by wheelchair travel than by inefficient walking. This emphasis on mobility over ambulation, particularly as the child nears adolescence, must be stressed to prevent parental dissatisfaction and unrealistic expectations.

Orthotic Aids

Because normal children do not attain upright posture until around 1 year of age, standing orthoses are not appropriate until this time. Before this age, crawling and sitting are encouraged and orthoses to facilitate these activities are prescribed. Occasionally a body jacket improves sitting in the child with severe kyphosis. A caster cart or other device (which the child mobilizes by use of the upper extremities) can enhance exploration in children with good trunk and head control who cannot crawl effectively.[1] At around 1 year of age, the ability to stand can be assisted by a "parapodium" or standing table. When the child expresses an interest in walking, other, more complex orthoses are employed depending on functional level. Proper fitting of these orthoses is contingent on the absence of musculoskeletal deformity.

Benefits of Early Ambulation

Early ambulation, even in patients with high level of involvement, has been noted to be beneficial, although essentially all of these patients will use a wheelchair by the time they are teenagers. In a study comparing these patients to peers in whom a wheelchair was prescribed early in life, the early ambulators were more independent, had fewer fractures and decubitus ulcers, and were better able to transfer.[12] Other benefits of upright posture are improvement in kidney, bladder, and pulmonary function. In addition, upright posture benefits sensorimotor development early in life, and there are positive effects on self-esteem.[1,6,7]

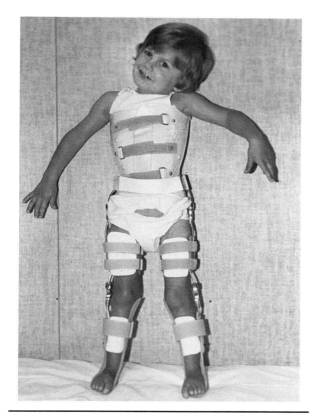

Fig. 40-2. An example of a thoracolumbar sacral hip-knee-ankle-foot orthosis, appropriate for standing and early ambulation in children with thoracic lesions. (Courtesy of Loren Saxton, c.p.o.)

Ambulation Patterns and Orthotic Types

Several types of ambulation are possible. Nonfunctional ambulators do so only during physical therapy sessions. Household ambulators are able to transfer and ambulate independently for short distances on level terrain. Community ambulators can walk with essentially unlimited capacity over any terrain.[1,7,8]

In children with thoracic level lesions, the goals must be clear to the parents and patients from the outset. Early ambulation can be encouraged, but by adulthood virtually all of these patients will use a wheelchair. Patients and family should be helped to understand that this "deterioration" is not unexpected, but rather the natural history. Appropriate orthoses for this level must stabilize the spine, hips, knees, ankles, and feet (Fig. 40-2). With this support, a swing-

through gait is feasible in a nonfunctional or household ambulatory capacity.

Children who have lesions at the L1, L2, and L3 levels have hip flexion but no hip extension. Reciprocating orthoses can be used in these patients, and they can usually attain household ambulatory status (Fig. 40-3). Ideally these children should be thin, have good balance, and be without hip or knee flexion contractures.

With L4 level lesions or lower, children frequently must be started in orthoses that stabilize the hips, knees, ankles, and feet. Usually they can progress to ankle-foot orthoses. It is psychologically better to start with more support and remove orthotic components as the patient progresses than to start with too little support and later have to add more.

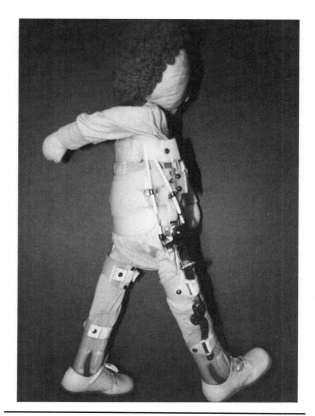

Fig. 40-3. An example of a reciprocating orthosis appropriate for children with high lumbar lesions with good hip flexors and poor extensors interested in early ambulation. (Courtesy of Loren Saxton, c.p.o.)

ORTHOPAEDIC PROBLEMS

Spinal Deformities

Spinal deformity in myelomeningocele can be kyphotic or scoliotic, often as a result of both paralytic (weak muscles) and congenital (wedge vertebra) causes. Paralytic curvatures are usually long and flexible, whereas congenital curvatures are often focal and rigid. The incidence of scoliosis is approximately 50 percent by adolescence,[13,14] but it may be as high as 85 percent in patients with thoracic-level lesions.[2]

Aside from vertebral abnormalities, other factors play a role in spinal deformities. Worsening scoliosis (especially at a young age), pain, change in neurologic level, or increasing spasticity may indicate worsening hydrocephalus, hydromyelia, or cord tethering.[1,2,11] In the work-up of progressive spinal deformity, these disorders must be considered and detected by a thorough neurologic examination and spinal imaging. Cord tethering is more frequent in lower lumbar lesions than in thoracic lesions.[2] Magnetic resonance imaging is effective in identifying syringomyelia and hydromyelia but less effective in clarifying cord tethering, which is better imaged by metrizamide myelography and computed tomography.[2] In clinically significant lesions, treatment by shunting or tethered cord release is indicated. Treatment may not correct progressive scoliosis but can arrest progression and facilitate nonoperative management.[2,15]

Treatment of Spinal Deformities

Treatment goals include producing a compensated spine over a level pelvis with as normal a height as possible. The indication for early arthrodesis in congenital curvature is documented progression, because these curves do not respond to bracing. In paralytic scoliosis a total contact thoracolumbosacral orthosis may control progression until puberty, thereby preserving height. At that time (10 to 14 years of age), if the curve is progressive the spine is fused. A translucent plastic orthosis can facilitate monitoring pressure-sensitive insensate skin. Chair inserts may be of benefit.

Congenital kyphosis may be so severe at birth that it may compromise skin closure and, if left untreated, can lead to pulmonary compromise and compression of abdominal viscera. Early vertebral resection and short fusion may be indicated, but usually the deformity progresses, requiring kyphectomy and fusion later.[16,17] Paralytic kyphotic deformity, as with paralytic scoliosis, may be amenable to orthotic treatment through childhood, similarly requiring fusion at puberty.

Spine surgery in patients with myelomeningocele is frequently complicated by sepsis, loss of correction, and pseudarthrosis, especially at the lumbosacral joint. The best results have been obtained with anterior and posterior fusion to the pelvis, including at least posterior instrumentation.[18,19] Infections with scoliosis surgery have been diminished by ensuring that there is intact stable skin over the lesion, by controlling urinary sepsis with either urinary diversion or a successful intermittent catheterization program, and by the use of prophylactic antibiotics selected to cover urinary tract flora.[19] Because spinal deformity surgery in myelomeningocele is far more difficult than in idiopathic cases, ideally only very experienced spine surgeons should tackle these cases.

Hip Deformities

Clinically pertinent hip deformities in patients with myelomeningocele include joint contracture and hip instability due to continued action of the flexors and adductors and paralysis of the abductors and extensors (Fig. 40-4). The result is progressive hip subluxation and dislocation. Abduction and external rotation contractures also occur, usually in patients with high lumbar or thoracic lesions. When it is unilateral, an abduction contracture frequently is associated with a contralateral adduction contracture and with pelvic obliquity. The hip with the abduction contracture usually remains located but the pelvic obliquity often leads to a contralateral hip adduction contracture, as a result of which hip subluxation or dislocation ensues owing to the "uncoverage" of the adducted femoral head. This phenomenon, widely recognized in the poliomyelitis era, is also common in myelomeningocele patients but often goes unrecognized.

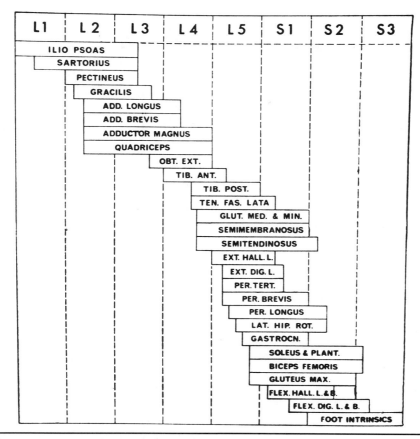

Fig. 40-4. Root innervation of lower extremity musculature. (From Sharrard,[22] with permission.)

Hip Contractures

Treating hip contractures without also treating hip instability per se is indicated for patients with high-level lesions (L3 or above) because hip instability is not a major determinant of ambulatory capacity in these patients, and, in contrast to patients with cerebral palsy, is rarely painful. Thus in patients with high lumbar level involvement, the hip radiographs can be ignored and the contractures addressed. The primary requirement for hips in these patients is to allow brace wear and wheelchair sitting.

Hip flexion and adduction contractures are most frequent with lesions at L3 or L4 in the presence of paralysis of hip abductors, hamstrings, and gluteus maximus, with hip flexors and adductors functioning partially unopposed (Fig. 40-4). An untreated hip flexion contracture causes a problem with standing because it tends to throw the trunk forward, requiring more support by the upper extremities (with crutches). Compensatory severe lumbar lordosis may result. Early treatment includes gentle passive stretching exercises and prone positioning. To prevent deformity, if the child has remained contracture free, total body bracing is employed at about 1 year of age. This orthosis allows standing. If contractures occur despite vigilant therapy, by 2 years of age or older, soft tissue releases (psoas and adductors) are indicated. If soft tissue releases are not sufficient, proximal femoral extension osteotomy may be required. Postoperatively it is important to minimize the time of cast immobilization (no more than 2 to 3 weeks) to limit the possibility of pathologic fracture from osteoporosis.[20] With osteotomy, rigid internal fixation facilitates early cast removal. After cast removal, the patient is encouraged to sleep prone and to stand or walk in an appropriate orthosis.

In patients with high-level lesions, abduction and external rotation contractures are usually the result of malpositioning. It is important to institute early physiotherapy and parental education concerning proper positioning. This should be started even while the neonate is still in the intensive care unit. If the contractures are not amenable to treatment by physiotherapy, soft tissue releases as described by Ober and Yount are indicated,[1] with the possible addition of release of the external rotators and hip capsule or proximal femoral derotational osteotomies.

Hip Instability

Hip dislocation in the child with myelomeningocele can be teratologic (fixed, high, prenatal), congenital (perinatal), and developmental (resulting from muscle imbalance after birth). Teratologic dislocations should not, in general, be treated by open means because this can lead to a stiff hip, which will later prove to be more of a handicap than the dislocation.[1] The following discussion concerns congenital and developmental subluxation and dislocation of the hip.

The primary cause of hip subluxation or dislocation is weakness of the hip abductors and extensors with unopposed intact hip flexion and adduction function. Thus, patients with very high (thoracic) or very low (sacral) lesions are less likely to have hip subluxation or dislocation because no imbalance is present about the hip joint (thoracic level—no hip muscles working; sacral level—all hip muscles working) (Fig. 40-4). It follows that the most troublesome group of patients are those with midlumbar lesions.[21,22] Carroll noted that, neonatally, 50 percent of hips in patients with high lumbar lesions were subluxated or dislocated; over the next 2 to 4 years of age this increased to 75 percent. In the group with L3 and L4 lesions, neonatally 65 percent of hips were unstable, progressing to 77 percent over the ensuing few years. In the group with L5 lesions, 19 percent were born with unstable hips and hip instability developed in 50 percent over the first few years.[23] Sharrard noted that at 1 year of age, patients with lesions at T12 or above did not have dislocated hips but 13 percent of hips

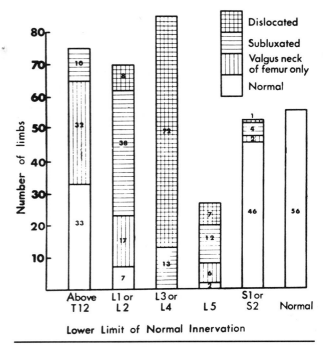

Fig. 40-5. Illustration of which neurologic levels are at most risk for hip subluxation and dislocation. (From Sharrard,[22] with permission.)

were subluxated; those with L1 and L2 lesions 63 percent of the hips were subluxated and 13 percent were dislocated; 15 percent of hips in patients with L3 or L4 lesions were subluxated but 85 percent of hips were dislocated; in children with lesions at L5 44 percent had subluxation of their hips and 26 percent had dislocation[22] (Fig. 40-5).

In the neonate with congenital subluxation or dislocation, closed reduction is usually possible. However, the need for surgery to close the skin over the defect or shunting procedures may delay splinting or casting. In neonates with hip instability and tight hip adductors, there may be a place for subcutaneous adductor release and closed reduction followed by splinting. Carroll, however, prefers to avoid splinting and to maintain range of motion with physiotherapy.[23] If splinting or casting is used, positions in which the hip is maintained in flexion are undesirable because patients will develop contractures. The preferred position is neutral with respect to flexion and extension (or no more than 20° to 30° of flexion), abduction (40° to 50°), and slight internal rotation.[1,23] Once reduced, maintenance of reduction is dependent on neurosegmental level of involvement. Those patients with thoracic lesions will usually maintain their reduction; those with lower lesions will have various degrees of muscle imbalance, with the worst imbalance in patients with L3 and L4 lesions. Goals in the care of the hips in patients with lesions above L3 are to optomize sitting and brace wear, and therefore specifically to maintain contracture-free, symmetrical (avoiding pelvic obliquity), and supple hips. These goals may not necessarily require reduction (especially if there are bilateral dislocations) and, in fact, performing open reduction in these patients may be detrimental if it is followed by stiffness[1,23] (which can occur in 20 to 30 percent even after only one operation.[24]

Aggressive attempts to obtain hip reduction are reserved for those patients with good quadriceps function and thus a good potential for walking,[1,2,23] although some authorities would say that ambulatory capacity is enhanced in patients with L3 lesions by reduced hips.[7] The best candidates for aggressive surgical correction are those with unilateral dislocations between 1 to 3 years of age, in good health, with a stable neurologic status, and a good potential for walking.[1,23]

Obtaining or maintaining hip reduction and stability requires not only correction of the bony abnormality but also improvement of the muscle imbalance. In patients with subluxation, this entails closed reduction followed by consideration of iliopsoas or external oblique muscle transfers to the greater trochanter.[1,2,22,23] These transfers probably do not provide functional hip abduction but may act by removing a deforming force or via a tenodesis effect.[23]

A less aggressive approach toward improving muscle imbalance includes adductor and psoas lengthening. Proximal femoral varization osteotomy may be indicated in cases of associated coxa valga, and in a study by Weisl and colleagues this was found to be equally successful (in concert with psoas release adductor tenotomy and obturator neurectomy) as iliopsoas transfer alone.[24]

Salter and Pemberton inominate osteotomies are considered inappropriate in myelomeningocele hip

problems, because these procedures improve anterolateral coverage, and anterolateral deficiency is usually not the problem in neuromuscular hip dysplasia. Rather, the acetabular deficiency in myelomeningocele is usually superior and posterior.[1] Therefore, in cases of acetabular deficiency, an acetabuloplasty,[1,23,25,26] a shelf procedure,[27] or Chiari osteotomy is recommended to provide coverage in the specific area of superposterior deficiency. In cases of dislocation, after careful consideration, open reduction and capsulorrhaphy are added.[23]

Knee Deformity

Knee deformity in patients with myelomeningocele includes flexion contracture, genu recurvatum, and genu valgum. Flexion contracture can result from or be associated with hip flexion contracture or calcaneus foot deformity. Treatment in these cases should also address the primary cause. As knee flexion contractures progress past 15° to 20°, greatly increased demand is placed on the quadriceps during ambulation,[1,28] and flexion contractures of more than 30° are difficult to brace. Because a patient's function as a community ambulator may depend on the efficiency of quadriceps function, the reason for preventing or correcting knee flexion contractures is obvious. Serial corrective casts (including dropout casts) are sometimes used, avoiding prolonged wear to forestall osteoporosis. In severe cases unresponsive to conservative measures, release of the hamstrings, the gastrocnemius-soleus origin, the posterior knee capsule, and occasionally the posterior cruciate ligament is indicated. Rarely, supracondylar femoral osteotomy is practicable, but only after soft tissue release has proved to be inadequate. In patients with associated hip flexion contracture, the hip is treated during the same operation.

Newborn infants with myelomeningocele and genu recurvatum are frequently born in the breech position and have an associated high incidence of congenital dislocation of the hip. The level of involvement is usually L3 or L4, although some patients can have higher lesions with flial extremities and quadriceps fibrosis. The deformity does not preclude standing, but walking is difficult,[10] and sitting in a car and at school desks is impaired. Initial treatment includes physiotherapy with stretching and serial night splinting. If the deformity is unresponsive to these measures, quadricepsplasty is indicated.[1,23]

Genu valgum most commonly occurs in patients with thoracic or high lumbar lesions with a tight iliotibial band. When the deformity impairs bracing or ambulation, section of the iliotibial band is performed.[1] Carroll has noted that genu valgum can be seen in the patient with lower lumbar lesions and weak hip abductors. In this case, during stance the hip adducts, the knee flexes owing to some quadriceps weakness, and the foot rotates externally to facilitate progression of the body over the front of the foot. Apparently this causes a valgus moment at the knee with a line of weight-bearing lateral to the knee. Appropriate treatment of the contracture and orthoses with rocker-bottom shoes are recommended.[23]

Foot and Ankle Deformities

Sixty to 90 percent of children with myelomeningocele have foot deformities, often present at birth.[1,2,10,23,29] Some feet, normal at birth, develop deformity later. Equinus, equinovarus, and cavus feet can be seen with lesions at all levels.[23] In patients with lesions above L3, the feet are usually flail. The most common foot deformity in patients with L4 and L5 lesions is calcaneus foot, as a result of an active tibialis anterior muscle and a weak triceps surae.[10] Pes cavus and claw toes are most frequently seen in patients with lesions at the upper sacral levels with functioning toe extensors and weak toe flexors and intrinsic muscles.[1]

The goal in the treatment of foot deformities associated with myelomeningocele is to achieve a plantigrade braceable foot with stable skin.[1,2,23]

Pes Calcaneus

A calcaneus foot deformity is a considerable disability. The area for weight-bearing on the plantary aspect of the foot is diminished such that the risk of pressure ulceration on an insensate foot is increased. This is exacerbated by abnormal development of the

os calcis (in the absence of the trophic effects of a functioning triceps surae) with a more vertical than normal attitude. Ambulation is less efficient without the normal control of ankle dorsiflexion during midstance resulting in a crouched gait and decreased step length.[30] Initial treatment is with stretching and careful casting or bracing. In applying casts or braces, it is important to avoid high-pressure areas, which can lead to decubitus ulcers.

To improve calcaneus deformity, many authors recommend transferring the anterior tibial tendon through the interosseous membrane to the os calcis, at 3 to 4 years of age.[1,23,31,32] Banta and coworkers have had good experience with this procedure with the addition of Achilles tenodesis to the fibula. Gait studies showed improved parameters, including decreased knee flexion during stance. The need for ankle-foot orthoses was not eliminated by the surgery, however. These authors did not have problems with progressive equinus deformity with growth.[33] It has been our experience that the posteriorly transferred anterior tibial tendon alone does not provide functional plantar flexion power as determined by manual muscle testing.[34] It has also been shown that the anterior tibial muscle does not change phase after the transfer and, therefore, cannot function as a plantar flexor of the foot during gait.[35] Despite these points, benefits of the anterior tibial transfer are the removal of the deforming force and provision of a favorable trophic influence on the calcaneus.[34]

Pes Cavus

If left untreated from birth, a calcaneus foot can develop into a calcaneocavus foot, which at about 6 years of age becomes a fixed osseous deformity. Treatment is with a posterior displacement osteotomy of the calcaneus,[36] usually done in concert with metatarsal or midfoot osteotomies and plantar release. In feet with weak toe flexors, gastrocnemius-soleus, and intrinsic muscles but with functioning toe extensors, pes cavus with claw toes usually develops. Mild cases are treated with stretching, and more severe cases are treated with proximal transfer of the toe extensors to the metatarsals and plantar fascia release. In patients with bony deformity, a similar approach to that already mentioned for calcaneocavus deformity is employed.

Valgus Ankle

Valgus ankle deformity is common in children with low lumbar lesions and is seen in approximately 10 percent of patients with myelomeningocele.[37] When severe, the foot is difficult to brace and pressure ulceration can result on the medial aspect of the foot. Usually the deformity is predominantly at the ankle; therefore, subtalar fusion is not appropriate.[23] Deformity results from relative shortening of the fibula, and, as valgus configuration progresses, pressure on the lateral portion of the distal tibial physis further accentuates the growth disturbance.[1] In patients younger than 6 years of age, Achilles tenodesis to the fibula is believed to arrest progression by stimulating fibular growth.[1,38] In older children, correction is best with distal tibial osteotomy.[39] For children in whom the deformity is below the ankle, some authors prefer calcaneal osteotomy.[23] On occasion we have combined both a distal tibiofibular osteotomy with a sliding calcaneal osteotomy to fully correct the deformity. Other authors have recommended triple arthrodesis.[37] However, in general, fusion of hindfoot and midfoot bones is not advised in patients with insensate feet. If the result is not perfectly balanced, the chances for skin ulceration may increase.

Neurogenic Clubfoot

Neurogenic clubfoot in patients with myelomeningocele is usually more rigid than is the congenital counterpart.[1,2,23] However, stretching and serial casting (taking care not to cause pressure ulceration) should be initiated as soon as possible. Although partial correction is obtainable, surgery is usually necessary and usually can be done when the patient is 6 months to 1 year of age. One-stage radical posteromedial release as described by Turco and others is the most successful. Most surgeons prefer the Cincinnati incision.[1,2,23] Surgery for the neurogenic clubfoot is more radical than for the congenital type; clubfeet in patients with myelomeningocele not only require release but also require excision of portions of tendons and sheaths, fibrosed muscle, and contracted joint capsules to prevent recurrence.[1] On occasion, talectomy is indicated to obtain correction of the hindfoot in severe or recurrent cases.[40]

Congenital Vertical Talus

Congenital vertical talus is a rare deformity most commonly seen in children born with myelodysplasia, in whom it is noted in 5 to 10 percent.[1,23] The pattern of muscle imbalance associated with this deformity is that seen with lesions at the first sacral segment, with intact peroneus muscles, anterior tibial muscle, and toe extensors and poor function of the toe flexors, triceps surae, and posterior tibial muscle. The deformity is very rigid and, although it may be partially benefited by stretching and serial casting, it virtually always requires surgical correction. This is best performed between 6 months and 18 months of age.[1,2,23] Surgery entails reduction of the talonavicular and calcaneocuboid joints and rendering the foot flail, as recommended by Carroll, by release of the toe extensors, the tibialis anterior and posterior, the peroneus muscles, and the tendo Achillis.[23] Other authors recommend transfer of the peroneus muscles to the insertion of the tibialis posterior and transfer of the tibialis anterior to the neck of the talus to correct muscle imbalance.[1,2]

In general, after surgical correction of foot deformity, ankle-foot orthoses are indicated at least until skeletal maturity to prevent recurrence, and often to enhance the efficiency of gait.

SUMMARY

Children with myelomeningocele are at a distinct disadvantage from birth, because they lack the mobility with which to experience the environment and consequently, even aside from intracranial defects, are predisposed to developmental delay. Psychosocial development, development of self-esteem, and emancipation are impaired. The goal of the multidisciplinary rehabilitation team is to enhance development by intervening at certain times and not interfering at other critical stages of development. One important early determination concerns whether the patient will be a functional ambulator. In general, this is possible in patients with lesions at L4 or lower. In all patients, achievement of a straight spine and level pelvis should be attempted. Supple symmetric hips and knees are important in all patients whether they are ambulators or sitters; however, reduced hips are important only in patients with lesions at L4 or lower. Hip reduction should not be achieved at the expense of stiffness, especially in patients destined to be wheelchair users. The goal in the care of the foot is to obtain a plantigrade posture that is braceable with intact skin.

REFERENCES

1. Tachdjian M: Pediatric Orthopedics. 2nd Ed. WB Saunders, Philadelphia, 1990
2. Beaty JH, Canale ST: Current concepts review: orthopedic aspects of myelomeningocoele. J Bone Joint Surg [Am] 72:626, 1990
3. Soare PL, Raimondi AJ: Intellectual and perceptual-motor characteristics of treated myelomeningocoele children. Am J Dis Child 131:199, 1977
4. Smith ED: Spina Bifida and the Total Care of Spinal Myelomeningocoele. p. 49. Charles C Thomas, Springfield, IL, 1965
5. Simons CR, Pardes H (ed): Understanding Human Behavior in Health and Illness. Williams & Wilkins, Baltimore, 1977
6. Nickel V (ed): Orthopaedic Rehabilitation. Churchill LIvingstone, New York, 1982
7. Asher M, Olsen J: Factors affecting the ambulatory status of patients with spina bifida cystica. J Bone Joint Surg [Am] 65:350, 1983
8. Hoffer M, Feiwell E, Perry R et al: Functional ambulation in patients with myelomeningocoele. J Bone Joint Surg [Am] 55:137, 1973
9. Huff CW, Ramsey PL: Myelodysplasia. The influence of the quadriceps and hip abductor muscles on ambulatory function and stability of the hip. J Bone Joint Surg [Am] 60:432, 1978
10. Lindseth RE: Treatment of the lower extremity in children paralyzed by myelomeningocoele. Instr Course Lect 25:76, 1976
11. Hall PV, Campbell RL: Kalsbeck JE: Meningomyelocoele and progressive hydromyelia. J Neurosurg 43:457, 1975
12. Mazur JM, Shurtleff D, Menelaus M: Orthopedic management of high-level spina bifida: early walking compared to early use of a wheelchair. J Bone Joint Surg [Am] 71:56, 1989
13. Banta JV, Whiteman S, Dyck PM et al: Fifteen year review of myelodysplasia. J Bone Joint Surg [Am] 58:726, 1976
14. Raycroft JF, Curtis BH: Spinal curvature in myelomeningocoele: natural history and etiology. In AAOS Symposium on Myelomeningocoele. p 186. CV Mosby, St. Louis, 1972
15. Hall PV, Lindseth RE, Campbell RL, Kalsbeck JE: Myelodysplasia and development scoliosis. A manifestation of syringomyelia. Spine 1:48, 1976
16. Leatherman KD, Dickson RA: Congenital kyphosis in myelomeningocoele. Vertebral body resection and posterior spine fusion. Spine 3:222, 1978
17. Lindseth RE, Selzer L: Vertebral excision for kyphosis in children with myelomeningocoele. J Bone Joint Surg [Am] 61:699, 1979
18. Fergusen RL, Allen BL: Staged correction of neuromuscular scoliosis. J Pediatr Orthop 3:555, 1983
19. Osebold WR, Mayfield J, Winter R, Moe J: Surgical treatment of paralytic scoliosis associated with myelomeningocoele. J Bone Joint Surg [Am] 64:841, 1982
20. Lock TR, Aronson DD: Fractures in patients who have myelomeningocoele. J Bone Joint Surg [Am] 71:1153, 1989
21. Carroll NC, Sharrard WJ: Long-term follow-up of posterior iliopsoas transplantation for paralytic dislocation of the hip. J Bone Joint Surg [Am] 54:551, 1972
22. Sharrard WJ: Posterior iliopsoas transplantation in the treatment of paralytic dislocation of the hip. J Bone Joint Surg [Br] 46:426, 1964
23. Carroll NC: Assessment and management of the lower extremity in myelodysplasia. Orthop Clin North Am 18:709, 1987
24. Weisl H, Fairclough J, Jones D: Stabilization of the hip in myelomeningocoele. Comparison of posterior iliopsoas transfer and varus-rotation osteotomy. J Bone Joint Surg [Br] 70:29, 1988
25. Albee FH: The bone graft wedge. Its use in the treatment of relapsing, acquired and congenital dislocation of the hip. NY Med J 102:433, 1915
26. Mubarak SJ, Mortenson W, Katz M: Combined pelvic (DEGA) and femoral osteotomies in the treatment of paralytic hip dislocation. Orthop Trans 11:526, 1987
27. Staheli LT: Slotted acetabular augmentation. J Pediatr Orthop 1:321, 1981
28. Perry J, Antonelli D, Ford W: Analysis of knee joint forces during flexed knee stance. J Bone Joint Surg [Am] 57:961, 1975
29. Schafer MF, Dias LS: Myelomeningocoele. Orthopedic Treatment. Williams & Wilkins, Baltimore, 1983
30. Sutherland DH, Cooper L, Daniel D: The role of the ankle plantar flexors in normal walking. J Bone Joint Surg [Am] 62:354, 1980
31. Bliss D, Menelaus M: The results of transfer of the tibialis anterior to the heel in patients who have a myelomeningocoele. J Bone Joint Surg [Am] 68:1258, 1986
32. Peabody CW: Tendon transplantation in the lower extremity. Instr Course Lect 6:178, 1949
33. Banta J, Sutherland D, Wyatt M: Anterior tibial transfer to the os calcis with Achilles tenodesis for calcaneal deformity in myelomeningocoele. J Pediatr Orthop 1:125, 1981
34. Abrams R, Odom J: Efficacy of early tendon transfer in the treatment of calcaneocavus foot deformity in L5 myelomeningocoele patients. Orthop Trans 12:37, 1988
35. Janda J, Skinner J, Barto P: Posterior transfer of tibialis anterior in low-level myelodysplasia. Dev Med Child Neurol 26:100, 1984
36. Mitchell G: Posterior displacement osteotomy of the calcaneus. J Bone Joint Surg [Br] 59:233, 1977
37. Nicol R, Menelaus M: Correction of combined tibial torsion and valgus deformity of the foot. J Bone Joint Surg [Br] 65:641, 1983
38. Westin G, DiFore R: Tenodesis of the tendo Achillis to the fibula for paralytic calcaneus deformity. J Bone Joint Surg [Am] 56:1541, 1974
39. Sharrard W, Webb J: Supramalleolar wedge osteotomy of the tibia in children with myelomeningocoele. J Bone Joint Surg [Br] 56:458, 1974
40. Trumble T, Banta J, Raycroft J, Curtis B: Talectomy for equinovarus deformity in myelodysplasia. J Bone Joint Surg [Am] 67:21, 1985

41 Inflammatory Arthritis

RICHARD F. SANTORE
KIM L. STEARNS

The inflammatory arthritides in general are chronic illnesses that, once established, usually last for the remainder of the patients' lives. Rheumatoid arthritis, the most prevalent of these, is defined as a systemic disease that involves not only joints but also other areas of the body and requires a multidisciplinary approach to therapy.[1] Approximately 2.1 million adults in the United States (1.5 million females and 600,000 males) have classic or definite rheumatoid arthritis.[2] The individual patient experiences chronic rheumatoid arthritis as a multidimensional problem that affects every aspect of the person's life from the physical, to financial, to social relationships, to personality. These physical, economic, and psychosocial problems will exist despite the best available medical and surgical treatment. Doctors and other health care professionals should anticipate these problems and help the patient and the family deal with them. It is important to make the proper diagnosis as early as possible so that appropriate treatment can begin immediately.

Rehabilitation in the broadest sense is that process that coordinates a broad range of efforts designed to help patients achieve their maximal potential for normal living.[3] This approach involves full utilization of a team of medical and surgical specialists, therapists and counselors, and community organizations such as the Arthritis Foundation, which together form the patient's total support system. The goals of therapy are pain relief, arrest or retardation of disease progression, and prevention and correction of deformity. The ultimate goal is the achievement of maximum function within the context of permanent partial impairment. Treatment begins with the initial assessment, which involves a complete physical examination, psychosocial evaluation, and vocational and socioeconomic assessments. Early referral of patients with newly diagnosed conditions to the Arthritis Foundation is extremely helpful to them. At little or no cost, patients have access to information brochures, support groups, and educational forums.

EVALUATION

The initial evaluation should always begin with a complete medical history and review of systems. Also important to obtain is a family history of related illnesses, because many of the inflammatory arthritides have a familial basis, with genetic predispositions. Ankylosing spondylitis is a good example and is related to the presence of the histocompatibility antigen HLA-B27, found in over 90 percent of persons affected. Each child of a person who carries the HLA-B27 antigen has a 50 percent chance of carrying the same antigen, which confers an overall 10 percent chance of developing ankylosing spondylitis.

Most diagnoses of rheumatoid arthritis are made according to the criteria developed by the American Rheumatism Association (ARA)[4] (Table 41-1). In addition, the ARA has developed a functional classification system based on the severity of the disease[5] (Table 41-2). In the general community, most patients are seen initially by their primary care physicians, who should be familiar with these diagnostic criteria. In most cases, early involvement of a rheumatologist is essential.

Table 41-1. American Rheumatism Association Criteria for Rheumatoid Arthritis[a]

Conditions:
1. Morning stiffness.
2. Arthritis in at least one joint.
3. Swelling of at least one joint.
4. Swelling of at least one other joint.
5. Symmetrical simultaneous swelling of two joints.
6. Subcutaneous nodules.
7. Typical roentgenographic changes.
8. Positive agglutination test.
9. Poor mucin clot test.
10. Characteristic synovial biopsy.
11. Characteristic nodule histology.

Ranking:

Classic:	7 criteria (criteria 1 through 5 must be present for at least 6 weeks)
Definite:	5 criteria (criteria 1 through 5 must be present for at least 6 weeks)
Probable:	3 criteria (criteria 1 through 5 must be present for at least 6 weeks)
Possible:	At least 2 of the following: morning stiffness, persistent or recurrent arthritis for at least 3 weeks, history or observation of joint swelling, subcutaneous nodules, elevated erythrocyte sedimentation rate or C-reactive protein.

[a] Adopted by the American Rheumatism Association, 1963.

The criteria for diagnosis of rheumatoid arthritis include morning stiffness, joint pain and swelling, presence of subcutaneous nodules, radiographic changes, rheumatoid factor, and certain histologic changes. The degree of confidence with which the diagnosis is made depends on how many of the criteria are present and how long the symptoms have been present. Possible causes are stimuli such as an infectious viral or bacterial agent, or some connective tissue constituents that trigger the host immune-response destructive process. Thus, it is important to question the patient thoroughly about prior febrile illnesses. The history should document prior episodes, first joint involvement, history of injury, pattern of symptoms, and prior medical treatment.

Rheumatoid arthritis affects the patient systemically as well. Extra-articular manifestations include rheumatoid nodules in 25 percent of cases, and eye, lung, heart, spleen, and kidney involvement.

A history of low back pain or symptoms referable to the sacroiliac joints may be early signs of ankylosing spondylitis. This disorder generally affects the patient in late adolescence or early adulthood.

Psoriasis can produce a profound inflammatory arthritis in addition to its cutaneous lesions. Psoriasis causes pitting of the nails and may produce an erosive arthritis in the distal interphalangeal joints of the hands.

PHYSICAL EXAMINATION

The physical evaluation usually concentrates on the musculoskeletal system, with attention to the number of inflamed joints and the extent of joint involvement. Inspection and palpation initiate the examination. The range of motion of each joint must be documented, as well as joint strength. Examination of the periarticular soft tissues is critical, because soft tissue contractures often precede or coexist with joint deformities. The integrity of the supporting ligamentous structures is assessed as well. Muscle strength testing is performed, with the muscles graded on five levels[6]: grade 5 correlates with normal strength, grade 4 means good strength with some loss of strength against resistance, grade 3 denotes muscle contraction that is antigravity, grade 2 signifies muscle contraction with gravity eliminated, and grade 1 means only slight muscle contraction occurs. Although grading muscle strength is essential, the results do not necessarily correlate with endurance and do not allow quantification of a sustained contraction, the true indicators of cardiovascular reserves. Involvement of a physical therapist can be enormously helpful in providing detailed information about muscle strength grading and range of motion after initial diagnosis and throughout the course of treatment. With respect to wrist and hand evaluation, involvement of an occupational therapist is especially valuable.

Table 41-2. Functional Classification of American Rheumatism Association

Class I	Complete Able to carry on all usual duties without handicap
Class II	Adequate for normal activities, despite handicap of discomfort or limited motion at one or more joints
Class III	Limited Can perform little or none of the duties of usual occupation or self-care
Class IV	Largely or wholly incapacitated Bedridden or confined to wheelchair; little or no self-care

CERVICAL SPINE

Cervical spine involvement may ocur in as many as 86 percent of patients with rheumatoid arthritis.[7] Three types of instability are seen, including atlantoaxial instability (the most common type), superior migration of the odontoid process, and subaxial instability. It is very important to question the patient about neck pain, clicking, and pain along the back of the occiput, such as occurs with greater occipital nerve irritation, because cases of sudden death in rheumatoid arthritis patients with cervical spine involvement have been reported.[8] A gentle cervical spinal examination with flexion and extension should be accompanied by a radiographic series in any patient with symptoms. Radiographs must reveal the cervical spine to the lower border of C7. All cervical flexion and extension must be actively performed by the patient; manipulation or passive range of motion of the neck by x-ray technologists or physicians is to be avoided. Radiographs are taken as the patient gently flexes and extends the neck until symptoms begin or an endpoint is reached. It is important from a technical point of view that the seventh cervical vertebra be included in all lateral radiographic projections.

When advanced cervical involvement is suspected, a complete neurologic study is required; however, the examination may be difficult owing to the presence of severe peripheral deformity or a past history of surgery. Electromyography (EMG) and somatosensory evoked potentials aid in diagnosis and in determining the presence and level of neuropathy.

LUMBAR SPINE

In ankylosing spondylitis, progressive stiffness of the entire spine develops over time, with pain especially in the region of the sacroiliac joints. Characteristically, there is decreased excursion of the lumbar spine during forward flexion with loss of the normal lumbar lordosis. The Shober test measures the distraction of two points placed 10 cm apart with the patient erect. Normal distraction is 5 to 10 cm, but this distance is greatly reduced in ankylosing spondylitis. Radiographs of the lumbar spine show the characteristic "bamboo spine" with bridging syndesmophytes and vertebral body fusions.

Several important laboratory tests are also available to aid in diagnosis of inflammatory arthritis. The erythrocyte sedimentation rate (ESR) is usually elevated in active disease. For this reason, ESR values are not helpful in testing for occult infections in rheumatoid arthritis patients. This also pertains to the white blood cell (WBC) count, which can be elevated as a result of long-term administration of corticosteroids. Patients with rheumatoid arthritis and other inflammatory arthritides are often anemic. A normocytic anemia, typical of anemia of chronic disease, occurs in the majority of patients.[9] The presence of elevated titers of rheumatoid factor (RF) is often diagnostic. RF is a circulating immunoglobulin (80 percent IgM) causing positive latex fixation, but correlating poorly with disease activity. IgM rheumatoid factor is found in approximately 75 percent of adult patients with rheumatoid arthritis. This is not diagnostic, however, because RF is also found in 1 to 5 percnet of the normal population. In the patient with a joint effusion, the synovial fluid should be analyzed. This is best done by submitting an aspirate obtained atraumatically for complete synovial fluid analysis, including examination for crystals. Classically, in inflammatory arthritis, the synovial fluid should have no bacteria and should have 10,000 to 40,000 WBCs, with 60 to 70 percent polymorphonuclear leukocytes. Crystal analysis will help diagnosis crystalline synovitis, such as gout or deposition of calcium pyrophosphate dihydrate (CPPD). A relationship between certain histocompatibility antigens and the inflammatory arthritides is known. For instance, over 90 percent of patients with ankylosing spondylitis are HLA-B27 positive, and there is a 50 percent association of rheumatoid arthritis with the HLA-DW4 locus.

Infection is a very important consideration in the differential diagnosis of any patient with acute onset of monoarticular arthritis. Gonococcal arthritis is a possibility, and questioning the patient about sexual habits is crucial. As mentioned previously, an aspiration of the joint under sterile conditions must be performed for culture and sensitivity tests. In general, infectious synovial fluid is cloudy, with a high polymorphonuclear leukocyte count, poor mucin clot, and low glucose concentration.

In a rheumatoid arthritis patient with new acute joint effusion, it is also important to rule out coexistent infection by means of joint aspiration. However, normal indicators of infection are questionable because those patients on a long-term corticosteroid regimen may have a consequently high white blood cell count and the ESR may already be elevated, owing to chronic inflammatory disease. Any primary care physician, family practitioner, or internist is capable of performing a diagnostic work-up; however, a rheumatologist can be consulted to advise, coordinate, and help interpret the results of these diagnostic tests.

PSYCHOSOCIAL EVALUATION

The psychosocial evaluation identifies the type of coping mechanisms employed by the patient. This is best done by a psychologist or psychiatrist with an interest in arthritis patients. Patients with chronic illnesses generally go through the common stages of adaptive behavior (i.e., denial, anger, bargaining, depression, and acceptance), similar to the established mechanisms of coping with the death of a loved one. Patients are asked about their perceptions of how the illness affects their lives. The patient's support system must be explored because family members and friends are often asked to participate in the evaluation. Psychologists and psychiatrists are available to deal with problems ranging from sexual concerns to prescribing medications for sleep or depression. Meenan and coworkers have developed a multidimensional index measuring the health status of the patient with arthritis, which contains a self-administered questionnaire that was constructed using two previously tested health status measures: Bush's Index of Well Being and The Rand Health Insurance Study Batteries.[10,15] The Health Assessment Questionnaire evaluates level of activity, social involvement, activities of self-care, and emotional factors.[11] An Occupational Therapy Behavioral Model evaluates function from a behavioral point of view by assessing a patient's values, habits, personal interactions, and interactions with the environment.[12]

SOCIOECONOMIC AND VOCATIONAL ASSESSMENT

The cost of a chronic illness can often have an impact that is overwhelming for a patient and the family. McDuffie reported that the average person with stage III rheumatoid arthritis suffers a 60 percent decline in earnings during the first 6 years after onset of the disease.[13] In 1978, Meenan and colleagues published a study on the costs of rheumatoid arthritis.[14] The direct medical costs per patient were reported to be three times the national average for health care in general. The indirect costs to the patient from lost income were three times the direct medical costs, and only 42 percent were covered by transfer payments. Thus, the unreclaimed income losses were the greatest economic burden to the patient. It is apparent, therefore, that when rheumatoid arthritis strikes the main wage earner of a family, the potential effects on the socioeconomic status of the entire family are enormous.

Pincus and Callahan found that intelligence was the best predictor of improvement in social adjustment.[15] Those patients with only a grade school education suffered more functional impairment and had a higher mortality rate over a 9-year period than those with a high school education. Patients with college educations had the most favorable outcome.

PHYSICAL THERAPY

A myriad of physical methods are available in the treatment of inflammatory arthritis. The program is individualized and may be categorized as either preventive or restorative. It is important for the clinician to maintain close contact with physical therapists who are monitoring the patient's progress. Compliance is a big issue, and the closer the patient-doctor relationship the more likely it is that the patient will be compliant with the therapy regimen.

Physical therapy is very important for alleviation of acute symptoms, but there is no evidence that it induces remission or alters the state of disease progression. The mainstays of rest, ice, compression, and elevation are still useful.

Ice packs or ice massage are helpful in reducing swelling of acutely inflamed joints. Cold can provide effective short-term analgesia and is often useful in treating acute hemarthrosis because it induces vasoconstriction.

Heat may be supplied superficially or deeply. Superficially, heat produces sedation, analgesia, and relaxation but does not penetrate more than a few millimeters and should not be used for extended periods or in patients with impaired sensation or circulation. Deep heat, in the form of ultrasonic waves, does penetrate to deeper soft tissue layers and, when given over the course of several days, can be very therapeutic.

Exercise

Exercises can be performed actively or passively, and the program is individualized according to the patient's needs. Passive exercise is used less often, being reserved for patients with severe weakness or peripheral neuropathy who otherwise cannot move the affected joints. Passive range of motion can also aid in the prevention of soft tissue contractures.

The active exercise programs employed most commonly are isometric (i.e., static muscle contraction) and isotonic (i.e., dynamic muscle contraction). Rest and immobilization for short periods of time in the acute situation are acceptable, but prolonged rest and inactivity lead to muscle atrophy and loss of function. Strict bed rest leads to disuse osteoporosis, joint contractures, or bony ankylosis. Total inactivity of muscle can result in loss of strength of 3 percent per day[16] and loss of muscle bulk of 30 percent in 1 week.[17] Specific upper extremity strengthening exercises are very important because the use of ambulatory aids (e.g., crutches or a walker) depends on competent upper extremities.

Isometric strengthening produces no joint motion and is excellent for maintaining muscle tonicity in acutely inflamed joints that may be very painful to move. Quadriceps strengthening can be performed both isometrically and isotonically and is useful in the treatment of the acute inflammatory stages as well as in the perioperative period. Nordemar showed the benefits of physical training in 23 patients with rheumatoid arthritis. Those patients who trained for 4 to 8 years had a higher activity of daily living capacity; there was more pronounced weakness in the controls.[18]

The early problems encountered in patients with ankylosing spondylitis are thoracolumbar and sacroiliac joint stiffness. Spinal deformity and morbidity may be improved with the institution of an early postural and exercise program.

The Arthritis Foundation has promoted and sponsored pool and land exercise programs throughout the country over the last decade. These programs can be accessed by individual patients easily, either at their own request or upon referral from their doctor or therapist. For the pool programs, a doctor's release is commonly requested.

OCCUPATIONAL THERAPY

Occupational therapists may perform many roles in the care of the patient with inflammatory arthritis. Their primary objectives are to rehabilitate the upper extremities through the use of various therapeutic regimens already mentioned. Occupational therapists are very involved in the performance training of activities of daily living (ADL). They provide instruction on the use of raised toilet seats and the processes of dressing and undressing. Also, a program has been developed to teach energy conservation behaviors to patients with rheumatoid arthritis using standard occupational therapy techniques.[19] Occupational therapists also function in the psychiatric community and provide individual and group therapy for those patients with psychiatric disorders.

SPLINTS

Splints, braces, and casts are popular in the management of the inflammatory arthritides and, when used properly, can improve function dramatically. Their main indications are to unweight joints, stabilize joints, and position extremities in a functional posture to achieve optimum usage. There are no objective data showing that splints (static or dynamic) correct deformities, and it is doubtful that they prevent the progression of deformity. Postoperatively, splints are helpful in maintaining anatomic alignment.

Upper Extremity Devices

The common upper extremity deformities in rheumatoid arthritis involve the wrist, carpus, and metacarpophalangeal and interphalangeal joints. These deformities are commonly related to muscle and ligament imbalances, with changes in ligament and tendon orientation and secondary deformation. Wrist synovitis can lead to ligamentous laxity, causing ero-

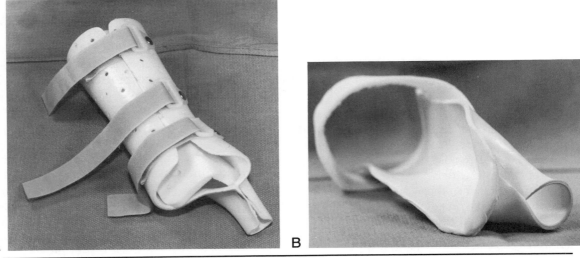

Fig. 41-1. Two types of hand splints. **(A)** Commercially produced. **(B)** Custom molded.

sion at the wrist with volar subluxation of the hand relative to the wrist. A resting splint may be worn to immobilize the wrist, reducing the inflammation and providing support, thus helping to compensate for the laxity in the ligaments. This can be effective long before surgery (such as a wrist fusion) is necessary. Two types of splints are available: (1) commercially produced splints and (2) custom-molded splints. Low-temperature thermoplastic materials (Polyform; Smith and Nephew, Rolyan) are commonly used by occupational therapists (Fig. 41-1) to custom make splints. This material softens when dipped into water at 160°F and will conform nicely to the patient's arm as it cures to a strong, rigid splint in the desired position.

In rheumatoid arthritis, deformities occuring at the metacarpophalangeal joints lead to volar displacement of the proximal phalanges with ulnar drift of the phalanges. Laxity of the volar plate at the proximal interphalangeal (PIP) joint with attentuation of the terminal extensor tendon at the distal interphalangeal (DIP) joint produces a swan-neck deformity. Attenuation of the lateral extensor bands over the PIP joint with volar displacement causes a flexion deformity force, which leads to a boutonnière deformity. The swan-neck orthosis will minimize extension at the PIP joint, thus stabilizing the lax volar

plate. The boutonnière arthrosis is essentially the same as the swan-neck arthrosis except it is worn rotated 180° to aid the instrinsic muscles in extending the PIP joint after the lateral bands have slipped volarly.

Commonly, patients with rheumatoid arthritis develop tendinitis of the first extensor compartment (abductor pollicis longus and extensor pollicis brevis), known as De Quervain's tenosynovitis. Functional wrist splints are useful in relieving pain and reducing synovitis by immobilizing the wrist and first carpometacarpal joint. Functional splints are also useful in treating carpal tunnel syndrome.

Dynamic outrigger splinting is used in the postoperative period as passive and active resistive devices for the metacarpophalangeal and interphalangeal joints or can also be used to prevent or to stretch contractures.

Lower Extremity Devices

As the foot becomes involved in rheumatoid arthritis there is a natural progression of deformity with associated pain and disability. Vainio reported that 89 percent of 955 adult patients with rheumatoid arthritis had foot problems.[20]

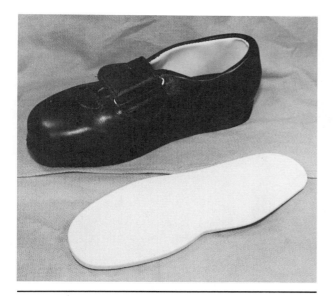

Fig. 41-2. Extra depth shoe with Plastizote insert and crepe rubber soles.

overemphasized in the patient with rheumatoid arthritis who has foot involvement. Devices need to be custom made for each patient. Early on, metatarsalgia can be relieved using metatarsal pads in the shoes. With increasing forefoot deformity an extra-depth shoe with Plastizote insert and crepe rubber soles may be prescribed (Fig. 41-2). A rocker bottom may also be added to further decrease the stresses in the metatarsal areas. For hindfoot instability and disability, a lightweight plastic ankle-foot orthosis (AFO) or molded leather ankle brace may be supportive.

Ambulatory aids such as crutches, canes, or walkers may be required. However, significant upper extremity involvement can preclude use of standard devices. Special cane hand grips and forearm crutches reduce the amount of stress on the upper extremities during usage. Walkers can be modified by adding forearm platforms and wheels to aid ambulation (Fig. 41-3).

According to Thompson and Mann, hallux valgus occurs in more than 60 percent of rheumatoid arthritis patients.[21] In the forefoot there is loss of soft tissue support of the first metatarsophalangeal joint with drift of the great toe into valgus angulation. This decreases the weight-bearing capacity on the great toe, thereby transferring increased stress to the lesser toes. This, combined with synovitis of the metatarsophalangeal joints of the lesser toes and distal displacement of the metatarsal fat pad, leads to subluxation or frank dislocation of the lesser metatarsophalangeal joints. Secondary lesser toe deformities, such as claw toe, hammer toe, and mallet toe are relatively common.

Hindfoot involvement progresses slowly in one-third of patients with rheumatoid foot problems.[21] Subtalar involvement produces hindfoot valgus deformity with secondary involvement of the midtarsal joints. The ankle joint and midfoot are affected less commonly, although ankle stiffness is a common finding in all rheumatoid arthritis patients with foot involvement.

It is important to have access to a pedorthotist, because custom-fitted shoes are required for each patient, and the importance of good shoes cannot be

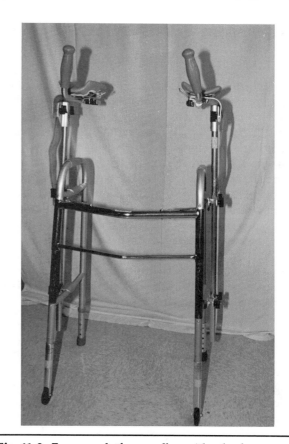

Fig. 41-3. Forearm platform walker with wheels.

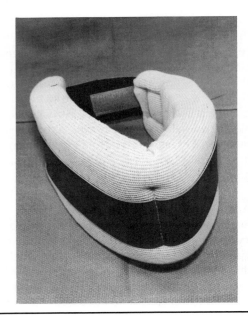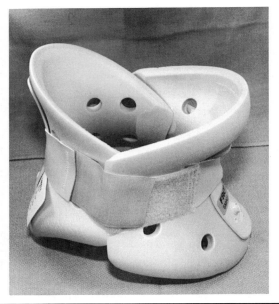

Fig. 41-4. Philadelphia collar and soft collar.

SPINAL ORTHOTICS

Spinal orthoses are used for relief of pain or to aid in stabilization. They are used mostly in the cervical spine owing to the high prevalence of cervical instability. Soft collars are used predominantly for pain relief because their ability to provide functional stabilization is minimal. A Philadelphia collar provides more support than a soft collar but still does not immobilize the upper cervical spine rigidly (Fig. 41-4). After operations, a four-poster or cervical halo may be necessary. The other spinal brace commonly used is a lumbosacral corset, which will provide limited support for low back pain and should be used in combination with a therapeutic exercise program. Reliance on a back brace or support alone leads to lumbar spine muscular atrophy.

MEDICAL MANAGEMENT

Drug therapy is the cornerstone in both the early and ongoing management of the inflammatory arthritides. Two basic categories of drugs are used. Agents that are used in the acute inflammatory period include the various analgesics, aspirin, and other non-steroidal anti-inflammatory drugs (NSAIDs). The drugs used to induce remission and also employed over long term include NSAIDs, corticosteroids, gold, antimalarials, and chemotherapeutic agents.

Aspirin

Long considered the most commonly used drug to treat inflammatory arthritis, aspirin is both inexpensive and effective. The usual starting dose is 600 to 900 mg four times a day with the aim of achieving a serum salicylate level of 20 to 30 μg/dl.[22] This provides analgesia as well as the proper levels of an anti-inflammatory agent. Common side effects are tinnitus and gastrointestinal upset; the latter can be minimized by taking enteric-coated tablets or by taking the drug with food. Poor compliance is a problem in long-term therapy because few patients remember or are willing to take the 10 to 14 aspirin tablets that are required daily for the optimal anti-inflammatory response.[23] It is very difficult to document increased efficacy with other NSAIDs, but problems with gastrointestinal upset and compliance are aspirin's biggest drawbacks.

Table 41-3. Daily Cost of the Most Commonly Used NSAIDs

Drug	Regimen	Daily Cost
Flurbiprofen (Ansaid)	100 mg tid	$2.54
Indomethacin (Indocin)	50 mg tid	$2.26
Indomethacin (Indocin SR)	75 mg bid	$2.23
Sulindac (Clinoril)	200 mg bid	$2.01
Ketoprofen (Orudis)	75 mg bid	$1.97
Naproxen (Naprosyn)	500 mg bid	$1.90
Piroxicam (Feldene)	20 mg qd	$1.70
Flurbiprofen (Ansaid)	100 mg bid	$1.70
Diclofenac sodium (Voltaren)	75 mg bid	$1.64
Ibuprofen (Motrin)	800 mg tid	$1.29

(From Cardinale VA [ed]: Redbook. William J Reynolds Publishing Company, 1990.)

Nonsteroidal Anti-inflammatory Drugs

If aspirin is not tolerated or if the desired response is not obtained with maximum dosage, another NSAID may be substituted. At the present time, many rheumatologists initiate treatment with other NSAIDs because of the problems with aspirin just outlined. In rheumatoid arthritis these drugs are virtually as effective as salicylates in full dosage and have a clinical response superior to that of aspirin in the seronegative spondyloarthropathies as well.[1] Most of the newer NSAIDs used to treat chronic arthritis are given either once, twice, or three times a day. However, their cost is much higher than that of aspirin, generally in the range of $1.00 to $2.50/day for therapy (Table 41-3).

Acting at the cyclo-oxygenase level, NSAIDs inhibit the formation of prostaglandins, which are thought to be very important in the inflammatory process. Several different compound classes of drugs are available, and it is common to switch to a drug in a different class if the response is poor or if the side effects are intolerable (Table 41-4). An initial analgesic effect occurs after oral administration, with the anti-inflammatory effect taking place after a therapeutic blood level is attained, usually in 5 to 7 days. Common side effects include gastrointestinal intolerance and exacerbation of peptic ulcer symptoms. More severe side effects are hepatic and renal dysfunction, leukopenia, and rash. Some newer oral agents (e.g., Pepcid) are available to offset some of the gastrointestinal symptoms. Because of their asso-

ciated risks of increased bleeding, these agents should be discontinued several days preoperatively. Salsalate (Disalcid) is an NSAID that is a dimer of salicylic acid. However, it is insoluble in acid gastric fluids but readily soluble in the small intestine, thereby diminishing the incidence of gastric ulceration. Unlike aspirin, Disalcid does not inhibit platelet aggregation.

Corticosteroids

Systemic corticosteroids are very potent anti-inflammatory agents and their use in the long-term management of inflammatory arthritis is common. Their use is not without major side effects, however, and the lowest possible dosage is desirable. An initial effect, known as steroid personality, is the feeling of well-being or euphoria experienced by many patients. Long-term usage may produce osteoporosis,

Table 41-4. Classes of Nonsteroidal Anti-inflammatory Drugs

Drugs by Chemical Group	Trade Name
Salicylates	
Aspirin	(Various)
Sodium salicylate and other salts of salicylic acid	Trilisate
Salsalate	Disalcid
Diflunisal	Dolobid
Indole derivatives and related components	
Indomethacin	Indocin
Sulindac	Clinoril
Tolmetin	Tolectin
Zomepirac	Zomax
Pyrazolones	
Phenylbutazone	Butazolidin
Oxyphenbutazone	Tandearil
Phenylpropionic acids	
Ibuprofen	Motrin
Naproxen	Naprosyn
Fenoprofen	Nalfon
Flurbiprofen	Ansaid
Ketoprofen	Orudis
Fenamates	
Mefenamic acid	Ponstel
Meclofenamate	Meclomen
Oxicams	
Piroxicam	Feldene
Phenylacetic acids	
Diclofenac	Voltaren

avascular necrosis, and thinning of the dermis. After being used over long periods, steroids must be tapered when decreasing the dose. Also, patients on systemic corticosteroid therapy must be covered with a steroid preparation in the perioperative period. Alternate-day dosing is desired for patients with ongoing long-term usage.

Intra-articular Corticosteroids

Localized synovitis in one or two affected joints may respond to intra-articular injection of corticosteroids. Fluid from an involved joint should be aspirated to rule out infection. Injection will often relieve pain and will be useful in the rehabilitation process, allowing earlier range of motion in painful joints.

Remission-Inducing Agents

Long-term administration of gold salts has been effective in inducing partial or complete remission. Details of administration are outlined in pharmacology textbooks, and only those physicians with proper training and experience in monitoring the usage of these agents should be involved in this form of therapy. Administration originally was provided by weekly intramuscular injections of an aqueous solution of gold salts. At present the most popular mode of administration is with the oral form of gold, auranofin (Ridaura). Gold salts are not without adverse side effects, however. Reactions include stomatitis, metallic taste in the mouth, pruritus, rash, vasomotor reaction, dermatitis, neuropathy, and rarely blood dyscrasias.

Antimalarial compounds such as hydroxychloroquine sulfate (Plaquenil) are effective in the treatment of rheumatoid arthritis. The most feared complication, retinotoxicity, is rare and dose related.

Cytotoxic Immunosuppressant Agents

Methotrexate, azathioprine, cyclophosphamide, and D-penicillamine are beneficial in treating protracted rheumatoid arthritis. Side effects can be severe. The use of these drugs required careful medical supervision and is ideally done by a rheumatologist. Recently, simultaneous multidrug therapy has emerged as a successful option in many patients, replacing the pyramid philosophy of sequential drug therapy.

SURGICAL TREATMENT

With progression of pain and deformity, surgery becomes inevitable in rheumatoid arthritis. Surgery can provide a variety of options, ranging from pain-relieving measures to life-saving procedures. The majority of these operations are elective procedures and are done to increase the function of the joint or reduce pain.

Soft Tissue Procedures

One of the more common surgical procedures in the patient with rheumatoid arthritis is soft tissue release. Releases may be performed for cases of peripheral nerve entrapment (e.g., carpal tunnel syndrome, ulnar and radial nerve entrapment), which are common disorders seen in rheumatoid arthritis. Joint contracture release may be performed either as a primary procedure or as a secondary procedure accompanying arthroplasty or tendon transfer. Releases may be performed in the shoulder joints, wrists, hips, knees, and hindfeet. Excision of rheumatoid nodules from the extensor surfaces is performed for pain, cosmesis, or nerve compression.

Synovectomy

Synovectomy is still considered very useful in patients with class I and class II disease. Synovectomy provides the most benefit in the knee and elbow. Benefits are mostly related to pain relief, with little effect on increasing motion. This procedure is considered if continuous symptoms of pain and swelling associated with synovial proliferation persist for longer than 6 months despite treatment. Synovectomy is contraindicated in the patient with advanced disease or with ankylosis of the joint and in a poorly motivated patient. Enthusiasm for arthroscopic synovectomy has developed,[24] because it is believed to decrease operative morbidity. However, complete synovectomy is difficult to achieve arthroscopically. Radiation synovectomy, which consists of an intra-articular injection of a radioactive material, is an alternative to surgical synovectomy. Results in patients with class I and class II disease after 2 years showed an 80 percent improvement.[25]

Osteotomy

Osteotomy is an excellent reconstructive alternative in the long bones of young, active patients with limited joint disease. However, this is rarely possible in inflammatory conditions, because often diffuse erosive changes involving the whole joint are present.

Cervical osteotomy is occasionally performed in the patient with advancing ankylosing spondylitis and severe cervical kyphosis.[26] Posterior osteotomies can be performed under local anesthesia, because it can be extremely difficult to intubate the patient with severe fixed kyphosis. This procedure is necessary to allow the patient to see straight ahead. No internal fixation is usually necessary, only external support being required owing to the strong propensity for new bone to form. Likewise, thoracolumbar osteotomy can correct severe kyphotic deformities in the lower spine.

Arthrodesis

In certain joints, arthrodesis is an excellent means of achieving stability, relieving pain, and improving function. Cervical spine involvement with resulting instabilities can occur, and cases of sudden death from cord compression have been reported with long-standing rheumatoid arthritis. Posterior cervical fusions are performed for symptomatic instability. Occipital cervical fusions stabilize the upper cervical spine when there is basilar invagination or superior migration of the odontoid process. Cervical fusion provide stability in cases of atlantoaxial and subaxial instabilities.[7]

The wrist may be fused when there is severe wrist involvement with volar subluxation of the carpus on the distal radius. The fusion allows the wrist to function as a fixed fulcrum. Interphalangeal fusions allow better function than individual joint arthroplasties. These fusions are performed in functional positions. Arthrodesis is very useful in the treatment of ankle and hindfoot disability. Arthroplasty has met with poor results in the ankle, for which arthrodesis is preferable. Subtalar and triple arthrodesis are performed for advanced involvement of the hindfoot unresponsive to conservative measures. First metatarsophalangeal joint fusions often accompany forefoot reconstructions in the lesser toes.

Arthrodeses of the hip and knee are rarely performed and are poorly tolerated by patients with inflammatory arthritis. Knee fusions are usually performed only as a salvage procedure after treatment of infected total knee arthroplasty.

Arthroplasty

The major joints in the extremities are served much better by arthroplasty than by arthrodesis in advanced cases. Owing to the nature of the joint involvement, diffuse erosion occurs on both sides of the joint, necessitating total joint arthroplasty. The hips, knees, shoulders, and elbows are the most commonly involved joints to require arthroplasty. Acetabular protrusion is common in rheumatoid arthritis, and patients undergoing total hip arthroplasty often require femoral head bone grafting to augment the acetabular component. Total knee arthroplasty is often more complex in rheumatoid arthritis because extreme soft tissue releases may be required in addition to the bony cuts. In the presence of bilateral severe fixed flexion contractures, it is preferable to perform the procedures simultaneously or serially within 2 to 3 weeks of each other to facilitate rehabilitation, because if only one side is done, there is a high incidence of recurrence. In the patient with polyarticular disease involving both upper and lower extremities, it is preferable, in general, to perform replacement of the lower extremity major joints before proceeding with the upper extremity reconstruction. This permits patients to walk and transfer effectively even in the presence of residual upper extremity disability.

The metacarpophalangeal joints and the lesser digits are also benefited by arthroplasty. Resection arthroplasty is the procedure of choice for forefoot involvement with subluxation or frank dislocations of the metatarsophalangeal joints. Rehabilitation of the major weight-bearing joints is covered in other chapters and will not be elaborated on here.

REFERENCES

1. Moskowitz R: Specific treatment of common rheumatologic disorders. p. 321. In Moskowitz R (ed): Clinical Rheumatology: A Problem Oriented Approach. 2nd ed. Lea & Febiger, Philadelphia, 1982
2. Lawrence R, Hochberg MC, Kelsey JL et al: Estimates of the prevalence of selected arthritis and musculoskeletal diseases in the United States. J Rheumatol 16:427, 1989
3. Krusen FH: The scope of physical medicine and rehabilitation. In Krusen FH, Kottke FJ, Ellwood PM (eds): Handbook of Physical Medicine and Rehabilitation. WB Saunders, Philadelphia, 1971
4. Ropes MW, Bennett GA, et al: 1958 revision of diagnostic criteria for rheumatoid arthritis. Bull Rheum Dis 9:175, 1958
5. Steinbrocker O, Traeger CH, Batterman RC: Therapeutic criteria in rheumatoid arthritis. JAMA 140:659, 1949
6. Gerber LH: Rehabilitation of patients with rheumatic diseases. p. 1769. In Kelly WN, Harris ED Jr, Ruddy S, Sledge CB (eds): Textbook of Rheumatology. Ed. WB Saunders, Philadelphia, 1985
7. Ranawat C, O'Leary P, Pellicci P et al: Cervical spine fusion in rheumatoid arthritis. J Bone Joint Surg [Am] 61:1003, 1979
8. Martel W, Abell M: Fatal atlanto-axial luxation in rheumatoid arthritis. Arthritis Rheum 6:224, 1963
9. Hardin JG Jr: Rheumatoid arthritis. p. 63. In Ball GV, Koopman W (eds): Clinical Rheumatology. WB Saunders, Philadelphia, 1986
10. Meenan RF, Yellin EH, Nevitt M, Epstein WV: The impact of chronic disease: a sociomedical profile of rheumatoid arthritis. Arthritis and Rheum 24:544, 1981
11. Fries JF, Spitz P, Kraines G, Holman H: Measurement of patient outcome in arthritis. Arthritis Rheum 23:137, 1980
12. Kielhofner G, Burke JP: A model of human occupation. Part I. Conceptual framework and content. Am J Occup Ther 34:572, 1980
13. McDuffie FC: Morbidity impact of rheumatoid arthritis on society. Am J Med 78:1, 1985
14. Meenan RF, Yellin EH, Henke CJ et al: The costs of rheumatoid arthritis: a patient-oriented study of chronic disease costs. Arthritis Rheum 12:827, 1978
15. Pincus T, Callahan LF: Formal education level predicts morbidity and mortality in rheumatoid arthritis. Arthritis Rheum 27:S26, 1984
16. Kottke FJ: The effects of limitation of activity upon the human body. JAMA 196:825, 1966
17. Muller EA: Influence of training and of inactivity on muscle strength. Arch Phys Med 51:449, 1970
18. Nordemar R: Physical training in rheumatoid arthritis: a controlled long-term study. II. Functional capacity and general attitudes. Scand J Rheumatol 10:25, 1981
19. Gerber L, Furst G, Shulman B et al: Patient education program to teach energy conservation behaviors to patients with rheumatoid arthritis: a pilot study. Arch Phys Med Rehabil 68:442, 1987
20. Vainio K: The rheumatoid foot: a clinical study with pathological and roentgenological comments. Ann Chir Gynaecol [Suppl] 1:45, 1956
21. Thompson FM, Mann RA: Arthritides. p. 158. In Mann RA (ed): Surgery of the Foot. 5th Ed. CV Mosby, St. Louis, 1986
22. Williams RC: Rheumatoid arthritis. Hosp Pract, p 57, June 1979
23. Katz WA: Modern management of rheumatoid arthritis. Am J Med 79:24, 1985
24. Highgenboten CL: Arthroscopic synovectomy. Orthop Clin North Am 13:399, 1982
25. Banet W, Zuckerman J, Sledge C: Synovectomy: its use in the treatment of rheumatoid arthritis. Res Staff Physician 32(10):34, 1986
26. Simmons EH: Kyphotic deformity of the spine in ankylosing spondylitis. Clin Orthop 128:65, 1977

42 Post-traumatic and Degenerative Arthritis

F. RICHARD CONVERY
MARTHA MINTEER CONVERY

ANATOMY

A diarthrodial (freely moving) joint consists of articular (hyaline) cartilage covering the ends of long bones, a surrounding capsular and ligamentous structure that connects the two epiphyses* enclosing the joint, and a synovial membrane lining the inside of the capsule. Articular cartilage has neither blood vessels nor nerves, and the synovial membrane is only very sparsely innervated.[1] Conversely the joint capsule and ligaments are very richly supplied with many larger nerve fibers.[2]

The innervation of a joint is easily recalled by remembering Hilton's law, which states that the motor nerve to a muscle tends to give a branch of supply to the joint that the muscle moves and another branch to the skin over the joint. Because all joints are moved by more than one muscle, joint innervation is from multiple nerves. For example, the hip joint is innervated by the obturator, femoral, and sciatic nerves.

The blood supply of joints is quite standardized. The capsule inserts at the point of the physeal scar, where the physis (epiphyseal plate) is or was. This insertion site has a very richly supplied circular anastomosis (the circulus vasculosus of Hunter), which provides an abundant blood supply to the epiphysis and synovial membrane.

---

* An epiphysis is the end of a long bone, the diaphysis is the center, and the metaphysis is the transitional flared area between. The physis is the secondary center of ossification that closes with maturity.

The blood supply of the proximal portion of the femur is significantly different from the standard arrangement just described.[3] The proximal femoral physis is at the junction of the head and neck of the femur (subcapital). The capsule of the hip joint inserts on the femur, along the intertrochanteric line, which is much removed (distally) from the subcapital area. According to design, the circular anastomosis is positioned at the site of the capsular insertion. The base of the femoral head receives some blood, but only a small amount from endosteal vessels of the neck. The blood supplying the femoral head comes primarily from the anastomosis, travels up the neck —outside the bone but within the capsule—and enters the epiphysis proximal to the old physis (an extraosseous but intracapsular blood supply). The artery of the ligamentum teres femoris provides a small source of supply to the region of the fovea, but this is a minimal source, and the artery is not patent in 12 to 15 percent of Caucasian adults.

Joint pain is caused by three distinctly different mechanisms. Loss of articular cartilage resulting in bone-on-bone contact causes severe pain. Subchondral bone is rich in sensory nerve fibers. One of the features of degenerative arthritis is subchondral bone sclerosis, which characteristically is highly vascular. The dull, boring pain of advanced joint disease, especially at rest, is thought to be related to vascular engorgement.[3] The richly innervated capsule is a mesenchymal tissue; like the gastrointestinal tract, also a mesenchymal tissue, it is exquisitely sensitive to

571

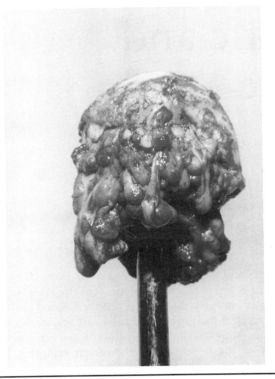

Fig. 42-1. Synovial inflammation in a hip with osteoarthritis. Many authors dislike the term "osteoarthritis," because the disorder is not an inflammatory arthritis, such as rheumatoid disease, and prefer "degenerative joint disease" (in the United States) or "osteoarthrosis" (in Europe). There is, however, a low-grade inflammatory component to osteoarthritis. Proliferative synovitis, as demonstrated in this figure, is not uncommon. White cell counts in the synovial fluid are three to four times normal and the nonsteroidal anti-inflammatory drugs are therapeutically helpful.

Table 42-1. Chemical Changes in Articular Cartilage

In Normal Aging	In Osteoarthritis
Decreased water content	Increased water content
Decreased hydrodynamic size of proteoglycan subunits	Decreased proteoglycan content
Probable decrease in collagen content	Decreased hydrodynamic size of proteoglycan subunits
	Increased proteoglycan extractability

weight) and proteoglycans (25 percent of the dry weight). The tightly enclosed chondrocytes cannot stimulate an antigenic response and therefore cartilage is "immunologically privileged," a feature that makes cartilage transplantation (allografting) feasible with only minimal concern for rejection. Chondrocytes, glycoproteins, and lipids account for the remaining 10 percent of the dry weight. The chemical changes that occur in normal aging and osteoarthritis are summarized in Table 42-1.

The arrangement of the collagen fibrils changes from the surface to the subchondral aspects of bone, an important feature in the pathogenesis of cartilage degeneration. The superficial tangential zone is composed of dense collagen fibers aligned parallel to the joint surface and is well labeled as the *armor plate*. In the middle zone the fibrils are less numerous and without specific orientation. In the deep zone adjacent to the subchondral bone the fibrils line up perpendicular to the subchondral bone, through which the cartilage is attached to the bone, and are perpendicular to the joint surface as well. This arrangement was first described by Benninghoff[4] in 1925 and is frequently referred to as Benninghoff's arcades (Fig. 42-2).

stretch. Aspiration of a tense, painful effusion, as in a traumatic hemarthrosis or hemophiliac effusion, eliminates the pain almost immediately. Irritation of the synovium, as by inflammation, also causes appreciable pain (Fig. 42-1).

ARTICULAR CARTILAGE

Chemistry

Water is the primary constituent of articular cartilage, constituting 70 to 80 percent of the total weight. The cartilage matrix tightly enclosing the chondrocytes consists primarily of collagen (65 percent of the dry

Joint Lubrication

Standard machine bearings are lubricated by a hydrodynamic mechanism in which a wedge of fluid forms at the junction of the bearing surfaces. Continuous high speed motion in a single direction is essential to maintain the wedge type of lubrication in a condition that is not present in human joints. Human joints oscillate slowly and reverse direction constantly, which prevents the formation of a hydrody-

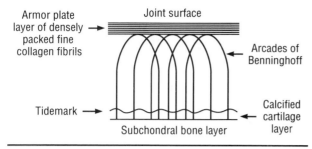

Fig. 42-2. A schematic drawing demonstrates the architectural orientation of collagen fibrils in articular cartilage. (From Benninghoff,[4] with permission.)

namic wedge; accordingly, they cannot be lubricated like a machine bearing.

Two major lubricating mechanisms function to lubricate articular cartilage, depending on the load and motion condition present.[5] In a low-load situation boundary lubrication predominates, whereas high-load, rapid motion conditions induce a self-pressurized hydrostatic weeping lubrication. Boundary lubrication (low load) occurs via the attachment of a layer of proteoglycan molecules to the articular cartilage on each side of the joint. Motion takes place between the two layers (the boundary) because the resistance to shear is much less between the layers of the proteoglycan molecules than in the attachment of those molecules to the articular cartilage. This mechanism is fragile; it will hold up only under low-load conditions and is not operational under high loads or rapid movement.

Under high loading and rapid motion conditions, weeping lubrication predominates. As the joint is loaded, interstitial fluid is squeezed out of the articular cartilage at the point of contact. A film of interstitial fluid separates the articular surfaces. When the load is released, the interstitial fluid returns to the cartilage by osmotic pressure. The combined interstitial fluid and synovial fluid lubricant is referred to as the squeeze-film.

The coefficient of friction in animal joints decreases as the load increases. It is thought that this occurs as a result of a proportionally greater contribution of the squeeze-film mechanism. Mechanical factors also contribute to the total lubricating mechanism. When

a load is applied, the articular cartilage surface flattens to decrease the frictional resistance. This mechanism is referred to as the elastohydrodynamic effect and operates in conjunction with the weeping lubrication mechanism.

To summarize, the two major mechanisms of joint lubrication are boundary and weeping lubrication, which are supplemented by the elastohydrodynamic effect, especially when large loads are applied.

Pathogenesis of Degeneration

The earliest gross change of degeneration in articular cartilage is a softening of the surface layer, initially in a focal area (chondromalacia), that is associated with an early loss of proteoglycans but no change in the collagen content. As the process continues, fissures and clefts develop in the armor plate layer and expose the collagen fibrils of the middle and deep layers, which, because of their orientation, are more susceptible to wear (Fig. 42-3). That is, they lack the wear-resistant feature of the surface layer in which the fibrils are more horizontal. The chondrocytes react by proliferation and increase the output of proteoglycans. However, despite this increase, there is still a net loss. The chondrocytes clump together in clones. Despite the loss of the hydrophilic proteoglycans, the water content of degenerating cartilage increases.

With further progresson of the degeneration, the body attempts to repair the joint. Articular cartilage lacks the inherent ability to repair itself and, since it cannot do so, nature responds by setting in motion processes that will ultimately eliminate the joint. Debris from the wearing away of the articular cartilage is absorbed by the synovial membrane, producing a low-grade irritative synovitis. The capsule thickens and becomes tighter, and motion decreases. Osteophytes proliferate at the periphery of the joint at the chondro-osseous junction and grow toward each other, in an attempt to join together from each side of the joint. The ultimate objective of these interrelated events is to eliminate the joint, first by a fibrous ankylosis and finally by an osseous ankylosis.* These processes, however, are very slow, pro-

---

* Ankylosis is complete loss of joint motion as a result of a disease process, in contrast to arthrodesis, which is a surgical procedure. Both result in an immobile, pain-free joint.

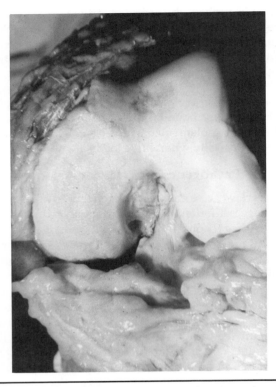

Fig. 42-3. Early degenerative arthritis of the knee showing the soft fibrillated cartilage on the lateral condyle and in the trochlea, which was in apposition to the patellar articular surface.

duce both pain and limitation of motion, lead to increasing disability, and cause the patients to seek treatment. In some respects the body's attempt at "repair" causes more disability than the loss of articular cartilage.

CLINICAL PRESENTATION

It is clinically useful, particularly with respect to the hip, to subdivide degenerative arthritis into either primary or secondary disease. Primary degenerative joint disease (DJD) is that which occurs in the absence of any recognized cause and in some patients and by some authors has been attributed to accelerated aging of the joint (malcem coxae senilis). Secondary DJD occurs in response to a preexisting problem such as acetabular dysplasia (i.e., a shallow acetabulum resulting from congenital hip disease. The clinical value of this subdivision is that the natural history of primary disease, in contrast to secondary disease, does

not necessarily involve a progressive disability. Furthermore, the age of onset in primary disease is later. The pain of degenerative joint disease is highly proportional to activity levels. With continued aging, functional requirements decrease and even though the disease may progress, the symptoms may remain constant because of the decreased functional requirements. Secondary disease usually first appears at an earlier age, most often is steadily progressive, occurs when functional expectations are much greater, and results in more significant disability. Accordingly, it is the patient with primary disease who is most likely to respond to conservative treatment, such as weight loss, the use of external support, and nonsteroidal anti-inflammatory drugs. Conservative treatment in secondary disease, although effective in the initial stages, quite rapidly becomes of limited value, and surgical intervention is required.

The concept of primary or idiopathic osteoarthritis of the hip has recently been challenged. It has been stated that, with careful radiographic assessment, clearly demonstrable abnormalities were seen in more than 90 percent of patients who had been considered to have idiopathic osteoarthritis of the hip. Furthermore, when these abnormalities were combined with known metabolic abnormalities, such as ochronosis, hemochromatosis, and calcium pyrophosphate disease, it seemed clear that either primary osteoarthritis of the hip does not exist or, if it does, it is extraordinarily rare.[6]

PATIENT ASSESSMENT

The presenting complaint in DJD most often is pain that is activity related and frequently worsens after the activity is completed, as in the evening or during the next day. When assessing the severity of pain, it is helpful to distinguish pain from suffering by an assessment of the functional limitations. There are no absolute pain units and clearly pain tolerance varies widely, depending on the psychologic makeup of the patient. To properly assess the effectiveness of conservative treatment, or to select patients for operative intervention, it is essential to quantitate, in objective terms, the pain severity. This is done most effectively by an assessment of functional limitations. The maximum walking distance is usually quantitated most easily, but it is equally important to determine not what the patient *can* do, but what actually *is* done. For example, a patient might report that he *can* walk six blocks but, when asked how often he does so, he will relate that he does this only rarely because of having to "pay for it" the next day. Pain at night, either preventing sleep or awakening the patient, is a distressing complaint; it is more common in the hip than in the knee, and it indicates more severe involvement. The quantity of analgesic medications required is frequently documented but is a subjective assessment that does not distinguish between pain and suffering. Inability to climb stairs or to get up from a chair is more meaningful information. The mechanical and symptomatic benefits of using external support (e.g., a cane) are well understood.[7] The willingness or reluctance to use a cane is a semiobjective measure for assessing the degree of pain.

The pain of DJD is a dull, aching type of pain that is poorly localized, directly related to activity, and frequently referred distally. The patient with low back disorders often will have "hip pain" with the pain actually being perceived in the buttocks. Patients with hip disease often refer to radiating thigh and knee pain. The classic example of a child with knee pain and repeated negative radiographs of the knee who has Legg-Calvé-Perthes disease of the hip is well known. Many older patients have concomitant degenerative disease of both the lumbar spine and hip, with pain that radiates beyond the knee to the foot. Although it is commonly believed that hip pain does not radiate beyond the knee, this belief is incorrect, as is known clinically and has been well documented in one unpublished clinical study.[8] In this study, the intra-articular injection of bupivacaine hydrochloride (Marcain) helped determine the most symptomatic region.

Restriction of motion is the other major complaint of patients with DJD; however, unless it is severe, it usually is not a major disability. Contractual deformities do develop and are to a degree disease specific. In the hip, external rotation and adduction contractures are usual, yet they are relatively uncommon in the patient with inflammatory joint disease (i.e., rheumatoid arthritis). In the knee, varus deformities predominate in degenerative arthritis, whereas in rheumatoid arthritis valgus and external rotation deformities are more common (Fig. 42-4). If restriction

of motion is severe, dressing of the lower extremity is made difficult. Slip-on shoes and dressing aids can be helpful.

Lower Extremity

The examination of lower extremity joint problems begins with a gait analysis. The specifics of gait analysis in the motion laboratory are reviewed in Chapter 22, but for routine clinical evaluations such sophisticated techniques usually are not required.

An antalgic (against pain) gait (i.e., a pain relieving gait) is characterized by a fast swing phase on the opposite side. The stance phase of the affected side is increased owing to an increase in the two periods of double limb support and a decrease in the period of single limb support. A normal gait is very symmetric and sounds like a metronome. An altalgic gait is asymmetric and sounds like a ticking clock. Many times — and especially in a subtle antalgic gait — the alteration can be heard better than it can be seen.

A Trendelenburg gait and the Trendelenburg sign are two different entities, but both are the result of weakness of the abductor muscles (the gluteus medius and gluteus minimus). The primary function of the abductors is not to abduct the leg but to maintain a level pelvis in single limb stance. In the presence of weak abductors on the right side, when the left foot is raised from the floor the pelvis will drop down on the left, a positive right Trendelenburg sign. The sign names the side being tested, not the side that drops. A Trendelenburg gait is compensation for weak abductor muscles; in this gait, the patient lurches over the involved side and shifts the center of gravity toward the weak side, in an attempt to shorten the body weight lever arm. A Trendelenburg gait is also sometimes called an abductor lurch.

The patient with a painful hip will also shift the center of gravity toward the painful side. Shortening the body weight lever arm decreases the amount of force needed from the abductors to maintain a level pelvis. Joint pain is directly proportional to the load applied. The load that joint receives, called the joint reaction force, is a summation of the moments of the two levers. Thus, an abductor lurch will result from two causes: weak abductors or a painful hip. The combination of an antalgic gait and a Trendelenburg gait — the coxalgia gait — indicates a painful hip.

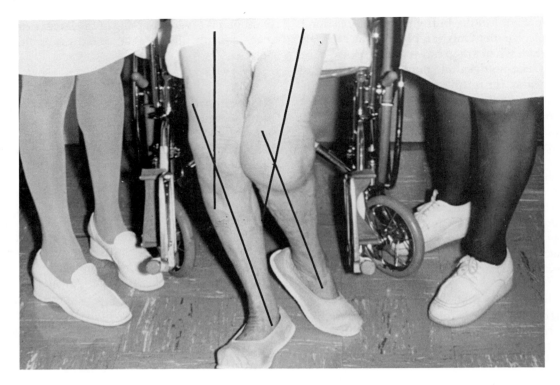

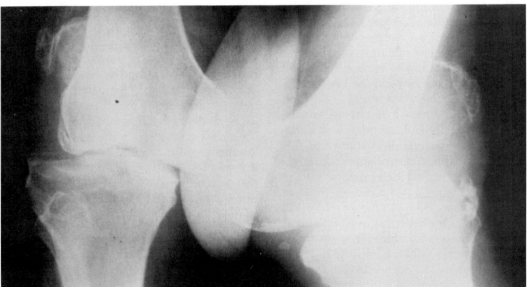

Fig. 42-4. A "windswept" deformity of the knees with a valgus deformity on the left and a varus deformity on the right. Angulatory deformities of joints are classified according to the deviation of the distal segment from the midline of the body.

The patient with DJD of the knee most usually has a varus deformity (bowleg) as the presenting feature, except when degeneration is secondary to old trauma (such as a lateral tibial plateau fracture) in which case a valgus (knockknee) deformity occurs (Fig. 42-4). Medial compartment (the articulation of the medial femoral condyle and medial tibial plateau) involvement frequently occurs secondary to old trauma, a previous meniscal injury, or a tibial shaft fracture, but most commonly it occurs because of a slowly progressive atraumatic varus deformity.

Frequently a degenerative knee in varus configuration will be unstable owing to prolonged stretching of the lateral collateral ligament. More commonly, however, the knee may seem unstable to the inexperienced examiner when a laterally directed force is applied. In this situation, the knee opens medially, giving the impression of instability. However, the opening stops at the point of physiologic valgus (5° to 7°) and is not due to laxity of the medial collateral ligament but results from loss of hard tissue (bone and cartilage) in the medial component. Ligamentous laxity causing instability is best recognized by observing a lateral thrust. Lateral thrust occurs when the tibia shifts horizontally on the femur in midstance.

A popliteal cyst is a common physical finding. A popliteal cyst is an outpouching or herniation of the posterior capsule and appears as a soft, fluid-filled cavity in the popliteal fossa between the hamstring tendons. In contrast to rheumatoid arthritis, in which rupture of a popliteal cyst is well recognized, rupture is a very rare event in degenerative arthritis although it is a common physical finding. In rheumatoid arthritis, synovial fluid flows into the cyst but does not return to the joint proper because of the so-called ball-valve effect.[9] Whether this occurs in degenerative arthritis is not known, but the size of the opening at surgery is quite large, and a two-way flow of synovial fluid in degenerative arthritis might explain the very low frequency of popliteal cyst rupture in this disease. The cyst is a secondary effect of the joint disease and treatment is directed to the joint, not the cyst. More specifically, the cyst need not be removed surgically and will resolve when the basic disease is treated, whether by conservative or surgical intervention.

Spontaneous osteonecrosis of the knee is a well-described but frequently missed diagnosis that occurs in the clinical setting of degenerative arthritis.[10] Most commonly occuring in the medial femoral condyle, the presentation is a spontaneous nontraumatic onset of pain in an elderly patient with localized pain at the medial joint line. Early in the disease process, radiographs are negative and the usual first diagnosis is a degenerative or torn meniscus. The very specific spontaneous onset, a characteristic presentation of osteonecrosis elsewhere, is an important diagnostic feature. A technetium bone scan is diagnostic if the physician orders one.

Degenerative arthritis of the ankle is quite unusual. Quite frequently, however, the ankle is a site of traumatic arthritis. Fractures and fracture dislocation that are not anatomically reduced, intraosseous loose bodies, and unstable ankles resulting from recurrent ankle sprains can all lead to traumatic arthritis. In some patients, progression to severe disability can be quite rapid.

Upper Extremity

Degenerative joint disease (osteoarthritis) is quite common in the hand. The distal and proximal interphalangeal joints and the carpometacarpal joints are the most commonly involved sites. Elbow involvement is quite rare and most usually has a traumatic cause. Degenerative arthritis of the shoulder, although not as common as in the hip or knee, is not unusual.

The shoulder is a complex of four joints working in concert. The glenohumeral joint, the scapulothoracic articulation (not a true joint), and the acromioclavicular and sternoclavicular joints all participate in shoulder motion and function. The scapulothoracic rhythm, in which approximately one-third of shoulder elevation occurs at the scapulothoracic articulation, provides for approximately 60° of motion, even if the glenohumeral joint is completely ankylosed. The acromioclavicular joint is a frequent site of degenerative arthritis, which must be distinguished from an impingement syndrome. The impingement syndrome occurs secondarily to chronic swelling and fibrosis of the supraspinatus tendon and the greater tuberosity, which, because of the swelling, becomes caught beneath the acromion and the arteriorly directed coracoacromial ligament. Classically, the patient has anterior shoulder pain as the shoulder is elevated. The pain occurs at about 60° to 90° of elevation and, once elevated beyond that point, the pain resolves. Likewise, the shoulder is usually pain free at rest. Degenerative arthritis of the acromioclavicular joint and the impingement syndrome frequently coexist. The diagnosis is established by the impingement test, in which pain is relieved by a local anesthetic injected into the coracoacromial ligament beneath the acromion.[11]

The shoulder is the most mobile joint in the body, and early loss of joint motion occurs early in the progression of DJD. The earliest change in degenerative arthritis is a loss of the range of external rotation. Although the functional need for a normal range of motion in the shoulder is not marked, it is important to institute an aggressive exercise program early in the conservative treatment of degenerative arthritis. Loss of motion due to pain tends to be self-perpetuating. When the shoulder is painful, a patient will rest the arm by the side, resulting in loss of motion. As time progresses, the contracture itself becomes painful, making an exercise program painful even though the arthritic process may be responding to conservative treatment. Especially in the older patient, a vicious cycle of pain, loss of motion, contracture formation, pain with exercise, further rest, and additional loss of motion is created.

The rotator cuff, although not a joint, is frequently a site of incapacitating degeneration. The vulnerability of the supraspinatus tendon beneath the acromion is so great that degeneration is almost a process of normal aging. In one autopsy series, the prevalence of complete rupture of the supraspinatus tendon was 26 percent in cadavers (average age, 65 years). An additional 20 percent of cadavers had partial ruptures.[12]

The supraspinatus tendon also is a frequent site of calcific tendinitis, a manifestation of attrition and degeneration facilitated by the relatively poor blood supply of the tendon. It is worth remembering that the calcification may be asymptomatic, and the radiographic presence of calcification alone does not establish the diagnosis in a painful shoulder.

A healthy rotator cuff — the conjoined tendons of the supraspinatus, infraspinatus, and teres minor muscles — that inserts on the greater tuberosity is essential for normal function and equally important for a successful shoulder joint replacement. The function of the rotator cuff is to stabilize the shoulder in abduction. Without this stabilization, when abduction is initiated by the deltoid muscle, the humeral head would sublux superiorly and abduction would not occur. The classic diagnostic test for loss of rotator cuff function is the ability to actively abduct the arm when it is first passively abducted to 90° but inability to abduct it from the zero position. If there is too little motion to allow testing, it is sometimes possible to observe superior subluxation of the humeral head with attempted abduction. Atrophy of the supraspinatus muscle, in the fossa superior to the spine of the scapula, also is an indication of little or no rotator cuff function. If there is any question of the diagnosis, an arthrogram will clarify the issue (Fig. 42-5).

The radiographic appearance of advanced destruction of the shoulder with degenerative arthritis is — in contrast to other joints — not so striking (Fig. 42-6). The relative paucity of osteophytes, the lack of marked sclerosis, and a poorly visualized cartilage space do not at all reflect the degree of degeneration or the significance of the disability.

In the hand, Heberden's nodes occuring over the distal interphalangeal joints are the most common form of osteoarthritis. These nodes are caused by an enlargement of the periarticular bone and the capsule and synovial proliferation. Progressive loss of cartilage and deformity follow. Although initially these nodes are quite tender, the long-term result is a painless deformity with flexion contractures, medial or lateral deviation, or combinations of both with subluxation.

Similar nodes occur with similar results over the proximal interphalangeal joint, but in this location they are designated Bouchard's nodes. They are frequently confused with rheumatoid nodules, which also have a predilection for the proximal interphalangeal joint.

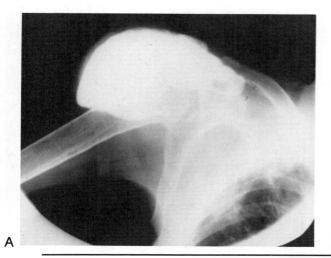
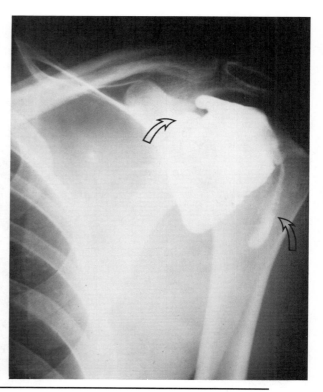

Fig. 42-5. Shoulder arthrogram demonstrating dye in the subdeltoid bursa, which is superficial to the rotator cuff and does not communicate with the shoulder, indicating a rupture. The amount of dye in the bursa does not correlate with the size of the rupture. **(B)** Normal shoulder arthrogram. The arrows indicate dye within the sheath of the long head of the biceps and the subscapularis bursa.

A special form of osteoarthritis—erosive osteoarthritis—occurs in the hands, which has inflammation as a very prominent feature. Erosive osteoarthritis is very common in females, is characterized by recurrent episodes of severe pain in the proximal and distal interphalangeal joints, and seems to have a familial pattern. The synovial membrane frequently is indistinguishable from that typically seen in rheumatoid arthritis, and the radiographs typically demonstrate characteristic erosive lesions that of the type expected to be present in rheumatoid arthritis.

Spine

Osteoarthritis of the spine is ubiquitous and is said to be universal in all patients over the age of 70 years. The presentation occurs in two forms, but both may progress to the point at which the spinal canal is compromised (spinal stenosis), with the potential for significant leg pain, sensory deficits, and even motor loss. In the diarthrodial (facet) joints, osteoarthritis develops in the same way as in synovium-lined joints elsewhere. The disk spaces are not diarthrodial joints but are syndesmoses in which there is no articular cartilage, synovial membrane, or fluid. DJD does develop, but most often it is secondary to disk disease earlier in life, previous trauma, malalignment, or metabolic abnormalities such as ochronosis.

Regardless of the initial locus of involvement, the potential for spinal stenosis exists for both forms, and it is stenotic symptoms that predominate in the elderly. In the elderly, the differential diagnosis between spinal stenosis and vascular insufficiency can be difficult, because the presenting feature of both is claudicating symptoms in the legs. Because of the

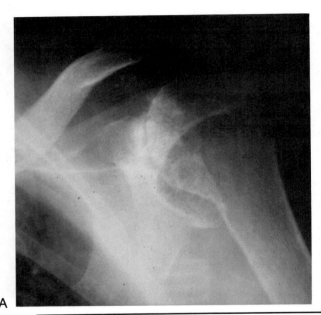

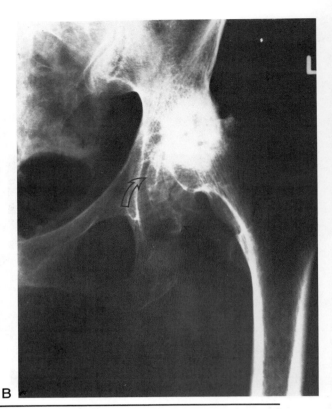

Fig. 42-6. Advanced degenerative arthritis of the shoulder **(A)** is compared to advanced destruction of the hip from the same disease **(B)**. Note the large medial osteophytes on the femoral head and the acetabulum (arrows). Such proliferative changes usually are absent in the shoulder, although superior subluxation, as in this hip **(B)**, also is demonstrated in the shoulder and indicates complete loss of rotator cuff function.

potential for serious complications, a careful vascular work-up and computed tomographic (CT) scans of the spine frequently are required.

Diffuse idiopathic skeletal hyperostosis (DISH), or Forestier's disease, is an unusual type of spine involvement that is characterized by a picture simulating ankylosing spondylitis. In addition, because approximately 30 percent of patients with two diseases are HLA-B27 positive, immunologic testing does not distinguish between the two. The ossification, however, is primarily anterolateral and occurs most frequently in the thoracic spine, is seen predominantly in elderly males, and has a characteristic "flowing" appearance. The flowing ossification anteriorly can be contrasted with the typical "bamboo" appearance of the spine in ankylosing spondylitis.

TREATMENT

Conservative Methods

In most patients, the progression of DJD from the initial minor annoyance to incapacitating disability is quite relentless, with waxing and waning of symptoms but still an increasing loss of function and increased pain. The response to therapeutic intervention will be directly related to the severity of the arthritis.

Nonsteroidal anti-inflammatory drugs (NSAIDs) are the mainstay of medical management,[13] but equally important in treatment are specific physical measures, which are much more successful than in rheumatoid arthritis. Aspirin is effective and usually is the first drug used because of cost. It is necessary to take aspirin on a regular schedule of six to eight tablets per day for it to be maximally effective. Aspirin allergy (asthma) is a recognized contraindication, and aspirin should not be used in patients with bleeding disorders. The most common side effect of aspirin is gastrointestinal intolerance or peptic ulcer disease. In part, because of this frequent side effect, a long list of new NSAIDs have been introduced. All of these are said to be less irritating to the gastrointestinal tract, but such irritation is still the primary reason for poor patient compliance. Aspirin is both an analgesic and an anti-inflammatory drug, whereas the NSAIDs have no analgesic properties. Many patients do not understand this difference and will take NSAIDs on a sporadic or an as-needed basis; consequently, they need to be educated about the need for regular administration. One of the peculiarities of NSAIDs is that although one agent may be effective in a specific patient, it may not be of help in another patient with the identical disease, but an alternative agent will be. Accordingly, when there is no response, it is frequently helpful to try several alternatives before declaring a failure to respond. There is no place in the medical management of degenerative arthritis for the use of systemic corticosteroids, antimalarial drugs, gold compounds, or antimetabolites, all of which are used in the treatment of rheumatoid arthritis.

In contrast to systemic corticosteroids, water-soluble corticosteroids given by local injection can be very beneficial in the conservative management of degenerative arthritis. Numerous studies have demonstrated the adverse effects of intra-articular steroids on cartilage metabolism, and a syndrome known as "steroid arthropathy" has been reported, characterized by accelerated joint destruction owing to the injudicious use of intra-articular corticosteroid injections. The rationed use of intra-articular injections, especially when there is an effusion or significant inflammation, can be most beneficial and can provide relief of pain for 3 months or more. Furthermore, if the alternative is surgical intervention, the known deleterious effects pale in comparison.

Physical measures are most important in degenerative arthritis. Weight reduction frequently is a major problem because reduced physical activity makes losing weight even more difficult than usual. Water exercise or swimming in a properly motivated patient can be beneficial. Even with severe joint disease most patient can use a stationary bicycle. However, as in all weight reduction programs, the reduction of calorie intake is the most essential component.

The use of a cane, although cosmetically unacceptable to many persons, can provide a major mechanical assist. Many patients who initially are unreceptive to using a cane will ultimately do so with enthusiastic counseling. Knowledge of the mechanics of the hip (see Chapter 55) is useful in understanding both the mechanical efficiency of a cane and why it must be used in the hand opposite to the affected side.

Assistive devices also serve as helpful tools. A pulley placed in the center of a door jamb through which a rope is passed can be used to increase shoulder motion. In unilateral shoulder disease a broomstick can be used in which the good side passively engages the involved side in the range of flexion and abduction motions. (Both hands grip the stick.)

Maintenance of muscle strength is equally important as maintaining range of motion. Isotonic exercise is not effective because of the pain produced, and it is particularly detrimental to a diseased joint because of the high shear forces produced. Alternatively, a resistive isometric exercise program should be taught. The goal is increased strength rather than endurance. Accordingly, maximal effort with low repetitions is appropriate, rather than a low-load, high-repetition program that increases endurance in preference to strength.

Indications for Surgical Intervention

The specifics of surgical management of degenerative arthritis will be covered in the chapters devoted to specific joints, but the indications for surgical intervention are similar regardless of which joint is involved. The goals of surgical treatment are relief of pain and improved function, but, with the exception of septic arthritis, surgery is an elective undertaking. The primary indication is disability unresponsive to conservative nonoperative treatment. Surgical treatment is a last resort, rather than a primary treatment. Once medical management has proved to be ineffective, the decision to recommend surgical treatment must be made on the basis of the risk-benefit ratio. No surgical procedure is risk free, and the possibility of a fatal outcome, although very rare, accompanies every operative undertaking.

The next consideration in making a decision for operative management is the joint involved. Replacements of the hip and knee routinely are quite successful, but 2 to 5 percent of cases do have a disastrous outcome from either postoperative sepsis or pulmonary embolism. In addition, there is a 5 to 10 percent chance of an adverse or unexpected outcome, such as dislocation, nerve or vascular damage, fracture, or leg length inequality; likewise, a number of medical complications accompany any major surgical procedure. In summary, the patient contemplating hip or knee replacement has an excellent chance (approximately 85 percent) of obtaining a perfect result. The important point is that the chance is 85%, not 100%.

Replacement of the shoulder joint when the rotator cuff is intact also usually is a very successful procedure. In the absence of an intact rotator cuff, pain relief can be expected, but very little improvement of range of motion occurs.

Replacements of the elbow and ankle have not, to date, achieved uniformly satisfactory results and still must be considered experimental. Alternative procedures, such as resection arthroplasty of the elbow and arthrodesis of the ankle, are available and as of this date are preferable, although each of these procedures has specific limitations.

Wrist replacement in properly selected patients—usually patients with rheumatoid arthritis—can be very helpful, but in patients with degenerative and traumatic arthritis, arthrodesis is probably preferable.

REFERENCES

1. Freeman MA, Wyke B: The innervation of the knee joint. An anatomical and histological study in the cat. J Anat 101:505, 1967
2. Kellgren JH, Samuel EP: The sensitivity and innervation of the articular capsule. J Bone Joint Surg [Br] 32:84, 1950
3. Trueta J: Studies of the Development and Decay of the Human Frame. WB Saunders Company, Philadelphia, 1968
4. Benninghoff A: Form und Bau der Gelenkknorpel in ihren Beziehungen zur Funktion. Z Anat Entwicklungsgesch 76:43, 1925
5. Radin EL, Paul IL: A consolidated concept of joint lubrication. J Bone Joint Surg [Am] 54:607, 1972
6. Harris H: Etiology of osteoarthritis of the hip. Clin Orthop 213:20, 1986
7. Blount WP: Don't throw away the cane. J Bone Joint Surg [Am] 38:695, 1956
8. Kleiner J, Thorne R, Curd J: The value of bupivicaine hip injection in the differentiation of coxarthroses from lower extremity neuropathy. Proceedings of the Resident Research Conference, University of California, San Diego, 1989
9. Jayson I, Dixon AS, Kates A et al: Popliteal and calf cysts in rheumatoid arthritis. Ann Rheum Dis 31:9, 1972
10. Ahlback S, Bauer GGH, Bohne WH: Spontaneous osteonecrosis of the knee joint. Arthritis Rheum 11:705, 1968
11. Neer CS II: Impingement lesions. Clin Orthop 173:70, 1983
12. Wilson CL, Duff GL: Pathologic study of degeneration and rupture of the supraspinatus tendon. Arch Surg 47:121, 1943
13. Brandt KD, Slowman-Kovacs S: Nonsteroidal antiinflammatory drugs in treatment of osteoarthritis. Clin Orthop 213:84, 1986

43 Hemophilic Arthropathy

JAMES V. LUCK, Jr.
CAROL K. KASPER

Hemophilia, which is inherited as a sex-linked recessive trait, occurs at a rate of in 1 in 10,000 male births in the United States. Two forms occur: hemophilia A, or factor VIII deficiency (approximately 85 percent of cases), and hemophilia B, or factor IX deficiency (about 15 percent). As many as 25 percent of cases of hemophilia A may be the result of de novo mutation, which is one of the highest rates for mutation for any genetic disorder.[1,2] These patients have a completely negative family history for hemophilia.

Hemophilia is associated with an arthropathy that commonly is symmetric and involves most often the knees, elbows, and ankles. The hips, shoulders, and subtalar joints are affected moderately frequently, and involvement of the wrists, fingers, and toes is rare. We have never seen a patient with primary spinal involvement.

The pathophysiology of hemophilic arthropathy has not yet been fully elaborated. It is known that articular cartilage is destroyed by direct synovial invasion and formation of subchondral synovial and degenerative cysts. As in other inflammatory arthritides, enzymatic degradation has been documented.[1,3] Iron pigment is deposited to a much greater extent than in other conditions with acute or chronic hemarthrosis and is presumed to be the precipitating cause of hemophilic synovitis.

The arthropathy all too often runs an unrelenting course from hemarthrosis to chronic synovitis with extensive erosion of joint surfaces and, ultimately, end-stage joint destruction (Fig. 43-1). However, the degree of response is not identical in all patients or even in all affected joints in the same patient. Bleeding into the joint may initiate a smoldering, low-grade synovitis and be followed by recurrent, subclinical bleeding that leads to steadily progressive arthropathy. Alternatively, one or more of the major joints may remain normal throughout the patient's adult life despite several hemorrhages in childhood and adolescence. Probably some type of autoimmune sensitivity is involved in this diversity of response. End stage is further complicated by arthrofibrosis and loss of motion as the hypertrophic synovium is replaced by dense, fibrous scar tissue. Often the patient develops severe contractures and deformity.

MANAGEMENT OF ACUTE HEMARTHROSIS

Before blood concentrates became available, treatment consisted of infusion of whole blood or plasma and prolonged immobilization and inactivity. Fibrosis is especially common in hemophilic arthropathy, and confinement to a wheelchair caused the joints to become frozen into position (Fig. 43-2). Equally severe were the accompanying muscle atrophy and concomitant joint destruction and deformity. Today the goal is to interrupt the progression of the arthropathy before it reaches an irreversible stage. The greatest chance of success is in the earliest phases of acute hemarthrosis.

As noted earlier, the mere presence of blood within the joint causes synovitis; this is the principal and perhaps the only etiologic factor. Unfortunately,

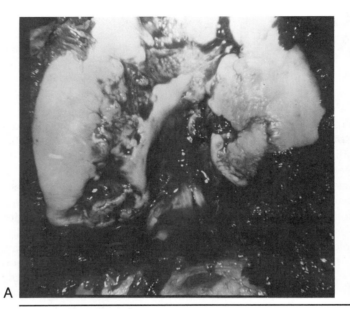
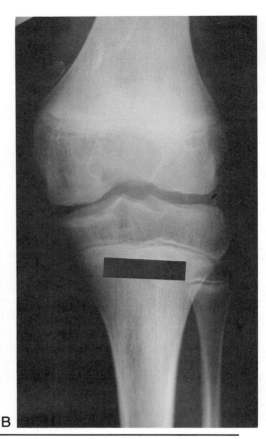

Fig. 43-1. (A) Chronic synovitis with chronic hemarthrosis in a hemophilic 14-year-old patient with severe factor VIII deficiency (type A). Note full-thickness erosion of most of the articular cartilage of both femoral condyles and the trochlea opposite the patella. **(B)** The patient's plain anteroposterior radiograph is deceptively benign, as is often the case, with minimal surface irregularity and good preservation of joint space.

once chronic synovitis develops, it is unlikely to resolve without causing arthropathy, and arthropathic joints in turn are unlikely to return to normal. With treatment, the rate of progression may be altered, but it seems inexorable. Treatment therefore must attempt to prevent synovitis before it can develop.

For this to be effective, parents and patients must learn the first signs of hemarthrosis—a limp in toddlers or a tingling sensation in older children. Because these signs must be learned, they probably are not feasible for recognizing the initial hemarthrosis early, but they may be useful for identifying subse-

quent hemarthroses or initial hemorrhages in other joints.

The goal of treatment is a return of the joint to normal. Management consists principally of early replacement of the deficient coagulation factor and restorative physical therapy (Fig. 43-2). For more significant hemarthroses, splinting may help reduce pain and inflammation in the initial 24 hours. Aspiration, although somewhat controversial, at times is clearly indicated (see later discussion). Close followup with careful examination is required to detect smoldering synovitis. Restorative physical therapy

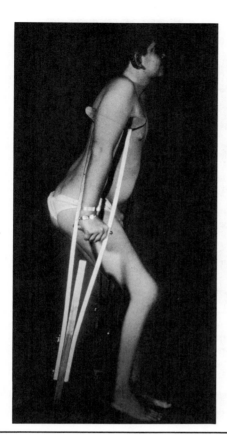

Fig. 43-2. Eleven-year-old patient with severe type A hemophilia who had marked contractures of his hips and knees as a consequence of hemophilic arthropathy and long periods sitting in a wheelchair. Today, with factor VIII coverage, physical therapy would be used a few days after a hemarthrosis to preserve joint range of motion and muscle strength.

and a conscientious, life-long exercise program are highly important in preventing rebleeding, chronic synovitis, and arthropathy.

As part of the annual comprehensive team evaluation, patients are examined by a physical therapist, who determines girth, strength (by both manual muscle testing and isokinetic analysis), and range of motion for all joints. These measurements provide baseline values for comparison when evaluating recovery from hemarthrosis.

ASPIRATION

Indications

The role of aspiration in the management of acute hemarthrosis remains contested, largely because it has never been proved to prevent chronic synovitis and consequent arthropathy. Nevertheless, several situations exist for which aspiration clearly is beneficial.

Painful Hemarthrosis

Aspiration may be very helpful in relieving a tense hemarthrosis, which often is accompanied by a severe pain that may not subside until after several days of splintage and blood factor replacement. This frequently requires hospitalization and parenteral administration of narcotics. In our experience, the amounts of potentially addictive analgesics needed by the patient are reduced and hospitalization sometimes can be avoided entirely by early aspiration. Other benefits include shortening of the duration of disability and possible prevention of elbow or shoulder hemorrhage by reducing the period of dependency on crutches.

Open Epiphyses and Hemarthrosis of the Hip

The need for aspiration is probably most urgent (and most definite) in a child or youth with open epiphyses who has an acute hemarthrosis of the hip. If the increased intra-articular pressure is not relieved, circulation to the femoral head will be impaired, leading to ischemic necrosis and ultimately degenerative arthritis (Fig. 43-3). Aspiration should be performed within 6 hours of onset of the hemorrhage. Unfortunately, many patients have been instructed on how to treat themselves with blood factor at home, and consequently they rarely are seen by a physician until the day after the bleeding began. Special patient and family education is needed in this area to prevent serious complications.

A hemophilic patient with severe groin pain whose hip is held in flexion, abduction, and external rotation and who is afebrile can be diagnosed with high prob-

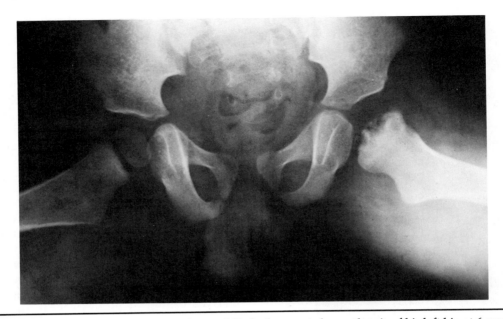

Fig. 43-3. This patient with type A severe hemophilia had an acute hemarthrosis of his left hip at 6 months of age, which resulted in avascular necrosis of the capital femoral epiphysis. As is evident on this radiograph at 18 months, the femoral head never developed. (From Luck JV Jr, Kaspar CK: Surgical management of advanced hemophilic arthropathy. Clin Orthop 242:60, 1989, with permission.)

ability to have hemorrhage, but it still remains to be determined whether the bleeding is retroperitoneal or intra-articular. Clues may be subtle, such as anterior thigh numbness in cases of retroperitoneal bleeding. Quadriceps muscle weakness is difficult to evaluate, but the patellar reflex may be diminished in severe retroperitoneal hemorrhage. An anteroposterior pelvic radiograph with increased femur-to-teardrop (FT) distance that had not been present previously indicates hip hemorrhage with significantly increased pressure, and aspiration should be performed immediately. With less severe hip bleeding and no increase in FT distance on radiographs, the patient is probably not at risk for ischemic necrosis. In addition, closure of the epiphyseal plate also is associated with a markedly diminished risk of necrosis.

Although ultrasonography and computed tomography (CT) are quite useful in defining retroperitoneal hemorrhage, they may consume valuable time that might better be spent in instituting treatment as early as possible. If lateral subluxation of the femoral head appears on the radiograph of a hip that heretofore

had been normal, aspiration should be performed before additional diagnostic studies are undertaken.

Pyarthrosis

Although hematogenous spread of infection is rare, it is a well-established phenomenon in cases of hemarthrosis. An additional strong indication for aspiration in acute hemorrhage into the joint is to rule out pyarthrosis.

Technique

An important consideration when employing aspiration is to minimize the pain and psychic trauma to the patient. If fears are aroused by the procedure, patients (especially children) may fail to report subsequent hemorrhages. Small children may benefit from sedation prior to aspiration, but older patients require only a careful, reassuring explanation. A local anesthetic will be effective in eliminating discomfort and can be given using a 27-gauge needle. Meticulous sterile technique is mandatory, and cultures should be obtained from the aspirate routinely.

Prevention of Synovitis

Will aspiration help prevent chronic synovitis and speed recovery in the patient with moderate hemarthrosis and a normal joint? At least in theory this would seem likely, because absorption of blood by the synovium leads to pigment deposition and is responsible for chronic hemophilic synovitis. Therefore, reducing the volume of blood in the joint through aspiration might well prevent irreversible changes. However, this is still speculative and requires further research.

GRADING OF HEMARTHROSIS

For convenience, a grading system for hemarthrosis would be valuable. Different joints may be graded differently; for example, in the knee, four grades are definable:

Grade I: Medial fluid wave only; patella not ballotable
Grade II: Patella ballotable on compression of the suprapatellar pouch
Grade III: Patella ballotable without compression of the suprapatellar pouch
Grade IV: Tense hemarthrosis; patella not ballotable

For other joints, such as the elbow and ankle, probably only three grades (mild, moderate, severe) are required.

Mild: Barely detectable fluid wave
Moderate: Easily ballotable
Severe: Tense hemarthrosis

Grading of hemarthrosis of deep joints, such as the hip and shoulder, depends on severity of symptoms and radiographic findings, including capsular distention and joint subluxation. Because these changes are difficult to quantify, involvement probably is definable only as moderate and severe. Slight degrees of hemarthrosis are very difficult to differentiate from other conditions that cause similar symptoms.

Decisions on aspiration often are made on the basis of the grading system. For example, our present guidelines for joint aspiration of the knee are shown in Table 43-1. If chronic synovitis develops, aspiration is no longer performed for grade II or III he-

Table 43-1. Guidelines for Joint Aspiration of the Knee

Grade	Normal Joint	Arthropathic Joint
I	No	No
II	Yes	No
III	Yes	Only if symptoms warrant
IV	Yes	Yes

marthroses unless symptoms warrant. The only strong contraindication is the presence of a blood factor inhibitor.

SURGICAL INTERVENTION

Operations for hemophilic arthropathy may be divided into three categories according to severity of the joint pathology: synovectomy is used in early to moderate arthropathy, synovectomy and débridement in moderate to advanced arthropathy, and arthrodesis or arthroplasty in advanced or end-stage arthropathy.

Before factor VIII concentrate became available in 1967, surgery was undertaken only very rarely for advanced hemophilic arthropathy, mainly in patients with mild hemophilia and higher blood levels of factor VIII or IX.[4-6] After the concentrate was introduced, surgeons at major hemophilia centers began treating patients with end-stage hemophilic arthropathy with reconstructive surgery.[5-9]

Over the past quarter century (from mid-1967 to the present), over 500 major operations for arthropathy were performed on hemophilic patients at our institution. A report was published earlier on the hematologic management of these patients for the years 1967 to 1983.[9] The frequency of postoperative hemorrhage was not reduced even when triple the amount of factor VIII concentrate was given. Rather, the frequency of bleeding after surgery correlated much better with site and type of surgery than with circulating levels of factor VIII at the time the bleeding began. For example, the rate of occurrence of postoperative hemorrhage at the surgical site was 40 percent for the knee compared with 15 percent for all other sites. Kay and colleagues[10] had reported similar results.

Careful screening is carried out preoperatively for presence of factor VIII inhibitor or any medical contraindication to an elective reconstructive procedure. Factor VIII concentrate is given so blood levels are above 100 percent of normal 1 hour before surgery. For 2 weeks postoperatively, bolus therapy with factor VIII is continued every 8 to 12 hours with the intent of reaching a trough of 60 percent of the normal level. If the patient requires vigorous phys-ical therapy to increase the joint range of motion, infusions are given before each session so that the blood level of factor VIII reaches 30 percent of normal.

At our institution, the practice for the past 5 years has been to maintain a constant level of factor VIII of at least 60 percent of normal for the first week by continuous infusion. In keeping with efforts at cost containment, selected patients—only those who have undergone lesser procedures (such as radial head excision and elbow synovectomy), who are on a self-infusion program, who live close by, and who are eminently reliable—are permitted to leave the hospital after the first week. No complications have been reported after discharge with this protocol.

In the following sections, we describe our experience with surgical intervention in advanced hemophilic arthropathy by specific anatomic regions.

Shoulder

Arthropathy of the shoulder has received relatively little attention, but there is no joint in the body in which muscle atrophy is of more crucial import. In addition, as with hip pain, pain in the shoulder can be intractable, interfering with daily activities and interrupting sleep.

Conservative measures frequently are of little use in chronic synovitis of the shoulder. Attempts at strengthening result in increased pain and bleeding. Radionuclide synoviorthesis, although used for 20 years in other countries for hemophilic synovitis, is just beginning to be used in the United States.[11-13] Other methods also lack effectiveness; open shoulder

synovectomy is no longer performed because it is associated with persistent pain and excessive loss of motion, and shoulder arthroscopy would be severely limited by the extreme fibrosis and hyperplasia that characterize synovitis in this joint.

Consequently, synovitis in the shoulder progresses inexorably to end-stage arthropathy. The patient usually has severe stiffness and muscle atrophy, and, as in other joints, hemarthrosis diminishes as fibrosis develops. Pain is the primary indication for surgery; the loss of shoulder motion by itself does not cause enough impairment of the activities of daily living to warrant surgical intervention.

Either arthroplasty or arthrodesis may be chosen; the patient must be involved in the decision after receiving careful counseling. Traditionally arthrodesis has been the approach used for end-stage arthropathy of the shoulder. This technique gives predictable and dependable long-term results, but results in a lesser range of motion for the joint, especially rotation. A concomitant impairment of elbow motion, which nearly all these patients have, makes the loss of motion of the shoulder even more serious.

Among the first three patients treated by arthrodesis at our institution, two did not achieve solid bony union, although clinical results were good (absence of pain and bleeding into the joints) because fibrous ankylosis was secure. Apparently the nonunions resulted from a combination of fixation using a single-plane glenohumeral screw and reactive sclerosis at the glenohumeral joint. No nonunions have occurred since our institution began using the three-plane screw fixation method developed by Vainio (Fig. 43-4), which involves AO screw fixation of the acromiohumeral and coracohumeral junctions in addition to the glenohumeral joint. Added stability is achieved with glenohumeral and acromiohumeral wire loops. In shoulder arthrodesis, the upper extremity is placed in a salute position with the shoulder in 20° to 30° of scapulohumeral abduction, 30° of forward flexion, and 30° to 40° of internal rotation. The shoulder is immobilized in a modified Bateman pillow support, which will allow periodic elbow motion, until fusion is apparent radiographically. All of the patients undergoing arthrodesis are able to reach the top of the

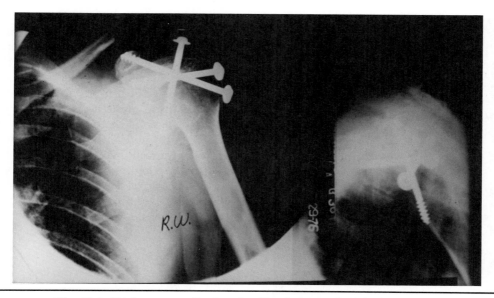

Fig. 43-4. Triplane screw fixation shoulder fusion as described by Vainio

head with the help of neck flexion, and all can reach the sacrum.

Over the past decade we have performed three prosthetic shoulder arthroplasties in hemophiliac patients using Neer II prostheses with cement fixation. Thus far, with 4 to 10 years' follow-up, the results in all cases have been satisfactory. Recurrent hemarthroses have not occurred in any of the patients, and two have remained pain free, with the remaining patient having occasional slight pain. The range of motion has been improved in all after the surgery. In addition, rotation is better than in the patients who underwent arthrodesis, although forward flexion and combined abduction are essentially the same after both procedures.

Elbow

Even in end-stage arthropathy of the elbow, symptoms are seldom severe enough to warrant surgical intervention. Only radial head excision and synovectomy have been found useful for these patients. Radial head excision with or without synovectomy is indicated if the patient has pain, chronic bleeding unresponsive to other methods of treatment, and loss of forearm rotation (mainly supination), to an extent that it causes disability. These complications are predominantly the result of derangement of the proximal radioulnar joint secondary to hypertrophy and irregularity of the margins of the radial head (Fig. 43-5). Typically the pain is posterolateral and the patient has focal tenderness over the posterior aspect of the proximal radioulnar joint; in addition, pain increases on forearm rotation, particularly supination. The level of resection is just below the ulnar facet, which eliminates impingement but preserves part of the annular ligament, which provides stability.

This procedure has produced excellent results; pain relief has been quite good even though most patients have advanced ulnohumeral joint degeneration, and recurrent or chronic hemarthroses have been eliminated in approximately 90 percent of patients. Preoperatively, loss of supination causes the most impairment to the patient, especially when supination is less than 45°. This degree of loss will impair the patient's ability to eat normally, accept coins when making purchases, and carry out personal hygiene tasks. Persons who had had limited ability to rotate the forearm preoperatively have gained an average of 30° of supination after radial head excision, which has significantly improved their ability to perform the activities of daily living.

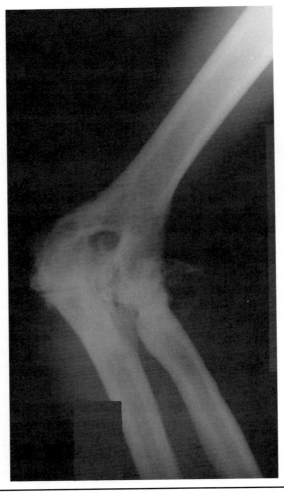

Fig. 43-5. Advanced hemophilic arthropathy of the elbow demonstrating marked hypertrophy of the radial head, which impinges on the ulna and restricts forearm rotation.

Flexion-extension range is a function of the ulnohumeral joint, its capsule, and the musculotendenosis units crossing the joint and is not significantly altered by excision of the radial head with synovectomy. In addition, loss of the flexion-extension range in chronic hemophilic arthropathy is a long-term process that is not significantly altered by débridement of the ulnohumeral joint, which is often performed in conjunction with radial head excision and synovectomy for smoother joint motion. Surprisingly, in one of our cases, flexion-extension range was improved dramatically by a combination of surgical and medical management. A 10-year-old boy with severe type A hemophilia developed heterotopic ossification after a hemorrhage in his right (dominant) brachialis muscle. The elbow flexion range was reduced from 135° to 10°. One year later, when the patient's alkaline phosphatase level had returned to normal, the finger of heterotopic bone extending from the distal humerus across the elbow was excised. This was followed by 6 weeks of therapy with indomethacin and diphosphonate, which was successful in preventing recurrence of the heterotopic ossification. Continued passive motion postoperatively and several weeks of physical therapy were successful in restoring the patient's elbow range of motion to normal.

Hip

Arthropathy of the hip occurs less commonly than arthropathy of the knee, ankle, or elbow in hemophilia. Children may develop a rapidly progressive, severe arthropathy after a single bleeding episode as a result of increased intracapsular pressure, which leads to osteonecrosis of the capital femoral epiphysis (Fig. 43-3). More commonly, however, the arthropathy results from chronic synovitis, as in other joints.

J. Vernon Luck, Sr., performed the first prosthetic arthroplasty of the hip in a hemophilic patient in the United States in 1968. This pioneering operation was a cup arthroplasty. At our institution, between 1968 and 1982 six different surgeons performed a total of three additional cup arthroplasties and 10 primary cemented hip replacements. The surgeons differed in their choice of prostheses, which included the Mueller (five cases), Aufranc-Turner (two cases), Charnley (one case), Harris (one case), and Wagner resurfacing (one case) prostheses. In addition, six primary hip replacements using cementless prostheses have been performed since 1982.

The long-term survival of these various types of hip replacement has been no better than fair (60 percent revision rate over a period of 22 years). Nevertheless, the clinical outcome has been entirely satisfactory in that patients without other major disabling conditions are substantially better off today than before their original surgery, and all are capable of unrestricted community ambulation without assistive devices.

Among the 16 patients treated surgically at our institution, nine have required revisions: three cup arthroplasties for pain and bleeding, five cemented hip replacements (three for loosening without infection and two for sepsis), and a repeat Wagner resurfacing 5 years after the original operation because of a fracture of the femoral neck sustained in a fall. In this last-mentioned patient, even though the cement-bone interface remained secure on both sides of the joint, the femoral head was avascular and the reactive membrane occupied approximately 50 percent of the cement-bone surface area on the acetabular side. One of the two septic cases required a Girdlestone resection arthroplasty for a *Pseudomonas aeruginosa* infection; he is free of pain and able to get about the community without the need for assistive devices.

At 8 to 18 years' follow-up, aseptic failures have been seen in 33 percent of primary cemented prostheses —a rate that would seem to be slightly higher than might be expected for another form of polyarthritis in comparable groups of patients. Loosening of cemented prostheses in hemophilic patients may be explained partially by increased stresses caused by the remarkably stiff-legged gait seen in advanced hemophilic arthropathy. This stiffness results from severe arthrofibrosis of the knee and ankle, which results in a lengthened lever arm and loss of normal shock absorption by the ankle and knee. All of the patients with aseptic failures had bilateral knee and ankle arthropathy, and none had had knee replacements.

Finally, among the six operations using porous coated uncemented hip prostheses performed at our institution since 1982, none has required revision. However, a longer follow-up period is needed to determine if this method does indeed provide significant improvement.

Knee

The knee is the only joint in which we have had experience with synovectomy as an isolated procedure. The indications for this operation are recurrent or chronic hemarthroses unresponsive to appropriate conservative management. A trial of conservative treatment usually requires 4 to 6 months. However,

by the time these patients come to surgery, they usually have a significant amount of full-thickness articular cartilage erosion, and the remaining articular surface certainly has sustained significant mechanical and biochemical stresses. For these reasons, synovectomy is rarely, if ever, curative but is often effective in resolving the chronic and recurrent hemarthroses and possibly slowing the progression of arthropathy. Resolution of the chronic hemarthrosis allows the patient to resume therapeutic exercises, often with marked improvement in function and significantly reduced requirement for clotting factor replacement.

Although it would seem reasonable to consider surgical synovectomy before joint surface derangement occurs, this is usually impractical. The erosion occurs very early in this process, often before the synovitis becomes symptomatic and before any radiographic changes become evident. In addition, usually the patients are in the age range of 3 to 8 years, quite young to consider for a major operation in the face of mild symptoms and uncertainty about long-term benefit.

Over the last two decades, several hemophilia centers around the world have used radionuclide synovectomy in the hope of resolving the synovitis before irreparable joint surface destruction occurs. In these cases as well, the early age of onset has posed an obstacle because physicians at most centers are reluctant to subject children under the age of 10 years to high-dose radiation even if it is well localized and contained. Radionuclide synovectomy is especially useful in the hemophilic patient with chronic synovitis who would be a candidate for surgical synovectomy but who must be turned down because of a high level of clotting factor inhibitor.

Severe pain and disability in hemophilic patients is most frequently the result of end-stage arthropathy of the knee. Although the ankle and elbow joints are involved about equally frequently, they require surgical intervention less often. We have had experience with five types of operations: débridement, débridement with patellectomy, osteotomy, fusion, and prosthetic arthroplasty. Currently only three of these are used, because the results of patellectomy and osteotomy have not been satisfactory.

Débridement may be either arthroscopic or open. Recurrent hemarthrosis unresponsive to conservative management and symptoms of impingement, usually associated with loss of extension, are the primary reasons for performing débridement. The impingement symptoms may be intermittent, but sometimes they are unrelenting, and vigorous exercise or even passive range of motion may result in hemarthrosis, in which case débridement is indicated. The pain usually responds to nonsteroidal anti-inflammatory drugs (NSAIDs) and analgesics. However, when pain is the predominant symptom in cases of advanced arthropathy, débridement is rarely of long-term benefit. In a series of 18 patients who underwent débridement, six later required total knee replacement. The follow-up period ranged from 7 to 21 years, and in four of the failures, the total knee replacement was needed within 1 year of the débridement. Patients in whom débridement failed had arthropathic pain as their primary symptom and were older at the time the procedure was performed (average age, 30.8 years) than those who gained lasting benefit (average age, 16.5 years).

Loss of range of motion was a problem more often with open than with arthroscopic débridement. The arthrofibrosis that often characterizes advanced hemophilic arthropathy is the primary cause of this complication.[1,14-19] For open débridement the range of motion decreased by an average of 28°, versus 9° for arthroscopic débridement. However, 50 percent of patients undergoing the arthroscopic procedure had postoperative hemarthrosis, whereas none in the open débridement group had bleeding. This is attributed to the lack of hemostasis with arthroscopic débridement.

In our institution, primary knee fusions have been performed in seven cases of end-stage arthropathy. In two cases the patients had infections (one a hematogenous pyarthrosis with *Pseudomonas aeruginosa* and the other a chronic *Staphylococcus aureus* osteomyelitis occurring after an osteotomy). In five of the patients, including the one with the *Pseudomonas* infection, solid fusion was obtained without complications. The sixth patient bled from the denuded bone surfaced and the knee swelled to such an extent that the Charnley external compression device had to be removed. Healing took place without infection, al-

though the patient has a stable but painless pseudarthrosis. He is fully ambulatory with a cylinder orthosis. In the seventh patient, who had chronic osteomyelitis, fusion was obtained but a draining sinus developed. Six of the seven patients have involvement of both ankles and limited motion in the contralateral knee, but they can rise from chairs (preferably armchairs) without the need for assistive devices. None of these patients has developed associated ipsilateral hip or low back problems.

The knee is the joint that most frequently requires replacement in hemophilic arthropathy. The indications are mainly pain and disability unresponsive to conservative management in patients with radiographic evidence of end-stage changes. Patients with hemophilia may have end-stage arthropathy of the knee as early as late adolescence; by the third or fourth decade severe pain and disability may be present. In our series, the patients ranged in age from 21 to 52 years, with most being in their third or fourth decade. The sole patient with factor IX deficiency underwent the knee replacement operation at the age of 72 years and probably had osteoarthritis unrelated to her coagulopathy.

Forty-six of the patients in this series had severe type A hemophilia (factor VIII less than 1 percent), one had type B hemophilia, and one had von Willebrand's disease. Because life-threatening thromboembolic complications have been reported in patients with hemophilia B undergoing major surgery, owing to activated clotting factors in factor IX concentrate, no elective operations were performed on patients with hemophilia B at our institution until purified factor IX became available.

At our center, 10 percent of all operations performed on hemophilic patients involve knee replacement. Since 1974, 50 prosthetic knee arthroplasties have been undertaken, with a minimum follow-up of 2 years. These included eight tibiofemoral replacements, 20 cemented three-compartment replacements, and 22 cementless three-compartment replacements.

In the first seven patients (eight knees), the prostheses were cemented two-compartment replacements; all had an average loss of 10° of range of motion, and three patients had residual patellofemoral pain. In sharp contrast, the 42 remaining patients, who had three-compartment replacements, gained an average of 25° of range of motion, and only one had patello-femoral pain, presumably owing to a loose patellar component. Although the primary factor responsible for the gain in range of motion is presumed to be inclusion of the patellofemoral joint replacement, other factors probably also have contributed, such as improvements in manipulation technique with balanced forces about the knee and use of continuous passive motion. Twelve patients were treated with manipulation, the most recent in 1981. Since then, continuous passive motion has replaced manipulation and is begun approximately 3 days after the knee replacement operation if the wound appears healthy. In one patient, continuous passive motion was attempted immediately postoperatively, but this option was dropped because it seemed to be associated with increased bleeding.

In 1982, our group began using press-fit, bone ingrowth knee prostheses in patients with adequate bone stock. Eighteen patients have received 22 such cementless prostheses (17 porous coated anatomic, and five Miller-Gallant); follow-up has ranged from 1 to 8 years. Because there were cystic defects that were too large for contained, impacted bone graft and a press-fit prosthesis, the patellar button was cemented in 18 cases and the tibial component in four. In 14 cases, both with and without cement fixation, local bone graft was used to fill surface defects.

The group receiving cementless (mostly cemented-cementless hybrids) ranged in age from 28 to 54 years, similar to the group of 20 patients who received cemented three-compartment prostheses (22 to 54 years). Because the pathologic conditions in patients in these two groups were virtually identical, this forms a good basis for preliminary comparison. The two groups had a similar blood loss at surgery (748 ml for cemented, 612 ml for cementless), but postoperatively the Hemovac output averaged 606 ml more for the cementless group (247 ml for cemented versus 853 ml for cementless). Both groups had a similar gain in range of motion (25.6° for cemented, 28.7° for cementless). Pain relief has been excellent in both groups.

Deficiency of bone stock occurs relatively frequently in patients with hemophilic arthropathy as a result of mechanical erosion or synovial cysts, or both (Figs. 43-6 and 43-7). In earlier years this problem was handled by filling in the defects with polymethyl-methacrylate cement or using specially designed, stemmed components. More recently, bone grafting has become the procedure of choice; this method is especially advantageous if future revisions are required because of its potential to improve bone stock (Fig. 43-8). The amount of bone removed is minimal. Although large defects require allografts, small and moderate-sized defects are grafted with local autogenous bone. However, autogenous grafts from the iliac bone are avoided because of the potential risk of recurrent hemorrhage at the donor site. Results have been good, with none of the patients receiving the grafts having developed clinical or radiographic evidence of prosthesis loosening or infection to date.

Among the early postoperative complications were massive hemarthrosis (one case), recurrent hemarthroses (one case), Coombs' positive hemolysis (one case), and wound dehiscence during manipulation (one case). Hematogenous infection (affecting five knees in three patients) and loosening (one case each of the tibial component, femoral component, and patellar component) were late-developing complications. The cases of infection and loosening are described in more detail in the following paragraphs.

In recent years, as concern has grown over the possibility of human immunodeficiency virus (HIV) infection, increased attention is being paid to sepsis involving joint prostheses. In our series of knee replacement operations, three patients developed infection, although none at an early stage after operation. All of the infections followed a primary sepsis elsewhere in the body. In one case the patient had had a protracted sinusitis and the knee became infected 5 years after the joint replacement surgery. Bacterial cultures from both the sinus and the knee yielded β-hemolytic streptococci. After treatment with lavage and intravenous penicillin the knee has remained free of infection for 6 years.

The two other cases were both bilateral. The first of these occurred 7 months postoperatively after the patient developed a tooth abscess due to *Staphylococ-*

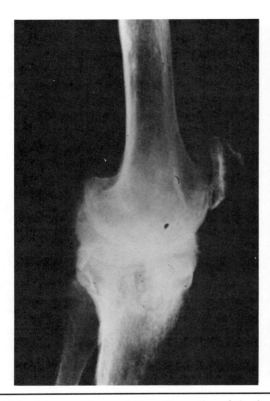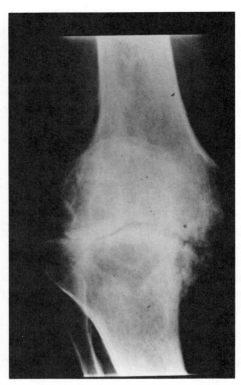

Fig. 43-6. Advanced hemophilic arthropathy of the knee, demonstrating complete loss of cartilage, lateral translation, fragmentation of the medial tibial plateau, and a large pseudotumorous synovial cyst in the proximal tibia.

cus aureus. This patient also was treated with lavage and intravenous antibiotics (clindamycin) and has remained free of infection for over 5 years. The remaining patient had multiple pyarthroses (involving the right sternoclavicular joint, the left elbow, and the right total knee prosthesis) as a consequence of *Staphylococcus aureus* septicemia. Open lavage and antibiotics failed to eliminate the infection, and removal of the prosthesis with subsequent knee fusion was required. At surgery all three bone ingrowth components were found to be solidly fixed to the host bone, and saws and osteotomes were needed to remove the prosthesis. This patient developed infection with various organisms in the left total knee and left total hip over the next 2 years.

In three patients aseptic loosening occurred, requiring additional surgery. The first patient had failure of the femoral component after a fall that resulted in a fracture of the distal femur about the component. In the second case, the tibial component of a Geomedic prosthesis failed; this patient had severe bone stock deficiency owing to a large pseudotumorous cyst in the upper tibia, which was filled with cement. In the third patient, the patellar component failed; the patella had been eroded so extensively that the patient did not have adequate bone stock for cement intrusion and fixation.

Two patients were treated by revision and one by patellectomy. The patient with the femoral component failure received a total condylar III prosthesis and at 7-year follow-up was doing well. The second patient, with the failure of the tibial component, had his prosthesis revised to a total condylar I and did well for 9 years, when he died from hepatic carcinoma. The patient with the patellectomy regained active motion over a range of 0° to 95°.

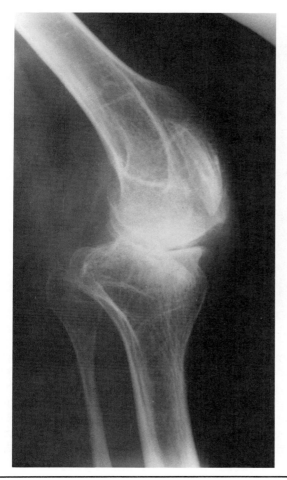

Fig. 43-7. Advanced hemophilic arthropathy of the knee with severe loss of bone stock of the lateral femoral condyle anteriorly due to lateral subluxation of the patella and erosion of the lateral trochlea. Also note the remodeling of the tibial articular surface, which occurred during childhood.

In addition, none of the 22 patients receiving bone-ingrowth prostheses at our institution in the past 8 to 10 years has shown clinical or radiographic signs of loosening.

The failure rate was four in 50 cases (8 percent) over a period of 2 to 16 years. Of the eight patients who had two-compartment prostheses inserted between 1974 and 1976, seven are still doing well and show no evidence of impending failure (including the first patient, who had a bilateral knee replacement in 1974 at the age of 24 years). These rates compare well with the long-term follow-up results reported by Insall and Kelley in 1986[20]; among the first 40 total condylar replacements inserted from 1974 to 1976 in patients with osteoarthritis and rheumatoid arthritis, their survival rate was 87.5 percent.

Search of the literature has yielded a total of 157 knee replacements in hemophilic patients.[1,14,15,17,21-29]

Ankle

The ankle is affected in hemophilic patients almost as frequently as the knee, and after the child begins to walk, this is usually the joint to be involved first. As a rule, the arthropathy is progressive. In end-stage joint disease, exostoses are found on apposing surfaces of the tibia and talus, and often there is associated arthropathy of the subtalar joint, manifested first at the posterior margin of the posterior facet (Fig. 43-9). As a result of the arthropathy, many patients develop equinus deformity and experience bleeding in the calf with muscle contracture.

Only a small percentage of patients require surgical procedures. The authors have performed 22 operations: 15 cases of tibiotalar arthrodesis, five cases of tibiotalar and subtalar arthrodesis, one case of pantalar arthrodesis, and one case of tibiotalar prosthetic arthroplasty. Internal fixation was used in 16 cases and Charnley external fixation in three cases. If the calcaneocuboid and talonavicular joints were normal they were not included in the fusion of the subtalar joint. Thus far none of the patients who have undergone this procedure over the past 7 years have shown signs of progressive degeneration of the unfused midfoot joints.

When the subtalar joint is involved along with the ankle (a common situation in hemophilia), we use two or three convergent cancellous screws to transfix the tibia, talus, and os calcis — a method also adopted independently by Wiedel at the University of Colorado (Fig. 43-9B).

Plaster casts are maintained in all patients for the first 6 weeks, during which time they are not allowed to bear weight on the ankle. During the second 6 weeks

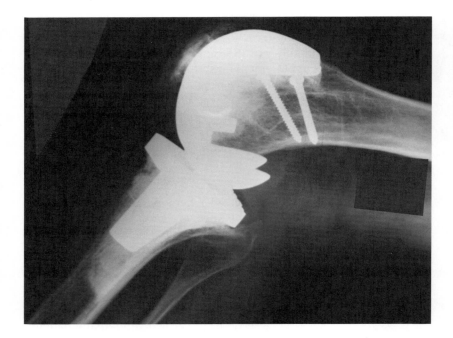

Fig. 43-8. Total knee replacement of the cemented three-compartment type, in which the worn-down lateral femoral condyle has been rebuilt with a local bone graft held in place until union occurs with two screws. (From Luck JV Jr, Kaspar CK: Surgical management of advanced hemophilic arthropathy. Clin Orthop 242:60, 1989, with permission.)

weight-bearing in a well-molded patellar tendon-bearing (PTB) cast is permitted. A molded polypropylene ankle-foot orthosis (AFO) is used even if the fusion appears solid at this time, until physicians are certain the fusion is strong enough to withstand all the stresses of daily activities.

External fixators have been used in three ankle fusions and one open tibial fracture. We believe they are safe for use in hemophilic patients and do not necessitate replacement of clotting factor for longer than the initial 2 weeks after surgery. Wilson and colleagues[29] and Patel and coworkers[30] have reported similar experience, but Trueta[31] and Arnold and Hilgartner[1] differ on theoretical grounds.

In one patient, external fixation of a tibiotalar joint led to painless nonunion, and one subtalar joint treated by internal fixation had delayed union. Often the tibiotalar joint unites earlier than the distal fibula. We now perform a distal fibular osteotomy to eliminate rotation stresses about the lateral malleolus. If this malleolus is unstable, it may be compressed against the talus with a single transfixing screw.

A review of the literature revealed only one article describing two cases of tibiotalar fusion in hemophilic patients.[8] Fusions occurred in both patients. One of the patients had only plaster immobilization and the other had a fibular on-lay graft with screw fixation. Because the rate of fusion has been similar in our series regardless of whether fixation is external or internal, it would seem that either option is suitable.

Only rarely are the talonavicular and calcaneocuboid joints involved. Among our cases a primary pantalar arthrodesis was required only in two patients, and only one additional case has been reported in the literature.[30] All three patients are capable of full weight-bearing without orthoses and have achieved solid fusions. In addition, combined ankle and subtalar fusions have been performed in four patients over a period of 5 years, and no signs of progressive arthritis have been found in any of the unfused hindfoot and midfoot joints. We believe that the ankle and subtalar joint are best treated by arthrodesis rather than prosthetic arthroplasty.

There has been only one tibiotalar joint replacement, performed in 1978. The patient now lives out of state and technically has been lost to follow-up. However,

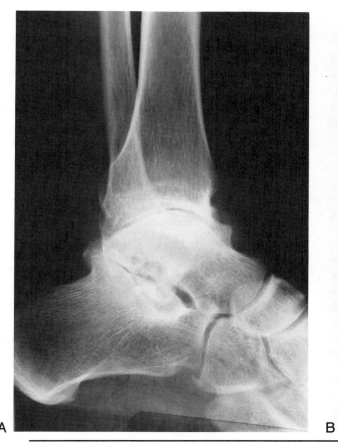
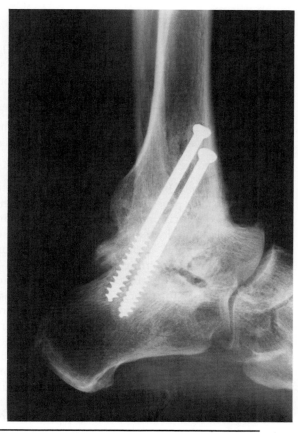

A   B

Fig. 43-9. (A) Advanced hemophilic arthropathy of the ankle and subtalar joint demonstrating erosive synovitis and loss of joint space of the posterior facet. Note preservation of the talonavicular and calcaneocuboid joints, which is usually the case in hemophilia. **(B)** Combined tibiotalar and subtalar fusion utilizing two converging screws traversing both joints. (A, From Luck JV Jr, Kaspar CK: Surgical management of advanced hemophilic arthropathy. Clin Orthop 242:60, 1989, with permission.)

his brother remains a patient at the same institution and states that he is without pain or hemarthroses.

HIV INFECTION AND ELECTIVE RECONSTRUCTIVE SURGERY

In recent years a question has arisen as to how the presence of acquired immunodeficiency syndrome (AIDS) or AIDS-related complex (ARC) has affected the indications for elective surgery in patients with these conditions. As in other situations, the risks versus benefits to the patient are weighed, and the

decision is made entirely on this basis. A comprehensive team evaluation, team conference, and multiple discussions with the patient are required before any decision is reached.

Patients with positive test results for HIV can be divided into three groups with respect to risks of elective operations. Patients in group I have antibodies to HIV but because they show no signs of disease, the risks for elective surgery are considered the same as for persons with negative HIV test results. The life expectancy of asymptomatic HIV-positive persons is unknown, but it is assumed to be long enough to make the elective procedures worthwhile.

Patients in group II have reduced numbers of CD 4 cells but do not have clinical AIDS and also have an unknown life expectancy, but this is more of a consideration than in group I patients. An absolute CD 4 cell count of less than 200 cells/ml points to an increased risk for development of postoperative complications, such as delayed wound healing or infection.

Patients in group III have AIDS, and rarely are elective orthopaedic procedures appropriate in this group. However, incision and drainage for active infection are occasionally required. Strict adherence to universal precautions, both in the operating room and in the patient's room or ward, is mandatory to minimize risks to health care personnel. Exposure of the skin and eyes to the patient's blood or body fluids is effectively prevented by use of face masks and impervious gowns and foot covers in the operating room. If power equipment that creates airborne blood droplets is used, such as saws or drills, space suits with both inflow and outflow hepafilters are employed. It is extremely important to avoid puncture injuries from needles, bone spicules, and other sharp objects commonly used in orthopaedic surgery. Other ways to minimize risk include no-touch surgical technique for suturing and the use of cut-resistant cloth gloves sandwiched between two pairs of latex gloves. A detailed description of these precautions is available elsewhere.[32]

REFERENCES

1. Arnold WD, Hilgartner MW: Hemophilic arthropathy. J Bone Joint Surg [Am] 59:287, 1977
2. Willert HG, Horrig C, Ewald W, Scharrer I: Orthopaedic surgery in hemophilic patients. Arch Orthop Trauma Surg 101:121, 1983
3. Stein H, Duthie RB: The pathogenesis of chronic hemophilic arthropathy. J Bone Joint Surg [Br] 63:601, 1981
4. DePalma AF, Cotler J: Hemophilic arthropathy. Clin Orthop 8:163, 1956
5. DePalma AF: Hemophilic arthropathy. Clin Orthop 52:145, 1967
6. Nilsson IM, Hedner U, Ahlberg A et al: Surgery of hemophiliacs—20 years' experience. World J Surg 1:55, 1977
7. Duthie RB: Reconstructive surgery in hemophilia. Ann NY Acad Sci 240:295, 1975
8. Duthie RB, Matthews JM, Rizza CR, Steel WM: The Management of Musculo-skeletal Problems in the Haemophilias. Blackwell Scientific Publications, Oxford, England, 1972
9. Kasper CK, Boylen AL, Ewing NP et al: Hematologic management of hemophilia A for surgery. JAMA 253:1279, 1985
10. Kay L, Stanisby D, Buzzard B et al: The role of synovectomy in the management of recurrent hemarthroses in hemophilia. Br J Haematol 49:53, 1981
11. Ahlberg A, Pettersson H: Synoviorthesis with radioactive gold in hemophiliacs: clinical and radiological follow-up. Acta Orthop Scand 50:513, 1979
12. Palazzi FF: Sinoviortesis radioactiva en hemophilicos. p. 225. In Palazzi FF (ed): Tratamiento Ortopedico de las Lesiones del Aparato Locomotor. FK Schattauer Verlag, Stuttgart, 1981
13. Rivard GE, Girard M, Lamarre C et al: Synoviorthesis with colloidal ^{32}P chromic phosphate for hemophilic arthropathy. Arch Phys Med Rehabil 66:753, 1985
14. Luck JV Jr: Prosthetic knee arthroplasty for advanced hemophilic arthropathy. p. 183 In Seligsohn U, Rimon A, Horoszowski H (eds): Haemophilia. Castle House Publications, Turnbridge Wells, England, 1981
15. Luck JV Jr: Surgical management of advanced hemophilic arthropathy. p. 145. In Dohring S, Schultiz KP (eds): Orthopedic Problems in Hemophilia. W Zuckschwerdt Verlag, Munich, 1986
16. Matsuda Y, Duthie RB: Surgical synovectomy for haemophilic arthropathy of the knee joint: Long-term follow-up. Scand J Haematol 33:237, 1984
17. McCullough NC III, Enis JE, Lovitt J et al: Synovectomy or total replacement of the knee in hemophilia. J Bone Joint Surg [Am] 61:69, 1979
18. Montane I, McCullough NC III, Lian EC-Y: Synovectomy of the knee for hemophilic arthropathy. J Bone Joint Surg [Am] 68:210, 1986
19. Wiedel JD, Gilbert MS, Berson BL, Hofmann A: Arthroscopy of the knee in hemophilia. p. 121. In Dohring S, Schulitz KP (eds): Symposium on Orthopaedic Problems in Hemophilia. W Zuckschwerdt Verlag, Munich, 1986
20. Insall JN, Kelly M: The total condylar prosthesis. Clin Orthop 205:43, 1986
21. Goldberg VM, Heiple KG, Ratnoff OD et al: Arthroplasty in classic hemophilia. J Bone Joint Surg [Am] 63:695, 1981
22. Lachiewicz PF, Inglis AE, Insall JN et al: Total knee arthroplasty in hemophilia. J Bone Joint Surg [Am] 67:1361, 1985
23. Magone JB, Dennis DA, Weis LD: Total knee arthroplasty in chronic hemophilic arthropathy. Orthopedics 9:653, 1986
24. Marmor L: Total knee replacement in hemophilia. Clin Orthop 125:192, 1977
25. Post M, Telfer MC: Surgery in hemophilic patients. J Bone Joint Surg [Am] 57:1136, 1975
26. Rana NA, Shapiro GR, Green D: Long-term follow-up of prosthetic joint replacement in hemophilia. Am J Hematol 23:329, 1986
27. Rovere GD, Webb LX, Nicastro JF et al: Knee replacement in the adult hemophilic patient. Contemp Orthop 11:15, 1985
28. Small M, Steven MM, Freeman PA et al: Total knee arthroplasty in haemophilic arthritis. J Bone Joint Surg [Br] 65B:163, 1983
29. Wilson FC, Mahew DE, McMillan CW: Surgical management of musculoskeletal problems in hemophilia. Instr Course Lect 32:233, 1983
30. Patel MR, Pearlman HB, Lavine LS: Arthrodesis in hemophilia. Clin Orthop 86:168, 1972
31. Trueta J: The orthopaedic management of patients with hemophilia and Christmas disease. p. 279 In Biggs R, Macfarlane

RG (eds): Treatment of Hemophilia and Other Coagulation Disorders. FA Davis, Philadelphia, 1966

32. American Academy of Orthopaedic Surgeons: Recommendations for the Prevention of Human Immunodeficiency Virus (HIV) Transmission in the Practice of Orthopaedic Surgery. American Academy of Orthopaedic Surgeons. Chicago, 1989

44 Major Fractures

VERT MOONEY
STEVEN BECKER

One of the most significant advances in musculo-skeletal care over the past several decades has been in the treatment of fractures. In the past, with so-called conservative care, significant deconditioning of soft tissues related to the skeletal injury occurred during the extended period of time necessary to achieve fracture union by natural means. However, in recent years, with the advent of greatly improved equipment and training, conservative care of most fractures is no longer the standard. A goal of fracture rehabilitation has always been to mobilize the injured tissues, both soft and skeletal, as rapidly as is consistent with the healing process. Now, with greatly improved internal fixation systems, delay in mobilization is reduced and early stretching and strengthening can occur. The most conservative approach is often surgical.

The purpose of this chapter is to supply some background information concerning concepts of care. A special note is made of the role of joint mobilization in fracture care. Finally, examples of current standard of care are provided to explain the rationale for early immobilization and principles of strengthening.

HISTORICAL CONSIDERATIONS

Rest and movement, those two diverse concepts, are the key factors that accelerate or confound fracture rehabilitation. For at least a century, the relative roles of each have been debated. Historically, fractures have been treated by . Rest was advocated primarily by members of the "English school," whereas motion was supported just as strongly in the European literature. This long-continued controversy was best summed up in the Robert Jones Lecture of 1952 by Perkins,[1] but a brief history is given here.

Prominent English physicians such as Hilton and Thomas[2] proclaimed the superiority of rest, and their views came to dominate the field. Perhaps because of their common language, Americans also adopted this viewpoint. For many years rest was the primary method of fracture care. Even recently the leading textbook on this subject[3] was based on the premise that fractures should be treated by rest followed by gradual mobilization.

Nevertheless other voices also were heard. As early as 1855, Smith of Philadelphia questioned the value of the prevailing practice of prolonged traction and plaster casts. He treated ununited femoral fractures by applying braces, which he called "artificial limbs." Smith wrote, "It is an inquiry worthy of note in passing whether in the treatment of fractures very perfect rest may not be one cause of the deficiency of the new bone union."[4] Similarly, perhaps the best proponent of the view that rest was not ideal was Lucas-Championiere in 1910,[5] who encouraged supervised active motion soon after injury, with the addition of friction massage to control discomfort. "Action is life" was the motto of this concept of care.

Nevertheless, despite these early voices, more than 100 years would pass before Smith's ideas were resurrected in America. While physicians on both sides of the Atlantic upheld the benefits of rest, concern for mobilization and rehabilitation led orthopaedists into the field of skeletal trauma care. The father of orthopaedics, Robert Jones, gained an impressive reputation in the early care of lower extremity fractures using the Thomas splint, a device invented by his uncle. This device was used during transport and eventually to suspend the limb in traction in cases of femoral fractures sustained by soldiers during World

War I. Later this same apparatus was adopted for management of industrial injuries. The splint had originally been used to allow walking while resting the tubercular knee. Because rest was the primary tool in treatment of tuberculosis, its adoption in the management of skeletal trauma is not surprising. It was the work of Robert Jones and his knowledge of bracing and mobilization that allowed orthopaedists to gain acceptance as qualified to provide fracture care, especially for workplace injuries. However, exercise to the joint was not advocated.

Finally, more than 100 years after it had been proposed, Smith's concept of ambulatory care of fractures was resurrected by Dehne,[6] who reported a perfect record of union in a large series using cast treatment for tibial fractures with immediate weight bearing. Dehne's father, an Austrian physician, had used Smith's braces, so the positive results of mobilization had become known to Dehne as a youth.

In the United States, the surgical care of fractures with internal fixation had been adopted initially by general surgeons; orthopaedists generally used plaster casts and braces. Such celebrated general surgeons as Sherman of Pittsburgh, Wade of New York Hospital, and McLaughlin of Columbia-Presbyterian were strong advocates of the surgical fixation of fractures during the 1940s and 1950s. However, high rates of failure and disastrous infections that occurred because of poor understanding of mechanical principles allowed the more conservative approach of the orthopaedists eventually to succeed that of the general surgeons for fracture care at most teaching institutions. The surgical approach was considered proper for skeletal reconstruction, but not for internal fixation of acute fractures; for the latter is was considered destructive to the principles of continued and prolonged rest so strongly held by the English-speaking orthopaedists.

In the 1970s the trend in fracture care began to swing toward the surgical fixation of skeletal trauma according to the Swiss AO technique. In an attempt to eliminate the "cast disease" caused by prolonged rest, Müller and colleagues[7] developed a whole new technique of fracture fixation based on sounder scientific principles than had hitherto been utilized. Far better engineering and biomechanical principles were provided to the surgeon.[7] From an administrative standpoint, fracture care had developed somewhat differently in Continental Europe than in England. In Europe the field of traumatology was more highly developed than that of orthopaedics; in many areas, the practice of orthopaedics remained strictly within the area of reconstruction (cold orthopaedics), whereas traumatology, which included all aspects of surgical care for trauma — including fractures — was the standard of care. Gradually the methods of rigid internal fixation, which forms the entire basis of the AO system of fracture care, gained increasing support until they are now very acceptable.

Thus, the two major aspects of care — rest and motion — have been combined in the Swiss method of fracture care. In this method, open reduction is followed by rigid internal fixation and profound rest to the skeletal system, which allows primary union of bone. In this system, the goal is sufficient stabilization of the skeletal system to allow rapid mobilization of joints and soft tissues and the return of normal function as soon as possible.

However, this approach is subject to two basic conceptual flaws: (1) the stabilization may be so efficient that it diminishes the stresses to the skeletal system so much that the repaired fracture is not strong enough to carry out its appropriate function when internal fixation is removed ("overkill"); and (2) failure is more likely when the treatment program is technically flawed; therefore, a higher level of surgical skill and mechanical understanding are necessary for the care of fractures. Although effective fracture rehabilitation is favored by the application of AO internal fixation methods, both the risks and the surgical skills needed are higher. Better training and more experience are necessary.

Probably the clinician who best stated the appropriate orthopaedic philosophy for fracture care was Goldthwaite,[8] who in the 1932 Robert Jones lecture suggested the principle on which fracture rehabilitation must be based: "The orthopaedic surgeon is most qualified to provide fracture care from acute onset through rehabilitation because it is a basic principle of this training that from the very beginning, he has the end result in mind." This keeping of the end result in mind is the principle that mandates mobilizing all resources in the rehabilitation program. Ironically, in this lecture Goldthwaite was speaking against operative care for fractures, or even for reconstructive chronic orthopaedic problems. However, even though his words are being taken out of context, the principles are sound for achieving the ideal end result.

PRINCIPLES OF SOFT TISSUE REHABILITATION

Specific techniques of achieving skeletal stabilization after fracture are not discussed here. They are, of course, quite detailed and vary according to the specific site. Attention to detail in surgical care in terms of technique equipment, and principles is an important component of fracture management and later rehabilitation of the patient. It is important, however, to recognize that once the fracture has been stabilized appropriately, the role of the soft tissues becomes increasingly important. The soft tissues include muscles, tendons and ligaments, and the joints, including articular surfaces and capsules. Each of them is discussed briefly.

What is definitely known about rehabilitation of muscles after injury? Certainly clinical experience has shown that inactivity rapidly results in muscle atrophy. In the days of cast care for extremity fractures, the cast had always loosened within a week of application owing to diminished dimensions of the nonfunctioning muscles. Fortunately, now that internal fixation and early mobilization are the rule, the length of time that elapses until muscles can be used actively is greatly shortened. Muscle strengthening must be consonant with the stability of the internal fixation, but certainly early active muscle function helps provide stresses to the fracture site as well as stimuli to muscle strengthening.

Muscle hypertrophy and increases in muscle strength are produced by high-tension, low-frequency contractions of skeletal muscle.[9] In the early stages of muscle rehabilitation, strength training sessions probably should not be on a daily basis because recovery from strength training requires perhaps 48 hours. Strength training programs, however, will increase the total muscle mass primarily by increasing the cross-sectional area of individual fibers (the

number of myofibrils per fiber). Type II fibers, used for bursts of energy, hypertrophy more than type I fibers, which are designed for lower tension but prolonged use. Actually exercise programs designed to increase muscle strength do not of themselves increase the maximum blood flow, and alternative exercise programs must be undertaken. Once sufficient muscle strength has been achieved to move the limb, a progressive training program focused on specific functions should be undertaken. Low-tension, high-repetition contractions performed for 30 to 60 minutes on a regular basis will certainly result in endurance training. The tension is low only in a relative sense; that is tension developed during the activity must be great enough to produce some overload. The intensity, duration, and frequency of endurance training are designed to stimulate an increased capacity for sustained effort without inducing chronic fatigue. Chronic fatigue is defined as impaired muscle function more than 24 hours after the exercise. Endurance training increases the oxidative capacity of the muscle system. It also increases the capillary density perhaps 20 to 50 percent over normal levels in persons without prior muscle injury.[10]

A major controversy still exists over the response of skeletal muscle to strength training or endurance training with respect to the role of hyperplasia. Whether fiber splitting occurs to a significant degree or the muscle increase is due completely to hyperplasia is not fully understood. Nonetheless, both endurance and hyperplasia increase specifically with training and thus must form part of a postfracture rehabilitation program.

Fortunately, in recent years a more efficient system for exercise performance and measurement of status has been developed. Isokinetic exercise devices were first introduced in the later 1960s.[11] These devices control rate but monitor torque throughout the entire range of the rate-controlled arc. Thus, efficient challenge of the muscle can be achieved throughout its range. Even very weak muscles can function with this equipment. Monitoring torque throughout the entire range can provide feedback for training and definition of status to the patient and therapist. Computer printouts allow a permanent record of performance. The pioneering program presented by Cybex has been the standard of muscle rehabilitation over the past several decades. Because the patents for this type of equipment have expired, other companies have begun to make similar equipment. Thus the current standard of care in postfracture treatment of major skeletal injuries is a progressive exercise program. The program must be monitored in some manner to evaluate function in terms of torque production and endurance. On the basis of functional measurement, much greater efficiency in rehabilitation can be expected.

Other limiting factors to soft tissue competence in postfracture care are the tendons and ligaments. It is well known that delay in mobilization of the collagenous soft tissues such as ligaments results in contracture (shortening). It is clear that much of this shortening is secondary to increase in cross-linking between various collagenous fibers.[12] In extensive animal studies, investigators found that alterations in collagen cross-linking, changes in collagen synthesis and degradation, and decrease in water and proteoglycan content occurred in immobilized joints. This seems to be a passive phenomenon related to disuse. An associated decrease occurs in strength of the collagenous tissues as well. In fact, the ligaments actually shorten when no stress is applied to them.[13] Indeed, in the shortened ligament, the contractile protein actin (the same protein responsible for muscle contraction) has been found; thus, there seems even to be an active component to contraction.

It therefore seems that joint stiffness associated with immobilization results from several factors. Certainly adhesions form between normal gliding surfaces, with loss of the normal areolar tissues. An increase in collagen cross-linking occurs in positions with limited lengthening potential. Active changes in length of the dense fiber components also occur.

One of the most important demonstrations of the role of inactivity versus activity was by Gelberman and associates.[14] In this canine study, repaired flexor tendon lacerations that had been subjected to rest were compared with mobilized tendons. In all of the mobilized groups, proliferation of the repair tissue was more efficient and, in fact, when the tendons were tested, those that were moved daily starting the day after repair were nearly twice as strong as those that were rested. One surprising aspect about this study was that adhesions did not form at the repair site, and

Table 44-1. Indications for Continuous Passive Motion Application (Parkland Hospital, 1982–1985)

Fractures	177		
Total joint replacement	35		
Infection	54		
Knee repair	17	Bilateral	13
Synovectomy	14	Unilateral	300
Open wound, knee	6		
Arthritis	10		
Patellectomy	3		
Total	316		313

thus the repair area did not become vascularized. This means that a major portion of the metabolic exchange at the fiber sites synthesizing collagenous tissues was on the basis of diffusion fluid exchange. This is extremely important when considering the clinical aspects of remobilization. Mobilization of collagenous tissues can occur even though the blood supply that accompanied the adhesions is obliterated. Although cellular activity is sparse in the collagenous tissues (tendons and ligaments), cellular metabolism can proceed without blood supply; mobilization itself can supply the mechanical pump to enhance diffusion. This certainly is justification for early mobilization.

How are these factors involved in the movement of joints themselves? Probably one of the most significant innovations in care of fractured limbs was the early application of continuous passive motion to these joints. Doubtlessly this advancement in care has emerged only recently because it required development of appropriate powered equipment.

In addition to Smith[6] and the Europeans mentioned earlier; there were other early voices encouraging motion as a therapeutic benefit to the injured joint. At

Table 44-2. Anatomic Location of Trauma and Sepsis

Fractures		Infection	
Hip	30	Hip	7
Knee	133	Knee	45
Ankle	3	Shoulder	1
Elbow	8		
Shoulder	3		
Totals	177		53

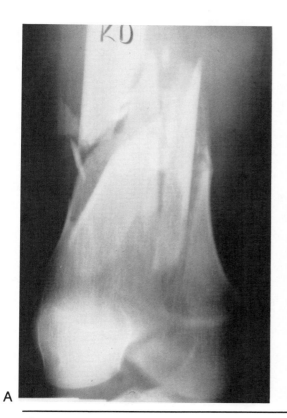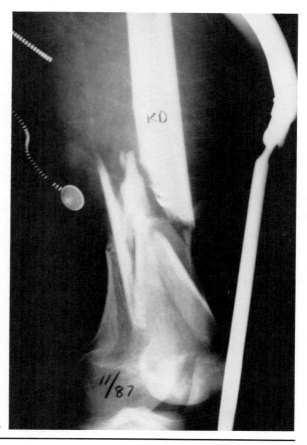

Fig. 44-1. Anteroposterior **(A)** and lateral **(B)** radiographs of a severely comminuted open fracture in Case 1. Conservative care may result in a union, but certainly significant stiffness of the knee would result even in this 19-year-old man.

the time of World War I, some surgeons advocated active motion for open septic knee injuries.[15,16] Achieving motion required a significant number of customized, counterbalanced, complex devices to encourage motion with minimal amount of muscle activity. It was recognized that muscles under poor control as a result of pain could not function smoothly. Nonetheless, despite the crude equipment, the early reports demonstrated significant improvement in joint function with diminished stiffness and deformity on the basis of early motion.

A surprising historical commentary on the use of devices for joint motion is appropriate here. The use of mechanical devices for improved function of the limbs certainly had been well established in the areas of athletic medicine and gymnastics, but the transfer

of these devices to the hospital environment seemed unfeasible.[17] Of course some clinicians gradually recognized that motion to the open injured, or infected joint could offer favorable results. This motion, however, was generally carried out actively by the patient, who was asked to stand at the bedside and go through an active assisted range of motion, which was usually accompanied by considerable pain. Various devices were developed that applied passive motion, actively powered by the patient to the injured limb. One of several orthopaedic surgeons who not only advocated motion but also developed a specific device was Perkins.[1] Perkins devised a system using a drop portion of the bed so that a patient with a fractured femur could sit and move the limb actively and passively. Another device applied specifically to the traumatized knee was designed by Apley.[18] Be-

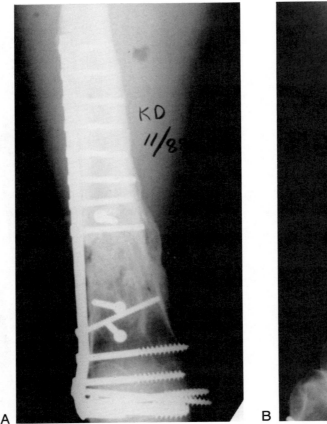 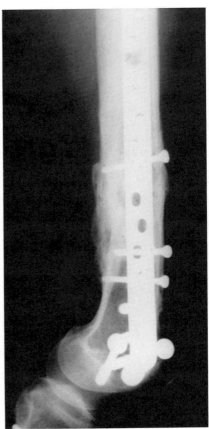

Fig. 44-2. Anteroposterior **(A)** and lateral **(B)** radiographs of patient in Case 1 showing status of fracture 1 year after onset. Open reduction and internal fixation have accomplished not only union but appropriate alignment and stability to allow early range of motion. By 3 months after injury, the patient was suffering no disability.

fore Apley's device was invented, the patient had to apply passive motion through a set of pulleys and slings.

The first application of powered motion to an injured joint for the purpose of improving range of motion was in 1967 by Nickel at Rancho Los Amigos Hospital.[19] An improved powered system for application to limbs was later devised by Coutts.[20] Initially these devices were intended for the treatment of total knee arthroplasties, but commercial equipment did emerge from these developments.

It was the work of this group that justified widespread clinical application. Salter conducted basic studies in the use of continuous passive motion (CPM) and it was he who coined the term.[21] Other basic studies were done by Shimizu and coworkers, who demonstrated that motion for 24 hours a day was not necessary to achieve effective results in the joints of animals. They also demonstrated, however, that application of CPM immediately was more effective than applying it after a delay.[22] CPM for 2 to 4 hours a day was not as effective as CPM for 8 hours a day. Therefore, a "dose-response" curve does seem to exist.

Results of extensive experience with CPM as applied to fractures about the joint and limbs over a 3-year period at Parkland Hospital have recently been published.[23] Tables 44-1 and 44-2 summarize this expe-

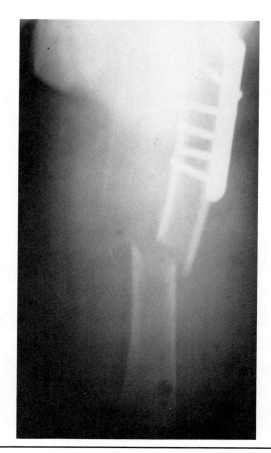

Fig. 44-3. This fracture has occurred in an osteoporotic femur distal to an old fracture repair site. The fracture occurred after minimal trauma. It could heal without internal fixation, but mobilization would be impossible.

rience. All patients were kept in the CPM device until they had near-normal range of at least 90°. The average time to achieve 90° range of motion after trauma was about 3 days. In the treatment of septic joints without the prior injury, however, the achievement of full range of motion took about 2 days. At Parkland Hospital patient compliance with CPM was sometimes variable. The majority of patients found the equipment comfortable and would remain in it for a prolonged period of time. One criterion for length of need of CPM is patient comfort when the CPM is stopped. Thus, if the CPM device has been stopped and the patient can go through a nearly normal range of motion, additional CPM is not necessary. Alternatively, the CPM device is needed when

the patient begins to have joint swelling after the discontinuation of CPM. Thus, we found that when the patient no longer had active pain or swelling and had a good active range of motion with the CPM device off, there was no longer a need to employ it. Contractures did not result after CPM discontinuation at this point.

EXAMPLES OF FRACTURE REHABILITATION

Case 1

A 19-year-old man who suffered injuries in a severe motor vehicle accident was brought to the emergency room with a grade 2 open fracture (Fig. 44-1). The day after injury he was taken to the operating room and had open reduction and internal fixation with a blade plate. He was placed in a CPM device in the recovery room, and this was continued for 2 days. He rapidly advanced to 90° of range of motion and at the time of discharge from the hospital 4 days after fracture he had 90° of range of motion actively. He was placed on a non-weight-bearing physical regimen for 6 weeks and partial weight-bearing for an additional 6 weeks. At the conclusion of 12 weeks he had achieved 140° of range of motion and was bearing full weight without pain. At follow-up 1 year later these achievements remained (Fig. 44-2).

This case is an example of the effect of early care and mobilization. The dimensions different in this type of case therefore a decade earlier are significant. The combination of early skeletal fixation and early motion allowed rapid return to normal function.

Case 2

A 90-year-old man with the past history of an old intertrochanteric fractured fixed 5 years earlier tripped while walking down the street and felt sudden pain in his right thigh. Radiographs obtained in the emergency room revealed a fracture below the old plate midshaft (Fig. 44-3). The bone was notably osteoporotic as well. The patient was taken to the operating room the following day and had an internal fixation using a femoral rod with distal cross-screw fixation (Fig. 44-4). He was placed in a CPM device for 2 days after surgery and started on pro-

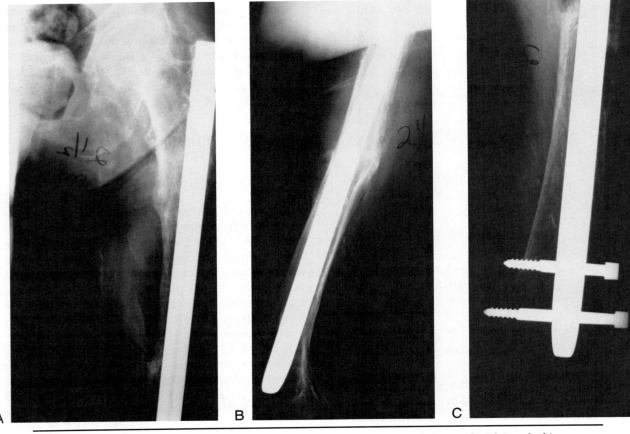

Fig. 44-4. (A–C) After removal of the old internal fixation, a large intramedullary rod with interlocking screws was used to stabilize the bone. Even though the canal was extremely wide, the interlocking screws offered sufficient stability to allow very early ambulation and range of motion. This would not have been possible without early internal fixation.

gressive weight-bearing. By 6 weeks he was bearing full weight with crutches and had 90° of range of motion at the knee. At 2.5 months' follow-up he was bearing full weight without crutches, although he did continue to have a mild limp.

This is a dramatic demonstration of advancements in fracture care. In an earlier era, this fracture would have been treated with traction or even a cast brace. Early immobilization would not have been available, and certainly a stiff knee would have resulted. The use of rod with interlocking screws to supply additional stability in the osteoporotic limb was a major benefit. Even in this aged gentleman mobilization

was possible within several days. Good range of motion at the knee could be expected.

Case 3

An 18-year-old man fell four stories and sustained a significant injury to the pelvis. Radiographs obtained in the emergency room revealed a Malgaigne type of fracture (Fig. 44-5A). Significant displacement was noted on the computed tomographic (CT) scan (Fig. 44-5B). Open reduction and internal fixation with specially designed pelvic plates allowed stabilization of the comminuted fracture. An ilioinguinal approach was used (Fig. 44-5C). The patient was able to

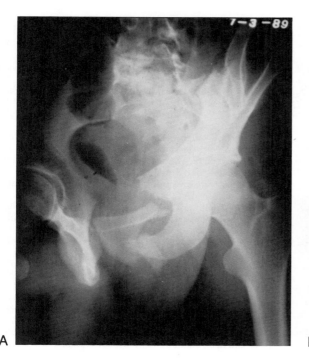

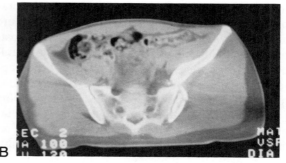

Fig. 44-5. **(A)** A severe comminuted fracture of the pelvis has occurred. Even in this youthful patient, prolonged bed rest would probably have resulted in death. Early immobilization is absolutely essential. **(B)** CT scan reveals the severity of a displacement, with the ilium on the left completely displaced anterior to the sacrum. Ambulatory function would be impossible with such an injury. **(C)** Open reduction–internal fixation was accomplished. This early stabilization allowed early mobilization. The patient had no long-term residual effects.

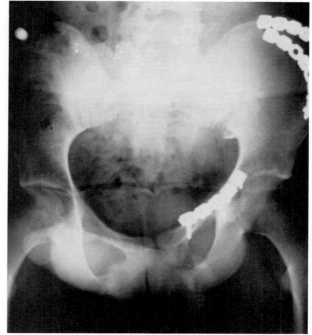

be mobilized within several days and had achieved full weight-bearing at 6 weeks. An early exercise program using an exercycle also contributed to the good result. At 6 weeks the patient had normal gait and full range of motion in the hips and in the back.

CONCLUSION

The principles of rehabilitation for major fractures are quite straight forward and simple. Rapid mobilization, including stretching, strengthening, and range-of-motion exercises, must occur or deterioration from scar formation, atrophy, and contracture will result. What used to be major problems in posttrauma rehabilitation have now been virtually eliminated with advances in fracture surgery. When appropriate skills and surgical teamwork are available, rapid mobilization can be expected. Understanding of pathophysiology and connective tissue repair has helped in designing rehabilitation programs. Certainly the addition of CPM has been of major influence in achieving improvement in posttraumatic range of motion at an early stage.

Today, for major fractures, duration of stay is usually dictated purely on the basis of medical and metabolic needs. Seldom is it necessary to have an inpatient rehabilitation program for fracture rehabilitation. In fact, the "sports medicine" attitude toward rehabilitation of the limbs after fractures is quite reasonable: Early aggressive challenge to neuromotor control and joint range. The rehabilitation process should be paced by measurement of function achieved by the joint. Because of the benefits of early expert surgery, minimal disability can be expected in the majority of major fractures.

REFERENCES

1. Perkins G: Rest and movement. J Bone Joint Surg [Br] 35:521, 1953
2. Thomas HO: Diseases of the hip, knee and ankle joints and their deformities treated by a new and efficient method. Clin Orthop 102:4, 1974
3. Watson-Jones R: Fractures and Joint Injuries. 4th Ed. Williams & Wilkins, Baltimore, 1960
4. Smith HH: On the treatment of ununited fracture by means of artificial limbs. Am J Med Sci, January, 1855
5. Lucas-Championiere JMM: Precis du Traitement des Fractures par le Massage et la Mobilisation. Steinheil, Paris, 1910
6. Dehne E: The ambulatory treatment of the fractured tibia. Clin Orthop 105:159, 1975
7. Müller ME, Allgower M, Willenegger H: Manual of Internal Fixation. Springer-Verlag, Berlin, 1970
8. Goldthwaite JE: The background and foregrounds of orthopedics. J Bone Joint Surg [Am] 15:279, 1933
9. Faulkner JA: New perspectives in training for maximum performance. JAMA 205:741, 1986
10. Saltin B, Gollnick P: Skeletal muscle adaptability: Significance for metabolism and performance. p. 555. In Geiger SR (exec ed): Handbook of Physiology: Section 10. Skeletal Muscle (Peachey LD, Adrian RH sect. eds.). American Physiological Society, Bethesda, MD, 1983
11. Thistle HG, Hislop HJ, Moffroid M, Lowman EW: Isokinetic contraction: a new concept of resistive exercise. Arch Phys Med Rehabil 48:279, 1966
12. Akeson WH, Woo SL-Y, Amiel D, Doty DH: Rapid recovery from contracture in rabbit hindlimb: a correlative biomechanical and biochemical study. Clin Orthop 122:359, 1977
13. Dahners LE: Ligament contraction: a correlation with cellularity and actin staining. Orthop Trans 11:56, 1986
14. Gelberman RH, Botte MJ, Spiegelman JJ, Akeson WH: The excursion and deformation of repaired flexor tendons treated with protected early motion. J Hand Surg [Am] 11:106, 1986
15. Everidge JA: A new method of treatment for suppurative arthritis of the knee joint. Br J Surg 23:566, 1919
16. Willems C: Treatment of purulent arthritis by wide arthrotomy followed by immediate active mobilization. Surg Gynecol Obstet 20:546, 1919
17. Zander JGW: The Apparatus for Medical-Mechanical Gymnastics and Their Use. Norstedt, Stockholm, 1894
18. Apley AG: Fractures of the lateral tibial condyle treated by skeletal traction and early mobilisation. J Bone Joint Surg [Br] 38:699, 1956
19. Fresno B Newspaper, June 17, 1967
20. Coutts RD: Continuous passive motion in the rehabilitation of the total knee patient, its role and effect. Orthop Rev 15:126, 1986
21. Salter RB, Simmonds DF, Malcolm BW et al: The biologic effect of continuous passive motion on the healing of full thickness defects in articular cartilage: an experimental investigation in the rabbit. J Bone Joint Surg [Am] 62:12, 1980
22. Shimizu T, Videman T, Shimazaki K, Mooney V: Experimental study on the repair of full thickness articular cartilage defects: effects of varying periods of continuous passive motion, cage activity, and immobilization. J Orthop Res 5:187, 1987
23. Mooney V, Stills M: Continuous passive motion with joint fractures and infections. Orthop Clin North Am 18:1, 1987

45 Amputation

HAROLD J. FORNEY

In no other field of orthopaedics is the team approach as important as in amputation surgery. The patient undergoes profound physical and emotional stresses, and successful rehabilitation requires the services of a variety of personnel from different disciplines. Amputation surgery is unique in that the functional loss is complete, instantaneous, extremely visible, and permanent. The goals of the rehabilitation team should be to maintain the very best possible residual limb and to restore limb function (and entire patient function) to as nearly normal as possible.

Therefore, amputation surgery should not be considered destructive; rather it is constructive and should result in the best end organ possible with which to control a prosthesis. This surgery requires great skill and attention to detail, and, at times, considerable ingenuity and creativity. It should not be delegated to an unsupervised junior surgeon, but rather is best done by a well-trained, experienced surgeon with the interest and ability to follow the patient through prosthetic fitting and complete rehabilitation. These skills can be learned by general surgeons, vascular surgeons, and plastic surgeons, but usually the task falls to the orthopaedic surgeon by virtue of training and general knowledge of the musculoskeletal system.

Historical and archaeologic records indicate that amputations were some of the very earliest surgical procedures, performed in very early times for ritual purposes, for punishment, or to remove a gangrenous or severely damaged limb. The development of amputation surgery paralleled the development of surgery in general. The earliest surgeons were military surgeons, and amputations were the most common operation because these were the only survivable procedures. Soldiers who suffered trauma to the head, chest, or abdomen were unlikely to survive.

Hippocrates performed and wrote about relatively sophisticated amputations in approximately 500 B.C. During the Dark Ages (A.D. 200 to 1500), medicine in general suffered a decline. Surgeons ceased using ligatures, again began treating amputations with hot oil or red-hot irons, and emphasized the importance of "laudable pus." In the 16th century, Ambroise Paré, a noted French battlefield surgeon ("I only dress the wounds; God heals them") reversed these trends and reintroduced the use of ligatures, stopped hot oil treatments, devised functional prostheses, and even advised revision surgery to allow better prosthetic fitting. In more recent times, the availability of safe anesthesia, roentgenology, asepsis, and antibiotics have all contributed to better results from amputation surgery.

The numbers are immense: There are currently 700,000 amputees of all types in the United States, with approximately 50,000 new operations being performed every year. However, these totals probably are not increasing because the majority of amputees are elderly with limited life expectancy (25 percent have died within 1 year and only half survive 3 years).[1] The ability of cardiovascular and neurologic surgeons to save the lives of patients who would have died a few years ago has produced some extremely difficult amputation problems. The treatment of peripheral vascular disease has occasionally produced such difficult situations as open hip disarticulations or simultaneous ablation of all four extremities.

Diabetes accounts for 45 percent of all nontraumatic leg and foot amputations in the United States.[2] With 500,000 new cases of insulin-dependent diabetes every year, and with an amputation rate of nearly 60 per 100,000 diabetic persons per year, it can be readily seen that the cost in terms of the human misery and economic expenditure is staggering. The relative

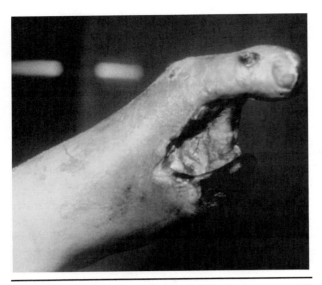

Fig. 45-1. Unsuccessful healing of diabetic gangrene will surely require below-knee amputation.

risk of amputation among diabetics appears to be the highest among younger people and occurs more commonly in males than in females (Fig. 45-1).

PRINCIPLES OF REHABILITATION

Ideally, rehabilitation of the amputee should begin before the surgery itself. However, time is frequently a factor and it is not always possible to make ideal preparations for the elderly patient who is extremely septic with diabetic gangrene or the young trauma victim who has lost, or soon will lose, a limb.

When possible, the services of an internist or endocrinologist should be engaged to assist with general medical care and especially with diabetic management during the hospitalization. Nutrition is especially important in healing the amputation wound.[3] Low serum albumin level and low lymphocyte counts are predictors of difficult wound healing and should be corrected preoperatively if possible.

The importance of the vascular laboratory will be discussed in more detail later. Arteriograms and noninvasive studies such as Doppler flowmetry may be of great value to the vascular surgeon in determining whether a reconstructive or limb-salvage procedure

can be performed. Frequently, a vascular bypass will make amputation possible at a more distal level.

Amputation surgery is best done by an orthopaedic surgeon, whose involvement should begin early in the course of treatment. The surgeon should evaluate the entire patient and thoroughly discuss the various alternatives. Frequently, amputation has not been mentioned to the patient previously, and the orthopaedic surgeon must draw on immense skill and expertise to present this in a positive manner while describing the proposed course of treatment.

Nurses and therapists can be a great help. If they are experienced in care of patients with amputations, they can explain the procedures and allay fear of the unknown. If there is enough time preoperatively, it is a good idea for the physical and occupational therapists to begin general strengthening and mobility exercises along with training and practice of activities of daily living.

Frequently, the prosthetist will begin involvement with the patient immediately in the operating room. A preoperative visit can be very helpful and reassuring, especially if the various prosthetic devices being considered can be demonstrated to the patient.

Most larger cities have an amputee support group, including volunteers who have had amputations themselves. These persons are available to visit the patient pre- and postoperatively to provide counsel and reassurance. A visit is even more effective if the volunteer and patient are matched by age, sex, and type of amputation.

Because the emotional impact of amputation can be quite severe, a visit by a psychologist or medical social worker is quite beneficial. Amputations are very disruptive to people's life-styles and their ability to work and care for themselves. Frequently, professional help is needed to get over the rough spots.

Postoperatively, most of the rehabilitation team will continue to work with the patient. In addition, a vocational rehabilitation specialist and recreational therapist may be added to complete the team. Recreation is very important for amputees. It seems as though some patients deliberately set out to prove

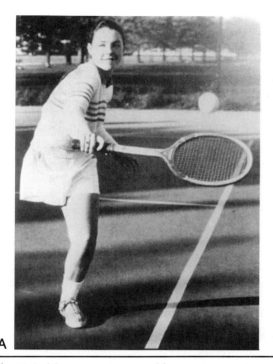 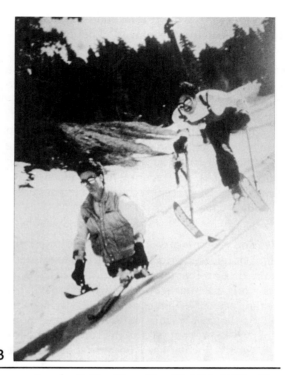

Fig. 45-2. Many amputees are able to engage in vigorous recreational activities (From Kegel B: J Rehabil Res Dev Clin Suppl #1. Rehabilitation Research and Development Service, Department of Medicine and Surgery Veterans' Administration, 1985.)

they are as good as they were prior to their amputation. With the use of newer socket-interface materials and energy-storing feet, amputees are now able to enjoy not only the less demanding sports, such as bowling, golf, and tennis, but also climbing, horse jumping, marathon running, and professional baseball. Downhill skiing is very popular, and many ski resorts have special centers for handicapped skiers (Fig. 45-2).

Rehabilitation of the amputee at home versus in an inpatient rehabilitation center is a highly individualized decision. In these days of cost containment and limited inpatient resources, many persons can be rehabilitated in their homes if they are sufficiently ambulatory for it to be safe and if there is sufficient support from family and others. However, when these conditions cannot be met, it is better for the patient to be hospitalized in a facility where care can be supervised by trained personnel. These decisions

can be best made with input from therapists, nurses, social workers, and others.

AMPUTATIONS OF THE LOWER EXTREMITY

Although this textbook is not intended as a manual of surgical technique, it seems appropriate to mention a few pertinent points about each amputation level in the lower extremity. Details of surgical technique are available in standard textbooks and atlases on the subject.[4-7]

Surgical technique in general is critical to a successful outcome. The basic principles of absolute asepsis, absolute hemostasis, and gentle handling of tissues are as applicable in amputation surgery as they are in other surgical specialties. If there is a question of sepsis in the operative area, the operation must be performed in stages. A second procedure for delayed closure or revision is far preferable to a questionable closure and risk of wound infection or breakdown, which might jeopardize the next higher level.

Whenever possible, an amputation should be done under tourniquet control. In dysvascular patients, the intitial skin incision is usually made without a tourniquet and, when adequate circulation has been established, the tourniquet is inflated. The operation can be done more quickly and accurately with less tissue damage than when a tourniquet is not used. One exception might be the patient who has recently undergone a vascular procedure, such as a bypass operation, on the same limb.

Muscles and tendons are stabilized as indicated, the tourniquet is released prior to closure, and hemostasis is obtained. Careful approximation of fascia and other layers is essential in limbs with marginal vitality and healing capacity. Nerves are sharply divided and allowed to lie away from suture lines and bony prominences to prevent painful neuromas. A suction drain is nearly always used because a hematoma, with its possibility of becoming infected, can make the difference between success and failure.

The majority of patients are elderly, frequently very ill, and in poor general health. As mentioned, a good medical and vascular surgical work-up is essential. When this has been accomplished and amputation determined to be appropriate and inevitable, the surgeon must determine the amputation level. The need for amputation is frequently obvious; however, level at which the amputation should be carried out is more difficult to judge though no less important. The surgeon must use great judgment and skill to leave the longest possible residual limb for functional purposes and yet avoid the discouragement and risk of repeated failure and revisions. For example, the value of preserving the knee is demonstrated by Volpicelli and co-workers,[8] who noted that no patients who underwent bilateral above-knee amputations for vascular disease were able to use prostheses for functional ambulation. Those with unilateral above-knee or below-knee amputations and those with bilateral below-knee ablations were progressively better walkers.[8]

Selection of Level

Physical examination is the simplest method of assessing limb viability. Skin color, hair growth patterns, skin temperature, and the presence of pulses are factors used for arriving at a decision on the level of amputation. Capillary filling time may also give some useful information.

Laboratory work-up may include arteriography, which is essential for the vascular surgeon if the possibility of vascular reconstruction exists. However, this procedure is invasive and carries some risk, and although it is useful in demonstrating the limb arteries it is of less value in predicting tissue viability at the level of the amputation wound.

Doppler systolic pressure measurements and the ischemic index, as developed by Wagner, hold some promise and may be very useful.[6] The reliability of this technique is reduced in the diabetic patient with rigid, noncompressible arteries (Fig. 45-3).

Transcutaneous measurement of skin oxygen saturation ($TCpO_2$) is fairly simple and reliable. No laboratory test is 100 percent reliable, however, and a $TCpO_2$ is no exception. Although some wounds will heal with a $TCpO_2$ of 0, the general consensus is that a reading of between 20 and 35 mm Hg is required for wound healing.[9,10]

Other laboratory tests, such as xenon-133 diffusion, plethysmography, laser Doppler flowmetry, electromagnetic flowmetry, and thermography, are either too unreliable or too cumbersome to be used routinely by the average practitioner.

The final decision regarding level of amputation is frequently made at the operating table. Although it is necessary to consider the laboratory tests, the final judgment depends on the actual condition of all tissues, especially the skin, as observed by the operating surgeon. If the skin bleeds well and the muscle is of good color and contractility, it is likely the wound will heal.

A final point regarding operative level concerns obtaining permission for the operation. It is always a good idea to have enough rapport with the patient so

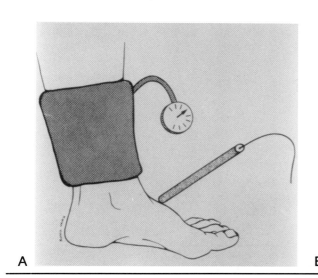
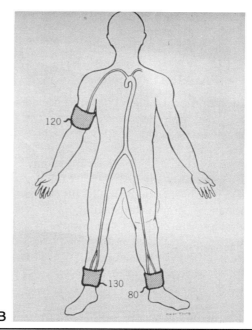

A   B

Fig. 45-3. Doppler flowmetry may be useful in determining amputation level. (From Kostuik,[6] with permission.)

that permission for the next higher level can be obtained if necessary. This gives the surgeon the option of revising the plan if unforeseen circumstances are encountered at the operating table.

Partial Foot Amputation

Less than 30 years ago, surgeons would not attempt anything less than an above-knee amputation in the diabetic patient, let alone consider a partial foot amputation. Today, with better surgical techniques, better general medical care, and more reliable predictors, the partial foot amputation is a very useful procedure.[11,12] Only a custom-molded shoe filler is necessary to restore function, and the functional difference between a foot amputation and above-knee amputation in the elderly patient is vast (Fig. 45-4).

The surgeon can and must exercise a great deal of creativity. Sometimes only a toe must be removed, but more commonly gangrene or infection is more extensive than it initially appears, necessitating a ray resection or transmetatarsal amputation. Amputa-

tion at the midtarsal (Lisfranc or Chopart) level is not recommended. The function is not much better than a Symes' amputation, and muscle imbalance and prosthetic fitting present real problems. The partial foot amputation is dressed with a rigid plaster dressing until wound healing is solid, and then a shoe filler

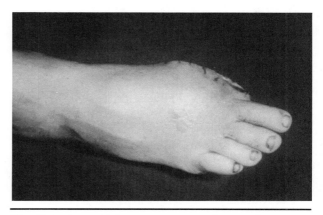

Fig. 45-4. A partial foot amputation is frequently successful.

is constructed. As with all amputations for vascular disease, weight-bearing is restricted until wound healing is complete.

Ankle Disarticulation

Amputation at the ankle level has traditionally been called a Symes' amputation. However, today few surgeons are doing a true Symes' procedure in the patient with vascular problems. The extra dissection required to free the distal tibia and fibula may be just enough to jeopardize the heel flap. Instability of this heel pad in the absence of the malleolus can present a real problem. A simple disarticulation is safer and more reliable. The surgeon can always resect the malleolus at a second stage as described by Wagner.[4] However, in most geriatric patients, cosmesis is not as important as function, making this second-stage procedure rarely necessary.

Ankle disarticulation has several functional advantages over the below-knee amputation. The longer lever arm provides better control of the prosthesis and requires less energy consumption. The end-bearing feature is durable, is less likely to be painful, and simplifies donning and doffing by the geriatric patient. Modern prosthetic techniques can now produce a lighter, more attractive, and more functional prosthesis than was previously possible.

In the face of forefoot infection or failure of a more distal amputation, the limb can be salvaged at the ankle level by resecting the involved foot through Chopart's joint, leaving the wound open. The ankle disarticulation is completed by resecting the talus and calcaneus at a second operation 5 to 7 days later.

Postoperatively, the wound is dressed with a rigid plaster dressing, which is usually left in place for 10 days unless systemic or local signs indicate a problem. The cast is then changed and left intact for another 10 days. At approximately 3 weeks postoperatively, the wound should have healed, and elastic wrapping and fabrication of a Symes' prosthesis can then begin. The prosthesis is usually a laminated plastic socket with a medial window for donning and a SACH foot. This initial prosthesis may last for 3 to 6 months, at which time the residual limb will have

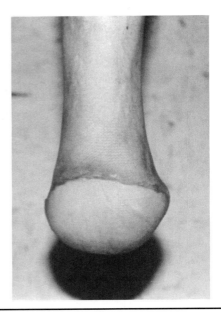

Fig. 45-5. Ankle disarticulation provides a stable, well-centered heel pad.

shrunken sufficiently to allow fitting of a more permanent prosthesis (Fig. 45-5).

Below-Knee Amputation

Thirty years ago ischemic limbs were rarely treated by below-knee amputation. Today, this is the most common operation performed in the elderly patient with vascular disease. The importance of preserving the knee has been demonstrated by many studies, including the one from Rancho Los Amigos revealing that useful ambulation by the geriatric patient with bilateral, above-knee amputation is virtually impossible, whereas approximately two-thirds of patients who had undergone bilateral below-knee amputations were able to walk[8] (Figs. 45-6 and 45-7).

Burgess and his associates in the 1960s developed surgical techniques and postoperative care that greatly enhanced the chances for success of below-knee amputations.[13,14] The operation is not especially difficult, and Burgess and his coworkers demonstrated that with good judgment, experience, and careful tissue management, successful healing could be obtained in a majority of cases using the long posterior flap technique. More recent experience

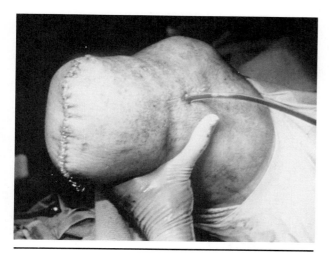

Fig. 45-6. A below-knee amputation using sagittal flaps results in a well-shaped, functional, durable residual limb.

shows that the sagittal flap technique is better than the posterior flap method.[15,16] The procedure is quicker, with less dissection of tissue planes required, and skin necrosis is less common. The shape of the residual limb is better for prosthetic fitting, and reduction of edema is more rapid.

The rigid postoperative dressing program developed by Burgess and colleagues is more applicable at the below-knee level than at any other, and is actually the key to success in many cases. This dressing is

applied in the operating room at the close of the procedure. Technical details are well documented.[4,6,7] Rigid dressings have the advantage of protecting the residual limb against trauma during early healing. Constant, even compression provided by the elastic plaster and waist belt suspension prevents edema, enhances wound healing, and makes the patient more comfortable.

Another important feature is prevention of flexion deformity at the knee, which can be a very troublesome problem with a nonrigid dressing. The rigid dressing is also useful in cases of potential sepsis when the wound must be left open pending a delayed closure in 5 to 7 days.

The suction drain is removed on the second postoperative day and the patient can be mobilized on crutches or a walker. Although a prosthetic foot unit can be attached to the cast and early weight-bearing initiated in the younger patient without vascular problems, this is not advisable for the patient with ischemia until the wound is securely healed. Usually the rigid dressing is left intact for approximately 10 days unless fever, foul odor, or excessive pain dictate earlier removal.

The wound is then inspected and the cast replaced for another 10 days. At that time, if the wound is healed, a compressive dressing may be started in preparation

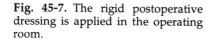

Fig. 45-7. The rigid postoperative dressing is applied in the operating room.

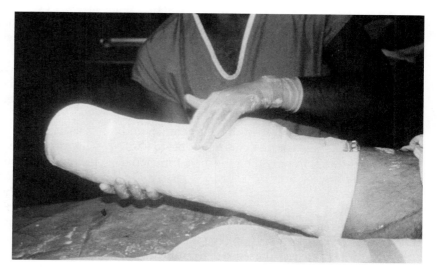

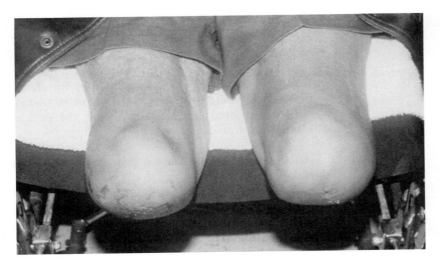

Fig. 45-8. Bilateral knee disarticulation.

for fitting with a preparatory prosthesis. Proper wrapping with elastic bandages is the best way to reduce the volume of the residual limb. This technique is not easy, but it can be learned from the standard textbooks of amputation. Patients should be taught to wrap the residual limb themselves, but if this is impossible, the next best approach is the commercial stump shrinker fitted by the prosthetist.

The patient's first prosthesis is a lightweight, inexpensive device with an adjustable shank and a simple SACH or single-axis foot. This is used for several weeks or months until the stump volume has stabilized and the patient has demonstrated readiness to proceed with a permanent prosthesis. Of course, general rehabilitation is continued during this interim, utilizing the team members deemed necessary.

Numerous different components are available for below-knee prostheses. The four basic decisions include socket type, shank design, suspension, and the foot-ankle complex. The operating surgeon should be familiar with these components to be able to work with the prosthetist in providing the most functional limb possible.

Knee Disarticulation

Historically, knee disarticulation (Fig. 45-8) has not enjoyed much enthusiasm because of the difficulty in prosthesis fitting. The thigh segment is too long and

the outside hinges are cumbersome and unsightly. Modern prosthetic techniques using such devices as four-bar and six-bar linkages and availability of better materials have solved some of these problems, and the through-knee amputation is now viewed as having several advantages over the above-knee procedures.[17]

The through-knee amputation is quickly and easily performed with minimal blood loss, which is an important factor in the geriatric patient in poor health. The end-bearing characteristic makes for a stable gait with good stump control, less energy consumption, and few problems of pain or skin breakdown. Finally, it is the amputation of choice in the nonwalking patient with a knee flexion contracture because it provides a longer lever arm and a broad thigh surface for sitting, and it avoids the problem of excessive pressure on the end of a below-knee residual limb with a knee flexion contracture.

This procedure is best done using the sagittal flap technique, leaving the patella in place and stabilizing the opposing muscle groups by suturing them into the center of the knee in the region of the cruciate ligaments. The limb is usually dressed with a plaster, sugar-tong splint, which is managed in the same manner as other rigid dressings. Early mobilization of the patient in accordance with good rehabilitation principles is then possible.

Above-Knee Amputation

When amputation at lower levels is not suitable because of unsolvable circulatory problems or failure of previous amputations, an above-knee amputation may be the only choice. It is actually the level of choice in the very sick, debilitated, nonambulatory patient in whom primary wound healing is the overriding concern. Bed care will be easier and complications fewer. In the absence of sepsis, an above-knee amputation is almost always successful from the circulatory standpoint.

The operation itself is simple. Flap design is not critical. Short, equal, anteroposterior flaps, sagittal flaps, or even a circular guillotine procedure will provide a satisfactory residual limb if care is taken to approximate muscle and fascia accurately and to cover the well-rounded bone end with good tissue. Complex myodesis or muscle-to-bone procedures are not indicated or necessary in most geriatric patients because they require more time and more dissection, which may be detrimental to the success of the operation. Postoperatively, a suction drain is used for 48 hours, and the wound is dressed with a bulky, elastic bandage. Rigid dressings are difficult to suspend properly and are usually not indicated in the older patient with vascular problems.

As with other amputations, rehabilitation begins immediately. The patient should be mobilized as soon as possible; however, prolonged sitting should be avoided because of the danger of developing a troublesome hip flexion contracture. This can be done by enforcing periods of lying prone several times a day. Elastic wrapping is continued until the stump volume has been reduced enough to allow for prosthetic fitting.

The decision on whether to prescribe a prosthesis for the geriatric patient with an above-knee amputation is not always an easy one, because it may be difficult to define specific goals. Nearly every patient (and family) wants a prosthesis, yet many insurance companies and government payors balk at providing a limb if the patient is a doubtful walker. To settle the issue, it may be necessary to prescribe an intensive trial of physical therapy or even a simple preparatory prosthesis with waist-belt suspension and manual-lock knee. If the patient progresses satisfactorily and demonstrates the motivation and physical ability to use a prosthesis, a more definitive limb can be ordered.

Perhaps more technical advances have been made in above-knee prosthetics than in any other field of prosthetics. The surgeon now has the option of prescribing anything from a simple lightweight prosthesis to be worn only a few hours a day for transferring and cosmesis to complex limbs with the newer reduced medial-to-lateral design, flexible suction sockets, hydraulic or pneumatic knees, ultralight carbon fiber construction, and energy-storing feet. Because this is not a textbook of prosthetic design, suffice it to say here that the selection is large and choices require careful consideration of many factors as well as a consultation with a skilled, experienced prosthetist.

Hip Disarticulation and Hemipelvectomy

In the past, amputation at the hip level was done primarily for malignant disease. However, today more patients are surviving major trauma, massive infections, and severe cardiovascular disease, so the amputation surgeon is presented with some very difficult problems, which push ingenuity to the limit. The younger patient undergoing elective hip disarticulation for malignant disease can be rehabilitated in the usual manner. Primary wound healing must be obtained, the patient mobilized on crutches, and a prosthesis constructed.

Frequently, the patient with trauma or infection will have other problems impeding progress, such as delayed wound healing. Long periods of dressing changes, hydrotherapy, skin grafting, and free tissue transfer may be necessary to effect wound closure and a satisfactory area for use of a prosthesis. Geriatric patients suffering from vascular problems usually have generalized disease rendering them bedridden or wheelchair bound. Long-term survival under these conditions is rare.

AMPUTATIONS OF THE UPPER EXTREMITY

Amputations of the upper extremity account for approximately 15 percent of all amputations in the United States. Although many of the basic surgical principles are the same for upper and lower extremity amputations (asepsis, hemostasis, and gentle handling of tissues), some very distinct differences exist between the two with regard to etiology, choice of level for amputation, prosthetic use, and rehabilitation technique.

Stability, durability, and equal limb lengths are essential features of lower residual limbs and the prostheses that substitute for them. In fact, without a suitable prosthesis, it is virtually impossible for the amputee to walk without an external aid. In contrast, the features that make the human hand such a valuable organ frequently eliminate the need for a prosthesis at all. Mobility, sensitivity, and cosmesis are much more important, and many patients function better one-handed than with attempts at making them bimanual via a complex, cumbersome, insensitive prosthesis. In these cases, rehabilitation first must be directed toward making the patient as functional as possible with one-handed skills.

Advances in the technology of upper extremity prosthetics have been truly miraculous. Some examples are described in this chapter as the various amputation levels are discussed. However, patients have a "gadget tolerance" limit, which is extremely variable from one person to another. In other words, the fact that a device can be made and fitted is no guarantee that it will applicable to all patients. This principle cannot be stated better than it was by the late Swedish bioengineer Forcheimer, when he said, "The most advanced application of technology is not necessarily the same as the application of the most advanced technology." Many upper extremity amputees will reject a complex, technically perfect prosthesis in favor of sensitivity and texture of their own residual limb.

Rehabilitation goals should be established early and include consideration of age, vocation, hobbies, gadget tolerance, and whether the amputation is on the dominant or nondominant side or is bilateral. The issue of dominance will greatly influence the patient's ability to function one-handedly. Some people are sufficiently ambidextrous that, with the help of a skilled therapist, they can convert their dominance.

Most upper extremity amputations are done for trauma and occur in a younger, healthier population than the lower extremity amputations in which patients vascular disease predominates. The amputation is frequently complete when the patient is first seen, although many persons struggle along with a stiff, deformed, painful, insensate extremity for a considerable length of time before amputation is considered.

In any event, early involvement of the entire rehabilitation team is important. If a patient's general condition permits, early mobilization and general rehabilitation procedures to maintain strength and mobility of all uninvolved parts should begin early. If the amputation involves the distalmost part of the limb, it is essential that the physician, physical therapist, and occupational therapist maintain mobility and strength in the shoulder. A key requirement for upper extremity function is the ability to position the hand or prosthetic terminal device in space. Without this ability, the limb is nearly useless. Rehabilitation nurses must be concerned with their patients' general medical condition and should strive to lead them toward independence in their activities of daily living.

Because of the traumatic nature of the amputation, the psychological impact may be great. The patient usually has no chance for preoperative preparation and the loss is painfully obvious immediately. Psychologists and medical social workers may be a great help in overcoming these problems. Inability to return to the same job may create a very stressful situation. Early vocational counseling may help to relieve this source of stress.

Amputation Level

As a general rule, when the upper extremity is involved, as much tissue as possible should be preserved. However, this can be carried to extremes, and the surgeon must be prepared to revise a residual limb early if the remaining part is painful, stiff, numb, or functionless. Wound healing is rarely a problem in the upper extremity, and sophisticated tests to assist with level determination are rarely necessary.

The principles of amputation already mentioned for the lower extremity apply in the upper extremity as well (absolute asepsis, absolute hemostasis, and gentle handling of the tissues). Scar placement is not so important because weight is not borne through the residual limb. There are pressure areas to avoid, however, including the volar and radial aspects of the forearm and the anterior aspect of the upper arm. Because of the very sensitive nature of the upper extremity and the paucity of subcutaneous tissue for padding, skin flaps and muscle repair should be designed so that neuromas are not in the scar or subject to pressure from bony prominences.

Partial Hand Amputation

By properly positioning the remaining parts of an injured hand, function can be maximized. Tender, insensitive, easily traumatized skin can be addressed surgically. Rarely is a prosthetic appliance necessary at this level. Amputations at the carpometacarpal level can be difficult because the patient frequently is reluctant to give up the tactile sensation of the residual limb in favor of a prosthesis, which may be too long in any event. Certain specialized prostheses can be fabricated for specific vocations or avocations, and occasionally a nonfunctioning, cosmetic hand may be indicated.

Wrist Disarticulation

Wrist disarticulation provides very good functional results. The lever arm is long, strength is adequate for a variety of heavy tasks, and the added supination and pronation adds to the usefulness of the prosthesis.

This operation is performed by making equal volar and dorsal flaps, dividing the muscles at the level to which the skin retracts, and then disarticulating the wrist without disturbing the distal radioulnar joint. This preserves approximately 50° of active supination and pronation within the prosthesis. The radial and ulnar styloid processes may be gently rounded and opposing muscles approximated. All nerves are gently pulled down and sectioned so that the neuroma will not be in an area of mechanical pressure.

Postoperatively, the limb may be fitted with a rigid dressing having the same advantages as in the lower extremity (protection of the wound, reduced edema, and pain control). Suspension is sometimes difficult and the cast may have to be changed to maintain compression. Malone and others have had good results with immediate prosthetic fitting.[18] A lightweight synthetic cast is applied and is fitted with a hook-terminal device and a standard body-powered, figure-of-eight harness.

The psychological advantage and early rehabilitation possibilities with this type of operation are a real benefit for the patient. Rehabilitation of the uninvolved body parts begins immediately. When the wound has healed and edema has subsided, a standard body-powered prosthesis is fitted with training conducted by the physical and occupational therapists.

After the patient becomes proficient with the prosthesis, and if motivation and funding are adequate, a more sophisticated prosthesis, such as a myoelectric device with a prosthetic hand, can be considered. The myoelectric device also has advantages and disadvantages. Although it is cosmetically attractive and requires no harnessing, it is heavier and not as dextrous as a more conventional prosthesis. In addition, the battery life is limited, the gloves are easily torn or stained, and the cost is quite high. Most amputees keep both types of prostheses and use them alternately depending on their needs.

Below-Elbow Amputation

Amputation through the forearm is possible at nearly any level. The design of the skin flap is not particularly important as long as the scar and neuroma are kept free of pressure areas. The prosthetic loading of the residual limb will be on the radial and volar aspects, and these areas must, therefore, have good skin. The muscles are closed in the routine manner.

One special point concerns the very short below-elbow amputation. If less than 2.5 cm of the radius will be covered by healthy skin, it is preferable to section the biceps tendon, allowing it to retract and depend on the brachialis muscle for flexion power. The patient can then be fitted as a below-elbow amputee and not require a prosthetic elbow. Prosthetic fitting and training follow the same principles mentioned in the preceding section. Further details regarding training procedures can be found in various textbooks.[4,6]

The bilateral below-elbow or wrist disarticulation presents a special problem. Although some of these patients function well with bilateral prostheses, another option is a Krukenberg operation. This is done by separating radius and ulna throughout their lengths and placing sensitive skin on the opposing surfaces. Supinator and pronator teres muscles are preserved for motor power. Patients become amazingly dextrous with this arrangement, although the appearance may be a disadvantage. The residual limb can still be placed in a prosthesis if desired. This is a very useful procedure in the bilateral or blind amputee.

Above-Elbow Amputation

Amputation at or above the elbow is accomplished by creating equal flaps, either anteroposterior or sagittal, allowing the skin to retract, and dividing the fascia and muscles at that level. The bone is divided at an appropriate level to allow closure without tension. The nerves are sectioned in such a way that neuromas will lie where they will not be traumatized. The anterior aspect of the residual limb will receive the most pressure inside the prosthetic socket; therefore, scars and neuromas should be kept away from this area.

Rigid postoperative dressings and immediate prosthetic fitting probably have some advantages, but it is very important that suspension be effective. The cast should never drop away from the residual limb. Physical and occupational therapy should begin immediately to maintain shoulder range of motion and overall physical fitness.

Restoring function to the above-elbow amputee is much more difficult and complex than when amputation is performed at the lower levels. The same problems exist at the elbow disarticulation level because a prosthetic elbow is necessary to position the terminal device in space.

A combination of motions is necessary to operate the elbow and terminal device in the conventional body-powered prosthesis. The elbow is usually locked and unlocked by humeral extension, whereas elbow flexion and operation of the terminal device depends on humeral flexion and scapular protraction. Today, one or both functions may be controlled by myoelectric components. Suspension is less difficult, but the prosthesis is heavier. Considerable diligent effort is required on the part of both the patient and the therapist so that the prosthesis can be used smoothly and effectively.

Amputations that result in 5 cm or less of humeral length (measured from the axilla) must be fitted as a shoulder disarticulation. Bone lengthening (to be discussed later) may have a real place in such circumstances.

A special situation in which an above-elbow amputation may be useful is the patient with a flail arm. Patients with brachial plexus injury resulting in disabling paresthesia and anesthesia of the hand can benefit greatly from amputation approximately 9 cm above the elbow and arthrodesis of the shoulder in approximately 25° of flexion and 25° of abduction. Frequently, it is difficult to convince the patient and family that this is the best therapy, and surgery must be delayed until thorough evaluation confirms the permanent absence of satisfactory function and adequate scapular motor power. The best results are obtained if surgery is done within 2 years after injury, before the patient has a chance to develop single-handed patterns of use. The patient is fitted as an above-elbow amputee.

Amputation at Shoulder Level

Amputation at the shoulder level is usually done for malignant tumors or very severe trauma. Surgical techniques are well described in standard textbooks.[4,5] Because the stresses are distributed over such a broad area, even split-thickness skin grafting is acceptable and satisfactory prosthetic fitting can be accomplished.

Because of the disfiguring loss of shoulder contour, a shoulder cap should be considered for cosmesis. Patients differ in functional needs, physical strength, and gadget tolerance; therefore, it is important to evaluate thoroughly all these factors before prescribing a complex, expensive prosthesis.

In a few cases, a prosthesis can be very functional. A body-powered prosthesis requires at least two, and perhaps three, joint controls. This regulation can be provided by a dual-control system (one cable, two functions), a nudge control, or a chest expansion control for the elbow lock. Another possibility is a control cable attached to a waist belt or perineal band. In contemporary prostheses, at least one function is controlled by an external power source and activated either by external switches or myoelectric relay. The mechanics of operating a shoulder disarticulation prosthesis can be extremely complex and will challenge the creativity and ingenuity of the surgeon, prosthetist, therapist, and the patient to the utmost.

AMPUTATION FOR NONVASCULAR PROBLEMS

Trauma, malignant tumor, severe uncontrollable infection, and benign deformity (congenital and acquired) probably account for most of the amputations done for nonvascular reasons. Patients can be spared complex, expensive, and hazardous surgery simply by the very definite procedure of amputation. The decision is not always easy, but once it is made, it can literally change a patient's life.

The feet illustrated in a Figure 45-9 are those of a middle-aged man with severe Charcot-Marie-Tooth disease. After multiple corrective operations on his feet, he was still virtually disabled by pain. His job and marriage were in jeopardy, and he was in danger of becoming an alcoholic. Bilateral ankle disarticulation turned his life around and he now works, travels, and participates in active sports such as bowling.

In many cases, the patient is extremely grateful when amputation is finally offered as a solution after many painful and fruitless operations. Such is the case with a child who underwent nine procedures on both feet for congenital absence of the fibula before the age of 13 years. The patient underwent bilateral Symes' amputations, and she now functions well as a below-

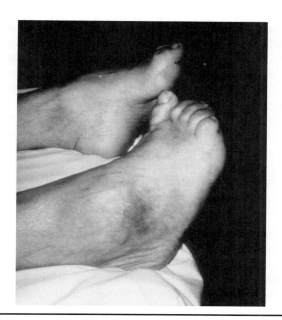

Fig. 45-9. Severe foot deformities due to peroneal muscle atrophy. Multiple previous operations had failed to relieve disabling pain.

knee amputee and has stated she wishes the operations had been done earlier.

Trauma

Miraculous advances in trauma surgery, such as internal fixation of fracture, soft tissue coverage by complex microsurgical techniques, and filling in of bone defects by vascularized bone grafts have made salvage of otherwise doomed limbs possible. However, the risks are great and sometimes after multiple operations, the patient finally comes to amputation anyway. Much patient suffering and disability—to say nothing of considerable expense—can be avoided by an early decision involving several consultants to amputate a severely traumatized limb rather than embarking on a long process of reconstruction.[19-21]

In grade III-C tibial fractures (those with the most severe soft tissue damage and involvement of one or more named vessels), the amputation rate varies from 20 to 75 percent. Although criteria exist for making such a decision, and Hansen has stated that orthopaedic surgeons should be able to make the decision without undue delay, it is not always that simple. Lange[21] indicated that even after consideration of all available criteria (massive crushing, ischemia or more than 6 hours' duration, severe fracture comminution or bone defect, infrapopliteal arterial injury, prolonged hypovolemic shock, and age of over 50 years), it is still very difficult to make an absolute, rigid recommendation. Most cases fall into an indeterminate prognostic group and it is difficult, if not impossible, to overcome the subjective feelings of the patient and family despite the existence of objective scientific evidence favoring one course or the other.

In any event, the pendulum seems to be swinging and traumatologists continue to define the criteria more accurately and to abandon the mind-set that amputation presents a therapeutic failure rather than a constructive procedure that may enable the patient to use modern prosthetics and get on with life.

Reimplantation has become more practical and more readily available in recent years as the criteria are better defined and more microvascular surgeons are available. Reimplantation is indicated only when definite improvement in function over prosthetic replacement can be predicted. The most common indications include a clean, sharp amputation of the thumb or multiple digits of the hand, or through a proximal portion of a limb. A team approach is definitely indicated owing to the complexity of the surgery and extremely long operating time. The team must not become so engrossed in re-establishing circulation that the skin, nerves, muscles, and bones are ignored. Rehabilitation can be prolonged and difficult as the team tries to balance restoration of function with healing of tissues. An excellent review of this subject is found in Kostuik's textbook on amputations.[6]

AMPUTATION IN CHILDREN

In most areas of medicine, care of children differs from that of adults, and amputation surgery is no exception. Limb deficiencies may be either congenital (70 percent) or acquired (30 percent). Because the needs of children are different from those of adults, care of their limb deficiencies requires great skill and

ingenuity from all members of the team. Mature adults are independent and most are reasonably responsible. The child, however, is immature, irresponsible, and quite dependent on others. Because of this, the team approach is highly recommended, even more so than for the adult.

In the traumatic amputation group, it has been shown by Galaway and others that social factors play a significant role.[6] Psychological and social service support can best be provided in a clinical setting. In addition, it is valuable for the patient and family to see and interact with others with similar deficiencies.

Three major points must be remembered when dealing with juvenile amputees, the first of which is growth. The surgeon must project toward the future maturity of the child, both in designing the operation and in planning for a prosthetic replacement. The second point relates to overgrowth. Amputations are done best through a joint rather than through the diaphysis of a long bone because the diaphysis runs a troublesome risk of bony overgrowth, which may require multiple revisions. Third, wounds heal more easily and rapidly in children because circulation is usually adequate, allowing more daring and creativity on the part of the surgeon in flap design and skin grafts.

Surgical revision is rarely necessary in the upper limb–deficient child. Nearly any residual limb can be fitted with a prosthesis, and frequently the vestigial digits can be used to activate portions of it. Surgery is more commonly performed on the lower limb because of the problems of leg length inequality and the requirement for a stable platform for weight-bearing (Figs. 45-10 and 45-11).

Extensive counseling for the parents is required because the decisions regarding treatment ultimately rest with them. Children are rarely able to participate to a significant extent in the decision making. In fact, if left to their own devices, children often develop tricky substitution maneuvers to ambulate or function single-handedly. Once these patterns are established, it is difficult to convert the children to be good

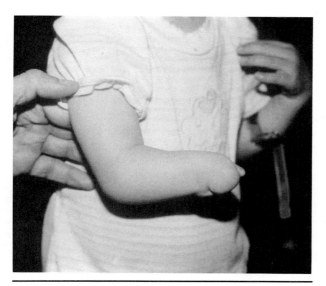

Fig. 45-10. Below-elbow limb defect is the most common defect in children.

prosthetic users. Excellent reviews of this subject are available.[4,6]

SHORT RESIDUAL LIMB

Advances in orthopaedic and plastic surgery have made it possible to revise residual limbs to allow function at the next level. For example, in past years the patient with a short, below-knee amputation complicated by adherent scar or skin graft would have had the extremity converted to a knee disarticulation or above-knee amputation to allow prosthetic fitting. Today, the below-knee level can be preserved by use of free tissue transfers, microvascular anastomoses (such as the latissimus dorsi muscle transfer), or tissue expanders.[7,22] In the last-mentioned technique, a bladder is inserted surgically under the skin and expanded gradually with periodic injections of saline solution until the skin is stretched enough to allow excision of the adherent skin and primary closure of the wound. Bone can then be lengthened, such as with the Ilizarov technique, to allow for satisfactory prosthetic fitting of persons with very short below-knee or short above-elbow amputations.

COMPLICATIONS

General Complications

The same complications that may be anticipated after any surgical procedure may also occur in amputation patients. General complications of surgery are perhaps more frequent in this group owing to the very nature of the patient population. The amputee with vascular problems is typically elderly and has cardiovascular disease frequently complicated by diabetes mellitus. The risks of anesthesia are higher, and wound infection and deep vein thrombosis are real concerns. These can be prevented with proper wound care, antibiotic prophylaxis, early mobilization, compression stocking, and anticoagulation in selected high-risk patients.

Overall function may be limited by problems unrelated to the amputation site itself. Generalized conditions such as chronic pulmonary or coronary artery disease may limit the patient's ability to walk. Most amputees and many physicians forget the increased energy consumption required for prosthetic use. This

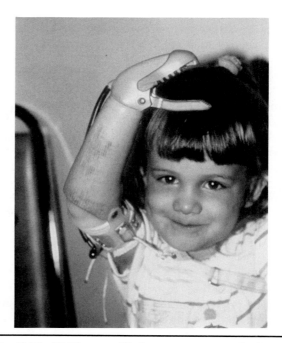

Fig. 45-11. Children readily learn to use a prosthesis.

demand becomes greater as the amputation level moves more proximally.

The use of a lower limb prosthesis may place excessive stress on the spine. Back pain may result from leg length inequality or other gait abnormalities. Ambulation may be limited by intolerable claudication in the contralateral leg in the patient with peripheral vascular disease. Instability or arthritis of the knee or hip above the amputation site may be aggravated by prosthetic use and must be addressed in the usual manner. Psychological complications are frequent. Evaluation and management of these complications are well covered in standard textbooks.[4]

Complications Involving the Residual Limb

When evaluating an amputee's situation, an early decision that needs to be made is whether it is a prosthetic or nonprosthetic problem. Nonprosthetic problems can be further broken down into medical versus surgical situations.

Wound healing is a sine qua non for successful amputation surgery. Hematomas, excessive edema, and infection all inhibit wound healing and can be prevented by absolute asepsis, careful hemostasis, prophylactic antibiotics, use of suction wound drainage, and attention to detail in postoperative care.

After secure wound healing, a variety of other complications involving the residual limb may occur, which impair function. Contractures may develop in the remaining joints. Once formed, they are very difficult to overcome and are better prevented by proper positioning, splinting, and exercising. Bony overgrowth or spur formation is usually seen in the child amputee but may be a problem in adults as well. Adherent skin may prevent proper use of a prosthesis. If this cannot be managed prosthetically with various interface materials, a surgical solution must be sought in the form of free tissue transfers or expanders.

Two complications from improper socket fit include choking or verrucous change in the distal end of the residual limb, usually due to lack of total contact with the socket. "Bottoming out" may result from further stump shrinkage and may be responsible for pressure ulcers on the residual limb.

Skin problems in the amputee are frequent. In addition to other skin conditions, such as allergic and circulatory problems, the residual limb is subject to a number of problems peculiar to it alone. When placed in a prosthetic socket for many hours, the residual limb is subjected to an abnormal environment of excessive heat and moisture, and it must endure unusual pressures and frictional stresses. It comes into contact with foreign interface materials, and bacterial flora may be changed drastically.

To prevent skin problems, the patient must be meticulous with hygiene, as it relates to both the residual limb and the prosthetic socket. The patient must also be alert to skin changes, and if these occur, the prosthetist or physician must be contacted promptly. Skin problems are so diverse and complex that entire books have been written on the subject.[23]

The evaluation and treatment of a painful residual limb can be difficult. Operative wound pain is to be expected, but it should subside within a week or so. Phantom sensations are always to be expected and may be present to some degree for the rest of the patient's life. Significant, disabling phantom pain, however, is rare but when present, it is very resistant to treatment. Neuroma pain is usually easily diagnosed. It may be present from the time the limb is amputated or may develop many years later. Ultrasound and electrical stimulation have been extremely effective in the treatment of neuroma pain; other measures include injection and surgical resection. Reflex sympathetic dystrophy syndrome can be treated by various medications and nerve blocks but occasionally is so troublesome it requires a higher amputation. However, even with this drastic measure, pain relief may be unsuccessful.

FUTURE DIRECTIONS

In addition to constant refinement of surgical technique, the future direction of amputation surgery will probably move toward better predictors. The need for better criteria to define indications for amputation, particularly in the trauma patient, is great. Much suffering can be prevented by more accurately predicting the level at which an amputation will succeed. Undoubtedly, some of the techniques now used in research will be refined and made available to the average clinician.

Rehabilitation efforts will be accelerated. These changes not only will make the amputee more functional in the long run but also will decrease the time involved, thereby saving a great deal of money and frustration. The goal must be to restore the amputee to as near normal function as possible and as quickly as possible.

Advances in prosthetics have been almost beyond the imagination in recent years. The goal has been, and must continue to be, the production of a prosthesis that will duplicate normal function as nearly as possible. One area for improvement is the development of better interface materials. Comfort and skin problems continue to plague the amputee, and there must be a continued search for better plastic, rubber, and silicone materials.

The trade-off of stability versus mobility of a prosthesis can be addressed by more creative biomechanical engineering research. The need for reducing the weight of a prosthesis while making it durable enough for long-term use is another problem that must be addressed. There is a need for better prosthetic hands, which are functional yet cosmetically accurate and durable enough to withstand mechanical and chemical insult. Another area for research is the development of an improved sensory feedback system for the upper extremity amputee.

Computer-assisted design and manufacture of prostheses holds some promise as it makes possible the extension of the service area of the certified prosthetist to areas now too remote for adequate coverage.

With attention to detail, a positive attitude, and involvement of a dedicated rehabilitation team, amputation surgery can be a satisfying and rewarding field for all those involved. Patients can be rehabilitated and restored to a surprising functional level, even in the advanced age groups. Many return to the work force, resume active avocations, and become productive members of society.

REFERENCES

1. Bodily KC, Burgess Em: contralateral limb and patient survival after leg amputation. Am J Surg 146:280, 1983
2. Diabetes in America. US Department of Health & Human Services, Washington, DC, 1984
3. Kay SP, Moreland JR, Schmitter E: Nutritional status and wound healing in lower extremity amputations. Clin Orthop 217:253, 1987
4. American Academy of Orthopaedic Surgeons: Atlas Of Limb Prosthetics: Surgical And Prosthetic Principles. CV Mosby, St. Louis, 1981
5. Crenshaw AH (ed): Campbell's Operative Orthopedics. Vol. I. 7th Ed. CV Mosby, St. Louis, 1987
6. Kostuik JP: Amputation Surgery and Rehabilitation. The Toronto Experience. Churchill Livingstone, New York, 1981
7. Murdoch G, Donovan RG (eds): Amputation Surgery And Lower Limb Prosthetics. Blackwell Scientific Publications, Oxford, England, 1988
8. Volpicelli LJ, Chambers RB, Wagner FW: Ambulation levels of bilateral lower extremity amputees. Analysis of 103 cases. J Bone Joint Surg [Am] 65:599, 1983
9. Oishi CS, Fronek A, Golbranson FL et al: The role of noninvasive studies in determining levels of amputation. J Bone Joint Surg [Am] 70:1520, 1988
10. Wyss CR, Harrington RM, Burgess EM, Matsen FA III: Transcutaneous oxygen tension as a predictor of success after amputation. J Bone Joint Surg [Am] 70:203, 1988
11. Pinzur M, Kaminsky M, Sage R, et al: Amputations at the middle level of the foot. J Bone Joint Surg [Am] 68:1061, 1986
12. Pinzur MS, Sage R, Schwaegler P: Ray resection in the dysvascular foot. A retrospective review. Clin Orthop 191:232, 1984
13. Burgess EM, Romano RL: The management of lower extremity amputees using immediate postsurgical prostheses. Clin Orthop 57:137, 1968
14. Burgess EM, Romano RL, Zettl JH: The management of lower extremity amputations. Publ. No. TR 10-6. US Government Printing Office, Washington, DC, 1969
15. Au KK: Sagittal flaps in below-knee amputations in Chinese patients. J Bone Joint Surg [Br] 71:597, 1989
16. Yamanaka M, Kwong PK: The side-to-side flap technique in below-the-knee amputation with long stump. Clin Orthop 201:75, 1975
17. Pinzur MS, Smith DG, Daluga DJ, Osterman H: Selection of patients for through-the-knee amputation. J Bone Joint Surg [Am] 70:746, 1988
18. Malone JM, Fleming LL, Roberson J et al: Immediate, early, and late postsurgical management of upper limb amputation. J Rehabil Res Dev 21:33, 1984
19. McAndrew MP (ed): The severely traumatized lower limb: reconstruction versus amputation (Section I). Clin Orthop 243:3, 1989
20. Hansen ST: Overview of the severely traumatized lower limb. Clin Orthop 243:17, 1989
21. Lange RH: Limb reconstruction versus amputation decision-making in massive lower extremity trauma. Clin Orthop 243:92, 1989
22. May JW, Sheppard J: Reconstruction of the stump after below-the-knee amputations. Soft tissue expansion and local muscle rotation flaps; a case report. J Bone Joint Surg [Am] 69:1240, 1987
23. Levy SW: Skin Problems of the Amputee. WH Green, Inc, St. Louis, 1983

SUGGESTED READING

Franzeck UK, Talke P, Bernstein EF et al: Transcutaneous pO_2 measurements in health and peripheral arterial occlusive disease. Surgery 91:156, 1982

Golbranson FL, Asbelle C, Strand D: Immediate postsurgical fitting and early ambulation: a new concept in amputee rehabilitation. Clin Orthop 56:119, 1968

Hadden W, Marks R, Murdoch G, Stewart C: Wedge resection of amputation stumps: a valuable salvage procedure. J Bone Joint Surg [Br] 69:306, 1987

Moore TJ, Barron J, Hutchinson F et al: Prosthetic usage following major lower extremity amputation. Clin Orthop 238:219, 1989

46 Compartment Syndrome and Ischemic Contracture

MICHAEL J. BOTTE
RICHARD H. GELBERMAN

Compartment syndrome is a pathologic condition of increased pressure within a closed fascial space (muscle compartment) that reduces capillary blood perfusion below a level necessary for tissue viability.[1] Acute compartment syndrome is the most severe form and usually develops after trauma.[2-7] Intracompartmental pressure can be elevated to a level and duration such that irreversible injury to muscle and nerve occurs. After necrosis takes place, muscle undergoes fibrosis and contracture, which can result in a dysfunctional limb known as *Volkmann's ischemic contracture*.[6,8-22] This permanent sequela often can be avoided or minimized with aggressive emergency muscle decompression via fascial incision (fasciotomy) performed in the early or acute stages, thus allowing reperfusion of ischemic muscle and nerve.[10,12,17,23-26]

Acute compartment syndrome should be considered a separate entity from chronic or exertional compartment syndrome.[6] Chronic compartment syndrome generally is a less severe condition that usually occurs after exercise and transiently raises intracompartmental pressure sufficiently to produce temporary ischemia, pain, and occasionally neurologic deficit. This less severe form usually is not associated with permanent sequelae and does not produce ischemic contractures. The chronic form often is treated with regulation of activity and occasionally requires elective fasciotomy. Chronic compartment syndrome is mentioned here only to avoid confusion with the acute form, and is not the subject of this chapter. It is acute compartment syndrome and its sequela of Volkmann's ischemic contracture (which usually require extensive rehabilitation efforts) that are discussed here.

HISTORICAL ASPECTS

von Volkmann described muscle ischemia and extremity paralysis resulting in contracture in 1881.[22] Paralysis and contracture were thought to be caused by the application of tight, constricting bandages to an injured limb. In 1914, Murphy reported an increase in pressure within a fascia-enclosed muscle space as a result of hemorrhage and edema, and he was first to suggest that paralysis and contracture might be prevented by fascial incision.[27] In 1926, Jepson first demonstrated the effects of early fascial decompression on injured muscle.[28] Since then, a number of authors have provided reports on the pathogenesis and sequelae of compartment syndromes. The theory now widely accepted is that microcirculatory impairment secondary to sustained increases in intracompartment interstitial pressure is the critical factor that causes compartment syndrome and, ultimately, Volkmann's ischemic contracture.[1,8,10,15-18,21,28-34]

COMPARTMENT SYNDROMES

Muscle Compartments of the Extremities

Each skeletal muscle is surrounded by its own thin fibrous sheath known as the epimysium. In addition to this fibrous sheath, muscles or groups of muscles usually are enclosed by an additional fascial sheath known as the deep fascia. Groups of muscles subsequently form discrete compartments, whose boundaries are composed of fascia, interosseous membranes, or bone. Major muscle compartments are listed in Tables 46-1 and 46-2.[35-39] It is this anatomic arrangement that predisposes muscle to formation of compartment syndrome. Because major nerves pass through or adjacent to these compartments, nerves are vulnerable to the effects of increased pressure from compartment syndrome.

Pathophysiology

Requirements for the development of compartment syndrome are a limiting envelope (fascial sheath) surrounding the muscles and increased interstitial tissue fluid pressure within the envelope (i.e., within the compartment). Usually an inciting event causes an initial increase in tissue fluid pressure from edema or hemorrhage.[6] This initial increase in tissue pressure decreases capillary flow and results in areas of muscle ischemia. Muscle ischemia promotes vasodilation and increased capillary permeability, causing additional edema within the compartment and resulting in a further increase in tissue pressure. Rising compartment pressure leads to compartmental tamponade and sustained ischemia. Muscle and nerve tissue are especially vulnerable to ischemia and will sustain irreversible damage if sufficient pressures are maintained.[11,15,16,32,40] Normal muscle tissue fluid pressure is usually less than 8 mmHg. Animal studies have shown that pressures maintained above 30 mmHg for 8 hours are able to cause irreversible damage to muscle and significant nerve conduction dysfunction.[11,15,16,32]

Table 46-1. Major Muscle Compartments of the Upper Extremity

Compartment	Principal Muscles
Shoulder	
Deltoid compartment	Deltoid
Arm	
Anterior compartment	Biceps brachii
	Brachialis
	Coracobrachialis
Posterior compartment	Triceps (three heads)
Forearm	
Mobile wad	Brachioradialis
	Extensor carpi radialis longus
	Extensor carpi radialis brevis
Anterior compartment	Pronator teres
	Flexor carpi radialis
	Flexor digitorum superficialis
	Flexor carpi radialis
	Flexor carpi ulnaris
	Flexor digitorum profundus
	Flexor pollicis longus
	Palmaris longus
Posterior compartment	Extensor digitorum communis
	Extensor carpi ulnaris
	Extensor digiti quinti
	Extensor pollicis longus
	Abductor pollicis longus
	Extensor pollicis brevis
Hand	
Thenar compartment	Abductor pollicis brevis
	Flexor pollicis brevis
	Opponens pollicis
Hypothenar compartment	Abductor digiti minimi
	Flexor digiti minimi
	Opponens digiti minimi
Interosseous compartments	Dorsal interosseous
	Palmar interosseous

Causes of Compartment Syndromes

The causes or inciting events leading to compartment syndromes are numerous and include fracture; soft tissue injury (crush or blunt trauma); spontaneous hematoma from hemophilia; prolonged limb pressure from unconsciousness secondary to drug overdose; edema occurring as a result of infection, burns, frostbite, revascularization of arterial injury, or snake bites; external pressure caused by unprotected limb placement during prolonged surgery; and ischemia induced by prolonged use of surgical tourniquets.[2,4,6,18,19,24,27,28,35,39,41,42]

Compartment syndrome from fractures occurs more often in closed fractures in which the facial sheath is maintained. Constricting casts or occlusive dressings placed on acute fractures or immediately after surgery do not allow for further swelling and add to the risk of compartment syndrome. In adults, tibial and forearm fractures are among the more common fractures that result in compartment syndrome.[2,4,6,12,20,24,25] In children, supracondylar fractures of the elbow have been shown to be a frequent cause, especially when compounded with application of tight-fitting casts, concomitant brachial artery injury, or arterial occlusion.[8,19,28]

After operative revascularization of an extremity, a postischemic edematous response occurs, resulting in possible compartment syndrome. Prophylactic extremity fasciotomy is usually performed after revascularization of a limb that has been avascular for more than 6 hours.

Burns can lead to compartment syndrome by causing intramuscular edema from the inflammatory response to the burn. In addition, the burned skin looses elasticity, especially if an eschar forms.[41] The constricted, burned skin acts similarly to an occlusive dressing, by not allowing the extremity to expand in response to the burn. The pressure in the muscle underneath the eschar thus increases.

Snake bites cause an intense inflammatory response that precipitates edema and can result in compartment syndrome, especially if the venom is injected deep to the muscle fascia and into a muscle compartment. In most cases, however, snake fangs do not reach deep enough to enter the muscle fascia and the venom is injected subcutaneously, which is less likely to produce compartment syndrome.[41]

Diagnosis of Compartment Syndrome

Diagnosis of compartment syndrome is usually made clinically and confirmed by measurement of intracompartment tissue fluid pressure (Fig. 46–1A).[41] Clinical findings include (1) a swollen, tense compartment; (2) pain (usually out of proportion to that expected from the existing injury); (3) sensory deficits; and (4) motor weakness or paralysis. Pain associated with compartment syndrome usually is accentuated with stretch of the muscle by manipulation of

Table 46-2. Major Muscle Compartments of the Lower Extremity

Compartment	Principal Muscles
Hip	
Gluteal compartment	Gluteus maximus
	Gluteus medius
	Gluteus minimus
	Tensor fasciae latae
Iliacus compartment	Psoas major
	Psoas minor
	Iliacus
Thigh	
Anterior compartment	Rectus femoris
	Vastus lateralis
	Vastus intermedius
	Vastus medialis
	Sartorius
Medial (adductor) compartment	Pectineus
	Adductor brevis
	Adductor longus
	Adductor magnus
	Gracilis
Posterior compartment	Biceps femoris
	Semitendinosus
	Semimembranosus
Leg	
Anterior compartment	Tibialis anterior
	Extensor hallucis longus
	Extensor digitorum longus
	Peroneus tertius
Lateral compartment	Peroneus longus
	Peroneus brevis
Superficial posterior compartment	Gastrocnemius
	Soleus
Deep posterior compartment	Flexor hallucis longus
	Tibialis posterior
	Flexor digitorum longus
Foot	
Lateral plantar compartment	Abductor digiti minimi
	Flexor digiti minimi
	Opponens digiti minimi
Medial plantar compartment	Abductor hallucis brevis
	Flexor hallucis brevis
Central plantar compartment	Flexor digitorum brevis
	Lumbricals
	Quadratus plantae
	Adductor hallucis
Interosseous compartments	Dorsal interosseous
	Plantar interosseous

the digits or distal extremity. The hypesthesias and anesthesia produced by compartment syndrome usually are located in the area distal to the compartment (i.e., in the sensory distribution of the nerves that course through the compartment). Sensibility

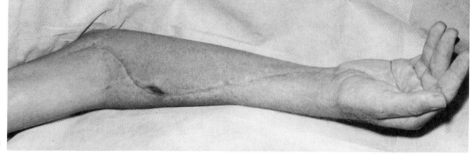

Fig. 46-1. (A) Upper extremity with compartment syndrome. Note swelling and tense-appearing flexor compartments of the forearm. Incision site is marked in preparation for fasciotomy. Other clinical findings in this patient included severe forearm pain, sensibility deficits in the thumb, index, and long fingers, and weakness with digital and thumb flexion. Pain was accentuated with passive extension of the digits. **(B)** Incision required for adequate flexor compartment release and median nerve decompression. **(C)** Intraoperative photograph after fasciotomy. **(D)** Forearm approximately 6 weeks after faciotomy. Symptoms had resolved and skin incision has healed. (Fig. B from Gelberman et al,[23] with permission.)

deficits usually precede motor dysfunction.[1,40] *Pulses usually remain intact* because systolic arterial pressure (normally 120 mmHg) usually is far above the pressure within the muscle afflicted with compartment syndrome (30 to 60 mmHg); thus, blood flow through the major arteries is not impeded and pulses remain intact.

Delay in the diagnosis of compartment syndrome can occur in the patient with pre-existing or concomitant central or peripheral nerve dysfunction. Patients with cognitive deficits from traumatic brain injury or drug or alcohol intoxication are difficult to examine and are at risk for missed diagnosis, especially if they are unresponsive, uncooperative, or show no appreciable pain. The diagnosis can also be delayed in the patient with concomitant peripheral nerve or spinal cord injury if motor and sensory deficits are incorrectly attributed solely to the nerve injury or if the patient shows little or no pain because of concomitant nerve injury.

Although the diagnosis of compartment syndrome is initially made clinically, confirmation is aided with measurement of intracompartmental tissue fluid pressure. Intracompartmental pressure measurement can be accomplished by a variety of methods. The most popular methods include the wick catheter technique, the slit catheter technique, continuous infusion techniques, and new transducers that report the pressure digitally.[1,5,6,12,24,43,44]

Treatment of Acute Compartment Syndrome

Initial treatment of acute compartment syndrome is removal of splints or any occlusive dressings or casts. If symptoms do not resolve quickly, fasciotomy remains the treatment for established compartment syndrome (Fig. 46–1B–D).[1,5,6,10–12,18,23,25,26,38] Fasciotomy releases the pressure of the involved compartment by interrupting the enclosed constricting envelope surrounding the muscle. Once the pressure is relieved, circulation within the compartment is restored and ischemia is alleviated. Release of edematous or constricting skin is often required. After decompression, the skin incision usually is left open in anticipation of further swelling. Delayed primary closure or split-thickness skin grafting is performed

after the swelling has subsided, usually 5 to 7 days after fasciotomy.

Reduction of skeletal muscle necrosis using intermittent hyperbaric oxygen has been reported as an adjunct to fasciotomy; however, its role in the management of compartment syndrome is not well established.[45]

Outcomes of decompression are variable and depend on amount of muscle and nerve damage prior to treatment.[6,12,24,40,46] The level and duration of pressure maintained on the muscle and nerve are related to final outcome. In addition, systemic blood pressure also may influence outcome, with systemic hypotension thought to result in less extremity compartment perfusion and possibly worsening the final outcome. Many patients treated promptly with appropriate fasciotomy will ultimately have minimal dysfunction, whereas others, especially those with delays in diagnosis or treatment, will develop the full sequelae of Volkmann's ischemic contracture with severe functional deficits.

VOLKMANN'S ISCHEMIC CONTRACTURE

Pathogenesis

Muscle is highly vulnerable to changes in oxygen tension. It undergoes necrosis after 4 hours of experimentally produced ischemia by tourniquet application.[15,16] With prolonged ischemia produced by sustained compartment syndrome, muscle necrosis (infarction) occurs. Subsequent fibroblastic proliferation within the muscle infarct occurs. The muscle mass undergoes a variable amount of longitudinal and horizontal contraction as it becomes a fibrotic mass. This process can progress over a 6- to 12-month period after the ischemic insult. The necrotic muscle often adheres to surrounding structures, which fix the muscle position and further reduce muscle mobility. Secondary compression of the surrounding structures occurs, with peripheral nerves being particularly vulnerable.[12] Primary limitation of muscle excursion and longitudinal contraction during fibrotic proliferation lead to loss of joint motion and subsequent joint contracture (Fig. 46–2). Peripheral nerve injury, stemming from both ische-

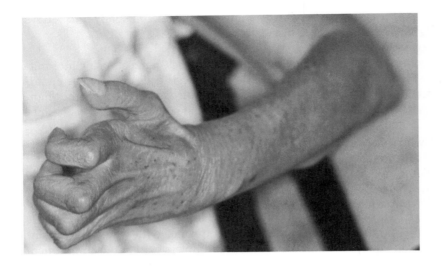

Fig. 46-2. Upper extremity demonstrating the devastating sequelae of untreated compartment syndrome. The patient now has established Volkmann's contracture. Unrecognized compartment syndrome had occurred originally after revascularization of a dysvascular extremity with arterial injury. The deformed extremity is now dysfunctional, with severe sensory and motor deficits. Fixed contractures are present at the elbow, wrist, and digits. The forearm muscle mass is fibrotic, with a firm "woody" consistency owing to severe muscle fibrosis. The flexor digitorum profundus, flexor pollicis longus, and flexor digitorum superficialis muscles are all severely involved.

mic insult from the original compartment syndrome and secondary compression owing to muscle fibrosis and limb contracture, further contributes to limb dysfunction and disability.

Deformity of the Upper Extremity

In the upper extremity, injury to forearm muscles that results in ischemic necrosis is usually most marked in the deep flexor compartment (Figs. 46 – 3 and 46 – 4). The flexor digitorum profundus and flexor pollicis longus muscles are most commonly affected. In the mildest contractures, only a portion of the flexor digitorum profundus muscle undergoes necrosis, usually involving the ring and long fingers. In severe contractures, all four digits are involved (Fig. 46 – 2). The flexor digitorum superficialis and pronator teres muscles generally are less severely affected. In the most severe cases, however, the wrist flexors and even the wrist and digital extensors may undergo varying degrees of fibrosis and contracture.[12,47]

The specific primary involvement of the deep flexors of the forearm is attributed to their deep location within the forearm compartment, a factor that is believed to increase their vulnerability to ischemia.[34] The deepest compartment areas, particularly those regions adjacent to the bone, have been found to have the highest interstitial pressures during compartment syndrome.[15] With compression from within, the circulation to the deep portions of the muscle belly is compromised, whereas collateral circulation to the more superficial portions of the muscle may be retained. When a compartment syndrome is untreated, swelling may eventually resolve, but the damaged muscle becomes fibrotic. The characteristic deformity of ischemic contracture may take many weeks or months to develop completely. When the arm, forearm, and hand are all involved, deformity in the upper limb usually consists of elbow flexion, forearm pronation, wrist flexion, thumb flexion and adduction, digital metacarpophalangeal joint extension, and interphalangeal joint flexion. The metacarpophalangeal joint extension and proximal interphalangeal joint flexion gives rise to a claw hand deformity (Fig. 46 – 2).

The pathomechanics of the Volkmann's ischemic claw hand deformity are complex. Although similarities exist between Volkmann's contracture and intrinsic muscle contracture, the actual mechanics of the deformities are considerably different. Intrinsic muscle contracture results in an "intrinsic plus" deformity, characterized by flexion at the metacarpophalangeal joints and extension at the proximal interphalangeal joints. Volkmann's ischemic contracture usually leads to an "intrinsic minus" deformity, characterized by hyperextension at the metacarpophalangeal joints and flexion at the interphalangeal joints. Although the two entities are asso-

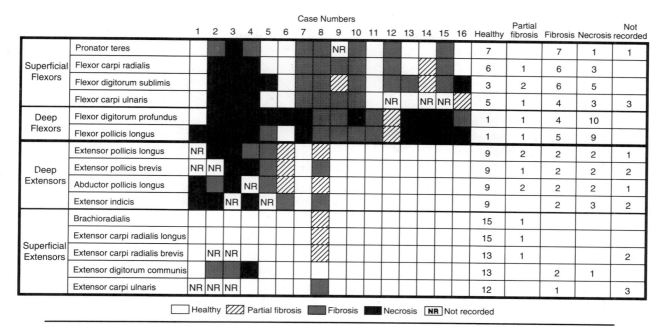

Fig. 46-3. The muscles affected in 16 cases of Volkmann's contracture of the forearm. (From Seddon,[34] with permission.)

ciated and may occur simultaneously, the resultant claw hand (intrinsic minus) is determined by contracture of the more powerful extrinsic finger flexors. A paradoxical situation of a claw hand deformity with intrinsic muscle tightness also exists.[12] The intrinsic muscle contracture may not become apparent until the extrinsic flexors have been released by tendon lengthening, muscle recession, or tenotomy.

An additional factor in the pathomechanics of upper extremity deformity is the amount of peripheral nerve injury superimposed on the muscle injury. Median and ulnar neuropathy may occur, both from the original ischemic insult and from subsequent compression that develops during muscle fibrosis. Ulnar and median neuropathy will add to dysfunction of intrinsic muscles of the hand, thereby contributing the intrinsic minus, or claw hand deformity.

Classification of Upper Extremity Contractures

In the upper extremity, ischemic contractures have been classified according to severity of involvement.[12,47,48] The simplest classification system, de-

scribing mild, moderate, and severe involvement, is useful for determining treatment options.

Mild or localized contracture of the upper extremity is limited to a portion of the deep intrinsic finger flexors, and usually involves only two or three fingers. Hand sensibility is normal, and strength is normal or minimally impaired. Intrinsic muscles are not involved, and fixed joint contractures do not occur. Most mild types of Volkmann's contracture are caused by fractures or crush injuries to the forearm or elbow, usually in young adults.[17,47]

Moderate contractures of the upper extremity are considered the classic type, primarily involving the flexor digitorum profundus and flexor pollicis longus muscles. Less frequently, the flexor digitorum superficialis, flexor carpi radialis, and flexor carpi ulnaris muscles are involved. The wrist and thumb become flexed, and the hand assumes an intrinsic minus deformity from contracture of the long finger flexors.

In moderate contractures, secondary compression neuropathies may develop, especially at specific anatomic sites where nerves pass beneath ligaments or

A

B

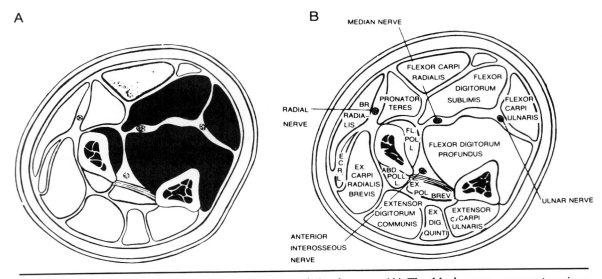

MEDIAN NERVE

MEDIAN NERVE

FLEXOR CARPI
RADIALIS

FLEXOR
DIGITORUM
SUBLIMIS

FLEXOR
CARPI
ULNARIS

PRONATOR
TERES

RADIAL
NERVE

BR
RADIA-
LIS

E
C
R
L

FL
POL
L

EX.
CARPI
RADIALIS
BREVIS

ABD
POLL
L.

FLEXOR DIGITORUM
PROFUNDUS

EX.
POL BREV

ULNAR NERVE

EXTENSOR
DIGITORUM
COMMUNIS

EX
DIG
QUINTI

EXTENSOR
C/CARPI
ULNARIS

ANTERIOR
INTEROSSEOUS
NERVE

Fig. 46-4. Cross section in Volkmann's contracture of the forearm. **(A)** The black areas represent various involved muscles (based on data provided in Fig. 46-3). **(B)** Key to muscles. The plane of section is through the upper third of the forearm. E and EX, extensor; Dig, digiti; FL, flexor; POL and POLL, pollicis; L, longus; BREV, brevis; BR, brachioradialis; ABD, abductor; C, capri; R, radialis. (From Seddon,[34] with permission.)

fibrous arcades, or through contracted muscles. The median nerve frequently is involved, compressed at either the lacertus fibrosus, pronator teres, or flexor digitorum superficialis muscle, or within the carpal tunnel. The ulnar nerve may be compressed at the elbow between the two heads of the flexor carpi ulnaris. The radial nerve, which is rarely involved, may be compressed at the arcade of Frohse or within the supinator muscle.

Many moderate contractures of the upper extremity are caused by supracondylar fracture of the humerus. These fractures commonly occur in the age group of 5 to 10 years.[17,19,28,47]

Severe contractures are those that involve both the forearm flexors and the forearm extensors. Secondary complications, such as neuropathy, malunion or nonunion of fractures, and cutaneous scarring with skin contracture, are often encountered. Common causes of severe contracture are prolonged ischemia secondary to brachial artery injury, prolonged external compression secondary to drug overdose, or severe devascularizing crush injuries.[6]

Rehabilitation and Reconstruction

Mild Contractures

Treatment of mild contractures of the upper extremity depends on the severity of deformity and time interval between injury and initiation of treatment. Contractures of the deep forearm flexors, with normal hand sensibility and preservation of remaining extrinsic muscle strength, often can be treated nonoperatively with a comprehensive hand rehabilitation program and team approach.[12] Hand therapy, employing active and passive mobilization, strengthening, and static and dynamic extension splinting, is employed to maintain or improve thumb web space width, strengthen weak thumb intrinsic muscles, and correct or improve digital flexion contractures. Serial digital casting is rarely required for mild contractures. Bivalved pancake plaster casts or splints can be alternated with low-profile digital extension and thumb opposition splints. A C-bar may be incorporated into the splint to maintain thumb position. Early in the rehabilitation program, static, and dynamic splinting is alternated at 2-hour intervals during the day. At night, plaster or custom synthetic extension splints are worn. Strengthening with progressive active mobilization against resistance is instituted. Splinting techniques for Volkmann's contracture are described in further detail by Goldner.[13] A satisfactory outcome can usually be expected when mild contractures are treated with these techniques soon after their development.

When mild contractures are encountered late or do not respond to a nonoperative rehabilitation program, operative treatment can be considered.[47] If the contracture is limited to one or two digits and a cord-like area of induration is palpable, simple excision of the infarcted muscle or lengthening of the involved flexor tendon can be performed.[47] The flexor digitorum profundus muscles to the ring and long fingers most often require infarct excision. If the contracture is localized to the pronator teres, muscle myotomy or excision can be performed. If the contracture and induration involve three or four digits, flexor tendon lengthening (employing Z-lengthening) may be required.[12]

Moderate and Severe Contractures

The treatment of moderate to severe contractures may be divided into four phases: (1) release of secondary nerve compression, (2) treatment of contractures, (3) tendon transfers for restoration or reinforcement of lost function, and (4) salvage procedures for the severely contracted or neglected extremity.[12,47]

Phase 1: Release of Secondary Nerve Compression.
Subsequent to muscle infarct, peripheral nerves can be compressed either by constricting fibrotic muscle or at specific anatomic locations where space is minimal. Because improvement of nerve function is related to the severity and duration of compression, early nerve decompression is required to minimize further dysfunction. Nerves may sustain compression for longer periods than muscle and still show some reversibility, particularly in sensibility function.[12,34] When nerve continuity is maintained, nerves may show signs of gradual recovery over a 12-month period.[34,46] In severe ischemic contracture, when fibrosis is extensive, all three major forearm nerves may become compressed. Careful clinical as-

sessment is essential, and appropriate nerve decompression is performed as indicated. The median nerve is especially at risk, because it lies in the center of the constricting cicatrix and may become compressed in four anatomic regions: the lacertus fibrosus, the pronator teres, the proximal arch of the flexor digitorum superficialis, and the carpal tunnel.[23,24] Ulnar nerve compression occurs at a much lower rate than median nerve compression. The ulnar nerve is often compressed at the elbow as it passes between the ulnar and humeral heads of the flexor carpi ulnaris muscle. Decompression is indicated if signs of ulnar motor and sensory loss are present. Although the radial nerve is rarely involved in compression neuropathies after ischemic contracture, it may require decompression as it passes under the tendinous origin of the supinator muscle (arcade of Frohse) or within the muscle itself. Radial nerve compression at this level is manifested by motor loss of the digital and thumb extensors and the ulnar wrist extensors. The radial wrist extensor muscle strength and radial nerve sensibility remain intact, because these nerve branches arise proximal to the area of compression.[12,23,24]

Nerve decompression should be performed as soon as the condition of the patient permits. A nerve stimulator may be helpful for verification of conductivity, especially in heavily scarred areas. Early return of sensibility and a decrease in pain occur when timely decompression is undertaken. Nerves that are damaged irreparably, or those with loss of continuity, will require secondary excision of damaged nerve segments and repair or reconstruction with microsurgical techniques.[12]

Phase 2: Release of Contracture.
Fixed contractures that develop over time usually produce characteristic deformities of elbow flexion, forearm pronation, wrist flexion, digital clawing, or thumb adduction.[12,47] When these deformities are refractory to passive mobilization and a splinting and serial casting program, surgical reconstruction can be performed. Seddon recommends at least 6 months of preliminary splinting prior to contracture release.[34] Common procedures employed to correct these established fixed contractures include infarct incision and flexor tendon lengthening, excision, or recession (flexor pronator slide).[20,49] A chief disadvantage of

tendon lengthening procedures is the additional weakening produced in these impaired muscles. However, release of a severe contracture usually is more functionally advantageous than maintenance of maximal strength. Tendon transfers, if needed, are performed at a later date.[12,14,24,26,47,50-53] In the nonfunctional, severely deformed extremity, contracture release may be useful to facilitate hygiene in the palm or antecubital fossa or to facilitate dressing.

Phase 3: Tendon Transfers to Restore or Reinforce Function. Among the most desirable functions to restore in the patient with ischemic contractures are finger and thumb flexion and thumb opposition.[50,53,54] Tendon transfers usually are delayed until nerve recovery has reached a plateau and the contractures have been maximally corrected with a mobilization and splinting program or with operative release. A series of tendon transfers designed to provide digital flexion and thumb opposition has been described.[12,47,50,53,54] Because the extensor muscles usually are involved the least in ischemic contractures, these muscles are used as donor muscles to provide digital and thumb flexion and thumb opposition. Examples of tendon transfers include the extensor carpi radialis longus transferred to the flexor digitorum profundus and the extensor carpi ulnaris (lengthened by a tendon graft) transferred to the thumb for opposition. The tendons of the flexor digitorum superficialis are excised if nonfunctional. The extensor pollicis brevis can be used to reinforce the extensor carpi ulnaris opponens transfer. Alternative transfers to augment thumb opposition include the extensor indicis proprius opponensplasty popularized by Zancolli[53] and Burkhalter and coworkers[50] and the abductor digiti quinti opponensplasty described by Huber.[54] The brachioradialis may be transferred to the flexor pollicus longus to reinforce thumb flexion.[47]

When flexor tendons have been weakened severely by previous lengthening, reinforcement by transfer of the extensor carpi radialis longus to the flexor digitorum profundus and transfer of the extensor carpi ulnaris to the flexor pollicis longus can be performed.[13]

Phase 4: Salvage of the Severely Contracted or Neglected Forearm. If the procedures of phases 2 and 3 do not provide satisfactory correction of contractures,

additional reconstructive surgery or salvage measures may be required.[12,47] Procedures that have proved useful for the severely contracted or neglected forearm include proximal or distal row carpectomy (which shortens the limb and allows wrist extension while maintaining flexibility), radial and ulnar shortening, wrist fusion, and digital joint fusion. Carpectomy may be performed prior to tendon transfer. Interphalangeal joint arthodesis in a more functional position can correct severe fixed contractures, especially when adequate muscles for transfer are not available. Arthrodesis can be combined with shortening of the digit to prevent stretching of the digital neurovascular structures when the digit is extended to a more functional position. After interphalangeal joint fusion, the limb can function as a hook, which is generally superior to a prosthesis, especially if some sensibility is retained.[13] Radial and ulnar shortening are rarely necessary or recommended.

The hand deformity associated with Volkmann's contracture is complex and requires a systematic, therapeutic approach. Intrinsic muscle contractures should be addressed only after extrinsic finger flexors have been released. Fixed contractures create a claw hand deformity. After extrinsic muscle release, an intrinsic plus deformity of the hand may occur. Complete release of intrinsic contractures may not be desirable, because retainment of some metacarpophalangeal joint flexion will prevent recurrence of the claw hand deformity. If the intrinsic contracture is severe, the oblique fibers of the extensor hood may be released to permit flexion of the interphalangeal joints.[12]

Thumb-in-palm deformity often accompanies the claw hand in ischemic contractures. The deformity results from both intrinsic and extrinsic contractures. Flexion contracture of the interphalangeal joint may be corrected with flexor pollicus longus release or lengthening. Residual deformity is attributable to intrinsic contracture, joint contracture, or skin contracture of the first web. Procedures recommended for correction of thumb-in-palm deformity include release of the adductor pollicis, deepening of the thumb web space, fusion of the metacarpophalangeal joint or interphalangeal joint, or excision of the trapezium.[13] Thenar origin release and release of the first dorsal interosseous muscle also may be necessary for full correction.

The most significant hand impairments are caused not by intrinsic contractures but by sequelae of extrinsic muscle contractures in the forearm. Problems resulting from these include loss of median and ulnar nerve sensibility (from nerve compression by fibrotic muscle masses), intrinsic paralysis secondary to median and ulnar motor nerve paralysis, and digital joint flexion deformities secondary to contracture of the extrinsic flexors. Proper management of these problems, as described in phases 1 and 2, should significantly improve hand function.

Deformity of the Lower Extremity

In the lower extremity, patterns of ischemic contractures and deformity depend on the specific compartments involved. Involved compartments that subsequently undergo muscle necrosis will develop joint contracture deformity as the muscle undergoes fibrosis with longitudinal contraction. Concomitant nerve compression results in weakness of the corresponding innervated muscles. Although compartment syndromes of the thigh and buttocks do occur, they are much less common than those that develop in the leg and foot (Fig. 46–5).

Any of the four compartments of the leg can be afflicted with compartment syndrome.[2,4,5,18,25,33,41,42] Unexpected claw toe deformity (characterized by flexion of the proximal and distal interphalangeal joints and extension of the metatarsophalangeal joints) occurring after treatment of fractures of the tibia and fibula has been thought to be due to unrecognized and untreated compartment syndrome of the deep posterior or anterior compartments of the leg.[41,55] Necrosis and fibrosis of the deep posterior compartment and anterior compartment of the leg cause contracture of the extrinsic toe flexor and extensor muscles, resulting in claw toe deformities. This is similar to contracture of the upper extremity, in which deformity is caused by contracture of the more powerful extrinsic muscles, resulting in an intrinsic minus (claw hand or claw toe) deformity. In addition, varus deformity often accompanies toe deformity from necrosis, fibrosis, and contracture of the tibialis posterior or tibialis anterior muscle. Compartment syndrome of the lateral compartment with subse-quent contracture can result in abduction deformity of the foot. Compartment syndrome with contracture of the anterior compartment can cause calcaneus deformity (dorsiflexion attitude of the foot). However, concomitant injury to the anterior tibial nerve or paralysis of the ankle dorsiflexors can result, conversely, in loss of dorsiflexion, resulting in a drop-foot gait. Compartment syndrome that produces fibrosis and contracture of the superficial posterior compartment of the leg results in equinus deformity. Unexpected cavus foot deformity occurring after fracture of the tibial and fibula also has been thought to be due to unrecognized compartment syndrome, resulting in injury to the posterior tibial nerve with loss of intrinsic muscle function, causing imbalance of the stronger extrinsic muscles.[55]

Compartment syndrome involving the intrinsic muscles of the foot can occur from crush injuries.[7,26,35,39] Because crush injuries to the foot are not uncommon, not surprisingly the intrinsic muscles, with their well-defined compartments and many rigid osseofascial boundaries, are particularly at risk.[37,38] The foot has four separate, easily identifiable compartments: medial, central, lateral, and interosseous (Table 46–2). The end product of untreated compartment syndrome of the foot is paralysis and contracture of the intrinsic muscles, resulting in dysfunction, deformity, and, frequently, chronic pain. The intrinsic muscles of the foot atrophy, the forefoot and toes develop contractures, and the foot becomes immobile from fibrosis of necrotic muscle.[7,26,35,39]

As with the digits in the hand, the pathomechanics of toe deformity are complex, and either "intrinsic minus" (claw toes) or "intrinsic plus" toes may develop. Intrinsic minus deformity (claw toes) is characterized by extension at the metatarsophalangeal joints and flexion at the proximal and distal interphalangeal joints. This occurs from loss of intrinsic muscle function, leading to muscle imbalance with overpull of the extrinsic toe extensors and flexors. The intrinsic muscles (i.e., the interosseous and lumbrical muscles) function to flex the metatarsophalangeal joints and extend the proximal and distal interphalangeal joints. Loss of function of these muscles leads to a deformity characterized by extension of the metatarsophalangeal joints and flexion of the interphalangeal joints. Therefore, paralysis of the intrinsic

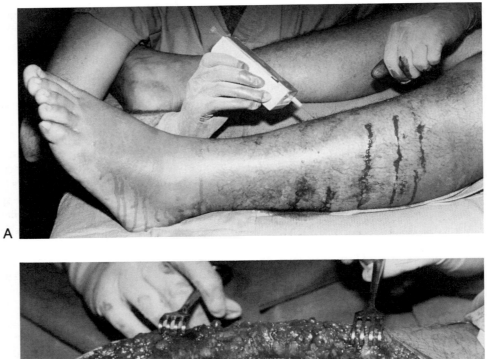

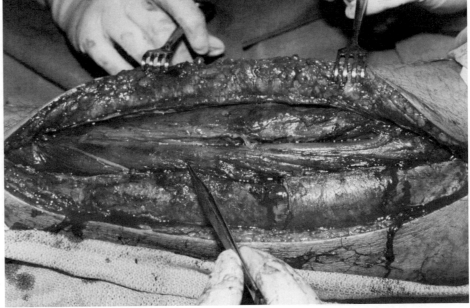

Fig. 46-5. (A) Leg with compartment syndrome. Patient had swollen, tense anterior compartment, severe pain, numbness of the dorsal portion of the first web space of the foot, and inability to extend the toes. Intracompartmental pressures are being determined. **(B)** Fasciotomy incision of leg for treatment of compartment syndrome of the anterior compartment.

muscles from compartment syndrome can produce an intrinsic minus foot with claw toes. Conversely, however, an intrinsic plus foot also can develop. The intrinsic plus foot is characterized by flexion at the metatarsophalangeal joints with extension at the proximal and distal interphalangeal joints. This is produced by shortening of the intrinsic muscles from fibrosis and contracture formation. Whether the toes will become clawed (intrinsic minus) or whether they will develop an intrinsic plus deformity probably depends on many factors, including the relative involvement of nerve dysfunction (from necrosis or compression by fibrotic muscle), the amount of muscle necrosis, and the relative amounts of muscle paralysis versus muscle fibrosis or contracture that develop. In addition, contributions to deformity from involvement of the extrinsic muscles with fibrosis, shortening, and contracture will contribute to claw toes. Cavus foot deformity results both from paralysis and contracture of the intrinsic muscles and from overpull of the extrinsics.

Compartment syndrome of the foot also may cause sensibility deficits from nerve necrosis or compression, thus compounding the disability.

Rehabilitation and Reconstruction

Compared to the upper extremity, less information is currently available concerning the results of reconstruction and rehabilitation of ischemic contractures of the lower extremity. The same philosophy as described for the upper extremity should generally be considered. This includes prevention and treatment of contractures by splinting and mobilization for mild involvement, and release of secondary nerve compression followed by operative treatment of contractures and foot reconstruction for more severe involvement.

Equinus deformity from contracture of the superficial posterior muscle compartment is often correctable with passive mobilization. Serial casting and dynamic splinting are effective adjuvants. Caution must be exercised with serial casting or dynamic splinting if previous nerve injury has resulted in sensibility impairment, since patients with such impairment are at high risk for skin breakdown or pressure ulceration. When contractures have been corrected, therapy can continue with further muscle strengthening and night splinting as necessary to maintain correction. When chronic muscle imbalance exists, the patient is susceptible to development of late deformity. Home exercise programs and intermittent splinting can be continued as needed for long-term management.

When more severe involvement is present, nerve decompression, as indicated, should be performed as soon as possible, with the aid of a nerve stimulator at the time of surgery for verification of nerve conductivity, especially in heavily scarred areas. Severe contractures that are not responsive to nonsurgical methods are treated with operative release or lengthening of tendons and soft tissues. Equinus deformity refractory to dynamic splinting or serial casting can be treated with tendo Achillis lengthening. For heavily scarred posterior compartments, open lengthening procedures of this tendon are preferable to percutaneous tenotomy. For flexible equinovarus, tendon transfers such as the split tibialis anterior tendon transfer (combined with tendo Achillis lengthening) can be performed if the tibialis anterior has adequate strength. Lengthening of the extrinsic tendons and soft tissues on the medial aspect of the ankle may be necessary as well. For paralysis of the anterior compartment with drop-foot, tendon transfer can be considered if an available donor muscle exists. Hindfoot arthrodesis as a salvage procedure can be considered to correct severe or rigid deformity. Claw toes and a cavus foot deformity can be treated with conventional methods of foot reconstruction, utilizing soft tissue procedures for flexible deformities or bony procedures for rigid or fixed deformities. It is preferable to obtain an arteriogram to further assess vascular status prior to embarking on reconstructive or salvage procedures, because many of these patients who have sustained severe injuries to the leg or foot may have sustained arterial injuries as well.

Free Vascularized Tissue Transfers

Microsurgical advances have allowed free transfer of vascularized skin, nerve, and muscle. Transfer of the lateral head of the pectoralis major to the forearm flexor for ischemic contracture has been discussed.[12,56] Satisfactory results also have been reported using a free vascularized superficial radial nerve graft transfer to an irreparably damaged median nerve.[12,47] Free vascularized tissue transfer has become increasingly popular, and reconstruction of forearm muscles using gracilis, rectus femoris, latissimus dorsi, and pectoralis muscles has been described. Although the early results of these procedures are promising, their role in the reconstruction of limbs with severe Volkmann's contracture remains to be determined.[47,56,57]

CONCLUSION

Compartment syndrome is a pathologic condition of increased tissue fluid pressure within a closed fascial space (muscle compartment) that reduces capillary blood perfusion below a level necessary for tissue viability. Muscle and nerve are particularly susceptible to permanent injury from increased pressure of compartment syndrome. Treatment of acute compartment syndrome is fasciotomy to relieve tissue pressure. Sustained intracompartmental pressures will lead to muscle and nerve necrosis and fibrosis. Fibrosis of muscle can cause secondary nerve compression. As the injured muscle undergoes fibrosis, it shortens and results in limb contracture, deformity, and dysfunction—a condition known as Volkmann's ischemic contracture. Treatment of mild ischemic contracture includes maintenance of motion, prevention or correction of mild contractures with splinting and mobilization, and muscle strengthening. Treatment of severe ischemic contractures includes surgical release of secondary nerve compression, prevention or correction of contractures through dynamic and static splinting, active and passive mobilization, and muscle strengthening. In addition, severe deformity often requires surgical release or lengthening of contracted soft tissues. Limb reconstruction can ultimately be performed using tendon transfers, muscle recession or lengthening, osteotomy, or arthrodesis. A team approach for these challenging rehabilitation problems will offer the patient the optimum method of management.

REFERENCES

1. Hargens AR, Akeson WH, Mubarak SJ et al: Kappa Delta Award Paper. Tissue fluid pressures: from basic research tools to clinical applications. J Orthop Res 7:902, 1989
2. Blick SS, Brumback RJ, Poka A et al: Compartment syndrome in open tibial fractures. J Bone Joint Surg [Am] 68:1348, 1986
3. Matsen FA: Compartmental syndrome. A unified concept. Clin Orthop 113:8, 1975
4. Mubarak SJ, Owen CA: Compartmental syndrome and its relation to the crush syndrome: a spectrum of disease. Clin Orthop 113:81, 1975
5. Mubarak SJ, Owen CA, Hargens AR et al: Acute compartment syndromes: diagnosis and treatment with the aid of the wick catheter. J Bone Joint Surg [Am] 60:1091, 1978
6. Mubarak SJ, Hargens AR (eds): Compartment Syndromes and Volkmann's Ischemic Contracture. WB Saunders, Philadelphia, 1981
7. Myerson M: Diagnosis and treatment of acute compartment syndromes of the foot. Orthopaedics 13:711, 1990
8. Benjamin A: The relief of traumatic arterial spasm in threatened Volkmann's contracture. J Bone Joint Surg [Br] 39:711, 1959
9. Brooks B: Pathological changes in muscle as a result of disturbances of circulation. An experimental study of Volkmann's ischemic paralysis. Arch Surg 5:188, 1922
10. Eichler GR, Lipscomb PR: The changing treatment of Volkmann's ischemic contractures from 1955 to 1965 at the Mayo Clinic. Clin Orthop 50:215, 1967
11. Gelberman RH, Szabo RM, Williamson RV et al: Tissue pressure threshold for peripheral nerve viability. Clin Orthop 178:285, 1983
12. Gelberman RH, Botte MJ: Management of Volkmann's contracture. p. 1131. In Chapman MW (ed): Operative Orthopaedics. JB Lippincott, Philadelphia, 1988
13. Goldner JL: Volkmann's ischemic contracture. p. 823. In Flynn JE (ed): Hand Surgery. Williams and Wilkins, Baltimore, 1975
14. Griffiths DL: Volkmann's ischemic contracture. Br J Surg 28:239, 1940
15. Hargens AR, Schmidt DA, Evans KL et al: Quantitation of skeletal-muscle necrosis in a model compartment syndrome. J Bone Joint Surg [Am] 63:631, 1981
16. Hargens AR, Romine JS, Sipe JC et al: Peripheral nerve conduction bock by high muscle compartment pressure. J Bone Joint Surg [Am] 61:192, 1979
17. Holden CE: The pathology and prevention of Volkmann's ischemic contracture. J Bone Joint Surg [Br] 61:296, 1979
18. Lipscomb PR: The etiology and prevention of Volkmann's ischemic contracture. Surg Gynecol Obstet 103:353, 1956
19. Meyerding HW: Volkmann's ischemic contracture associated with supracondylar fracture of humerus. JAMA 106:1139, 1936
20. Rergstad A, Hellum C: Volkmann's ischemic contracture of the forearm. Injury 12:148, 1980
21. Sorokhan AJ, Eaton RG: Volkmann's ischemia. J Hand Surg [Am] 8:806, 1983
22. Volkmann R von: Die ischaemischen Muskellahmungen und Kontrakturen, Zentralbl Chir 8:80, 1881
23. Gelberman RH, Zakaib GS, Mubarak SJ et al: Decompression of forearm compartment syndromes. Clin Orthop 134:225, 1978
24. Gelberman RH: Volkmann's contracture of the upper extremity: pathology and reconstruction. p. 183. In Mubarak SJ, Hargens AR (eds): Compartment Syndrome and Volkmann's Contracture. WB Saunders, Philadelphia, 1981
25. Mubarak SJ, Owen CA: Double-incision fasciotomy of the leg for decompression in compartment syndromes. J Bone Joint Surg [Am] 59:184, 1977
26. Myerson M: Experimental decompression of fascial compartments of the foot—the basis for fasciotomy in acute compartment syndromes. Foot Ankle 8:308, 1988
27. Murphy JB: Myositis. JAMA 63:1249, 1914
28. Mubarak SJ, Carroll NC: Volkmann's contracture in children: etiology and prevention. J Bone Joint Surg [Br] 61:285, 1979
29. Ashton H: The effect of increased tissue pressure on blood flow. Clin Orthop 113:15, 1975
30. Ashton H: Critical closure in human limbs. Br Med Bull 19:149, 1963
31. Dann I, Lassen A, Westing H: Blood flow in human muscles during external pressure on venous stasis. Clin Scil 32:467, 1967
32. Hargens AR, Akeson WH, Mubarak SJ et al: Fluid balance within the canine anterolateral compartment and its relationship to compartment syndromes. J Bone Joint Surg [Am] 60:499, 1978
33. Rorabeck CH, Macnab I: The pathophysiology of the anterior tibial compartmental syndrome. Clin Orthop 113:52, 1975
34. Seddon HJ: Volkmann's contracture: treatment by incision of the infarct. J Bone Joint Surg [Br] 38:152, 1956
35. Bonuti PM, Bell GR: Compartment syndrome of the foot. A case report. J Bone Joint Surg [Am] 68:1449, 1986

36. Garfin SR: Anatomy of the extremity compartments. p. 17. In Mubarak SJ, Hargens AR (eds): Compartment Syndromes and Volkmann's Ischemic Contracture. WB Saunders, Philadelphia, 1981
37. Grodinske M: A study of fascial spaces of the foot. Surg Gynecol Obstet 49:739, 1929
38. Loeffler RD, Ballard A: Plantar fascial spaces of the foot and proposed surgical approach. Foot Ankle 1:11, 1980
39. Myerson M: Acute compartment syndromes of the foot. Bull Hosp Joint Dis Orthop Inst 47:251, 1987
40. Botte MJ, Rhoades CE, Gelberman RH et al: Peroneal nerve function in acute anterior compartment syndrome. Orthop Trans 10:206, 1986
41. Clawson DK: Claw toes following tibial fracture. Clin Orthop 103:47, 1974
42. Rorabeck CH, Macnab I: Anterior tibial compartment syndrome complication fractures of the shaft of the tibia. J Bone Joint Surg [Am] 58:549, 1976
43. Mubarak SJ, Hargens AR, Owen CA et al: The wick catheter technique for measurement of intramuscular pressure: a new research and clinical tool. J Bone Joint Surg [Am] 58:1016, 1976
44. Whitesides TE Jr, Hanes TC, Morimoto K, Harada H: Tissue pressure measurements as a determinant for the need of fasciotomy. Clin Orthop 113:43, 1975
45. Strauss MB, Hargens AR, Gershuni DH et al: Reduction of skeletal muscle necrosis using intermittent hyperbaric oxygen in a model compartment syndrome. J Bone Joint Surg [Am] 65:656, 1983
46. Sundoraraj GD, Mani D: Pattern of contracture and recovery following ischemia of the upper limb. J Hand Surg [Br] 10:155, 1985
47. Tsuge K: Treatment of established Volkmann's contracture. J Bone Joint Surg [Am] 57:925, 1975
48. Benkeddache Y, Bottesman H, Hamdani M: Proposal of a new classification for established Volkmann's contracture. Ann Chir 4:134, 1985
49. Page CM: An operation for the relief of flexion-contracture in the forearm. J Bone Joint Surg 5:233, 1923
50. Burkhalter WE, Christensen RC, Brown P: The extensor indicis proprius opponensplasty. J Bone Joint Surg [Am] 55:725, 1973
51. Parks A: The treatment of established Volkmann's contracture by tendon transplantation. J Bone Joint Surg [Br] 33:359, 1951
52. Peacock EE, Madden JW, Trier WC: Transfer of median and ulnar nerves during early treatment of forearm ischemia. Ann Surg 169:748, 1969
53. Zancolli E: Tendon transfers after ischemic contracture of the forearm. Classification in relation to intrinsic muscle disorders. Am J Surg 1098:356, 1965
54. Huber E: Hilfsoperation bei median Uslahmung. Dtsch Arch Klin Med 136:271, 1921
55. Karlstrom G, Lonnerholm T, Olerud S: Cavus deformity of the foot after fracture of the tibial shaft. J Bone Joint Surg [Am] 57:893, 1975
56. Ikuta Y, Kubo T, Tsuge K: Free muscle transplantation by microsurgical technique to treat severe Volkmann's contracture. Plast Reconstr Surg 58:407, 1976
57. Tamai S, Komatsu S, Sakamoto H et al: Free muscle transplants in dogs with microsurgical, neurovascular anastomoses. Plast Reconstr Surg 46:219, 1970

47 Reflex Sympathetic Dystrophy

HARRIS GELLMAN

Reflex sympathetic dystrophy (RSD) is the most frequently used term for a disorder that has previously appeared in the literature under a confusing array of designations since Mitchell and associates[1] first related the findings of causalgia ("burning pain") due to gunshot injuries to major mixed nerves during the Civil War. Causalgia, minor causalgia, Sudek's atrophy, posttraumatic pain syndrome, sympathalgia, shoulder-hand syndrome, and chronic traumatic edema are among some of the other names that have been commonly used.

CLINICAL ASPECTS

The most prominent feature of RSD is pain, usually much greater than would be expected for the degree of injury. The pain is constant and can be exacerbated by emotional factors. Severe hyperalgesia is often poorly localized, frequently progressing to a diffuse distribution. Swelling is the most constant physical finding, which if not treated early is often followed by the rapid onset of stiffness (Fig. 47-1). Clinicians with experience treating RSD agree that early diagnosis is of paramount importance.[2] The most perplexing feature is how a trivial injury can produce pain that far surpasses the magnitude of the initial injury, and persist long after the injury has healed.

Secondary signs that are variably present depending on the type and stage of RSD include osseous demineralization, sudomotor changes, temperature changes, trophic changes, vasomotor changes, discoloration, palmar fibrosis, and hyperhidrosis.[2]

Course of the Syndrome

Reflex sympathetic dystrophy usually evolves in three stages, all dominated by severe burning or aching pain. The course varies depending on the severity of the disorder and whether proper treatment is started. Without treatment the disorder will usually pass through the following stages.

Stage I

The first stage begins anytime from the injury to several weeks thereafter. An increase in edema, erythema, and warmth, reflecting an increase in the superficial blood flow of the injured part may occur. Hyperhydrosis, muscle wasting, and increased hair and nail growth may also be seen. Pain is constant and is aggravated by movement and weight-bearing. Disuse of the painful part occurs voluntarily to minimize pain, or therapeutically, as with a fracture treatment. Radiographic changes of osteopenia can occur as early as 4 to 8 weeks after the onset of pain. In mild cases this stage may last only a few weeks, then subside spontaneously or respond rapidly to treatment if it is initiated early. The average duration of stage I is 3 months, but it can last as long as 6 months.[2]

Stage II

Stage II appears about 3 months after the onset of pain. In this stage, pain becomes even more severe and diffuse. The skin becomes cool and pale and may be cyanotic. Edema spreads and changes from a soft to a brawny type. Hair is lost, and nails become brittle and cracked and they may even be grooved. Joint motion becomes limited with thickening of the joint. Stage II may last from 3 to 6 months.

Stage III

For many patients, pain becomes intractable in stage III and may spread proximally to involve the entire limb. Joints become rigid and finally ankylosed. De-

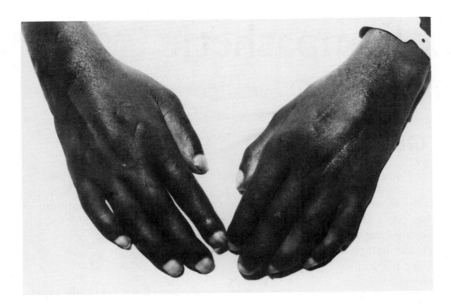

Fig. 47-1. Hands of a patient with reflex sympathetic dystrophy. Note swelling and glossy, mottled skin.

crease in the superficial blood flow results in marked trophic changes of the skin. Contraction of the flexor tendons occurs and may lead to joint subluxation. Radiographs now consistently show marked and diffuse disuse osteoporosis.

Some of the problems and effects of the prolonged pain of RSD include family disruption and divorce, family sorrow for loved ones, temporary and often permanent unemployment, and misdiagnosis and disbelief by physicians, leading to improper treatment and multiple surgeries. There is a decrease in quality life for the patient in addition to greatly increased health care costs.

DIAGNOSIS

The diagnosis of reflex sympathetic dystrophy is based primarily on clinical criteria.[3] The patient should have a history of recent or remote trauma, either accidental or iatrogenic, with persistent pain that is burning, aching, or throbbing in character. One or more of the following signs is seen: vasomotor or sudomotor disturbances, edema of the limb, sensitivity to cold, trophic changes, and muscle weakness or atrophy. Relief of pain and modification of signs after regional sympathetic blockade is virtually diagnostic of the disorder. Many subtle cases of mild RSD are accompanied by only one or two of the symptoms

and signs, or the entire symptom complex may be vague and confusing, making a differential diagnosis difficult. In addition, certain medical problems such as traumatic brain injury may make obtaining a detailed history impossible. In these cases advanced radiographic techniques and thermography may help to confirm the diagnosis.

The most reliable aid to diagnosis, in addition to the physical examination, has been the three-phase radionuclide bone scan (TPBS). MacKinnon and Holder[4] have reported 96 percent sensitivity and 98 percent specificity in the diagnosis of RSD using this scan. Prior to the use of the TPBS, the finding of periarticular or diffuse mottled osteoporosis on plain radiographs (Fig. 47-2) was used as an aid in the diagnosis of RSD.[5]

Andrews and Armitage[6] studied 19 patients with traumatic quadriplegia using a correlation of radiographic and clinical findings. Mottled osteoporosis was noted in the hands of five patients, four of whom complained of pain in the affected hands. Radiographs, unfortunately, are much less sensitive and specific. Because calcium content must be altered by 30 to 50 percent to be demonstrable on conventional bone radiographs, the TPBS will be positive earlier than conventional radiographs. Similarly, patchy demineralization is not specific for RSD and has been

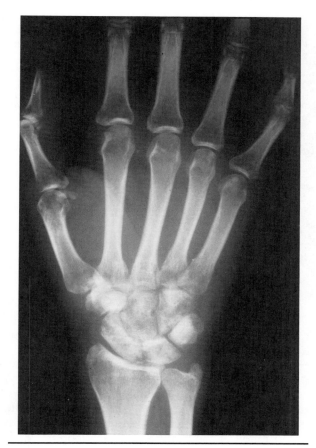

Fig. 47-2. Radiograph demonstrating macular and periarticular osteopenia seen in reflex sympathetic dystrophy.

reported as a positive finding in 30 to 80 percent of cases.[6-9] Demineralization may also result from the disuse atrophy associated with muscle paralysis.[10] Thus, radiographs in quadriplegic or hemiplegic patients generally are not helpful in differentiating atrophy occurring as a result of disuse from RSD.[9,11-14] In addition, spasticity in the brain-injured patient may mask or prevent the development of osteoporotic changes that might otherwise occur.

Three-phase scanning consists of a radionuclide angiogram (sequential 5-second images obtained over a span of 40 seconds in both hands) (Fig. 47-3), followed by a blood pool phase obtained using 500,000-count images (Fig. 47-4); a third or delayed metabolic bone phase image is then obtained 3 to 4 hours after injection (Fig. 47-5). Delayed-phase scans

are evaluated using the criteria of MacKinnon and Holder.[4] Results are graded as normal (Fig. 47-5), focally or multifocally abnormal (Fig. 47-6), or diffusely abnormal (Fig. 47-7). For a scan to be considered diagnostic of RSD, the delayed phase must show diffusely increased activity in the involved radiocarpal and ulnocarpal joints, intercarpal joints, carpometacarpal joints, metacarpolphalangeal areas, and juxtaarticular regions of the digits.[4] Periarticular accentuation in the delayed phase of the TPBS has been a characteristic finding in RSD, occasionally even preceding clinical symptoms. The blood flow and pool image changes have not been as useful in hemiplegic and quadriplegic patients, because both increases and decreases in flow have been seen in patients with characteristic findings in the delayed phase.[14] Brain-injured patients usually require sedation and close observation during the scan. The diagnostic accuracy, however, has been shown to exceed that of clinical examination alone in this patient population. This is especially important in neurologically impaired patients, for whom the goal is early and rapid rehabilitation. A delay in diagnosis and treatment could result in permanent stiffness, contractures, and loss of function in the hands of patients who must rely solely on their upper extremities.

Thermography has also been reported to play a significant role in confirming the diagnosis in the more subtle cases of RSD.[15-18] Using liquid contact thermography, Low and colleagues[17] studied 121 patients with chronic pain and noted a 21.5 percent incidence of previously undiagnosed RSD. Uematsu and colleagues[18] studied patients with RSD using electronic telethermography. With this technique, they found that the condition is not as rare as previously believed. Hendler and associates[15] evaluated 224 consecutive patients who had complained of chronic pain but who did not have positive radiologic, neurologic, orthopaedic, or laboratory evidence; these patients had been referred to them for psychiatric evaluation. Abnormal thermographic results in the affected limb (reduction in temperature of 1°C or more) were found in 43 (19 percent) of the patients. Of this group, 32 (74 percent) patients had evidence of RSD. The diagnosis was confirmed by sympathetic block, which in some patients was followed by sympathectomy, resulting in permanent pain relief.

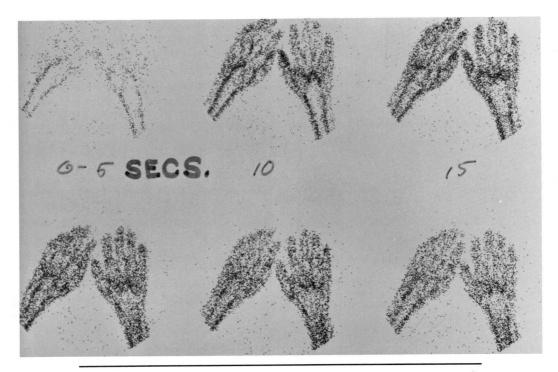

Fig. 47-3. Radionuclide angiogram phase of three-phase bone scan (normal).

Sylvest and coworkers[19] have described the use of resting blood flow and muscle temperature to help confirm the diagnosis of RSD. Temperature and blood flow measurements were carried out on both extremities of 51 patients. On clinical evidence 25 patients were believed to have RSD. The temperature of the brachioradialis muscle and resting blood flow of the same segment of the forearm were significantly elevated in the reflex dystrophic arms as compared with the healthy side, whereas the control patients revealed no such differences. Blood flow and muscle temperature measurements may prove useful not only as an aid to diagnosis but also in following the patient's response to treatment.

ETIOLOGY

Several theories of the pathogenesis of RSD have been formulated, with overactivity of the sympathetic nervous system resulting in an abnormal feedback mechanism being the common denominator.[20-24] Whether the overactivity is a result of an artificial peripheral synapse formed between sensory afferents and sympathetic efferents, or the central excitation within the spinal cord of gate-opening small pain (C) fibers, treatment goals are aimed at interruption of the positive feedback loop.[20-23,25-27] For this reason, surgical as well as chemical sympathectomy has been recommended as treatment.[20,25,26]

The exact mechanism whereby the sympathetic response becomes abnormal is not known. Normally, in response to injury there is an activation of the sympathetic nervous system. Sympathetic outflow, initiated by the pain of injury, causes vasoconstriction in the limb, leading to decreased blood loss and swelling. After injury, sympathetic tone decreases and blood flow to the limb increases, allowing entry of constituents for repair as well as the removal of waste products from the site of injury. If sympathetic tone persists inappropriately, an abnormal feedback mechanism and an atypical sympathetic reflex results. This causes tissue edema, resulting in capillary collapse and ischemia, which in turn causes local pain in the injured limb. This pain signal re-excites the sympathetic nerves and thus a positive feedback circuit becomes established.[2] Successful treatment of RSD is contingent on interruption of this abnormal

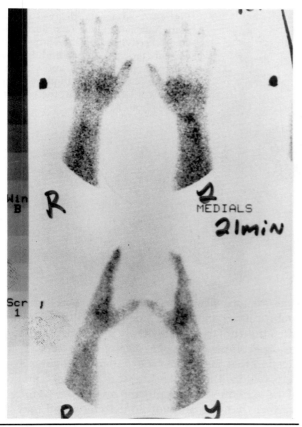

Fig. 47-4. Blood-pool phase of three-phase radionuclide bone scan (normal).

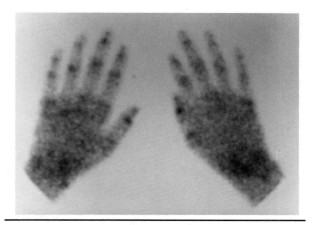

Fig. 47-5. Normal delayed-phase of three-phase bone scan.

continuous feedback loop. One method of accomplishing this is by sympathectomy, accomplished either surgically, systemically by medication, or locally by the instillation of anesthetics.

It has also been postulated that a short circuit develops between the pain-bearing nerve fibers and those of the sympathetic nervous system and could lead to the development of RSD after nerve injury. The arrangement of the motor, sensory, and sympathetic fibers in the proximal nerve trunk and spinal cord favor the formation of artificial synapses after injury. It has been postulated that these artificial synapses permit efferent impulses in adjacent sympathetic nerves to be relayed across to fine sensory fibers and that this abnormal activity results in reflex sympathetic dystrophy.[20,27] In retrospect, it should not be

surprising, therefore, to see RSD in spinal cord–injured patients.

SIGNIFICANCE OF RSD IN REHABILITATION

A severely painful upper extremity in patients who become paraplegic or quadriplegic as a result of a cervical spinal cord injury can present a major obstacle to rehabilitation. Complaints such as poorly localized pain, swelling, hypersensitivity to touch, and edema of the hands with glossy, mottled skin (Fig.

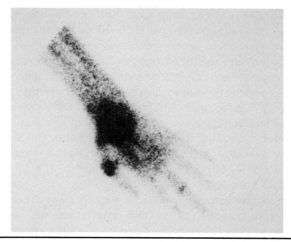

Fig. 47-6. Focally abnormal (left wrist) delayed phase of three-phase bone scan.

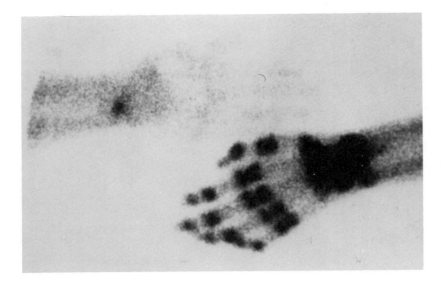

Fig. 47-7. Abnormal delayed phase scan (left hand) demonstrating increased activity in the intercarpal and carpometacarpal joints and in the metacarpophalangeal and juxta-articular regions of the digits. (Palms are down, left hand is at the bottom of the photo.)

47-1) should make the physician suspect RSD as the cause. Attempts at joint motion are usually resisted by the patient because of the intense pain. Although RSD is not commonly thought of in the differential diagnosis of upper extremity pain in the cervical spinal cord–injured patient, it has been well recognized in the hemiplegic patient.[5,6,12,24,28,29]

Sixty consecutive patients admitted to the spinal cord injury unit at Rancho Los Amigos Medical Center, Downey, CA, were interviewed for complaints of upper extremity pain and examined for hand tenderness, swelling, and/or stiffness. Patients with these findings underwent upper extremity evaluation with standard radiographs and TPBS. Symptomatic spinal cord–injured patients were examined an average of 9 months after the injury (range, 2 months to 3 years). No correlation was found between the incidence of RSD and the level of spinal cord injury or whether the injury was complete or incomplete. Many patients had bilateral involvement, which should be a clue to the observer that RSD may be the cause of the pain. The overall incidence of RSD in spinal cord–injured patients was found to be 10 percent.[30]

Upper extremity pain and hyperpathia are also frequently observed in patients after traumatic brain injury. These symptoms often pose a diagnostic dilemma, because most of these patients are cognitively unable to express or localize pain or participate in examination. Diagnosis of pain in the traumatic brain-injured patient is frequently difficult. More often than not these patients are unable to vocalize or localize complaints of pain. Many times the only indication that the patient is experiencing pain is a severe, rapid withdrawal response to attempted motion of the extremity. Frequently the involved extremity is warmer than the uninvolved extremity and may be mildly swollen or edematous, with mottled, glossy skin. Joint stiffness may occur rapidly in this patient population whether or not RSD is present. Careful examination may make the astute physician suspicious of the presence of RSD. Unfortunately, the differential diagnosis of upper extremity pain in the brain–injured patient with multiple injuries involves a large number of entities.

The rate of RSD in 100 consecutive admissions for rehabilitation to Rancho Los Amigos Medical Center was found to be 12 percent. All patients with RSD had an average Rancho Cognitive Level[31] of V, and all had Glascow Coma Scale scores less than 8, requiring 3 months or more of inpatient rehabilitation, reflecting the severity of their central nervous system injury. The mean time from injury to diagnosis of RSD was 3.9 months (range, 1 to 16 months). Without exception, RSD was present in the extremity with spasticity or patterned movement. There was a statistically significantly higher incidence of associated injury in the group of patients with RSD ($P < 0.01$).

Seventy-five percent of the patients with RSD had an associated upper extremity injury, compared with only 32 percent in the group without. Finally, it is apparent that patients with RSD attain a poorer outcome on the basis of Glasgow Outcome Scale scores and require longer periods for rehabilitation than patients without RSD. This fact is likely due to both the severity of the brain insult in the RSD patients and the RSD itself. With early diagnosis and prompt treatment, the physician can minimize the contribution of RSD to delay in rehabilitation. With approximately 50,000 persons with brain injuries annually requiring extended rehabilitation in the United States, a 12 percent incidence of RSD could theoretically result in 6,000 of these patients developing some form of RSD. If the patients are left untreated, many of these cases may progress to unnecessary, permanent disability.

Similarly, an incidence of RSD of 12.5 to 25 percent is reported after stroke.[5,6,12,24,28,29] Certainly, maintaining a high index of suspicion for RSD is indicated when caring for the neurologically impaired patient.

TREATMENT

Most physicians would agree that, if possible, relief of the initiating painful lesion should be obtained to control and to prevent the recurrence of RSD. This may involve elimination of painful pressure points under a cast, injection of trigger points, resection of neuromas, or decompression of a nerve entrapment.[32] The importance of early diagnosis cannot be overemphasized. Delay in treatment not only results in prolonged rehabilitation but also may allow the pain and physical alterations due to the RSD to become established and refractory to treatment. Poplowski and colleagues,[33] in a review of 126 patients with a diagnosis of posttraumatic dystrophy, found that the most important factor in predicting improvement with treatment was a short interval (less than 6 months) between the onset of dystrophy and the initiation of therapy.

Physical Therapy

The role of physical therapy for patients with established RSD syndrome remains an area of controversy. Several authors have reported the successful use of physical therapy alone in milder cases. Buker and associates[34] reported six patients with causalgia who were managed effectively with physical therapy alone. They emphasized the importance of early aggressive physical therapy; the sooner that therapy can be started the better the success. The therapist must be aggressive and initiate enthusiastic treatment, urging the patient to move actively. Omer and Thomas[35] also reported that 14 (20 percent) of their 70 patients with causalgia were treated successfully with physical therapy, which included elevation, traction, splinting, and general body conditioning. Although some form of physical and occupational therapy seems to be essential in the treatment of RSD, used injudiciously either of these can make existing symptoms worse. Most forms of therapy employ heat or ice packs but extremes of temperature should be avoided, because this may increase afferent transmission and exacerbate the condition.[36] A similar situation may occur if the extremity is permitted to be dependent. Early active motion is the goal of therapy.

Splinting is an integral part of the treatment program to prevent contracture formation. Passive ranging of joints may also be used, but the therapist should caution the patient about the risk of intensifying pain, swelling, and stiffness by forcing motion. Elevation is an important part of the treatment, and patients are encouraged to do exercises with the extremity elevated, and also to mobilize the shoulder because they frequently develop stiff, painful shoulders. Leach and coworkers[37] have recommended continuous elevation by spica cast as an adjunct to physical therapy to aid in reduction of edema and to better allow aggressive therapy. Range of motion and stretching exercises are used to counteract the tendency toward contracture formation. Motor re-education, relaxation, and strengthening exercises are added as the condition allows.

Prior to discontinuing formal therapy, the patient should always be instructed in a home exercise program to maintain gains. If pathologic changes such as shortening of tendons or fixed contractures are present in advanced cases, orthopaedic care is necessary for restoration of function.

Drug Therapy

Oral medications most commonly used include muscle relaxants, α and β blockers, analgesics, anti-inflammatories, tricyclic antidepressants and related compounds, tranquilizers, and calcium channel blockers.

Of the many actions of the sympathetic nervous system, the α-adrenergic action is the most important in its effect of vasoconstrictor in the skin and subcutaneous tissues of an extremity.[2] Phenoxybenzamine (Dibenzyline)[38] is the most effective α-blocking agent and has the fewest undesirable side effects. The initial recommended starting dose is 10 mg/day.[2] This dosage should be maintained for at least 5 days before any attempt is made to increase the dosage. If the patient complains of "fuzzy vision," dizziness, or lightheadedness at the end of the 5-day period, the dosage should not be increased until the symptoms decrease to a safe level. Each increase in dosage should be monitored for at least 5 days before another increase is made. Most patients can tolerate two to three doses per day, with three being an average. Ghostine and colleagues[39] reported the results of 40 cases treated with phenoxybenzamine. They noted that all 40 patients obtained complete relief but recommended dosages as high as 80 mg/day. Phentolamine (Regitine) is also an α-blocking agent, but its use is contraindicated in several types of cardiac conditions.[2]

Oral guanethidine in a single dose of 20 to 30 mg/day for 8 weeks has been suggested by Tabira and coworkers.[40] The drug acts orally on the postganglionic sympathetic neurons and depresses the function of the postganglionic adrenergic nerves, thus blocking sympathetic nerve–mediated impulses.[2,40] Disadvantages of oral guanethidine include the possibility of inciting mental depression, loss of appetite, impotence, and despondency. Because considerable orthostatic hypotension may occur, care must be exercised in its use.

The β-blocking agent propranolol (Inderal) also has been used in the treatment of RSD. Simpson[41] has reported good results with 40 mg orally every 4 hours and then increasing to 240 mg/day in relieving pain and other symptoms of causalgia. Tahmoush[42] also reported effective relief of the pain, hyperalgesia, and hyperpathia of causalgia with propranolol administered in doses of 320 mg/day. In some medical conditions propranolol is contraindicated because its β-adrenergic blocking action may negate the vasodilator effect of the β-catecholamines. There are many cardiac contraindications to the use of Inderal, and it should not be used in patients with asthma or a history of bronchospasm because of its broncho constrictive action. I personally use a modest dose of Inderal of 10 mg three to four times daily as part of the adjunctive treatment regimen for patients referred for the treatment of RSD. In addition, I include one of the nonsteroidal anti-inflammatory medications that can be taken on a twice-a-day basis because this makes it easier for patients to comply. Amitryptyline (Elavil) in a 25-mg starting dose is given at bedtime. The Elavil dosage is raised in increments of 25 mg weekly up to 200 mg as needed to decrease anxiety, aid the patient in getting a full night's sleep, and treat the depression, which many patients develop as a result of the RSD.

Mood-modifying drugs such as chlorpromazine (Thorazine), trifluoperazine (Stelazine), chlordiazepoxidl (Librium), diazepam (Valium), and Elavil[43] have been reported to be helpful in the control of RSD. It should be noted that their role is only adjunctive to the primary treatment, which involves interruption of the abnormal sympathetic reflex.[2]

Calcium channel blockers are a recent addition to the drug armamentarium for the treatment of RSD. Calcium entry blockers represent a means of inducing peripheral vasodilation without specifically interfering with the peripheral sympathetic nervous system.[44-46] They inhibit the movement of calcium ions into cells, and the resulting inhibition of excitation-contraction coupling causes relaxation of the arteriolar smooth muscle and vasodilation.[47] Calcium channel blockers have little effect, however, on the smooth muscles of veins. Nifedipine, a calcium entry blocker, relaxes smooth muscle,[45] increases peripheral blood flow,[44] and antagonizes the effects of norepinephrine on arterial and venous smooth muscle.[45] These effects have been exploited in the treatment of Raynaud's phenomena, with moderate success.[48,49] Nifedipine may not only interrupt the pain cycle in patients with RSD but may also reverse signs of vasomotor instability.[50] Prough and associates[50] reported the use of oral nifedipine in the treatment of 13 patients with RSD. Seven patients had complete relief of symptoms, two had partial relief; three withdrew because of headache; and one patient failed to obtain relief. Of the 10 patients who tolerated the nifedipine therapy, one died and two continued the medication for partial palliation of symptoms. The medication was successfully withdrawn from three of the remaining seven patients and their symptoms did not return. The other four patients noted recurrence of pain with weaning from the drug.

Sympathetic Interruption

The rationale for sympathetic blockade in patients with RSD is the interruption of the abnormal reflex arc mediated by the autonomic nervous system. Sympathetic interruption can be either chemical (local or regional) or surgical. If symptoms are not relieved promptly by oral medications combined with aggressive physical and occupational therapy, or if they become worse, treatment should proceed directly to sympathetic blocks.[51] Blocks are both diagnostic and therapeutic. Early, the relief of pain may last well beyond the duration of the block and even be curative. Blocks should be repeated (to a maximum of 8 to 12 blocks) until pain is controlled. If the results of the block are equivocal, a control block with normal saline solution may be performed. If relief becomes less effective after repeated sympathetic blocks and the initial response was a good one, surgical sympathectomy should be considered. Early sympathectomy will prevent the occurrence of irreversible trophic changes, as well as the establishment of fixed pain patterns, which may become refractory even to sympathectomy if the syndrome is allowed to continue untreated.

For the upper extremity, stellate ganglion blocks are performed using either 1 percent lidocaine or 0.25 percent bupivicaine (Marcaine). The stellate ganglion, which lies at the level of C7–T1, is bathed in the local anesthetic. The direct anterior approach to the stellate ganglion is recommended because it has a low complication rate and is easily performed.[52] A satisfactory technique for stellate ganglion block of the upper extremity is as follows[51]: With the patient's head extended and turned away from the physician the needle is inserted at a point 4 cm lateral to the midline and 4 cm up from the clavicle to a depth of 4 cm in the neck. The needle is directed medially and somewhat inferiorly toward the lateral bony mass of C7–T1. An injection of 10 ml of local anesthetic is customary. If the block is successful, a profound Horner's syndrome, with warming and drying of the hand as well as relief of pain, should follow immediately.

Lumbar block is more difficult than stellate ganglion block.[51] The preferred technique involves three needles placed 5 cm laterally to the midline opposite the transverse processes of L1, L2, L3, and L4. When the transverse processes are encountered, the needles are redirected above or below and inserted to a depth of 3.5 to 4 cm, so that their tips encounter the sympathetic trunk, lying along the anterolateral border of the lumbar vertebrae. Ten milliliters of 1 percent lidocaine are then injected through each needle. If the block is successful, within a few moments a sympathetic effect is apparent, with warming and drying of the foot and relief of pain.

Following stellate ganglion block or block of the lumbar sympathetic ganglia, minor or major complications may occur.[53,54] After stellate ganglion block, minor complications include dizziness, ringing in the ears, a feeling of blacking out, pain at the site of injection, and nerve block of the recurrent laryngeal, vagus, or phrenic nerves as well as part or all of the brachial plexus; major complications include severe systemic toxic reaction resulting in respiratory and cardiovascular collapse, total spinal anesthesia, pneumothorax, or cerebral air embolism. Minor complications after lumbar sympathetic block include paralysis of lumbar nerves from overflow or epidural block; major complications include severe systemic toxic reaction from high blood level of local anesthetic drug, resulting in respiratory and cardiovascular collapse with or without seizures, or total spinal anesthesia. The physician performing the block must be aware of the potential for these complications and recognize their signs and symptoms immediately. The equipment and drugs should be readily available to treat any complication that may arise. Moore[54] reported no serious complications after performing over 2,000 stellate ganglion blocks and close to 500 lumbar sympathetic blocks over a 15-year period.

Kleinert and associates[43] reported that 80 percent of their patients who were resistant to other medical management and physical therapy experienced pain relief from one or more stellate ganglion blocks. Of these, 81 percent required no further treatment during 1 to 5 years of follow-up. Nineteen percent of patients experienced a temporary response but ultimately required surgical sympathectomy. Only 17 percent of the patients in their group did not obtain permanent improvement. Lankford and Thompson[55] also reported favorable results after sympathetic blockade. They found that 89 percent of their patients with a diagnosis of causalgia and 80 percent of those with other dystrophic variants reported complete long-term palliation. Wang and coworkers[56] reported that at 3-year evaluation, 65 percent of patients treated by sympathetic block continued to show improvement, compared with only 41 percent of those managed by conservative means. When treatment was started within 6 months of onset, 70 percent of patients maintained improvement over the 3 years, compared with only 50 percent in the group whose treatment was not initiated until 6 to 12 months after onset of symptoms. Linson and colleagues[57] treated 29 patients with continuous stellate ganglion blockade using bupivicaine every 8 hours for an average of 7 days. Improvement during treatment was documented in all but two patients with regard to joint motion and pain relief and in two-thirds with regard to trophic and vasomotor changes. Long-term follow-up demonstrated a 25 percent relapse rate, but marked improvement persisted in the remainder.

Provided the procedure is done properly, response to regional sympathetic block is prompt and dramatic, with relief of pain, allodynia, and hyperpathia. If the patient has evidence of vasoconstriction, block results in an increase in the temperature of the limb, disappearance of cyanosis, and decrease in swelling over the next several hours and improved function in a few days.[3] The duration of the response produced by local sympathetic block varies from a few hours to several days, whereas after intravenous regional sympathetic blockade using guanethidine the duration of response is considerably longer. The experience of many authors would suggest that sympathetic blockade, when used properly early in the course of the disease and combined with physical therapy, cures approximately 80 percent of the patients with RSD.[3,19,22,23,26,58] Proper use requires correct diagnosis, early treatment, and *complete* sympathetic interruption of the limb, promptly followed by physical therapy.[3]

Alternatively, intravenous infusion of reserpine or guanethidine, agents that effectively produce a transient chemical sympathectomy, have also been used.[36,59-61] The technique of intravenous infusion of guanethidine described by Hannington-Kiff[61] is based on the principle that guanethidine functions as a false transmitter, being actively taken up by the sympathetic nerve endings and displacing norepinephrine from its storage sites. Glynn and coworkers[60] demonstrated significantly greater pain reduction after blocks with intravenous infusion of guanethidine than with physiologic saline solution. Several patients treated with intravenous saline solution also experienced pain relief, however, suggesting a strong placebo effect.

Duncan and associates[59] have reported improvement in both range of motion and pain relief in 20 patients in the later stages or RSD, with associated joint stiffness after joint manipulation during Bier block with reserpine or guanethidine and prednisolone. The injected agents for Bier block in their study consisted of 35 to 45 ml of 0.5 percent lidocaine, 1.5 to 2 mg of reserpine or 5 to 10 mg of guanethidine, and 80 to 100 mg of prednisolone. The block is allowed to become established for 10 to 15 minutes before the stiff joints are taken through a full range of motion. The block is left in place for a total of 20 to 30 minutes to allow for tissue binding of the reserpine or guanethidine and the prednisolone. At the end of the procedure, ice packs are applied, the tourniquet is deflated, and the extremity is elevated. Blocks may be repeated every 48 to 72 hours. Discontinuation of the blocks is dictated by a plateau in the patient's response. Usually no more than four to eight blocks should be used. It should be emphasized that extreme care must be taken when manipulating stiff joints to prevent fracture. In their study group, mean range of motion improved from 46.3 percent of normal before the blocks to 81 percent of normal after the blocks, and patients reported a mean of 80 percent reduction in their pain. Although reported complications that can occur after reserpine or guanethidine Bier block have been few, they include orthostatic hypotension, dizziness, somnolence, nausea, and vomiting.

Surgical or chemical sympathectomy is indicated primarily in those cases in which repeat sympathetic blocks produce relief, but the relief is only temporary or transient.[3,26] The choice for a chemical or a surgical procedure depends on the patient's attitude toward the two techniques, physical condition, and stage and severity of the RSD. Chemical sympathectomy with 6 percent aqueous phenol or 50 percent alcohol produces sympathetic interruption for several weeks to several months and is especially useful in older or poor-risk persons.[3] In patients who are younger and in good physical condition, surgical sympathectomy is preferable. Traditionally, the posterior approach of Smithwick[62] to the sympathetic ganglia has been used. Atkins[63] described the transaxillary approach, entering the pleural cavity through the second intercostal space, a technique that has become very popular. This approach has the advantage of providing excellent exposure and direct access to the proximal thoracic chain (the first to fourth thoracic ganglia along with the distal stellate ganglia), but because it requires a thoracotomy it has potentially greater morbidity than is associated with the traditional posterior approach. Whichever approach is used, the operation is highly technical and demanding and requires special training for its effective and safe use.

Corticosteroids

Currently, the area of greatest controversy in the treatment of RSD concerns the efficacy of systemic corticosteroids.[8,36,64-67] Kozin and associates[67] reported that 63 percent of patients studied had a good response to systemic corticosteroid therapy, and this figure was increased to 82 percent and 63 percent in subsets with definite and probable RSD respectively. Five patients who were given stellate ganglion blocks after corticosteroid therapy showed no improvement in this study. In most cases, patients received 60 to 80 mg of prednisone for 2 to 4 days and then the dosage was decreased by 10 to 20 mg every 2 to 4 days, with the dose later being tapered rapidly from 40 mg to 5 mg. The dosage was maintained at this level for several additional weeks. The mechanism of action of corticosteroids in the treatment of RSD is not clear. Kozin and associates[67] demonstrated

chronic perivascular inflammatory infiltrate on synovial biopsy specimens from involved extremities. The potent anti-inflammatory properties of prednisone may account for some of the therapeutic effect. It has also been hypothesized that corticosteroids, by their stabilizing effects on basement membranes, can reduce capillary permeability and therefore decrease the plasma extravasation that is commonly associated with the early stage of RSD.[36,67]

Mention is rarely made of the side effects of corticosteroid therapy. Glick[66] reported objectionable weight gain and moon facies in two patients and dyspepsia in three. The high frequency of bilaterality of RSD, however, suggests one potential advantage of using systemic corticosteroids, in contrast to the unilateral beneficial effects of sympathetic blockade.[8]

Alternative Treatment Modalities

Stilz and coworkers[58] described success in treating RSD in a child with the use of transcutaneous nerve stimulation. Electrical stimulation for the relief of pain had been advocated from the late 1800s. This method fell into disrepute for a long while and it was not until the gate control theory of pain was advanced by Melzak and Wall[68] that interest in this type of therapy was rekindled. Over the ensuing years, electrical nerve stimulation has been used for treatment of a variety of pain states by a variety of techniques (dorsal column stimulation, skin electrodes, implanted electrodes) with varying degrees of success. Shealy and Maurer[69] described treatment of pain, including causalgia, by electrical stimulation. In the patients studied they reported 25 percent complete and 60 percent partial relief of chronic pain. Meyer and Fields[70] reported a series of eight patients who were treated for causalgia with transcutaneous nerve stimulation; six had relief for varied periods of time after discontinuation of the stimulator. Unfortunately, in their series, stimulation was used only for short periods of time, and there was no long-term follow-up. Loeser and colleagues[71] reported 13 patients with RSD, 9 of whom had initial relief of pain, although only 2 of these 9 achieved long-term relief. Transcutaneous electrical stimulation has been used successfully in children and may be the second line of defense when physical therapy alone fails to control symptoms.[58] The apparent lack of associated morbidity with this treatment has been offered as a major advantage. Kesler and associates[72] treated 10 children with RSD using physical therapy and transcutaneous electrical nerve stimulation. All children were treated as outpatients. Seven children had complete remission within 2 months. Two other improved, and only one had no response. Abrams,[73] however, reported increased sympathetic tone associated with the use of transcutaneous electrical stimulation.

Blanchard[74] has reported successful use of temperature biofeedback in one patient with upper extremity RSD. Using biofeedback, the patient was able to learn to attain a reliable hand-warming response of $1°$ to $1.5°C$. Coincident with his learning to increase the temperature in the extremity, the pain in his hand and arm decreased markedly and remained absent at 1 year follow-year. Although this represents only one case, biofeedback has been used successfully in other situations in which pain control was needed and may provide a valuable adjunctive tool in the management of these difficult patients.

PSYCHOTHERAPY

Many patients with long-standing, chronic RSD undergo emotional and psychologic disturbances as a result of their long suffering and disability. Intense psychologic support and encouragement to undertake a vigorous program of physical therapy and exercise of the limb should be a part of all treatment. The patient should be continuously encouraged to use the involved limb. The need to allay fear, anxiety, and apprehension is essential. Depression should be treated with tricyclic antidepressants. If severe psychopathology is deemed to be present, psychiatric counseling and a course of psychotherapy should be instituted. The importance of this goes far beyond support for just the patient, because often the family members need psychologic support as well to deal with their problems and prevent the sad complication of divorce and dissolution of the family.

REFERENCES

1. Mitchell SW, Morehouse GR, Keen WW: Gunshot Wounds and Other Injuries of Nerves. JB Lippincott, Philadelphia, 1864
2. Lankford LL: Reflex sympathetic dystrophy. p. 539. In Green DP (ed): Operative Hand Surgery. Churchill-Livingstone, New York, 1982
3. Bonica JJ: The Management of Pain. 2nd Ed. Lea and Febiger, Philadelphia, 1990
4. MacKinnon SE, Holder LE: The use of three-phase radionuclide bone scanning in the diagnosis of reflex sympathetic dystrophy. J Hand Surg [Am] 9:556, 1984
5. Moskowitz E, Bishop HF, Pe H, Shibutani R: Post hemiplegic reflex sympathetic dystrophy. JAMA 167:836, 1958
6. Andrews LG, Armitage KJ: Sudek's atrophy in traumatic quadriplegia. Paraplegia 9:159, 1971
7. Arnstein A: Regional osteoporosis. Orthop Clin North Am 3:585, 1972
8. Kozin F, Genant HK, Bekerman C, McCarty DJ: the reflex sympathetic dystrophy syndrome. II. roentgenographic and scintographic evidence of bilaterality and of periarticular accentuation. Am J Med 60:332, 1976
9. Kozin F, Soin JS, Ryan LM et al: Bone scintigraphy in reflex sympathetic dystrophy syndrome. Radiology 138:437, 1981
10. Panin N, Gorday WJ, Raul BJ: Osteoporosis in hemiplegia. Stroke 2:41, 1971
11. Chu DS, Petrillo C, Davis SW, Eichberg R: Shoulder-hand syndrome: importance of early diagnosis and treatment. J Am Geriat Soc 29:50, 1981
12. Davis SW, Petrillo CR, Eichberg RD, Chu DS: Shoulder-hand syndrome in hemiplegic population: five year retrospective study. Arch Phys Med Rehabil 58:353, 1977
13. Genant HK, Kozin F, Bekerman C et al: The reflex sympathetic dystrophy syndrome. A comprehensive analysis using fine detail radiography, photon absorbtiometry, and bone and joint scintigraphy. Radiology 117:21, 1975
14. Greyson ND, Tepperman PS: Three-phase bone studies in hemiplegia with reflex sympathetic dystrophy and the effect of disuse. J Nucl Med 25:423, 1984
15. Hendler N, Uematesu S, Long D: Thermographic validation of physical complaints in "psychogenic pain" patients. Psychosomatics 23:283, 1982
16. Perelman RB, Adler D, Humphreys M: Reflex sympathetic dystrophy: electronic thermography as an aid in diagnosis. Orthop Rev 16:561, 1987
17. Low PA, Neumann C, Dyck PJ et al: Contact thermography in diagnosis of reflex sympathetic dystrophy: a new look at pathogenesis. Thermology 1:106, 1985
18. Uematsu H, Hendler N, Hungerford D et al: Thermography and electromyography in the differential of chronic pain syndromes and reflex sympathetic dystrophy. Electromyogr Clin Neurophysiol 21:165, 1981
19. Sylvest J, Jensen EM, Siggard-Andersen J, Pedersen L: Reflex dystrophy. Resting blood flow and muscle temperature as diagnostic criteria. Scand J Rehabil Med 9:25, 1977
20. Barnes R: The role of sympathectomy in the treatment of causalgia. J Bone Joint Surg [Br] 35:172, 1953
21. Bonica JJ: The Management of Pain with Special Emphasis on the Use of Analgesic Block in Diagnosis, Prognosis, and Therapy. Lea & Febiger, Philadelphia, 1953
22. De Takats G: Causalgic states in peace and war. JAMA 128:699, 1945
23. Evans JA: Reflex sympathetic dystrophy: report of 57 cases. Ann Intern Med 26:417, 1947
24. Rusk HA: Rehabilitation of patients with stroke. p. 625. In Rehabilitation Medicine. 3rd Ed. CV Mosby Co, St. Louis, 1971
25. Kwan ST: The treatment of causalgia by thoracic sympathetic ganglionectomy. Ann Surg 101:222, 1935
26. Shumacker HB, Spiegel IJ, Upjohn RH: Causalgia. The role of

sympathetic interruption in treatment. Surg Gynecol Obstet 86:76, 1948

27. Sunderland S: Pain mechanisms in causalgia. J Neurol Neurosurg Psychiatry 39:471, 1976

28. Ohry A, Brooks ME, Steinbach TV, Rozin R: Shoulder complications as a cause of delay in rehabilitation of spinal cord injured patients. Paraplegia 16:310, 1978

29. Wainapel SF, Freed MM: Reflex sympathetic dystrophy in quadriplegia: case report. Arch Phys Med Rehabil 65:35, 1984

30. Gellman H, Eckert RR, Botte MJ, Sakimura I, Waters RL: Reflex sympathetic dystrophy in cervical spinal cord injured patients. Clin Orthop 233:129, 1988

31. Garland DE, Hanscom DA, Keenan MA, et al: Resection of heterotopic ossification in the adult with head trauma. J Bone Joint Surg [Am] 67:1261, 1985

32. Stein AH Jr: The relation of median nerve compression to Sudek's syndrome. Surg Gynecol Obstet 115:713, 1962

33. Poplowski ZJ, Wiley AM, Murray JF: Posttraumatic dystrophy of the extremities. A clinical review and trial of treatment. J Bone Joint Surg [Am] 65:642, 1983

34. Buker RH, Cox WA, Scully TS et al: Causalgia and transthoracic sympathectomy. Am J Surg 124:724, 1972

35. Omer G, Thomas S: Treatment of causalgia: a review of cases at Brooke General Hospital. Texas Med 67:93, 1971

36. Schutzer SP, Gossling HR: Current concepts review. The treatment of reflex sympathetic dystrophy. J Bone Joint Surg [Am] 66:625, 1984

37. Leach RE, Clawson DK, Caprio A: Continuous elevation by spica cast in treatment of reflex sympathetic dystrophy. J Bone Joint Surg [Am] 56:416, 1974

38. Fowler FD, Moser M: Use of hexamethonium and dibenzyline in diagnosis and treatment of causalgia. JAMA 161:1051, 1956

39. Ghostine SY, Comair YG, Turner DN et al: Phenoxybenzamine in the treatment of causalgia. Report of 40 cases. J Neurosurg 60:1263, 1984

40. Tabira T, Shibasaki H, Kuroiwa Y: Reflex sympathetic dystrophy (causalgia) treatment with guanethidine. Arch Neurol 40:430, 1983

41. Simpson G: Propranolol for causalgia and Sudek atrophy. JAMA 227:327, 1974

42. Tahmoush AJ: Causalgia: redefinition as a clinical pain syndrome. Pain 10:187, 1981

43. Kleinert HE, Cole NM, Wayne L et al: Post-traumatic sympathetic dystrophy. Orthop Clin North Am 4:917, 1973

44. Eklund L-G: Ca-blockers and peripheral circulation — physiological viewpoints. Acta Pharmacol Toxicol 43(Suppl 1):33, 1978

45. Mikkelsen E, Andersson K-E, Pedersen OL: The effect of nifedipine on isolated human peripheral vessels. Acta Pharmacol Toxicol 43:291, 1978

46. Anderson K-E: Effects of calcium and calcium antagonists on the excitation-contraction coupling in striated and smooth muscle. Acta Pharmacol Toxicol 43(Suppl 1):5, 1978

47. Goodman LS, Gilman AG: The Pharmacologic Basis of Therapeutics. 7th Ed. Macmillan, New York, 1985

48. Rodeheffer RJ, Rommer JA, Wigley F, Smith CR: Controlled double-blind trial of nifedipine in the treatment of Raynaud's phenomenon. N Engl J Med 308:880, 1983

49. Smith CD, McKendry RJR: Controlled trial of nifedipine in the treatment of Raynaud's phenomenon. Lancet 2:1299, 1982

50. Prough DS, McLesky CH, Poehling GG et al: Efficacy of oral nifedipine in the treatment of reflex sympathetic dystrophy. Anesthesiology 62:796, 1985

51. Thompson JE: The diagnosis and management of post-traumatic pain syndromes (causalgia). Aust NZ J Surg 49(3):299, 1979

52. Carron H, Litwiller R: Stellate ganglion block. Anesth Analg 54:567, 1975

53. Moore DC: The use of stellate ganglion block and lumbar sympathetic block in orthopaedics: indications, technique, and complications. Clin Orthop 100-111

54. Moore DC: Regional Block. 3rd Ed. Charles C Thomas, Springfield, 1961

55. Lankford LL, Thompson JE: Reflex sympathetic dystrophy — upper and lower extremity: diagnosis and management. Instr Course 26:163, 1977

56. Wang JK, Johnson KA, Ilstrup DM: Sympathetic blocks for reflex sympathetic dystrophy. Pain 23:13, 1985

57. Linson MA, Leffert R, Todd DP: The treatment of upper extremity reflex sympathetic dystrophy with prolonged continuous stellate ganglion blockade. J Hand Surg 8:153, 1983

58. Stilz RJ, Carron H, Sanders DB: Case history number 96. Reflex sympathetic dystrophy in a 6 year old: successful treatment by transcutaneous nerve stimulation. Anaesth Analg 56:438, 1977

59. Duncan KH, Lewis RC, Racz G, Nordyke MD: Treatment of upper extremity reflex sympathetic dystrophy with joint stiffness using sympatholytic Bier blocks and manipulation. Orthopaedics 11:883, 1988

60. Glynn CJ, Basedow RW, Walsh JA: Pain relief following postganglionic sympathetic blockade with intravenous guanethidine. Br J Anaesth 12:1297, 1981

61. Hannington-Kiff JG: Pharmacological target blocks in hand surgery and rehabilitation. J Hand Surg [Br] 9:29, 1984

62. Smithwick RH: the rationale and technique of sympathectomy for the relief of vascular spasm of the extremity. N Engl J Med 222:699, 1940

63. Atkins HJB: Sympathectomy by axillary approach. Lancet 1:538, 1954

64. Bulgen D, Hazelman B, Ward M, McCallum M: Immunological studies in frozen shoulder. Ann Rheum Dis 37:135, 1978

65. Christensen K, Jensen EM, Noer I: The reflex sympathetic dystrophy syndrome response to treatment with systemic corticosteroids. Acta Chir Scand 148:653, 1982

66. Glick EN: Reflex dystrophy (algoneurodystrophy): results of treatment by corticosteroids. Rheum Rehabil 12:84, 1973

67. Kozin F, Ryan LM, Carrera GF et al: The reflex sympathetic dystrophy syndrome: III. Scintigraphic studies, further evidence for the therapeutic efficacy of systemic corticosteroids, and proposed diagnostic criteria. Am J Med 1:23, 1981

68. Melzak R, Wall PD: Pain mechanisms: a new theory. Science 150:971, 1965

69. Shealy CN, Maurer D: Transcutaneous nerve stimulation for control of pain. Surg Neurol 2:45, 1974

70. Meyer GA, Fields HL: Causalgia treated by selective large fiber stimulation of peripheral nerve. Brain 95:163, 1972

71. Loeser JD, Black RG, Christman A: Relief of pain by transcutaneous stimulation. J Neurosurg 42:308, 1975

72. Kesler RW, Saulsbury FT, Miller LT, Rowlingson JC: Reflex sympathetic dystrophy in children: treatment with transcutaneous electrical nerve stimulation. Pediatrics 82:728, 1988

73. Abrams SE: Increased sympathetic tone associated with transcutaneous electrical stimulation. Anesthesiology 45:575, 1976

74. Blanchard EB: The use of temperature biofeedback in the treatment of chronic pain due to causalgia. Biofeedback Self-Regul 4:183, 1979

48 Chronic Osteomyelitis

EPHRAIM M. ZINBERG

Chronic osteomyelitis has classically been one of the most difficult problems to deal with in orthopaedic surgery. In the past, frustration with failed attempts at cure has often led to limb amputation. Greater understanding of the prevention and cure of osteomyelitis and new reconstructive procedures utilizing microsurgical techniques have resulted in both definitive eradication of infection and limb salvage. This chapter focuses on pathogenesis and prevention of chronic osteomyelitis, principles of treatment, and reconstructive options.

PATHOGENESIS AND PREVENTION

Several factors contribute to the development of osteomyelitis in open fractures. Some are inherent characteristics of these wounds, whereas others are iatrogenically introduced; all can be minimized or eliminated through prudent surgical judgment. Open fractures are by definition contaminated. Wound hematoma provides an excellent culture medium for the proliferation of bacteria and subsequent infection. The presence of a "dead space" after soft tissue and bone débridement further aids this process. Devascularized skin, muscle, and bone is often present, especially in high energy type II and type III open fractures. If inadequately débrided, these will undergo necrosis and contribute further to infection. Primary wound closure can promote the collection of a deep hematoma, can prevent the egress of bacteria and purulent material once formed, and can make it difficult to inspect muscle tissue, which may subsequently become necrotic. Additionally, closure under tension can lead to further skin necrosis. Finally, the introduction of foreign substances in primary internal fixation can, in the presence of a contaminated wound, lead to wound infection, wound dehiscence, and osteomyelitis.

The following principles of management of open fractures are subject to some debate; in my opinion, however, they represent the "safe" approach to open fractures, and if rigidly adhered to, should lead to a reduction of the incidence of chronic osteomyelitis.

1. First and foremost, *a meticulous and complete débridement* must be carried out. All devascularized soft tissue and bone should be removed, with particular emphasis on the excision of nonviable or even questionably nonviable muscle. Most bone fragments completely stripped of soft tissue attachments should be discarded to prevent subsequent formation of a sequestrum. Large fragments may be retained initially for stability, although in my experience these often undergo delayed necrosis and lead to deep infection even after wound coverage with vascularized tissue. If this occurs, further bone débridement and late bone grafting become necessary.
2. *A thorough wound irrigation* should follow débridement.
3. *Primary closure should probably be avoided* in most type II and all type III wounds to prevent wound infection and dehiscence. Primary closure may be considered if the following "ideal" wound conditions are met:
   a. Complete débridement has been done.
   b. Contamination is minimal.
   c. Minimal soft tissue injury has occurred.
   d. A tension-free closure is possible.
   e. The wound has been open less than 6 hours.
   It should be clear that open fractures rarely meet these prerequisites; therefore, in my opinion, primary closure should rarely be done for such injuries. Rather, the wound should be inspected two or more days later ("second look"), further débridement done if necessary, and delayed primary closure accomplished.
4. *Fracture stabilization is performed.* Although orthopaedic

659

surgeons are often tempted to provide definitive primary stabilization with internal fixation, this is to be discouraged in open fractures, particularly types II and III. Heavy reliance should be made on primary external fixation and proper wound care with *delayed internal fixation* if necessary.

DIAGNOSIS

The diagnosis of osteomyelitis is made by history, physical examination, and radiographs, often supported in questionable cases by radioisotopic bone scans and confirmed by microbiologic and histologic data. The history is usually clear, involving an open fracture that was closed primarily, was inadequately débrided, or underwent primary internal fixation, or a closed fracture that underwent internal fixation. The patient will complain of increasing pain in the involved area, swelling, redness, and often purulent drainage from the wound. Examination may reveal a febrile patient with tenderness, swelling, erythema, and purulent drainage. In very chronic cases the surrounding skin may be indurated and scarred and exhibit brawny edema. Radiographs show an irregular or moth-eaten area, subperiosteal new bone formation, or frank bone destruction. In some cases a sequestrum, or retained avascular bone fragment, may be present. If radiographic changes are not revealing, radioisotopic imaging may be helpful. Newer methods, such as sequential technetium-99m (^{99m}Tc) and gallium scans or the indium-labeled leukocyte scan, have been shown to have a greater specificity for the diagnosis of osteomyelitis than the ^{99m}Tc scan alone.[1]

The diagnosis is made at the time of surgical treatment: The bone appears irregular, sclerotic, and avascular, and purulent drainage is present, often in the medullary canal. Cultures and histologic studies of the affected bone are confirmatory.

TREATMENT

Treatment of established osteomyelitis is the complete elimination of all infected tissues. In the past, serial débridements and sequestrectomies formed the standard surgical protocol, removing only that amount of soft tissue and bone obviously infected or necrotic. Reluctance on the part of surgeons to create

a large soft tissue or bone defect that would be difficult to reconstruct only delays definitive eradication of infection. This is probably one of the primary reasons for the chronicity of osteomyelitis. An aggressive or even radical débridement of soft tissue and bone is often necessary for cure. Once this is accomplished, with subsequent wound inspection and cultures confirming successful elimination of infection, efforts are directed toward limb reconstruction. Reconstructive goals will depend on the needs for wound coverage and skeletal restoration.

WOUND COVERAGE

Three primary aims should be met in consideration of the options for wound coverage in osteomyelitis: (1) coverage per se, to prevent further ingress of bacteria and desiccation of deep tissues; (2) obliteration of dead spaces to minimize hematoma formation; and (3) optimizing the healing environment, preferably by bringing new, well-vascularized tissue to the area. These wounds are usually walled off by scar tissue and are relatively avascular; coverage by vascular tissue not only can increase antibiotic access but can actually improve both soft tissue and bone healing.

Wound Coverage Options

The simplest method of wound coverage that will meet the aims just noted should be chosen.

Direct Wound Closure

Direct wound closure may be carried out if it can be done without tension and if it does not create a dead space. These wounds rarely have sufficient viable skin and subcutaneous tissue to allow for closure, and the surgeon should resist the temptation to close them under tension, which can lead to necrosis of skin margins. Furthermore, if, despite successful skin closure, a dead space overlying bone remains, bacterial colonization, infection, and wound dehiscence often result.

Split-Thickness Skin Grafting

Split-thickness skin grafting can be performed only on a well-vascularized bed (e.g., subcutaneous fat, granulation tissue, muscle, tendon covered by paratenon, or bone covered by periosteum). After débridement of an osteomyelitic wound, bare bone is exposed; this will naturally not support a skin graft. Occasionally a wound of small diameter may be allowed to undergo granulation from surrounding vascular soft tissues; after adequate granulation tissue has covered the exposed bone it is covered by skin graft or allowed to epithelialize.

Open Cancellous Bone Grafting

Open cancellous bone grafting utilizes cancellous bone chips to fill a bone defect associated with overlying skin loss. This was first described by Mowlem [2] in 1944, and other reports followed.[3-7] It was popularized by Papineau and coworkers[8,9] in Europe and is often referred to as the "Papineau technique." This technique consists of three stages. In the first stage, devascularized bone and soft tissue are excised. Dressings are then changed frequently until the cavity is covered with healthy granulation tissue. This process is complete an average of 3 weeks later. At the second stage, the defect is filled with small cancellous iliac bone chips. Frequent dressing changes are resumed while the bone graft becomes vascularized by granulation tissue over a period of several weeks. In small wounds, epithelialization often occurs spontaneously; in larger wounds, split-thickness skin grafting is performed at a third stage. The major advantage of this procedure is its predictability. In one report from the Mayo Clinic,[10] 18 consecutive patients had eradication of infection and bone healing with this technique. There are, however, significant disadvantages. Open cancellous bone grafting is time consuming, involves prolonged hospitalization, is limited to relatively small bone defects, and often exhibits complications. In the same series, overall hospitalization time was 51 days, three patients required additional bone grafting, and two patients had recurrent infection.

Pedicled Muscle Flaps

Pedicled muscle flaps are muscles that are mobilized and transposed locally for wound coverage, leaving the vascular pedicle intact. The concept behind this procedure is coverage by highly vascular tissue. The use of muscle flaps meets all of the aims listed previously, providing coverage, obliteration of dead space, and an improved healing environment. Experimental studies have shown that a muscle transposed into a contaminated wound increases local blood

Table 48-1. Donor Muscles for Pedicled Muscle Transfer

Muscle	Zone of Coverage
Rectus femoris	Hip, femur
Vastus lateralis	Hip, femur
Gastrocnemius	Knee, proximal one third of tibia
Soleus	Midde one third of tibia

(From Zinberg EM: Free-muscle transfer for chronic osteomyelitis. Surg Rounds Orthop 3:26, 1989, with permission.)

supply and provides resistance to infection.[11] More recent studies demonstrated that an avascular segment of bone can become revascularized by coverage with a muscle flap, in contrast to control segments covered with skin.[12] This increased vascularity logically provides access to the area for the blood-borne elements involved in host defense and for systemic antibiotics. This is a particularly advantageous factor in wounds that are sequestered from blood supply by necrotic, avascular tissue. Pedicled muscle flaps are indicated for coverage of defects that cannot be covered by simpler means. This includes the following:

Wounds with exposed bone devoid of periosteum or tendon devoid of paratenon
Wounds with deep dead spaces that require obliteration
Wounds beneath which subsequent reconstructive procedures may be required (e.g., bone grafting, nerve grafting, tendon transfers)

The use of pedicled muscle flaps in chronic osteomyelitis was first described in 1946,[13] and indications, donor sources, and technique have since been refined.[14-19]

Table 48-1 lists the lower extremity muscles available for transposition and their zones of coverage. The most common lower extremity bone involved in osteomyelitis is, by far, the tibia, owing in part to the high incidence of open fractures in this area. Additionally, a relatively thin layer of soft tissue covers the tibia, consisting anteromedially of only skin and subcutaneous tissue. Thus, the gastrocnemius and soleus have become the "workhorses" in the lower extremity for pedicled muscle transfer. Defects of the proximal one-third of the tibia can be readily covered with the gastrocnemius muscle. Because it is the anteromedial surface of the tibia that most often requires coverage, the medial head of the gastrocnemius is

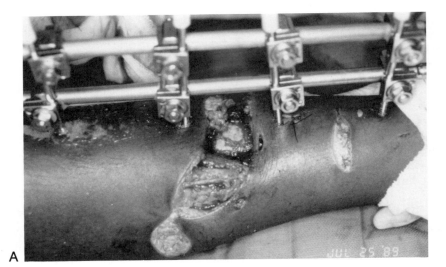

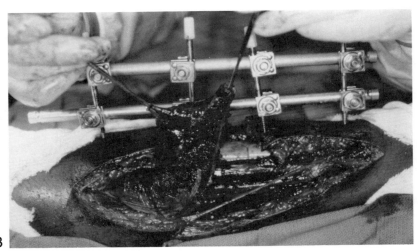

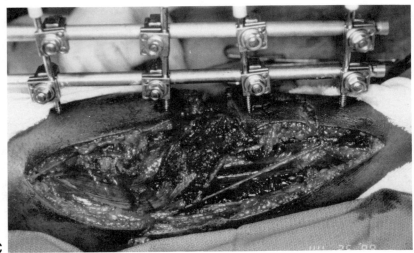

Fig. 48-1. (A–F) Pedicled muscle flap coverage of tibial defect using soleus muscle.

Fig. 48-1 *(Continued).*

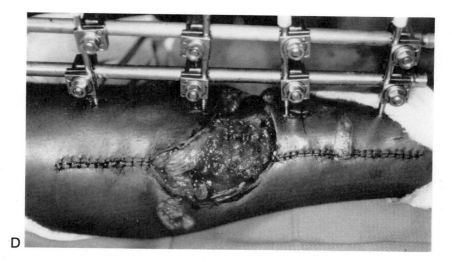

D

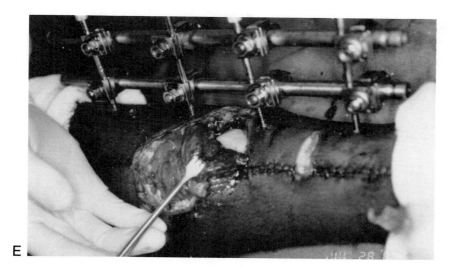

E

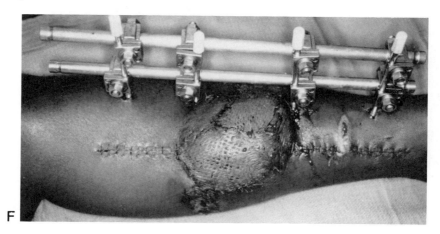

F

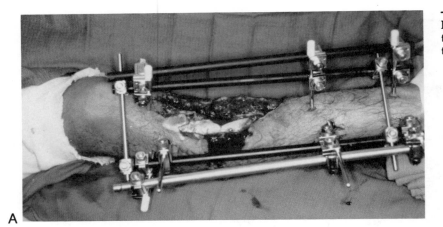

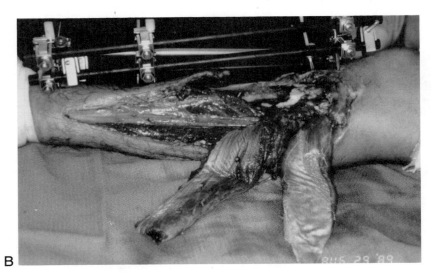

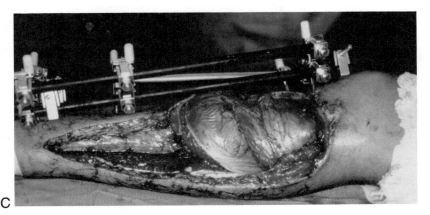

Fig. 48-2. (A–E) Coverage of large tibial defect with combined gastrocnemial-soleus flap.

Fig. 48-2 *(Continued).*

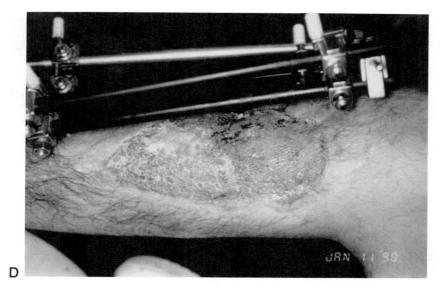

D

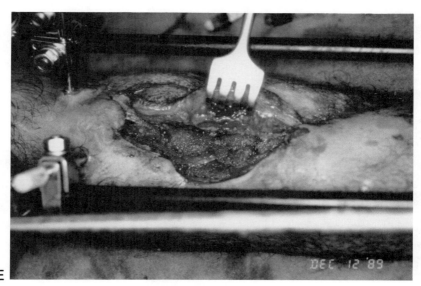

E

usually used. The anterolateral tibial surface, which is covered by muscles of the anterior compartment (tibialis anterior, extensor hallucis longus, and extensor digitorum longus), usually has adequate intrinsic soft tissue cover in this area; however, if significant soft tissue loss has left this surface exposed, it may be covered by the lateral head of the gastrocnemius. Defects of the middle one-third of the tibia can usually be covered with the soleus muscle. The soleus is a bipennate muscle, and the medial one-half will cover most defects. However, in many of these extremities

the initial trauma, often with a crushing component, has extended to muscles of the posterior compartment, rendering them marginally vascular. Additionally, the soft tissue induration that accompanies chronic infection can cause these muscle to be less pliable than normally. Thus, when the soleus is being mobilized, the distal end, detached from the Achilles tendon, may become avascular and undergo necrosis. This muscle may, under these circumstances, be useful for coverage only as far distally as the midshaft of the tibia.

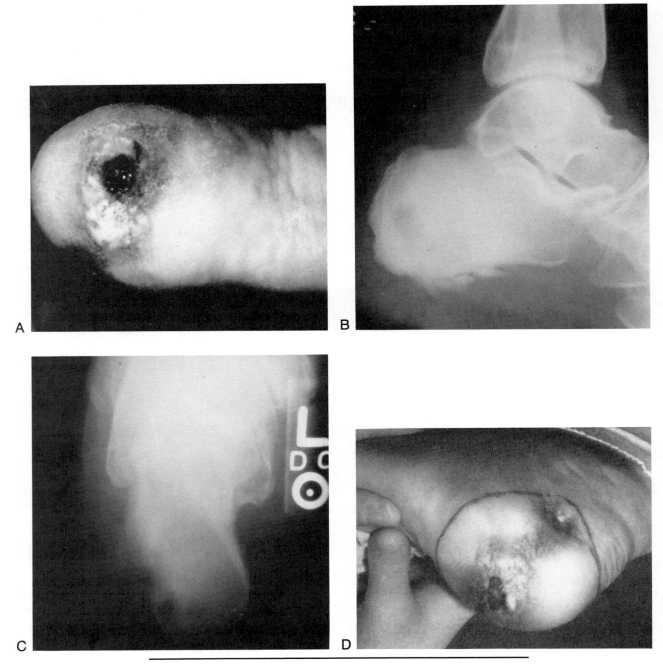

Fig. 48-3. (A–K) Coverage of heel with free latissimus dorsi muscle flap.

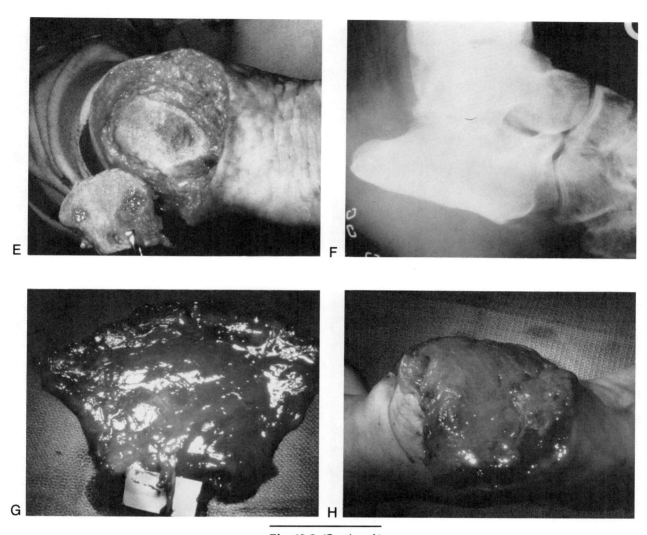

Fig. 48-3 *(Continued.)*

Figure 48-1 illustrates the use of the soleus flap for coverage of a defect of the midshaft of the tibia. After adequate soft tissue and bone débridement, an area of bone measuring 5 × 5 cm is exposed (Fig. 48-1A). The medial one-half of the soleus muscle is detached from its insertion into the Achilles tendon and from the lateral one-half of the soleus (Fig. 48-1B). This dissection requires ligation and division of the distal vascular perforators from the posterior tibial artery and vein; care is taken to preserve the proximal perforating vessels. The muscle is then transposed anteriorly to provide bone coverage and is partially inset (Fig. 48-1C&D). The peripheral one-third to one-half

of the muscle is not completely inset to provide adequate drainage from beneath the flap. Two or 3 days later, the patient is returned to the operating room, the flap is lifted, and the underlying bed is inspected (Fig. 48-1E). At this time the bed should be clean; the flap is then completely inset and covered with split-thickness skin graft (Fig. 48-1F). If there is evidence of purulent drainage or further tissue necrosis, another débridement and irrigation are performed and the flap is simply replaced on its underlying bed. Wound inspection is again carried out 48 to 72 hours later. This process may have to be repeated several times before final insetting and skin grafting. One

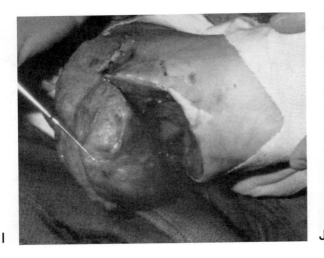

I

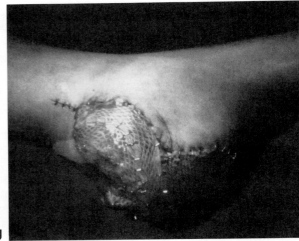

J

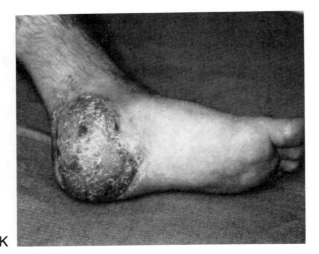

K

Fig. 48-3 (Continued).

useful guide to successful eradication of infection in these instances is the degree to which the muscle adheres to the underlying bone (M. B. Wood, personal communication, 1985); when it adheres well, infection is usually controlled and insetting may be completed.

For defects of the proximal one-half of the tibia, the gastrocnemius and soleus muscles may both be required. After substantial bone excision (Fig. 48-2A), the medial head of the gastrocnemius and medial one-half of the soleus are transposed (Fig. 48-2B&C) and covered subsequently by split-thickness skin graft (Fig. 48-2D). Four months later, the flap is raised and the bone cavity filled with iliac bone graft (Fig. 48-2E).

In a review of 42 patients with osteomyelitis treated with a pedicled muscle flap, 39 had successful eradication of infection (29) at 2-year follow-up.[20] However, 25 of the 42 had complications that required additional surgery, including muscle flap revision (four patients), repeat skin grafting (nine patients), excision of marginal skin ulcers (five patients), evacuation of hematoma (three patients), and excision of retained sequestra (five patients).

Free Muscle Flaps

When soft tissue defects cannot be closed directly or by coverage with skin graft, and no local muscle flaps are available, free muscle flaps may be required. These are muscles transferred with their vascular pedicles to a distant site, inset, and revascularized by microvascular anastomoses. Success of these flaps is dependent on patency of the anastomosed vessels and requires microsurgical expertise. Assuming continued vessel patency, free muscle flaps equal pedicled flaps in terms of viability and therefore provide all the advantages of pedicled flaps. The uniqueness of these flaps lies in their versatility. They can be transferred to any distant site that has an artery and at least one vein in good condition. They can be used, then, in areas "out of range" of local muscle flaps. These include the distal one-third to one-half of the tibia, the ankle, the heel, and the upper extremity. Furthermore, because of their free nature, they can be contoured to a wound more easily than pedicled flaps. They can, in fact, be folded, rolled, split longitudinally, or even pushed into a bone cavity to obliterate the dead space. This quality is not shared by the other popular class of free flaps, fasciocutaneous flaps, which consist of skin, subcutaneous fat, and underlying fascia.

Free muscle flaps were first employed for wound coverage per se. Only in the past decade has their usefulness in the treatment of chronic osteomyelitis become apparent.[21-24] The following muscles are the most commonly used donor muscles for free muscle transfer: (1) latissimus dorsi, (2) rectus abdominis, (3) serratus anterior, and (4) gracilis.

The latissimus dorsi has been the "workhorse" of free flaps, especially for lower extremity wounds. It is a large, flat muscle that can cover an area as large as 25×35 cm. It has a long pedicle (thoracodorsal artery and vein) of excellent caliber. It may be transferred alone or with an island of overlying skin (myocutaneous flap).

The rectus abdominis is a smaller muscle than the latissimus dorsi but is very useful for small to moderate-sized defects up to 5×20 cm. It has a long pedicle (inferior epigastric vessels) of excellent diameter.

It is harvested with the patient in a convenient supine position and leaves a very acceptable hidden donor scar.

The serratus anterior consists of several slips arising from the upper eight or nine ribs; the lower two or three slips may be used as a free muscle flap, thus preserving donor muscle function and preventing winging of the scapula. The vascular supply is a branch of the thoracodorsal artery, an excellent pedicle. This muscle can cover an area as large as 10×12 cm.

The gracilis is a long, strap-like muscle situated along the medial aspect of the thigh. Although it is quite expendable in terms of its function, its small width and short vascular pedicle limit its usefulness.

The following case reports illustrate the use of free muscle transfer in the treatment of chronic osteomyelitis.

Case 1: A 47-year-old man with long-term sensory impairment in the lower extremities secondary to a lumbar spinal disorder unknowingly sustained a deep puncture wound to the left heel when he stepped on a nail. He subsequently developed a deep wound infection, which progressed to advanced osteomyelitis (Fig. 48-3A–C). At the initial surgery, wide débridement of the infected soft tissue (essentially the entire heel pad) and the plantar aspect of the calcaneus was done (Fig. 48-3D–F). The dressing was changed in the operating room 3 days later and revealed a clean wound with no further purulence or necrotic tissue. One week after débridement a latissimus dorsi free muscle flap (Fig. 48-3G) was transferred to the heel (Fig. 48-3H) and revascularized by anastomosing the thoracodorsal vessels to the posterior tibial vessels. The flap was inset around one-half of its periphery, leaving the remainder free for drainage. Three days later inspection of the underlying bed revealed no further drainage and no necrotic tissue (Fig. 48-3I). Insetting was completed and the flap was covered with a split-thickness skin graft (Fig. 48-3J). The graft "took" nicely, the muscle atrophied as expected, and there has been no recurrence of infection in 3 years (Fig. 48-3K).

Case 2: This patient is a 44-year-old man who sustained a closed spiral fracture of the distal tibia, which was initially treated by closed reduction and casting (Fig. 48-4A). After delayed union the patient

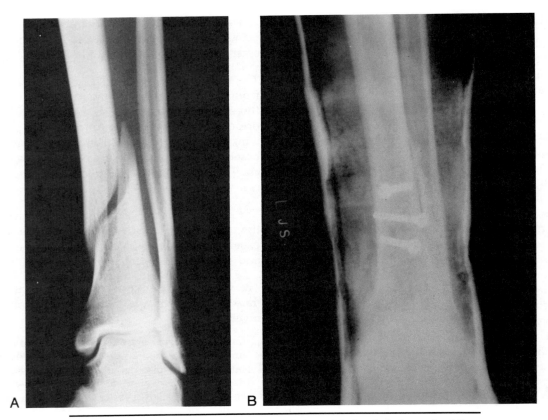

Fig. 48-4. (A–E) Coverage of distal tibial defect with free latissimus dorsi flap.

underwent open reduction and limited internal fixation with A-0 screws (Fig. 48-4B). Deep wound infection, dehiscence, and osteomyelitis developed, necessitating wide débridement of bone and soft tissue (Fig. 48-4C). Cultures yielded *Staphylococcus aureus*. One week after the final débridement (with one "clean" intervening dressing change) the patient underwent free latissimus dorsi transfer (Fig. 48-4D) followed by split-thickness skin grafting 3 days later. Complete insetting of the flap was done at the time of skin grafting; persistent drainage, however, necessitated subsequent flap elevation and irrigation of the underlying bed on two occasions (Fig. 48-4E). The drainage ceased thereafter, the flap began to adhere to the underlying bed, and 5 months later the patient underwent cancellous iliac bone grafting.

Case 3: This case illustrates the use of the rectus abdominis flap for coverage of a tibial defect. After débridement of infected soft tissue and bone (Fig. 48-5A), the defect is covered with a free rectus ab-

dominis flap (Fig. 48-5B&C), which is in turn covered with a split-thickness skin graft (Fig. 48-5D). In this case no subsequent bone grafting was necessary.

To date, the two largest series of free-tissue transfers for chronic osteomyelitis were reported by Weiland and coworkers[23] and Irons and colleagues.[24] In Weiland and associates' series an immediate flap failure occurred in 19 percent (7/37) owing to vessel thromboses. Of the 30 initially successful cases (in terms of survival), six (20 percent) were complicated by recurrent sepsis. In Irons and coworkers' series, five of 31 initially successful flaps (16 percent) were complicated subsequently by sepsis.

MANAGEMENT OF BONE DEFECTS

After adequate débridement of osteomyelitic bone, an assessment must be made of the adequacy of remaining bone and the need for bone grafting. Be-

Fig. 48-4 *(Continued).*

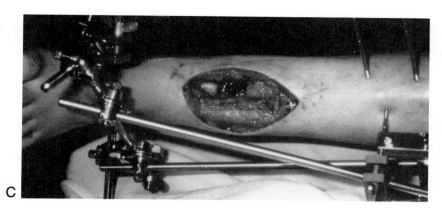

C

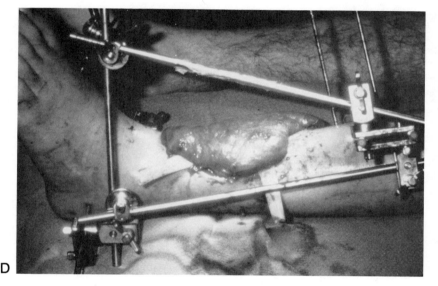

D

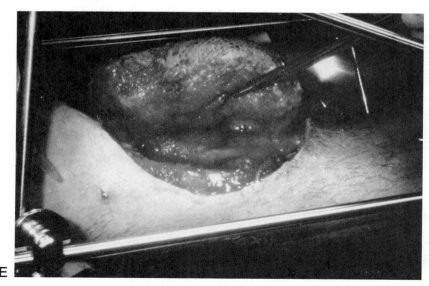

E

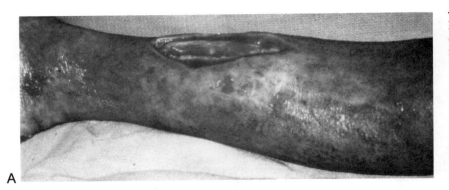

A

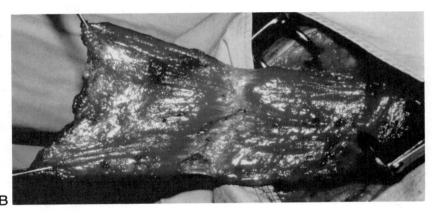

B

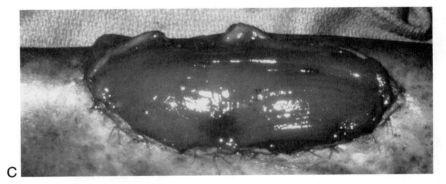

C

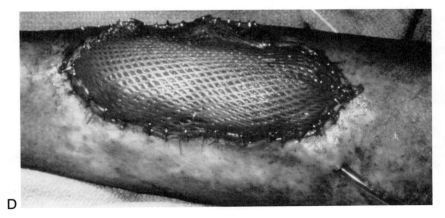

D

Fig. 48-5. (A–D) Coverage of tibial defect using free rectus abdominis muscle flap.

cause most of these cases are complications of fractures, even after relatively little bone is débrided bone grafting is usually indicated not only to replace lost bone mass but also to aid in fracture union. Indeed, the bone defect after débridement is usually significant, with only 50 percent or less of the circumference remaining. Conventional cancellous iliac bone grafting is the procedure of choice, usually performed 3 months or more after definitive soft tissue coverage.

Extensive long-bone osteomyelitis may require wide or even radical bone excision to ensure complete eradication of infection. If a segmental defect results, it may be amenable to conventional iliac bone grafting. The surrounding soft tissue bed must have adequate vascularity to revascularize the grafted bone. It is precisely in such situations that transferred muscle flaps, pedicled or free, are so helpful in increasing local vascularity and improving the healing environment.

Vascularized Bone Grafting

Most segmental defects that measure less than 6 cm in diameter will eventually incorporate the conventional bone graft and exhibit bony union. Problems arise with larger defects, measuring 6 to 8 cm or greater. Complications include delayed union (often 12 to 18 months), nonunion, and late fracture of the graft. In these large defects, vascularized bone grafting may be indicated. In this procedure a segment of bone, usually the fibula, is transferred along with its vascular pedicle to the recipient site, stabilized, and revascularized by microvascular anastomoses. The advantage of this procedure is that the transferred bone already has vessels; unlike the conventional bone graft, which is initially avascular and must heal by the slow process of "creeping substitution," a vascularized bone graft is a viable segment of bone, which should heal at both ends by standard fracture healing. Experimental studies have shown that the viability of a vascularized bone graft is greater than that of a conventional bone graft but somewhat less than that of normal undisturbed bone.[25] This may explain why some cases result in nonunion at one or both junctures, requiring additional procedures. In one report on 20 patients who underwent vascularized bone transfer for chronic osteomyelitis, 12 (40 percent) attained primary healing with no additional

procedures, and an additional four healed after a second operation, for an overall eventual union rate of 60 percent.[26] Although this may not appear to be a very high success rate, it must be borne in mind that these patients required radical bone excision to achieve cure of infection, leaving very little in the way of reconstructive options for limb salvage; indeed, without vascularized bone grafting many of these limbs would have required amputation.

The most common donor source for vascularized bone grafting is the fibula. As much as 30 cm of fibula can be transferred, with the peroneal vessels. The other readily available source is the iliac crest, with a pedicle of the deep circumflex iliac vessels. This may be transferred together with a large amount of overlying soft tissue (composite free-tissue transfer) in cases of combined bone and soft tissue loss.

The use of the vascularized fibula in chronic osteomyelitis of the tibia is illustrated in Figure 48-6. This 44-year-old man had long-standing chronic osteomyelitis of the tibia resulting from an open fracture. He had already undergone several surgical procedures, including sequestrectomies, open reduction and internal fixation, conventional bone grafting, and pedicled muscle transfer for coverage. He was left with chronic drainage and a short, bowed extremity (Fig. 48-6A&B). At initial surgery, radical bone resection was performed (Fig. 48-6C&D). One week later, vascularized fibular transfer was done (Fig. 48-6E). Six months subsequently, union had been achieved at the distal junction (Fig. 48-6F), but the proximal juncture was ununited (Fig. 48-6G). Secondary open reduction and internal fixation with plate and screws along with iliac bone grafting was required on two occasions to achieve proximal union (Fig. 48-6H).

SUMMARY

Although chronic osteomyelitis remains one of the more difficult problems in orthopaedic surgery, greater understanding of the need for radical débridement has improved cure rates. Newer reconstructive techniques, some involving microsurgery, have allowed salvage of many limbs that otherwise would have required amputation.

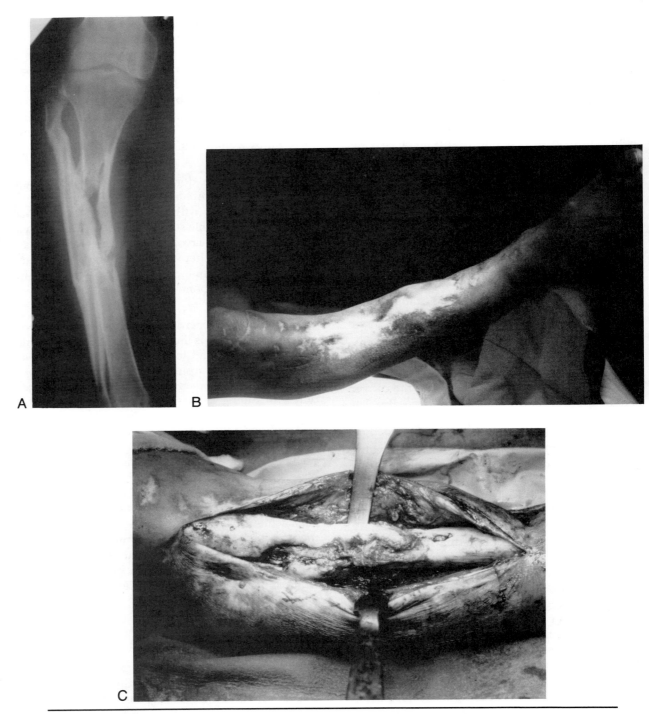

Fig. 48-6. (A–H) Reconstruction of tibial defect, after radical bone excision, with vascularized fibular graft.

Fig. 48-6 *(Continued).*

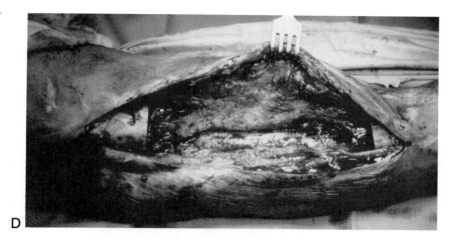

D

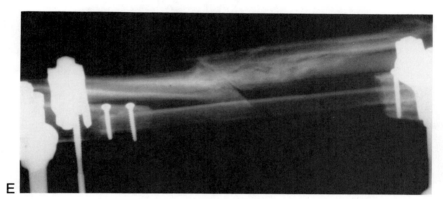

E

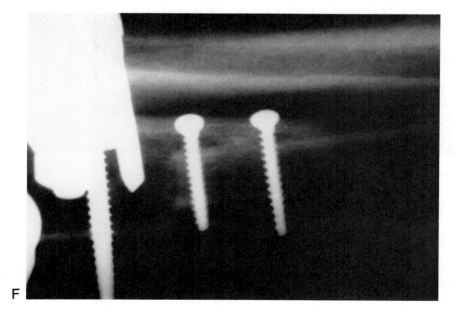

F

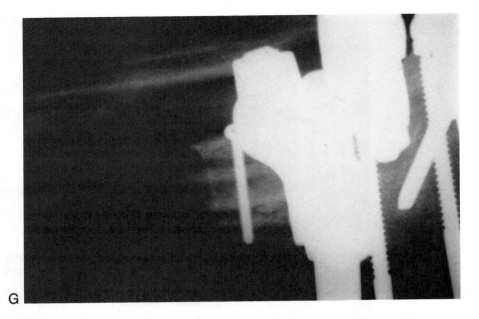

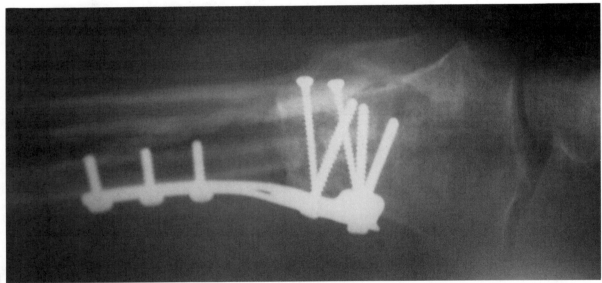

Fig. 48-6 *(Continued).*

REFERENCES

1. Merkel KD, Fitzgerald RH, Brown ML: Scintigraphic evaluation in musculoskeletal sepsis. Orthop Clin North Am 15:401, 1983
2. Mowlem R: Cancellous chip bone-grafts. Lancet 2:746, 1944
3. Coleman HM, Bateman JE, Dale GM, Starr DE: Cancellous bone grafts for infected bone defects. Surg Gynecol Obstet 83:392, 1946
4. Higgs SL: The use of cancellous chips in bone grafting. J Bone Joint Surg [Am] 28:15, 1946
5. Hageman KE: Treatment of infected bone defects with cancellous bone-chip grafts. Acta Clin Scand 98:576, 1949
6. Mazlett JW: The use of cancellous bone grafts in the treatment of subacute and chronic osteomyelitis. J Bone Joint Surg [Br] 36:584, 1954
7. DeOliveira JC: Bone grafts and chronic osteomyelitis. J Bone Joint Surg [Br] 53:672, 1971

8. Papineau LJ: L'excision-greffe avec fermeture retardée délibérée dans l'ostéomyélite chronique. Nouv Presse Med 2:2753, 1973
9. Papineau LJ, Alfageme A, Dalcourt JP, Pilon L: Ostéomyélite chronique: excision et greffe de spongieux à l'air libre après mises à plat extensives. Int Orthop 3:165, 1979
10. Cabanela ME: Open cancellous bone grafting of infected bone defects. Orthop Clin North Am 15:427, 1984
11. Chang N, Mathes SJ: Comparison of the effect of bacterial inoculation in musculocutaneous and random pattern flaps. Plast Reconstr Surg 70:1, 1982
12. Richards RR, Schemitsch EH: Effect of muscle flap coverage on bone blood flow following devascularization of a segment of tibia: an experimental investigation in the dog. J Orthop Res 7:550, 1989
13. Stark WJ: The use of pedicled muscle flaps in the surgical treatment of chronic osteomyelitis resulting from compound fractures. J Bone Joint Surg 28:343, 1946
14. Ger R: The techniques of muscle transposition in the operative treatment of traumatic and ulcerative lesions of the leg. J Trauma 11:502, 1971
15. Ger R: Muscle transposition for treatment and prevention of chronic posttraumatic osteomyelitis of the tibia. J Bone Joint Surg [Am] 59:784, 1977
16. Briggs JG Jr, Huang TT, Lewis SR: Use of muscle flaps in the treatment of osteomyelitis of the tibia. Tex Med 74:82, 1978
17. Mathes SJ: The muscle flap for management of osteomyelitis. N Engl J Med 306:294, 1982
18. Mathes SJ, Albert BS, Chang N: Use of the muscle flap in chronic osteomyelitis: experimental and clinical correlation. Plast Reconstr Surg 69:815, 1982
19. Arnold PG, Irons GB: Lower-extremity muscle flaps. Orthop Clin North Am 15:441, 1984
20. Fitzgerald RH Jr, Ruttle PE, Arnold PG et al: Local muscle flaps in the treatment of chronic osteomyelitis. J Bone Joint Surg [Am] 67:175, 1985
21. May JW Jr, Gallico GG III, Lukash FN: Microvascular transfer of free tissue for closure of bone wounds of the distal lower extremity. N Engl J Med 306:253, 1982
22. Irons GB, Fisher J, Schmitt EH III: Vascularized muscular and musculocutaneous flaps for management of osteomyelitis. Orthop Clin North Am 15:473, 1984
23. Weiland AJ, Moore JR, Daniel RK: The efficacy of free tissue transfer in the treatment of osteomyelitis. J Bone Joint Surg [Am] 66:181, 1984
24. Irons GB, Wood MB, Schmitt EH: Experience with 100 consecutive free flaps. Am Plast Surg 18:17, 1987
25. Arata MA, Wood MB, Cooney WP: Revascularized segmental diaphyseal bone transfers in the canine: an analysis of viability. J Reconst Microsurg 1:11, 1984
26. Wood MB, Cooney WP III, Irons GB: Skeletal reconstruction by vascularized bone transfer: indication and results. Mayo Clinic Proc 60:729, 1985

49 Sports Injuries

ROBERT T. BURKS

There is far too much information on sports injuries than can fit into one small chapter. The greatest difficulty in this type of undertaking is to pare down information so as to make it useful, but at the same time not be so brief that too much is lost. Consequently, only common sports injuries that occur to the knee, ankle, and shoulder are described here. It should be noted that if all sports injuries are considered, overuse injuries, strains, contusions, and similar types of trauma are most common. In this chapter, however, the focus is more on common injuries of the joints.

Because most of the topics discussed here are true injuries, it is important to mention the timing of the examination. One of the unique aspects of sports medicine is the opportunity for a physician to be available at or near the time an injury occurs. There is usually a "golden period" of an hour or so once the initial pain from an injury recedes in which an examination is very revealing. Complete examination of the knee or ankle at this time, for example, can be almost as good as an examination under anesthesia. A few hours later, after hemorrhage and edema have taken place, the extremity is so painful that the examination can be difficult. It is important for sports medicine specialists who are fortunate enough to be at the site of an injury to do a detailed examination and not wait for "better surroundings" such as an emergency room or office. This first examination is usually the best and the opportunity should not be wasted.

THE KNEE

The knee is a frequent site of injury in sports. It is also an area where diagnoses are missed because they may be more subtle than the examiner appreciates.

Ligament Injuries

The knee's four important ligaments are the anterior cruciate ligament (ACL), posterior cruciate ligament (PCL), medial collateral ligament (MCL), and lateral collateral ligament (LCL).

Anterior Cruciate Ligament

The ACL runs from the posterior inner wall of the lateral femoral condyle to the anterior central aspect of the tibial plateau. This ligament is the primary restraint to anterior translation of the tibia with respect to the femur.[1] Damage to it is detected by anteriorly displacing the tibia with respect to the femur to determine a change in excursion compared to the opposite knee, or a change in the "endpoint." This change in endpoint is a relative feeling, when the practitioner is performing an anterior drawer–type maneuver, that the limit of translation is soft or "spongy" if there is a tear of the ACL. The Lachman test, the most sensitive test for an ACL tear, is an anterior drawer maneuver of the tibia with the knee flexed only 20° to 30°. Commonly textbooks on physical examination recommend the test for the ACL at 90° of flexion, but this diminishes sensitivity of the test and many ACL injuries will be undetected if a Lachman test is not performed.[2]

An important point is that acute injuries of the ACL are most often noncontact injuries. Frequently a "clipping"-type injury is thought to be necessary to tear an ACL. However, far more commonly an ACL tear occurs without contact, such as when a person comes down from a rebound and twists the knee or plants a foot on an unforgiving surface at high speed and causes excessive torsion at the knee. With an acute injury the patient will frequently describe a "pop" or "snap" and an inability to continue in the activity. Swelling also occurs rapidly, which is the hemarthrosis that is seen with almost all acute ACL tears. If the examiner ascertains that a patient has had a twisting injury of the knee, felt a "pop," experienced an inability to continue the activity, and had fairly immediate onset of swelling, an ACL tear must be ruled out.

At the time of an ACL tear other ligaments may be damaged, a meniscus may be torn, or other injuries such as an osteochondral fracture can occur. Associated injuries can be ruled out by physical examination, radiographs, and perhaps magnetic resonance (MR) imaging or even arthroscopy. For an "isolated" ACL tear, it is necessary to counsel patients on whether ACL reconstructive surgery should be carried out. In general, one-third of patients will adapt reasonably well to the lack of an ACL, and one-third of patients will have to give up activities or modify their life-styles in some way, but will otherwise get along without reconstructive surgery. The other one-third of patients will have difficulty even with activities of daily living and routine recreation.[3] Age of the patient, activity level, associated injuries or disabilities, and so forth all play a role in surgical decision making. For those patients who choose a nonoperative approach, rehabilitation of the leg will be important. Focus should be on return of leg strength not only to the quadriceps and hamstring groups but also to the hip and calf muscles. Range-of-motion exercises of the knee should be carefully monitored to be sure steady improvement toward a normal range of motion is accomplished. ACL functional braces, of which there are many types, may also play a role in returning a patient to sports activities.

In a chronic setting of ACL insufficiency the patient will be easier to examine. These patients will most likely have had a few episodes in which the knee "gave out" or buckled during a twisting-type activity. These injuries will frequently be followed by swelling but with progressively less disability time than with an acute injury. As the length of time increases from the index injury, the percentage of patients with meniscal tears increases significantly as well. Frequently a patient is seen who has had an ACL tear at some point in the past and because of knee instability (giving-way) episodes has subsequently had a meniscec-

tomy. This knee is then on a long downward road toward continued disability and degenerative changes.

Reconstructive techniques for ACL deficiency have expanded exponentially in recent years. Many different types of reconstructions are available to the patient at this time, but this topic goes beyond the scope of this chapter. Suffice it to say that almost all techniques employ arthroscopy as an assist in the procedure, in addition to early motion and more aggressive physical therapy.[4] In times past, a knee might be in a cast for about 6 weeks after ACL reconstruction. This would be rare today, and most programs institute early motion of the knee to protect the articular surface, improve early range of motion, apply some stress to the graft for remodeling, and minimize adhesions. Although surgeons may differ on techniques and type of graft material used, the principles of using a high-strength graft,[5] accurate graft placement, secure fixation, and early motion are fairly universal.

Posterior Cruciate Ligament

The PCL runs from the inner wall of the medial femoral condyle and roof of the intercondylar notch and attaches intracapsularly over the proximal posterior aspect of the center of the tibia. The PCL is the primary restraint to posterior translation of the tibia with respect to the femur.[1] The mechanism of a PCL disruption classically is a blow to the tibial tubercle, which drives the tibia posteriorly. This can be seen with a fall directly onto a flexed knee, or as in a hockey player sliding into the boards or a goalpost with the force directed posteriorly on the tibial tubercle. A skin laceration or contusion over the anterior aspect of the tibia should therefore alert the examiner to the possibility of a PCL disruption. However, PCL injuries can occur with torsion as well.

A PCL rupture is a much easier diagnosis to miss than that of the ACL tear. The increased laxity that occurs with the PCL tear is most detectable with the knee flexed to 90°. The examiner applies a posterior force to the tibia and feels the resulting posterior displacement of the tibia. With an acute injury, patients may not be comfortable with this much motion and hence the examination can be more difficult. In addition, the large hemarthrosis that is seen with an ACL injury is not the norm with a PCL tear, which can lead to a false sense of security that a major injury is not present. To complicate matters further, a PCL tear can frequently be mistaken for an ACL disruption, because the tibia is positioned posteriorly owing to the absence of the PCL. (Remember the PCL is the primary posterior restraint. Without it the tibia sags into a more posterior position in relation to the femur.) The examiner then pulls the tibia forward and interprets this as a positive anterior drawer and mistakes the injury for an ACL disruption. To help resolve this potential dilemma the quadriceps active drawer maneuver can help position the patient's knee appropriately[6] (although this again can be difficult acutely). With a normal knee flexed to 90°, a contraction of the quadriceps muscle alone will actually displace the tibia posteriorly 1 to 2 mm in relation to the femur. However, if the PCL is incompetent, the tibia will already be positioned posteriorly relative to the femur and a quadriceps contraction will pull the tibia anteriorly. Therefore, at 90° of flexion, anterior motion of the tibia caused by quadriceps contraction is abnormal and is diagnostic of a PCL injury.

Late PCL reconstruction is a more difficult operation than an ACL reconstruction and the results are not as uniformly favorable. Therefore, in the acute setting the presence of a PCL injury that is reparable would be a significant advantage. For example, the PCL can be avulsed with a fragment of bone, which is ideal for repair. In the setting of multiple injuries this is frequently missed on initial radiographs and again a high index of suspicion is necessary. This is important for the physical medicine and rehabilitation professional because this injury can be lost among head, chest, and abdominal injuries and major fractures. The significance of early intervention in the setting of a reparable PCL rupture cannot be overstated.

There is much debate about the natural history of a chronic PCL disruption.[7] Many authors believe that with appropriate rehabilitation disability is minimal with disruption of this ligament. However, patients are seen with late onset of arthrosis primarily in the medial compartment and in the patellofemoral joint as a result of PCL disruption. It is frequently stated that with a PCL disruption the patient experiences "disability," whereas with an ACL disruption the patient experiences "instability." With gross posterior laxity of the knee, patients can benefit from reconstructive procedures. However, the current capability of restoring a knee to its preinjury status is simply not as good for a late PCL reconstruction as with a late ACL reconstruction. This must obviously temper surgical judgment.

Medial Collateral Ligament

The MCL is the primary restraint to valgus stress at the knee.[1] It is probably the most common of the ligaments about the knee to be injured, and the classic injury is that seen with a lateral blow to the knee in football. The patient has tenderness over the course of the MCL, which most likely will be centered over the actual area of disruption. This may be over the medial epicondyle where the ligament originates, or over the joint line, which would represent an insubstance tear, or perhaps distally near its tibial attachment. With a valgus test of the knee, in approximately 20° of flexion, an examiner can palpate opening of the medial joint line as the tibia and femur separate. For valgus or varus tests I prefer the method of cradling the leg between the examiner's humerus and thorax. This leaves the hands free to palpate the actual joint line. Valgus or varus stress can be applied gently by manual pressure at the knee while palpating the joint line. A useful system for grading MCL injuries is that a grade I injury has pain over the MCL but no instability on valgus testing compared to the contralateral knee. A grade II injury shows some increased joint space opening on stress but there is a definite stop or endpoint. A grade III injury is complete and shows no endpoint on valgus stress. Stress radiographs are usually not necessary for diagnosis of MCL injuries. However, if the patient is skeletally immature a physeal (growth plate) injury can be mistaken for an MCL tear and radiographs can be helpful.

The current state of MCL injuries is that most are treated nonoperatively if they are isolated injuries.[8] It has been shown that with bracing of the knee to prevent valgus load and early rehabilitation aimed at muscle strengthening and gradual return of range of motion of the knee, patients will have just as acceptable a result as with operative intervention. They also avoid the risks and complications of surgery. However, what becomes more paramount in treating this injury conservatively is to be sure that associated ligamentous disruptions have been ruled out because a combined ligament injury, such as an ACL and MCL disruption, would necessitate operative intervention in most settings.

Lateral Collateral Ligament

The LCL attaches to the lateral femoral epicondyle and runs to the proximal lateral aspect of the fibular head. At times it has been thought of as a vestigial ligament, but it is now known to be the primary restraint to varus stress of the knee. Similar to the MCL with a valgus test, the LCL is identified by feeling the lateral joint line and applying a varus load to the knee in approximately 20° of flexion.

The LCL presents a difficult repair or reconstruction dilemma, whether the injury is acute or chronic. Fortunately, the mechanism of injury to the knee to produce a rupture of the LCL is such that this is a far less common injury than injuries to the MCL. It is uncommon for a blow to be delivered to the medial side of the knee that would stress the LCL. In addition, it is uncommon to have an LCL rupture as an isolated injury, and this is much more commonly associated with an injury to one or both of the cruciate ligaments. Because of the difficulty in late reconstructive surgery and because LCL injuries are usually associated with other injuries, the diagnosis and treatment should be vigorously pursued if there is any question that an LCL injury exists. If at all possible, these injuries should be repaired soon after occurrence to try to optimize later knee function.

Meniscal Tears

The knee menisci have received a tremendous amount of attention in the orthopaedic literature. It has been determined that the menisci perform very important functions of load bearing, shock absorption, provision of stability in the presence of an ACL deficit, and possibly lubrication of the knee. The medial meniscus rests on the medial plateau and is shaped like the letter C. The lateral meniscus rests on the lateral plateau but is more completely circular in shape. Both deepen their respective sides of the tibial plateau and make it more concave. The anterior and posterior horns of the menisci are attached to the tibial bone and the remainder is attached to the knee capsule. The lateral meniscus does have a bare area through which the popliteus tendon traverses. Because of the importance of meniscal function in the knee, arthroscopy has become established in recent years to minimize meniscal removal and leave behind as much normal meniscal tissue as possible at the time of surgery. Now the era of meniscal repair has arrived and when possible, meniscal tears are being repaired surgically to eliminate any meniscal tissue removal.

When a meniscus is torn, many patients will relate a twisting injury of the knee and perhaps even hearing a "knuckle-crack" at the time of their twisting injury. They may describe catching, popping, or perhaps even true locking of the knee at times after the index injury. However, it is equally common that patients do not remember exactly how their symptoms started but describe the same clicking and popping. Usually the patients are able to localize their pain to either the medial or the lateral joint line. On-and-off, slight effusions are also common with meniscal tears. True locking of the knee related to a meniscal tear results in a physical inability of the patient to extend the knee the final 20° to 30° because of a block within the knee. Patients sometimes describe pain in the knee when extending or an inability to flex the knee, but this does not represent mechanical locking. Many provocative tests have been described to elicit symptoms when doing a physical examination for a meniscal tear. The McMurray test is the best known of these. In this test, the examiner flexes the knee, externally rotates the tibia, applies light valgus pressure and extends the knee. Most of the times when this is performed in the presence of a meniscal tear, the examiner will elicit joint line area pain, but not a pop or clunk, as originally described.

Meniscal tears differ from ligament tears in that treatment is seldom needed emergently. Even with a truly locked knee it is no longer the normal approach to teach that this should be treated as an emergency, as might be expected for an open fracture. Many times a capsular sprain or patellofemoral pain can masquerade as a meniscal tear and, therefore, appropriate time and conservative measures are indicated before rushing in to treat every knee that might possibly have a meniscal tear. The treatment of meniscal tears is now universally by arthroscopy. Deciding on whether the tear is reparable or not is made by direct visualization of the meniscus. MR imaging is becoming more popular as a diagnostic aid for meniscal tears. This would seem to be redundant if a patient has classic findings, but it can be of help in doubtful cases.

Patellar Dislocation

Acute patellar dislocation is a common injury of young sports participants. A football lineman can plant his foot to change directions and the femur internally rotates with respect to the tibia, which creates an increased "Q angle." The Q angle is formed by the line of action of the quadriceps from the anterior superior iliac spine to the patella and a line from the patella to the tibial tubercle. The more extended the knee the less stable the patella, because the depth of the femoral sulcus that articulates with the patella is least in full extension. As the knee flexes, the patella sinks deeper into the sulcus, which increases its stability owing to greater joint congruity and contact. With contractions of the quadriceps muscle, the patella is put under a significant lateral force, particularly with an increasing Q angle, and can be actually pulled out of the sulcus and dislocated laterally, as in the example of the football lineman. A direct mechanism of dislocation with a blow to the knee is possible as well.

At the time a patellar dislocation occurs, an osteochondral fracture of the patella or lateral femoral condyle can occur and become a loose body in the joint (Fig. 49-1). The patellar dislocation will frequently become reduced before the patient or the examiner learns the exact nature of the injury, and when a hemarthrosis occurs it can make differential diagnosis more difficult. Normally tenderness at the medial border of the patella, patellar apprehension, and radiographs can be of help in making this diagnosis. Patellar apprehension is the uneasy feeling and guarding a patient exhibits when the examiner pushes the patella laterally, beginning to reproduce the injury. The reduction of a dislocated patella is quite easy; if the knee is extended slightly and gentle lateral to medial pressure applied to the patella, reduction can be accomplished (Fig. 49-2).

Many times patellar dislocation can be managed nonoperatively in patients with normal-appearing extremities and an excellent result obtained.[9] However, in a patient with passive lateral hypermobility of the patella, dysplastic vastus medialius obliquus (VMO), proximal and/or lateral position of the patella, or history of prior subluxation or dislocation, the tendency for another dislocation may be significant and acute surgery for repair might be the recommended choice. No matter what method of treatment is selected after a patellar dislocation, rehabilitation of the quadriceps, in particular, with emphasis on the VMO is very important for future knee function. One favorite method of rehabilitating the quadriceps is on a knee extension device, in which the resistance is applied to the ankle or distal part of the tibia and the patient forcefully extends the knee. Although this is good resistance for the quadriceps muscle, it places undue stress on the patellofemoral articulation.[10] These types of rehabilitation devices for patellofemoral problems should be discouraged. Straight leg raises, which use no knee flexion at all, or terminal extension exercises, using only the last 20° to 30° of extension, are good exercises with which to start. Short arc (meaning flexion less than approximately 40°) leg presses or squats can be added as the patient can tolerate them. Knee support sleeves made out of neoprene with a hole cut out for the patella are also popular in dealing with these patellofemoral problems.

THE ANKLE

The ankle is probably the most frequently sprained joint in the body. Because of this, ankle injuries occupy a significant focus whenever sports injuries are discussed. Yet, as common as ankle injuries are, many times there is a significant difference in how certain injuries are treated. The anterior talofibular ligament, which runs from the anterior distal aspect of the tip of the fibula to the neck of the talus, is the most commonly injured of the ankle ligaments. Normally this occurs in a plantar flexion, inversion-type injury. The calcaneofibular ligament, which runs from the distal anterior aspect of the fibula posteriorly to the calcaneus, is one of the few ligaments in the body that crosses two joints and therefore lends stability not only to the ankle joint but also to the subtalar joint. One of these is injured to some degree

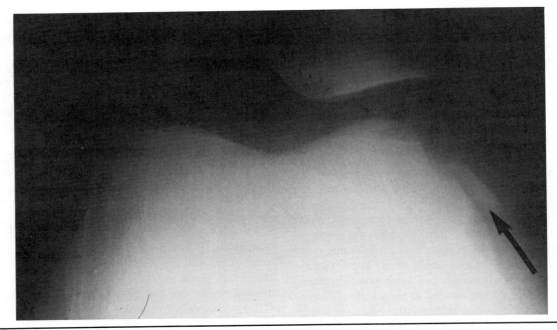

Fig. 49-1. Patellofemoral view of a knee after a patellar dislocation. An osteochondral fragment is on the lateral aspect of the knee and is shown by the arrow. Small dash marks on the apex of the patella show the lucent region from which the fragment came. Note that the patella is still positioned laterally in relation to the femoral groove.

when the lateral complex is sprained with an inversion-type injury. The posterior talofibular ligament attaches to the inner distal fibula and to the posterior talus at the articular margin. Injury to this ligament is difficult to detect and is not discussed to a great extent in the ankle sprain literature.

It is the difficulty in defining exactly which ligament is injured, and to what extent, that can make ankle sprains so hard to quantitate precisely. There is a vast amount of material in the literature on how "loose" an ankle can be and still be normal. Obviously quantitating injury is difficult if "normal" is hard to define. Some investigators divide ankle sprains into mild, moderate, and severe, depending on swelling, pain, and abnormal laxity on examination. However, what one person judges to be mild another considers moderate, and so precision in diagnosis is lacking. Other investigators divide sprains into single or double ligament, but this frequently requires stress radiographs or invasive studies to diagnose, which are difficult to obtain with a painful, swollen ankle. Most often the presenting features consist of diffuse swelling, ecchymosis, restricted motion, and somewhat diffuse

lateral tenderness, making a precise diagnosis difficult.

The anterior talofibular ligament can be tested with an anterior drawer maneuver, whereby the examiner restricts the anterior translation of the tibia and with the same hand feels the anterolateral corner of the talus. With the examiner's other hand holding the calcaneus and pulling it forward, anterior translation of the talus in relation to the tibia can be palpated and compared to that on the opposite side. Similarly, if the calcaneus is cupped and inverted, the corner of the talus can be found to displace gradually out of the ankle mortise if calcaneofibular ligament incompetence is present. This is felt as an increasing distance from the anterolateral talus to the distal lateral tibia. Stress radiographs to evaluate the laxity of the ankle can be obtained with the examiner performing the stress tests as just described and then having a radiograph made. Displacements can then be evaluated and compared to those on the opposite side.

Great controversy exists over the treatment of ankle sprains.[11] Some authors advocate early surgery and repair, but it is probably safe to say that most ankle

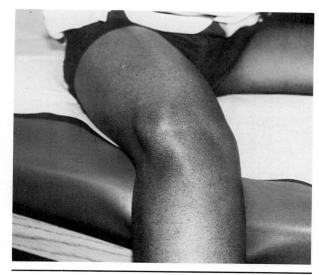

Fig. 49-2. Patellar dislocation. Note the lateral position of the patella.

sprains are managed conservatively. Treatment should include compression, ice, and elevation to minimize swelling, which will help with obtaining earlier motion and in diminishing pain as well. Depending on severity, crutches are used as pain dictates. Many types of ankle orthoses are available now, which provide the patient with the convenience of removability for personal hygiene and comfort, but they also have adequate stability to keep the patient more mobile early on in the course of the injury. Casts are preferred by some physicians, but with casts it is difficult to control swelling and stiffness becomes a greater problem when the cast is removed and rehabilitation begins.

As the initial swelling and pain recede, improvement in ankle motion should be sought. Strengthening of the dorsiflexors, plantarflexors, inverters, and everters of the ankle is emphasized, as is proprioceptive training as the ankle continues to recover. A testimony to the fact that conservative management works fairly well for most of these patients is that the ankle is the most common joint to be sprained and yet late reconstructive surgery for recurrent instability is a fairly infrequent procedure. In fact, Snook and co-workers, who designed a reconstructive procedure, reported only 60 cases over a 23-year experience.[12] Part of the explanation for this finding may lie in the

fact that with weight-bearing most of the stability of the ankle comes from its bony architecture, not from the ligaments.

What can cause difficulty with ankle sprains is to be lulled into a sense of complacency by thinking that every ankle sprain is a minor injury and will improve rapidly with time. There are many associated injuries that can masquerade as ankle sprains and should be sought to be sure that they are not missed. These injuries include osteochondral fractures of the talus, lateral talar process fractures, a fracture of the base of the fifth metatarsal, and syndesmosis injuries. Osteochondral fractures will frequently be revealed on plain radiographs but can be missed owing to the domed nature of the talus. Sometimes plantar flexion mortise views or even computed tomographic (CT) scans are necessary. To help direct attention to the area of pathology, a bone scan can be of help in the case of an ankle sprain that simply does not seem to get better to help look for subtle fractures. Lateral talar process fractures are easy to miss on initial films if strict attention is not paid to this area. The lateral talar process articulates with the fibula above and the posterior calcaneal facet below. The injury is best seen on the mortise view of the ankle. When the radiographic appearance is in doubt, associated imaging methods such as CT scans can be of help (Fig. 49-3). Fractures of the base of the fifth metatarsal occur with inversion-type injuries and represent avulsion by the peroneus brevis tendon. Normally when these patients have point tenderness over the base of the fifth metatarsal the diagnosis is easy. However, on occasion when the patient reports having "sprained the ankle," this area may not be addressed with appropriate attention. Syndesmosis injuries occur when the connection between the tibia and fibula is disrupted but in the absence of a fracture. The deltoid ligament is ruptured and the talus can be displaced into a more lateral position. The subtle widening of the mortise may be present on plain films or on stress views, and it is important to detect these injuries because late treatment can be difficult. Frequently, tenderness is localized over the anterior distal tibiofibular joint more than around the lateral ankle ligament complex, and swelling over this area can be a clue to the injury. At times a bone scan has been advocated to assist when the diagnosis is in doubt.[3] With deltoid area pain and tenderness,

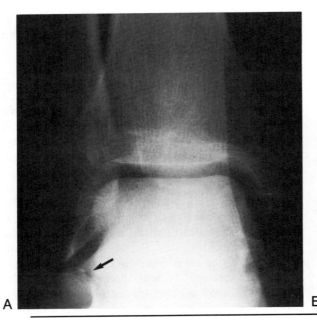
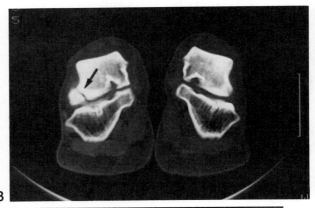

Fig. 49-3. (A) Anteroposterior view of an ankle. Note area of suspected irregularity at the tip of the arrow. (B) CT scan of the talus and calcaneus shown in **A** demonstrating the fracture in the talus.

but no fractures on plain radiographs, this injury should be considered.

THE SHOULDER

Afflictions of the shoulder girdle are common in sports and represent a significant percentage of athletic injuries.

Acromioclavicular Joint Injury

The acromioclavicular (AC) joint joins the axial skeleton to the upper extremity. It is held together by a stout capsule and the coracoclavicular ligaments. The coracoclavicular ligaments run from the base of the coracoid to the undersurface of the clavicle. Because the joint is subcutaneous, examination for displacement or tenderness is easy.

The AC joint can be a problem as an isolated entity, such as in a weight lifter with degenerative changes of this joint. It can also become painful after type I and II AC joint separations, which are discussed later. The diagnosis is helped by noting direct tenderness over the AC joint on physical examination and increased pain with cross-body adduction of the shoul-

der. An injection of lidocaine into the joint should temporarily relieve pain and ensure the diagnosis. In those athletes who have degenerative changes in the AC joint and pain, resection of the distal portion of the clavicle usually provides complete relief of symptoms if conservative measures fail.[14]

Acute injury to the AC joint is common and would be typified by a defensive lineman unceremoniously dumping a quarterback onto the point of his shoulder, causing a separation of the AC joint. AC joint injuries sustained in this fashion are typically classified into three grades.[15] In grade I injury, the capsule of the AC joint is damaged but the coracoclavicular ligaments remain intact and there is still stability of the AC joint. This is typified by pain and swelling over the AC joint, but no other abnormalities are noted on physical examination or on radiographs. In a grade II injury there is disruption of the AC joint capsule and partial injury of the coracoclavicular ligaments, allowing a slight separation of the true AC joint. These patients similarly have pain and swelling over the AC joint, but a slight step-off at the joint may be palpated and, on a weight-bearing radiograph of the shoulder (10 to 15 lb suspended from the wrist), asymmetry of the AC joint may be noted with slight

Fig. 49-4. Note the grade III AC separation on the left shoulder with the significant difference in contour compared to the right shoulder.

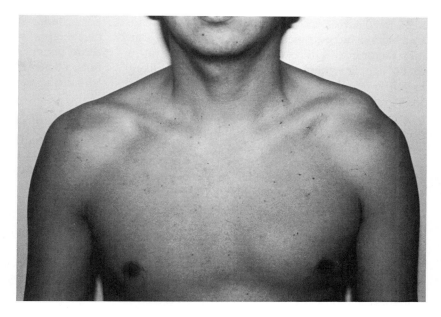

widening of the coracoclavicular space. In a grade III injury the AC capsule has been disrupted, the coracoclavicular ligaments have been totally disrupted, and the clavicle may completely dislocate from its articulation with the acromion. This may be readily determined on physical examination when a significant step-off is present at the joint (Fig. 49-4). Radiographs frequently show the complete separation but occasionally a weight-bearing view may be needed to demonstrate the extent of the injury.

In grades I and II injuries the athlete is treated expectantly with ice, rest, and a sling for comfort in the initial setting, and then with early motion and rehabilitation. Treatment for grade III injuries is more controversial and may be a choice between conservative management, as with grade I or II, and operative intervention for repair of the joint. Many studies have been done to compare the results of conservative treatment with operative repair. However, no consensus has yet been reached, and treatment still varies. To complicate matters further, late repairs can be performed and good results expected, so some physicians may treat these injuries conservatively and undertake surgery only for those patients who seem to have problems with conservative care. Determination of treatment will be made on the basis of patient preference, physician preference, activity, and so forth.

Shoulder Dislocation

Another very common problem in the athletic population is shoulder dislocation. As an example of this injury, picture a linebacker reaching out to tackle a running back with his arm in abduction and external rotation, being involved in a pileup, and ending up with an anteroinferior traumatic dislocation. These patients are in great pain, and prompt medical attention is needed. The arm is held in a position of slight abduction and in external rotation. There is fullness of the anterior shoulder, and the acromion seems prominent because the humeral head is anterior and not in its usual position beneath the acromion. Although experienced sports medicine personnel might prefer to do an immediate shoulder relocation, those not experienced in this treatment should have the patient transported rapidly to an emergency room for evaluation and reduction. It is important to document the neurologic status of any patient with a shoulder dislocation, and in particular to pay attention to the axillary nerve and therefore deltoid muscle function. After reduction, the usual treatment is a sling or shoulder immobilizer to allow the injured anterior structures to heal.

After a traumatic anterior dislocation, the long-term problem for the athlete is that of recurrence. Studies have estimated that an anterior dislocation will recur in 50 to 90 percent of young athletes and they therefore have to be counseled accordingly. The one common factor in all studies discussing recurrence rate is that of age. The younger athletic person is more likely to suffer another dislocation than a middle-aged weekend sports participant. Therefore, for conservative management a general recommendation based on age would be 3 to 6 weeks of immobilization for persons less than 20 years old, 1 to 3 weeks for patients over 40, and no more than 1 week for those over 60.[15] Braces are available for shoulder dislocaters to help minimize this problem during an athletic season, and these are primarily used in football. However, because they restrict range of motion, braces become impractical for athletes in skills positions or in other sporting events for which full motion of the shoulder may be necessary.

The surgical treatment of recurrent anterior shoulder dislocation currently is undergoing something of an evolution, particularly with increased emphasis on arthroscopic repairs. Suffice it to say that, whether the approach is open or arthroscopic, the most common method is to attach the glenohumeral ligaments back to the anterior aspect of the glenoid. Traditionally, this type of repair is termed a Bankart repair.

Some shoulders do not actually become dislocated but only subluxated. Owing to abnormal laxity or a tearing of the capsule, the humerus can slide partially out of the glenoid but become reduced spontaneously. This is frequently referred to as the "dead arm" syndrome and can occur with forceful overextension of the arm, as in throwing, a tennis serve, and similar actions.[16] Some patients may feel the arm slipping out of place and others may have only pain. The symptoms are normally transient and related to the inciting activity, with some activities being well tolerated. In the athletes who do not feel the shoulder slipping out, this can be a very difficult diagnosis. On physical examination, a positive apprehension sign is usually seen. This sign is noted when the examiner abducts the shoulder to approximately 90° and rotates it externally as the shoulder is extended. The patient feels some discomfort but, more importantly, feels the shoulder may "come out of joint" or at least reproduce the symptoms. Conservative measures are aimed initially at avoiding the aggravating activity and at instituting shoulder strengthening exercises.

For anterior subluxations, strengthening adduction and internal rotation are especially emphasized. In those patients in whom conservative management fails, a Bankart type of repair is performed as with the true dislocations.

Posterior dislocations of the shoulder are far less common than anterior dislocations, constituting perhaps only 2 to 4 percent of all shoulder dislocations. The mechanism is frequently a direct posterior blow, such as occurs when an offensive lineman with his arm elevated forcibly hits a defensive lineman, driving the humeral head posteriorly. These injuries can be easier to miss than might be expected. Because posterior dislocations are seen most frequently with electrical shock or seizures, it is important for professionals in physical medicine and rehabilitation to consider the diagnosis. In the athletic population it is recurrent posterior instability or subluxations that predominate as problems, not repeated dislocations as are common with anterior dislocations (Fig. 49-5). On physical examination in cases of posterior dislocation, a major clue is the patient's lack of external rotation. Again, any posterior dislocation that is acute would best be managed by transporting the patient to a medical facility for reduction of the dislocation and radiographic evaluation. It is most important with all of these types of shoulder injury that an axillary radiograph be obtained to document the location of the humeral head, because other views can sometimes be misinterpreted or simply be inadequate (Fig. 49-6).

Shoulder Impingement

One of the more frequent sports diagnoses currently being made is that of shoulder impingement.[17] This is a dilemma primarily for athletes participating in sports that involve overhead arm movement, such as tennis and swimming, and is also a phenomenon of athletes as they age. Normally the rotator cuff tendons fit intimately under the coracoacromial arch. The arch is made up of the coracoacromial ligament and acromion itself. The rotator cuff is composed of the subscapularis tendon, which originates on the anterior scapula and inserts on the lesser tuberosity, the supraspinatus muscle which originates from the supraspinatus fossa and inserts on the greater tuberosity of the humerus, the infraspinatus and teres

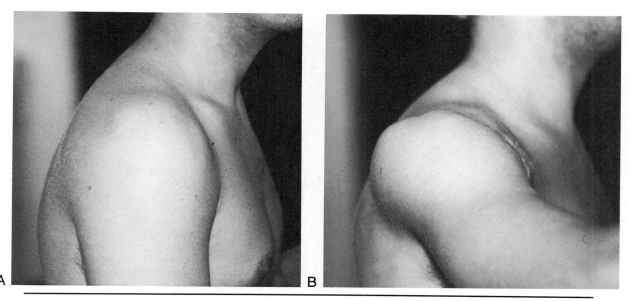

Fig. 49-5. (A) Posterior subluxation of the right shoulder. At rest the shoulder appears normal. **(B)** As the patient elevates his arm the posterior aspect of the shoulder shows fullness where the humeral head has subluxed posteriorly.

minor muscles which originate from the scapula as well and insert distal to the supraspinatus muscle on the greater tuberosity. The long head of the biceps tendon runs between the lesser and greater tuberosities and inserts on the superior glenoid cavity. In impingement of the shoulder, the rotator cuff "rubs" or "impinges" on the anterior edge of the acromion, primarily during forward elevation of the arm and internal rotation. The principal cuff tendon involved in this impingement is the supraspinatus tendon. Frequently patients will describe pain in the lateral deltoid region and also have night pain. For most patients the pain occurs with the activity for which they sought medical care, such as throwing, blocking in volleyball, and so forth. On examination, the impingement sign is noted when the examiner passively elevates and internally rotates the humerus and pain is produced in the periacromial area. Repeated internal and external rotation of the shoulder in an abducted position can cause similar pain. Because the rotator cuff muscles depress the humeral head, if they weaken or tear, the humeral head can be displaced more superiorly, causing a vicious cycle of impingement, because this displacement allows the humeral head to come closer to the acromion and further aggravates the impingement.

Neer[17,18] developed the concept of impingement and recognized three stages. Stage I impingement is characterized by inflammation and edema, which subsides when the aggravating activity is stopped and is managed conservatively. This is typically seen in patients less than 25 years old. In stage 2 inflammation, fibrosis and thickening occur in the rotator cuff and cause the patient discomfort even when the aggravating activity has been stopped. Typically, these patients are more often in the 25 to 40-year-old group. Again, attempts are made to handle this stage conservatively, but operative intervention may be necessary. In stage 3, a rotator cuff tear has developed and most likely the patient will require operative intervention. This stage is normally seen in patients over 40 years of age.

The conservative management of impingement centers on avoidance of the aggravating activity, administration of nonsteroidal anti-inflammatory agents, shoulder stretching, and muscle strengthening. Stretching is aimed primarily at the posterior capsule and cuff. Physical therapy with modalities is frequently useful to help decrease pain. Exercises are aimed at internal and external rotation strengthening with the arm in an adducted position.[19] In abduction

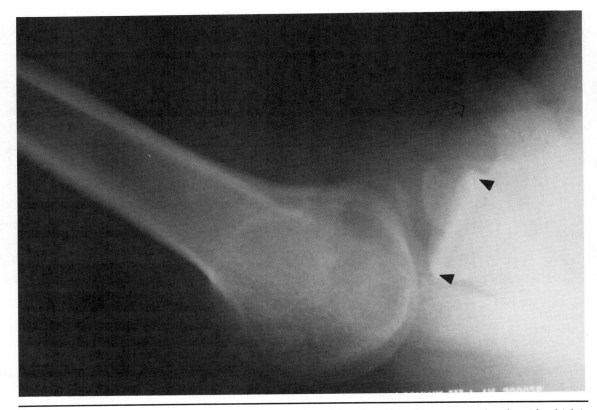

Fig. 49-6. An axillary radiograph demonstrating posterior subluxation of the humerus on the glenoid, which is demonstrated clearly on this radiograph but may be missed on standard anteroposterior radiographs. The arrowheads outline the anterior and posterior edges of the glenoid cavity. The open arrow is on the coracoid process at the anterior aspect of the shoulder.

exercises the arm is kept below the horizontal to minimize impingement. If after several months the patient fails to improve, removal of the undersurface of the anterior acromion, resection of the coracoacromial ligament to decompress the space, and attending to any cuff pathology may be indicated. This can be performed arthroscopically or by open means. Not all shoulder pain occurring with overhead activity is impingement, and frequently the differential diagnosis can be taxing. Chronic calcific tendinitis, mild frozen shoulder, AC joint arthritis, cervical radiculopathy, old humerus fracture, and other entities can be present to one degree or another.

The biceps tendon, as already described, runs in close proximity to the anterior rotator cuff. Frequently pain in the area that is truly impingement is confused as biceps tendinitis. Although biceps tendinitis can occur as an isolated entity, most authors believe this is related to impingement. Therefore, treatment should be aimed at the impingement rather than at the biceps itself. In fact, as impingement advances and a rotator cuff tear is perhaps seen, it is not uncommon to see a rupture of the long head of the biceps.

REFERENCES

1. Noyes FR, Grood ES: Classification of ligament injuries: why an anterolateral laxity or anteromedial laxity is not a diagnostic entity. p. 185. Instr Course Lect 36:185, 1987
2. Torg JS, Conrad W, Kalen V: Clinical diagnosis of anterior cruciate ligament instability in the athlete. Am J Sports Med 4:84, 1976
3. Noyes FR, Matthews DS, Mooar PA, Grood ES: Symptomatic anterior cruciate deficient knee. J Bone Joint Surg [Am] 65:163, 1983
4. Noyes FR, Mangine RE, Barber S: Early knee motion after

open and arthroscopic anterior cruciate ligament reconstruction. Am J Sports Med 15:149, 1987

5. Noyes FR, Butler DL, Grood ES et al: Biomechanical analysis of human ligament grafts used in knee ligament repairs and reconstructions. J Bone Joint Surg [Am] 66:344, 1984

6. Daniel DM, Stone ML, Barnett P, Sachs R: Use of the quadriceps active test to diagnose posterior cruciate-ligament disruption and measurement of posterior laxity of the knee. J Bone Joint Surg [Am] 70:386, 1988

7. Parolie JM, Bergfeld JA: Long-term results of nonoperative treatment of isolated posterior cruciate ligament injuries in the athlete. Am J Sports Med 14:35,38, 1986

8. Indelicato PA: Non-operative treatment of complete tears of the medial collateral ligament of the knee. J Bone Joint Surg [Am] 65:323, 1983

9. Cash JD, Hughston JC: Treatment of acute patellar dislocation. Am J Sports Med 16:244, 1988

10. Hungerford DS, Barry M: Biomechanics of the patellofemoral joint. Clin Orthop 144:9, 1979

11. Cox JS: Surgical and nonsurgical treatment of acute ankle sprains. Clin Orthop 198:118, 1985

12. Snook G, Chrisman OD, Wilson TC: Long-term results of the Chrisman-Snook operation for reconstruction of the lateral ligaments of the ankle. J Bone Joint Surg [Am] 67:1, 1985

13. Marymont JV, Lynch MA, Henning CE: Acute ligamentous diastasis of the ankle without fracture. Evaluation by radionuclide imaging. Am J Sports Med 14:407, 1986

14. Cook FF, Tibone JE: The Mumford procedure in athletes. Am J Sports Med 16:97, 1988

15. Neer CS II, Rockwood CA Jr: Fractures and dislocations of the shoulder. p. 675. In Rockwood CA Jr, Green DP (eds): Fractures in Adults. JB Lippincott, Philadelphia, 1984

16. Rowe CR, Zarins B: Recurrent transient subluxation for the shoulder. J Bone Joint Surg [Am] 63:863, 1981

17. Neer CS II: Impingement lesions. Clin Orthop Rel Res 173:70, 1983

18. Neer CS II: Anterior acromioplasty for the chronic impingement syndrome in the shoulder. A preliminary report. J Bone Joint Surg [Am] 54:41, 1972

19. Jobe FW, Moynes DR: Delineation of diagnostic criteria and a rehabilitation program for rotator cuff injuries. Am J Sports Med 10:336, 1982

Section V

REHABILITATION ACCORDING TO ANATOMIC REGION

50 Rehabilitation of the Hand

JOHN M. RAYHACK
JOY N. LANGWORTHY

GENERAL CONSIDERATIONS

Rehabilitation of the hand after injury or disease has become a highly specialized art. Three components are essential to the success of such a program: a cooperative and motivated patient, a skilled and compassionate therapist, and open communication among the patient, therapist, and physician.

The patient who is referred for hand rehabilitation may need nothing more than a simple splint or instructions for a gentle home exercise program. Alternatively, the therapist may find a tearful, frightened, and confused patient with a devastating hand injury. The challenge of such a case to the therapist is enormous. As with any rehabilitation situation, a caring attitude and patient education are vital to the success of the overall program. In this chapter, an attempt is made, whenever possible, to focus on basic principles rather than trying to detail the treatment of specific disease or injury states. For example, the section on desensitization deals with an issue that is common to the treatment of the fingertip amputation site, the carpal tunnel incision, and the isolated radial sensory neuroma. The treatment principles are the same, but the application must be individualized to the patient's needs. Not to be understated is the importance of therapist's skill and experience in choosing the most appropriate treatment regimen.

EDEMA CONTROL

After trauma, infection, and surgical intervention, a serofibrinous exudate will often form in the subcutaneous tissues, in the fascial spaces, and around collateral ligaments and the joint capsule. The potential danger of this physiologic response to tissue trauma is that the swelling may be excessive or unduly prolonged. A chronic condition of pain, joint stiffness, and joint contractures can ensue owing to thickening and organization of this protein-rich exudate. To avoid this disastrous result, a prevention program is of paramount importance.

Well known is the need to elevate the involved extremity above the level of the heart. This may be accomplished by using a sling suspended by an intravenous pole or by propping up the extremity on several pillows with the forearm placed in a vertical position. In conjunction with elevation, splinting is important to keep the hand in an intrinsic plus position.

With digit involvement, the splint should hold the wrist extended 30° to 40°, the metacarpophalangeal (MCP) joints flexed 60°, and the interphalangeal (IP) joints fully extended. This position keeps the MCP and IP ligaments on maximum stretch and prevents ultimate joint contractures. If the digits are uninvolved by the initial injury, they should be left unimpeded to permit active movement. Full motion of the digits provides a pumping action that propels edema fluid and lymph from the injured tissues. An additional benefit of digit motion is the maintenance of tendon gliding, which is so crucial to ultimate motion. Care must be taken to avoid constriction of the dorsal venous structures when using a splint that employs a dorsal shell.

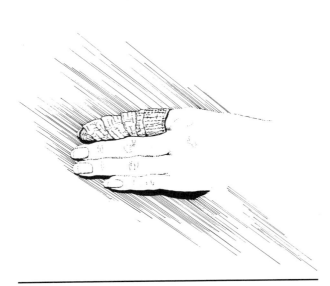

Fig. 50-1. Coban wrap is used to apply gentle compression to reduce edema.

In addition to motion of the digits, other uninvolved joints should also be included in the therapy process. If possible, elbow and shoulder motion should be stressed. This assists limb circulation and avoids the potentially disastrous shoulder-hand syndrome.[1]

Continued edema at 10 to 14 days is usually reversible but could be a serious threat if left untreated. At this point, the therapist must employ more aggressive means to thwart this potentially serious situation. Measurement of hand volume with a volunteer is an important means of monitoring a therapy program aimed at reducing edema. Circumferential measurements of the digits, wrist, and forearm are more time consuming, but accurately pinpoint the contribution of each body part to the overall edema problem.

To assist the outflow of extracellular fluid in the digits, light compression can be applied in a distal to proximal direction through the use of Coban (3M), a self-adherent elastic tape (Fig. 50-1). However, care must be taken to guard against excessively tight application. The patient must be carefully instructed as to the proper technique and, once this is well understood, a home program of wrapping can be followed. A major advantage of this modality is that active range of motion exercises can be performed with the Coban in place.

Similar, but less widely used today, is the technique of string wrapping. With this technique, a soft cord is wrapped around the digits for 5 minutes three times daily. This is followed by range-of-motion exercises, which may be supplemented by retrograde massage. This should be performed with firm, deep pressure directed distal to proximal. Skin friction should be minimized with the addition of a lanolin lotion during the implementation of this technique.

When the entire hand is involved, an Isotoner glove can provide effective continuous external compression (Fig. 50-2). It is often helpful to turn the glove inside out to avoid localized pressure from the seams. Tubigrip is also a good form of compression for hand, wrist, and forearm swelling. Involvement of the entire extremity, or the presence of refractory pitting edema, an intermittent mechanical pump with pneumatic sleeves may be employed. Use of these commercially available devices must be carefully supervised to avoid excessive pressures and possible vascular embarrassment. This is especially true in the insensate extremity. Use of a custom made garment after these measures will help prevent the reaccumulation of extracellular fluid.

It is clear that chronic edema may lead to very serious functional deficits. Prevention through education and constant vigilance must remain the primary concern of the hand therapist and surgeon.

STATIC SPLINTING

Although it is similar in general to dynamic splinting, static splinting is used early in treatment and has as its goal protection and optimal positioning of an injured structure while preserving motion of adjacent joints. With the use of such a splint, the injured part is immobilized and supported. Dynamic splinting in contrast utilizes traction to facilitate joint changes.

Classic examples of static splinting are the Stack splint for mallet deformity and Bunnell's splint for protection of central slip repairs. Both maintain a low-profile design and allow motion of adjacent units. Unique to these particular splints is their capacity to diminish tension on the repaired structure while concurrently permitting motion of the adjacent joint. Each has the effect of pulling the extensor tendon origin distally with active flexion, thereby di-

Fig. 50-2. Isotoner glove provides external compression to the entire hand thus reducing edema.

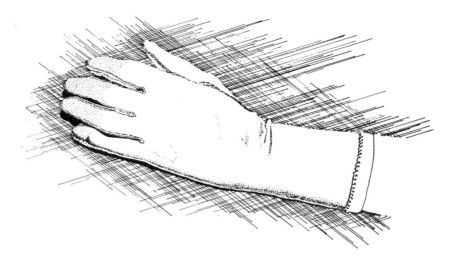

minishing the tension on the injured extensor structure. Splints to protect rheumatoid joints are yet another version of static splinting. Designed to avoid the unrelenting pull of unbalanced tendons and joints, these "resting splints" provide immeasurable comfort and slow the process of joint deformation. A custom metal ring (Fig. 50-3) is an example of a static splint designed to prevent proximal interphalangeal joint (PIP) joint hyperextension. The use of static

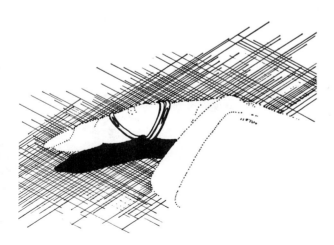

Fig. 50-3. A cosmetically appealing and comfortable metal splint can prevent PIP joint hyperextension while allowing flexion.

splinting in burn rehabilitation is discussed later in this chapter.

The advantages of low-profile static splinting are evident. Individual joints can be protected with the least amount of interference to adjacent joints so that hand function can be permitted. The short radial thumb shell for carpometacarpal degenerative joint disease and the volar wrist support splint for carpal tunnel syndrome are good examples. Stable fractures and nerve repairs can be statically immobilized through the use of lightweight splints, thereby facilitating patient comfort, guarding against skin bruising in pressure areas, and preventing fracture displacement or tension on the nerve repair. The therapist's intervention to ensure proper fit of the splint as swelling subsides is an important aspect of fracture care.

DYNAMIC SPLINTING FOR JOINT CONTRACTURE

Chronic edema, coupled with prolonged immobilization and subsequent ligament shortening and capsular contracture, often results in refractory joint contractures. Skin contracture and adherence to injured local tissues also contribute to this problem. The rehabilitation of such a contracture requires gentle stretching of the involved tissues. Although too much stress can lead to localized bleeding, subsequent pain, and further inhibition of joint motion, too little stress

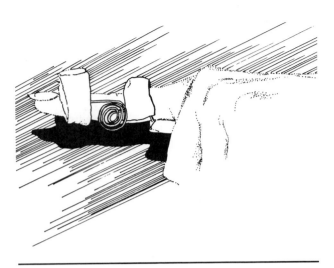

Fig. 50-4. Capner splint is used to apply gentle, adjustable extensor tension to treat PIP joint contractures.

can be equally ineffective owing to the lack of requisite stretching of contracted tissues.

An important principle of such a splint is the maintenance of a low-profile design, which encourages splint wear through improved cosmesis and minimal interference with clothing. Moreover, adjacent uninvolved joints remain free for mobilization.

Dynamic splinting plays a major role in the rehabilitation of joint contractures; however, problems can arise from a lack of sufficient knowledge regarding the appropriate tension under which the rubber bands should be placed. In this situation the experience of the occupational therapist is valued. It is the clinical judgment of this therapist that determines not only the lowest profile splint to employ, but also the appropriate tension under which the splint should be placed. This often requires gentle splint modification as well as determination and maintenance of the elusive "appropriate" tension. The dynamic nature of this splint is further complicated by the ever-changing elasticity of the rubber bands as well as the alterations resulting from diminished contracture as the joint motion improves. Springs with variable forces are now available that provide constant tension. Further research will, it is hoped, provide more objective data to guide and improve the application of dynamic traction in the future.

Joint contractures may also be treated by commercially available spring-loaded dynamic splinting. For example, PIP joint contractures may be treated by Capner splints (Fig. 50-4), Joint Jacks (Fig. 50-5), and LMB springs (Fig. 50-6). As in locally fabricated thermoplastic splints, these commercial splints apply different degrees of tension and require the same degree of clinical judgment by the therapist to determine not only the appropriate splint to use but also the necessary tension. In addition, duration of splint use and accurate positions require the constant vigilance of the therapist.

Sustained elastic pressure is yet another mode of dynamic splinting that can be applied easily to increase finger flexion. Rubber glove finger sleeves (Fig. 50-7) and elastic strap traction are examples of this method of treatment. Their main disadvantage is often a function of the limited tolerance of the adjacent skin, which shortens the length of time sustained elastic pressure can be used.

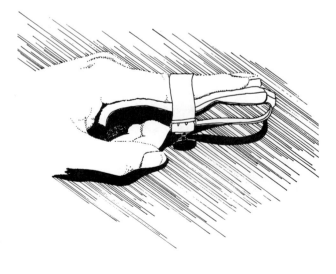

Fig. 50-5. Use of a Joint Jack to apply passive stretch to the PIP joint.

Dynamic splinting, regardless of the specific type employed, should be followed by a specific active range-of-motion program whenever possible. This will help maintain the gains in motion made possible through the passive program.

Dynamic splints may be ineffective in overcoming chronic joint contractures, which may then require surgical releases (e.g., checkrein ligament release). However, the pain, local bleeding, and voluntary joint motion limitation that result from surgical procedures may then require the reimplementation of many of the methods outlined previously.

DYNAMIC SPLINTING TO PROTECT REPAIRED TENDONS

In the same way that elastic bands can provide the sustained tension necessary to overcome the elasticity of shortened ligaments or muscle-tendon units in joint contractures, they can also be used to replace the function of a recently repaired tendon. Dynamic rubber band traction for repaired flexor tendons is perhaps the best known example of this use.[2]

This technique has subsequently been modified with the addition of a distal palmar bar to block MCP flexion.[3] This modification emphasizes PIP and distal

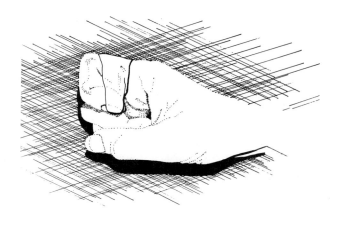

Fig. 50-7. Rubber glove sleeves provide gentle stretch to increase PIP and DIP flexion.

interphalangeal joint (DIP) joint motion and tendon excursion. The dynamic rubber band traction procedure involves the use of a posterior plaster splint applied at surgery. This splint initially acts as the fulcrum against which the elastic bands are applied and is subsequently replaced by a thermoplastic splint fabricated by the therapist. The wrist is flexed 35° and MCP joints are flexed 70° to avoid tension on the repaired flexor tendon. A hook applied to the nail is attached to a rubber band or elastic thread and attached to a safety pin or hook applied to the volar wrist area. Degree of tension and line of pull are factors that need careful surveillance by both surgeon and therapist. By actively extending the finger, passive gliding of the repaired flexor tendon is achieved, thus avoiding the spot welding that is so detrimental to subsequent tendon gliding. PIP flexion contractures are a well-recognized complication of such a splinting program and require the rehabilitation team to be on constant alert to prevent them. For this reason, many surgeons and therapists prefer intermittent application of the rubber band with strapping of the finger against the dorsal splint through the use of a Velcro strap. Alternatively, passive finger flexion can be used in lieu of the rubber band traction technique by employing a modified Duran technique.[4]

Moreover, dynamic passive extension splinting for extensor tendon repair in zones V, VI, and VII has been added to the rehabilitation armamentarium.[5]

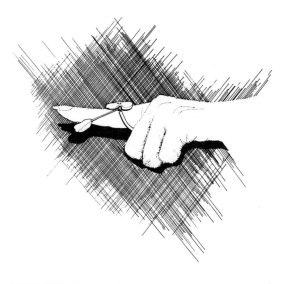

Fig. 50-6. LMB splinting applies gentle passive stretch to the PIP joint.

Making allowance for the same need to protect a repaired tendon, this splint enables the extensor tendons to be passively mobilized while permitting active finger flexion. A dorsal forearm–based static splint is fashioned to keep the wrist in slight extension. Dynamic traction applied through an outrigger passively extends the MCP and PIP joints to 0°. Active flexion is permitted to 30° of MCP flexion. This may be blocked by an overlay static splint to impede excessive pull through this splint. The splint is removed after 3 to 4 weeks and active extension is then begun.

DYNAMIC AND STATIC SPLINTING FOR MCP ARTHROPLASTY

Postoperative hand rehabilitation after MCP arthroplasty is critical during the period of joint capsule formation. This "encapsulation process" is based on the concept that the formation and development of collagen can be guided by a specific therapy program. The goal is to achieve mobility by stressing the scar in the volar and dorsal planes to develop sufficient laxity for flexion and extension to occur. Stability is provided by constant early splinting to eliminate excessive lateral motion and to foster capsular tightness in the mediolateral plane.

After removal of the bulky surgical dressing at 3 to 5 days following surgery, the patient is placed in a dynamic MCP joint extension splint. The static forearm-based component of this splint maintains the wrist in slight dorsiflexion and radial deviation. Slings attached to dorsal outriggers are positioned at the proximal phalangeal level to maintain the MCP joints in 0° to 10° of extension and approximately 10° of radial deviation. A pronation tendency of the index finger can be overcome through the use of two slings, which form a "force couple" that results in slight supination.[6]

The dynamic extension splint is worn at all times for 3 weeks. Active flexion and extension exercises are performed within the splint for 15 minutes every waking hour. An intrinsic minus position (MCP extension, IP flexion) facilitates maximal extensor tendon and extensor hood gliding through the dorsal scar. Passive range of motion is also performed gently with avoidance of any lateral motion. After 3 weeks,

flexion splinting may be incorporated into the treatment program for short periods of time if needed. The final goal for MCP motion is 70° of MCP flexion actively and 90° passively.

Dynamic extension splinting can be supplemented at 3 to 6 weeks with a static resting splint maintaining the digits in extension for night use. Daytime splinting may be discontinued as early as 6 weeks postoperatively. Static night splinting is indicated for 3 to 6 months or longer. Light, nonresistive prehension tasks can be commenced at 4 weeks and gentle strengthening should be initiated at 6 weeks after the removal of the daytime splint.

In the arthroplasty patient, deterioration of function is not uncommon, and the therapist must assess activity of daily living needs and recommend appropriate assistive devices to increase patient independence. The patient should also be instructed in methods of joint protection and energy conservation.

HAND REHABILITATION IN RHEUMATOID ARTHRITIS

The patient with rheumatoid disease represents a particular challenge to the therapist and physician. Often multiple joints are involved concurrently, and this may complicate the formidable task of rehabilitation.

The initial patient assessment is often quite time consuming but extremely important. It is imperative that the therapist understand the patient's normal daily activities, degree of pain, relative muscle strengths and weaknesses, general medical condition, and emotional status. The therapist must determine if deterioration in patient function is temporary or permanent. If temporary, it is often possible to return the patient to the previous level of activity. A temporary flare-up often benefits from rest, splinting, and a structured exercise program. Through the use of moist heat or paraffin, much of the patient's pain and stiffness may be alleviated prior to embarking on an exercise program. This can consist of active assistive or active exercises occasionally followed later by gentle active resistive exercises.

Resting splints are frequently helpful to immobilize inflamed joints, which helps to decrease muscle spasms and reduces inflammation and pain. Equally beneficial are assistance devices that permit activities of daily living to be performed with less effort and more comfort. Such aids can be as simple as a circular rubber disk that allows easy removal of the lid from a jar.

As more advanced inflammatory changes occur, the therapist needs to individualize the treatment according to the stage of involvement of the patient.[7] For example, patients with more advanced synovial involvement requiring dorsal tenosynovectomy will need active assistive exercises in their postsurgery therapy protocol. With increasing involvement of the MCP joints (e.g., with subsequent subluxation and dislocation) necessitating MCP arthroplasty, therapy will shift in focus to dynamic passive extension splints and joint capsule remodeling.

The therapist's continued monitoring of the rheumatoid patient over an extended time will help identify early setbacks and possibly identify areas in need of additional prompt attention.

DUPUYTREN'S CONTRACTURE

Despite numerous attempts, little objective evidence has been obtained to prove that dynamic splints, ultrasonography, scar massage, and application of pressure molds are effective in the nonoperative treatment of Dupuytren's contracture. Hence, the therapist's intervention in the treatment of this palmar and digital connective tissue disease is virtually always limited to the postoperative period. Close supervision and constant encouragement are practically prerequisites to ensure successful results in moderately and severely involved extremities.

From the moment that the postoperative dressing is removed at 1 to 3 days after surgery, often revealing an open palmar wound,[8] the patient and therapist are faced with several concurrent problems. Despite accurate preoperative warnings, patients still tend to be surprised by the enormity of the open wound. Reassurance that the open palmar wound will in fact eventually close, as unbelievable as it seems, is the beginning of the overall educational process, which

must be spearheaded by the therapist. Most surgeons and therapists agree that all the work that ensues after the open palm surgical technique is justifiable if it prevents one hematoma and its serious secondary effects of increased pain and potential hand stiffness.

The initial evaluation of both the active and passive motion of the digits and the condition and location of the associated digital incisions will guide the formulation of the individualized rehabilitative program. In addition, the MCP and PIP joint extension achieved during surgery must not be forgotten through postoperative inattention. Clearly, communication with the surgeon regarding realistic expectations for an individual patient based on results achieved at surgery is quite important.

Wet-to-dry saline dressings, whirlpool treatments, home soaks, and sterile dressing applications to treat open wounds coexisting with closed surgical skin incisions complicate the rehabilitative task. As in other areas of therapy, a balancing act must be maintained between protecting sensitive soft tissues, splinting previously contracted joints in extension, and alternating active flexion and extension exercises of the digits to preserve motion. In addition, edema control and desensitization techniques as described in this chapter must be applied until skin softening and tolerance for functional use is achieved.

Static extension splints are required for nighttime use for as long as 3 to 6 months. Careful follow-up at this time will often demonstrate a loss of some of the extension achieved and maintained previously. This may be a harbinger of refractory areas that may ultimately require reoperation at a later date. The thumb, thumb web, and index finger are particularly prone to this refractory phenomenon, as clearly shown by Tubiana and Defrenne.[9]

REHABILITATION OF THE BURNED HAND

The mainstay of treatment of the burned hand is prevention of soft tissue contractures, avoidance of hypertrophic scarring, and maintenance of range of motion of digits. In the acute phase, limb elevation and early range of motion to provide a pumping action to the burn edema must be stressed. Splinting is employed at about 3 to 5 days, when the vessels regain their normal permeability. Because the dorsum of the hand and wrist is frequently involved, every attempt should be made to avoid the "position of deformity" characterized by wrist flexion, MCP joint extension, and IP joint flexion.[10] By keeping the MCP joints flexed with IP joints extended in the intrinsic plus position, maximum stretch to collateral ligaments is achieved. Splinting should be initiated at the first sign of decreased joint mobility or skin tightness.[10] Splinting may also be necessary to immobilize fractures that cannot be practically casted or internally fixed owing to the increased risk of infection. Gauze wrapping should be used to maintain the splint in place to avoid the compressive effect of straps. In the child under 3 years of age, large, bulky dressings should be used in lieu of splints. Splinting may also be necessary after split-thickness skin grafting. This should be initiated immediately and maintained until all skin tightness is gone. Frequently, splinting in the operating suite at the time of correction is warranted. This is especially true in the young child. In circumferential digital burns, longitudinal fingernail traction may be necessary to control rotation and keep the fingers abducted. This is also beneficial after skin grafting to avoid traction on the graft.

The therapist must work closely with the burn team to perform range-of-motion exercises during dressing changes. These short exercise periods are vital to the prevention of deforming contractures and to avoid the subsequent need for secondary reconstructive procedures. The addition of topical antibiotics is unimpeded by the use of thermoplastic splints, which can easily be cleaned and reapplied. As early as physically possible, the patient is urged to commence with self-care and activities of daily living. One of the first activities is that of self-feeding, which stresses the concept of self-reliance. With an improving medical condition, motor activities are initiated to increase strength, mobility, and fine motor skills. Gradually increasing demands of the therapy program are instituted on the basis of the patient's joint motion, overall strength, coordination, and sensation, which must be continually monitored. Scar stabilization and maturation is a very protracted event that can take up to $1\frac{1}{2}$ years in hypertrophic scars. It is important to minimize the hypertrophic potential of deep second- and third-degree burns to improve the ultimate cosmetic appearance and functional result. Helpful in this regard is the use of initial compression wraps (Fig. 50-1) followed by custom elastic gloves. Zippers can be added to assist ease of glove application, and open fingertips can be permitted to increase sensory input. To maximize compression, inserts can be placed inside the gloves over concave surfaces. These pressure garments are worn continuously and may be placed over oil- or water-based lubricants. Each of these has inherent disadvantages. Oil-based lubricants may cause excessive soiling and do not add moisture, and water-based lubricants need to be reapplied frequently and do not prevent evaporative water loss. Because the majority of healing occurs at home, constant surveillance of a home-based program is crucial to the overall success of the burn program. As with other therapeutic endeavors, patient motivation and compliance need to be monitored to maximize the benefits of this demanding overall rehabilitative program.

SENSORY RE-EDUCATION AFTER NERVE INJURY

Improvement in sensory results after nerve repair remains one of the major challenges of therapists and physicians alike. From a morphologic point of view, it is clear from the classic work of Sunderland[11] that a physical barrier can exist at any level between the neurons and the end organ of sensitivity. Clearly, despite the most meticulous surgical technique, only a certain number of injured axons actually reach the proper end organs. Confounding this problem of the anatomic impediment is the impaired cortical interpretation of stimuli generated in this altered afferent system.

Re-education programs rely on one's general ability to compensate for various deficits through the process of adaptation. Such a program stresses the use of various forms of sensory stimuli and the relearning of the cortical representation for a given stimulus. The ultimate goal of such a program is to maximize hand function to permit the return to activities of daily living as well as to permit the performance of work tasks. The injured worker is thus more quickly returned to productive employment.

Paradoxically, perhaps, the desired goal of functional sensation is achieved only through the persistent use of the sensory-impaired extremity. Although the therapist cannot control a patient's motivation or basic intelligence level, the therapy environment can be controlled so as to maximize the effectiveness of the sensory reeducation program.

Localization, tactile gnosis, and two-point discrimination are specific sensory skills that are first evaluated by the therapist. It is through these evaluations that the therapist defines a program of protective sensory education in the severely involved or insensate hand. Alternatively, a program of discriminative sensory re-education is appropriate for the extremity that lacks tactile gnosis but already possesses protective sensation.

As the name implies, protective sensation is made possible by those stimuli that provide feedback regarding potential danger to the individual (pain, heat, cold, sharpness, pressure). Given the lack of such stimuli, the patient must be made more aware of the need to provide constant surveillance to the injured part. Avoidance of noxious stimuli and constant visual checks become an important part of the retraining process. Tool modifications that provide less pressure per surface area of skin are examples of the adaptive maneuvers that can be equally effective in reducing the stress to a localized insensate area.

Discrimination sensory re-education is possible in the patient who possesses protective sensation and at least touch perception to the fingertips — a vital key to the localization component of sensory re-education. Initiating such a program too early may lead to frustration and failure. *Localization training*[12] is begun with moving touch using a wide pressure application, such as a pencil eraser. The stimulus progresses from moving to constant pressure applied with smaller and lighter stimuli. By excluding visual stimuli, the patient is forced to concentrate solely on the tactile perception. If incorrect, the patient is allowed to watch as the stimulus is reapplied, thus reinforcing visual and tactile perceptions. With repetition of this process, localization learning is gradually enhanced. The second and more advanced component of sensory re-education in the hand is *discrimination training*. This facet stresses the ability to discern differ-

ences between objects based on texture, shape, hardness, and general dimensions.

The goals of such a program are directed toward functional use of the hand. Not unexpectedly, the functional gains achieved can be lost over time if the hand is not used. Stressing the importance of continuing the home program learned during the formal re-education therapy process reinforces the success of the program and maintains the gains over a longer period of time.

DESENSITIZATION

Hypersensitivity is a condition of extreme irritability to touch and should not be confused with sensory re-education for insufficient sensory input (discussed previously). A hypersensitive state may exist when there is quick retraction after stimulation by external contact, as for example, in a painful amputation site with an associated superficial neuroma. An extremity containing such a sensitive area poses a formidable challenge to the therapist and patient alike. The bond of trust and reassurance created between the therapist and patient is crucial to the success of coaxing a patient to stimulate the very area that is understandably being consciously protected. It is only through the use and stimulation of the hypersensitive area that the noxious stimuli can become more tolerable.[13] This is a learned response, and patient education must become an integral part of the therapeutic process if functional use of the extremity is to be achieved.

The basic element of treatment of a hypersensitive area is the concept of progressive contact of the involved part with increasingly irritating stimuli. Various textures (felt, Velcro, burlap) and small particles (rice, popcorn, macaroni) are gradually introduced into contact with the injured area. Quite interestingly, what constitutes an irritant varies in severity from one patient to another. Given the theoretical scenario of two patients with an identical hypersensitivity problem, individual responses may vary greatly for a given noxious stimulus. For this reason, standardized treatment programs are probably less effective than individualized programs based on initial patient responses to various applied stimuli.

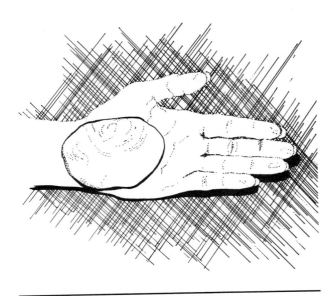

Fig. 50-8. Silicone elastomer pad used to provide constant extreme pressure to flatten an actively maturing scar.

Another effective means of applying a progressive irritating stimulus to a hypersensitive area is through use of an electric vibrator. A vibratory impulse is brought into contact with the uninvolved area surrounding the injured part and gradually approaches the sensitive area. By increasing the frequency of the vibrations and the duration of application, a graded noxious stimulus can be applied. The application should first be intermittent and later be modified to be constant as patient tolerance increases. Alternatively, a given stimulus can be gradually increased by applications that spatially approach direct contact with the maximally sensitive area.

Less intense but equally as deserving of attention is the sensitive incision site. A recently made carpal tunnel incision provides a widely seen example of this problem. Although this is not thought of as possessing quite the sensitivity of a superficial neuroma, it is nevertheless quite irritable and amenable to treatment with desensitization techniques. Massaging the scar with a light lubricant (cocoa butter, aloe vera, vitamin E) is an effective means of softening the scar and initiating patient contact with the sensitive area. Subsequently, various textures can be rubbed over this scar as tolerance increases. Another effective means of softening such a scar is through the use of a silicone elastomer pad (Fig. 50-8), which is

molded over the incision and secured with an elastic wrap. This effectively provides a constant external pressure that flattens the new actively maturing scar, helping to realign the collagen fibers. While it is worn, the elastomer has the added benefit of protecting the injured area from additional injury. Care should be taken to avoid prolonged use, however, because maceration of soft tissues could result.

PAIN CONTROL

Uncontrolled pain can be both physically and emotionally debilitating. Pain can severely limit function, and the patient's complaint of pain must be respected and every attempt made to relieve it must be initiated early.

Transcutaneous electrical nerve stimulation (TENS) is a useful method in minimizing both acute and chronic pain.[14] The gate control theory postulates that peripheral afferent impulses facilitate or inhibit the gateway to the brain; however, the exact mechanism is still not completely understood. Iontophoresis is a noninvasive method of administering medication for pain relief into superficial layers of intact skin. It is based on the principle of ion transfer.

Heat application is especially beneficial when used prior to exercise. Heat may be applied in various forms, including moist hot packs, fluidotherapy, whirlpool, paraffin, or ultrasound. Improper use of heat will increase edema and of course is contraindicated for an insensate extremity or when there is insufficient vascular supply. Ice packs constrict veins and decrease edema temporarily, thus increasing pain thresholds. Contraindications are the same as for heat.

PAIN DYSFUNCTION—REFLEX SYMPATHETIC DYSTROPHY

The superficial position of the sensory nerves and the high concentration of nerve endings make the hand unusually vulnerable to pain. While the majority of patients will react to a painful stimulus in an appropriate manner, a small percentage will develop a pain dysfunction. This pain, which is out of proportion to the injury, is associated with vasomotor instability, muscle atrophy, joint stiffness, osteoporosis, and disturbance in sweat production. Crush injuries, gunshot wounds, and burns frequently are associated with pain dysfunction, although relatively minor procedures such as a carpal tunnel release or distal radial fracture can trigger this potentially devastating complication.

Lankford and Thompson have divided the syndrome of reflex sympathetic dystrophy into various subgroupings.[15] Of these, the types most often necessitating rehabilitation of the hand are (1) shoulder-hand syndrome, which usually starts in the shoulder, and is seen with myocardial infarctions and strokes; and (2) minor and major traumatic dystrophy, which are associated with minor and major crush injuries to the hand and fingers or to the entire extremity, respectively. Reflex sympathetic dystrophy is discussed more fully in Chapter 47.

The therapist's role in reflex sympathetic dystrophy involves the basic techniques of desensitization, edema control, gentle range-of-motion exercises, and splinting. More recently, a promising concept of "stress loading" has been instituted, which provides stressful stimuli to the extremity without necessitating joint motion.[16]

RANGE OF MOTION

Early motion is essential in re-establishing tendon gliding and joint mobility if normal hand function is to return. The effects of immobilization on connective tissues can severely affect the final outcome of therapy. The timing of the initiation of range-of-motion exercises after hand injury and surgery varies depending on sufficient soft tissue healing and adequate skeletal fixation. Immediate attention should be given to proximal uninvolved joints to restore preoperative mobility and prevent secondary complications.

Active range of motion facilitates the gliding of tendons between soft tissues. It increases tensile strength of repaired structures. Active motion effectively decreases edema by displacing excessive interstitial fluid, improves circulation, and aids in preserving anatomic structures. Joint motion is maintained and increased and muscles gain in strength. Active motion promotes articular cartilage nourishment and healing.

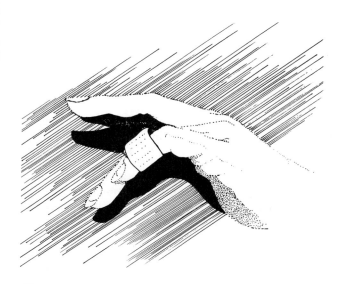

Fig. 50-9. A buddy strap is used to protect an injured finger by securing it to an adjacent uninjured finger.

Passive range of motion maintains and increases joint mobility and prevents adhesions.[17] It assists in preventing and reducing contractures. In this regard, digital buddy strapping (Fig. 50-9) is often used to maintain mobility and to protect injured collateral ligaments. Passive stretching of excessively tight tissues assists in regaining normal anatomic position. Forceful manipulation is contraindicated because soft tissues may tear, resulting in increased scarring and stiffness. Passive range of motion should be performed slowly and smoothly. The stretch should be prolonged, with a low amount of stress. Joints should first be gently distracted to avoid compression of the structures being moved. Passive motion should be followed by active motion when possible to maintain mobility gains. Specific exercises and modalities are outlined as follows.

1. *Tendon gliding exercises* promote maximal excursion and differential gliding of both flexor digitorum superficialis (FDS) and profundus (FDP) tendons in relation to each other and to flexor sheath and bone. This set of exercises includes the "fist" (MCP and IP flexion), the "straight fist" (MCP and PIP flexion with DIP extension) and the "hook" (MCP extension with IP flexion) positions. The FDP attains maximal gliding with the fist position and the FDS with the straight fist. The hook position promotes maximal glide between both flexor tendons.
2. *Blocking exercises* allow isolated gliding of FDS and FDP

tendons. Blocking of the FDS is performed by maintaining all other fingers in extension. Blocking of the FDP is performed by stabilizing flexed digital joints in extension. Tendon excursion is limited in this type of exercise.

3. In *passive place and hold exercises,* the therapist flexes the fingers into the palm and the patient holds this position isometrically for 10 seconds. The therapist then holds the fingers in extension, gradually decreasing support as the patient holds the position.

4. In *putty stretches,* the patient presses flexed MCP joints into putty with the wrist at neutral. PIP joints are flexed into the putty with the wrist and MCP joints in neutral. The DIP joints are next flexed into the putty with the wrist and MCP joints at neutral and PIP joints flexed. For extension stretches, the patient drags the extended fingers over putty toward the body. Each exercise is repeated 10 times.

5. *Dynamic splinting* provides controlled passive range of motion when therapeutic exercise alone is not sufficient.

6. *Continuous passive motion* (CPM) may decrease adhesion formation and joint stiffness. It stimulates the repair and regeneration of articular tissues (cartilage, tendon, ligaments).[18] CPM has been found to increase cartilage nutrition and to clear enzymes and exudate from infected joints. It may enhance synovial fluid circulation. A decrease in pain has been reported with its use. The true effects of CPM are not yet known, and it has not been proved that greater range is achieved. CPM is useful as an adjunct to therapy.

7. *Functional electrical stimulation* is an external excitation that artificially produces a contraction of innervated muscle. It may be used for muscle re-education, to prevent atrophy, to increase range of motion and strength and to decrease edema, muscle spasms, and spasticity.

8. *Biofeedback* is used to isolate and coordinate specific muscle groups. It assists the patient in relaxing antagonistic muscles. It provides both auditory and visual feedback of muscle contractions. Biofeedback has been shown to be beneficial in prosthetic training.

9. *Moist heat* is an effective method used prior to exercise to alter viscoelastic properties and improve results of range of motion. Other beneficial forms of heat used prior to exercise are fluidotherapy and paraffin with a prolonged passive stretch. Heat is contraindicated when sensation or vascularity is impaired.

STRENGTH AND ENDURANCE

Maintaining and increasing muscle strength are vital for return of function after hand injury. They should not be initiated until adequate healing has taken place and sufficient joint mobility has been obtained.

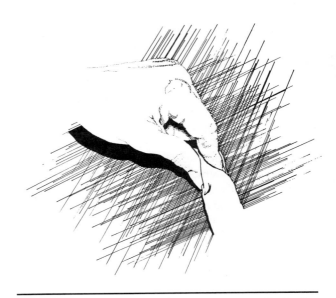

Fig. 50-10. Therapy putty—a moldable silicone rubber compound used to increase strength and range of motion in the hand.

Maximum contraction of weak muscles is necessary to increase strength. Isometric, isotonic, and isokinetic exercises are three methods of strengthening muscles. Isometrics produce static muscle contraction around a joint by working against an immovable object or by use of a sustained grip. Isotonics involve active contraction with range of motion. Isokinetics involve use of the force exerted by a patient governed by the speed of a machine in which force is exerted by the patient, but speed is controlled by equipment.

Increased endurance is gained through the use of moderately resistive graded activity that requires a steadily greater number of repetitions. A progressive resistive exercise program promotes the return of strength and endurance. Pain and swelling should not increase. Strengthening techniques include the use of therapy putty (Fig. 50-10), the hand gripper (Fig. 50-11), theraband, weights, and light crafts.

BTE WORK SIMULATOR

The BTE (Baltimore Therapeutic Equipment Company) Work Simulator[19] is a commercially available device designed to permit the assessment and rehabilitation of patients' upper extremity disorders. A

Fig. 50-11. The Hand Helper Exercise Aide allows graded gripping exercises through the use of a variable number of rubber bands.

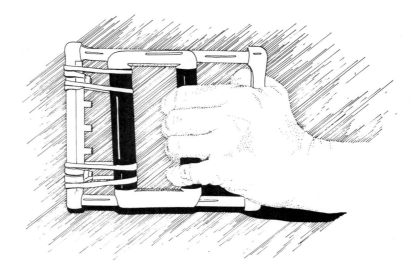

multitude of job tasks and activities of daily living can be simulated with this compact device, thus permitting the development of comprehensive programs to address particular functional deficits in patients. The main component of this device is the axial head and shaft, whose resistance to rotation and amount of distance achieved can be measured and plotted with respect to time by the attached computer console. Through manipulation of the various attachments and control of the force distance and time, a specifically designed rehabilitation program can be created by the hand therapist. Strength and endurance training are possible and adaptable to a patient's varying rate of progress and changing needs over time.

Now available is the Quest, a BTE software program that automatically calculates objective bilateral comparisons of maximum strength, power, and endurance, including coefficient of variations. Grafts and standardized reports are produced. The readily available feedback is important to both the patient and therapist and has led to much of the success of this novel therapeutic and evaluation tool.

WORK THERAPY/HARDENING/ TOLERANCE

Several terms have been applied to the challenge of returning the injured worker to previous employment after injury to the upper extremity. *Work ther-apy, work hardening,* and *work tolerance* are terms that apply to a structured program that must be formulated individually by the occupational therapist. Variables that are modified according to the patient's work demands and injury status include the amount of weight or resistance applied, the type of muscle contraction, and the general goals for each of the five levels of the therapy process.[20] These are summarized in Table 50-1.

Knowledge of the patient's injury, status of the healing process, and previous occupational tasks are prerequisites to determining at what level a particular patient enters the work hardening program. In many instances, levels 1 and 2 have been initiated in a previous therapy setting in the recent postinjury phase. Often the patient can enter the formal work hardening program at the second, third, or fourth level. Clearly, the designations of *work hardening* and *early occupational therapy* often overlap in the early phases.

The challenge to the occupational therapist is to formulate a plan that avoids further injury, encourages tolerance for increasing hand usage, and facilitates the ability to perform functional work tasks. Because of the number of variables involved, this complex task presents a formidable challenge to the therapist and patient alike. As in other therapy modalities,

Table 50-1. Levels of Work Hardening Therapy

Level	Resistance	General Goals	Example Activities	Contraction
1	0–1 lb	Obtain early motion Facilitate coordination and prehension	Dowel or block manipulation	Light prehension
2	1–3 lb	Strengthening initiated	Leatherwork, ceramics, wax sculpture	Isometric (no change in muscle length)
3	3–30 lb	Promote near-maximal contraction of weak muscles	Wood working—sanding, sawing	Isotonic (change in length without changing tension)
4	30–60 lb	Superior physical endurance	Simulation of work tasks	Isokinetic (change in length and tension)
5	60–150 lb	Maximum strength and endurance	Extreme heavy lifting	Isokinetic (change in length and tension)

communication and patient education are of paramount importance to the overall success of the program.

When the patient attains increasing strength and endurance, a home program can be incorporated into the overall plan, thus permitting maximal rehabilitation to occur outside the formal therapy environment. Weekly evaluations to assess performance are important to monitor progress and to alter the therapy program as needed. The BTE work simulator has proved very effective as an aid in increasing the actual strengthening and endurance of the extremity, during formal therapy sessions, and in evaluating and recording the patient's progress during various phases of a home-based program.

HAND REHABILITATION CENTER

The infrastructure of a "hand rehabilitation center" can vary greatly depending on geographic location, population density, and a myriad of other complex variables. The center can be complex, as in the traditional large hospital-based unit encompassing a team of physical and occupational therapists working in conjunction with industrial rehabilitation specialists.[21] Alternately, it can be as simple as a single (physician-employed) office-based therapist. Intermediate to these two extremes is the free-standing independent therapy corporation.

The key element linking these types of centers is the highly individualized and sophisticated care offered to the hand-injured patient, which is made possible by the carefully coordinated effort by the physician, the therapist, and the patient. The benefits of the one-on-one interaction that occurs between therapist and patient go well beyond the formal rehabilitation plan. For example, the therapist in such a center is in an ideal position to assess the psychological and personal impact of a hand injury in a particular patient. Ease of communication and a feeling of closeness are facilitated by the on-site therapy of the office-based therapist. However, some of the more specialized tasks, such as formal work hardening programs, may be more suited to the hospital-based rehabilitation center or the free-standing therapy corporation specializing in this service. Today, legislators are embarking on legislation to limit any perceived abuses due to potential conflict of interest between physicians and therapists, particularly with regard to the physician-owned practice.[22] It remains incumbent on hand rehabilitation centers to continue to stress the quality of their multiple services and to demonstrate fiscal responsibility to the satisfaction of legislators and insurers alike.

Acknowledgment. This chapter was illustrated by D. Cooper Katz.

REFERENCES

1. Steinbrocker O: The shoulder-hand syndrome: associated painful homolateral disability of the shoulder and hand with swelling and atrophy of the hand. Am J Med 3:402, 1947
2. Lister GD, Kleinert GE, Kutz JE: Primary flexor tendon repair followed by immediate controlled mobilization. J Hand Surg 2:441, 1977

3. Strickland JW: Biologic rationale, clinical application, and results of early motion following flexor tendon repair. J Hand Ther 2:71, 1989
4. Duran RH, Houser RG, Stover MG: Controlled passive motion following flexor tendon repair in zones 2 and 3. In: Proceedings of the American Academy of Orthopaedic Surgeons Symposium on Flexor Tendon Surgery in the Hand. CV Mosby, St. Louis, 1975
5. Evans RB: Therapeutic management of extensor tendon injuries. Hand Clin 2:166, 1986
6. Swanson B, Swanson G, Leonard J, Boozer J: Postoperative rehabilitation programs in flexible implant arthroplasty of the digits. p. 912. In Hunter JM, Schneider LH, Mackin EJ, Callahan AD (eds): Rehabilitation of the Hand. 3rd Ed. CV Mosby, St. Louis, 1990
7. Millender LH, Nalebuff EA: Early rheumatoid hand involvement. Orthop Clin North Am 6:697, 1975
8. McCash CR: The open palm technique in Dupuytren's contracture. Br J Plast Surg 17:271, 1964
9. Tubiana R, Defrenne H: Les localizations de la maladie de Dupuytren à la partie radiale de la main. Chirurgie 102:989, 1976
10. Salisbury RE, Reeves SU, Wright P: Acute care and rehabilitation of the burned hand. p. 831 In Hunter JM, Schneider LH, Mackin EJ, Callahan AD (eds): Rehabilitation of the Hand. 3rd Ed. CV Mosby, St. Louis, 1990
11. Sunderland S: Nerves and Nerve Injuries. 2nd Ed. Churchill-Livingstone, New York, 1978
12. Callahan AD: Methods of compensation and re-education for sensory dysfunction. p. 611. In Hunter JM, Schneider LH, Mackin EJ, Callahan AD (eds): Rehabilitation of the Hand. 3rd Ed. CV Mosby, St. Louis, 1990
13. Barber LM: Desensitization of the traumatized hand. p. 721. In Hunter JM, Schneider LH, Mackin EJ, Callahan AD (eds): Rehabilitation of the Hand. 3rd Ed. CV Mosby, St. Louis, 1990
14. Lee VH, Reynolds CC: Clinical application of the transcutaneous electrical nerve stimulator in patients with upper extremity pain. p. 538. In Hunter JM (ed): Rehabilitation of the Hand. 2nd Ed. CV Mosby, St. Louis, 1984
15. Lankford LL, Thompson JE: Reflex sympathetic dystrophy, upper and lower extremity: diagnosis and management. Instr Course Lect 26, 1977
16. Watson HK, Carlson LK: Treatment of sympathetic dystrophy with an active stress loading program. J Hand Surg 12:779, 1987
17. Frank C, Akeson WH, Woo SL et al: Physiology and therapeutic value of passive joint motion. Clin Orthop 185:113, 1984
18. Salter RB, Simmonds DF: The biological effect of continuous passive motion on the healing of full thickness defects in articular cartilage: an experimental investigation in the rabbit. J Bone Joint Surg [Am] 62:1232, 1980
19. Curtis RM, Engalitcheff J: A work simulator for rehabilitating the upper extremity—preliminary report. J Hand Surg 6:499, 1981
20. Ballard M, Baxter P, Bruening L, Fried S: Work therapy and return to work. Hand Clin 2:247, 1987
21. Schlegel R, Clark G: Hand rehabilitation unit in a hospital setting. p. 1230. In Hunter JM, Schneider LH, Mackin EJ, Callahan AD (eds): Rehabilitation of the Hand. 3rd Ed. CV Mosby, St. Louis, 1990
22. Stark P: Ethics in Patient Referral Act. "Congressman Stark Amendments," Omnibus Budget Reconciliation Act of 1989.
23. Wehké MA, Hunter JM: Flexor tendon gliding in the hand, Part II differential gliding. J Hand Surg 10A:575, 1985.

51 Rehabilitation of the Wrist

WILLIAM P. COONEY III
ANN H. SCHUTT

Injuries of the wrist are among the most common of those involving the upper extremity. The majority occur as a result of a fall onto the hand or from a direct blow.[1] Fractures of the radius more commonly occur in elderly persons,[2] whereas scaphoid fractures or fracture-dislocations are seen in younger persons.[3] Pure ligament injuries, such as dislocations of wrist bones, are less common.

The rehabilitation of wrist injuries must be delayed for a required period of time to allow for fracture and ligament healing, usually in a cast or splint. When surgical treatment is performed, the rehabilitation process may be longer because the integrity of additional soft tissues must be violated to gain surgical exposure for definitive joint injury or fracture treatment. Occasionally surgery to fix fractures rigidly can speed up the recovery period, allowing earlier motion and strengthening.[4]

In this chapter, the basic pathophysiology of fractures, ligament injuries, and inflammatory diseases that affect the wrist are reviewed, and the preferred rehabilitation programs to regain maximum function are discussed. Distal radius fractures, scaphoid fractures, wrist sprains (scapholunate ligament dissociation), and wrist dislocations or fracture-dislocations are reviewed. The overall approach to rehabilitation after surgery for rheumatoid arthritis is presented.

REHABILITATION AFTER FRACTURES OF THE RADIUS

Fractures of the distal radius can be classified as (1) simple extra-articular, nondisplaced fractures (Colles' type fractures); (2) intra-articular, moderately displaced fractures (Frykman type fractures); or (3) complex comminuted, displaced fractures (burst fractures).[2] They often include injury to the distal radioulnar joint (Table 51-1). For the undisplaced or minimally displaced distal radius fracture, the usual treatment is closed reduction and either long-arm or short-arm cast immobilization. If the distal radioulnar joint is significantly injured, a long-arm cast to control forearm pronation-supination is preferred. The period of treatment for most distal radius fractures is 6 to 7 weeks of cast immobilization followed by 2 to 4 weeks of supportive static splinting (Fig. 51-1). The splint is removed intermittently for mobilization of the joints and strengthening of muscles. As with other fractures involving the wrist, often the patient has associated soft tissue injury with hematoma formation and swelling involving the distal forearm and dorsal aspect of the hand. The amount of initial fracture displacement and the amount of energy involved in producing the original injury determine the extent of soft tissue involvement.[5] If a delay has occurred in initial treatment or if cast immobilization is improperly applied in a constricting or forced position,[6] further soft tissue damage, persistent swelling, and increased soft tissue compartment pressures may result. An improperly applied plaster cast, which extends beyond the metacarpophalangeal joint blocking finger flexion (Fig. 51-2) or which crosses on the dorsal surface of the hand proximal to the metacarpophalangeal joint, will often produce a constricting effect on the fingers and result in considerable swelling within the fingers and soft tissue edema in the hand.

For most undisplaced or minimally displaced fractures, the patient is placed in a supportive splint as early as 3 to 4 weeks after injury and most certainly

Table 51-1. Classification of Distal Radius Fractures

Type	Treatment
Extra-articular	
Undisplaced	Closed reduction Cast
Displaced	
Stable	Closed reduction Cast
Unstable	Closed reduction Percutaneous pins External fixation
Intra-articular	
Undisplaced	Closed reduction Cast
Displaced (reducible)	Closed reduction Percutaneous pins Rush rods External fixation
Displaced (unreducible)	Open reduction—limited External fixation Internal fixation
Complex	Open reduction—bone graft External fixation Internal fixation

by 6 weeks after injury (Fig. 51-1). Hand physical and occupational therapy is prescribed with the goal of developing active assisted range of motion and strengthening exercises for the wrist and forearm.[7] Efforts should be made while the patient's hand is in the cast to encourage active bending of the fingers (flexion-extension) and to perform "six-pack" hand exercises (full range of motion of the digits) (Fig. 51-3). When possible, elbow flexion-extension, forearm pronation and supination motions, and especially shoulder flexion, abduction, and external rotation exercises are encouraged. As it does in other fractures of the upper extremity, the shoulder can serve as a venous pump that helps prevent accumulation of traumatic edema fluid within the hand and distal forearm. Moberg has emphasized the importance of shoulder motion in preventing postinjury and dependent edema.[8] Shoulder motion combined with elevation of the hand and wrist above the heart can prevent unwanted limb swelling.

On the basis of this concept, active shoulder motion is started the day after the distal radius fracture, and the patient is asked to perform shoulder range-of-motion exercises with three to five repetitions every hour for

5 minutes. Antiedema measures of extremity elevation, digital decongestant massage, and digital elastic supports are similarly recommended. After the distal radial fracture has healed, an aggressive exercise therapy program is almost always required. Approximately 70 percent of patients need some assistive therapy. Some patients need even greater assistance and professional therapy for as long as 3 to 4 months after fracture of the distal radius. The average recovery period after a distal radius fracture is nearly 6 months, and grip strength only becomes maximal at 9 months.[9]

With more displaced distal radius fractures, different treatment options may be chosen, including external fixation with pins placed through the metacarpals of the hand and through the distal one-third of the radius.[9] After this type of treatment, early referral for hand physical or occupational therapy is indicated to prevent binding of the finger extensor tendons, for assisted finger range of motion exercises, and for antiedema measures (Fig. 51-4).[10] If there has not been an injury to the distal radioulnar joint, forearm pronation-supination can be started. The "six-pack" (range of motion) hand exercises are prescribed for these patients, and elbow and shoulder motion are encouraged.

External fixation is generally maintained for a period of 8 weeks after treatment of distal radius fractures, with a minimum of 6 and a maximum of 10 weeks. After removal of the external fixation, joint capsular stiffness of the wrist is usual. In general, patients need about 9 months to regain maximum wrist motion. The patients' wrist should be in a supportive static splint[11,12] immediately after removal of external fixation, and a program of wrist and hand range-of-motion exercises, hand strengthening, friction massage at the pin sites, and decongestant massage is prescribed. Occasionally the use of a compression pump, such as the elastic Jobst pump, or supportive wrapping, such as Coban or Tubigrip of the digits of the hand and wrist, is needed to control posttraumatic swelling. Most patients require a hand gripper, soft sponge, or therapeutic putty for strengthening (Fig. 51-5). At least once weekly, professional therapy is needed to review, update, and remind the patient of the need for assisted and active motion, grip strengthening, and functional activities.

Fig. 51-1. Splinting for distal radius fractures. **(A)** Combined dorsal and volar shell coaptation splint. This type is useful for early mobilization of minimally displaced stable fractures while maintaining rigid immobilization. **(B)** Volar wrist support splint: an all-purpose splint for use after removal of either cast or external fixation. A volar "keel" increases rigidity for manual labor. **(C)** Dorsal-based splint. This type is useful for light labor or for a white-collar worker who needs protective stability but freedom for full thumb and finger motion.

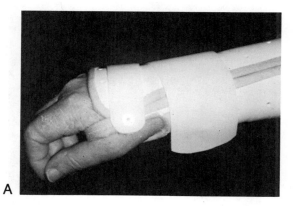

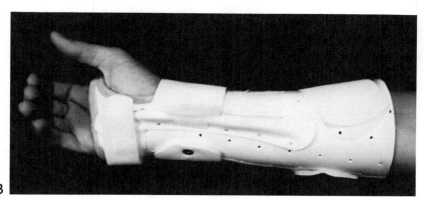

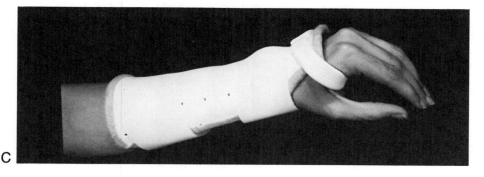

For the more comminuted intra-articular fractures of the distal radius, treatment has recently included open reduction with combinations of internal and external pin fixation.[13,14] Because these fractures result from high-energy injuries and can be accompanied by extensor tendon damage, carpal tunnel syndrome, and intracapsular wrist ligament injuries, rehabilitation is longer and more intensive than for most other distal radius fractures. Some surgeons have recommended early bone grafting of these injuries in combination with internal plate or external pin fixation in an effort to speed fracture healing.[15] With such techniques, it may be possible to remove the external fixator at 3 to 4 weeks and initiate early active range of motion of the wrist. After these types of injuries, it has occasionally been necessary to include dynamic wrist flexion-extension splints (Fig. 51-6) in the rehabilitation program to facilitate improved wrist motion.[12,16,17] These splints may be started as early as 10 weeks after the original fracture. In young

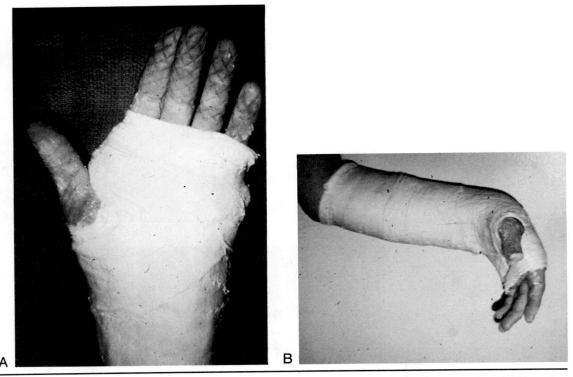

Fig. 51-2. Improper cast applications. **(A)** Cast extends across the palm, blocking finger motion. **(B)** Excessive wrist flexion constricting venous return.

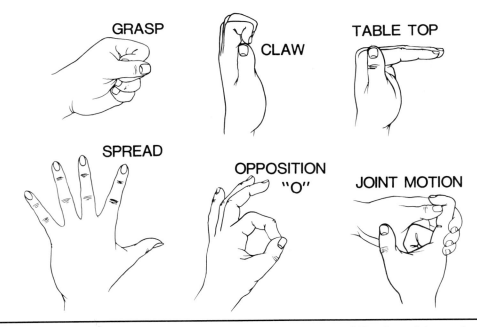

GRASP

CLAW

TABLE TOP

SPREAD

OPPOSITION "O"

JOINT MOTION

Fig. 51-3. "Six-pack" hand exercises are an effective exercise program to mobilize finger joints and soft tissues. (Courtesy of J. H. Dobyns, M.D., Emeritus Staff, Mayo Clinic.)

Fig. 51-4. Low-profile external fixation frame (Ace-Colles). Early finger range of motion permits continued light active functional use of the hand.

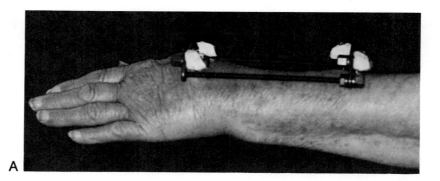

A

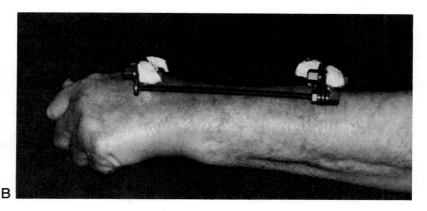

B

adults with such injuries, the Baltimore Therapeutic Exercise machine (BTE)[18] (Fig. 51-7) has been a valuable tool in encouraging rehabilitative exercises and for following the progress of rehabilitation strengthening. These types of devices and work capacity evaluations have been helpful in determining when a working adult may return to previous employment or should seek new types of employment. Because wrist motion and strength may not return to normal after distal radius fractures, reassessment of the work environment and the patient's ability to return to the previous form of work is important.

Injuries to the Distal Radioulnar Joint

When distal radius fractures are associated with injury to the distal radioulnar joint, support cast or splint immobilization of the elbow is required.[2] The forearm should be placed in a neutral rotation position halfway between pronation and supination to maximize joint articular cartilage contact. At 3 weeks after injury, the immobilization can be changed to a below-elbow forearm splint or cast to allow gentle assisted forearm pronation and supination exercises. The amount of rotation should be controlled primarily by the patient with a gradual increase in proportion to symptoms. A nearly full return of forearm rotation can be expected. In certain patients, particularly those referred late or those who have not had early range-of-motion exercises, loss of forearm rotation may be significant. We have found that, in this group, dynamic forearm rotation splints[12,19] (Fig. 51-8) stressing either pronation or supination can be designed to provide improved forearm rotation. These types of dynamic splints are preferable to isolated passive stretching because they provide a gradual prolonged stretch over time and tend to avoid problems of sudden excessive stretch, pain dystrophy and the difficult rehabilitation often associated with muscle co-contraction, guarding, overprotection, and spasm.[20]

Pain Dysfunction Syndromes

We have found after fractures of the distal radius and distal radioulnar that joint rehabilitation may be necessary for up to 3 months. An occasional patient has

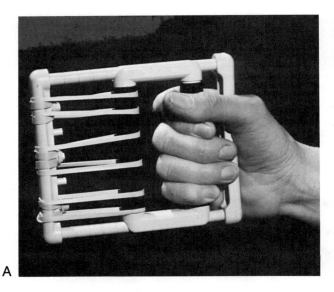

A

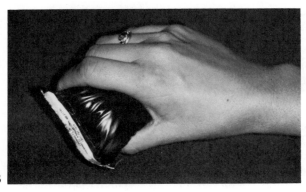

B

Fig. 51-5. Hand gripping modalities to improve strength. **(A)** Rubber band tension hand gripper. **(B)** Mississippi Mud Gripper. **(C)** Dyna gripper.

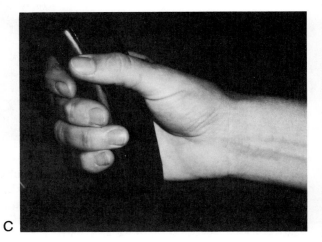

C

been seen who has required as much as 6 months of professional therapy. The most significant challenge to the therapist is the patient with a fracture of the distal radius who has endured a painful postfracture rehabilitation treatment program with extended use of narcotic analgesics.[6] These patients often have the most severe presentation of pain dystrophy that rehabilitation specialists see in their practice (Fig. 51-9). If the patient has an abnormal pain response with use, burning, dysesthetic pain at rest, and painful guarding of normal motions, physicians and therapists should be alerted to an impending problem of upper limb pain dysfunction syndrome (upper limb reflex dystrophy).[21,22] Pain dysfunction can occur with simple, undisplaced fractures as well as with more comminuted fractures.[6] When the patient's complaint of fracture pain is ignored, when the pain-

ful limb is suppressed by narcotics, or when the rehabilitation program is excessive or inappropriate, pain dystrophy will result that will defer limb rehabilitation long after the fracture is healed. Routine prescriptions of narcotic pain medication—including codeine—for any longer than 48 hours after the original fracture has occurred—are not recommended. Patients need instructions regarding elevation, relaxed active range-of-motion exercises, and caution against muscle co-contraction and guarding; when these are provided, pain syndromes are usually prevented.

Pain dystrophy occurring after distal radius fractures can be associated with local signs and symptoms related to flexor or extensor tendinitis, median neuritis (carpal tunnel syndrome), cutaneous neuritis, or

Fig. 51-6. Dynamic wrist flexion-extension splints. The hinge is located in line with the center of rotation in the head of the capitate. **(A)** Wrist extension splint with optional degrees of rubber band dynamic traction. **(B)** Wrist flexion splint. Flexible rubber tubing allows for adjustable tension. **(C)** Wrist flexion splint. The moment arm of the rubber band traction can be modified by location of the attachment keel to the distal, hand-based component.

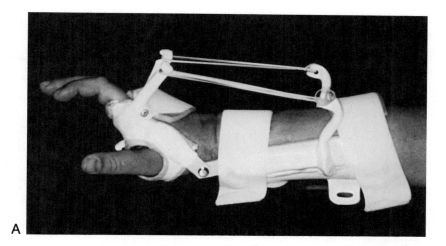

A

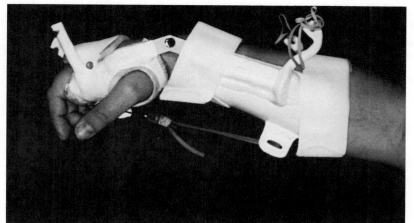

B

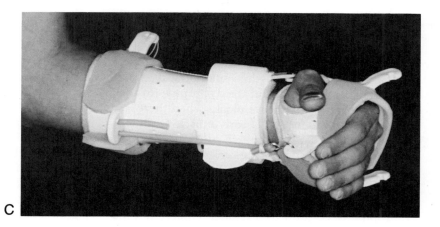

C

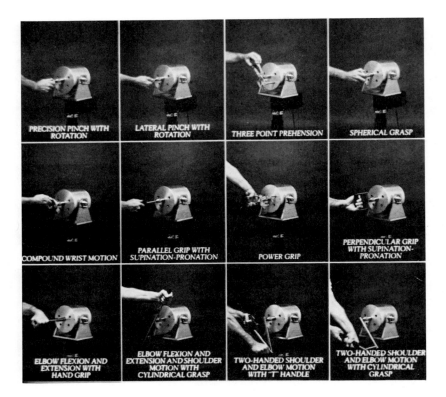

Fig. 51-7. Baltimore Therapeutic Exercise (BTE) machine. This device allows dynamic exercises for compound wrist motion, parallel grip with pronation-supination, power grip, and different types of prehensile grasp combined with wrist motion for both strengthening and work hardening. (From Pendergraft et al,[18] with permission.)

posttraumatic vascular hyperactivity.[23,24] Occasionally, pain dystrophy can be generalized, affecting the entire upper extremity.[21] When the hand and shoulder are involved primarily, the condition is called the "shoulder-hand syndrome."[8] The treatment program for these difficult cases consists of the following components: (1) rest with a supportive splint; (2) non-narcotic pain medication, (3) usually a nonsteroidal anti-inflammatory medication; (4) local trigger point injections with lidocaine and bupevacaine; (5) sympathetic nerve blocks when autonomic dysfunction is a major component of the dystrophy; (6) axillary or supraclavicular nerve blocks when there is a diffuse pain component; (7) early muscle re-education to prevent guarding, muscle co-contractions, or spasms; and (8) antiedema measures. Relaxed active range-of-motion exercises of the digits, elbow (when possible), and shoulder (when properly performed) must be carried out once the pain component of the dystrophy is controlled. Peripheral nerve blocks (performed with diluted concentrations of analgesics) can diminish sensory feedback and autonomic

input while preserving motor function. Some physicians have recommended reserpine or guanethedine blocks alone or reserpine in combination with prednisolone.[12] We have had little experience with these pharmaceutical agents and rely more on selective local nerve blocks or high stellate, intraclavicular, or axillary nerve blocks.

Once the elements of pain have been relieved by appropriate blocks and supportive splints, immediate hand physical and occupational therapy measures should be coordinated. Stress loading, controlled and repetitive, can be initiated. Patients must be persuaded that it is their responsibility to rehabilitate themselves by active and active-assisted exercise programs.[10] Passive motion alone is not adequate and often is contraindicated in cases of dystrophy. Appropriate applications of hot-cold contrast baths, fluidotherapy, ultrasonography with cortisone phonophoresis, and nondependent whirlpool can help the patient regain an active range of motion.[12,25]

Fig. 51-8. Dynamic forearm rotation splints. A distal ulnar gutter forearm splint with wrist support is combined with an above-elbow proximal support. Dynamic traction is provided by outriggers placed perpendicular to the longitudinal axis of the forearm. **(A)** Pronation splint with ulnarly placed outriggers joined by adjustable rubber tube traction. **(B)** Supination splint with radially placed outriggers joined with rubber band tube traction. The amount of force (torsional load) can be adjusted by either the length of the outrigger or tension on rubber tubing. (From Brand,[20] with permission.)

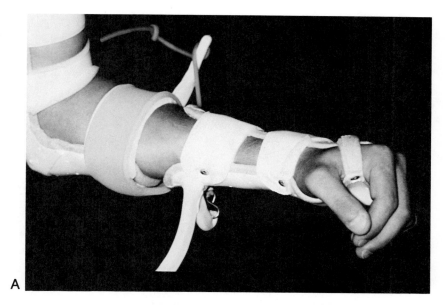

A

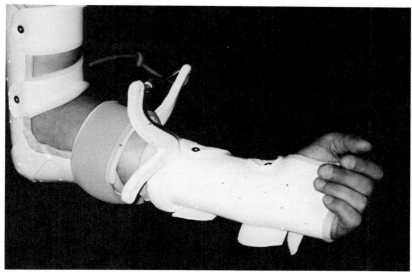

B

The methods used during this period must be *pain free*, and the common expression *"no pain, no gain" does not apply* in the rehabilitation of these conditions. A combination of treatment methods often is necessary. In addition to the local or systemic blocks mentioned earlier, we include oral anti-inflammatory medication, non-narcotic pain medication, and nerve tranquilizers. In severe cases, a short course of prenisolone (Medrol dose pack), which helps control swelling and counteracts tendon and joint adhesions,

can be helpful in getting the patient started on the rehabilitation program.

Surgical Treatment

Surgical treatment of upper limb dystrophies is contraindicated, because the additional insult of surgery can produce more pain, muscle guarding, and protective dysfunction than originally was present, thus limiting the efforts at hand and occupational or

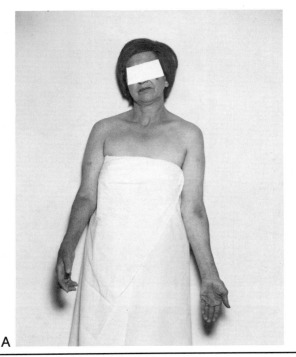 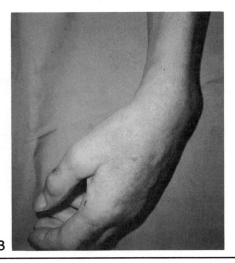

Fig. 51-9. Pain dysfunction occurring after Colles' fracture. **(A)** Right upper limb dysfunction with loss of forearm rotation; protective elbow muscle spasm, and dependent edema. **(B)** Hand-wrist deformity. This patient has malangulation of distal radius with dorsal edema, and arthrofibrosis of fingers with complete loss of finger motion. (From chapter 7, Fig. 18a,b. In Rockwood and Green's Fractures in Adults. 2nd ed. JB Lippincott, Philadelphia, 1984, with permission.)

physical therapy rehabilitation.[22] An acute median neuropathy is the single exception to this rule. In the patient with an acute median nerve compression occurring after a distal radius fracture, a carpal tunnel release may provide dramatic improvement in the patient's symptoms and facilitate the rehabilitation program. When other surgical indications are present (e.g., fracture nonunion or malunion), surgery is best avoided until pain can be relieved, some degree of normal function restored to the extremity, and the major components of dystrophy adequately reduced or eliminated.

Some cases of post-traumatic dystrophy are distinctly iatrogenic, having occurred as a result of unwise or unwarranted treatment by well-meaning physicians and therapists.[6] The effort to gain increasing range of wrist motion must be limited by the patient's response to pain and swelling. Clearly, slow, gradual improvements of motion are more easily tolerated and are more beneficial to the patient than aggressive

therapy, which often leads to neurogenic pain, protective guarding, and decreased active use of the extremity. Once present, these unfortunate effects seriously prohibit a good rehabilitation program and may lead to permanent limb impairment.

Cutaneous Neuralgia: A Special Problem Associated with Wrist Injuries

A special, localized type of upper limb dystrophy that can be particularly resistant to treatment after wrist fractures is cutaneous sensory nerve irritation or neuralgia.[21,24] The most common form is radial neuralgia.[23] Radial neuralgia (or neuritis) may be present alone or may be accompanied by lateral antebrachial cutaneous neuralgia. In this condition, the radial side of the wrist and forearm, in addition to the volar side of the wrist and thumb, are hypersensitive to touch. Often increased discomfort is present on motion of the wrist. This entity may be confused with deQuervain's tenosynovitis. The differential diagnosis is made by lightly stroking the dorsal aspect of the hand or thumb, which produces a dysesthetic sensation, or by noting hypersensitivity (Tinel's sign) with percussion over the radial nerve or lateral antebrachiocutaneous nerve. Occasionally the palmar cutaneous nerve can be involved. In most distal radius fractures, it is unusual for the ulnar cutaneous nerves to be symptomatic.

The treatment of localized nerve pain (neuralgia) usually consists of a series of local lidocaine or bupivacaine and cortisone nerve blocks performed on an every-other-day basis and combined with desensitization massage. A course of three to five nerve blocks spaced 48 to 72 hours apart is recommended. Employing transcutaneous electrical nerve stimulation (TENS) in between the nerve blocks can augment the effect of blocking dysesthetic nerve pain. After nerve blocks, physical and occupational therapy programs that stress active use of the hand and wrist are necessary. Static supportive splints should be used to protect the hypersensitive area. The splint should be applied carefully over the radial side of the wrist because local hypersensitivity can be aggravated by a tight or compressing splint. Velcro straps need to be placed away from the site of irritation. At home, the patient needs to assist in decreasing the area of sensitivity by running a stream of warm (definitely not hot) water over the affected area,[26,27] by ice massage, or by desensitization massage with the application of different textures of varying degrees of firmness. Fluidotherapy[28] can be helpful in certain patients. These methods provide a positive sensory stimulus to the central nervous system. Hand physical and occupational therapy must once again be done cautiously and carefully to avoid aggravating pain. The majority of patients will respond to this type of treatment program, although it may take up to 6 to 8 weeks before hypersensitivity is resolved.

Tendon Injuries Associated with Wrist Fractures

Flexor and extensor tendon injuries may occur directly as a result of wrist fracture-dislocations or fractures of the distal radius, or they may occur later, particularly after distal radius fractures.[5,6,29] In most circumstances, tendon repair is appropriate if it is recognized within the first 7 to 10 days after injury.

Extensor tendon injuries are commonly associated with distal radius fractures,[6] whereas flexor tendon injuries result from displaced scaphoid fractures or fracture-dislocations.[30] Tendon injuries are more common after undisplaced than displaced fractures and occur in closed compartments, such as the extensor retinaculum or carpal tunnel. Late presentation of flexor and extensor tendon injuries appears to result from a loss of blood supply and fraying of tendon over bone. Direct repair of tendon injuries generally is not possible when patients come to medical attention at a late stage. In cases in which tendon injuries occur after fractures of the wrist, it is important first to rehabilitate the hand and wrist before recommending any tendon reconstruction procedures. Maximum range of motion of the wrist and fingers must be achieved through hand and physical or occupational therapy, and all associated local or regional dystrophies must be treated and resolved before surgical treatment. Overly aggressive treatment of tendon injuries before the hand and wrist are fully rehabilitated compromises the end result and on occasion makes necessary further operative intervention in the form of either tenolysis or further tendon reconstructive procedures. Hand, physical and occupational therapists should be communicating with the hand surgeons to help determine the ideal time for tendon reconstructive procedures.

Malunion of Distal Radius Fractures

Undertreatment of fractures of the distal radius by incomplete fracture reduction, particularly in middle-aged or elderly patients, is an unfortunate occurrence.[6,31] Repeat reduction can be obtained up to 3 weeks after injury. When malalignment of a distal radius fracture is recognized later than this time, often both the patient and the surgeon desire immediate reconstructive surgery (e.g., corrective osteotomy) in an effort to place the wrist back in proper alignment. *This temptation should be resisted.* A minimum of 6 months, and preferably 9 to 12 months, should pass after the fracture had occurred before any reconstructive surgery is considered. Often the patient has considerable soft tissue injury as well as the potential for local dystrophy associated with distal radius fractures. These injured tissues (tendons, nerves, ligaments) must be given adequate rehabilitation and time to heal before a surgeon embarks on efforts to provide anatomic and radiographic improvement.

For some patients, the benign neglect of a malunited distal radius fracture may be the treatment of choice until sufficient time has passed during which trial of function can determine the amount of disability. In many patients, no further treatment will be required as they adjust to the wrist injury. In other patients, a Darrach resection of the distal ulna will be sufficient to restore forearm rotation, and the malalignment of the distal radius may be compatible with good wrist motion and strength.[32] However, in many patients, a corrective osteotomy of the distal radius with interposition of the iliac crest is required to restore radial length and correct the excessive dorsal tilt of the distal radius.[31] During the waiting period before surgery, the therapist should maximize finger and wrist range of motion and strengthen functional use of the hand. The patient can be instructed in performing activities of daily living and in how to use assistive devices. Surgical treatment should rarely be performed on the basis of the radiographic appearance of the wrist alone, and a careful assessment of the functional demands of each patient should be considered and weighed, bringing into play important factors such as age, occupation, and the home environment.

REHABILITATION OF NONTRAUMATIC ARTHRITIS OF THE WRIST

Patients with rheumatoid arthritis will commonly have involvement of the wrist as a major component in their disease. Rheumatoid deformities of the wrist characteristically involve radial deviation and ulnar subluxation. Collapse or zig-zag malalignment of the wrist potentiates the ulnar drift deformity of the finger metacarpophalangeal (MCP) joint and instability of the distal radioulnar joint. Rupture of extensor tendons also may occur. To prevent these progressive deformities, early static night and day splint immobilization of the rheumatoid patient is recommended to counteract the forces that produce collapse deformity of the wrist (Fig. 51-10B). Rheumatoid splints should be placed proximally on the forearm and extend down across the wrist to include the hand, using the principles of three-point pressure to help correct the deformity. Efforts should be made

to place the wrist in ulnar deviation and extension, with pressure applied on the ulnar side of the wrist to counteract the tendency of the carpus to slide ulnarly down the inclined plane of the distal radius.[12,33] With resting splints, we prefer to have the MCP joints placed in nearly full extension and radial deviation. The distal (DIP) and proximal (PIP) interphalangeal joints are placed in slight flexion. To counteract adduction deformities of the thumb, a position of interphalangeal (IP) and MCP extension and slight abduction and opposition is recommended. A daily static resting splint for the wrist (Fig. 51-11) is very beneficial in many rheumatoid arthritis patients, with the preferred position being 20° to 25° of wrist extension and slight ulnar deviation to counteract the tendency toward radial displacement of the carpus but also to place the wrist in maximum position for stronger grasp.

After reconstructive surgery of the wrist, rehabilitation is an important part of the patient's return to recovery. Synovectomy (and tenosynovectomy) of the wrist, either alone or in combination with tendon transfers, is still a valuable treatment option early in the course of the disease.[34,35] Through a dorsal incision, the extensor tendons are cleared of excessive tenosynovium and a dorsal T-shaped incision is performed to expose the midcarpal and radiocarpal joints. After completion of the synovectomy, the wrist capsule closure is performed and a portion of the extensor retinaculum is placed beneath the extensor tendons to protect them from later invasion of wrist synovial tissues. After such procedures, a static supportive wrist splint with dynamic extensor support is usually necessary for a period of 3 to 4 weeks and must be combined with active and active assisted finger range of motion in the splint to prevent development of adhesions of the extensor tendons.[35]

Occasionally synovectomy of the radiocarpal joint is performed simultaneously with synovectomy of the distal radioulnar joint. Additional soft tissue procedures may be needed to stabilize dorsal subluxation of the distal ulna and prevent damage to the ulnar extensor tendon. Finally, transfer of the extensor carpi radialis longus over to the extensor carpi ulnaris is performed in combination with synovectomy to provide a dynamic force bringing the wrist into ulnar deviation and extension. Tendon

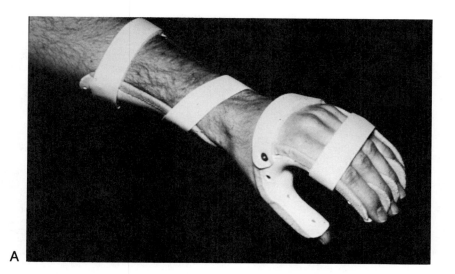

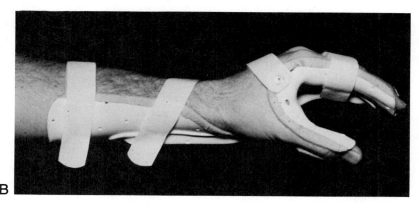

Fig. 51-10. Rheumatoid arthritis: static splinting. (A) Dorsal view. The splint is designed to immobilize the wrist in extension and ulnar deviation to correct the tendency for volar carpal subluxation, ulnar translation, and radial deviation. (B) Lateral view. The wrist in extension balanced by nearly full metacarpophalangeal extension (10°, 15° of flexion); the proximal interphalangeal joints are in slight flexion, and thumb is in abduction-extension. Instability patterns of the thumb may require variation in thumb position.

transfers require approximately 6 weeks to heal and, therefore, continuous static splint immobilization for a minimum period of 4 weeks with intermittent splinting for 8 to 12 weeks is necessary. Wrist range-of-motion exercises can be initiated gently at this time under the supervision of a therapist. The patient generally is weaned from the supportive splint over the next 3 to 6 weeks. Retraining of the tendon transfer occasionally is necessary under the guidance of the hand therapist.

Total Wrist Arthroplasty

In many patients with rheumatoid arthritis of the wrist, total wrist replacement may be necessary because of the extent of destructive disease and associated carpal instability.[36,37] Often wrist arthroplasty

is performed on the nondominant wrist, whereas arthrodesis is preferred on the dominant wrist. In those patients who have had a wrist arthroplasty, the rehabilitation program is similar whether the surgeon has chosen a Silastic wrist replacement or a total wrist replacement.[37] Because the soft tissue reconstruction involved in both of these procedures is extensive, a period of immobilization of 3 to 4 weeks is recommended, with the wrist in slight extension and ulnar deviation. From this position a more controlled rehabilitation can be initiated. In general, the goal of the surgeon and therapist is to achieve 35° to 40° of wrist extension, 25° to 30° of wrist flexion, and a total of 40° of combined radioulnar deviation. Studies from our laboratory[38] have demonstrated that 40° of wrist flexion and extension is satisfactory for most activities of daily living (meals and food preparation, per-

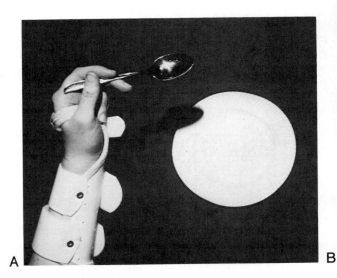

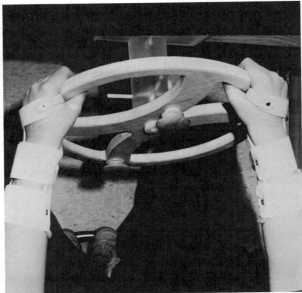

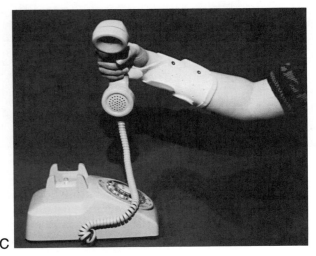

Fig. 51-11. Rheumatoid arthritis day resting splints. **(A)** Static wrist extension–ulnar deviation resting splint allows for activities of daily living while providing wrist support and stability. **(B)** Bilateral resting splints are quite functional in a position of wrist extension and ulnar deviation. **(C)** Wrist-neutral resting splints may be necessary on the dominant wrist to perform certain daily activities, such as typing, telephone reception, and personal hygiene. Splints can and should be adapted to the functional needs of the patient.

sonal hygiene, other work and functional activities) and that motion greater than this generally is unnecessary. A second reason for avoiding excessive wrist motion is because instability of the wrist and particularly of the wrist implant has been associated with the presence of a lax wrist and loose ligaments.[39] With total wrist arthroplasty, immediate movement of the wrist after surgery may lead to excessive joint laxity,[36] and a period of rest is preferred to improve soft tissue equilibrium and healing.

In the rheumatoid arthritis patient, once the rehabilitation program has been started, the goals of treatment are to keep the wrist in ulnar deviation and extension with a daytime supportive wrist splint and to maintain the wrist in a neutral position with a resting splint at night (Fig. 51-10). The resting night splint includes the fingers and thumb as well as the wrist. Gradual return of strength should occur over this time period, beginning initially with light gripping exercises and, after 3 months, progressing to the use of weights or elastic devices for isometric and isotonic strengthening exercises.

Total wrist arthroplasty and Silastic wrist arthroplasty can be accompanied by an unstable distal radioulnar joint.[35] Surgical options include excision of the distal ulna (Darrach procedure), fusion of the distal radioulnar joint with proximal pseudarthrosis (Kapandjii procedure), or partial resection of the distal ulna. After these procedures, hand physical or occupational therapy is indicated not only to regain limited wrist range of motion as described earlier but also to restore forearm pronation-supination. The goal is to regain approximately 60° of supination and 45° to 50° of pronation. In the rheumatoid arthritis patient, more motion may occasionally be desired if the shoulder cannot compensate with abduction and external rotation. In general, rehabilitation of the wrist and forearm is carried out in the same time frame whether the operation involves total wrist arthroplasty, Silastic wrist arthroplasty, or treatment of the distal radioulnar joint.

Tendon transfers after treatment of the rheumatoid arthritis may be necessary to rebalance the wrist into a position of ulnar deviation and extension.[34,36] Occasionally, they are necessary after rupture of finger extensor tendons. When tendon transfers have been performed in the rheumatoid arthritis patient, the period of splint immobilization is longer than in post-traumatic conditions. Initial immobilization is for 6 weeks, followed by a gradual restoration of motion and dynamic supportive splinting for an additional period of 4 weeks. The total period of splint immobilization may extend to 10 weeks, with retraining of the tendon transfers in the dynamic splint starting at approximately 6 weeks. When total wrist surgery has been accompanied by tendon transfers or tendon grafts to replace ruptured finger extensor tendons, the period of rest is longer to avoid excessive stress on the tendon transfers. Rather than commencing motion at 4 weeks, generally it is necessary to immobilize the wrist for approximately 6 weeks.[37] Then, gradually, the therapist initiates range-of-motion exercises and retraining of the tendon transfers while continuing support of the wrist and digits in a night static resting splint.

After both tendon transfers and synovectomy of the wrist, a supportive resting splinting is recommended for a maximum period of 8 weeks at night and 3 to 4 months during daytime activities.

REHABILITATION AFTER FRACTURES OF THE SCAPHOID

Fractures of the scaphoid bone are the result of high-impact stress on the wrist.[3] Hyperextension injuries will fracture the scaphoid either alone or in association with ligament damage. Undisplaced fractures are treated in a thumb spica cast for 6 to 12 weeks. Tomograms may be necessary to show fracture healing and are required in any questionable cases. Displaced scaphoid fractures usually require open fracture fixation. The Herbert screw and AO screw are popular devices to achieve rigid fixation, and early motion at 2 to 3 weeks is advocated.[4] K-wire fixation is the more traditional treatment with fixation maintained for up to 8 to 10 weeks. Without internal fixation, immobilization may be required for up to 6 months, a time that will significantly affect wrist rehabilitation.

Rehabilitation after cast removal involves assisted wrist motion and thumb motion. Heat and ultrasonography with cortisone phonophoresis may be needed to soften contracted joint capsules. Gentle distraction-stretch exercises of the wrist also may be beneficial. A supportive static thumb spica splint (Fig. 51-12) is preferred once the cast or pins have been removed. Fracture union must be confirmed by tomograms of the wrist before aggressive stretching is initiated. Return to full strength and motion may take up to 6 months. As a result of the prolonged rehabilitation required after closed treatment of displaced fractures, we recommend early compression screw fixation with wrist motion to start within 3 weeks, while maintaining a protective splint until the fracture has healed.

REHABILITATION AFTER SCAPHOLUNATE DISSOCIATION

Ligament injuries of the wrist can be partial or complete and involve either the radial or the ulnar side of the wrist.[30,40] Scapholunate dissociation involves a

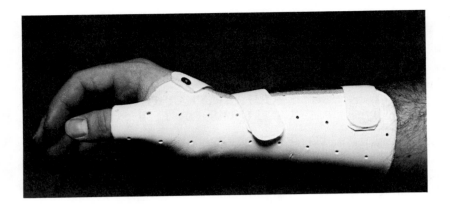

Fig. 51-12. Thumb spica splint is preferred for protection of scaphoid fractures during the period of rehabilitation. The wrist is placed in slight extension and radial deviation to "unload" the scaphoid.

tear of scapholunate interosseous ligaments that connect the very mobile scaphoid to the lunate.[41] When a ligament tear is *complete,* a direct repair is performed with injuries less than 6 months old. Fusion of the scaphoid to the distal row of carpal bones (STT or SC fusions) is required for established scapholunate instability.[40] If the ligament tear is partial (incomplete), direct repair usually is indicated for all injuries (acute and chronic).[41] With repair or fusion, immobilization for 8 to 12 weeks is necessary to allow for solid bone or ligament healing. Rehabilitation while in a cast support consists of finger and thumb exercises, active range-of-motion (six-pack) exercises, and light gripping (strengthening). No lifting of weights or firm gripping should be allowed.

Formal rehabilitation starts after the cast and pins are removed. Once again, a static supportive wrist splint to protect the healing tissues and to prevent injury to atrophic muscles from disuse is advised. Wrist motion usually is quite limited initially after ligament repair. With fusion, at least one-third of wrist motion will be lost. Careful return of motion can be achieved with gentle active assistive stretch, up to the point of mild discomfort but not enough to provoke swelling or pain that persists after the treatment program has concluded. Once motion is recovering, stengthening with hand gripper (Fig. 51-5) and resistant weights or elastics can be started. The BTE (Fig. 51-7) may be helpful to simulate work or avocational pursuits. Rarely is a dynamic splint for prolonged stretching considered.[20] Strength and functional use without pain is a more important goal than return of full motion. A minimum period of 4 months—commonly 6 months—is needed before patients who have had ligament repair are ready to return to work.

REHABILITATION OF FRACTURE-DISLOCATION OF THE WRIST

The most severe wrist injuries are fracture-dislocations of the wrist.[29,42] These injuries involve not only a fracture of a carpal bone but also significant ligament damage. Thus, they are at least twice as severe as a scaphoid fracture alone or isolated ligament injuries of the wrist. Although conservative cast treatment is advocated by some physicians, more surgeons now prefer open reduction, internal fixation of fractures, and primary ligament stabilization.[43] Occasionally, both a dorsal and a volar incision are required to repair the torn ligaments or to provide pin or screw fixation of carpal bone fractures.[44] The surgical procedure, therefore, adds to the considerable soft tissue injury that is already present.

After surgical treatment of fracture-dislocations of the wrist, cast or static splint immobilization may be necessary for as long as 3 to 4 months because of the nature of the original injury.[42] Considerable joint stiffness is always present after these injuries. The goals of rehabilitation are correspondingly limited considering the degree of original injury and the delay before therapy can be started. A good result in such injuries is reestablishing 50 percent of normal strength and 40 to 60 percent of normal motion—results are attained in only 72 percent of patients. Therefore, therapy initially will be mainly supportive and only later will be applied to maximize the end results with respect to motion and strength. Active assisted motion is begun as soon as fracture healing is confirmed and ligament repair is assessed. Forceful motion and passive stretching is contraindicated. Dynamic splints have not been helpful to date in these patients. Ultrasonography, ultrasonography with cortisone phonophoresis, heat, and other soft tissue adaptive therapies may prove beneficial.[45] Strengthening programs are helpful but often are prolonged. Full rehabilitation will not be evident before 1 year. Patients should be so warned and instructed not to expect either a rapid or a full recovery. Much of the rehabilitation must be done by the patients themselves, slowly and over time. The therapist needs to be supportive and ready to change to new modes of treatment once progress has plateaued. Occasionally intra-articular steroids can be helpful to relax restrictive adhesions or treat localized arthritis. Unfortunately, the prognosis for fracture-dislocations is not good, with over 35 percent of patients having post-traumatic arthritis and 40 percent going on to require further wrist surgery, such as partial or complete fusions. With the stimulus of more rigid primary fracture fixation and the potential benefit of continuous passive motion,[46] early physical therapy programs may be warranted considering the generally poor prognosis associated with many of these injuries.

BASIC PROCEDURES AND TECHNIQUES OF REHABILITATION OF THE WRIST

Goals

The primary goal of rehabilitation of the wrist is to maximize the residual functional capacity of a person with an injured, operated, or diseased wrist, hand, and/or upper extremity and to return the patient quickly and effectively to an appropriate level of employment and activity. Patients are usually referred for rehabilitation shortly after completion of a surgical procedure or casting for fractures. Essentially, rehabilitation starts while the patient's wrist is in a cast. It is recommended that therapy be initiated at the earliest possible stage so that rehabilitation can be maximized and residual contractures and complications can be minimized. Specifically, the goals of

therapy are the prevention or reduction of edema, assistance in tissue healing, relief of pain, assistance in relaxation, prevention of misuse, disuse, or overuse of the muscles, avoidance of muscle spasms, and improvement of coordination by re-education.[10] At appropriate times, desensitization of hypersensitive areas can be initiated. Rehabilitation measures can maintain increased range of motion as well as improved independence, endurance, and performance of daily functional activities: it can also increase strength, evaluation of work capacity, and initiation of work hardening programs.[7]

Static and Dynamic Splinting

Often in the rehabilitation process, a splint is prescribed. The two basic types of splints are static and dynamic.[11,47] Static splints for the wrist, hand, or elbow are used to protect soft tissues from overstretching, to prevent contractures, and to support the wrist after a fracture or surgical repair to facilitate the healing of bone and soft tissues. A static splint does not allow movement. The wrist in the static splint can be placed in a resting position or in the position of support for the wrist during grasp. When it is adjusted serially, the static splint may maintain increases that are achieved after range-of-motion exercises. Static splints help to provide rest.

Dynamic splints allow movement. They may be hinged or have external joints.[17,33,48] These splints usually have a power source such as rubber bands, electric motors, or springs. Dynamic splints can be driven by muscles, and synergistic wrist and hand movements can result. Dynamic splints help to resist, assist, or stimulate movement and allow the mobility of joints in a specific direction to be controlled.[17,47] They can provide the force that substitutes for weak or absent muscle power. Dynamic splints can be used for prolonged passive stretching in the case of contracted capsules or ligaments in the wrist, which result from prolonged immobilization or which occur after wrist reconstruction surgery. Dynamic splints for prolonged gentle stretching can be worn periodically for a prescribed length of time several times per day, with the static splint holding the range of motion gained from prolonged stretching.

Edema Control

After an injury or operation, edema must be prevented or treated early to maintain effective rehabilitation.[27] Edema that is allowed to persist may become chronic and can cause fibrosis of connective tissues around muscles, vessels, and nerves.[49] Joint ankylosis can result, with secondary ligament and capsule contractures. Gliding of tendons and muscles, the prerequisite for active hand and wrist rehabilitation, will be lost.

Elevation and early relaxed active range-of-motion exercises of the extremity can be effective in preventing edema and many of its complications. When possible, range of motion should always be started in the joints that can be moved postoperatively and after trauma. Even small amounts of motion help. The patient should be instructed to keep the limb elevated above the level of the heart to promote venous and lymphatic drainage. Shoulder forward elevation, abduction, and rotation combined with movement of the fingers is a time-honored method of maximizing the benefit of gravity and the fluid dynamic pump.

Decongestant massage is helpful in treating edema. The massage is performed from distal to proximal to facilitate the movement of the edema fluid out of the fingers. Once the cast is removed, the decongestant massage can be extended to the wrist and forearm to help eliminate the edema of the fractured or surgically injured wrist. (The decongestant massage is usually done before the application of the elastic wraps or Tubergrip.)

Elastic wraps such as Coban or Exban, or thick string wraps around the fingers from distal to proximal, can aid in temporarily decreasing the edema. Ace wraps or Tubigrip can help decrease the swelling around the traumatized wrist, forearm, or hands. Active range-of-motion exercises of the digits and wrist during and after the wrapping can help diminish swelling, and the pumping action of active muscle contractions can decrease edema.

The intermittent pneumatic compression pump is useful in cases of edema caused by soft tissue injury, in cases of reflex sympathetic dystrophy if the extremity is not painful, and in cases of dependent or chronic edema.

Range-of-Motion Exercises

Remobilization of injured tissues is extremely important and its timing was discussed in the previous sections. However, the purpose of remobilization is for muscle re-education so that purposeful, voluntary, and acceptable movement can be established.[10] Re-education with range-of-motion exercises is extremely important when abnormal motor patterns are present. These are often seen in wrist fractures when the patient attempts to use the finger extensor muscles for wrist extension. Much of the therapist's time is spent in re-education for active relaxed range of motion. The course of treatment progresses from gentle, relaxed, active assistive motion to active range-of-motion exercises followed by strengthening. Biofeedback during re-education can be helpful in enhancing motor control. Muscle electrical stimulation also can help achieve muscle pull-through and aid re-education in tendon transfers when applied appropriately after healing. Myostimulation can also be used occasionally for active stretching.[50]

Co-contraction, guarding, misuse, disuse, and overuse of the muscles must be prevented if rehabilitation is to be accomplished. Careful guidance and monitoring of progress from light to moderate to heavy activities is an important part of rehabilitation of patients. The loss of active motion is a frequent complication after a wrist fracture, arthritic disease, or operation. Early physical or occupational therapy of the hand is imperative. Capsular and ligamentous tightness after immobilization of the wrist is a cause of loss of range of motion. This immobilization, which is necessary to allow healing of bone and soft tissue structures, should not interfere with motion of adjacent joints, and any joint that does not require immobilization should be started without delay on active range-of-motion exercises. Gentle active assisted range of motion should be performed without force. The shoulder and elbow, as well as the digits when possible, should be included in early range-of-motion exercises. The shoulder may require assisted movement in the initial stage as active assisted or passive relaxed exercises but should never be forced.

If the degree of permissible range of motion is limited, this must be communicated by the surgeon to the therapist, who should be informed of the appropriate course of healing of fractures, the type of operative procedure, and the structural results that are to be achieved and are necessary.[7] This communication is imperative after surgical procedures for tendon repair and reconstruction, ligament and capsular repair, stabilization for fractures of the bone about the wrist, and wrist arthroplasties.

Passive relaxed range of motion does not mean strongly stretching and when performed should be done slowly without pain. Stretching is rarely necessary after a fracture or after surgical repair of a tendon. Active assisted range of motion is done to increase or maintain the range of motion without muscle misuse, disuse, or overuse. Active range-of-motion exercises are the exercises used most commonly in wrist rehabilitation.[10] However, gentle prolonged stretching is used when there are adhesions after tendon healing or when the moving plane places restrictions on the tendons. Stretching can also be employed after wrist capsule repair (at 6 weeks). Appropriate healing should be accomplished before this type of prolonged stretching is done. The gentle prolonged passive stretch by an external force, such as dynamic splinting, often is done 20 to 30 minutes four times per day. Applying a gentle stretching force over a prolonged period of time is much more effective and safe than applying a high force over a short period of time. Stretching should be performed without pain, swelling, or fatigue.

Various passive range-of-motion devices[17] can be helpful if they are fitted properly, if proper alignment is assured, and if the extremity is comfortable and relaxed during the passive range of motion.

Adjuncts to Range of Motion

Adjunctive methods of treatment, in addition to range of motion, strengthening exercises, and stretching, include the application of heat (such as the whirlpool without dependency), hotpacks with the extremities elevated, radiant heat, fluidotherapy, phototherapy, paraffin baths, or contrast baths with hot and cold water.[25-28,51,52] Other adjuncts to rehabilitation can be friction massage to improve range of

motion of the scar tissue or to loosen skin over adhesions around an incision. Deep sedative massage can be soothing and can help bring about relaxation in preparation for exercises. Also, constant firm pressure from an elastomer pad, iodoform pad, or elastic wraps, garments, or sleeves can aid in softening the scar.

To enhance movement, ultrasound with gentle prolonged stretching has been used over areas that are restricted.[25] Ultrasound with phonophoresis of 10 percent cortisone in Aquasonic or Aquaphore is especially helpful in capsular or ligamentous tightness. Periosteal pain should be avoided. Ultrasound is contraindicated in children who have an open physes. Sonography has been used after silicone wrist joint arthroplasties but is contraindicated for metal implants. Iontophoresis can be used to infiltrate localized areas with cortisone or other drugs.[51]

Joint Jacks, knuckle benders, and reverse knuckle benders may be effective methods to provide prolonged gentle stretching of contractures of fingers or wrist, if the direction of motion is correct. These devices should fit the patient well and have an effective angle of pull without causing undue pressure or circulatory problems.[20] They should be used in multiple repetitions for short periods of time and not at night.

Strengthening

Once the desired range of motion is achieved, muscle strengthening and endurance training can begin. Progressive resistive exercises of gradually increasing weights, or elastics for resistance, can be helpful. Exercises for strengthening can be isotonic, isometric, or isokinetic. Devices that can be helpful in a graded exercise program include a hand helper, hand exercises, various spring-resisted weight devices, therapeutic putty, and elastic straps. Functional activities of progressively increasing difficulty and resistance also can be helpful in strengthening.

Machines such as the Cybex isokinetic machine, the BTE, or the Lido work set are helpful for strengthening and endurance training as well as recording progress.[18,53] Endurance training should be done slowly in gradual increments of exercise.

Work Rehabilitation

Work rehabilitation and retraining are extremely important and should be the ultimate goal of rehabilitation efforts. Work hardening programs of gradually increasing increments, whether performed in a therapy department or at the work site, have been helpful. Work capacity evaluations that assess capabilities of work and the limitations of the patient after an injury allow recommended changes at jobs when necessary and have proved to be extremely important in rehabilitation of the patient back into the work environment. The work hardening can be achieved through the Lido work set or BTE machine or with stress loading.

Sensory Re-education

Sensory re-education may be necessary if there has been traumatic injury to the nerves about the wrist. This technique is used to develop a conscious perception and proper interpretation of a distorted or insufficient sensation in a patient with impaired sensory perception. The use of various forms of TENS before and during exercises can be considered if pain is a common problem.[54] This technique helps patients with cutaneous hypersensitivity and may aid in pain relief in patients with causalgia or pain dysfunction syndromes.

SUMMARY

Pain should be controlled without the use of narcotics. Control of edema and assurance of relaxed active range of motion are extremely important so that the patient can regain proper movement of the hand and wrist. When dystrophy occurs posttraumatically, it will prolong the rehabilitation immensely. Prevention is the desired course, but sometimes that is not possible. Relaxed gentle active and active assisted range-of-motion exercises are essential to prevent the complications of joint contractures, but these should not cause pain or result in prolonged discomfort after the exercise is stopped. It is important that the patient move actively and be reassured that movement is not going to make the discomfort worse. Gentle prolonged stretching can be helpful if it is not pain producing. A gradual work hardening program, once a sufficient and pain-free range of motion has been attained, may be necessary. Delays in initiating reha-

bilitation often result in less than optimal recovery. Cooperation and communication among the patient, hand surgeon, hand physical or occupational therapists, and other health professionals must be maintained to gain the best recovery possible.

REFERENCES

1. Johnson RP: The acutely injured wrist and its residuals. Clin Orthop 149:33, 1980
2. Cooney WP, Agee JM, Hastings H, Melone CP: Symposium: management of intra-articular fractures of the distal radius. Contemp Orthop 21:71, 1990
3. Cooney WP, Dobyns JH, Linscheid RL: Fractures of the scaphoid: a rational approach to management. Clin Orthop 149:90, 1980
4. Herbert TJ, Fisher WE: Management of the fractured scaphoid using a new bone screw. J Bone Joint Surg [Br] 66:114, 1984
5. Chapman DR, Bennett JB, Bryan WJ, Tullos HS: Complications of distal radius fractures. J Hand Surg 7:509, 1982
6. Cooney WP, Dobyns JH, Linscheid RL: Complications of Colles' fractures. J Bone Joint Surg [Am] 62:613, 1980
7. Knapp ME: Aftercare of fractures. In Krusen FN (ed): Handbook of Physical Medicine and Rehabilitation. 2nd Ed. WB Saunders, Philadelphia, 1971
8. Moberg E: The shoulder-hand-finger syndrome. Surg Clinic North Am 40:367, 1960
9. Cooney WP: External fixation of distal radius fractures. Clin Orthop 180:44, 1983
10. Kottke FJ: Therapeutic exercises to maintain mobility. In Kottke FJ, Stillwell GK, Lehmann JF (eds): Krusen's Handbook of Physical Medicine and Rehabilitation. 3rd Ed. WB Saunders, Philadelphia, 1982
11. Fess EE, Philips CH: Hand Splinting: Principles and Methods. 2nd Ed. CV Mosby, St. Louis, 1987
12. Schutzer SF, Gossling HR: The treatment of reflex sympathetic dystrophy. J Bone Joint Surg [Am] 66:625, 1984
13. Bradway JK, Amadio PC, Cooney WP: Open reduction and internal fixation of displaced comminuted fractures of the distal radius. J Bone Joint Surg [Am] 71:839, 1989
14. Melone CP: Open treatment of displaced articular fractures of the distal radius. Clin Orthop 202:103, 1986
15. Leung KS, Shen WY, Leung PC et al: Ligamentotaxis and bone grafting for comminuted fractures of the distal radius. J Bone Joint Surg [Br] 71:838, 1989
16. Bunnell S: Active splinting of the hand. J Bone Joint Surg 28:732, Oct 1946
17. Calditz JC: Low profile dynamic splinting of the injured hand. Am J Occup Ther 37:183, 1983
18. Pendergraft KJ, Cooper JK, Clark GL: The BTE work simulator. p. 1210. In Hunter JM, Schneider LH, Mackin EJ, Callahan AD (eds): Rehabilitation of the Hand: Surgery and Therapy. 3rd Ed. CV Mosby, St. Louis, 1990
19. Bunnell S: Spring splint to supinate or pronate the hand. J Bone Joint Surg [Am] 31:664, 1949
20. Brand P: The forces of dynamic splinting. In Hunter JM, Schneider LH, Mackin EJ, Callahan AD (eds): Rehabilitation of the Hand. 2nd Ed. CV Mosby, St. Louis, 1984
21. Bonica JJ: Causalgia and other reflex sympathetic dystrophies. Postgrad Med 53:143, 1973
22. Kleinert NE, Cole NW, Wayne L, et al: Post-traumatic sympathetic dystrophy. Orthop Clin North Am 4:917, 1973

23. Dellon AL, Mackinnon SE: Radial sensory nerve entrapment in the forearm. J Hand Surg [Am] 11:119, 1986
24. Hosman J: Minor causalgia: a hyperesthetic neurovascular syndrome. N Engl J Med 222:870, 1940
25. Miller LE, and others: Sequential use of hot packs and ultrasound. Phys Ther 59:559, 1979
26. Mullins PA: Use of therapeutic modalities in upper extremity rehabilitation. In Hunter JM, Schneider LH, Mackin EJ, Callahan AD (eds): Rehabilitation of the Hand: Surgery and Therapy. 3rd Ed. CV Mosby, St. Louis, 1990
27. Walsh M: Relationship of hand edema to upper extremity position and water temperature during whirlpool. J Hand Surg [Am] 9:609, 1984
28. Borrell RM, Henley EJ, Ho P, Hubbell MK: Fluidotherapy: evaluation of a new heat modality. Arch Phys Med Rehabil 58:69, 1977
29. Bilos ZJ, Pankovich AM, Yelda S: Fracture-dislocation of the radiocarpal joint. J Bone Joint Surg [Am] 59:198, 1977
30. Linscheid RL, Dobyns JH, Beckenbaugh RD et al: Instability patterns of the wrist. J Hand Surg 8:682, 1983
31. Amadio PC, Botte MJ: Treatment of malunion of the distal radius. Hand Clin 3:541, 1987
32. Ekenstam FW, Engkvist O, Wadin K: Results from resection of the distal end of the ulna after fractures of the lower end of the radius. Scand J Plast Reconstr Surg 16:177, 1982
33. DeVore GL: Preoperative assessment and postoperative therapy and splinting in rheumatoid arthritis. p. 942. In Hunter JW, Schneider LH, Mackin EJ, Callahan AD (eds): Rehabilitation of the Hand. CV Mosby, St. Louis, 1990
34. Flatt AE: Care of the Rheumatoid Hand. 4th Ed. CV Mosby, St. Louis, 1987
35. Nalebuff EA, Millender LH: Reconstructive surgery and rehabilitation of the hand. In Kelley WN, Harris ED Jr, Ruddy S, Sledge CB (eds): Textbook of Rheumatology. 2nd Ed. WB Saunders, Philadelphia, 1985
36. Beckenbaugh RD: Implant arthroplasty in the rheumatoid hand and wrist: current state of the art in the United States. J Hand Surg 8:675, 1983
37. Beckenbaugh RD: Arthroplasty of the wrist. p. 194. In Morrey BF (ed): Joint Replacement Arthroplasty. Churchill Livingstone, New York, 1991
38. Ryu J, Cooney WP, Askew L et al: Functional range of motion in the wrist joint. J Hand Surg (in press)
39. Cooney WP III, Beckenbaugh RD, Linscheid RL: Total wrist arthroplasty: problems with implant failure. Clin Orthop 187:121, 1984
40. Taleisnik J: Carpal instability: current concepts. J Bone Joint Surg [Am] 70:1262, 1988
41. Cooney WP, Linscheid RL, Dobyns JH: Carpal instability: ligament repair and reconstruction. p. 125. In Neviaser RJ (ed): Controversies in Hand Surgery. Churchill Livingstone, New York, 1990
42. Green DP, O'Brien ET: Classifications and management of carpal dislocations. Clin Orthop 149:55, 1980
43. Moneim MS, Hofammann KE III, Omer GF: Transscaphoid perilunate fracture-dislocations: result of open reduction and pin fixation. Clin Orthop 190:227, 1984
44. Linscheid RL, Dobyns JH: Complication of treatment of fractures and dislocations of the wrist. p. 339. In Eppo CN Jr (ed): Complications in Orthopedic Surgery. JB Lippincott, Philadelphia, 1986
45. Griffin JE, Echternach JL, Price RE et al: Patients treated by ultrasonic driven hydrocortisone and with ultrasound alone. Phys Ther 47:594, 1967
46. Saltee RB, Harris DJ: The healing of intra-articular fractures with continuous passive motion. Instr Course Lect 28:102, 1979
47. Schutt A: Splint Manual for the Upper Extremity. Department of Physical Medicine and Rehabilitation, Mayo Clinic, 1988
48. Dimick MP: Continuous passive motion for the upper extremity. In Hunter JM, Schneider LH, Mackin EJ, Callahan AD (eds): Rehabilitation of the Hand. 3rd Ed. CV Mosby, St. Louis, 1990
49. VanDemark RE, Koucky RE, Fischer FJ: Peritendinous fibrosis of the dorsum of the hand. J Bone Joint Surg [Am] 30:284, 1948
50. Benton LA, et al: Functional electrical stimulation. Rancho Los Amigos Hospital Bulletin, Downey, CA, 1980
51. Harris PR: Iontophoresis: clinical research in musculoskeletal inflammatory conditions. J Orthop Sports Phys Ther 4:109, 1982
52. Lehmann JF, Warren LG, Scham SM: Therapeutic heat and cold. Clin Orthop 99:207, 1974
53. Curtis R, Engalitdeff J: A work simulator for rehabilitating the upper extremity. J Hand Surg 6:499, 1981
54. Ersek RA: Pain Control with TENS: Principles and Practice. Warren H Green, St. Louis, 1981

52 Rehabilitation of the Elbow

ROBERT N. HOTCHKISS
SYLVIA DAVILA

Painless, stable motion of the elbow, gives an individual the ability to position the hand in space for manipulation of the environment. Any condition that limits motion, causes pain, or results in instability of the elbow, in turn, compromises the function of the hand.

The goal of rehabilitation of the elbow joint following injury or reconstructive surgery is to maximize function without damage to the reconstructed or repaired structures. Optimal care balances vigor with prudence, timing the progression of treatment by the biologic signposts of healing and inflammation.

Head injury and paralysis also impair elbow function by creating muscle imbalance and secondary contracture. Treatment of these conditions requires careful individual assessment and a comprehensive approach to the patient's situation.

REQUIREMENTS OF ELBOW FUNCTION

The requirements of elbow function can be divided into four separate but dependent features: motion, stability, strength, and comfort. Each of these plays a role in the function of the elbow and, therefore, the entire upper extremity. Most rehabilitation protocols correctly focus on improving motion and strength, but stability and comfort should not be ignored. In most cases, it is not possible to advance concurrently on all four fronts. For example, a patient with a recent unconstrained total elbow replacement should not be immediately placed in full extension, for fear of causing a posterior dislocation. In this instance, striving to improve the range of motion should not be ignored, but it should be deferred until the healed anterior capsule can accept the stress without dislocation. The goal of rehabilitation is to apply the appropriate therapy at the opportune time.

Motion

Morrey[1] studied the range of motion and the range of position required to perform many of the tasks of daily living. Based on this study, most activities required a range of 30° to 130° of flexion (for simplicity, full extension is 0° of flexion) (Fig. 52-1). Fifty degrees of pronation and 50° of supination was required in forearm rotation (Fig. 52-2). It is important to emphasize that not only a wide range of motion was used by the subjects, but a *wide range of positions* (100° arc). Tying shoes required the greatest extension (nearly 20°), and eating and drinking the most flexion.

The data from this study should serve as guidelines but not goals. There are some patients who seek or require greater motion either because of limitations in adjacent joints, or because of a particular occupation or avocation. There are also instances in which gains in motion are not achievable without extensive, unwelcome surgery. In these situations, the therapist can assist the patient with adaptive techniques and tools.

This study also underscores the quandary in describing the optimal position for elbow arthrodesis, because there seems no best position—not even 90° of flexion.

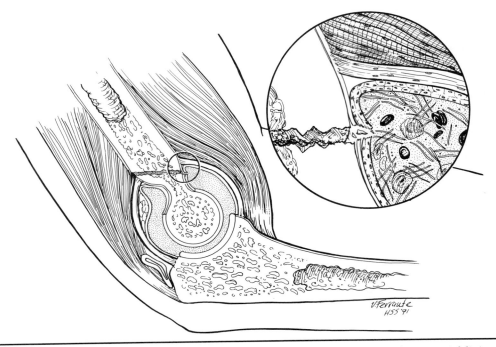

Fig. 52-1. The joint is distended by hematoma after acute injury to the elbow. The synovial lining may be disrupted. Note that the joint capsule is quite thin.

Stability

Anterior-Posterior Stability

A combination of muscle tension, articular anatomy, and ligaments stabilizes the elbow, making it one of the most constrained joints in the body.[2-7] The ulnohumeral articulation is hemicircumferential and nearly mimics a true hinge, with only minor movement in the instant center of rotation during flexion and extension.[8] With the brachialis/biceps and triceps under tension, the elbow is usually quite stable to anterior-posterior stress, even after injury to the collateral ligaments, as occurs in posterior dislocation.[9-12]

Valgus Stability

Because of the natural carrying angle of the elbow, away from the trunk, longitudinal load creates a valgus moment at the elbow. Tension develops in the stout medial collateral ligament and prevents valgus displacement or axial ulnohumeral rotation. If the medial ligament is at all strained or mechanically incompetent, compression at the radiocapitellar joint occurs, making the radial head an important secondary stabilizer[3,5,7] (Fig. 52-3).

After injury or reconstruction of the medial ligaments, it may be important to provide protection from valgus stress, allowing both the anterior capsule and the medial ligaments to heal. This is discussed in more detail subsequent sections (see "Elbow Dislocation").

Throwing activities can also exert enormous valgus stress. Stabilization of the elbow of the throwing athlete is highly specialized, and surgical reconstruction may be required. A specific rehabilitation program for the throwing athlete is out of the realm of this chapter, but such programs can be found in texts that address sports medicine and the throwing athlete.[13]

Strength

Strength and endurance requirements are individual and have not been standardized. "Normal strength" is difficult to define unless specifically tied to a particular activity or job. It is sometimes reasonable to

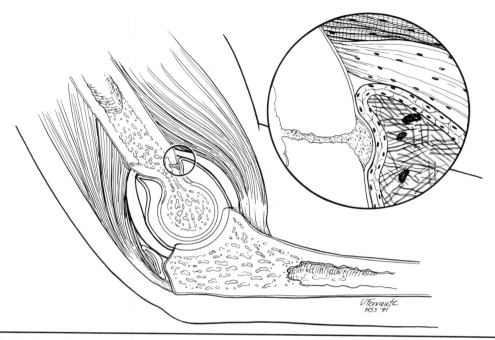

Fig. 52-2. In the early reparative phase, the inflammatory cells and fibroblasts produce collagen, emeshing the capsule and synovial lining. The exact mechanism for the beginning of capsular thickening is not understood.

use the unaffected side as a comparison, but this is not always feasible, as in cases of polyarthritis. In most cases, the rehabilitation program will maximize both endurance and power in the later phases of recovery.

Comfort

The presence of disabling pain, with or without motion, will preclude any significant gains in motion or strength. The surgeon must work closely with the therapist to manage the pain with appropriate analgesics and secondary modalities. In most instances, if adequate skeletal stability is achieved a comfortable rehabilitation program can be commenced.

Any use of passive manipulation or stretching has been condemned by many out of fear that such motion leads to heterotopic ossification or reflex dystrophy. To date, there is no definitive proof that passive motion causes heterotopic bone formation. However, we believe that overzealous passive stretch causes microtears and perhaps hemorrhage, restarting the inflammatory process. By contrast, gentle,

sustained passive stretch seems to remodel the soft tissue without causing inflammation. If the therapist encounters increasing or sudden pain and discomfort, out of proportion to what is expected, the treating physician should be notified. A failure of fixation or an unrecognized dislocation can occur during rehabilitation.

THE PHASED RESPONSE TO TRAUMA (OR SURGERY)

Following trauma, a predictable sequence of cellular events occurs at all levels of the injury. The basic reparative cell—the fibroblast—synthesizes collagen as fibrous tissue with a differing phenotypic potential depending on the mechanical environment and location of the cell. Skin, tendon, muscle, joint capsule, and bone have the potential to form a single scar, binding each layer to the next. If left undisturbed, this bound mass of fibrous tissue can prevent independent excursion of each layer, disabling the limb. However, mechanical stimuli can alter the biology and, perhaps, gene expression of the reparative cell. With protected motion during healing, the "sin-

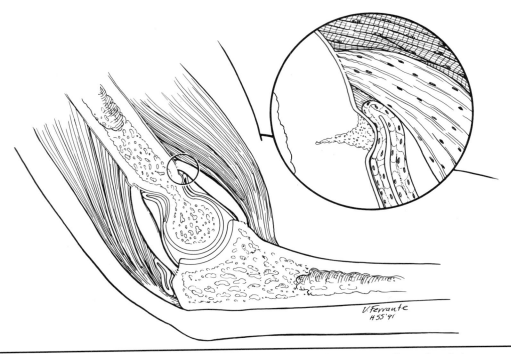

Fig. 52-3. In the late phase of post-traumatic stiffness, the synovial space has collapsed and the surrounding capsule has significantly thickened, both anteriorly and posteriorly.

gle scar'' can be modulated. Healing tendons can lose their adherence to overlying skin, and muscle can regain its appropriate resting length. The ligaments and capsule surrounding the joint usually adapt to the shortest length required. If stressed and elongated, the capsule can adjust and lengthen gradually, without tearing. *The essence of rehabilitation is to create the optimal mechanical environment for the responding reparative cells.*

Although there is a temporal continuum of the cellular response, it is helpful to divide the healing into three phases: *inflammatory, early remodeling, and late remodeling.* These phases can be monitored clinically and reflect the underlying progression of cellular events. The ability to judge which phase a patient is in comes from listening to and examining the patient during rehabilitation. There is no absolute demarcation between each phase, and patients respond differently depending on their own biology and the severity of injury. Some are so-called scar formers, in whom every layer of the injury binds to the next despite the most timely care. Others seem to sail through with few adhesions, pain, or disability.

The elbow joint is particularly sensitive to trauma and inflammation. Relatively minor injuries or inflammatory conditions seem to create more stiffness and loss of motion than in other joints. Nirschl and Morrey[14] have speculated that the anterior joint capsule is especially sensitive to inflammation and rapidly thickens. When this occurs in the flexed position, which is most comfortable, active motion exercises and everyday use of the arm may not necessarily overcome the contracture. The triceps does not have the mechanical advantage of the flexors, the biceps, and the brachialis.

The Inflammatory Phase (0 to 2 Weeks)

Biology

Inflammation is a necessary initiative event in healing soft tissues and bone. The cells of inflammation—polymorphonuclear leukocytes, monocytes, and macrophages—contribute a variety of chemical mediators that influence platelet activity, edema, and vasodilation. In the first few hours after injury or surgery, clotting blood, white blood cells, and plate-lets aggregate, laying the foundation for reorganization of the injured area. Any devitalized tissue is consumed by macrophages. There is also increased blood flow in the zone of injury, partially mediated by prostaglandins, which explains the hyperemia of injury. The concomitant injury to blood vessels, especially draining veins, further contributes to swelling.

Unfortunately, the presence of the inflammatory cells and their associated products also causes pain, inhibiting movement of the limb. From a teleologic view, there was probably some survival value in limiting the use of an injured limb. Unfortunately, evolution could not anticipate rigid internal fixation or total elbow arthroplasty. The pain associated with inflammation is usually at cross-purposes to rehabilitation of the elbow, because it limits motion in the early phases.

Clinically, pain and swelling dominate the injury in the first 2 weeks; the severity of each is proportional to the size of the zone of injury.

Treatment

In this phase the immediate goals are to control pain, minimize edema, and maintain range of motion. Any repaired structure must also be protected, including the skin wound until sufficiently healed.

Before seeing the patient, the therapist and treating surgeon should mutually understand the goals and limitations of the therapy program. If there is even slight discrepancy in instruction, the patient can become confused or hostile. The surgeon should explain either by note or verbally, the injury, surgery, and treatment goals. The therapist, with this information, can then design a program based on appropriate restrictions.

Patient education should begin at the first visit and continue at each appropriate point. An informed patient is likely to be less anxious and more cooperative.

Pain Control

Pain in the early phase is an expected and natural part of the inflammatory response. The patient should be reassured of this and encouraged to distinguish between acceptable, tolerable discomfort and pain that is a warning sign of impending damage. The patient should also understand that much of the pain comes from edema and stiffness. As these resolve, the pain should subside. If the pain interferes with the patient's efforts or emotional well-being, it should be controlled with either medication or transcutaneous electrical nerve stimulation (TENS). TENS may be more acceptable because it has the advantage of being in the patient's control and does not interfere with alertness. The value of TENS varies with each patient.

Edema Control

During the inflammatory phase edema contains fibroblasts that synthesize collagen, producing scar tissue. Edema reduction minimizes scar formation, both at the elbow and at the hand. Initially, the edema is "pitting" and can be treated with compression and elevation techniques. If left untreated, this swelling becomes more "brawny," filled with adherent scar. Minimizing the swelling at this later stage is more problematic since the modulation of scar tissue takes more time than reducing fluid and inflammatory cells in the "pitting" stage.

Initially, *elevation* effectively limits edema, and the patient is encouraged to keep the arm on a pillow while sleeping and in a sling when up and about. If wounds and external hardware allow them, *compression sleeves* or wraps can reduce edema. Tubigrip (Moorestown, NJ) can be purchased in different widths and cut to the appropriate length so as to include the entire arm to the axilla or cover only the elbow area. An elastic bandage wrapped spirally can also work as a compression device. However, this is awkward for the patient to apply.

During office visits, *decongestive or retrograde massage* of the edematous elbow can be applied with the patient supine and the arm elevated. The strokes should be long and firm, milking the edema from interstitial tissues distal to proximal. Decongestive massage should be performed for 5 to 10 minutes several times a day, especially before exercise and after the application of ice packs. The initial massage is gentle, avoiding tension to healing wounds.

Severe edema, involving the entire upper extremity, may require *intermittent compression units* such as those made by Jobst or Flowtron. In some regions smaller units can be rented for home use, increasing the frequency of application. General guidelines for use in the upper extremity are a limit of 55 mm Hg pressure and a ratio of inflation to deflation time of 3:1.

Ice or cold packs can reduce swelling and pain during rehabilitation. The cold seems to control the swelling following range-of-motion (ROM) exercises and provides analgesia. The ice packs should be applied for 10 to 30 minutes depending on the depth of the tissues being treated. Analgesia begins about 15 minutes after application. Cold packs can be applied several times per day, depending on the frequency of exercise sessions.

In many therapy clinics phonophoresis and iontophoresis are commonly used treatments for inflammatory conditions. These modalities deliver anti-inflammatory and/or analgesic medication into tissue. Scientific rationales and the rate of drug delivery have not been well studied or documented. Scientific evidence of drug penetration is inconclusive and fragmentary.

High-voltage galvanic stimulation (HVGS) has been reported to be effective in eliminating or minimizing fibrotic or chronic edema. Its use is also indicated in the treatment of organized hematoma. HVGS stimulates muscle contraction, which facilitates blood flow by the action of a muscle pump. This muscle activity alleviates edema and helps resolve hematomas. HVGS should not be used if active muscle contraction is contraindicated. An additional benefit of HVGS is its TENS effect in pain control. Its wave form is similar to those of some TENS units.

Wound Care

Some open wounds require débridement and can be cleansed by the whirlpool. Because the arm sits in a dependent position in warm water during treatment, edema can temporarily increase.[15] To reduce edema during whirlpool cleansing, limit each session to 15 minutes. The patient should raise the hand overhead every 5 minutes for 5 minutes and make a fist repetitively during treatment.

Motion

Gentle active and active-assisted ROM exercises should begin as soon as postoperative pain permits, usually 3 to 5 days after surgery. Elbow extension, flexion, supination, and pronation may be performed with the patient lying supine or sitting with the upper arm well supported on a table. To decrease pain and muscle spasm while maintaining or increasing ROM, use gentle oscillatory joint play movements in grades I and II. As the patient is able to tolerate the exercises, progress to active and active-assisted motion in a gravity-eliminated position and then against gravity. Supination and pronation exercise should be done with the patient's elbow touching the side to ensure pure radioulnar joint motion without substitution.

Active and passive ROM exercise of uninvolved joints is important to prevent loss of motion and weakness caused by disuse and protective posture. Frozen shoulder syndrome and reflex sympathetic dystrophy are not uncommon in elbow injuries and may be prevented in the inflammatory phase with careful management. ROM of the shoulder and hand should be evaluated periodically throughout the period of elbow rehabilitation to ensure that it is not deteriorating.

Flexion and extension movements of both the hand and wrist maintain musculotendinous length and prevent flexor and extensor tenodesis. Tenodesis exercises combine composite finger flexion with simultaneous wrist flexion followed by combined finger extension and wrist extension.

Active and passive ROM exercise should not exceed the limits of repaired tissue. The exercises should be individualized according to the specific needs of the tissues, balancing the goal of avoiding inflammation.

During the inflammatory phase the frequency and duration of exercise is dependent upon the goals of treatment. If maximizing mobility is the primary goal, exercise should be performed every 1 to 2 hours with 10 repetitions. The patient should be instructed to hold each position for 3 to 5 seconds. If maximizing stability while maintaining mobility is the primary goal, exercise should be performed only two to three times per day, gently and slowly holding each position for several minutes.

Continuous Passive Motion. There are many advocates of continuous passive moton (CPM) following surgical procedures and contracture release of the elbow.[16-18] However, there is no compelling evidence that CPM improves the ultimate range of motion or enhances outcome. The rationale for its use in the inflammatory phase of elbow rehabilitation is to minimize edema and joint effusion while maximizing mobility. The available CPM devices for the elbow are limited and require abduction and external rotation of the shoulder. The axis of motion must be adjusted carefully.

Splinting

The purpose of splinting during the inflammatory phase is to provide protective positioning to prevent injury and deformity, while resting and supporting structures during healing. The protective splint is fabricated of perforated, thermoplastic material that is light and conforming yet rigid enough to provide support. The optimal protective position of the elbow and upper extremity will be dictated by the injury. It may be necessary to limit or prevent motion in one direction but not another (e.g., allow free wrist motion or eliminate it). For maximum support of the upper extremity the splint should extend proximally to the axilla and distally to the palmar flexion crease to support the wrist. The splint should be contoured, adjusted, and/or padded to avoid contact with exposed hardware and prevent undue pressure over bony pominences, wounds, and subcutaneous hardware.

During the inflammatory phase, the splint should be worn full time day and night, removing it only for wound care and exercises.

Early Remodeling Phase (2 to 8 Weeks)

Biology

During the second phase of wound healing (weeks 2 to 8), the fibroblasts and myofibroblasts synthesize collagen at a rapid pace. Initially the collagen production is vigorous and somewhat disorganized,

principally providing wound closure. Gradually, this bulk of disorganized collagen will be reworked by the macrophages and fibroblasts to construct a more purposeful structure, enhancing the tensile strength without increasing the bulk of the tissue. The scar remodeling process, whether at the skin surface or deep in the wound, is greatly influenced by its mechanical environment. Length adaptation in the musculotendinous units begins with compensatory shortening, depending on position. Although these changes are not necessarily permanent, once established, they are difficult to ameliorate.

At this point the acute inflammatory symptoms have begun to recede, and the patient begins to tolerate more passive stretch during this phase. Any overzealous stretching in this phase is extremely deleterious. If the therapy program produces injury rather than the adaptive remodeling sought, the acute inflammatory response recurs, creating pain and what seems to be an exaggerated inflammatory response. This can lead to devastating dystrophic response in the elbow and the adjacent wrist and shoulder.

Treatment

Edema Control

Decongestive massage should now be applied with deeper pressure with continued use of compression sleeves and wraps. Brawny or chronic edema can be effectively eliminated or minimized with HVGS by electrically stimulating a muscle pump. The treatment guidelines for edema control include using a negative polarity. Blood and plasma cells are negatively charged; therefore, negative current will repel them from the edematous tissue. HVGS should be used with caution. Avoid an intensity that produces muscle contraction if active muscle contraction is contraindicated in the postoperative protocol.

Scar Management

Once the wounds have healed, friction massage should be instituted to stretch superficial adhesions. Friction massage should be gentle initially to prevent tissue damage. As the scar matures it becomes thicker and more dense. The massage should then be applied with more pressure to affect deeper adhesions. Massage will also be beneficial in desensitizing the hypersensitive scar.

Other Therapeutic Modalities

Heat, moist heat, and fluidotherapy relieve muscle spasm, enhance circulation, and augment ROM and passive stretching. Heat is most effective when used before each therapy session.[19,20] Fluidotherapy allows active ROM exercises during its application and also provides desensitization. Whirlpool is limited to wound care because of dependency and increased swelling.

Ice or cold packs are applied after exercise to minimize inflammation and reduce spasm.

Motion

Active ROM exercises for the elbow and forearm are continued but now emphasizing more forceful contraction and increased number of repetitions to increase strength and endurance. Resistive strengthening exercise of the elbow and forearm are deferred. Depending on the posttraumatic or postsurgical precautions, gentle passive stretching may be initiated in this phase. It is extremely important that the therapist discuss each case with the attending physician and/or obtain as much information as possible from the medical records and x-rays before initiating passive ROM.

Passive ROM exercises should be applied as a gentle prolonged stretch with the patient completely relaxed to avoid co-contracting. Low force should be used to stretch the tight structures and gain motion rather than cause microtears in the tissues and provoke an inflammatory response. The patient should be instructed that mild discomfort should result from the stretch but not significant pain, which is the body's warning sign of tissue damage.[21,22] Passive ROM exercise should also be continued as needed for the uninvolved joints of the hand, wrist, and shoulder.

In this phase joint mobilization techniques are restricted to grades I and II for the elbow and radioulnar joints. Tensile strength of ligaments and tendons in this phase is still very low, and excessive stress can cause microtrauma. If there are no contraindications,

strengthening exercise for grip and the shoulder may be initiated. The use of light functional activities should also be included because they provide an excellent means of increasing strength and endurance and maintaining hand functon. These may be performed with the arm elevated to control edema. The activities can be carefully chosen and designed to encourage as few or as many motions of the upper extremity as possible, and they are less boring and tedious than ROM exercises.

Active use of the arm in light activities of daily living is now encouraged, using adaptive techniques where there are limitations.

Splinting

Because of the low tensile strength of the soft tissue, splints in this phase may provide only light stress. The decision to use splints is dictated by the condition of the healing structures. Healing unstable fractures, ligament injuries, tendon and nerve repairs, and skin grafts may be damaged by prematurely applied stress. However, if motion in a particular plane and direction does not jeopardize a healing structure, early light stress may be applied within 1 to 2 weeks within a safe ROM arc. If the purpose of the splint is only to provide support to intact but healing structures, it may be removed frequently for exercise but still used during functional activities and activities of daily living.

To gently increase ROM, serial splinting may be considered. An adjustable hinge is used for this purpose. It also provides good lateral stability. The thermoplastic splint may be changed to increase or free the desired motion and/or possibly trimmed back to allow free use of the hand and wrist. During this phase the splint may need periodic adjustments as edema decreases to accomodate the decrease and provide optimal support.

Late Remodeling Phase (2 to 6 Months)

Biology

The process of scar maturation in all tissues of the injury lasts for several months. The precise mechanisms of this process are poorly understood. Collagen cross-links and fiber orientation as well as bone remodeling continue to be influenced by the mechanical environment. The rehabilitation program should continue as long as the goals have not been met and the maturation phase has not ceased.

Clinically, the maturity of the process can be judged by the "plasticity" of the ROM. If the patient seems to lose ROM between stretching sessions, or loses ground when not wearing a splint, the remodeling process is not complete. Likewise, if gains continue to be made, even on a temporary basis, after each session, therapy should not be discontinued unless all goals have been achieved.

Assuming all structures have healed, the home program and sessions with the therapist will concentrate on increasing motion and strength. By 8 weeks, the restrictions against passive ROM and resistive exercises have been removed. If CPM has been used, it is discontinued. Pain is now usually only experienced at the extremes of motion and with excessive stress. The therapist must continue to carefully monitor the patient's status in response to the treatment.

Treatment

Therapeutic Heat

Therapeutic heat prior to passive stretching is now crucial to increase tissue extensibility, influencing plastic deformation of connective tissue. Because of its greater depth of penetration, *ultrasound* may be the best choice, allowing the therapist to selectively heat the tight capsular tissues of the elbow along with and prior to capsular stretching and joint mobilization. If the restriction of motion is due to muscular restriction, the ultrasound is applied to the tight muscle prior to and during stretching.

Both therapeutic heat and cold relieve pain and spasm. Some patients will respond better to one than the other and prefer one over the other before and after exercise and activity.

Neuromuscular Electrical Stimulation

Neuromuscular electrical stimulation (NMES) facilitates muscle contraction for muscle re-education and increased strength after immobilization. Because NMES can produce a strong muscle contraction, its

use should be deferred until 8 weeks after surgery or trauma. Care should be taken to avoid overuse, which can elicit an inflammatory response.

Motion

Progression of the passive ROM exercise program now includes more aggressive, prolonged stretching of involved muscle groups, but only as tolerated and indicated. Passive ROM exercises may include the use of contraction-relaxation exercises for musculotendinous stretching of elbow flexor-extensor and supinator-pronator muscles. If there are no contraindications, the therapist may progress to the use of joint mobilization techniques for stretching of capsular structures.

Various forms of passive motion and joint mobilization may be used for the stiff elbow and are well described in the literature. It is beyond the scope of this chapter to discuss them, and they should only be performed by a well-trained, experienced therapist.

Strength

Resistive exercise should not be initiated until fracture union is stable and/or soft tissue has adequately healed, usually 6 to 8 weeks after surgery or trauma. In patients with arthritis, strengthening is limited by pain. Isometric exercise and gradual resumption of activity is the best option for these patients. The isometric exercise should include elbow flexion, extension, supination, and pronation and wrist extension and flexion. Grip strengthening using putty of progressive resistances allows strengthening without excessive joint motion.

Progressive resistive exercises with free weights or wall pulleys is another excellent means of providing strengthening exercises. Wall pulleys may be used in proprioceptive neuromuscular facilitation (PNF) patterns to allow general strengthening of the entire upper extremity. Elastic resistance, such as the Theraband, allows strengthening of specific muscles utilizing concentric and eccentric muscle contraction. Its versatility allows isolation of specific muscles or motions of the elbow or general strengthening of the entire upper extremity when used in PNF patterns. The Theraband comes in various resistances, allowing the patient to be progressed. It may be used as part of the home program, reserving the use of sophisticated objective exercise equipment for the clinic.

Isokinetic exercise is optimally used in the rehabilitation of individuals requiring high-rate muscle contraction in their work or sport activities. Most isokinetic exercise machines can isolate all the elbow, forearm, and wrist motions.

Work Simulation/Work Hardening

The final stage in elbow rehabilitation should include work simulation and work hardening. The emphasis for the patient should include lifting, pushing, and pulling.

Splinting

Splinting may be needed for mobilizing either the humeroulnar joint in extension and flexion or the radioulnar joint in supination and pronation or both. The limitation of motion that developed during the first and second phases is a result of immature scar that in the third phase can be favorably altered and modified by judiciously applied mechanical stress to maximize articular glide and soft tissue excursion. Static or dynamic splints may accomplish this either alone or in combination. Each has its advantages depending on the amount of scar, the structures involved, and the preference of the physician and therapist. With all forms of splinting, the stress applied should stretch to the point of discomfort but not pain and should be carefully monitored to avoid undue compression or distraction. The force should be low but continuous and prolonged to effectively elongate adhesion.

Dynamic splinting of elbow flexion and extension is more appropriate for application of a low force to mild contractures such as those seen after a total elbow replacement or after surgery or trauma where there is little soft tissue involvement. Dynasplint (Baltimore, MD) has developed a splint for elbow extension and flexion contractures that provides a low, constant force.[23,24] Our results with these devices have not been good. Compliance with this device has been lower than with the custom-molded orthotic. In addition, the patients have difficulty aligning the splint without assistance. Without accurate alignment, the resultant mechanical force is less than optimal.

Conversely, dynamic splinting for forearm supination and pronation has been beneficial in our experience. Our design uses force perpendicular to the axis of motion of the radioulnar joint, with proximal and distal bases providing congruous fit to distribute pressure.

We have found the custom-fabricated turnbuckle splint to be the most effective orthosis for mobilizing flexion and extension contractures of the elbow. Because the distal and proximal cuffs are molded to the patient, an accurate fit is obtained. This allows the patient to don the splint and adjust it with ease.

Splints for increasing more than one plane of motion can be used in combination. For example, the patient may alternate between the flexion and extension turnbuckle splints every other night and use the supination-pronation splint every other hour during the day.

Further discussion of splint principles and methods is beyond the scope of this chapter. If the therapist is not experienced in splinting, it is important that they be informed about splinting options and timing, so as to be able to refer the patient to an experienced therapist or orthotist.

SPECIFIC PROBLEMS, INJURIES AND OPERATIONS

Flexion Contracture

Early

Flexion contractures are extremely common after any elbow injury. An early contracture, one occurring before 6 months after injury, can often be improved. Structural limitations may be present and must be investigated before assuming the contracture is due to muscle-tendon shortening or capsular contracture. Heterotopic bone formation or intrarticular incongruity will limit mobility and may not necessarily be seen on plain radiographs. Often there is a firm endpoint when these are present, but not always.

Not all flexion contractures require treatment. Those of less than 30° are usually not disabling. However, the first months after surgery or injury are the optimal time to minimize the contracture.

For patients who are not improving with gentle passive stretching and active ROM exercises, we use turnbuckle splinting based on the description of Green and McCoy.[25] Instead of plaster, however, we use custom-molded thermoplastic material. This material can be easily molded to maximize soft tissue contact and can be removed for bathing and other exercises. The mechanical axis should be located over the epicondyles for the hinges. Green and McCoy[25] showed that a turnbuckle splint could improve the ROM as late as 6 months after injury, and this has been our experience with the removable thermoplastic turnbuckle orthosis. As the contracture resolves, the turnbuckle loses its mechanical advantage, and improvement with this device for contractures of less than 30° is difficult.

Once the splint is fabricated, the patient wears it for periods of 4 hours, gradually extending the elbow as tolerated. Rest periods in comfortable, unstressed positions are taken every 2 hours for 15 to 30 minutes. Compliance with particular schedules is dependent on the individual patient. Frequent communication between the therapist and the treating physician is important.

Established

Established flexion contractures of the elbow are those that have not improved with static or dynamic splinting and have occurred at least 6 months after injury. Most of these patients require surgical release, both of the anterior capsule and, with exploration, of the olecranon fossa. The postoperative rehabilitation of these patients requires great diligence. Urbaniak et al.[26] recommended splinting for at least 6 months after release. Ilizarov has used a hinged construct fabricated from ring-based external fixations system, slowly, passively extend the contracted elbow, but there are no reported series. Other devices using this method are currently being tested and hold promise.

Severe contracture from soft tissue loss or burns requires transferred tissue from a distant source.[27]

Injuries

Elbow Dislocation

Simple posterior elbow dislocation is one of the most common injuries to the elbow. In most instances the first phase of injury persists for 1 to 2 weeks. The principle risk in this early phase is redislocation from excessive extension, but this is rare. The goal of the therapist is to maximize motion without jeopardizing stability. It is helpful for the surgeon, at the time of reducton, to assess stability in extension. For example, if the elbow seems to redislocate at 30° of extension, a program with extension to 45° can commence in the first 2 weeks. At 2 to 3 weeks extension to 30° is allowed, with steady progression to full extension over 6 to 8 weeks. Most patients, despite a vigorous program of rehabilitation, will have a remaining flexion contracture of 20° to 30°, which is seldom disabling.[11,28-30]

Occasionally, a patient will have an associated radial head fracture requiring excision. In this situation, the elbow can be extremely unstable if allowed to extend even beyond 60° to 90°. If signs of brachialis injury or coronoid fracture (another "terrible triad") are present, repair of the fracture or reattachment of the brachialis may be necessary. A hinged orthosis with mechanical extension stops can prevent excessive extension. As the capsule heals in the first few weeks, the stops can be adjusted to allow increasing extension. Most of these patients can expect a flexion contracture of at least 20°.

Radial Head Fracture

Fractures of the radial head seldom require any immobilization.[31-38] If operation is not required, a simple sling can be used. Forearm rotation exercises should begin as soon as possible. These can often be started by the first week. Full supination seems more difficult to achieve than pronation, and we concentrate on this in the early phases. Flexion and extension is also important. Although these fractures often seem minor and have little initial swelling or pain, the time for rehabilitation can last several months.

Fractures of the Distal Humerus

Intrarticular fractures of the distal humerus treated with open reduction and internal fixation require early and vigorous rehabilitation. If skeletal stability is in question, early motion is precluded for fear of loss of fixation and fracture displacement. The surgical approach employed also can influence postoperative therapy. If a triceps splitting approach was used, stress of the repair may cause tendon disruption. For those patients with an olecranon osteotomy, early motion is feasible. We employ the Bryan approach for these fractures, and active motion exercises can be initiated within days of surgery without fear tendon injury.

Before bone healing, sustained passive stretch can be started after the first 2 weeks. Care should be taken to watch for any fracture displacement. Ballistic motion, active or passive, is forbidden. We use a removable custom-molded thermoplastic splint 1 week after surgery. This facilitates hygiene (the patient can shower without the splint) and home exercises.

After the bone is healed, we use a more vigorous program combining hanging weights for extension and assistive active motion for flexion. If at 6 weeks the patient has not achieved motion to 30° short of full extension, a turnbuckle splinting program is started. As long as progress is made and the patient exhibits plasticity during the therapy sessions, the program continues. The duration of therapy in these injuries is quite variable and is influenced by the amount of associated soft tissue injury. If the zone of injury is quite large, the remodeling process can persist for months.

Strengthening usually begins 8 weeks after injury, when bone healing is complete.

Head Injury

Severe trauma that results in both head and elbow injury usually requires a delayed approach with limited goals. Three factors stack the deck against a satisfactory result[39,40]: (1) delayed treatment of the elbow injury, (2) spasticity resulting from the head injury, and (3) extensive heterotopic bone formation secondary to the head injury. Each patient must be evaluated carefully for each stage of treatment. A comprehensive assessment of needs, from hygiene to function, should guide each stage of care.

Arthroplasty

Distraction/Fascial

Rehabilitation following distraction/fascial arthroplasty depends on the method used. If the device used for distraction arthroplasty is a simple hinged device such as that described by Walker and Deland[41] and later modified by Morrey,[18] or the Volkov type, attention to active and passive motion should begin immediately after surgery. Some begin with CPM in the recovery room, but this can lead to hematoma formation. Swelling about the axis pin is also increases pain in the immediate postoperative period.

Once drains are out, usually 2 days after surgery, we begin active motion with passive assist. When not moving, the patient is held in as much extension as possible, using a plaster splint initially. This is later converted to a thermoplastic splint when swelling decreases and the wounds have healed. The greatest difficulty after distraction arthroplasty is reformation of the flexion contracture. There is a reflexive inhibition, probably prompted by posttraumatic inflammation, that limits extremes of motion and active muscle contracture.

Morrey[18] has described the use of the turnbuckle orthosis in combination with the hinged-distractor device in distraction arthroplasty patients. This is usually necessary for several months.

Total Elbow Replacement

Constrained and "Sloppy Hinge" Replacement

After operation the patient's elbow is placed in 80° of flexion and held there with a plaster splint. Two weeks after operation this is changed to a thermoplastic splint, and active ROM exercises with a passive assist are started. With the cemented prosthesis, active motion should not lead to loosening. The triceps mechanism should be protected by extension exercises with a gravity assist until 6 to 8 weeks.

Regaining strength is usually the most difficult aspect of rehabilitation, because most of these patients have had such chronic pain and disability that the muscle atrophy is difficult to overcome. Strengthening exercises continue for 6 months.

Unconstrained Replacement

Unconstrained total elbow replacements require more attention to stability. The surgeon must communicate with the therapist. The risk of posterior dislocation increases as the elbow is extended in the early phases of healing. It is sometimes helpful for the surgeon to record the point of instability at the time of operation and restrict extension movement until the capsule heals. Each prosthesis comes with recommendations for postoperative management. With so many designs presently available the therapist should refer to these resources.

If the therapist detects a sudden change in the ROM, or sudden pain develops, the surgeon should be notified, because it is possible that a dislocation has occurred.

TREATMENT FAILURES

Some patients will not improve despite the best effort. If progress is not being made, then the therapist must review the potential reasons for failure.

Psychology

Poor Compliance

Some patients do not understand biologic concepts. It is the responsibility of the surgeon and the therapist to educate the patient to the best of their ability. A consistent treatment regimen also increases confience and understanding.

The perception of pain varies enormously from patient to patient. Some simply do not tolerate vigorous rehabilitation.

Secondary Gain

Workmen's compensation or pending liability cases often interfere with the patient's motivation toward optimum recovery. It is sometime helpful to counsel the patient about this dilemma, openly recognizing the mixed message sent by society.

Biology

Heterotopic Bone Formation

Heterotopic bone formation after injury can block motion about the elbow after trauma or surgery. The location seems somewhat dependent on the injury itself, although this is not always predictable. Bone can form posteriorly, anteriorly, and around the radial head, blocking forearm rotation. After elbow dislocation, calcification of the collateral ligaments is often seen, but is usually not of any clinical significance.

The formation of heterotopic bone can be quite insidious, or it may be rapid and massive, as in the case of the head-injured patient. It is useful to warn the patients of this possibility. Most patients with severe elbow injuries or large reconstructive procedures probably benefit from the use of oral indomethacin during the first 6 weeks following injury or surgery.[42]

Although low-dose radiation has been used to treat heterotopic bone formation in the hip, we have not used this about the elbow.[43]

Reflex Sympathetic Dystrophy

Reflex sympathetic dystrophy can occur in the hand after elbow injury. In our experience, this is more commonly associated with severe injuries that required or were treated with long periods of complete immobilization, without attention to the hand or fingers. As in all injuries to the upper extremity, it is important to attend to the adjacent joints. Discussion of the use of sympathetic blockade, TENS, and other modalities for reflex sympathetic dystrophy is beyond the scope of this chapter.

REFERENCES

1. Morrey BF, Askew LJ, An KN, Chao EY: A biomechanical study of normal elbow motion. J Bone Joint Surg [Am] 63:872, 1981
2. London JT: Kinematics of the elbow. J Bone Joint Surg [Am] 63:529, 1981
3. Morrey BF, An KN: Articular and ligamentous contributions to the stability of the elbow joint. Am J Sports Med 11:315, 1983
4. Morrey BF, An KN, Stormont TJ: Force transmission through the radial head. J Bone Joint Surg [Am] 70:250, 1988
5. Hotchkiss RN, Weiland AJ: Valgus stability of the elbow. J Orthop Res 5:372, 1987
6. Morrey BF: Biomechanics of the elbow. p. 43. In The Elbow and Its Disorders. WB Saunders, Philadelphia, 1985
7. Sojbjerg JO, Ovensen J, Nielsen S: Experimental elbow instability after transection of the medial collateral ligament. Clin Orthop 218:186, 1987
8. Schwab GH, Bennett JB, Woods GW, Tullos HS: Biomechanics of elbow instability: the role of the medial collateral ligament. Clin Orthop 146:42, 1980
9. Josefsson PO, Gentz CF, Johnell O, Wendeberg B: Surgical versus non-surgical treatment of ligamentous injuries following dislocation of the elbow joint. J Bone Joint Surg [Am] 69:605, 1987
10. Josefsson PO, Johnell O, Wendeberg B: Ligamentous injuries in dislocations of the elbow joint. Clin Orthop 22:221, 1987
11. Mehlhoff TL, Noble PC, Bennett JB, Tullos HS: Simple dislocation of the elbow in the adult. J Bone Joint Surg [Am] 70:244, 1988
12. Fess EE, Philips CA: Hand Splinting: Principles and Methods. p. 2. CV Mosby, St. Louis, 1900
13. Mikic ZD, Vukadinovic SM: Late results in fractures of the radial head treated by excision. Clin Orthop 181:220, 1983
14. Nirschl RP, Morrey BF: Rehabilitation. p. 147. In The Elbow and its Disorders. WB Saunders, Philadelphia, 1985
15. Magness J: Swelling of the upper extremity during whirlpool baths. Arch Phys Med Rehabil 51:297, 1970
16. Breen TF, Gelberman RH, Ackerman GN: Elbow flexion contractures: treatment by anterior release and continuous passive motion. J Hand Surg [Br] 13:286, 1988
17. Salter RB: The effects of continuous passive motion on healing full thickness defects in articular cartilage. J Bone Joint Surg [Am] 62:1232, 1980
18. Morrey BF: Post-traumatic contracture of the elbow. J Bone Joint Surg [Am] 72:601, 1990
19. Lehman J: Therapeutic heat and cold. p. 404. In Therapeutic Heat & Cold. Williams & Wilkins, Baltimore 1982
20. Michlovitz SL: Thermal Agents in Rehabilitation. FA Davis, Philadelphia, 1986
21. Maitland GD: Peripheral Manipulation. Appleton-Century-Crofts, New York, 1970
22. Mennell JM: Joint Pain: Diagnosis and Treatment Using Manipulative Technique. Little, Brown & Company, New York, 1964
23. Hepburn GR, Crivelli K: Use of elbow Dynasplint for reduction of elbow flexion contracture: a case study. J Orthop Phys Ther 5:269, 1984
24. Richard RL: Use of the Dynasplint to correct elbow flexion burn contracture: a case report. J Burn Care Rehabil 7:151, 1986
25. Green DP, McCoy H: Turnbuckle orthotic correction of elbow-flexion contractures after acute injuries. J Bone Joint Surg [Am] 61:1092, 1979
26. Urbaniak JF, Hansen PE, Beissinger SF, Aitken MS: Correction of post-traumatic flexion contracture of the elbow by anterior capsulotomy. J Bone Joint Surg [Am] 67:1160, 1985
27. Stern PJ, Law EJ, Benedict FE, MacMillan BG: Surgical treatment of elbow contractures in postburn children. Plast Reconstr Surg 76:441, 1985
28. Borris LC, Lassen MR, Christensen CS: Elbow dislocation in children and adults. A long-term follow-up of conservatively treated patients. Acta Orthop Scand 58:649, 1987
29. Josefsson PO, Johnell O, Gentz CF: Long-term sequelae of simple dislocation of the elbow. J Bone Joint Surg [Am] 66:927, 1984
30. Linscheid RL: Elbow dislocations. p. 414. In The Elbow and Its Disorders. WB Saunders, Philadelphia, 1985
31. Coleman DA, Blair WF, Shurr D: Resection of the radial head for fracture of the radial head. J Bone Joint Surg [Am] 69:385, 1987
32. Gerard Y, Schernburg F, Nerot C: Anatomical, pathological and therapeutic investigation of fractures of the radial head in adults. J Bone Joint Surg [Br] 66:141, 1984
33. Goldberg I, Peylan J, Yosipovitch Z: Late results of excision of the radial head for an isolated closed fracture. J Bone Joint Surg [Am] 68:675, 1986
34. Morrey BF: Radial head fracture. p. 378. In The Elbow and its Disorders. WB Saunders, Philadelphia, 1985
35. Radin EL, Riseborough EJ: Fractures of the radial head. J Bone Joint Surg [Am] 48:1055, 1966
36. Stephen IBM: Excision of the radial head for closed fracture. Acta Orthop Scand 52:409, 1981
37. Swanson AB, Jaeger SH, La Rochelle D: Comminuted fractures of the radial head. J Bone Joint Surg [Am] 63:1039, 1981
38. Weseley MS, Barenfeld PA, Eisenstein AL: Closed treatment of isolated radial head fractures. J Trauma 23:36, 1983
39. Garland DE, O'Hollaren RM: Fractures and dislocations about the elbow in the head injured adult. Clin Orthop 168:38, 1982
40. Roberts JB, Pankratz DG: The surgical treatment of heterotopic ossification at the elbow following long-term coma. J Bone Joint Surg 61A:760, 1979
41. Deland JJ, Garg A, Walker PS: Biochemical basis for an elbow hinge distractor design. Clin Orthop 215:303, 1987
42. McLaren AC: Prophylaxis with indomethacin for heterotopic bone after open reduction of fracture of the acetabulum. J Bone Joint Surg [Am] 72:245, 1990
43. Coventry MB, Scanlon PW: The use of radiation to discourage ectopic bone. A nine year study in surgery about the hip. J Bone Joint Surg [Am] 63:201, 1981

53 Rehabilitation of the Shoulder

MICHAEL J. SKYHAR
THOMAS C. SIMMONS

GENERAL CONSIDERATIONS

The shoulder is the most mobile of all the joints in the body. The inherent bony constraints present in the glenohumeral joint are minimal. The stability, strength, and function of the glenohumeral articulation depend directly on ligaments, tendons, muscles, and surrounding joints. In addition to the glenohumeral joint, the scapulothoracic, acromioclavicular, and sternoclavicular joints are integral components of a normally functioning shoulder. It is the combined normal actions of all of these structures that allows the shoulder to act as a platform from which the upper extremity can perform all its functions.

The biomechanics of the shoulder have been poorly understood historically. In the past 5 years, research on basic science of the shoulder has proliferated. This new knowledge has allowed shoulder rehabilitation to become more specific and scientific.

The shoulder is, perhaps, the most challenging portion of the body to rehabilitate. Traumatic, degenerative, and surgical lesions of this region generally are perceived as being inordinately painful. The shoulder also has a propensity toward soft tissue fibrosis and contracture after injury and surgery.

The goals of shoulder rehabilitation are to relieve pain, restore muscle strength, and maximize dynamic function. The therapist must realize that there are no "cookbook" approaches to rehabilitation of the shoulder. The disease process and goals of the patient must be considered when planning a rehabilitation approach. Most importantly, realistic expectations must be accepted by the patient, surgeon, and therapist regarding the potential outcome of the particular shoulder problem. Patients must be encouraged to assume an active role in both understanding and carrying out their own shoulder rehabilitation. Patients cannot be expected to perform shoulder exercises with ease if they do not, or cannot, understand rehabilitation objectives. Likewise, therapists must understand the specific anatomic problem, current objectives, and limitations to complete their jobs safely and effectively.

When the patient has had surgery, only the surgeon knows the quality and limitations of the repair and whether the rehabilitation goal is joint stability, mobility, or both. In general, exercises to regain joint mobility are given priority over strengthening exercises.

ASSESSMENT OF SHOULDER FUNCTION

Subjective Assessment

Pain and consequential diminished range of motion are the most common presenting complaints about the shoulder. Knowing the patient's age and shoulder pain history can often lead to the diagnosis. The onset, site, character, periodicity, and radiation of the pain as well as associated symptoms (such as weakness) and aggravating or relieving factors are very important. It is sometimes very difficult to differentiate neck or radicular pain from a primary pathologic condition of the shoulder. In general, referred pain to the shoulder from the cervical spine is maximal over the top of the shoulder, radiates in a specific distribution (usually below the elbow), and is relieved by rest. This type of pain often diminishes at night and is aggravated by cervical spine motion or stress testing. Primary shoulder pathologic states usually are manifested as poorly defined pain over the anterolateral aspect of the shoulder, which is aggravated by moving the shoulder through the range of motion, and which worsens at night. Although radiation of pain below the elbow can occur, this is very uncommon in primary pathologic conditions of the shoulder.

Pain is a subjective complaint, and evaluators of shoulder function must be able to quantitate objectively the amount of pain a patient is experiencing. This is very important in assessing results of shoulder rehabilitation. Several factors can be assessed to acquire an objective evaluation of a patient's shoulder pain:

1. Quantification of anti-inflammatory, analgesic, and narcotic requirements and their effects
2. Presence or absence of night pain
3. Specific amount of interference with sports, work, or activities of daily living
4. Use of a linear pain scale, such as a scale of 1 to 10

Objective Assessment

Inspection

Examination of the shoulder should begin with a general visual inspection of the entire shoulder girdle and upper extremity on both sides. Four general features must be evaluated.

Attitude of Shoulder and Upper Extremity

Many patients with chronic shoulder pain will elevate the involved shoulder, and hold the arm stiff during ambulation. Patients in acute pain often will cradle the injured upper extremity with the opposite arm in an adducted and internally rotated position.

Deformity or Atrophy

Masses, bumps, and lumps must be discovered. Specific and generalized muscle atrophy can be diagnosed by comparison to the opposite, normal ex-

tremity. Specific muscle atrophy can be due to a pathologic condition of the rotator cuff or be of neurogenic origin, as with scapular winging. Specific sites of swelling may assist in the diagnosis of acute injuries. The biceps must always be inspected for evidence of long head rupture.

Skin

The skin must be inspected for scars, erythema, ecchymosis, and other evidence of disease.

Palpation

Palpation for specific sites of pain in the shoulder is not as rewarding as at other anatomic sites because the glenohumeral joint is located so deeply beneath layers of muscles. The examiner can readily palpate the superficial areas for tenderness, however. The acromioclavicular and sternoclavicular joints can be palpated for effusions, instability, and pain. Tenderness in the bicipital groove can indicate biceps tendinitis or impingement. The scapula and acromion can be palpated for masses and fractures. The area of the greater tuberosity is a common site for rotator cuff tears and calcific tendonitis.

Range of Motion

Assuming a maximal arm elevation potential of 180°, the glenohumeral joint contributes about 120° and the scapulothoracic approximately 60°. The glenohumeral joint allows all the humeral rotation.

Virtually all functional glenohumeral motion, including elevation, occurs in the plane of the scapula. Most routine arm functions are performed with the humerus in the plane of the scapula. The concept of *total shoulder elevation* is based on the fact that the plane of the scapula provides the easiest path for the arm to reach its maximal elevation potential. Most systems for recording shoulder motion dwell on pure maximal forward flexion and abduction. However, total elevation is a much more meaningful and functional measurement. The extent of shoulder motion in any person depends on multiple factors, including age, sex, ligamentous laxity, and body habitus. The best example of "normal motion" in any patient is the motion in the opposite, asymptomatic shoulder.

THE SOCIETY OF AMERICAN SHOULDER AND ELBOW SURGEONS BASIC SHOULDER EVALUATION FORM

Name _____

Shoulder: R/L
Hospital No. _____

Date of Examination: _____
(Circle choice)

I. Pain: (5 = none, 4 = slight, 3 = after unusual activity, 2 = moderate, 1 = marked, 0 = complete disability, and NA = not available) _____
II. Motion
   A. Patient sitting (enter motion or NA if not measured):
      1. Active total elevation of arm: _____degrees
      2. Passive internal rotation:
         (Circle segment of posterior anatomy reached by thumb)
         (Enter NA if reach restricted by limited elbow flexion)

1 = Less than trochanter	8 = L2	15 = T7
2 = Trochanter	9 = L1	16 = T6
3 = Gluteal	10 = T12	17 = T5
4 = Sacrum	11 = T11	18 = T4
5 = L5	12 = T10	19 = T3
6 = L4	13 = T9	20 = T2
7 = L3	14 = T8	21 = T1

      3. Active external rotation with arm at side: _____ degrees.
      4. Passive external rotation at 90° abduction: _____ degrees.
         (enter "NA" if cannot achieve 90° of abduction)
   B. Patient supine:
      1. Passive total elevation of arm: _____ degrees.*
      2. Passive external rotation with arm at side: _____ degrees.

III. Strength (5 = normal, 4 = good, 3 = fair, 2 = poor, 1 = trace, 0 = paralysis, and NA = not available) (Enter numbers below)
   A. Anterior deltoid _____
   B. Middle deltoid _____
   C. External rotation _____
   D. Internal rotation _____

IV. Stability (5 = normal, 4 = apprehension, 3 = rare subluxation, 2 = recurrent subluxation, 1 = recurrent dislocation, 0 = fixed dislocation, and NA = not available)
(Enter numbers below)
   A. Anterior _____
   B. Posterior _____
   C. Inferior _____

V. Function (4 = normal, 3 = mild compromise, 2 = difficulty, 1 = with aid, 0 = unable, and NA = not available) (Enter numbers below)
   A. Use back pocket (if male); fasten bra (if female) _____
   B. Perineal care _____
   C. Wash opposite axilla _____
   D. Eat with utensil _____
   E. Comb hair _____
   F. Use hand with arm at shoulder level _____
   G. Carry 10 to 15 lb with arm at side _____
   H. Dress _____
   I. Sleep on affected side _____
   J. Pulling _____
   K. Use hand overhead _____
   L. Throwing _____
   M. Lifting _____
   N. Do usual work _____ (Specify type of work) _____
   O. Do usual sport _____ (Specify sport) _____

VI. Patient Response:
(Circle choice)
(3 = much better, 2 = better, 1 = same, 0 = worse, and NA = not available/applicable)

*Total elevation of the arm is measured by viewing the patient from the side and using a goniometer to determine the angle between the arm and the thorax.

Fig. 53-1. The shoulder evaluation form adopted by the American Society of Shoulder and Elbow Surgeons.

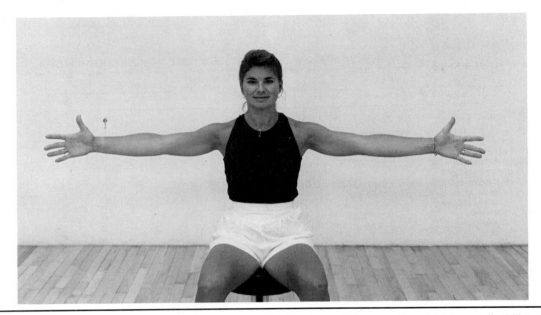

Fig. 53-2. Total elevation of the shoulder is measured in the plane of the scapula, which is usually 20° to 30° anterior in relation to the plane of pure abduction.

Therefore, it is very important to observe and document range of motion in both shoulders at the initial evaluation.

To facilitate more uniform reporting, the Society of American Shoulder and Elbow Surgeons has adopted a simplified reproducible system for evaluation of shoulder range of motion (Fig. 53-1). The Society has agreed that the following components represent a minimum that needs to be reported.

Total Elevation, Both Active and Passive (Fig. 53-2)

The plane of motion for total elevation usually occurs about 20° to 30° from the sagittal plane, but that may be influenced by the presence of shoulder disorder. Total active elevation is measured by asking the patient to raise the arm against gravity in the scapular plane while seated. The seated position allows both unrestricted motion of the scapula and function of its muscles. It also eliminates compensatory lumbar spinal, pelvic, and leg motions, which may confuse the measurements, as occurs in the standing position (Fig. 53-3).

Measurement of passive total elevation of the arm is accomplished with the patient supine. The examining table can serve as a reference point from which to measure, and the presence of the table effectively eliminates lower extremity and spinal motion. Total shoulder elevation is measured in the range of 0° to 180°. During initial evaluation of total elevation, it is important to note the relative contributions of scapulothoracic and glenohumeral motions. Shrugging of the shoulder during attempted arm elevation is a sure sign of a pathologic shoulder condition. (Fig. 53-4).

External Rotation

External rotation of the arm is measured in two different arm positions. Active and passive external rotation is measured with the arm at the side. Active and passive external rotation should also be measured with the arm in 90° of abduction. It is not unusual to see abnormalities in one position of external rotation that might not be present in the other position. For instance, a patient with anterior instability will have limited external rotation at 90° of abduction but will have normal external rotation, both active and passive, with the arm at the side.

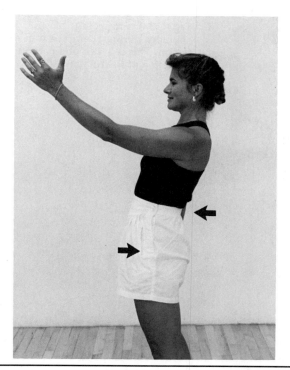

Fig. 53-3. Apparent arm elevation can be increased in the standing position by compensatory lumbar lordosis and hip extension. The seated position allows a more accurate measurement of true total active elevation.

Another example would be a baseball pitcher, who would have excess external rotation at 90° of abduction compared to the opposite side. Therefore, it is very important to compare the range of external rotation of both upper extremities, in both positions.

To record external rotation with the arm at the side, the elbow should be flexed to 90° and the forearm should be in the sagittal plane. The patient should be seated to measure active range of motion. The upright position eliminates the effects of gravity and allows easy comparison to the opposite side. Passive external rotation of the arm should be measured with the patient supine, which eliminates thoracic motion and provides relaxation (Fig. 53-5A). External rotation at the side is recorded from a range of 0° at the neutral position to 90° of maximum external rotation.

External rotation with the arm abducted 90° should be measured with the patient seated, observing this motion in both upper extremities simultaneously. Again, the seated position will eliminate compensatory motions, which confuse the reading. Passive external rotation with the arm abducted to 90° should be measured with the patient supine, noting apprehension in the terminus of motion (Fig. 53-5B).

Internal Rotation

Internal rotation of the arm has typically been awkward to measure because the trunk gets in the way with the forearm moving in the cross-sectional plane. It is much more meaningful to document how far the patient can reach the thumb up the back. This maneuver requires some extension of the shoulder but gives a much more meaningful and reproducible way to measure internal rotation. To accomplish this measurement, active or passive, the patient should be seated and the examiner must have free access to the patient's back.

When measuring active motion, the patient is asked to move the hand around to the back by internally rotating the arm and then placing the thumb in the hitch-hiking position as far up the spine as possible (Fig. 53-6). The maneuver is then repeated with the opposite extremity. Passive motion is performed much the same way, with the patient seated, except that the examiner is moving the extremity to the point of pain tolerance or motion limitation. The vast majority of patients are able to raise the hand at least to the level of the greater trochanter. Useful anatomic landmarks for measuring and documenting internal rotation start at the greater trochanter. The following landmarks can be used to document progressive internal rotation: gluteal region, sacrum, and each vertebral spinous process from L5 through T1.

Muscle Strength

The standard grading system (0 to 5) for motor strength should be used. All motor groups of each upper extremity should be tested systematically during the initial evaluation. This becomes especially salient when a pathologic condition of the cervical spine or radiculopathy is suspected.

The majority of shoulder problems encountered by physicians are caused by lesions of musculotendinous units. These lesions will invariably be mani-

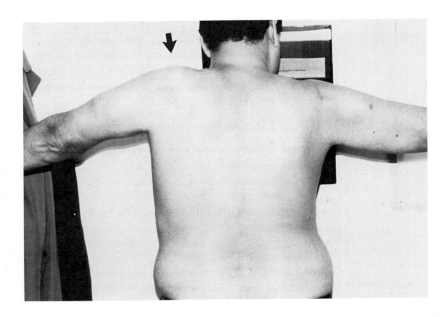

Fig. 53-4. Shrugging of the left shoulder during attempted arm elevation. This is a sign of a pathologic condition of the rotator cuff.

fested as a significant motor weakness about the shoulder. Assuming no neurologic involvement, the following motor tests should be performed, because they usually indicate a primary pathologic condition of the shoulder.

1. *External rotation at the side.* Weakness of external rotation at the side usually indicates a significant rotator cuff tear.
2. *Abduction.* Weakness in initiating and sustaining pure abduction of the shoulder usually occurs with rotator cuff incompetence.
3. *Deltoid muscle.* Anterior, middle, and posterior bundles of the deltoid muscle should always be tested, because weakness of this muscle is a sensitive indicator of a shoulder disorder, much like the quadriceps is for the knee.

Stability

Stability of the glenohumeral joint depends mainly on intact and normally functioning glenohumeral ligaments and rotator cuff. Shoulder instability can be classified according to the system developed at the Hospital for Special Surgery, New York (Table 53-1). A combination of a good history and physical examination usually is all that is necessary to classify a shoulder instability. Being able to correctly classify shoulder instability is crucial to initiating proper treatment and to subsequent rehabilitation. The primary direction of instability is perhaps the most diffi-

cult determination for physicians and physical therapists to make. Although most instability is anteroinferior, instability can occur in any direction or combination of directions. Determining arm position at the moment of instability is mandatory when obtaining a history. Anterior instability is usually associated with the abducted and externally rotated arm position. Posterior instability is manifested with the arm in flexion, internal rotation, and adduction. Inferior laxity is noted with axial downward traction on the arm, manifested by an asymmetrical sulcus sign. Inferior laxity is usually associated with multidirectional instability.

Examination of the glenohumeral joint for stability should be performed routinely in any shoulder evaluation. This can easily be done in the operating room under anesthesia, with the patient fully relaxed. It is much more difficult to perform with the patient fully awake, however. Many patients with symptomatic instability are apprehensive with any type of stress testing and exhibit protective reflex muscle recruitment. This makes evaluation of stability impossible. The key to successful evaluation of glenohumeral stability is complete patient relaxation. The patients also must have confidence that the examiner is not going to hurt them. The technique for examination is identical in the office and under anesthesia.

Fig. 53-5. External rotation should be measured at the side **(A)** and at 90° of abduction **(B)** while supine.

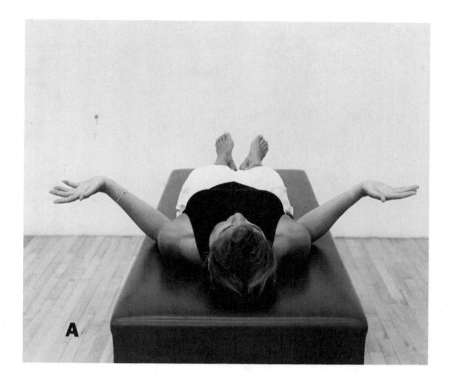

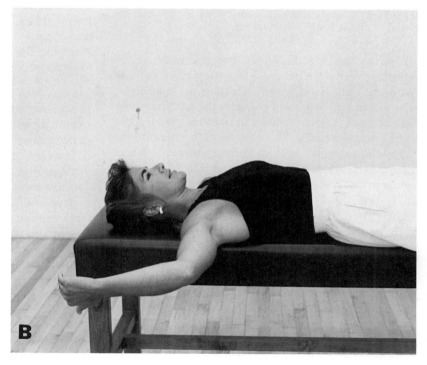

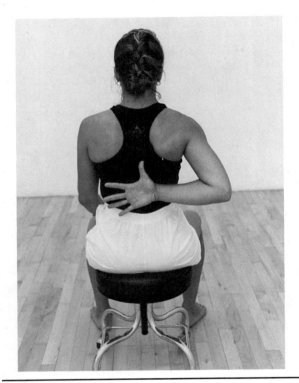

Fig. 53-6. Internal rotation is measured by placing the "thumb up the back" while seated.

To stress the right shoulder, the examiner, while kneeling next to the patient, holds the patient's elbow with the right hand, gently applying an axial load. The examiner's left hand palpates the humeral head and acts as a fulcrum to lever the patient's head anteriorly or posteriorly. The degree of humeral head translation is noted with the arm abducted 90° and neutrally rotated. Flexion or extension of the arm while in this position can be utilized to amplify instability (Fig. 53-7). Increasing external rotation will tighten the anterior capsule, preventing the examiner from noting the degree of anterior translation. Similarly, internal rotation will tighten the posterior capsule, decreasing perceived posterior laxity. By altering the degree of rotation and axial load, the optimum arm position for provoking maximal glenohumeral translation can be found. Shoulder instability is graded according to the system developed at the Hospital for Special Surgery. Grade I, or subluxation, implies greater than 50 percent humeral head translation on the glenoid without dislocation. The presence of grinding in the labrum should be noted.

Table 53-1. Hospital for Special Surgery Shoulder Instability Classification

A. Frequency
  1. Acute
  2. Recurrent
  3. Fixed
B. Etiology
  1. Traumatic (macrotrauma)
  2. Atraumatic
    a. Voluntary
    b. Involuntary
  3. Microtrauma (repetitive use)
  4. Congenital
  5. Neuromuscular (cerebral palsy, Erb's palsy, seizures)
C. Degree
  1. Dislocation
  2. Subluxation
  3. Micro
D. Direction
  1. Anterior
  2. Posterior
  3. Inferior
  4. Multidirectional

Grade II is frank dislocation without locking. Grade III is dislocation associated with the ability to lock the humeral head over the edge of the glenoid. Generalized ligamentous laxity should be factored in when assessing the outcome of any shoulder stability examination.

In addition to supine stability testing, inferior laxity of both glenohumeral joints should be tested with the patient standing. With the patient fully relaxed, equal downward traction is applied to both arms. A "sulcus" will form just inferior to the anterior edge of the acromion. The sulcus sign is measured in centimeters and should be symmetrical. A significant (greater than 1 cm) unilateral increase in the sulcus sign on one side indicates inferior glenohumeral laxity, which is usually associated with multidirectional instability (Fig. 53-8).

Infrequently, the stability profile cannot be obtained in an awake, apprehensive patient. In these cases, the history is extremely important. If in doubt, examination under anesthesia can be performed and, in fact, should always be performed immediately prior to operating on any shoulder.

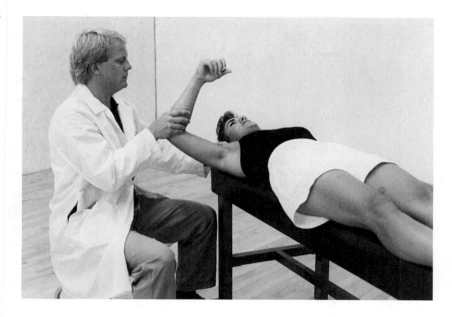

Fig. 53-7. Technique for supine shoulder stability assessment. The technique is the same whether in the office or under anesthesia.

The mastery of shoulder stability testing requires patience and practice. When performed properly, there is no indication for diagnostic radiologic adjunctive studies.

Functional Assessment

Finally, it is very helpful to document specific functional capabilities of the shoulder. Improvement in levels of functional capabilities after treatment and rehabilitation of the shoulder is the goal for most patients. The shoulder evaluation form from the Society of American Shoulder and Elbow Surgeons lists multiple activities that indicate general shoulder health (Fig. 53-1). Both the medical team and the patient can monitor functional abilities as treatment proceeds.

BASIC RULES OF SHOULDER REHABILITATION

1. *Exercises to regain range of motion have priority over exercises to strengthen.* It makes no sense to try to regain strength when motion is still abnormal. Strengthening exercises near the terminus of any range of shoulder motion generally are associated with pain. The major goal in the rehabilitation of all types of shoulder problems, including surgical problems, is maintenance and restoration of motion.

2. *There is nothing wrong with scapular elevation.* Normal motion of the shoulder requires elevation of the scapula. If this did not occur, there would be impingement of the greater tuberosity on the underside of the acromion. It is unwise to force patients to keep their scapulae immobilized when attempting to restore arm motion and elevation.

3. *Record motion and functional capabilities at each rehabilitation session.* Graphic records give the medical team, as well as the patient, good feedback regarding progress of a particular shoulder problem.

4. *Early passive motion is not unsafe.* Passive range of motion exercises performed by the physician or therapist at any time postoperatively are safe, provided that the ranges used correspond to those limitations determined by the orthopaedist at surgery.

5. *Establish realistic functional goals.* Patients, physicians and therapists who have unrealistic goals often end up frustrated. In certain shoulder problems, such as end-stage cuff disease, the functional goals may be very limited. If the medical team and the patient understand this from the outset, there will be fewer hard feelings in the end. It is very important to give the patient as much positive feedback as possible, as in any rehabilitation setting.

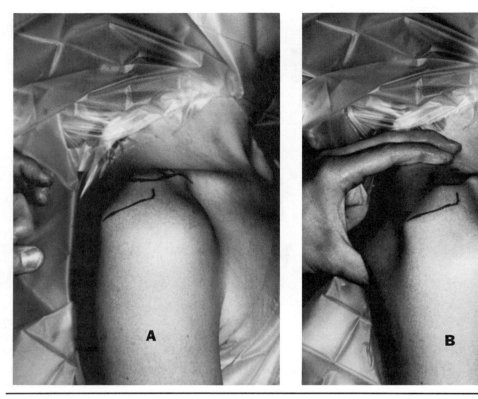

Fig. 53-8. The sulcus sign is produced by downward traction on the arm. **(A)** Shoulder without downward traction. **(B)** Large sulcus sign. Comparison of the two sides must be performed and differences quantitated.

6. Avoid those activities or modalities that markedly increase pain. Some pain is normal, but pain can become a negative reinforcement if consistently inflicted by a therapist.

7. Start functional treatments early with appropriate dosage being the key. Communications between physician and therapist should occur early and often. The therapist should not worry about reporting negative findings or lack of progress but should stress to patient's a determination to help them improve. The need for complete compliance also is stressed.

REHABILITATION OF SPECIFIC SHOULDER PROBLEMS

Rotator Cuff

Rotator cuff disorders are the most common cause of shoulder pain. The muscles of the rotator cuff are tonic and are therefore highly dependent on an ade-

quate blood supply and oxygen tension. A watershed area for the blood supply exists in the marginal supraspinatus tendon.[1] The key to rotator cuff rehabilitation is to provide a pain-free environment for revascularization of the tendons of the rotator cuff. Our approach to rotator cuff rehabilitation is based on the teachings of Ola Grimsby, M.N.F.F., M.N.S.M.T. The initial goal is to facilitate tendon revascularization through isolation and reinforcement of high repetition, nonresistive tonic cuff musculature activity.[2]

Nonsurgical Rotator Cuff Rehabilitation

Treatment should always begin as soon as possible. During episodes of acute inflammation, the weight of the arm alone is enough to aggravate pain. Eliminating the weight of the arm, which must be done before initiating therapy, can be accomplished by any method provided that the humerus can rotate on its own axis. The patient progresses from 50 to 100 repetitions a day of simple pain-free, active internal and

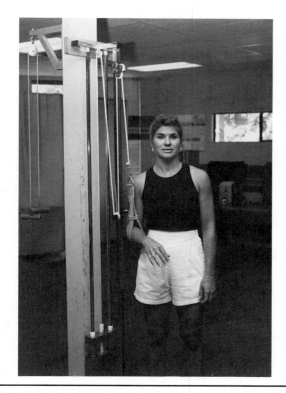

Fig. 53-9. Technique for performing unweighted axial humeral rotation.

external rotation to three sets of 100 repetitions a day (Fig. 53-9). The cumulative total of repetitions should be 5,000 to 6,000. Next, abduction followed by forward flexion can begin gradually. This should be initiated by moving the body, not the arm, with a tilt table. For forward flexion, the prone position may be used. Axial rotation is again stressed in varying degrees of abduction and forward flexion, in pain-free arcs of motion. Once satisfactory increases in forward flexion and abduction have been gained with the arm unweighted, active forward flexion may begin. The biceps and eventually the coracobrachialis muscles are used to create humeral head depression during forward flexion. Once active forward flexion becomes easier, abduction may begin. The program must continue without irritating the involved muscle or muscles. If high-repetition adduction cannot be performed, pain-free active assisted exercise is started using a pulley system. Muscle oxygenation and coordination will improve, allowing pain-free active motion.

The regimen for progression of resistive exercises and repetitions is patterned after Odvar Holten's 1-RM (100 percent resistance maximum) pyramid[3] (Fig. 53-10). This allows the therapist to assess and treat any stage of muscle rehabilitation objectively. Finally, sport-specific exercises may begin.

Rehabilitation of the scapular stabilizer muscles should begin simultaneously with that of the rotator cuff. If these muscles are weak or elongated, their ability to facilitate phasic activity diminishes, resulting in decreased rotator cuff efficiency. Instruction in scapular positioning is imperative for developing increased rotator cuff tension and strength. Average conservative treatment time for the rotator cuff varies but typically lasts 1 to 3 months.

Rehabilitation after Rotator Cuff Surgery

At the time of rotator cuff repair, it is imperative that the surgeon determine the "safe zone" for shoulder range of motion. This should be communicated to the therapist, because the pain-free range of motion is not always synonymous with the safe zone of range of motion. The safe zone is that range of motion that does not place stress on the rotator cuff repair. In most stable repairs, the safe zone is full range of motion. As long as the safe zone is respected, early passive and/or active motion may begin immediately or as soon as the patient can tolerate it. Early passive range of motion starts 1 to 2 days postoperatively. Codman's exercises are used first to facilitate patient relaxation. Passive stretching within the safe zone is then performed, gradually increasing the range as pain permits. Unweighted axial rotation of the arm, as mentioned earlier, may also begin. This is performed five times a day until the patient is ready to perform these exercises actively. The therapist can teach a friend or relative of the patient to continue these exercises at home.[4]

Initiation of active motion depends on the size and quality of the repair of the rotator cuff tear. Generally, passive and active assisted range-of-motion exercises are continued for a full 6 weeks postoperatively. Many patients obtain pain relief early on by placing a pillow between the body and arm, especially at night, which takes tension off the cuff. Gentle active motion may begin, using the protocol for

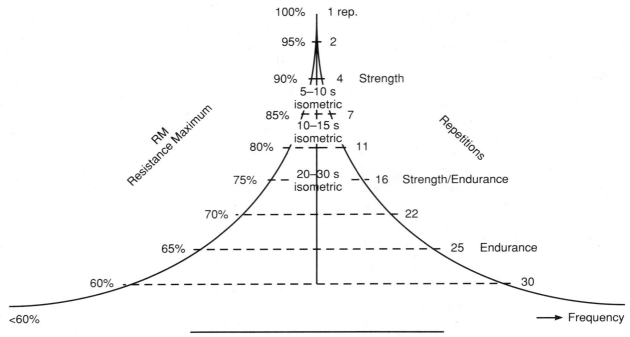

Fig. 53-10. The Odvar Holten pyramid diagram.

conservative rotator cuff rehabilitation, including isometrics. Placing of large, unexpected loads on the shoulder should be avoided for 6 to 9 months after surgery. Proper rehabilitation after rotator cuff surgery is mandatory and usually needs to be controlled directly by the surgeon.

Adhesive Capsulitis

Many criteria have been advanced for the diagnosis of adhesive capsulitis. Any case of chronic diminished passive and active range of motion of the shoulder joint that is not the result of a neurogenic, tendinous, or biomechanical cause probably is adhesive capsulitis. It has a multifactorial etiology and is definitely phasic in nature. The basic pathologic process is diminished volume and elasticity of the joint capsule.

Adhesive capsulitis is a very difficult problem for both physician and therapist and should be avoided through early physical therapy intervention. Prolonged immobilization is destructive to tissue and obviously nonfunctional. Therapists perform an essential role as teachers, instructing patients about the natural history of their condition and directing rehabilitation.

Regardless of the length of time symptoms have been present or the phase of the disease, physical therapy should be the initial mode of treatment. Numerous other adjunctive treatments have been advocated. Gentle, slow stretching of the joint capsule should be performed using joint mobilization techniques, with high-repetition active or active assisted range-of-motion exercises. Attempts at forced stretching of the adhering capsule only provoke a more vigorous inflammatory response, causing pain and diminishing the patient's confidence in the therapist. Any gains in motion attained by forceful maneuvers in therapy generally are short lived and frustrating. Patients must be told to be persistent and patient because results will be slow. Modalities such as heat, ice, and ultrasound, are useful for pain control, but have no utility for increasing range of motion. At least 6 weeks of physical therapy should be attempted.

When it becomes clear that the patient's range of motion has plateaued, closed manipulation of the shoulder under anesthesia should be performed, if indicated. This normally is an outpatient procedure. After manipulation, physical therapy is performed daily to maintain range of motion for up to 2 weeks, if necessary. Techniques carried out after manipulation are similar to those used before manipulation but are more aggressive. Use of a continuous passive motion machine at home is sometimes helpful. Restraining the arm in an overhead position while sleeping at night helps to maintain motion. Once range of motion is nearly normal, strengthening exercise may begin, making use of any method. The need for a second manipulation is very uncommon.

Instability

When true glenohumeral laxity is present, muscle strengthening is of limited utility for preventing glenohumeral laxity during dynamic functions. Remember that masculature about the shoulder contributes to only a minor degree to stability of the glenohumeral joint, as opposed to the joint capsule and glenohumeral ligaments.[5] Instability in any direction resulting from ligamentous laxity (nontraumatic) responds to rehabilitation more consistently than any instability of traumatic origin. However, we highly recommend a trial of conservative treatment prior to embarking on any more definitive treatment. The goals of instability rehabilitation are the strengthening of specific muscle groups and, more importantly, increasing their sensitivity to stretch.

Grimsby's three-stage program is useful for accomplishing this rehabilitation.[3] Stage I begins with low-speed, high-repetition, minimum-resistive exercise in the beginning and middle ranges of motion. Stage I is meant to increase muscle endurance and circulation, avoiding overexertion. Stage II involves increasing resistance and adding isometrics in the inner ranges of motion. This will increase strength and sensitivity to stretch. Stage III continues to increase resistance (usually 80 percent 1-RM) and adds isometrics through a full but not maximal range of motion. Increasing the stretch sensitivity of the rotator cuff musculotendinous units may be protective in the outermost ranges of shoulder motion, where instability typically occurs. When treating anterior instability, rehabilitation should concentrate on the internal rotators and adductors (pectoralis, subscapularis, latissimus dorsi, anterior deltoid muscles). For poste-

rior instability, the external rotators are emphasized (posterior deltoid, infraspinatus, and teres minor and major muscles). Multidirectional instability requires comprehensive rotator cuff rehabilitation.

After Surgery for Instability

As with rotator cuff surgery, the surgeon must determine the safe zone for range of motion at the time of surgery. Early passive motion exercising may usually begin immediately within the safe zone. Active biceps and triceps, forearm, and wrist exercises may begin immediately. After surgery for instability, the goal is full shoulder range of motion and eventual return to unrestricted sporting activities.

Developing a set routine for rehabilitation after instability surgery is ill advised. For example, a young woman with ligamentous laxity should progress much more slowly than an elderly man who begins with a moderate degree of stiffness.

After Anterior Stabilization

The motions to be protected after anterior stabilizations are external rotation and abduction. Early passive motion may begin within the safe zone immediately. At 3 to 4 weeks postoperatively, the shoulder is checked for stiffness and a formal physical therapy program started. If the surgeon believes that stiffness is imminent, slow passive stretching beyond the safe zone may begin right away. Usually a shoulder immobilizer is worn for 6 weeks. Beyond 6 weeks postoperatively, passive stretching beyond the safe zone may definitely begin. For the next full 6 weeks, passive, active assisted, and active exercises should be used to gain nearly full range of motion. During this time strengthening within the safe zone may begin, including isometrics. Beyond 3 months postoperatively, Grimsby's third stage of rehabilitation may begin. Contact sports are not allowed for 9 months postoperatively. The rehabilitation is performed exactly the same way whether the stabilization was performed in an open operation or arthroscopically.

After Posterior Stabilization

An orthosis designed to maintain the shoulder in external rotation at the side is worn for 6 weeks after posterior stabilization. During this time, internal rotation beyond neutral is not allowed. However, unlimited wrist and elbow active exercises and shoulder isometrics may begin. During the second 6 weeks, range of motion is regained slowly using passive and active assisted exercises. Strengthening may begin when range of motion is nearly full, using Grimsby's approach. Maximal internal rotation and adduction are attained slowly. Unlimited strengthening may occur from 3 to 6 months postoperatively. Easy throwing may begin at 6 months postoperatively and contact sports can be resumed at 9 months.

After Surgery for Multidirectional Instability

Depending on the direction and degree of laxity, an anterior, posterior, or combined capsular shift type of procedure will be performed. The main goal of this type of surgery is elimination of inferior capsular laxity. A well-fitting shoulder immobilizer is worn for 6 weeks to prevent the weight of the arm from causing inferiorly directed shear across the capsulorrhaphy. Recall that multidirectional instability is usually associated with generalized ligamentous laxity, so that rehabilitation must progress more slowly after surgery. Permanent rotational contractures are unusual after this type of operation. Beyond the initial 6-week period of complete shoulder immobilization, gentle passive, active assisted, isometric, and active range-of-motion exercises may begin and continue for 3 to 4 months. Joint mobilization techniques using inferior gliding and traction on the arm must be avoided. At 4 months postoperatively, comprehensive rotator cuff and shoulder girdle muscular rehabilitation may begin. Contact sports and throwing are not allowed for 1 year.

Rehabilitation of Protective Reflexes

The longer patients have had shoulder instability, the more likely it is that they have developed "apprehensive mental contractures" and reflexive protective shoulder mechanics. A very important aspect of rehabilitation in cases of shoulder instability is helping patients overcome these apprehensions. Restoration of normal shoulder biomechanics takes a great deal of patience on the therapist's part and may require a year or longer.

Impingement Syndrome

The impingement syndrome progresses through a series of stages, regardless of cause. Etiologic factors include trauma, abnormal acromial morphology, acromioclavicular joint prominence, proximal humeral fractures, overuse syndromes, parascapular muscle weakness, rotator cuff tears, and glenohumeral instability. The cause will determine the length and severity of the disease. The basic pathologic process is diminished volume in the subacromial space, also known as a diminished supraspinatus outlet. Normally the outlet volume diminishes with shoulder elevation and rotation in abduction. When the resting volume of the space is decreased as a result of any of the reasons given earlier, these motions create impingement of the rotator cuff tendons on thickened bursa or acromion, or on both, resulting in pain. The eventual outcome is altered shoulder biomechanics in the short run and ultimately an attritional rotator cuff tear. Adhesive capsulitis may result at any point. Regardless of the stage of the disease, rehabilitation can restore the shoulder to an acceptable functional level.

During the phase of acute inflammation, range of motion must be maintained with passive and active assisted range of motion. Joint mobilization techniques using inferior gliding are very useful to relieve stenosis of the subacromial space. Recruitment of the humeral head depressor muscles (biceps, coracobrachialis, subscapularis, infraspinatus) also is mandatory during range-of-motion exercises. When the inflammatory phase diminishes (1 to 2 weeks), rotator cuff and scapular stabilizer rehabilitation may begin. High-repetition and low-resistance exercises should be used. They should be performed exclusively with the shoulder below the horizontal (90° of abduction, 90° of flexion) (Fig. 53-11). This is carried out for 6 weeks, and during this time all unnecessary overhead activities are avoided. If symptoms are markedly diminished, gentle slow rotator cuff rehabilitation above the horizontal may begin. Sports and other activities using overhead motion usually can be performed at about 3 to 6 months after the onset of treatment. If symptoms persist, further conservative treatment is unlikely to be helpful.

After Acromioplasty

Acromioplasty usually can be performed as an open procedure or arthroscopically without releasing the deltoid muscle from its insertion onto the acromion. However, some surgeons still prefer to release the anterior deltoid as part of an open approach. This has

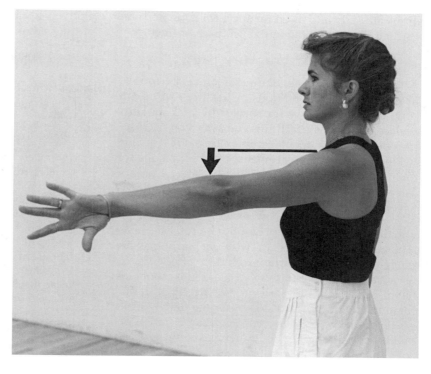

Fig. 53-11. Initial rotator cuff muscle rehabilitation for the impingement syndrome must be performed below the horizontal arm position (90° of abduction or 90° of flexion).

obvious implications for rehabilitation after acromioplasty. If the deltoid muscle has been released, active forward flexion of the shoulder must be avoided for 3 to 4 weeks to allow the insertion to heal. Failure of deltoid repair is a serious complication. If the deltoid muscle was not released, active range of motion may begin immediately. Full range of motion should be gained over 3 to 4 weeks prior to starting resistive exercises. Rotator cuff rehabilitation below the horizontal is then initiated and continued for 3 months. After 3 months, if overhead motion is not painful, rotator cuff rehabilitation above the horizontal and resisted exercise may begin. The subacromial bursa usually takes about 3 months to re-form after surgery, which is why patients remain symptomatic for so long after a seemingly innocuous procedure. If patients try to perform overhead motions in sports prior to 5 to 6 months postoperatively, the recovery course will be prolonged. If the deltoid muscle was released, passive forward flexion is performed for the first 3 to 4 weeks; otherwise the program is the same.

Shoulder Fractures

Shoulder fractures are either stable or unstable from the outset, and generally the unstable fractures require surgical intervention. The goal of any fracture fixation is to allow early motion. In either type, the rehabilitation program is similar. Shoulder fractures are extremely painful, and the patient should be allowed 2 weeks of immobilization prior to starting rehabilitation. This will also allow some early fracture healing to occur. At about 2 to 3 weeks, an early passive motion program may begin if radiographs show no change in fracture position. Passive and active assisted exercises and pulleys are used until 6 to 8 weeks after the fracture, at which time most fractures are healed sufficiently to start a full rotator cuff rehabilitation program. Beyond 8 weeks, any lost motion may be regained with daily gentle stretching exercises without fear of disrupting the fracture.

When severe fractures require proximal humeral replacement, an aggressive early passive range-of-motion program is started 2 to 3 days postoperatively. This situation is believed to differ from other types of fracture fixation because this procedure is associated with a high rate of contracture postoperatively. Once the tuberosities have started to unite to the humeral shaft, an aggressive, full rehabilitation program is maintained until range of motion is nearly normal. It is very important that the surgeon and therapist communicate early and often for specific instructions regarding the rehabilitation of each type of fracture.

Arthroplasty

Arthroplasty of the glenohumeral joint is performed in many different conditions. A healthy rotator cuff complex is mandatory for successful total shoulder replacement. In osteoarthritis and avascular necrosis, the bone and rotator cuff complex are of ideal quality for total shoulder replacement. The best results for total shoulder arthroplasty generally occur in cases of osteoarthritis and avascular necrosis, and these patients are the easiest to rehabilitate.

Rehabilitation after an uncomplicated total shoulder replacement should begin with an early passive range-of-motion program 2 to 3 days after surgery. Because the subscapularis tendon and the rotator interval are violated to perform the surgery, external rotation should proceed slowly for the first 4 weeks postoperatively. Otherwise, aggressive range-of-motion and strengthening exercises should proceed as in the previously described protocol.

Sometimes osteoarthritis is associated with a deficient posterior glenoid or patulous posterior capsule, or both. This predisposes the total shoulder replacement to posterior instability. In these situations, forward flexion with the arm in adduction above the horizontal and elevation of the arm when supine should be avoided for 6 weeks. Similarly, if the total shoulder replacement is performed for arthropathy associated with chronic anterior instability, rehabilitation should proceed very similarly to that for routine anterior stabilization procedures.

When rheumatoid arthritis is the reason for total shoulder replacement, the rotator cuff muscles and tendons usually are of poor quality. Rehabilitation will progress much more slowly and should be directed by the surgeon because of special problems encountered at surgery. In certain situations of rheumatoid arthritis, cuff arthropathy, and posttraumatic deformities, total shoulder replacement is performed for pain relief only, and functional goals are very limited. Appropriate rehabilitation can always help these patients, however.

After total shoulder replacement, no upper extremity weight-bearing activities, such as crutch use and transfers, should be performed for 6 months postoperatively to allow complete healing and rehabilitation of the rotator cuff.

Neuromuscular Problems

A large number of neuromuscular problems can affect the shoulder girdle. A general classification gives an indication of the range of possible pathologic conditions:

1. *Upper motoneuron diseases:* stroke, tumors of brain and spinal cord, head injury, multiple sclerosis, cerebral palsy
2. *Lower motoneuron diseases:* brachial plexus injuries, infectious or idiopathic myelopathy or neuropathy, idiopathic brachial neuritis, spinal cord tumors, cervical radiculopathy, cranial nerve injury, compression neuropathy, peripheral nerve injuries
3. *Myopathies:* muscular dystrophy, inflammatory myopathies, metabolic myopathies, endocrine myopathies, toxic and drug-induced myopathies
4. *Miscellaneous:* reflex sympathetic dystrophy, arthrogryposis, other congenital defects

Most of these problems result in either spasticity, flaccidity, weakness, or specific nerve lesions. Permanent flaccid paralysis generally cannot be helped much with rehabilitation. Passive joint range-of-motion exercises can reduce edema, prevent contractures, and provide some pain relief. After a stroke, the shoulders typically develop internal rotation and adduction contractures because of neglect. Most of these contractures are very painful, and aggressive therapy is necessary to prevent them until the patient regains some volitional control. The use of supportive pillows and splints while in bed is advantageous. Prone positioning with the shoulder abducted and rotated externally is a good stretching maneuver. Forceful stretching should not be performed in any setting, because pain and spasticity may increase. When rehabilitation fails, open surgical release of contractures may be necessary.

The main goal in treating any neuromuscular shoulder problem is prevention of contractures and facilitation of neuromuscular reeducation through high-repetition, low-stress painless therapy. In the future, selective neural and muscular electrical stimulation with computer-enhanced proprioceptive biofeedback may be very useful in this regard. The therapist must always remember that shoulders with neuromuscular problems are susceptible to all of the aforementioned diagnoses, and when treating the patient for shoulder pain, a complete differential diagnosis must be considered.

REFERENCES

1. Rathbun JB, Macnab I: The microvascular pattern of the rotator cuff. J Bone Joint Surg [Br] 52:540, 1970
2. Grimsby O: Manual Therapy of the Extremities. A Course Workbook. Sorlandets Institute, Everett, WA, 1986
3. Grimsby O: Fundamentals of Manual Therapy. A Course Workbook. Sorlandets Institute, Everett, WA, 1985
4. Neer CS: Shoulder Reconstruction. WB Saunders, Philadelphia, 1990
5. Schwartz RE, O'Brien SJ, Torzilli PA, Warren RF: Capsular restraints to anterior-posterior motion of the shoulder. Trans Orthop Res Soc 12:78, 1987

54 Rehabilitation of the Spine

VERT MOONEY

This chapter focuses on nonsurgical care for back and neck problems. The majority of the discussion is focused on the soft tissue causes of back and neck pain, rather than rehabilitation after fractures and other major trauma. Certainly the principles to be described are applicable to these entities as well.

The great majority of neck and back pain must emerge from some soft tissue "injury." Unhappily, physical examination and even imaging studies seldom identify the specific location of this injury. Thus, rational rehabilitation is difficult to advocate in a specific sense: the "weak link" is not known. Thus, some assumptions must be made as to the specific entity being treated with rehabilitation procedures.

Probably the best framework on which to build a rehabilitation program was proposed by the Consensus Committee, which was commissioned by the Quebec government in an effort to curb costs of industrial back injuries and develop mechanisms for a rational treatment program. The Committee reported on the assessment and management of what they called "activity-related spinal disorders." Table 54-1 presents the classification of spinal disorders identified by this committee. As is noted in this table, the first three classifications are based purely on pain location; the other classifications have physical examination or imaging corroboration. A classification of pain without physical signs applies to the majority of back pain patients (and neck pain patients as well) seen in physician's offices. This emphasizes that the majority of spine soft tissue injuries do not have a precise medical diagnosis and prognosis. Thus, a treatment plan focused on rational soft tissue injury care is reasonable. The initial discussion deals with the treatment of acute soft tissue injuries identified by location in the back, buttocks, or legs without radiculopathy. However, many of the other classifications of back disorders, such as spinal stenosis and herniated discs, will also benefit from the rehabilitation procedures advocated later in this chapter.

It should also be noted from Table 54-1 that classification of spinal disorders by duration is advocated by the Committee. Acute injury is identified as 1 week in duration, and subacute 2 to 7 weeks. Anything over 7 weeks in duration is identified as chronic injury. This is quite a departure from previous traditional classifications in which "chronic" usually has been identified as any condition 3 to 6 months in duration. However, it is very reasonable to suggest that chronicity emerges in back injuries after 7 weeks in that little spontaneous recovery of soft tissue can be expected after 7 weeks. Thus, the treatment program must be focused on measures aimed at the health of already deteriorating soft tissues.[1]

ACUTE AND SUBACUTE BACK REHABILITATION

When the pain complaint manifests itself as back pain with limited range of motion, located either in the low back, buttock, or posterior thigh and calf without radiculopathy, it is assumed that there has been some soft tissue injury to the disc, surrounding ligaments, or perhaps even the muscle. No study has been able to differentiate the specific anatomic location based on physical examination. Changes seen by various imaging studies do not suggest the cause in that degenerative changes occur equally in individuals with and without back pain throughout their

Table 54-1. Activity-Related Spinal Disorders

Classification	Symptoms	Duration of Symptoms from Onset	Working Status at Time of Evaluation
1	Pain without radiation		
2	Pain + radiation to extremity, proximally	a (<7 days)	W (working)
3	Pain + radiation to extremity, distally[a]	b (7 days–7 weeks)	I (idle)
4	Pain + radiation to upper/lower limb + neurologic signs	c (>7 weeks)	
5	Presumptive compression of a spinal nerve root on a simple roentgenogram (i.e., spinal instability or fracture)		
6	Compression of a spinal nerve root confirmed by Specific imaging techniques (i.e., computer tomography, myelography, or magnetic resonance imaging) Other diagnostic techniques (e.g., electromyography, venography)		
7	Spinal stenosis		
8	Postsurgical status, 1–6 months after intervention		
9	Postsurgical status, >6 months after intervention 9.1 Asymptomatic 9.2 Symptomatic		
10	Chronic pain syndrome		W (working) I (idle)
11	Other diagnoses		

[a] Not applicable to the thoracic segment.

various decades of life.[2,3] Single-level disc space narrowing may be associated with back pain, but this entity is also present in persons without back pain. For instance, in the study by Frymoyer and colleagues, although 37 percent of those subjects with severe pain had single-level disc space narrowing, 19 percent of those with no pain also had single-level narrowing.[4] Thus, it is reasonable to expect that soft tissue injury, which is the source of back pain, may be at locations other than those that deteriorate into degenerative disc disease. This serves as justification for using pain location and duration as the chief mechanism of classification rather than radiographic studies. As noted previously, the physical examination is not at all helpful in that the soft tissue injury location is not usually reflected by any specific findings.

What is the rational form of treatment of these soft tissue injuries? Should it be bed rest? Fortunately scientific studies have looked at the role of bed rest as a treatment mode for back problems. One study randomized subjects into those restricted to bed rest versus those permitted immediate activity. At 1-year follow-up there was no detectable difference in the speed or extent of pain resolution. In fact, those subjects who were placed at bed rest for at least 4 days took 42 percent longer to return to normal activities.[5] Another study by Deyo et al., which now ranks as a

classic report, demonstrated that those patients assigned to brief bed rest treatment had 45 percent fewer days of work loss than those on prolonged bed rest of 7 days or more. No differences were observed in the course of pain resolution, functional recovery, or satisfaction with care.[6] These results, of course, are quite reasonable from a physiologic standpoint. Proteoglycan and collaginous connective tissues are poorly supplied with blood, and the nutrition to these tissues is achieved primarily by activity and mobilization rather than rest. Assuming that the injury has been to such tissues, their repair would require exchange of fluids that is enhanced by physical changes in posture and position. Thus, there is no rational reason to expect that bed rest in itself will be of benefit to the injured soft tissues that are the source of pain.

What can be done? Assuming that the pain has emerged from some injury to the soft tissue— probably the disc—how can its location be assessed so as to develop a rational treatment plan? Perhaps the best approach to treating the soft tissue injury is the McKenzie method. The majority of persons with soft tissue back injuries are classified in this conceptual scheme as having a syndrome of derangement (Table 54-2). These are individuals who typically feel pain throughout the range of motion, not just at the

Table 54-2. McKenzie Mechanical Syndromes

	Postural	Dysfunction	Derangement[a]
Definition	End-range stress of normal structure	End-range stress of shortened structure (scarring, fibrosis, nerve root adherence)	Anatomic disruption and/or displacement within the motion segment
Findings with repeated movements	Full ROM[b] No pain during, or as a result of, movements (pain only with prolonged end-range stress)	Pain at limited end range only No pain during motion No radiation (except nerve root adherence) *No centralization occurs* Does not progressively worsen or improve Pain stops shortly No rapid changes occur	Pain during movement (mid-range) Peripheralization occurs *Centralization occurs* Progressively worsens or improves Remains worse or better Rapid changes occur
Requirements of treatment	Requires posture correction Correction obtained only by patient	Requires remodeling Remodeling requires regular, frequent stretching achieved only by patient	Requires reductive procedures Should be achieved only by patient whenever possible to educate for prevention of recurrences

[a] The Derangement category can be further broken down into subcategories according to the location of the patient's pain and the presence or absence of acute spinal deformity.
[b] ROM, range of motion.

end of the range. However, while they are performing end-range movements, there may be a change in location of the pain. Typically, movements can be identified in which end-range bending in one direction will shift the pain, which is usually asymmetric at the start of the movement, further peripherally (down the leg or into the buttock), whereas end-range bending in the opposite direction will tend to centralize the pain to the midline low back. In some patients these movements are in the sagittal plane and in others, in the lateral plane. Identification of a direction of end-range spinal movement that causes "centralization" of referred pain has been shown to be of significant value as an outcome predictor of treatment success using the McKenzie principles.[7] In the McKenzie treatment program cyclic range-of-motion exercises, usually in extension, are an integral part of the rehabilitation plan. These are exercises the patient must do without assistance. The patient first learns to hold postures that tend to centralize the pain, and then learns to frequently cycle among these postures, which also tends to centralize the pain. The efficacy of these treatment plans is far greater in the acute setting. In the study by Donelson et al.,[7] of 53 patients with referred symptoms in the lumbar spine of less than 4 weeks' duration, 89 percent demonstrated centralization during assessment. Of those

with centralization, 98 percent had good or excellent treatment outcomes. In another study of 300 low back and neck patients (W. Rath and J. D. Rath, Spine Center of New Jersey, Somerville, NJ, unpublished data, 1989), 64 percent of whom had symptoms for longer than 6 weeks, 90 percent of those with or without referred symptoms and without neurologic deficit had good or excellent outcomes. The average number of physical therapy treatments was 6.8. In those patients with less than 7 days of symptoms, however, 100 percent had good or excellent results and all returned to work. Of those with symptoms between 7 days and 6 weeks in duration, 87 percent had good or excellent results. Thus, with the passage of time there is some deterioration in efficacy of the McKenzie program.

Various studies have compared this mode of treatment to other maneuvers. For instance, when compared to Williams flexion exercises, the McKenzie extension program was found superior.[8] When compared to 90/90 traction or to back school, the McKenzie program was also found to be superior.[9] Even when compared to mini back school, the McKenzie treatment program seems to be superior in perspective randomized studies.[10]

Some sources of pain are apparently not due to soft tissue injury but rather merely due to postural stresses. In the McKenzie classification these pain sources have been identified as producing postural syndrome and dysfunction syndrome. These syndromes occur in more chronic settings, but are easily treated by instruction in appropriate postures (Table 54-2).

In short, the McKenzie approach is a treatment plan based on evaluation of pain location and maneuvers that change the pain location from referred to centralized. It focuses on repetitive exercises that centralize the pain and on postures that prevent end-range stress (Rath and Rath, unpublished data, 1989).[11] It is an activity-oriented program best applied early after the onset of back and leg pain produced by soft tissue injuries. Active patient participation is a necessity for the success of this program.

SUBACUTE AND EARLY CHRONIC SPINE REHABILITATION

Once pain has been present for several weeks, additional factors other than the failure of the injured soft tissue to repair itself come into play. It seems probable that neuromotor control becomes deranged, with associated early fatigue to musculature. In an effort to counteract this phenomenon, a group of exercises have been advocated that achieve stabilization of the torso through increased muscle tone.[12] An outline of this lumbar stabilization program is presented in Table 54-3. This method is based on the assumption that a lumbar motion segment, once injured, is at risk for repetitive injury because of the existence of a "weak link" in the kinetic chain and the inability of the body to defend against this. The lumbar stabilization program expects that the acute pain has been controlled by methods such as steroid injections and use of various other medications, manipulations, and traction, all of which are short lived. The main goal of this program is building musculature to achieve stabilization of the torso, according to the concept that a muscle "fusion" occurs via the co-contraction of abdominal muscles that provides a corseting effect to the lumbar spine. Of course, before any stabilization routine is undertaken, flexibility of the motion segments must be guaranteed.

Table 54-3. Exercise Training in the Lumbar Stabilization Program

I. Soft tissue flexibility
  1. Hamstring musculotendinous unit
  2. Quadriceps musculotendinous unit
  3. Iliopsoas musculotendinous unit
  4. Gastrocnemius-soleus musculotendinous unit
  5. External and internal hip rotators
II. Joint mobility
  1. Lumbar spine segmental mobility
    a. Extension
    b. Flexion (unloaded)
  2. Hip range of motion
  3. Thoracic segmental mobility
III. Stabilization program
  1. Finding neutral position
    a. Standing
    b. Sitting
    c. Jumping
    d. Prone
  2. Prone gluteal squeezes
    a. With arm raises
    b. With alternate arm raises
    c. With leg raises
    d. With alternate leg raises
    e. With arm and leg raises
    f. With alternate arm and leg raises
  3. Supine pelvic bracing
  4. Bridging progression
    a. Basic position
    b. One leg raised with ankle weights
    c. Stepping
    d. Balance on gym ball
  5. Quadruped
    a. With alternating arm and leg movements
  6. Kneeling stabilization
    a. Double knee
    b. Single knee
    c. Lunges
      1. Without weight
      2. With weight
  7. Wall slide quadriceps strengthening
  8. Position transition with postural control
    a. Abdominal program
      1. Curl-ups
      2. Dead bug
        a. Supported
        b. Unsupported
      3. Diagonal curl-ups
      4. Diagonal curl-ups on incline board
      5. Straight leg lowering
    b. Gym program
      1. Latissimus pull-downs
      2. Angled leg press
      3. Lunges
      4. Hyperextension bench
      5. General upper body weight exercises
    c. Aerobic program
      1. Progressive walking
      2. Swimming
      3. Stationary bicycling
      4. Cross-country ski machine
      5. Running
        a. Initially supervised on a treadmill

The important element of the stabilization program is the achievement of dynamic control of the lumbar spine forces to eliminate repetitive injury to the intervertebral disc, facet joints, and related structures. Thus, flexibility training that focuses on the important muscle-tendon units is the initial phase of treatment. Inherent in this treatment program, however, is an emphasis on positioning the spine so that it is in a nonpainful orientation called the neutral spine position. The stretching and range-of-motion exercises must be carried out on a daily basis and supervision by an appropriately oriented trainer is important. Active assisted stretching is often necessary.

In the second phase of treatment the patient is trained in active joint mobilization methods such as extension exercises in prone and standing positions as well as alternating midrange flexion extension while in a four-point stance. Abdominal muscle strengthening is also achieved with simple curl-ups. The patient then progresses to more dynamic abdominal raising, such as in the "dead bug" exercises, exercises that use alternate arm and leg movements while lying supine, and exercises that use diagonal curl-ups and even exercises on an inclined board. Following this the patient progresses to aerobic exercises, exercises using a ball, and weight training (Table 54-3). Decisions as to advancement into more challenging exercises are based on functional progress and achievement of one exercise level compared to another, not on the basis of pain level. The program endpoint is determined by maximum functional improvement, the point beyond which the patient's function will not improve further through additional exercise training or pain control.

The effectiveness of this stabilization method has been well demonstrated in patients with severe disc abnormalities that were demonstrable by computed tomography or magnetic resonance imaging. In a study of patients with herniated disc, abnormal neurologic test results, and clinical evidence of radiculopathy, 96 percent had an excellent outcome using the stabilization exercises and epidural injections.[12] In this study 92 percent of patients returned to work, with sick leave lasting an average of 3.9 months. Even those patients with extruded fragments had an 86 percent success rate.

"Back school" was originally proposed as a mechanism to provide education in anatomy and the relationship of pain control to exercises. In the original study presented by Bergquist-Ullman, this method of education was found to be quite successful for acute problems in an industrial setting as compared to manipulation and other treatment modalities.[13] However, the effectiveness of this type of program does depend upon patient compliance and attitude toward the benefits in that it is largely a passive treatment method wherein a structured educational program is provided to the patients to increase their knowledge and understanding of low back pain and spine function. When a back school treatment program is applied to patients with chronic low back pain it is not very successful.[14]

The same is true for nearly every other method of passive treatment. No documentation of efficacy has ever been recorded for such mechanisms of treatment as transcutaneous electrical nerve stimulation or electrical muscle stimulation.[15] A comparison of electrical stimulation and ice massage shows that the ice seems to be better.[16,17] The lack of efficacy of such techniques makes sense if physical stresses are assumed to be necessary to align connective tissue and to supply nutrition to collaginous tissues which are poorly supplied with blood; in that case only mobilization techniques, even if done passively, have the opportunity to be of benefit. Passive manipulation, even if successful, will not involve patients in their own care. Thus, rehabilitation of the spine in acute as well as subacute settings requires patient participation in an active exercise program.

REHABILITATION FOR CHRONIC BACK PAIN

There is a changing standard of care for the treatment of back problems. Since the specific site of injury is seldom known, palliative care was considered appropriate in the past. Up until perhaps the last decade, rest and physical therapy modalities such as ultrasound were utilized because they seemed to reduce pain and provided muscle relaxation. The emerging concepts of sports medicine, however, have led to the realization that soft tissue injuries are not best treated in a passive way. For injuries to extremity joints other than fractures or dislocations, gradual progressive exercise programs to enhance the organization of repair components in the strained connective tissues have become the standard method of care. A combination of exercise with treatments such as the applications of ice to reduce pain reaction is now the standard of care for ankle sprains and similar injuries. It is therefore reasonable that exercise is also the recommended appropriate treatment for even chronic low back injuries. No matter where the soft tissue injury might be—in the disc, ligament, or osseous tendon attachment—progressive exercises should be of benefit. When exercises are used as a major treatment tool, an added benefit emerges in that the measurement of functional capacity replaces the patient's own assessment of pain as the basis for evaluating progress.

Rest produces deconditioning not only of the connective tissue but of the cardiovascular system as well. Information based on the detriments of lack of physical stress has emerged from the space program. In studies conducted in reduced gravity conditions, major deficits in cardiovascular and connective tissue and neuromotor function have been measured.[18] Thus, delay in initiating physical stresses to the connective tissue is not just neutral care, but is destructive to the patient's best interests.

Objective measurement of function is fairly easily accomplished in the realm of sports testing. Performance levels in the athlete are measureable. There are norms, which have been established by previous performance, against which to assess current performance. Athletic performance is a summation of many physical characteristics, including strength, endurance, and neuromotor function. To make the best use of performance measurements, specific components must be tested. It is recognized that no test can reliably predict performance, yet multiple testing is often of great significance in predicting successful treatment.

Approaches to Testing

Very early in the analysis of performance, range of motion was recognized as simply a measureable entity useful, in the absence of a normal range, as a possible predictor of deficit performance. Measure-ment of range of motion of the extremities is easily accomplished with goniometers, and the validity of such measurements can easily be verified by comparison to the opposite limb. Therefore range of motion became a standard of physical therapy assessment for extremity function. For the back, however, it was recognized that range of motion of the hips must be separated from that of the lumbar spine. Therefore, in the late 1960s specific discrimination of lumbar range was established using inclinometers.[19] This method of evaluating lumbar capacity is now the standard in the third edition of the American Medical Association's guidelines for impairments.[20] In fact, the delineation of lumbar range of motion is the only objective measurement of functional capacity currently cited for the assessment of spinal impairment in these guidelines. No one suggests that it gives a total picture, but no other functional capacity test for the spine has yet been judged reliable and valid by consensus.

Isokinetic Testing

It has long been recognized that range of motion testing is insufficient to evaluate the functional capacity of the extremities. A significant innovation occurred in the late 1960s when the capacity to control the variable of speed in muscle function was developed. By limiting the speed of performance to an adjustable constant rate, a new form of performance measurement was developed, which its innovators called *isokinetic.*[21] Isokinetic testing allows an individual to create as much torque as feasible while allowing force to be measured throughout the range of motion by controlling velocity. This type of measurement proved to be an excellent guide for sports medicine physicians trying to evaluate the relative strength of flexors and extensors and the status of rehabilitation after injuries to various joints.

It was not until the early 1980s that the concept of isokinetic testing was applied to the back. Using converted extremity equipment and normal subjects, the first study to be reported came from Japan in 1980.[22] Although the investigators did not have a method of normalizing the torque curves and the equipment required that subjects be tested in a recumbent position, several points emerged that have been confirmed by more recent studies. In normal subjects, the extensors of the back are stronger than its flexors, and the difference is more significant in men than in women. Aging has a definite influence upon the strength of trunk muscles: older subjects are notably weaker than young ones. The relative strengths of extensors and flexors, however, remains the same during the aging process.

To take measurements while subjects were in a more realistic posture in terms of back performance, Smidt et al. (also using converted equipment) utilized a sitting position.[23] The results confirmed that men are significantly stronger in torso musculature than women and that the back extensors in normal individuals are significantly stronger than the flexors. As in most of the early studies, the number of subjects was quite small. Furthermore, factors such as fitness and patient size were not considered. Nonetheless, testing performed in the sitting posture could isolate trunk musculature from hip musculature.

The first study using equipment specifically designed to isokinetically test back performance was by Mayer et al.,[24] who compared significant numbers of normal subjects (125) and chronic back pain patients (286). The patients were tested standing, which probably permits a more realistic evaluation of back performance. This study also used the weight of the subject as a method of normalizing the data, to make comparison among subjects more valid. Extensor musculature was again found to be stronger than flexor in normal subjects, but extensor muscles proved significantly weaker than flexor muscles in individuals suffering from chronic back pain. At higher speeds, torque production was significantly less in individuals with back pain than in normal subjects. The study also pointed out the extreme variability of initial evaluation in back pain patients. Consistency of performance, however, can be expected when the patients are familiar with the machine. Pain does not limit consistency when the patients are making maximal efforts and are used to the test equipment. Thus the equipment became available as a method for identifying submaximal or misleading performance on the part of the patients. The concept that only maximal effort could provide consistent performance was proposed in this study.

Another variation in the objective evaluation of back muscle performance was the assessment of trunk rotatory performance with isokinetic torque measurement equipment.[25] Torque measurement was accomplished with the subject sitting. Rotational torque in normal backs was about 50 percent of extensor torque, and torque production was significantly decreased in back pain patients to about 55 to 65 percent of extensor torque. Patients were not tested until they had achieved a normal range, which was easily definable by this equipment. The authors of this study also attempted to compare myoelectric performance with dynamic performance using isokinetic equipment, but they could make few correlations. No published study has yet been able to use electromyography as a specific predictor or discriminator of individuals with low back pain.

All of these studies used equipment from Cybex (Ronkonkoma, NY), the pioneer manufacturer of such devices. Other manufacturers have emerged since the expiration of some isokinetic equipment patents, and this has led to a virtual explosion in the marketing of functional testing equipment.

A flaw of all the early studies was that, in an effort to achieve repeatable data, the individual was constrained to the same position on each occasion of testing. Each person has a specific strategy for lifting and lowering that is based on a unique configuration of biomechanical factors. When strapped into a sitting or standing position, people do not lift the way they normally would. Another isokinetic test has since emerged that allows lifting to be performed in any posture desired. This simulated lifting task was performed from a standing position. In the initial report of this test, low back pain patients could lift only two-thirds of the weight lifted by normal patients.[26] Again, at higher speeds, patients performed more poorly in comparison with normal subjects. The equipment was quite safe, and the results of isokinetic performance testing were more consistent than those of isometric testing. Whereas patients tested isometrically sometimes complained of pain, those tested isokinetically did not. Finally, there was a very poor correlation between isokinetic performance and isometric performance. Isokinetic testing was therefore advocated as a safer, more reliable method of testing lifting performance. It has the potential to provide specific numeric measures of torque and work production.

Isoinertial Testing

An alternative to isokinetic testing is a computerized system known as *isoinertial* testing. Manufactured by Isotechnologies (Hillsborough, North Carolina), this constant-load device simultaneously measures change in torque and velocity in all three planes of motion (sagittal, frontal, and transverse). With so many variables operating at the same time, comparison from one day to another and from one individual to another is more difficult than with isokinetic equipment. Nonetheless, normal levels of function have been published.[27] Once again the results showed women to have lower torque and velocity measures than men. One of the most important contributions from studies using this equipment is that speed of performance is a major discriminator between individuals with back pain and those without back pain.[28] Investigators using this equipment have also observed that, with increasing fatigue, substitution and greater deviation in the arc of motion occur.

Such evaluation of lateral bending and rotation simultaneously with flexion and extension is a unique property of this equipment.[29] This is an excellent demonstration of how different systems of measurement can provide alternative perspectives on human performance. It also underscores the emerging awareness that one specific measure cannot summarize or diagnose with certainty the incapacity resulting from soft tissue injury in the back. One of the most useful aspects of tests with this equipment is the ability to monitor fatigue. Deviation from sagittal performance through muscle substitution, and slowing of rate of performance, correlates with fatigue in flexion-extension exertion against fixed resistance.

Unconstrained Lift Testing

Various other methods have become available to evaluate free lifting. The Lido lift is a variation of the Cybex lift task device already described. The subjects are tested in such a way that they can lift or lower any weight that the computerized equipment defines. They can lift straight or in a twisting mode to various heights. Numeric representation of performance, graphic feedback, and a printout of performance are available. An important additional advantage of this equipment is its ability to monitor acceleration compared to torque while lifting in an unconstrained manner. Deviation in the speed of performance seems to be an important discriminator of back pain patients.

Simpler methods of evaluating free lifting involve having the individual lift graduated weights. Thus performance can be measured in terms of increasing amounts of weight lifted over time. For safety, limits on performance can be identified to prevent overexertion. For instance, in the Pile test (Progressive Isoinertial Lifting Evaluation) the subject lifts and lowers a milk carton containing weights four times in 30 seconds, and 5- or 10-pound weights are added at 30-second intervals.[30] This type of test provides an alternative to methods requiring expensive equipment. Normal standards and comparisons of the performance of back pain patients against such standards have been published for these tests.

Isometric Testing

Although isometric testing was the first functional test method to assess lumbar performance and compare it with the expected performance of workers, this single-dimension method has not maintained its primacy in lumbar assessment.[31] In simple isometric testing, the posture of the test subject is difficult to control. In addition, the significant weak link in the back cannot be easily identified. Successful isometric testing depends upon arm strength, trunk strength, and leg strength, but standard test methods cannot readily separate the contribution of each of these.

Equipment has been developed, however, that very specifically segregates lumbar isometric performance from that of the arms and legs. This equipment, made by Medx (Ocala, FL), identifies isometric performance at various points in the range of lumbar extension by restricting the subject's position. Performance feedback and hard copy printout are available.[32] Thus, there still seems to be a place for isometric testing in lumbar functional capacity evaluation. Not only does the equipment monitor strength at various points in constrained lumbar extension but it can be used as a therapeutic device for strength training. Because of the very specific nature of the exercise on this equipment, very rapid improvement in isometric strength can be demonstrated. This is correlated with a high rate of symptom improvement as well. This equipment is also available for cervical spine testing and treatment both in the sagittal and in the rotation mode. Medx is the only computerized equipment for cervical spine testing. One other isometric lumbar test known as the Sorenson test has emerged. It requires the subject to hold the trunk parallel to the floor while unsupported. In industrial populations in Denmark, the inability to hold such a posture for 1 minute or more correlated with an increased incidence of back injury.[33]

NEED FOR FUNCTIONAL ASSESSMENT

Given the frequent inability to specifically locate the soft tissue injury in back or neck pain, quantitative assessment of function seems to be a reasonable way to obtain objective data at least as to the patient's current status. In a recent paper by Hasson and Wise, most earlier papers were criticized for not breaking the patient groups down into diagnostic categories; however, the diagnostic categories suggested by the authors are nonverifiable (i.e., sacroiliac strain versus facet syndrome versus disc pathology).[34] This is the very problem that plagues the treatment of chronic back pain: most of the sources of pain are nonverifiable. Pain in the back usually is without representation of specific nerve root dysfunction. The role of deconditioning — the impairment of physical capacity that may result from prolonged pain-limited behavior — cannot easily be evaluated with a simple physical examination. Such barriers to understanding have led to the development of pain clinics with a focus on the perception of pain rather than on the sources of pain. Behavioral control of pain has been the project in these centers, but restoration of functional capacity and return to work have not been measured goals.

The focus on treating the pain alone has led to a general suspicion — particularly among third-party payers — that rehabilitation for chronic pain may be ineffective, and in fact may be no better than a placebo, in attaining specific societal goals, such as return to work.[35] Fordyce and colleagues noted that pain clinics tend to treat the experience of pain but not the disability associated with pain behavior. Often pain is associated with the deconditioning syndrome, and technology now allows us to measure this. In the case of the back, objective lumbar function testing has been shown to significantly assist the treatment and rehabilitation of individuals with chronic back pain.[36]

Basing evaluation on functional capacity testing certainly is a great improvement over basing it on simple alteration in the patient's report of pain and function. With this more objective methodology, the focus is on returning the patient to work and normal life activities.

ORGANIZATION OF A SPINE REHABILITATION PROGRAM

It must be recognized that not only are there a wide array of structural diagnoses that create disability in the back and neck, but there are three major confounding factors. One was discussed earlier to some extent — the duration of the pain complaint. Another factor that bears emphasis is the relationship of behavioral problems to the structural abnormality. The third factor is the degree of physical deconditioning associated with chronicity. Thus, a spine rehabilitation program cannot expect to be the same program for all people. Patients need to be separated on the basis of chronicity (degree of deconditioning) as well as the degree to which behavioral problems enhance the pain complaint. Behavioral problems encompass a wide array of psychological disorders such as anxiety, hysteria, and depression. Interwoven among these may be frank psychotic problems such as personality disorders and schizophrenia. Anyone developing a rehabilitation program for spine dysfunction that has pain as the major complaint must expect the presence of these behavioral problems.

Thus, for spinal dysfunction that has not become chronic, exercise programs as discussed earlier should be quite sufficient. These may even be sufficient for spinal dysfunction in which the spinal impairment is purely structural, without any hint of deconditioning or behavioral problems. The troublesome spinal dysfunctions, however, are those that are so chronic that deconditioning has occurred and various elements of behavioral limitations are notable.

It is difficult to define the specific role of behavioral factors as they relate to patient motivation to participate in a progressive rehabilitation program. Depending on the sophistication of the rehabilitation center, various tests and various experts become available. There are standardized tests that are helpful in defining the level of psychological barriers, including the Minnesota Multiphasic Personality Inventory (MMPI), the Beck Depression Inventory, the McGill Pain Questionnaire, and the pain drawing.[37] A psychologist is valuable in interpreting these tests and should play a role in implementing programs that can assist the treatment program. The psychologist's role can vary from merely the interpretation of the test to active participation in a short-term treatment program. Basically there are five areas of treatment that can be provided by psychological services:

1. Individual and group counseling emphasizing a crisis intervention model (e.g. overcoming family problems, unemployment).
2. Family counseling, during which family members are encouraged to take an active part in the rehabilitation process and are provided with information about the philosophy of a psychologically oriented treatment program.
3. Behavioral stress management training using stress relaxation techniques such as biofeedback.
4. Cognitive-behavioral skills training that includes instruction in assertiveness, rational versus irrational thinking, and the management of stress and time.
5. Occupational work analysis and job matching, which looks at the physical capacity gains made by the patient and compares them to physical job demands as well as job stress.

The psychologist can assist in the education of the patient about issues such as work reinjury, compensation systems, and retraining options that can provide a viable plan for return to productivity.

A more pertinent issue for the context of this chapter is the mechanism by which to supply efficient and effective spine rehabilitation. There seems no question that the primary means to achieve this goal is the use of milestones of progress. Measurement of progress in exercise training is the basic maneuver by which effective rehabilitation can be attained.

This is a functional restoration approach, which should be distinguished from a pain clinic approach. Rather than focusing on pain, self-report, and related dysfunctional behavior, the restoration aims directly at the physical deconditioned syndrome. Decreased range of motion, weakness of spine musculature, decreased cardiovascular capacity, and impaired lifting capacity are the elements of physical dysfunction that must be measured. Pain is acknowledged and associated fear of activity is approached in a supportive and directive way. Also, psychosocial factors such as depression, anxiety, substance abuse, family dysfunction, and compensation litigation should be identified at the very beginning of rehabilitation and treated in an aggressive manner. Nonetheless, the major thrust is to correct the deconditioning that has occurred and facilitate return to work with functional limitations as identified by testing of these areas of dysfunction.

The measurement of physical function must fulfill certain criteria to be valid. It must be reproducible and comparable by the same evaluator at different times and by different evaluators independently. There must be an existing normative data base by which pathologic values may be clearly identified, since there is no comparable "normal side" in the spine. In each test, an assessment of effort must be available so that the objective validity of the particular test effort can be identified. The following paragraphs describe the type of measures that can be used as milestones of progress toward functional restoration.

Measurement of spinal range of motion is the most specific test and the most widely used. The best method is the two-inclinometer technique, as described earlier, which has been adopted by the American Medical Association in its revised *Guides to the Evaluation of Permanent Impairment.*[20] An important characteristic of this test is that it can assess poor effort by a discrepancy of greater than 10° to 15° between the most impaired straight leg raising and hip flexion as measured on the sacrum. Even when suboptimal effort is present, an abnormal ratio of true lumbar hip flexion can be identified at any point along the lumbar curve.[38]

Measurement of trunk strength is available from a wide array of computerized equipment that has been described earlier. To date no specific equipment has been definitely identified as superior to any other. Probably the most important factors in the use of such equipment is that those individuals who are performing the test should be thoroughly familiar with the equipment and that the patient should be comfortable in its use. The equipment is fairly complex, and a simple description of its use will not suffice in providing the tester with adequate expertise to carry out the test. Several weeks to months of experience are probably necessary before effective use of the equipment is obtained and valid testing can be expected. Of course, measurement of trunk strength is available from many other types of test. The use of isotonic equipment such as that made by Eagle gives a reliable definition of strength. The amount of weight lifted and the repetitions accomplished are objective milestones. Stabilization exercises are also reliable quantifiers of trunk strength, and the various steps in progress through this program are another set of objective milestones. Thus, it is certainly possible to carry out a very appropriate rehabilitation program without the use of expensive equipment. The important aspect is measurement of function, which allows both the trainer and the patient to be aware of progress.

Measurement of lifting capacity is an important aspect of functional measurement. Testing devices available that utilize isometric or isokinetic technology include the Cybex Lift Task, the Lido Lift, and the Biodex Lift Simulation. Additionally, there are simpler tests that merely measure the amount of weight that can be lifted in a standardized manner. An example is the Pile test, described earlier, in which the patient lifts a plastic milk carton containing weights from the floor to bench height and secondarily to a height at shoulder level; standards for this test have been published.[30] Certainly specialized tests can be developed and internal standards of performance determined. Tests like the Pile test can easily be standardized and present an inexpensive way to evaluate progress.

Assessment of cardiovascular endurance is certainly important in any setting in which function and restoration are the goals. Aerobic capacity is an important factor in disability. Physical inactivity certainly leads to loss of cardiovascular function, particularly in older individuals spending unusual amounts of time reclining in order to protect painful spinal segments. Aerobic capacity tests can be performed using a variety of protocols attached to a treadmill or bicycle ergometers. If lumbar function is so disturbed that use of a bicycle ergometer is not possible, upper extremity aerobic testing can be accomplished using specific ergometers designed for upper body challenges (UBEs). This area of testing is by far the most advanced, and oxygen consumption and fitness level norms can be attained from standardized tables.

Positional and activity tolerance is an important area of testing that is difficult to standardize. This type of testing is probably most important to assess whether the person can return to work at a job that requires some specific physical activity. Some centers focus their total attention on this phase of functional restoration, wherein various job tasks are re-created and the patient is challenged to improve tolerance of these tasks (work hardening or work simulation centers). Some centers have devised obstacle courses that require multiple positions in an attempt to assess the patient's tolerance of a variety of positions during daily living activities.

It should be recognized that preparation for participation in a very vigorous program is necessary. Someone who has been disabled for many months or even years cannot immediately jump into a stressful exercise program. Recently it has been pointed out that a pre-program period merely focusing on education and stretching offers great potential to enhance physical performance in a rehabilitation program. In a recent study two groups of chronic low back pain patients were evaluated. One group's pre-program treatment phase lasted 1 to 2 weeks and that of the second group lasted 2 to 6 weeks. Flexibility was the criterion of readiness to be involved in a more exhaustive program. Improvement of range of motion was identified as a significant mechanism to enhance function; those patients who had gone through the longer entry program of education and stretching when tested, performed nearly as well at entry into the rehabilitation program as those who had gone through the shorter pre-program performed at the *conclusion* of their rehabilitation time.[39]

WORKERS' COMPENSATION ISSUES IN REHABILITATION OF THE BACK

There are some unique characteristics to back rehabilitation that are engendered by workers' compensation issues. Probably the best summary of the difference between workers' compensation benefits and alternative care for spine injuries emerged from a recent study by the Minnesota Department of Labor and Industry.[40] This study was initiated to evaluate the rapid increase in costs of medical care specifically as related to Minnesota expenses. According the 1989 study, medical benefits account for 40 percent of the incurred workers' compensation benefits. The workers' compensation health care costs appeared to be rising faster than the general health care costs; between 1982 and 1987, health care expenditures in Minnesota rose 96 percent whereas health care expenditures in the United States as a whole rose 55 percent. Workers' compensation pays a small share (2 percent) of medical care costs both in Minnesota and nationally. Nonetheless, it is the fear of workers' compensation insurers that better cost control is achieved in the private insurance system and therefore that additional costs may be shifted to the workers' compensation system. This study not only analyzed the sources of the cost but compared the cost to that the state's largest private health insurer, Blue Cross/Blue Shield–Minnesota, for similar injuries.

This study found that 41.2 percent of the total costs to workers' compensation were due to back disorders. An additional 17 percent were due to sprain and strains to the extremities and 8.8 percent to contusions of various types. Only 6.2 percent of the costs to workers' compensation in 1989 in Minnesota were for care of fractures. In a comparison of the two systems, the cost per case for fracture care to Blue Cross/Blue Shield was about the same as that to workers' compensation, but the cost per case for back disorders to Blue Cross was 2.2 times less than that to workers' compensation. This supports the conclusion that, in verifiable conditions such as fractures, wherein the diagnosis and prognosis are clearly identified, medical costs are essentially the same. In nonverifiable conditions such as back disorders, the care may be extended for prolonged periods of time without clear understanding as to resolution. Moreover, the fact that over 40 percent of the costs to workers' compensation are attributable to back disorders emphasizes the peculiar incidence of back disorders in industrial medicine contrasted to disease incidence as a whole. Because compensation is available, back complaints are more common.

This study also pointed out that mechanisms of cost containment utilized by Minnesota and other states were equally ineffective in controlling the escalation. Some states achieved cost containment by limiting employee choice of provider. Others impose medical fee schedules on providers. Neither strategy has been successful in controlling medical costs. Finally, in an effort to reduce litigation relative to workers' compensation "injuries," 1984 legislation in Minnesota allowed compensation solely on the basis of medical diagnosis. Because of the inexact nature of medical diagnosis, especially as applied to back injuries, this strategy has been demonstrated to be flawed. No reduction in settlement cost has indeed occurred in Minnesota, and thus new legislation is about to be passed that repeals the diagnosis-based system and returns to a subjective system, which in general is the mechanism used throughout the other states.

Moreover, when efforts are made to try to reduce work injuries, and thus the cost of medical care, other barriers to progress emerge. In a recent study that searched for predictors of back complaints, physical characteristics were in general of no benefit in predicting incidence of back injuries.[41] In this prospective longitudinal study, over 3,000 volunteers in the aircraft industry underwent an extensive examination that included a thorough physical evaluation as well as evaluation of multiple other characteristics. This group was tracked for over 4 years and the incidence of back "injuries" was identified. The only physical variables that had a predictive value for back pain were age and weight in women and history of previous back problems and age in men. Back symptoms elicited by a positive straight leg raising test were associated with subsequent back pain in both men and women, but four out of five of those individuals with positive straight leg raising tests did not have an incidence of back pain in the ensuing 4 years. This extensive study conducted at the Boeing plant has shown that by far the most significant predictor of back injury is at a personnel relations level rather than a physical level. Those workers who had an adverse supervisor report in the 6 months prior to their back complaint had the greatest incidence of back problems. Joint range of motion, including lumbar range, and isometric strength testing were of no predictive value in this study.

The implications of the Minnesota study and the Boeing study are clear. Efforts to improve back rehabilitation, especially in the workers' compensation field, must be directed at both the psychological and the physical components of the problem. Early care certainly is an important aspect of this problem. The injured worker must be brought into rehabilitation before deconditioning and psychological dependency begin to emerge. Measurement of function, rather than searching for a diagnosis, is a most important strategy. Progress of the patient through a back rehabilitation program using milestones of functional measurement would seem to be the only strategy available to ensure efficient, effective care. The factors that hinder progress—anxiety in the workplace, assumed potentials for significant financial awards on the occasion of declared disability, and an attitude that one can "beat the system"—all work together to create a treatment scenario far worse than the realities of the problem. Rational care depends upon utilization of physiologic principles in the care of the injured worker, as is the case with any other injury. Rehabilitation essentially must be focused on reactivation and demanding the participation of the patient in the rebuilding of the injured connective tissues. Insistence upon these elements essentially is the "backbone" of spine rehabilitation.

REFERENCES

1. Spitzer WO, LeBlanc FE, Dupuis M et al: Scientific approach to the assessment and management of activity related spinal disorders. A monograph for clinicians: report of the Quebec Task Force on spinal disorders. Spine 12:7(suppl 1), 1987
2. Lawrence JS: Disc degeneration: its frequency and relationship to symptoms. Ann Rheum Dis 28:121, 1969
3. LaRocca H, MacNab I: Value of pre-employment radiographic assessment of the lumbar spine. Can Med Assoc J 101:49, 1969
4. Frymoyer JW, Newberg A, Pope MH et al: Spine radiographs in patients with low back pain. An epidemiological study in men. J Bone Joint Surg [Am] 66:1048, 1984
5. Gilbert JR, Taylor DW, Hildebrand A et al: Clinical trial of common treatments for low back pain in family practice. Br Med J 291:791, 1985
6. Deyo RA, Diehl AK, Rosenthal M: How many days of bed rest for acute low back pain? A randomized clinical trial. N Engl J Med 315:1064, 1986
7. Donelson R, Silva G, Murphy K: The centralization phenomenon: its usefulness in evaluating and treating referred pain. Spine 15:211, 1990
8. Nwugag V: Relative therapeutic efficacy of the Williams and McKenzie protocols in back pain management. Physiother Prac 1:99, 1985
9. Vanharanta H, Videman T, Mooney V: McKenzie exercises, back trac and back school in lumbar syndrome. Orthop Trans 10:533, 1986
10. Stankovic R, Johnell O: Conservative treatment of acute low back pain: a prospective randomized trial: McKenzie method of treatment vs. patient education in "mini back school". Spine 15:120, 1990
11. McKenzie RA: The Lumbar Spine: Mechanical Diagnosis and Therapy. Spinal Publications, Waikanae, New Zealand, 1981
12. Saal JA: Nonoperative treatment of herniated lumbar intervertebral disc with radiculopathy: an outcome study. Spine 14:431, 1989
13. Bergquist-Ullman M: Acute low back pain in industry: a controlled prospective study with special reference to therapy and vocational factors. Acta Orthop Scand [Suppl] 170:1, 1977
14. Lankhost GJ, Vanderstadt RJ, Vogelaar TW et al: The effect of Swedish back school in chronic idiopathic low back pain. Scand J Rehab Med 15:141, 1983
15. Kahanovitz N, Nordin M, Verdermane R et al: Normal trunk muscle strength and endurance in women and the effect of exercises and electrical stimulation. Part II: comparative analysis of electrical stimulation and exercises to increase trunk muscle strength and endurance. Spine 12:112, 1987
16. Melzack R, Jeans ME, Stratford JG et al: Ice massage and transcutaneous electrical stimulation: comparison of treatment for low back pain. Pain 9:209, 1980
17. Rutkowski B, Neidzialkowska T, Otto J: Electrical stimulation in chronic low back pain. Br J Anaesth 49:629, 1977
18. Lamb L, Johnson R, Stevens P: Cardiovascular conditioning during chair rest. Aerospace Med 35:646, 1964
19. Loebel W: Measurements of spinal posture and range in spinal movements. Ann Phys Med 9:103, 1967
20. Engleberg AL (ed): Guides to the Evaluation of Permanent Impairment. 3rd Ed. American Medical Association, Chicago, 1988
21. Thistle H, Hislop H, Moffroed M et al: Isokinetic contraction: a new concept of resistive exercise. Arch Phys Med Rehabil 48:279, 1967
22. Hasue M, Fujiwara M, Kikuchi S: A new method of quantitative measurement of abdominal and back muscle strength. Spine 5:143, 1980
23. Smidt G, Amundsen L, Dostal W: Muscle strength at the trunk. J Orthop Sports Phys Ther 1:165, 1980
24. Mayer T, Smith S, Keeley J et al: Quantification of lumbar function. Part 2: sagittal plane trunk strength in chronic low-back pain patients. Spine 10:765, 1985
25. Mayer T, Smith S, Kondraske G et al: Quantification of lumbar function. Part 3: preliminary data on isokinetic torso rotation testing with myoelectric spectral analysis in normal and low-back pain subjects. Spine 10:912, 1985
26. Kishino N, Mayer T, Gatchel R et al: Quantification of lumbar function. Part 4: isometric and isokinetic lifting simulation in normal subjects and low-back dysfunction patients. Spine 10:921, 1985

27. Seeds R, Levene J, Goldberg H: Normative data for Isostation B-100. J Orthop Sport Phys Ther 9:141, 1987
28. Seeds R, Levene J, Goldberg H: Abnormal patient data for the Isostation B-100. J Orthop Sports Phys Ther 10:121, 1988
29. Parnianpour M, Nordin M, Frankel VH et al: Triaxial coupled isometric trunk measurements. Occupational and Orthopaedic Center, Hospital for Joint Diseases Orthopaedic Institute, New York, NY. Presented at the Orthopaedic Research Society Meeting, Atlanta, Georgia, January 1988
30. Mayer T, Barnes MA, Kishino ND et al: Progressive isoinertial lifting evaluation: I. A standardized protocol and normative database. Spine 13:993, 1988
31. Chaffin DB, Park KS: A longitudinal study of low back pain as associated with occupational weight lifting factors. J Am Ind Hyg Assoc 10:513, 1973
32. Graves JE, Pollock ML, Carpenter DM et al: Quantitative assessment of full range-of-motion isometric lumbar extension strength. Spine 15:289, 1990
33. Biering-Sorenson F: Physical measurements as risk indicators for low back trouble over a one year period. Spine 9:45, 1984
34. Hasson SM, Wise DD: Instrumented testing of the back. Surg Rounds Orthop 10:28, 1989
35. Fordyce W, Roberts A, Sternbach R: The behavioral management of chronic pain: a response to critics. Pain 22:113, 1985
36. Mayer T, Gatchel RJ, Kishino N et al: A prospective short-term study on chronic low back pain patients utilizing novel objective functional measurement. Pain 25:53, 1986
37. Capra P, Mayer T, Gatchel R: Using psychological scales to assess back pain. J Musculoskel Med 7:41, 1985
38. Mayer T, Tencer A, Kristofersson S et al: Use of noninvasive techniques for quantification of spinal range of motion in normal subjects and chronic low back pain dysfunction patients. Spine 96:588, 1984
39. Kohles S, Barnes D, Gatchel RJ et al: Improved physical performance outcomes following functional restoration treatment of chronic low back pain patients: early versus recent training results. Presented in part at the annual meeting of the North American Spine Society, Colorado Springs, Colorado, July 1988
40. Report to the Legislature on Health Cost and Cost Containment in Minnesota Workers' Compensation. Minnesota Department of Labor and Industry, Minneapolis, 1990
41. Battie MC, Bigos SJ, Fisher LD et al: Anthropometric and clinical measure as predictors of back pain complaints in industry: a prospective study. J Spinal Disord 3:195, 1990

55 Rehabilitation of the Hip

CHARLES E. LOWREY
RICHARD D. COUTTS

Surgery of the hip joint is an extremely rewarding area in orthopaedics and rehabilitation. Over the past 30 years an explosion in interest and research has occurred, stimulated by the development of successful total hip replacement by Charnley of England in 1962. The indications for total hip arthroplasty (THA) have been defined more clearly, but older operations for hip disease, including hemi-arthroplasty, osteotomy, arthrodesis, and resection arthroplasty, have retained a place in the treatment of specific problems. Treatment of hip fractures has been revolutionized by new internal fixation techniques that provide immediate and stable fixation and allow early ambulation. The new surgical technology has made possible a more aggressive rehabilitative philosophy that emphasizes early ambulation and avoidance of prolonged bed rest. This philosophy has led to significantly lower rates of complications and mortality after major surgery of the hip joint.

Two general goals should be kept in mind during the rehabilitation that follows hip surgery. The first goal is to *prevent* or *avoid complications*. Such complications as dislocation, infection, or thromboembolism can be devastating in terms of functional outcome and can even cause the patient's death. The second general goal is to *maximize the outcome* of the surgical intervention. Re-establishing a normal gait pattern, regaining muscular strength, and learning to cope with residual disability will lead to better function and better quality of life in the long run.

Lately another stimulus for efficient and timely rehabilitation has emerged as an important factor. The establishment of payment systems based on diagnosis-related groups has resulted in hospital reimbursement for a limited number of in-patient days. Thus, economic incentives exist to achieve rehabilitative goals in a shorter number of hospital days. As a consequence, the average hospital stay for THA has decreased from over 20 days in the early 1970s to less than 10 days in 1991. The great satisfaction generated by this very significant reduction in hospital stay must be tempered by the knowledge minimum standards of care, including hospital stay, must be enforced to reliably avoid complications.

A team approach is taken to hip rehabilitation. The rehabilitation team is made up of a group of professionals, each with a specific area of interest, competence, and responsibility. The *orthopaedic surgeon* serves as the team leader. In this role, the orthopaedist provides general direction and goals to the other members and assumes overall responsibility for the patient's well-being. Other physicians, particularly internists and physiatrists, should be consulted as needed. *Nurses* interact intensively with the patient during the hospital stay. In the operating room and on the hospital ward, nurses monitor the patient and provide minute-to-minute evaluation and treatment. In some instances a home visiting nurse visits after hospital discharge. *Physical therapists* have responsibility for ambulation and transfer training, exercises for joint range of motion and muscle strengthening, and patient instruction concerning precautions, particularly dislocation precautions after THA. *Occupational therapists* teach patient skills for resuming the activities of daily living with disability after hip surgery. Occupational therapists educate and instruct patients in the use of aids for walking, bathing, and dressing. The *orthopaedic technician* serves as a surgical assistant in some hospitals. The technician also is responsible for the daily management of traction, slings, continuous passive motion (CPM) devices, braces, and casts that may be used with hip disorders. Finally, at the conclusion of an acute hospital admission, *social services* employees or the discharge coordinator is consulted to evaluate the patient's home environment and support systems. Hospital social workers are familiar with community health care resources, including skilled nursing care facilities and home programs. They can recommend programs to help in the patient's transition from the hospital environment to independent living. These services have had a profound impact on the length of hospital stay. Care that previously required continued hospitalization can now be provided in an outpatient setting.

This chapter is organized by the type of surgical procedure performed. Total hip replacement is discussed first, and relatively greater emphasis is placed on it as an example for hip surgery in general. Other surgical procedures discussed include hip fractures, osteotomy, athrodesis, and resection arthroplasty. Care is taken to highlight the similarities of these procedures to THA as well as their differences. Three rehabilitative time periods are examined: the preoperative period, the perioperative or hospital period, and the postoperative or recovery period. Examples of each rehabilitation team member's role are included where appropriate. The general goals of avoiding complications and maximizing functional outcome are broken down into specific recommended techniques and procedures.

TOTAL HIP ARTHROPLASTY

Total hip replacement (arthroplasty) is a mechanical solution to a biologic problem. In several diseases, most frequently osteoarthritis and rheumatoid arthritis, the articular cartilage lining the hip joint is destroyed. This causes pain and leads to decreased range of motion and muscle strength. Abnormal or substitution gait patterns may develop in response to the pain and decreased motion. Nonoperative treatments are used initially and include periods of rest, weight reduction, gentle exercises, nonsteroidal anti-inflammatory medications, and a cane held in the contralateral hand to help unload the affected hip. If

hip pain remains disabling despite these treatments, THA is undertaken. In this major operative procedure, the diseased joint tissues are excised and replaced with a metal and plastic hip joint.

Although scores of THA components are being marketed at the present time, they can be categorized into several major groups. The first consideration is the method of skeletal fixation. The components can be attached to the skeleton in one of two ways: either with bone cement or by press-fit supplemented with bone ingrowth. Bone cement, or methylmethacrylate, is a biocompatible acrylic plastic. It is purchased as a powdered polymer that is mixed with liquid monomer to form a doughy mass. This material is placed into the bone in the doughy state, the component is then inserted into the cement, and both are held securely in place until the cement hardens, in 12 to 15 minutes. When the methylmethacrylate has hardened, the implant is rigidly fixed to bone. Bone ingrowth fixation is obtained when living bone grows into and around a metal prosthesis, holding it in position. This type of fixation is obtained most reliably when a porous metal surface (pore size 100 to 400 μm) is held rigidly (micromotion less than 50 to 100 μm) in contact with cortical bone for 6 to 12 weeks. This allows bone ingrowth to occur into the pores of the metallic component, a process very similar to fracture healing. Initial fixation of the component is obtained by press-fit, using a component slightly larger than the prepared defect in the bone, or by screw fixation.

Materials used to construct THA components have been refined over the years. Components have been made modular to afford the surgeon a greater number of options during the operation, particularly to adjust leg length and femoral head size. Femoral components are made of strong superalloys of chromium-cobalt-molybdenum or titanium-aluminum-vanadium. The articulating surface of the acetabular component is made of ultra-high molecular weight polyethylene, a very durable plastic. The acetabular cup often is backed with metal alloy where it contacts the skeleton. Head-neck components come in four standard sizes: 22, 26, 28, and 32 mm in diameter. the larger size is more stable to dislocation but can result in increased acetabular wear.[1] Three or four sizes of neck length usually are available. Most femoral heads used at present are made of chrome-cobalt alloy, because titanium alloys have been shown to have some inferior wear characteristics.[2] Aluminum oxide and zirconium ceramics have been used to manufacture femoral heads with improved wear properties. Another new development has been application of a thin layer of calcium ceramic, such as hydroxyapatite, to the metallic component to improve or accelerate bone ingrowth.

Surgical approaches for THA generally involve an incision going anterior or posterior to the hip abductor musculature. The posterior approach is used more frequently. The joint capsule is either incised or removed and the hip is dislocated, giving exposure to the acetabulum. In some instances the greater trochanter (attachment site of the gluteus medius and gluteus minimus muscles) is osteotomized for exposure. This technique provides improved acetabular exposure and allows the surgeon to adjust the tension on the abductor musculature according to where the trochanter is reattached. Reattachment of the trochanter is accomplished with cerclage wires to hold the bone fragment in place until the osteotomy site has healed.

Over 120,000 total hip replacements are performed yearly in North America.[2] Early results of this procedure are good or excellent in over 90 percent of patients, making this the most reliable surgical treatment for arthritic hip disease. Patients should be informed that a good result after THA includes significant pain relief and good, although not necessarily normal, function. Some lifelong limitations must be accepted by the patient after THA. Prophylactic antibiotics must be used for dental or other invasive procedures in which the risk of bacteremia is present. This prevents hematogenous spread of bacteria to the artificial hip joint. A decreased range of motion should be accepted or the patient runs the risk of dislocation. High-impact sports such as jogging, tennis, or basketball should be abandoned because these activities probably increase the likelihood of failure by loosening.[2]

Long-term follow-up results indicate that the rates of aseptic loosening and other complications are low when modern cementing techniques for fixation of femoral components are used. Unfortunately, the frequency of loosening of cemented acetabular components rises precipitously at approximately 8 years after surgery and may be as high as 20 to 30 percent. Thus, many surgeons have adopted the "hybrid" hip as the primary method of fixation—a cemented femoral component combined with a press-fit acetabular component.[3] An uncemented femoral component is reserved for the younger patient, usually less than 60 to 65 years of age. In this group, a theoretical longevity advantage is traded for a slightly higher rate of early complications, including thigh pain, limp, and revision surgery.

Preoperative Period

THA is a major surgical procedure that carries the risk of major complications. Much can be accomplished in the preoperative period to prepare for surgery, reducing the likelihood of complications, and maximizing the eventual outcome.

First, to justify the risks of a major operation, the indications for surgery must be clear. The primary indication remains severe, disabling hip pain unresponsive to nonoperative treatment. Arthritic hip pain most often originates in the groin and radiates to the thigh and knee. The pain is worse with activity but may be present continuously. Rotation of the hip joint will usually reproduce the symptoms. In some instances, pain from a lumbar spine or intra-abdominal pathologic condition can be referred to the hip. In confusing cases an injection of local anesthetic solution into the hip joint, using sterile technique and fluoroscopic control, can clarify the source of discomfort. Range of motion of the hip may be decreased, particularly internal rotation. A preoperative hip evaluation and score, such as the one proposed by the Hip Society, should be used.[4] This provides a single number and a standard terminology for comparison. Radiographs are made of the hip. Typical changes of osteoarthritis include joint space narrowing, sclerosis, and osteophyte formation.

Orthopaedic evaluation and clearance just prior to surgery are standard. A diligent search for preexisting infection should be undertaken. A bladder infection or an infected ingrown toenail can become the source of a postoperative wound infection. This is a devastating and entirely preventable complication. The site of the proposed incision should be examined. Recent trauma or dermatitis may necessitate postponement to avoid wound healing problems. Preoperative screening laboratory tests should include complete blood count, chemistry screen, coagulation screen, urinalysis, and blood type and cross-match. A brief nutritional assessment should be made, including serum protein levels, because nutritional supplements are sometimes in order. Radiographs are obtained in at least two planes with a magnification marker taped to the patient. These are used for surgical planning, including templating components.

The elderly population undergoing total hip replacement frequently has preexisting medical problems along with hip arthritis. Such problems as diabetes, hypertension, or coronary artery disease should prompt preoperative evaluation by the appropriate specialist in internal medicine. The patient with inflammatory arthritis should have the arthritis under good medical control. The stress of surgery can exacerbate rheumatoid arthritis and other inflammatory arthritides. For patients on a chronic steroid regimen, a booster dose is given in the perioperative period. If dental hygiene is marginal, preoperative dental evaluation should be sought. Dental caries or gingivitis can cause bacterial seeding of the wound. These conditions should be corrected prior to hip replacement.

To prepare for total hip arthroplasty, patients can maximize their general health. Weight reduction is often part of conservative treatment and may decrease postoperative complications. Patients who smoke cigarettes should be encouraged to stop in the strongest possible manner. Not smoking for only 2 or 3 days prior to surgery will improve pulmonary capability. Nicotine chewing gum may be prescribed if this is helpful. Nonsteroidal anti-inflammatory medications should be discontinued 1 week prior to surgery, if this is possible. These medicines interfere with platelet function and prolong bleeding time. Preoperative physical therapy consultation is often obtained. Instruction prepares patients for therapy and familiarizes them with the physical therapy environment. Exercises can be started to improve muscle tone and strength.

Autologous Blood Donation

Most hospitals now have an autologous blood donation program through which patients can donate their own blood prior to THA. The blood is then given back during or after surgery, if needed. Fresh blood can be stored for 35 days. If longer storage is desired, the blood must be frozen and then thawed prior to administration. Freezing blood extends the shelf life for 6 to 12 months. Autologous blood donation has been shown to reduce the need for homologous blood transfusion.[5] This reduces the risk of transmission of viral diseases, including hepatitis and acquired immunodeficiency syndrome. The cost of an autologous unit of blood is comparable to that of a homologous unit. Patients should be offered the option of predonating blood for elective major surgery, including THA.

Preoperative Teaching

A preoperative teaching conference has been tremendously helpful in educating patients about hip replacement and alleviating anxiety about surgery. The conference can be held in a hospital classroom and may even include a tour of the hospital ward, physical therapy department, or operating rooms. The nursing service often takes a leadership role in organizing patient education. Operating room and ward nurses should try to attend the conference to meet patients scheduled for surgery and answer their questions. Other rehabilitation team members should attend or contribute to the conference. A videotape format has been useful if team members are unable to attend conferences in person. The orthopaedic surgeon, occupational therapist, physical therapist, discharge coordinator, and technician all have a unique role in the patient's care. Explaining each person's role "up front" will head off many questions and concerns.

Printed instructional materials also are important. These can be retained by the patient and reviewed in a leisurely fashion at home. Doctors and other rehabilitation team members may wish to develop their own instructional pamphlets. In addition, materials are available from the American Academy of Orthopaedic Surgeons (222 South Prospect Avenue, Park Ridge, IL 60068) and the National Arthritis and Musculoskeletal and Skin Diseases Information Clearing House (Box AMS, 9000 Rockville Pike, Bethesda, MD 20892).

Perioperative Period

Surgery

The most critical period, in terms of the patient's ultimate outcome, is during surgical placement of the THA components. If the proper components are selected, positioned correctly, and rigidly fixed to the skeleton, excellent function will usually be the outcome. If the components are inappropriately sized, malpositioned, or loose, the result will be poor.

Most total hip replacements are done through a posterior approach, sparing the abductor attachment. If a *trochanteric osteotomy* is necessary, the postoperative regimen must be modified. No active abduction exercises or passive adduction stretching is allowed until the trochanter has healed. If exercises are started too soon, the attachment wires will break and the trochanter will migrate proximally. This results in abductor weakness, a limp, and a positive Trendelenburg's sign.

The acetabular cup is positioned with approximately 30° to 45° of abduction from the transverse plane and 15° to 20° of anteversion from the sagittal plane. If screws are used for fixation, the safest area for placement is in the posterior-superior quadrant. The femoral stem is placed with 0° to 15° of anteversion. A trial range of motion is then examined. The hip should be stable to dislocation posteriorly at 90° of flexion, 45° of internal rotation, and neutral abduction. The joint should not dislocate anteriorly at full extension and 45° of external rotation. If the components are not stable, the cup is repositioned and stability is retested. The component neck length is selected on the basis of soft tissue tension and leg length. Often it is desirable to lengthen the extremity approximately 1 cm. The goal is to equalize the leg lengths. Lengthening of more than 3 cm risks creating a sciatic nerve palsy owing to stretching the nerve. If the patient has a fixed pelvic obliquity, leg length equalization will be more difficult to obtain. This is a difficult diagnosis to make preoperatively, but suspi-

cion should be aroused if the back range of motion is limited and scoliosis is present.

To reduce the risk of infection, prophylactic antibiotics are given intravenously. The incision is left open for as short a period of time as possible, and it is frequently irrigated with antibiotic-saline solution. Many surgeons use filtered body exhaust "space suit" operating gowns. Some operating rooms are equipped with filtered laminar air flow systems or ultraviolet light to reduce the level of bacteria in the air.

Postoperative Protocol

A standard protocol for the management of patients after routine total hip replacement should be established. This facilitates communication and minimizes errors. Standard orders should be written for the management of intravenous fluids, diet, activity, bowel and bladder function, medications, drains, laboratory tests, and so forth.

A radiograph is made of the hip in the recovery room. Because many dislocations occur between surgery and the recovery room, the surgeon should supervise transfers and the taking of radiographs. If a dislocation, fracture, or other problem is noted, it should be addressed immediately. The extremity that has been operated on is placed in a sling or an abduction pillow. This keeps the hip abducted to help prevent dislocation. A sling also helps venous drainage and facilitates the performance of some simple exercises (knee flexion-extension, hip abduction-adduction).[6]

Antibiotics are continued for 48 to 72 hours postoperatively. Because the rate of thromboembolism is high in unprotected patients after THA, some form of prophylaxis against deep vein thrombosis must be instituted. This may take the form of leg exercises, compression stockings, elevation, aspirin, heparin, warfarin, or some combination of these. The ideal regimen is not yet known.[7]

The surgeon removes the drain, if one is present, after 24 to 48 hours. The wound is inspected and the first dressing change is done by the surgeon on the second or third postoperative day. Blood transfusion is given as needed. We have been using reinfusion drains, which allow blood from the wound to be filtered and immediately transfused as an added method to avoid the use of homologous blood.

Deep breathing exercises and ankle pump exercises are started immediately. The patient sits at the bedside or in a chair the first day after surgery. Physical therapy treatment generally is started the first day. *Dislocation precautions* are taught early and repeated frequently. Patients must know that they may not flex the hip to a greater extent than 90°, raise the knee above the hip, bring the knee past the midline of the body, or rotate the extremity that has been operated on excessively inwardly or outwardly. Orthostasis is common after surgical blood loss and being in the supine posture. A tilt table occasionally is helpful initially to regain the upright posture.

Physical Therapy

The ideal physical therapy program should include several elements.[8] *Transfer training* from bed, chair, and toilet should be included. The patient must be taught how to get into and out of a car safely. *Gait training* is a key aspect of physical therapy. Patients should be taught to walk independently on level surfaces and to navigate stairs. On stairs the patient should lead up with the unoperated extremity. Most patients will use crutches or a walker for approximately 6 weeks after THA, particularly if a press-fit component is used. The orthopaedic surgeon should specify the weight-bearing status: (i.e., 25 percent of body weight, for example). The patient can then step on a scale with the extremity that we operated on to learn what 25 percent of body weight "feels" like. Partial weight-bearing is accomplished with the foot flat on the floor using a normal heel-to-toe transfer of weight. "Non–weight-bearing" results in more force being generated across the hip joint owing to muscle contractions. The physical therapist should pay close attention to the gait patterns. The patient must be taught to abandon any abnormal or substitution gait patterns present before surgery. A normal "step-through" gait can be achieved even when using a four-point walker. *Exercises* are the third component of a good physical therapy program. Isometric quadriceps and gluteal sets can be started in bed right after surgery. Ankle pumps also are started to improve blood flow from both legs and help prevent clot for-

mation. Later hip flexion, extension, and abduction exercises can be added. Active abduction is avoided if a trochanteric osteotomy has been done. A stationary bicycle with minimal resistance and the seat adjusted high to avoid excessive hip flexion has been useful for gentle range-of-motion exercises of the hip.

Occupational Therapy

Occupational therapists instruct the patient on activities of daily living and the use of aids. Most patients will require walking aids, either crutches or a walker. Forearm supports may be helpful for patients with inflammatory arthritis and upper extremity involvement. Patients should be reminded that they may stand unsupported with body weight distributed equally to both lower extremities, such as at the sink or stove. However, crutches must be used when walking, because single stance results in a magnification of body weight across the hip 2.5 times. Useful bath aids include a raised toilet seat, a tub or shower seat, and a long bath sponge. Frequently used dressing aids include a reacher/grabber, long shoehorn, sock cone, and elastic shoelaces to convert laced shoes into slip-ons.[9]

Discharge Criteria

A set of discharge criteria should be developed and applied to each patient before hospital release. These criteria can be relaxed if the patient is being transferred to a skilled nursing care facility where assistance is available. Prior to release the patient's condition should be stable medically. The patient's temperature should be below 100°F for at least 24 hours. The incision should be healing well with no sign of infection. The patient should demonstrate independent transfers from a bed and a chair and independent ambulation using a walker or crutches. If stairs are present in the home, the patient should be able to navigate them. Finally, the patient should be quizzed and demonstrate knowledge of dislocation and gait restrictions. The home exercise program and aids for activities of daily living should be understood thoroughly.[10]

Postoperative Period

After discharge from the hospital, there is a period of gradual recovery after hip replacement. Exercises started in the hospital are continued at home. A stationary bicycle may be used. A daily walk is recommended to gradually increase endurance. When press-fit components are used, most surgeons recommend protected weight-bearing for at least 6 weeks after surgery. With cemented components, weight-bearing can be advanced more rapidly. Dislocation precautions can be relaxed 6 weeks after the operation. The patient can stop sleeping with an abduction pillow at this time. Approximately 3 to 6 months are required to recover fully after THA.

Follow-up appointments are scheduled on a regular basis. The patient is instructed to contact the doctor immediately if signs of wound problems, including drainage, discoloration, or fever, develop. Otherwise, the patient is seen 2 weeks, 6 weeks, 3 months, and 12 months after surgery. A yearly examination and hip score should be recorded thereafter. This helps the surgeon to critically evaluate results and may help pick up problems early, when they can be corrected.

Some restrictions are permanent. High-impact sports should be avoided. Dislocation can occur years after THA, so it is prudent to avoid extremes of motion. Prophylactic antibiotics are used with dental work and some invasive procedures, such as cystocopy. These restrictions can be recorded conveniently on a wallet-sized card for the patient.

HIP FRACTURES

Hip fractures are numerically a larger problem than hip degenerative disorders. The number of hip fractures that occur yearly in the United States is estimated to be over 200,000.[11] Most of these fractures occur in older patients with weak, osteoporotic bone. Thus, the incidence of hip fractures is expected to gradually increase, because population demographics indicate the U.S. population is aging.

Historically hip fractures have had an extremely poor prognosis and often have resulted in the patient's death. Most elderly patients cannot survive prolonged bed rest, which was the traditional treatment many years ago. Complications (including thromboembolism, decubitus ulcers, pneumonia, and urinary sepsis) have frequently been responsible for mortality. Newer treatments emphasizing stable internal fixation of fractures or femoral head replacement with a prosthesis have eliminated prolonged bed rest and traction as a viable treatment. These surgical treatments have allowed early mobilization and weight-bearing ambulation. Getting the patient up out of bed early has been proved to reduce the complication rate significantly. The mortality rate, although decreased, remains high if patients are followed for 1 year after fracture.[12] This highlights the fact that patients are generally elderly and often have significant medical problems prior to hip fracture.

Classification

Classification of hip fractures is accomplished according to anatomic location and fracture pattern.[12] Fractures of the hip occur in one of three distinct anatomic areas: the femoral neck, the intertrochanteric femur, and the subtrochanteric femur. Subtrochanteric fractures are least common and will be discussed further. Femoral neck fractures carry a poorer prognosis for healing than intertrochanteric fractures, primarily because of two features. First, femoral neck fractures are located inside the hip capsule and thus are bathed in synovial fluid, which seems to slow healing. Intertrochanteric fractures, in contrast, are extracapsular. Second, intertrochanteric fractures seem to have a better blood supply. The ascending retinacular vessels that supply most of the arterial blood to the femoral head are very susceptible to injury by femoral neck fractures. Thus, complications such as nonunion and avascular necrosis of the femoral head are more likely with fractures of the femoral neck.

Subclassification of hip fractures can be complex. Many different classification systems have been proposed and used. Only two basic factors must be understood, however. First, is the fracture displaced or nondisplaced on radiographs? Displaced fractures do more poorly, particularly femoral neck fractures, in which the blood supply is more likely to be disrupted. Second, is the fracture stable when reduced? Significantly comminuted fractures and certain fracture patterns are inherently unstable, even when anatomically reduced. This is important for determining weight-bearing status for surgery. A stable fracture can accept more weight safely.

Treatment

Treatment of hip fractures in young patients is a separate issue. Young patients with normal bone sustain hip fractures only when exposed to violent injury, such as in a motor vehicle accident or a fall from a height. They are more likely to have associated injuries along with the hip fracture. A thorough investigation must be made for associated spinal fracture, pelvic fracture, or other injuries. In treating the fracture, every possible attempt should be made to salvage the femoral head. A primary hemi-arthroplasty is rarely a good choice in a young, active patient.

The typical patient with a hip fracture is elderly, however. Most commonly the injury occurs in a simple fall. Usually there are no significant associated injuries. These patients often have other medical problems. Early internal medicine consultation should be obtained to assist with the management of congestive heart failure, coronary artery disease, hypertension, chronic pulmonary disease, electrolyte abnormalities, diabetes, or other pre-existing medical problems. Although early surgery is preferable, in individual cases surgery should be postponed until the general medical condition is optimized. While awaiting surgery, patients often are more comfortable with 5 pounds of traction applied to a well-padded traction boot on the injured leg.

Intertrochanteric hip fractures often are best treated with a sliding hip screw. First an anatomic reduction should be obtained and verified on biplanar fluoroscopy. A large screw is placed across the fracture, through the center of the femoral neck, and into the femoral head. A barrel and side plate are placed over the hip screw and attached to the femur. The hip screw can "slide" in the barrel, allowing the fracture to collapse, compress, and seek a controlled, stable position.

Femoral neck fractures are considered in two groups —displaced and undisplaced. Undisplaced fractures may be fixed internally with screws or a sliding hip screw. Displaced femoral neck fractures, however, have a very high risk of developing complications, including avascular necrosis or nonunion. In the elderly patient these are best treated with hemi-arthroplasty. The femoral neck and head are excised and replaced with a prosthesis. Two general types of prostheses are in use at present, a fixed head or unipolar prosthesis and a bipolar prosthesis. The bipolar prosthesis has a small femoral head that articulates with a polyethylene liner inside a large metal cup. The outside of the cup articulates with the acetabular cartilage. Theoretically, motion occurs between the head and the liner, and between the cup and the acetabulum. Total hip replacement, using a femoral prosthesis and an acetabular prosthesis, is performed for femoral neck fracture under some circumstances. The primary indication is pre-existing hip disease, such as osteoarthritis.

Rehabilitation

Early mobilization is the key to avoiding complications associated with hip fracture. Patients are out of bed, standing or sitting in a chair, the day after surgery. Physical therapy treatment begins immediately. As with THA, ankle pumps and deep breathing exercises are started right away. Complications are similar to those seen after THA, including venous thrombosis, infection, prosthesis dislocation, and others. Antibiotics and anticoagulation regimens are used postoperatively. Weight-bearing status must be individualized. The surgeon is in the best position to evaluate fracture stability and should specify the amount of weight-bearing allowed. Recommended weight-bearing can vary from full weight to bed-to-chair transfers. Excellent nursing care is mandatory to avoid decubitus ulcers and to maximize nutrition and other medical needs. Recovery can be slow. Many patients will require temporary placement in a skilled nursing care facility after hospital discharge. The goal is to achieve preoperative functional status. If the patient was a limited household ambulator before the hip fracture, it is unrealistic to expect improvement to community or unlimited ambulation.

OSTEOTOMY

When the patient is likely to outlast the hip replacement, osteotomy should be considered. In this operation, bones near the hip joint—either the proximal femur or the pelvis—are cut, realigned, and allowed to heal. This can achieve several goals. Pre-existing deformity is corrected, improving hip mechanics. The weight-bearing surface can be increased, spreading the load over a larger area. Muscular forces, which account for the majority of the load across the hip, are relaxed. Although osteotomy does not increase overall motion, a more functional range of motion is created. Unfortunately, pain relief is not as predictable as with THA.[13]

Intertrochanteric osteotomy of the femur was introduced in 1894 for treatment of congenital dislocation of the hip. The procedure was refined by Pauwels, who described varus and valgus angulation of the osteotomy in the coronal plane in the 1950s. With the advent of THA in the 1970s, the indications for osteotomy diminished. However, as arthroplasty results were studied in the 1970s and 1980s, it became clear that younger, active patients did not do as well as older or less active patients. Attention has now returned to osteotomy as a surgical treatment for young, active patients with certain degenerative hip conditions.

If the primary problem is acetabular insufficiency, pelvic osteotomy is considered. Numerous specific procedures have been described by Salter, Sutherland, Steel, and others. However, the Chiari medial displacement osteotomy is probably the most useful for degenerative hip disease in adults. In this procedure, the pelvis is cut just above the hip capsule insertion. The acetabulum is then displaced medially and proximally. This improves hip mechanics, reduces muscle forces, and, most importantly, increases the volume of the acetabulum and acetabular coverage of the femoral head.

Fixation goals with osteotomy are similar to those of fracture fixation. Stable, rigid internal fixation is the key to allowing early mobilization. For proximal femoral osteotomies, we use a blade plate with screws. Pelvic osteotomies are fixed with lag screws and pins. If fixation is not adequate, cast immobilization is added. Cast immobilization is always used with children because they will not reliably cooperate with the rehabilitation program.

Postoperative rehabilitation is similar to that for THA, with some important differences. CPM is used preferentially in the early period to help promote cartilage healing. The patient is partially weight-bearing (about 20 to 25 pounds of force) on crutches until the

osteotomy has healed. This amount of weight-bearing serves simply to offset the distraction force provided by the weight of the extremity. No active hip exercises, other than walking, are started until the osteotomy has healed. The risk of losing fixation and causing an osteotomy malunion or nonunion is too great to begin early exercises or bicycle riding. However, isometric exercises such as quadriceps sets and gluteal sets are started to maintain muscle tone.

Abductor weakness is expected after Chiari osteotomy or varus intertrochanteric osteotomy. When the bone cuts have healed, an aggressive abductor strengthening program is started. Abductor exercises are done with gravity eliminated, then against gravity, and finally against gravity with weights. In a few cases abductor weakness persists despite adequate exercises. In these cases, removal of hardware 18 to 24 months after surgery can be combined with advancement of the greater trochanter to strengthen the abductors.

Satisfactory pain relief can be expected in over 80 percent of well-selected patients after osteotomy around the hip joint. Range of motion cannot be increased reliably by osteotomy, but the motion arc generally is in a more functional location after the procedure. Once the bone has healed, the hip is durable and will withstand sports activities and strenuous occupations. After removal of hardware the patient must return temporarily to crutches for 6 to 8 weeks. This precaution is intended to avoid a fracture through stress risers created by empty screw holes. The permanent restrictions of total hip replacement do not apply after osteotomy. Additionally, conversion of an osteotomy to a THA is much easier and has better results than revision total hip replacement.

ARTHRODESIS

Arthrodesis, or fusion, of the hip joint was introduced in the United States by Albee in 1908. This procedure usually results in a painless, stable joint. The goal of the operation is to achieve solid bony healing between the femoral head and acetabulum, thus obliterating the hip joint. Intra-articular and extra-articular bone grafting are variations in the technique employed to achieve fusion. Initially, prolonged postoperative immobilization of the joint was necessary, often from 3 to 18 months in a spica cast. More recently, improved internal fixation techniques have led to reduction in the time of immobilization needed.

Before hip arthrodesis is decided on, several criteria should be met. First, the hip problem should be unilateral. Bilateral fused hips prevent a functional gait and make perineal care difficult. The patient must have a normal lower back and ipsilateral knee because the fused hip places abnormal stresses on these structures. Additionally, patients should not be candidates for more functional procedures, including total hip replacement or intertrochanteric osteotomy. Practically, this limits hip arthrodesis to younger patients in whom life span exceeds the expected longevity of THA. Patients with heavy physical needs, such as laborers and sports enthusiasts, are good fusion candidates.

The present technique for hip fusion involves obliteration of any remaining articular cartilage and exposure of bleeding bone on the femoral head and acetabulum. The fusion area is grafted with bone and rigid fixation is obtained. Usually screws or bolts are passed across the joint. The ideal hip position is 30° of flexion, neutral rotation, and neutral abduction and adduction. Because of the long lever arm created by the extremity, great stress is placed on the fusion site. For this reason, it must be protected with spica cast immobilization until bone healing is radiographically evident.

External immobilization is utilized for at least 6 weeks. Immobilization is continued until healing is seen on radiographs. Patients can be partially weight-bearing on crutches during this time. When healing is complete, patients can expect a stable, painless, and durable hip. The gait after hip arthrodesis is relatively normal. A few patients experience difficulty with sports, bending, sitting, or sexual activity.[14] Because of the extra stress placed on the low back and knee, pain and degenerative changes can develop in these areas after hip fusion. Knee and back problems may respond to physical therapy treatment. If these problems become severe, the fusion can be converted to a total hip replacement. Therefore, it is essential that the technique employed to produce the hip fusion does not destroy any structures that would be necessary for conversion of the fusion to total hip replacement, such as the abductor muscles.

RESECTION ARTHROPLASTY

Resection arthroplasty of the hip was introduced by White in 1849 and popularized by Girdlestone for the treatment of septic arthritis and tuberculosis of the hip. The procedure involves removal of the femoral head, a portion of the femoral neck, and part of the acetabulum. The joint is left in a flail state, but it gradually stabilizes with scarring and muscle conditioning. In 1943, Girdlestone reported that the operation successfully controlled infection of the hip. Taylor reported in 1950 that resection arthroplasty for osteoarthritis reliably relieved pain and restored some mobility and function.[15]

At the present time, resection arthroplasty is a salvage procedure reserved for treatment of severe deep infection of the hip joint. Primary septic arthritis is best controlled with extensive surgical débridement, including resection arthroplasty if necesssary, and intravenous antibiotics. Most commonly this procedure is performed after removal of an infected total hip replacement. Occasionally a prosthesis may be salvaged by simple irrigation and débridement of the acute infection. More frequently, however, all components and cement must be removed to eradicate the infection. A total hip arthroplasty can be reimplanted immediately. If reimplantation is delayed, however, the incidence of recurrence of infection is diminished.[2]

The present regimen for treatment of infected THA begins with immediate irrigation, débridement, and removal of all components and cement. Culture and antibiotic sensitivity tests are performed. A 6-week course of culture-specific antibiotic treatment is given. Serial laboratory tests, including white blood cell count and erythrocyte sedimentation rate (ESR) are monitored. When the ESR has returned to normal, specimens from needle biopsies of the acetabulum and proximal femur are sent for culture. If cultures are negative while the patient is not taking any antibiotics, reimplantation of THA components can be scheduled.

Rehabilitation after resection arthroplasty of the hip is time consuming. Skeletal traction is standard for 3 to 6 weeks after surgery to help minimize shortening of the extremity. Usually a distal femoral traction pin is used with 10 to 15 percent body weight continuous traction in line with the femur. A CPM device can be incorporated into the treatment, set for 0° to 40° of flexion during the first several weeks. One or 2 weeks postoperatively, the patient may be removed temporarily from traction for physical therapy and gait training. The traction pin is left in place and traction is returned after each session.

Good pain relief and eradication of infection may be expected in nearly all patients after resection arthroplasty of the hip.[15] The procedure results in shortening of 1 to 5 inches, averaging 2.5 inches. Abductor insufficiency is always present, resulting in a Trendelenburg limp. Patients usually require cane or crutch support after resection arthroplasty. Most patients can function as limited community ambulators after this operation.

REFERENCES

1. Livermore J, Ilstrup D, Morrey B: Effect of femoral head size on wear of the polyethylene acetabular component. J Bone Joint Surg [Am] 75:518, 1990
2. Harris WH, Sledge CB: Total hip and total knee replacement. N Eng J Med 323:725, 1990
3. Harris WH, Maloney WJ: Hybrid total hip replacement. Clin Orthop 249:21, 1989
4. Johnston RC, Fitzgerald RH, Harris WH et al: Clinical and radiographic evaluation of total hip replacement. J Bone Joint Surg [Am] 72:161, 1990
5. Woolson ST, Watt JM: Use of autologous blood in total hip replacement. J Bone Joint Surg [Am] 73:76, 1991
6. Von Schroeder HP, Coutts RD, Billings E et al: The changes in intramuscular pressure and femoral vein flow with continuous passive motion, pneumatic compressive stockings, and leg manipulations. Clin Orthop 266:218, 1991
7. Sharrock NE, Brien WW, Salvati EA et al: The effect of fixed-dose heparin during total hip arthroplasty on the incidence of deep-vein thrombosis. J Bone Joint Surg [Am] 72:1456, 1990
8. Opitz JL: Total joint arthroplasty: principles and guidelines for postoperative physiatric management. Mayo Clin Proc 54:602, 1979
9. Seeger MS, Fisher LA: Adaptive equipment used in the rehabilitation of hip arthroplasty patients. Am J Occup Ther 36:503, 1982
10. Wong S, Wong J, Nolde T: Total hip replacements: improving post-hospital adjustment. Nurs Manage 15:34C, 1984
11. Nepomuceno C, Baker G, Shaddeau S et al: Rehabilitation of geriatric patients with Austin-Moore prostheses. Ala Med 56:28, 1986
12. DeLee JC: Fractures and dislocations of the hip. In Rockwood CA, Green DP (eds): Fractures in Adults. 2nd Ed. JB Lippincott, Philadelphia, 1984
13. Tronzo RG: Surgery of the Hip Joint. Vol II. 2nd Ed. Springer-Verlag, New York, 1987
14. Sponseller PD, McBeath AA, Perpich M: Hip arthrodesis in young patients. J Bone Joint Surg [Am] 66:853, 1984
15. Grauer JD, Amstutz H, O'Carroll PF, Dorey F: Resection arthroplasty of the hip. J Bone Joint Surg [Am] 71:669, 1989

56 Rehabilitation of the Knee

STEPHEN C. SHOEMAKER
MICHAEL J. SKYHAR
THOMAS C. SIMMONS

GENERAL PRINCIPLES OF KNEE REHABILITATION

The knee is one of the most frequently injured joints in the human body. The bipedal configuration radically increases the demands and risks placed on this joint. Consequently, restoration of function after injury or surgery is paramount.

Unlike a true hinge joint, the knee is an unstable construct in the absence of its soft tissue stabilizers. Osseous and ligamentous integrity is mandatory for optimal knee function and rehabilitation.

Physical Examination of the Knee

The physical examination of the knee must be performed in a concise, systematic manner. It should begin with a visual inspection of the joint. The presence of swelling should be noted. The examiner should be able to determine if the swelling is from an intra-articular effusion or an extra-articular source. The temperature, color, and uniformity of the skin should be examined. Scars should be noted and determined to be either post-traumatic or postsurgical in nature. Varus-valgus alignment of the lower extremity while bearing weight with the knee in full extension should be quantitated. Muscle atrophy in the thigh and calf musculature should be quantitated and compared to the opposite extremity. Perhaps most importantly, the patient's gait should be observed.

Range of motion of the knee should be recorded and compared to the opposite knee. Full extension is recorded as 0°. Hyperextension (or genu recurvatum), when present, is recorded as the number of degrees beyond 0 that the knee extends. Maximal flexion of the knee is recorded in absolute degrees with a goniometer along the lateral aspect of the leg, centered at the knee. Flexion can also be measured as the distance between the posterior aspect of the heel and the posterior thigh with the foot in the neutral position. Both active and passive range of motion of both knees should be recorded. Flexion contractures of the knee are best measured with the patient prone on the examining table. The patellae should be just distal to the edge of the table. The patient is asked to let both knees extend fully with gravity. The difference in heel height in the horizontal plane should be recorded. This is an accurate and reproducible method for following the progress of a flexion contracture. Extension contractures should be measured with the patient supine on the examining table. The hips are flexed to 90°. Both feet are allowed to fall with gravity. The absolute angles on each side or the difference in distance between the posterior heel and thigh can be measured. When contractures are present, particular attention should be paid to the type of endpoint that is present. Spongy and extremely painful endpoints can be indicative of a locked meniscal tear. Firm endpoints with minimal degrees of pain are more consistent with capsular contracture and scar tissue formation.

The knee should then be palpated systematically. All ligamentous structures, bony anatomic landmarks, and joint lines should be palpated according to a set routine during each examination. The precise location and degree of tenderness to palpation should be noted. An effusion, if present, should be quantified.

Testing of ligamentous stability should be performed on both knees. Integrity of the medial and lateral collateral ligaments is assessed by applying a valgus and varus stress with the knee both in extension and at 25° to 30° of flexion. The amount of joint space opening with stress testing is estimated in millimeters. Both knees are examined and the side-to-side difference in millimeters is recorded. The anterior cruciate ligament stability is best tested with the Lachman test. This is usually performed with the knee in 20° to 30° of flexion. Several variations of this test exist. The main goal is to obtain a side-to-side comparison with the patient completely relaxed. Devices such as the KT-1000 knee ligament arthrometer can accurately quantitate side-to-side differences in anteroposterior translation. Many tests are available for rotatory instability resulting from anterior cruciate ligament laxity. The most common is the pivot-shift test. The pivot-shift phenomenon can be amplified by performing the test in hip abduction. The test requires very gentle manipulation and complete patient relaxation. It takes a great deal of practice to master the pivot-shift or other rotatory instability testing. Spending time with someone proficient at performing these tests is the best way to learn the technique, as opposed to learning it from a textbook. Posterior cruciate ligament laxity can be detected as posterior sagging of the proximal tibia with the knee in 90° of flexion. The posterior drawer test is the most familiar screening test for posterior cruciate ligament laxity. A much more reliable and quantifiable maneuver for posterior cruciate laxity is the quadriceps active drawer test described by Daniel and coworkers.[1]

The patellofemoral joint constitutes perhaps the most difficult aspect of the knee examination from both a subjective and an objective standpoint. The overall rotational alignment of both limbs needs to be assessed from the hips to the ankles. Proximal femoral version needs to be determined and differences recorded. The Q- (quadriceps) angle is a clinical measurement recorded as the angle between two lines bisecting the center of the patella emanating from the anterior superior iliac spine and the tibial tubercle. The normal Q-angle in males is 10° to 11° and in females 13° to 15°. Distal to the knee, tibial torsion should be measured as well as the presence of pes planus. The tracking of the patellae should be observed throughout a full passive and active range of motion of both knees. Any abnormal axial tilting, mediolateral deviation, or symptomatic crepitus during range of motion should be noted. The relative tightness of the lateral retinacular structures may be checked in the supine position by having the patient cross the legs at the ankles. With the knees fully extended and the patient completely relaxed, the patella is simply pushed medially. The medial patellar displacement can be quantitated in millimeters. This is a simple, reliable, reproducible test for lateral retinacular tightness. Likewise, lateral patellar laxity must be evaluated when patellofemoral instability is a concern. This is done with the same sort of test, only pushing the patella straight laterally. In instances of acute patellofemoral lateral instability, there will be medial retinacular tenderness and apprehension when the patella is moved laterally.

Palpation all the way around the patellofemoral joint is important, but patellofemoral compression is not a reliable physical sign and will cause pain in many asymptomatic patients. A suprapatellar plica may be felt in the medial aspect of the patellofemoral joint. These plicae are rarely symptomatic. The examiner must also remember that the diagnosis of anterior knee pain is not always synonymous with chondromalacia. Chondromalacia is a pathologic diagnosis and not a clinical diagnosis. Many other causes of anterior knee pain exist besides chondromalacia.

Evaluation of the lateral and medial meniscus should begin with complete palpation of the entire tibial-femoral joint line. Meniscus pathology will usually cause very localized joint line tenderness. However, extreme anterior joint line tenderness usually is not specific for meniscus pathology. Functional tests for meniscus pathology, such as the McMurray sign and other tibial axial rotational maneuvers, by themselves are usually not that specific or reliable. When a patient has a true locked knee as a result of meniscal pathology, specific medial or lateral joint line tenderness will be present with inability to fully straighten the knee. Typically the patient has a 15° to 20° extensor lag with a spongy endpoint. A locked knee with ability to fully extend the leg but blocks in flexion is less common. The most reliable signs of meniscus pathology are patient history, joint line tenderness, effusion, and true locking of the knee.

Finally, the physical examination of the knee should include an assessment of the general neurovascular status of both lower extremities. Pulses and sensation of the skin need to be checked. Trophic changes, as seen in reflex sympathetic dystrophy, should also be noted. The popliteal fossa should never be overlooked on routine examination of the knee.

Basic Rules of Knee Rehabilitation

1. Osseous and ligamentous integrity must be present to restore optimum knee function.
2. The development of limited range of motion must be recognized early and treated aggressively when present.
3. In general, the sooner a patient is referred to physical therapy after injury or surgery the better the ultimate result is likely to be.
4. Patellofemoral problems should not be created or aggravated by knee rehabilitation procedures.
5. Functional exercises are mandatory for restoration of optimal knee function.
6. After injury or surgery, full unassisted weight-bearing should not begin until there is return of near-normal range of motion, gait, and cadence.
7. Reflex inhibition of the extensor and/or flexor mechanism after injury or surgery must be recognized and treated with the appropriate modalities.
8. Hamstring muscle rehabilitation is an integral part of any knee rehabilitation program.
9. Prior to any major knee reconstructive procedures, a preoperative consultation with a physical therapist is very helpful. This will facilitate the patient's understanding of the rationale behind the specific rehabilitation approach.
10. Free-flowing communication between the physician and therapist is mandatory to ensure an efficient and effective rehabilitation process.

Basic Physical Therapy Modalities Used in Knee Rehabilitation

Most of the physical therapy modalities used in rehabilitation of the knee are similar to those used for other joints. However, there are certain exceptions, as described in the following paragraphs.

Wall slides are performed with the patient lying supine. The affected heel is placed onto a wall in an elevated position. Range-of-motion exercises can be performed as passive, active, or active assisted. The range of motion that is used should be pain free. This type of exercise is very beneficial because the elevation assists in edema resorption. Elevation also provides some pain relief to the patient during the early phases of knee rehabilitation.

Hamstring and quadriceps co-contractions are very useful in anterior cruciate ligament reconstruction. Initially, these are performed with the knee in 45° to 60° of flexion. The patient is instructed to contract the hamstrings isometrically and hold them. The quadriceps is then fired isometrically without changing the angle of knee flexion. Theoretically, anterior tibial translation owing to quadriceps force is diminished by performing co-contraction exercises in this fashion.

Eccentric quadriceps loading can be very useful in the early treatment of patellofemoral disorders and overuse syndromes of the extensor mechanism. Eccentric quadriceps loading is best performed by manual hands-on techniques. Typically, a force is applied to the tibia with the knee near full extension. As this force creates knee flexion, the patient exerts quadriceps contraction against the force as the knee moves into further flexion. The initial force is applied with the quadriceps muscle in a shortened position and resistance is applied as the quadriceps is lengthened. This is in contrast to concentric exercises, in which the force is applied with the muscle initially in the lengthened position and resistance is continued as the quadriceps muscle shortens. This exercise should always be performed within the patient's pain-free range of motion.

Joint mobilization is a manual hands-on technique that increases joint mobility and decreases pain. This is accomplished by placing the joint in its resting (open pack) position. The proximal bony anatomy is fixed. A combination of distraction and gliding forces is then applied within the pain-free ranges of motion.

Functional weight-bearing exercises are meant to simulate normal knee loading situations. Examples include wall squats, knee dips, eccentric touchdowns, step-ups, and forward lunges. These exercises are typically started once weight-bearing is tolerated or allowed. Initially, these are performed isometrically, causing weight-bearing through both lower extremities. Range of motion, selective weight-bearing, resistance, speed, and repetitions are added as pain diminishes and strength increases. Agility training involves increasing functional weight-bearing exercises to increase speed and power. These would include cutting, jumping, one-legged hop, and similar exercises.

ANTERIOR CRUCIATE LIGAMENT

Nowhere else in the rehabilitation of orthopaedic problems will one find a wider variety of treatment methods than in anterior cruciate ligament (ACL) rehabilitation. Well-controlled, randomized studies with objective measurement of outcome are difficult to perform. Our approach to ACL rehabilitation is founded on clinical and biomechanical data available. It should not be construed as the definitive approach but rather as a rational one based on available information.

A basic understanding of joint mechanics is critical to ACL surgery and rehabilitation. The human knee is a diarthrodial ginglymus joint and, therefore, does not function as a true hinge. Knee flexion entails translation in combination with rotation of the joint surfaces. The ACL and posterior cruciate ligament (PCL) form a four-bar linkage, which, along with joint surface anatomy, dictates these motions.[2] Isometric graft placement results in the same graft length and tension in full flexion as that seen in full extension. Graft lengthening of 1 to 3 mm between 120° and full extension is considered ideal. Extreme graft lengthening (i.e., greater than 5 mm between 120° and full extension) will increase the likelihood of flexion contracture. Any amount of graft shortening with extension will increase graft tension as the knee flexes and will predispose the patient to graft failure or flexion loss. Ideal graft placement permits patients to obtain full range of motion early without fear of causing extraordinary tension on the newly placed graft.[3] Tension in isometrically placed grafts and in intact ACLs has been shown to be lowest at 20° to 40° of flexion and increases as the knee is extended.[4-9] These findings support the view that hyperextension

should be avoided in the early postoperative period. They do not, however, support avoiding terminal extension in isometrically or ideally placed grafts.

Equally important is an understanding of muscle-ligament interactions. The quadriceps, acting through the patellar tendon, creates an anterior drawer force on the proximal tibia from 70° of flexion to full extension. The maximum effect is seen between 40° and 20° of flexion.[10] Most biomechanical studies on quadriceps-cruciate ligament interaction have used a model that simulates sitting long-arc knee extension exercises with resistance or weights placed at the ankle. Changing the placement of the resistance or pad during long-arc knee extension exercises has been shown to alter anterior-posterior shear forces at the tibiofemoral joint.[11] A more proximal pad placement tends to decrease the amount of anterior shear that occurs at the tibiofemoral joint. Therefore, ACL-deficient or ACL-reconstructed knees should have a more proximal pad placement to decrease the anterior shear forces at the joint surfaces. Nonetheless, long-arc quadriceps knee extension exercises increase the likelihood of patellofemoral pain and anterior tibial displacement, in both ACL-deficient and ACL-reconstructed knees. It is our opinion that these exercises should be minimized, if used at all.

The contribution of hamstring forces toward stabilizing ACL-deficient knees was popularized through anecdote and poorly controlled studies. Recent biomechanical experiments and gait analysis have supported the contention that hamstring forces can control anterior tibial translation.[12] In vitro experiments have demonstrated that the increase in strain on the ACL due to isolated quadriceps force can be greatly reduced when both hamstring and quadriceps forces are applied (i.e., simulated isometric co-contraction).[13,14] Therefore, the emphasis in rehabilitation of both ACL-deficient knees and postoperative reconstructions should be placed on hamstring strengthening.

A controversial feature of rehabilitation following ACL reconstruction is the length of time patients are kept from participating in sports. On the basis of canine studies, the process of graft incorporation is presumed to take approximately 12 months. Anterior laxity measurements in patients after ACL reconstruction show that 25 percent of graft failure occurred between 6 and 12 months after operation. Few patients experience graft failure between 12 and 24 months after reconstruction.[12] In light of these findings, it is difficult to justify sending patients back to contact sports prior to 12 months postoperatively. The patients often feel as if they could return to sports sooner. One investigator has, in fact, determined that a high percentage of postoperative ACL reconstruction patients "cheat" by returning to sports without informing the surgeon until afterward.[15] Between 6 and 12 months postoperatively, we place tremendous emphasis on progressive activities (muscle training, agility) in preparation for return to sports at 12 months.

Bracing is another topic of controversy. Cadaver studies have shown braces to be effective in preventing anterior tibial displacements resulting from low levels of applied force.[16] Forces capable of producing injury are not well prevented by braces. Furthermore, no one brace fares any better than another in biomechanical testing. Bracing may have a role in postoperative care to aid in controlling tibial translations against low levels of applied force. Theoretically, this may protect the graft during the period in which it is remodeling.

Specific features of our postoperative ACL reconstruction protocol are included in Table 56-1. Based on biomechanical and postoperative in vivo studies, several general principles can be formed and used as guidelines:

1. Full passive range of motion can be achieved immediately without placing undue stress on the ACL graft.
2. Hamstring force protects the graft and, therefore, emphasis is placed on active knee flexion early.
3. Quadriceps force tends to displace the tibia anteriorly and, therefore, quadriceps training should be started after hamstring function is established. Long-arc quadriceps extension exercises are forbidden.
4. Patients engage in a progressive-activity rehabilitation program but are kept out of contact sports for 12 months postoperatively.

POSTERIOR CRUCIATE LIGAMENT

The posterior cruciate ligament (PCL) is the primary ligamentous restraint to posterior tibial displacements from 45° of flexion to full flexion.[17] This ex-

plains while PCL tears are best detected with patients supine and the knee flexed 90°. At full extension, posterior capsular structures share a considerable portion of ligamentous force, preventing posterior tibial displacements. Consequently, patients with isolated PCL tears generally function well during weight-bearing stance activities. Problems of instability are more apt to occur during activities involving flexion, such as rising from a seated position, squatting, and stair climbing.

One clinical study on isolated PCL-deficient knees found that patients with normal function and no symptoms had symmetrical quadriceps strength. Patients with symptoms of pain, instability, and decreased function had quadriceps strength less than 80 percent of that seen in the normal knee.[18] Long-term studies indicate that PCL-deficient knees are at higher risk for degenerative changes in the patellofemoral and medial compartments.[19] No clinical studies are available that demonstrate whether or not surgical reconstruction alters the long-term results in the isolated PCL-deficient knee. Therefore, the first approach to an isolated PCL-deficient knee is rehabilitation.

In the acute phase after PCL injury, various therapeutic modalities are used to control swelling and pain. Range of motion exercises should be done in the sitting position to minimize posterior sag of the tibia. Wall slides and active hamstring strengthening will exacerbate posterior tibial displacements, especially if quadriceps tone and function are poor. Long-term rehabilitation efforts are designed to improve quadriceps strength and minimize abnormal tibiofemoral motion without placing extraordinary stresses at the patellofemoral joint. Isometric quadriceps sets in full extension, short arc (20° of flexion to full extension) quadriceps exercises, and stationary biking are mainstays of treatment. Endurance is preferred to absolute strength. Patients should be encouraged to use less resistance and a greater duration of exercise. Currently, there are no braces that control posterior tibial translation satisfactorily and, therefore, bracing does not play a role in treatment of PCL-deficient knees.

PCL reconstructions are considered in patients with multiple ligament injuries or in patients with isolated PCL tears in whom conservative treatment efforts

Table 56-1. Protocol for Reconstruction of Anterior Cruciate Ligament

	Week 1	2	3	4	5	6	Month 3	4	6	8	10	12
Range of motion												
CPM	├──┤											
Passive flexion/extension	├──────────→											
Wall slides		├──────────→										
Active flexion		├──────────→										
Protection												
Knee immobilizer	├──────┤											
Crutches	├──────┤											
Partial weight-bearing	├──────┤											
Full weight-bearing					├────→							
Functional brace					├──────────────────────────→							
Exercises												
Hamstring curls			├────────────────────────→									
Isometric curls				├────→								
Stationary bike					├──────────────────────→							
Wall squats (45–90)						├────→						
Stairmaster						├────→						
Nordic track						├────→						
Activity												
Walking					├────→							
Swimming						├────→						
Street bike							├────→					
Fast walking							├────→					
Jumping rope								├────→				
Track/jogging								├────→				
Agility drills									├────→			
Running									├────→			
Running sports										├──→		
Cutting sports											├──→	
Jumping sports											├──→	

have failed. Because of the tendency for the tibia to sag posteriorly, both the patient and therapist must take extreme efforts to avoid the effects of gravity on hamstring pull on the proximal tibia.

After PCL reconstruction, patients are usually immobilized in full extension to avoid posterior sag and early graft stretch. Patients are encouraged to do isometric quadriceps contractions during this time. After 4 to 6 weeks of immobilization in full extension, efforts are directed to achieve full range of motion. This must be done in a way that avoids posterior sag. Passive flexion exercises should be done sitting rather than supine or with wall slides. If a continuous passive motion (CPM) machine is used, the pad is placed beneath the proximal calf instead of the distal calf. Quadriceps strengthening follows the same guidelines as outlined for conservative treatment. If patients are to do long-arc quadriceps sets, they should

be done with a distal pad and restricted to an arc of flexion from 45° to full extension. These exercises run the risk of precipitating patellofemoral pain and should be done with some caution.

PATELLOFEMORAL REHABILITATION

Anterior knee pain is characterized by retropatellar pain with activity, particularly stair climbing and descending. Crepitus with active knee extension is common particularly around 30° to 40° of flexion. Patients may occasionally complain of mild swelling.

Anterior knee pain is influenced by a combination of structural and functional factors. Alignment of the extensor mechanism is determined by the position of the tibial tubercle, the patella captured in the trochlea, and the pull of the quadriceps muscle. Tibial-femoral alignment and location of the tibial tubercle greatly influence the Q-angle. The presence of genu valgum or a laterally placed tibial tubercle will increase the Q-angle. Increased Q-angle is also associated with patellofemoral mistracking and pain. Hyperpronation of the feet can lead to external tibial torsion and genu valgum, thereby resulting in patellofemoral mistracking. Functionally, each of the four quadriceps muscles contributes stability to the patella in the trochlea during knee extension. Excessive strength in the vastus lateralis or relative weakness in the vastus medialis can lead to subtle abnormalities in patellar tracking in the trochlea during knee extension. The same effect can occur owing to tightness in the iliotibial band and lateral retinaculum.

Successful treatment of anterior knee pain demands that all contributing factors be identified and addressed. A thorough history and physical examination are critical. The majority of patients with anterior knee pain respond to conservative treatment. Many patients with structural abnormalities (i.e., genu valgum, high Q-angle) can obtain satisfactory relief by quadriceps strengthening. Conservative (i.e., nonoperative) treatment of anterior knee pain relies on a two-pronged approach. First, the patient must avoid or minimize aggravating activities such as squatting, stair climbing, and running up and down hills. A detailed history will often reveal activities that increase the patellofemoral contact forces and exacerbate the patient's complaints of pain. Second, quadriceps strengthening performed in a manner that minimizes the contact forces between patella and trochlea is necessary to cause improvement in the patient's symptoms.

Specific features of the quadriceps strengthening program should consider the patient's symptoms and physical signs. In patients with synovitis and exquisite patellofemoral irritability, initial efforts must be directed toward decreasing inflammation through ice, ultrasound, medication, and other therapeutic modalities. In patients with significant quadriceps inhibition, transcutaneous electrical stimulation may be useful. Tight soft tissue structures, such as the iliotibial band and lateral retinaculum, should be addressed through stretching exercises. Isometric quadriceps contraction in full extension is the most basic exercise in a quadriceps strengthening program. With

the knee in full extension, the patellofemoral contact forces are minimized. The patella enters the trochlea at approximately 20 to 30° of knee flexion. At flexion angles greater than 30°, quadriceps activity leads to increased patellofemoral contact force and, therefore, should be avoided. A patient with anterior knee pain should never, under any circumstances, do long-arc quadriceps extension exercises (i.e., extend the knee from 90° of flexion to full extension with a weight at the ankle).

After mastering isometric quadriceps sets in full extension, the patient may begin straight leg raises in full extension and short-arc quadriceps exercises (20° of knee flexion to full extension). When symptoms allow, exercises should be started on a stationary bike. Resistance should be minimal at first. When 20- to 30-minute sessions are achieved without discomfort, resistance is gradually increased. Quadriceps exercises such as Stairmaster, half squats, and half leg presses should be used with caution and stopped immediately if retropatellar pain is experienced. Other pain-free weight-bearing functional exercises are allowed. Patellofemoral taping is a relatively new technique that can be effective for proprioceptive training. Biofeedback is another modality useful for changing or enhancing the timing of selective quadriceps contraction.

Patellofemoral disorders that require surgical intervention and subsequent postoperative rehabilitation include instability (mistracking, subluxations, dislocations) and fractures. The approach to knee rehabilitation after patellofemoral surgery is generally the same as that for anterior knee pain. However, a few aspects deserve special attention, such as protection of the surgical repair, early passive range of motion, and quadriceps inhibition.

Care must be taken to protect the surgical repair, whether soft tissue repair or internal fixation was done. Communication between therapist and surgeon is critical to define the "safe limits" of rehabilitation. If possible, early passive range of motion is desired and should be achieved as soon as possible. Pain-free wall slides and passive knee flexion are basic exercises. CPM machines can relegate the patient to the role of passive observer rather than active participant if used too long. Quadriceps atrophy and inhibition invariably result after patellofemoral surgery. Therefore, emphasis on early quadriceps retraining and long-term quadriceps strengthening is mandatory.

MEDIAL COLLATERAL LIGAMENT (MEDIAL SUPPORTING STRUCTURES)

The medial collateral ligament (MCL) is a long, broad, fan-like structure, originating from the medial epicondyle of the femur. Deep and superficial portions have distinctly separate insertions. The deep MCL attaches just below the joint line via the coronary (meniscotibial) ligament. The superficial MCL inserts into the medial aspect of the proximal tibia metaphysis, deep to the pes anserinus. The deep MCL is, in effect, a capsular structure. This has prompted some authors to divide medial supporting structures of the knee into anterior, middle, and posterior thirds.[20] The superficial MCL is considered part of the anterior one-third, the deep MCL is the middle one-third, and the posterior oblique ligament and adjoining capsular structures make up the posterior one-third.

Injury to medial supporting structures can be classified by severity as grade I, II, or III. Confusion over nomenclature sometimes arises owing to differences in physiologic, anatomic, and biomechanical criteria used by various authors. It should be recognized that each classification scheme offers certain insights into injuries to medial supporting structures, yet all are somewhat arbitrary. We have found that a useful grading system takes many of the varied factors and criteria into consideration while helping to guide clinical decisions.

A grade I strain is a stretch injury without disruption of the collagen fibers of the ligament. Typically, patients will have a twist or a valgus-type mechanism of injury. Point tenderness at the MCL origin or insertion is common. An effusion is usually not present. Ligament testing fails to reveal increased medial joint space opening to valgus stress but may elicit pain. Depending on which fibers of the MCL are injured, the patient may have pain when the knee is fully extended.

In grade II strains, some but not all collagen fibers are disrupted. In addition to tenderness over the insertion or origin, or over both, large portions of the MCL can be painful to palpation. Mild effusion can occur. Ligamentous testing reveals an increase in the medial joint space opening to valgus stress with the knee in 20° of flexion. There is, however, a firm and definite endpoint. At full extension, a subtle increase may be seen. Stress radiographs under anesthesia will show that a 10-pound valgus stress with the knee flexed 20° results in a side-to-side difference in medial joint space opening of 5 mm or less. Range of motion will be limited, in both flexion and extension, as a result of pain.

In a grade III injury, the MCL by definition is totally disrupted. Considerable energy is required to produce such an injury. In addition, displacements involved are usually sufficient to damage other structures, such as the ACL. Hence, isolated grade III MCL strains are uncommon. There will be tenderness to palpation, but usually less severe than that seen in grade II injuries. Because the capsule has been disrupted, any effusion that might have accumulated will extravasate into the subcutaneous soft tissues. Global swelling of the knee and the leg results. Range of motion will be limited as a result of pain. The ligamentous testing reveals marked increase in the medial joint space opening with a soft endpoint at 20°. Clinically, instability can be demonstrated at full extension if the patient is relaxed.

Knowledge of combined injury facilitates diagnosis and treatment. Injuries to the MCL often occur in association with ACL tears. Usually, when there is a complete ACL disruption, a grade I or grade II MCL strain is also seen. The fabled "unholy triad"—anterior cruciate ligament, medial collateral ligament grade III, and medial meniscus tear—does occur, but is less common. The prevalence of medial meniscus tear in combination with isolated grade I MCL strains is extremely low. Although medial meniscus tears can occur in the face of grade II MCL strains, this too is uncommon. Medial meniscus tears are common in ACL-MCL injuries, but this seems to be more a function of the anterior instability than the medial injury.

Distinguishing a pathologic condition of the meniscus from MCL strain may, at times, be difficult. Both conditions may be manifested by limited motion in flexion or extension. Meniscal provocative tests also may elicit pain in patients with MCL strains who otherwise have normal menisci. Signs that aid in distinguishing MCL strains from other pathologic conditions of the knee can be elicited through careful physical examination. Tenderness over the MCL origin or insertion decreases the likelihood of meniscal pathology. Tenderness over the pes anserinus bursa also is uncommon with pathologic conditions of the meniscus. Medial joint line tenderness in combination with tenderness over the proximal tibia or distal femur is more likely to be of MCL origin. True mechanical signs are absent in patients with MCL injuries.

Treatment and rehabilitation of MCL injuries has been greatly simplified with the recognition that nonoperative intervention results in outcome equivalent, if not superior, to surgical repair.[21] Patients with grade I injuries should refrain from twisting or lateral movement activities for 4 to 6 weeks from the time of injury. Therapeutic modalities are useful to control pain and soft tissue swelling, if present. Isometric contractions of hamstrings and quadriceps can be started immediately. Gentle pain-free passive and active assisted range-of-motion exercises should be performed as tolerated. Stationary bike exercises facilitate range of motion as well as improving quadriceps tone and function. Weight-bearing is encouraged. Bracing is not necessary.

Grade II injuries may be treated similarly to grade I strains. Bracing plays a greater role and should be considered when instability is a factor. Grade III injuries that occur in isolation are uncommon. In these, bracing is mandatory. A short course (5 to 10 days) of immobilization in a knee immobilizer may be useful for pain control. Casting for prolonged periods is associated with a significant risk of flexion contractures and should be avoided. Because most grade III MCL injuries occur in combination with other injuries, the knee rehabilitation is often dictated by the surgical procedure on other injured ligaments. The use of bracing to prevent valgus stress on the MCL is usually included in this regimen.

REHABILITATION OF MENISCAL INJURIES

The vasculature of the human meniscus has been the subject of numerous studies. It is well known that the periphery of each meniscus has a vascular supply to a variable depth. Tears within the vascular portion of the meniscus usually have excellent healing potential with minimal intervention needed. However, the majority of the meniscus is avascular and has limited potential for healing. To make the diagnosis of a meniscus tear a combination of physical signs and symptoms must be present. These will usually include a combination of joint line tenderness, effusion, "giving way" of the knee or locking, positive meniscal provocative tests, and thigh atrophy. Acute meniscal injuries are often hard to diagnose. When acute meniscal injuries are suspected in the absence of knee ligamentous laxity or true locking, the patient should be sent to physical therapy for evaluation and treatment. A significant percentage of patients with this type of injury will improve sufficiently that they will not need any further treatment. Unless a knee is truly locked and cannot be unlocked over a couple of days, rapid surgical intervention for these types of injuries is not necessary. Rehabilitation of acute and chronic meniscal injuries follows basically the same approach. Pain must be the guide for the patient and the therapist. Specific ranges of motion or maneuvers that recreate pain should be avoided. In the absence of pain, all other physical therapy modalities, including functional ones, can be started immediately in these patients. If a meniscus tear is not going to heal, a lot of the aforementioned symptoms will persist and operative intervention becomes necessary.

After arthroscopic partial meniscectomy, the initial therapy is aimed at pain control. Once postoperative pain subsides, a full unlimited rehabilitation program can begin, working within the patient's limits of comfort.

Meniscal repair can be performed either arthroscopically or as an open procedure. A variety of rehabilitation protocols have been espoused for use after meniscal repair. We treat meniscal repairs in a cast or knee immobilizer with the knee in full extension for 4 weeks. Full weight-bearing is allowed. No resistive or shear-producing exercises should be performed for 4 weeks.

After 4 weeks, a full knee rehabilitation program can start. Functional and agility-type drills can begin at 3 months postoperatively. Sports should not be allowed for the first 6 months after operation. When meniscal repair is performed in conjunction with ligament repair or reconstruction, priority should be given to the specific rehabilitation involved with the ligament in question. Range of motion should not be limited after ligament reconstruction because of fears of developing contractures.

OVERUSE INJURIES

The most common overuse syndromes occurring about the knee include quadriceps tendinitis, patellar ligament inflammation (proximal and distal), iliotibial band syndrome, pes anserinus bursitis, and lateral and medial hamstring tendinitis at the joint line. All overuse injuries should be treated first with rest and activity modification.

Quadriceps tendon and patellar ligament inflammation can be treated in much the same way as described in the patellofemoral rehabilitation section. It has been well shown that eccentric-type loading of the extensor mechanism is valuable in treating these problems.

Iliotibial band syndrome is manifested as pain localized over the lateral femoral condyle. The pain may radiate toward the lateral joint line and proximal lateral tibial area. The pain generally tends to worsen with increased activities. There should be no sign of an intra-articular pathologic condition such as an effusion. Downhill running or stair climbing seems to aggravate the symptoms. This syndrome usually occurs after an inadequate stretching program and acute changes in training intervals. Often there is a tight iliotibial band, which can be diagnosed using the Ober test.[22] Anatomic factors associated with iliotibial band syndrome include hip abduction contracture with positive Ober test, genu varum, heel or foot pronation, tight heel cords, and internal tibial torsion. Irritation of the iliotibial band can occur at the lateral epicondyle, at the joint line, and at Gerdy's tubercle. Initial treatment of the iliotibial band syndrome includes rest, ice, activity modification, and stretching. The iliotibial band can be stretched with hip adduction motions with the knee both in flexion and in extension. These can be done in a lateral decubitus position or standing against a wall. Once medical therapy has diminished some of the pain, specific strengthening of the iliotibial band can begin. This can be accomplished through eccentric and concentric contraction of the hip abductors and extensors. The gluteus medius and gluteus maximus muscles can be isolated and strengthened separately.

The pes anserinus is the confluence of the sartorius, gracilis, and semitendinosus tendons on the proximal tibia, just medial to the tibial tubercle. A bursa located immediately beneath the confluence of these three tendons can become acutely inflamed. Usually exquisite tenderness to palpation and swelling occur in this area. Active adduction of the leg and internal rotation of the hip will aggravate the symptoms. Once medical therapy has reduced the acute inflammation, rehabilitation should consist first of localized treatment of pain. Stretching of the anserinus muscles can be accomplished by maneuvers involving hip abduction and knee extension combinations. Likewise, strengthening of the anserinus muscles can be performed with hip adduction and knee flexion with the tibia rotated internally.

The judicious use of rest and anti-inflammatory medications is mandatory in treating all the overuse type syndromes about the knee. All exercises must be performed in pain-free ranges of motion. Ultrasound and iontophonophoresis may be beneficial to treat localized areas of pain.

REHABILITATION OF FRACTURES ABOUT THE KNEE

Patellar fractures are common. Usually they involve some displacement of fracture fragments and disruption of quadriceps mechanism. However, a small percentage of patellar fractures are displaced minimally with no disruption of the quadriceps mechanism. In this type of stable fracture, full rehabilitation of the knee can begin as early as pain allows. When unstable patellar fractures have been fixed surgically, the patients can generally be started on range-of-motion exercise when the surgical pain is tolerable. The stability of the fixation must be confirmed with the treating surgeon. Typically, rehabilitation with range-of-motion exercises starts within one week of open reduction and internal fixation.

Many different types of fractures can occur in the distal femur and proximal tibia. Some of these fractures involve the articular surface of the joint. The criteria that most surgeons use to determine whether operative fixation is necessary include joint surface displacement of more than 2 mm and inherent instability as a result of the fracture. The vast majority of intra-articular fractures about the knee will be fixed surgically to allow early range-of-motion exercises and rehabilitation to begin. In each case, the therapist must check with the surgeon to determine safe limits of range of motion and weight-bearing status, and to decide when to start performing resistive exercises. It is often very helpful for therapists to see radiographs taken before and after fracture fixation. Most surgeons treat intra-articular fractures of the knee with CPM machines for a variable period of time. The majority of intra-articular fractures about the knee will heal within 5 to 6 weeks if fixed properly. Once the pain of the fracture and surgery has subsided, rehabilitation should begin as soon as possible with at least passive range-of-motion exercises. Intra-articular fractures that do not require fixation are generally stable enough to start range-of-motion exercises within 2 weeks. Communication among the therapist, surgeon, and patient is mandatory to ensure optimal results after fractures about the knee.

DEGENERATIVE JOINT DISEASE

Degenerative joint disease of the knee is a very common condition, usually affecting an older population. The disease is cyclical, associated with periods of exacerbations and remissions. The conservative treatment of this disease is with nonsteroidal anti-inflammatory medications and physical therapy. The approach to patients with symptomatic flare-ups of their degenerative joint disease consists of rest modalities and modified activity. Range-of-motion exercises are important but should not be done to the point of aggravating the patient's pain.

After symptoms of acute pain and swelling have improved, motion exercises and muscle strengthening

should be done on a maintenance basis. Ultimately, when the patient's symptoms have regressed, total knee replacement is indicated. Multiple factors go into deciding the timing of this operation, and this aspect is beyond the scope of this chapter.

REFERENCES

1. Daniel DM, Stone ML, Barnett P, Sachs R: Use of the quadriceps active test to diagnose posterior cruciate ligament disruption and measure posterior laxity of the knee. J Bone Joint Surg [Am] 70:386, 1988
2. Muller W: The Knee: The Form, Function, and Ligament Reconstruction. Springer-Verlag, New York, 1983
3. Penner DA, Daniel DM, Wood P, Mishra D: An in vitro study of anterior cruciate ligament graft placement and isometry. Am J Sports Med 16:238, 1988
4. Hoogland T, Hillen B: Intra-articular reconstruction of the anterior cruciate ligament. An experimental study of length changes in different ligament reconstructions. Clin Orthop 185:197, 1984
5. Markolf KL, Gorek JF, Kabo M, Shapiro MS: Direct measurement of resultant forces in the anterior cruciate ligament. An in vitro study performed with a new experimental technique. J Bone Joint Surg [Am] 72:557, 1990
6. Sapega AA, Moyer RA, Schneck C, Komalahiranya N: Testing for isometry during reconstruction of the anterior cruciate ligament. Anatomical and biomechanical considerations. J Bone Joint Surg [Am] 72:259, 1990
7. Schutzer SF, Christen S, Jakob RP: Further observations on the isometricity of the anterior cruciate ligament: an anatomical study using a 6 mm diameter replacement. Clin Orthop 242:247, 1989
8. Sidles JA, Larson RV, Garbini JL et al: Ligament length relationships in the moving knee. J Orthop Res 6:593, 1988
9. Yadsuda K, Sasaki T: Exercise after anterior cruciate ligament reconstruction. The force exerted on the tibia by separate isometric contractions of the quadriceps or the hamstrings. Clin Orthop 220:275, 1987
10. Grood ES, Suntay WJ, Noyes FR, Butler DL: Biomechanics of the knee extension exercise. Effect of cutting the anterior cruciate ligament. J Bone Joint Surg [Am] 66:725, 1984
11. Mandt PR, Daniel DM, Biden E, Stone ML: Tibial translation with quadriceps force: an in vitro study of the effect of load placement, flexion angle and ACL sectioning. Trans Orthop Res Soc 12:243, 1987
12. More RL, Kanas BT, Neiman R et al: Hamstrings — an anterior cruciate ligament protagonist. An in vitro study. Am J Sports Med (in press)
13. Arms SW, Pope MH, Johnson RJ et al: The biomechanics of anterior cruciate ligament rehabilitation and reconstruction. Am J Sports Med 12:8, 1984
14. Renstrom P, Arms SW, Stanwyck TS, Johnson RJ, Pope MH: Strain within the anterior cruciate ligament during hamstring and quadriceps activity. Am J Sports Med 14:83, 1986
15. Shelbourne KD, Nitz P: Accelerated rehabilitation after anterior cruciate ligament reconstruction. Am J Sports Med 18:292, 1990
16. Martensen W, Foreman K, Focht L et al: An in vitro study of functional orthoses in the anterior cruciate disrupted knee. Trans Orthop Res Soc 13:520, 1988
17. Shoemaker SC, Daniel DM: The limits of knee motion. p. 153.

In Daniel D, Akeson W, O'Connor J (eds): Knee Ligaments: Structure, Function, Injury and Repair. Raven Press, New York, 1990

18. Dandy DJ, Pusey RJ: The long term results of unrepaired tears of the posterior cruciate ligament. J Bone Joint Surg [Br] 64:92, 1982

19. Parolie JM, Bergfeld JA: Long term results of non-operative treatment of isolated posterior cruciate ligament injuries in the athlete. Am J Sports Med 14:35, 1986

20. Hughston JC, Andrews JR, Cross MJ, Mo Schi A: Classification of knee ligament instabilities. Part I. The medial compartment and cruciate ligaments. J Bone Joint Surg [Am] 58:159, 1976

21. Jokl P, Kaplan N, Stovell P, Keggi K: Non-operative treatment of severe injury to the medial and anterior cruciate ligaments of the knee. J Bone Joint Surg [Am] 66:741, 1984

22. Ober FR: The role of the iliotibial band and fascia lata as a factor in the causation of low back disabilities and sciatica. J Bone Joint Surg [Am] 18:105, 1936

57 Rehabilitation of the Ankle

A. AMENDOLA
I. J. ALEXANDER

THERAPEUTIC OBJECTIVES IN ANKLE REHABILITATION

Achieving the desired outcome in the rehabilitation of any musculoskeletal disorder is dependent on choosing modalities, exercises, and aids that will most rapidly and reliably bring patients to their individualized therapeutic goals. It is therefore important that this therapeutic objective be clearly defined at the initiation of the treatment program and that it is understood and agreed upon by both the therapist and the patient. The therapeutic objective established will depend on a number of factors: the nature and severity of the condition being treated; the age, activity level, and general health of the patient; and the patient's expectations and attitude.

Therapeutic objectives, in general terms, may include pain relief, resolution of edema, improved function, and return to previous activity level. Pain relief may be the benefit of treatment designed to eliminate the cause of the pain, protect the painful part, or inhibit the transmission of afferent pain impulses to the central nervous system. Resolution and control of edema is in itself an important objective but also results in both decreased pain and functional gain. Functional improvement occurs most rapidly once pain and edema are both under control. Increased range of motion, strength training, and improved joint stability all contribute to the restoration of function.

THERAPEUTIC MODALITIES

Heat and Cold Modalities

Surface cooling and warming, as well as deep heating with ultrasound and diathermy, are important modalities in rehabilitation of the ankle joint.

Cryotherapy

The use of cryotherapy is accepted by most practitioners as the initial treatment of choice for most syndromes that produce pain and swelling.[1,2] This is based upon the effect of cold in causing superficial vasoconstriction, which decreases blood flow and, therefore, hemorrhage in the traumatized area. Lowering the temperature decreases cell metabolism, which decreases oxygen and other nutrient consumption and thus contributes to decreased local blood flow. As a result, subcutaneous edema and resultant swelling is reduced.[3] In addition, cooling has an analgesic effect that may be the result of superficial receptor stimulation. According to the gate theory of pain modulation, these cutaneous impulses compete with pain impulses for afferent pathways, effectively blocking some of the noxious transmission or, in part, decreasing the local release of chemical mediators.[4,5] An accentuated deep vasodilatation that occurs in response to surface cooling may help clear toxic by-products of catabolism in the injured muscles and deep soft tissues.[6] Care must be exercised in the use of surface cooling, particularly with ice. Prolonged application may cause temporary damage to normal tissue. Paralysis may be a consequence of thermal trauma to superficial nerves, such as the peroneal nerve at the fibular head.

Icing produces certain stages of sensation. First, the cold feeling is noted for 1 to 3 minutes. This is followed by a burning or aching sensation occurring 2 to 7 minutes after application. Local numbness, or anesthesia, resulting from slowed nerve conduction, is noted at about 5 to 12 minutes. Reflex deep tissue vasodilatation without an increase in metabolism sometimes occurs as a fourth stage. Cold application should be limited to 12 to 15 minutes per treatment.[3,4] Care must be taken not to perform unreasonable activity under the anesthetic effect of icing, possibly inducing further injury. However, early controlled mobilization under these conditions allows earlier rehabilitation, clears debris, and prevents scarring.[3,7]

The most efficient methods of cold application include ice packs, chemical packs, ice massage, ice whirlpool, and iced wet towels. Coolant sprays have a limited application since their effect is only superficial. The use of ice is contraindicated in diseases that are exacerbated by cold, including Raynaud's phenomenon, peripheral vascular disease, cryoglobulinemia, and paroxysmal cold hemoglobinuria.[8]

Thermotherapy

Heat used therapeutically can be transmitted to the tissue by conduction, convection, or radiation. Heat modalities may be further classified into those that induce a superficial (less than 1 cm) or deep (1 cm or more) increase in tissue temperature. Superficial modes include the classical whirlpool, contrast baths, hot packs, paraffin baths, hydrocollater packs, and infrared heat. Deep modes include diathermy (shortwave and microwave) and ultrasound. In general, heat modalities are used in chronic arthritic and inflammatory conditions, in contrast to cold, which is used in acute inflammation or injury. The acute phase following an injury usually refers to the first 48 to 72 hours, but the benefit of using ice rather than heat during the rehabilitation phase of the injury is well supported.[9]

Numerous physiologic effects of heat have been documented. Analgesia is produced by the action of heat on nerve endings to increase pain threshold, the relief of muscle spasm through the gamma fibers of muscle spindles, the activation of descending pain inhibitory systems, and, in part, the removal of the by-products of injured tissue via increased blood flow.[10,11] Heat increases nutrient and/or oxygen delivery to the tissues, probably as a response to the increased metabolism.[12] In addition, with the increased temperature, the flexibility of soft tissues is enhanced and joint stiffness is reduced.[9]

Superficial Heat Modalities

Superficial heat modalities are used to reduce pain and stiffness, alleviate spasm, help resolve consolidating hematomas, and help in treating joint contractures. Caution should be exercised in patients with impaired sensation (i.e., neuropathic diabetics) and in acute injury, where heat is contraindicated.

Contrast baths, or alternating hot and cold, are used in situations of chronic pain and swelling (e.g., reflex sympathetic dystrophy). By alternately inducing vasodilatation and vasoconstriction, this method creates a "pumping" phenomenon that reduces swelling.[7] In addition, these baths interrupt the autonomic nerve dysfunction that accompanies dystrophy.[13]

Deep Heat Modalities

Diathermy. Diathermy uses high-frequency electromagnetic currents to produce deep heating of tissue through the induction of molecular movement. Heating with shortwave diathermy occurs to a depth of 3 to 4 cm, whereas microwave penetration is more superficial.[14] Using these modes, muscle and subcutaneous fat preferentially absorb most of the energy. Numerous papers have reported on the safety and effectiveness of diathermy.[15-17] Some authors question its therapeutic value, suggesting a considerable "placebo" clinical effect.[18] Use of diathermy in patients with neuropathy, arteriopathy, open wounds, and metallic implants is contraindicated.

Ultrasound. Ultrasound is a unique modality that uses high-frequency sound, inaudible to the human ear, to produce deep heat. Depth of penetration varies inversely with frequency and may reach up to 10 cm.[19,20] Effects of ultrasound include the alteration of cell permeability, local analgesia, decrease of neuroma-related pain, acceleration of healing, and decrease of scar formation.[21-24] Some of these changes are not related to the thermal effect of ultrasound.

The use of ultrasound energy to drive larger molecules through the skin into deeper tissues is referred to as phonophoresis. Corticosteroids, salicylates, and local anesthetics are commonly used as substrates. Penetration of significant amounts of these medications may occur as deep as 10 cm into the tissues.[19,20,25]

Corticosteroid Therapy

During rehabilitation of the ankle, particularly in overuse syndromes, corticosteroids are commonly used as an adjunct to other treatment modalities. The superficial location of the affected structures about the ankle allows easy access for phonophoresis, iontophoresis, and occasionally, peritendinous steroid injection. Phonophoresis and iontophoresis are both efficient means of corticosteroid delivery into tissue. These modalities are employed frequently, particularly in the management of chronic resistant tendinitis. Local steroid injection is used mainly when the tenderness is well localized.

Corticosteroids may also be an adjunct to differential injections used to determine origin of a specific pain. Temporary relief related to the local anesthetic may be extended by the anti-inflammatory effect of the corticosteroid. Adverse effects of corticosteroid injections include reduced local tendon strength, predisposing to rupture in the postinjection period, and articular cartilage damage with repetitive injections into joints.[26,27]

The use of oral corticosteroids for disorders involving the ankle is limited in our experience to treatment of reflex sympathetic dystrophy. Numerous investigators have shown the effectiveness of short-term high-dose and tapering doses of steroids in treating reflex sympathetic dystrophy.[28]

Electroneural Modalities

Current electrotherapy modalities include electrical muscle stimulation, transcutaneous electrical nerve stimulation (TENS), iontophoresis, electromyography (EMG), and biofeedback. EMG and biofeedback are modalities used specifically for assessment and

training purposes during functional rehabilitation. Electrical currents are used mainly in two clinical situations: to alter pain perception (TENS) or to produce contraction of a muscle, or a group of muscles, as an adjunct to exercise, primarily to retard muscle atrophy. Iontophoresis refers to the delivery of charged molecules into deep tissues through the use of continuous direct current stimulation.

Electrical Muscle Stimulation

Several studies have suggested that strength increases with electrical stimulation.[29-31] However, numerous papers indicate that electrical stimulation is no better than resistive exercise in maintaining or increasing strength.[29,31] Stimulators function through alternating current (AC) or direct current (DC), with variable frequency, waveform, and amplitude. Data documenting the differential effects of these variables is lacking. Electrical stimulation may be more beneficial postoperatively or postinjury if limb immobilization is necessary. In these situations, strength loss and the characteristic biochemical changes that occur in the muscle are retarded by the electrical current.[32-34]

Transcutaneous Electrical Nerve Stimulation

TENS is the application of current through the skin to peripheral nerves for the management of pain. Theories to support this effect include the gate theory of pain relief, which states that larger excitable sensory fibers are overstimulated to flood the afferent pathways to the brain and close the pathways to the smaller pain-sensory fibers.[35] Additional support derives from the finding that TENS stimulates the release of natural opiates—endorphins and enkephalins—from sensory nerves, further contributing to pain control.[36,37] The effectiveness of TENS appears to be maximal immediately after injury and decreases as time from injury increases.[38-40]

Exercise Modalities

Stretching

The beneficial effects of stretching are widely acknowledged. Stretching is generally recommended to prevent injury, improve performance, and enhance rehabilitation.[41-43] In addition, stretching improves the flexibility of musculotendinous units, increases joint range of motion, and reduces activity-induced muscle soreness.[44,45]

There are a number of different stretching techniques. Ballistic stretching involves repetitive bouncing movements but is considered less efficient than other techniques because of the inhibition induced by the stress reflex.[46] Static stretching is most often advocated because these inhibitory reflexes are minimized by the gradual lengthening of the muscles in the absence of pain. Static stretching also takes advantage of the viscoelastic properties of muscle that allow the musculotendinous units to experience stress relaxation and creep. These mechanical phenomena are essential to increase flexibility and joint range of motion. The optimal period of each stress was addressed by Taylor et al., who demonstrated in a rabbit model that the greatest muscle lengthening increases occurred in the first four stretches and in the first 12 seconds of each stress.[45] Little risk of injury accompanies static stretching, and generally it is not difficult to perform (Fig. 57-1).

Post-tetanic facilitation is a derivation of the static stretching techniques that utilizes sustained contraction against resistance to enhance stress relaxation with the subsequent stretch. Passive stretching refers to the external application of a stretching force by another individual in either a static or ballistic fashion. Again, the static application of this force is most effective.

Proprioceptive Training

Proprioception—the body's ability to vary contractile muscular forces in response to external forces—may be an important factor in the stability of joints and the likelihood of injury.[47] Functional joint instability after injury may be due to the loss of proprioception.[48] To appreciate the importance of proprioception, an understanding of muscle and joint receptors and their function is required.

Proprioceptive input originates in muscle spindles, Golgi tendon organs, and articular stretch receptors. Muscle spindles are found parallel to the muscle fibers and relay information concerning muscle length and amount and rate of stretch applied to that particular muscle. This information determines the recruitment of muscle fibers.[49] Golgi tendon organs are found at the musculotendinous junction and are very sensitive to stretch. The purpose of these sensory units is to prevent injury through activation of inhibitory neurons that will not allow excessive contraction.[49] Articular stretch receptors convey information regarding joint position, acceleration, and joint pressure.[50]

In general, the degree of proprioceptive loss is directly proportional to the length of time that the individual is withheld from activity.[47] Early rehabilitation will minimize this sensory deficit. Both stretching and electrical muscle stimulation may reduce proprioceptive loss.[47,51] To improve coordination, neuroreceptive training is performed on balance (wobble) boards.[52] This type of training prepares the proprioceptive system for more vigorous activity and sudden angular stresses to joints. Plyometrics, another form of proprioceptive rehabilitation, involves repetitive functional movement that requires coordination combined with horizontal and vertical propulsion. This may begin with double-leg forward hopping progressing to single-leg hop, vertical jump, and so forth. The final aspect of proprioceptive rehabilitation is sport-specific training, which focuses on the cardiovascular, neuromuscular, and proprioceptive requirements of a particular sport.

Strength Training and Assessment

Muscular strength is an important factor in performance. Strength training plays a significant role in rehabilitation after trauma or surgery and in injury prevention. Other terms used interchangeably with strength training include progressive resistance exercise, weight training, and resistance training.

Strengthening does not necessarily have to occur with the use of resistance or weight. Using strengthening exercises in rehabilitation requires a knowledge of the different types of muscle contraction. Concentric contraction occurs when a muscle is contracted from the extended to the shortened position. Eccentric contraction involves the gradual elongation of a contracted muscle. Muscular contraction may also be isometric, isotonic, isokinetic, or induced by electrical stimulation. *Isometric exercises* are performed with-

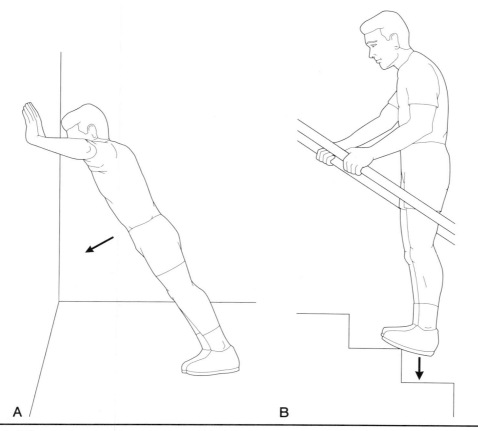

Fig. 57-1. Achilles tendon stretching program. **(A)** The position shown here is achieved by leaning forward, dropping the pelvis toward the floor, until tension is felt in the calf. The position is maintained for a count of 10 seconds without bouncing. A series of 10 stretches is performed twice daily, as well as prior to physical activities. **(B)** Alternative technique of Achilles tendon stretching. The ball of the foot is placed on the edge of the step, keeping the knees straight. Heels are allowed to drop to the floor until tension is felt in the calf. This position is maintained as described for **A**.

out joint movement with the muscle maintaining a constant length. *Isotonic exercises* are performed with a fixed or variable resistance and a change in the length of the muscle through a range of motion. Variable resistance usually occurs when using a barbell with a constant weight, because the force required by a muscle to move that weight varies with the change in length of the muscle. However, newer equipment systems utilize cans that produce a fixed resistance to the muscle even though a constant weight is being moved through the range of motion. Isotonic exercise may utilize either concentric or eccentric muscle contraction. *Isokinetic exercise*, used extensively in rehabilitation, is performed at a fixed speed with accom-

modating resistance and a change in muscle length. Accommodating resistance refers to the mechanical variation of applied resistance in proportion to the force generated by the muscle at each point through the range of motion.

The effectiveness of different exercise programs in bringing about strength gains varies considerably. Isokinetic exercises, which maintain maximal muscle tension throughout the range, produce optimal results in terms of the rate and magnitude of strength change.[53,54] Isometric exercise is the least efficient in improving muscle strength and endurance and does not help to restore or maintain joint range of motion.[53,54] Eccentric exercise is more efficient than concentric but must be closely supervised because eccentric contractures are associated with increased risk of muscle injury.[53,55] These factors should be kept in mind in designing a therapeutic exercise program. Early in the rehabilitation phase, isometric exercise should be considered. Isometric strengthening is often most effective when joint motion is limited by pain, protection of healing tissues is necessary, or muscle force is insufficient to move a load through a range. Custom programs of isokinetic and isotonic exercises are introduced when appropriate in the recovery phase and are the mainstays of any strength maintenance program.

Strength Assessment

Patients on a strengthening exercise program should have their progress monitored regularly to assess the therapeutic response and to time the return to preinjury activity. There are a number of means of carrying out such an assessment, but clinical evaluation is probably the most practical. This assessment should include the recording of subjective complaints and activities of daily living, and the periodic documentation of range of motion and anthropometric measurement (i.e., calf girth). Objective assessment of the patient's progress is possible on isokinetic equipment, which accurately records muscle strength, power, and endurance. These systems may be used as a direct measurement of the athlete's ability to return to sport. The addition of EMG to the isokinetic study also allows the clinician to look at patterns of muscle firing during specified activities.[31]

External Support Modalities

Ankle Stabilizers

Varying degrees of ankle stabilization to angular and rotatory stress are provided by casting, air stirrups, laced-up ankle stabilizers, and strapping or taping (Fig. 57-2). Indications for the use of these external aids include acute ligamentous injury or instability with recurrent chronic injuries. In the acute setting, total immobilization in casts is inferior to more functional treatment that allows early mobilization. Fewer residual symptoms and recurrent injuries accompany the use of removable devices that allow early mobilization.[48,56]

The prophylactic use of ankle taping and ankle supports is controversial. Advocates of ankle taping provide evidence that taping limits lateral ankle mobility and decreases risk of injury.[57] Others have questioned the effectiveness of ankle taping and the duration of its effect.[58] According to this group, tape loosens with time and mechanical stress, offering no advantage over other types of support. In a recent report, ankle stabilizers, in particular the laced-up brace, were more effective in preventing ankle injury and reinjury.[59]

Orthoses

In-shoe orthoses (insoles), custom or prefabricated, are used to redistribute weight under the foot, usually to unload high-pressure areas, absorb impact, or realign the foot to improve its mechanical function. The design of the orthosis and the materials used in its fabrication depend upon a number of patient factors, including body weight, activity, sensibility of the foot, condition of the skin, and, in particular, nature of the mechanical or medical problem being treated.

Characteristics of the ideal orthosis include effective load redistribution and impact attenuation, durability (of the properties), ease of fabrication, and affordability. Over-the-counter or custom rigid orthoses (plastic or acrylic) are extremely durable and best suited for patients with mild mechanical deformities and without focal areas of high pressure. The absence of a shock-dissipating component sometimes results in poor patient tolerance. Rigid orthoses should be avoided in the elderly, and in patients with diabetes mellitus or rheumatoid arthritis. An additional problem with rigid orthoses is that effective modification of the device delivered to the patient is quite difficult.

The opposite extreme is a soft unidensity shoe inlay of uniform thickness. The greatest attribute of this type of device is its affordability, if it is made of a resilient material that will not bottom out with good impact absorption. Although they disperse focal high pressures well, soft inlays are generally not easily molded and do not effectively redistribute high loads to unloaded areas. The optimal orthosis combines the support of the moldable, more rigid materials with the cushioning of the resilient foam or rubber (Fig. 57-3). These composite orthoses are best fabricated

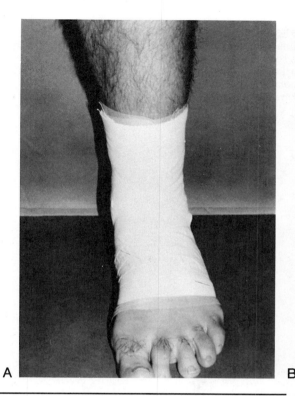

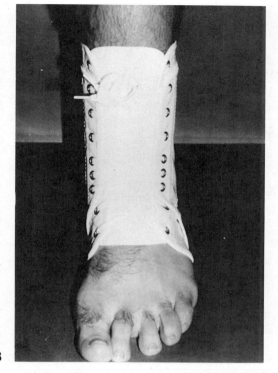

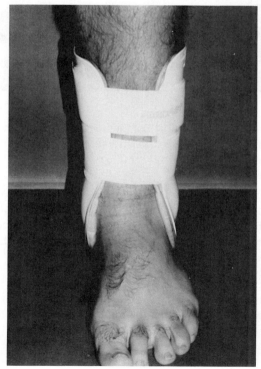

Fig. 57-2. Examples of various methods of ankle stabilization. **(A)** Ankle taping. **(B)** Lace-up ankle brace (AOA Sports Ankle Brace, AOA/Chick, Marlowe, OK). **(C)** Air Stirrup (Aircast, Incorporated, Summit, NJ).

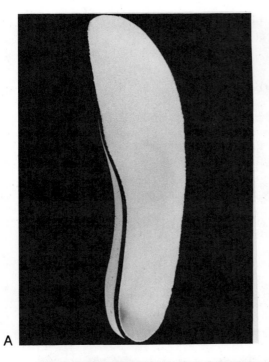

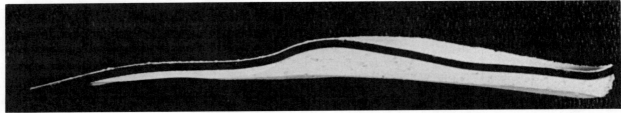

Fig. 57-3. Composite orthotic. **(A)** Orthotic with good longitudinal arch support and shock-absorbing properties. **(B)** Cross section demonstrates the various materials used in the orthotic: the softer, shock-absorbing materials are near the foot while the more dense, durable materials are further away from the foot.

by well-trained pedorthists who have experience treating foot problems and understand the materials and how to work with them.

With respect to the ankle, an orthosis can effectively reduce stress on the joint by providing impact absorption and by limiting torsional and bending forces transmitted to the ankle by a rigid, deformed foot.

Ankle-Foot Orthoses

Control of the ankle and hindfoot with rigid bracing is necessary in a number of circumstances, including arthritis, flexible deformities, articular instability, and neuromuscular disorders resulting in weakness. Occasionally, ankle-foot orthoses (AFOs) are used after acute injury, bony or ligamentous, to permit functional use of the limb while preventing further damage. The basis of these devices is a plastic shell fitting the lower leg and the foot with or without an ankle articulation. Prefabricated braces are less expensive and do not produce as good a fit as custom AFOs, but will often suffice, and are frequently used after tibial or ankle fractures.

Custom AFOs are easily modified to fit the specific needs of the patient. Examples of this include patellar tendon bearing to unload the ankle and a variety of shell modifications to provide more or less tibial stabilization. Extensive modification of the foot portion is also possible. A UCBO (University of California Berkeley Orthosis)–type foot component will provide excellent heel control and the desired degree of

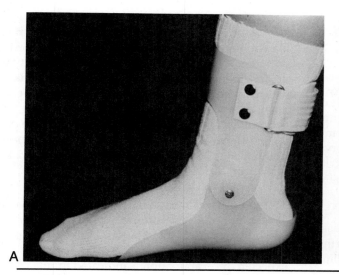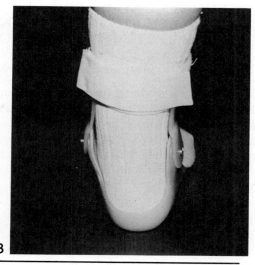

Fig. 57-4. (A & B) Articulated ankle-foot orthosis (AFO) with rear-entry design. This may be modified to a nonarticulated AFO.

arch support. In skilled hands, shock-absorbing materials can be fabricated into the plantar surface of the device when impact attenuation is necessary. A short articulated rear-entry AFO designed by the senior author (IA) and Roger Marzano, C.Ped., has been used extensively to control pain originating in the subtalar region (Fig. 57-4). The tibial and calcaneal fixation provided by the rear-entry design of the device effectively blocks subtalar motion and the low profile results in good patient compliance. Solid ankle AFOs are particularly useful for patients with a footdrop and after fusion for a Charcot ankle.

Shoes and Shoe Modifications

Selection of the most appropriate footwear is one of the most important aspects of preventive rehabilitation of the foot and ankle. There has been a great increase in athletic footwear in response to popular demand. Although this expanded market has improved the availability and selection of comfort footwear, the quality of the products conceived to rapidly meet the demand is sometimes poor. Careful evaluation is necessary to ensure proper fit and to meet the patient's specific requirements. Although each individual's requirements may differ, certain factors in shoe design should be considered.

Shoes should provide optimal shock absorption and heel control. Training shoes should have adequate compressibility of the heel to cushion the heel strike. Good shoes also have adequate medial support to prevent hyperpronation but are flexible enough to prevent stress on the Achilles tendon from a rigid lever arm. The inner aspects of the shoes should be inspected for protrusions or undulations causing pressure areas. Shoes should be fitted to the larger foot and have a minimum of 5 to 15 mm in front of the longest toe for adequate room. Waffled or studded soles are important for runners to provide cushion, good traction, and torsional control.

Shoe modification often obviates or may complement the use of orthoses. Modifications may include a myriad of possibilities such as more shock absorption, heel lifts, arch supports, supplemental medial or lateral support, high tops, or an extended heel counter.

Overall shoe quality has improved, but it is important that the characteristic of the shoe meet the patient's specific needs, primarily to prevent repetitive injury or aggravation of existing or recurrent problems such as overuse syndromes.

CLINICAL INDICATIONS FOR ANKLE REHABILITATION AND THERAPEUTIC INTERVENTION

Acute Ligamentous Ankle Injury

The majority of acute ligament sprains of the ankle do well without operative intervention. Residual symptoms of pain and instability have been found in a significant number of patients treated both conservatively and operatively.[60] Proper rehabilitation is critical in preventing and treating the late sequelae of these injuries.

The treatment program is divided into three phases. Initially, measures should be taken to prevent further injury and reduce and minimize pain and swelling. Depending upon the severity of the sprain, one may initiate partial weight-bearing, with or without crutches, using a prefabricated air splint, a lace-up brace, a compression dressing, or, occasionally, short-term cast immobilization. Cast immobilization has been shown to prolong functional recovery but is occasionally indicated in elderly patients or in instances of a sprain that makes weight-bearing impossible.[59] Cold modalities are used early and extensively during this phase.

The second therapeutic phase begins about 24 to 48 hours after the injury. Timing of its implementation depends upon the severity of the injury and tolerance of the patient. In this phase, range-of-motion exercises are performed actively or in an active assisted manner using body weight to provide the external force (e.g., with a tilt board). Calf and Achilles tendon stretching, only in the sagittal plane, is allowed. Cold therapy is continued before and after range-of-motion and stretching exercises. Eversion and inversion stress is avoided.

The third phase, which focuses on functional rehabilitation, begins when the patient is ambulating without pain, with minimal swelling, and near the full range of motion. A removable ankle support should be used. During this phase, range-of-motion exercises are continued but strengthening exercises are added. These include eversion, inversion, dorsiflexion, and plantar flexion against resistance. Proprioceptive training is performed on the wobble board. In those patients planning to return to recreational or athletic activity, proprioceptive training may be augmented with one-leg and two-leg vertical hopping. As pain settles and subjective stability improves, jogging and straight-ahead running may be incorporated into the program. Patients may be progressed to side-to-side hopping and running with patterned changes in direction as they near the point of return to their desired activity. Sport-specific training may also be undertaken with little risk of further injury.

Assuming an accurate diagnosis has been made, time to recovery and return to full activity may vary depending on patient tolerance and the severity of the ligamentous injury. If the patient is not progressing as expected, re-examination is indicated to rule out pathology that may have been overlooked. Frequently missed injuries include talar dome fractures, anterior process fractures of the calcaneus, fractures of the base of the fifth metatarsal, and injuries to the os trigonum (Fig. 57-5). In addition, reflex sympathetic dystrophy can occasionally complicate the resolution of a simple ankle sprain.[13]

Chronic ankle instability will often benefit from a course of conservative treatment, particularly if the initial rehabilitation was inadequate. Therapy for these patients should focus on recovering full range of motion if it is restricted, strengthening the muscles about the ankle, and proprioceptive training. An external support may be a useful adjunct in these individuals to prevent recurrent injuries, which usually result in significant setbacks in the recovery process. The patient can be gradually weaned from the device as inherent stability improves.

Tendinitis

Tendinitis is a frequent cause of pain about the ankle joint. Tendons crossing the ankle joint are subjected to repetitive loading, which can lead to stress injuries. The tendons most often involved include the Achilles, tibialis posterior, and peroneal tendons.[61] Careful clinical evaluation should identify etiologic and aggravating factors in these conditions. Optimal therapeutic outcome can be expected if these factors are corrected, in addition to locally treating the inflamed tendon.

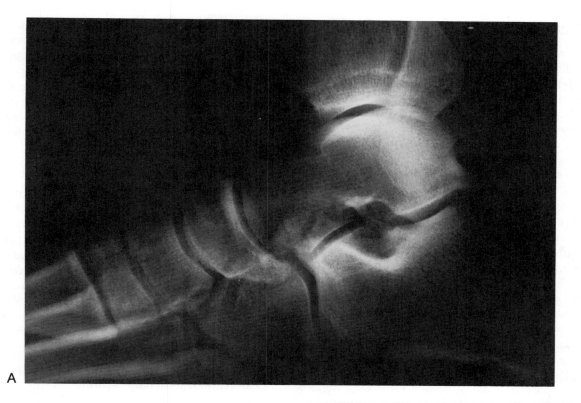

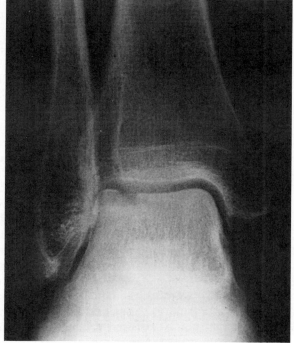

Fig. 57-5. Commonly missed occult fractures about the ankle mimicking ankle sprains. **(A)** Anterior process fracture of the calcaneus. **(B)** Osteochondral talar dome fracture.

Achilles Tendinitis

The management of Achilles tendinitis will vary depending upon the severity of the condition. In mild to moderate cases in which the patients do not limp and are still performing activities of daily living, a program consisting of decreased activity, anti-inflammatory medication, and shoe modification is initiated. Rigid-soled shoes have been shown to predispose to this injury[62]; therefore, a flexible-soled shoe with a heel lift is prescribed to decrease tendon stress. A simple home program is initiated using ice before and after stretching at least twice a day. Icing is best accomplished by laying the inflamed tendon area on a bag of crushed ice or frozen peas for 5 to 10 minutes before and after the stretching exercises. The key to the stretching technique is static prolonged stretches without bouncing, as shown in Figure 57-1. This program will also help strengthen the gastrocnemius-soleus complex.

In the very chronic or refractory cases, ultrasound using 10 percent hydrocortisone ointment is prescribed for at least 10 treatments for a concentrated local anti-inflammatory effect. In severe cases in which the patient limps with walking, attrition of the tendon may be present. These patients require prolonged protection utilizing a below-knee cast or brace for a period of 4 weeks or longer. Subsequent to immobilization, physical therapy is immediately resumed with an intense program of icing, stretching, and ultrasound.

Achilles tendon rupture probably occurs as a result of attrition but is almost always a traumatic event, commonly in middle-aged males.[61] Whether treated surgically or nonoperatively, Achilles tendon ruptures are initially immobilized in a plantar-flexed position to allow tendon healing. Initial therapy after cast removal is directed at restoring dorsiflexion at the ankle. Restoration of dorsiflexion should be gradual to avoid rerupture or attenuation of the repair. It may be helpful to gradually return the ankle to the neutral position with serial cast changes in the final stages of immobilization. Another alternative is to use a dorsal extension block splint to protect the ankle from dorsiflexion while allowing plantar flexion.[63] If equinus is present, a plantigrade foot can be restored by gradually reducing a heel lift until a normal shoe can be worn. A stretching program is started once the repair is considered to be secure and the patient is walking without pain. The goal of this program should be to regain full dorsiflexion and hindfoot inversion and eversion. Once full range of motion is obtained, a strengthening and proprioceptive training program for the ankle is initiated. Functional rehabilitation is not allowed until at least 5 months after injury or after repair of the Achilles tendon.

Tibialis Posterior Tendinitis

Walking or running places great mechanical demands on the tibialis posterior tendon, predisposing it to overuse and secondary inflammatory tendinitis. Tibialis posterior tendinitis is a disease spectrum whose manifestations range from an isolated tendinitis without any secondary tendon pathology in its early stages to rupture and complete collapse of the longitudinal arch in the later stages (Fig. 57-6). Inflammation and attrition of the tendon are usually well localized posteriorly and inferiorly to the medial malleolus.

In the early phase, when inflammatory tendinitis exists without secondary deformity or rupture, initial therapy consists of a stretching program using ice before and after exercises, anti-inflammatory medication, and modification of activity. Shoes should provide good medial support to prevent collapse of the longitudinal arch. Ultrasound with 10 percent hydrocortisone ointment is also very effective since the tendon pathology is well localized. In resistant cases of tendinitis, short-term cast or brace immobilization may be used as an adjunct.

In severe cases, partial or complete rupture of the tendon, resulting from attrition, may be present as a continuum of the disease process. Treatment of tibialis posterior tendon rupture is usually directed at providing medial support and preventing further deformity. One method of accomplishing this is with a custom-made, semirigid orthotic device augmented by a medial stabilizer on the shoe (Fig. 57-7). If these measures are unsuccessful, reconstruction may be considered in the appropriate patient.

Peroneal Tendinitis

Peroneal tendinitis may occur as an isolated phenomenon caused by mechanical stress as the tendon lies in the retrofibular sulcus or may result from ten-

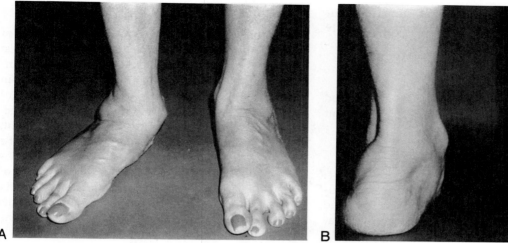
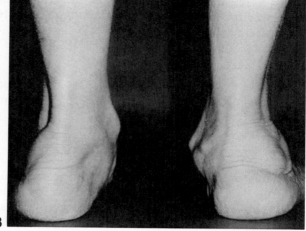

Fig. 57-6. **(A & B)** Clinical appearance of a patient with tibialis posterior tendon rupture; obvious collapse of the longitudinal arch with medial swelling is demonstrated **(B)**.

don subluxation. Peroneal tendinitis not associated with subluxation may be treated, as usual, with decreased activity, anti-inflammatory agents, and ice before and after exercises. A peroneal strengthening program with resisted eversion dorsi- and plantar-flexion exercises is strongly recommended. Local ultrasound with hydrocortisone in refractory cases may also be indicated. Shoewear may be modified with a

lateral heel flare to prevent chronic inversion reinjury.

In those cases in which the tendinitis is secondary to tendon subluxation, treatment should be directed at preventing instability in addition to addressing the inflammatory component. A tendon strap incorporating a pressure pad over the distal fibula may be

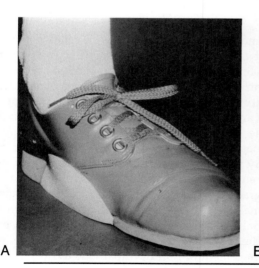
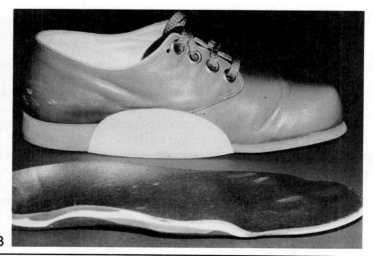

Fig. 57-7. **(A & B)** Shoe modification with in-shoe insert for conservative treatment of a tibialis posterior tendon rupture (Fig. 57-6).

used to prevent subluxation. Before surgery is considered for chronic tendon subluxation, particularly in post-traumatic cases, a 4- to 6-week period of immobilization in a cast may be beneficial.

Peroneus longus tendon rupture has been reported infrequently, and repair is recommended to prevent recurrent instability.[61]

Inflammatory Arthritis

Rehabilitation is a very important aspect in the management of inflammatory arthropathies. Foot and ankle involvement occurs in over 80 percent of patients with rheumatoid arthritis.[64] Therapy is indicated for improvement of pain symptoms and chronic fatigue and for restoration of unrestricted motion. Various splints and orthoses can be utilized to promote maximal function of the foot and ankle, as discussed previously. The rheumatologist involved should have the patient under optimal medical anti-inflammatory and analgesic management.

In acute inflammation of the ankle joint or soft tissue structures about the ankle, therapy initially is directed toward resolving pain and edema. Cryotherapy is utilized as in acute injuries. In severe inflammation a period of splinting or immobilization may be required before any further therapy. In general, patients with inflammatory arthritis should be counseled to engage in a practical modified activity-exercise program to maintain muscle tone and strength, help modulate pain symptoms, and promote a feeling of well-being. Once the pain and swelling have subsided, the patient may return to the previous exercise program if restriction of motion does not exist. Stretching exercises, manipulation, and occasional massage are useful modalities to help restore loss of motion. Fatigue is also a common finding in chronic inflammatory arthritis. Although it is usually the axial, shoulder, and pelvic girdle muscles that are affected by muscle atrophy and weakness, the leg muscles may also benefit from a regular ankle strengthening program. With chronic inflammation, heat modalities rather than ice are useful in relieving pain and joint stiffness. TENS has been effective for pain management in some of these patients.[65]

Osteoarthritis

The value of a therapy program for osteoarthritis of the ankle is limited. Principles similar to those used for other ankle disorders should be followed to maintain range of motion, good muscle strength, and pain control. Heat modalities are most effective in improving pain and stiffness in these patients. Protection of the arthritic ankle from overuse is important, and use of a cane or crutches during flare-ups may be indicated. A weight reduction program may be beneficial in obese patients. By reducing impact loading of the ankle, a viscoelastic heel pad may alleviate pain and slow progressing of the degeneration. If patients have disabling pain with only a jog of motion at the ankle joint, management with a nonarticulated ankle brace with a rocker-bottom sole on the shoe may alleviate their pain.

Reflex Sympathetic Dystrophy

The early diagnosis of reflex sympathetic dystrophy and institution of appropriate therapy are critical in achieving rapid resolution of symptoms. Therefore, in the assessment of a patient with poorly defined, chronic foot and ankle pain the possibility of a sympathetic dystrophy should always be suspected. Late diagnosis and failure to institute effective management lead to prolonged disability and difficulty obtaining complete resolution of this condition.

In the management of patients with reflex sympathetic dystrophy, cast immobilization or prolonged static splinting and forceful passive motion exercises are contraindicated.[13] Effective analgesia, particularly during therapy sessions, will avoid the development of an aggravated pain cycle. Contrast baths and a gentle range-of-motion program are effective. TENS has been shown to be effective, especially in the early phases of the syndrome. Physical therapy may be supplemented with high-dose prednisone tapered gradually over 10 to 14 days.[13] Encouraging functional use of the extremity will accelerate return to normal activities of daily living. In refractory cases sympathetic ganglion blocks have been effective in the management of reflex sympathetic dystrophy in the lower extremity.

REFERENCES

1. McMaster WC: A literary review of ice therapy in injuries. Am J Sports Med 5:124, 1977
2. Meeusen R, Lievens P: The use of cryotherapy in sports injuries. Sports Med 3:398, 1986
3. Hocutt JE, Jaffe R, Rylander CR, Beebe JK: Cryotherapy in ankle sprains. Am J Sports Med 10:316, 1982
4. Knight KL: Cryotherapy: Theory, Technique, and Physiology. p. 12. Chattanooga Corp., Chattanooga, TN, 1985
5. Waylonis GW: The physiological effects of ice massage. Arch Phys Med Rehabil 48:37, 1967
6. Yackzaw L, Adams C, Francis KT: The effects of ice massage on delayed muscle soreness. Am J Sports Med 12:159, 1984
7. Davies GJ: Physical therapy. p. 359. In: Sports Medicine of the Lower Extremity. Churchill Livingstone, New York, 1989
8. Grana WA, Curl WL, Reider B: Cold modalities. p. 25. In Drez D (ed): Therapeutic Modalities for Sports Injuries. Year Book Medical Publishers, Chicago, 1989
9. Baldwin FC, Vegso JJ, Torg JS, Torg E: Management and rehabilitation of ligamentous injuries to the ankle. Sports Med 4:364, 1987
10. Fischer E, Solomon S: Physiological response to heat and cold. p. 126. In Licht S (ed): Therapeutic Heat and Cold. E. Licht, New Haven, CT, 1964
11. Lehman JF, de Lateur BJ: Therapeutic heat. p. 404. In Lehman JF (ed): Therapeutic Heat and Cold. 3rd Ed. Williams & Wilkins, Baltimore, 1982
12. Abramson DI, Mitchell RE, Tuck S: Changes in blood flow, oxygen uptake and tissue temperature produced by topical application of wet heat. Phys Med 42:305, 1961
13. Alexander IJ, Johnson KA: Reflex sympathetic dystrophy Syndrome. p. 2187. In: Disorders of the Foot. 2nd Ed. WB Saunders, Philadelphia, 1991
14. Lehman JF, McMillan JA, Brunner GD et al: Temperature distributions as produced by microwaves in specimens under therapeutic conditions. Ann Phys Med 7:121, 1963
15. Law RWM, Dunscombe PB: Notes: some observations on stray magnetic fields and power outputs from shortwave diathermy equipment. Health Phys 46:939, 1984
16. Mosely H, Davison M: Exposure of physiotherapists to microwave radiation during microwave diathermy treatment. Clin Phys Physiol Med 2:217, 1981
17. Stuckly MA, Repacholi MH, Leeuyer DW et al: Exposure to the operator and patient during shortwave diathermy treatments. Health Phys 42:341, 1982
18. Gibson T, Grahame R, Harkness J: Controlled comparison of shortwave diathermy treatment with osteopathic treatment in low back pain. Lancet 1:1248, 1985
19. Griffin JE, Touchstone JC: Low intensity phonophoresis of cortisol in swine. Phys Ther 48:1336, 1968
20. Griffin JE, Touchstone JC: Effects of ultrasonic frequency on phonophoresis of cortisol into swine tissue. Am J Phys Med 51:62, 1972
21. Griffin JE, Karselis TC: Physical Agents for Physical Therapists. 2nd Ed. p. 52. Charles Thomas, Springfield, IL, 1982
22. Dysun M, Suckling J: Stimulation of tissue repair by ultrasound: a survey of mechanisms involved. Phys Ther 64:105, 1978
23. Currier DP, Greathouse D, Swift T: Sensory nerve conduction: effect of ultrasound. Arch Phys Med Rehabil 59:181, 1978
24. Farmer WC: Effect of intensity of ultrasound on conduction velocity of motor axons. Phys Ther 48:1233, 1968
25. Kleinkort JA, Wood F: Phonophoresis with one percent vs ten percent hydrocortisone. Phys Ther 55:1320, 1975
26. Ohira T, Ishikawa K: Hydroxyapatite deposition in articular cartilage by intraarticular injections of methyl prednisolone. J Bone Joint Surg [Am] 68:509, 1986
27. Kennedy JC, Willis RB: The effects of local steroid injections on tendons: biomechanical and microscopic correlative study. Am J Sports Med 4:11, 1976
28. Malkin LH: Reflex sympathetic dystrophy syndrome following trauma to the foot. Orthopedics 13:851, 1990
29. Drez D (ed): Therapeutic Modalities for Sports Injuries. Year Book Medical Publishers, Chicago, 1989
30. Laughman RK, Youdas JW, Garrett TR, Clao EYS: Strength changes in normal quadriceps femoris muscle as a result of electrical stimulation. Phys Ther 63:494, 1983
31. Lucca JA, Recchiati SJ: Effect of electromyographic feedback on isometric strengthening programs. Phys Ther 63:200, 1983
32. Stanish WD, Valiant GA, Bonen A et al: The effects of immobilization and of electrical stimulation on muscle glycogen and myofibrillar ATPase. Can J Appl Sports Sci 7:267, 1982
33. Eriksson E, Haagmark T, Kiessling KH et al: Effects of electrical stimulation on human skeletal muscle. Int J Sports Med 2:18, 1981
34. Morrissey MC, Brewster CE, Shields C et al: The effects of electrical stimulation on the quadriceps during postoperative knee immobilization. Am J Sports Med 13:40, 1985
35. Melzack R: Prolonged relief of pain by brief intense transcutaneous somatic stimulation. Pain 1:357, 1974
36. Sjolund B, Eriksson E: Endorphins and analgesia produced by peripheral conditional stimulation. Adv Pain Res Ther 3:587, 1979
37. Hughes GS, Lichstein PR, Whitlock D et al: Response of plasine beta-endorphins to transcutaneous electrical nerve stimulation on healthy subjects. Phys Ther 64:1062, 1984
38. Jensen JE, Conn RR, Hazelrigg G et al: The use of transcutaneous neural stimulation and isokinetic testing in orthoscopic knee surgery. Am J Sports Med 13:27, 1985
39. Smith MJ, Hutchins RC, Hehenburger D: Transcutaneous neural stimulation use in postoperative knee rehabilitation. Am J Sports Med 11:75, 1983
40. Arvidsson I, Eriksson E: Postoperative TENS pain relief after knee surgery: objective evaluation. Orthopedics 9:1346, 1986
41. Hubley-Kozay CL, Stanish WD: Can stretching prevent athletic injuries. J Musculoskel Med 1(9):25, 1984
42. Komi P: Neuromuscular biomechanics: selective correlates between structure and function. p. 60. In Machlum S, Nilsson S, Renstrom P (eds): An Update on Sports Medicine: Proceedings from the Second Scandinavian Conference in Sports Medicine. Sona Moria, Oslo, 1986
43. Stanish WD: Neurophysiology of stretching. p. 135. In D'Ambrosia R, Drez D (eds): Prevention and Treatment of Running Injuries. Slack, Thorofare, NJ, 1982
44. Devries HA: Prevention of muscular distress after exercise. Res Q 32:177, 1961
45. Taylor DC, Dalton JD, Seaber AV et al: Viscoelastic properties of muscle-tendon units: the biomechanical effects of stretching. Am J Sports Med 18:300, 1990
46. Davis VB: Flexibility conditioning for running. p. 147. In D'Ambrosia, Drez D (eds): Prevention and Treatment of Running Injuries. Slack, Thorofare, NJ, 1982
47. Day RW, Wildermuth BP: Proprioceptive training in the rehabilitation of lower extremity injuries. Adv Sports Med Fitness 1:241, 1988

48. Freeman MAR, Dean MRE, Hankam IWF: The etiology and prevention of functional instability of the foot. J Bone Joint Surg [Br] 47:678, 1965

49. Hason Z, Enoke RM, Stuart DG: The interface between biomechanics and neurophysiology in the study of movement: some recent approaches. Exerc Sport Sci Rev 13:169, 1985

50. Newton RA: Joint receptor contributions to reflexive and kinetic responses. Phys Ther 62:22, 1982

51. Beck JL, Wildermuth BP: The female athlete's knee. Clin Sports Med 4:2, 1985

52. Gray GW: Rehabilitation of running injuries: biomechanical and proprioceptive considerations. Top Acute Care Trauma Rehabil 1:67, 1986

53. Drez D (ed): Therapeutic Modalities for Sports Injuries. Year Book Medical Publishers, Chicago, 1989

54. Cahill BR (ed): Proceedings of the Conference on Strength Training and the Prepubescent. American Society for Sports Medicine, Chicago, 1988

55. Lieber RL, Friden JO, McKee-Woodburn TG: Selective damage of fast glycolytic muscle fibers with eccentric exercise of the rabbit tibialis anterior. Trans Orthop Res Soc 13:337, 1988

56. Brostrom L: Sprained ankles v. treatment and prognosis in recurrent ligament ruptures. Acta Chir Scand 132:551, 1966

57. Garrick JG, Regue RK: Role of external support in the prevention of ankle sprains. Am J Sports Med 5:241, 1977

58. Myburgh KH, Vaughan CL, Isaacs SK: The effects of ankle guards and taping in joint motion before, during, and after a squash match. Am J Sports Med 12:441, 1984

59. Rovere GD, Clarke TJ, Yates CS et al: Retrospective comparison of taping and ankle stabilizers in preventing ankle injuries. Am J Sports Med 16:228, 1988

60. Lassiter TE, Malone TR, Garrett WE: Injury to the lateral ligaments of the ankle. Orthop Clin North Am 20(4):629, 1989

61. Frey CC, Shereff MJ: Tendon injuries about the ankle in athletes. Clin Sports Med 7(1):103, 1988

62. Baxter DE: The foot in running and dancing. p. 502. In Mann RA (ed): Surgery of the Foot. CV Mosby, St. Louis, 1986

63. Carter TR, Fowler PJ, Blokker K: Functional post-operative treatment after Achilles tendon repair, abstracted. Am J Sports Med 18:544, 1990

64. Gerber LH: Primer on Rheumatic Diseases. p. 301. Arthritis Foundation, Atlanta, 1988

65. Kumar UN, Redford JB: Transcutaneous nerve stimulation in rheumatoid arthritis. Arch Phys Med Rehabil 63:596, 1982

58 Rehabilitation of the Foot

MARK S. MYERSON

Rehabilitation of the foot embraces many concepts already elaborated on in this text, and because many of the therapeutic modalities have already been discussed, these are not reiterated here. Instead, this chapter focuses on clinical conditions and their treatment, as well as static and dynamic disorders and deformities of the foot and their potential for rehabilitation. It deals specifically with chronic diseases and has been divided into three sections: the neuropathic foot, post-traumatic conditions of the foot and ankle, and the use of orthoses in rehabilitation of the foot.

THE NEUROPATHIC FOOT

The insensate foot presents a problem whose impact is enormous. The incidence of gangrene is approximately 80 times more common in patients with diabetes than in nondiabetics, and the rate of diabetes-related amputations in the United States is approximately 80 per 100,000.[1-4] The cost of these amputations is quite staggering, and, owing to prolonged hospitalization, amounts to approximately $400 million dollars annually. To a large extent, these amputations result from a combination of neuropathy and deformity, which ultimately leads to ulceration and infection. Although vascular disease is approximately 30 times more common in diabetics than in patients in a general nondiabetic population, it is my impression that neuropathy and deformity are the precursors of ultimate infection. Consequently, patient education and the prevention of foot- and ankle-related problems are of paramount importance. I have demonstrated, in a carefully controlled program of diabetic education, that the rate of ulceration and infection in these patients decreased dramatically when particular attention was paid to

shoewear. This has similarly been demonstrated by Davidson and colleagues, who showed that, through an appropriate foot care program, the amputation rate could be decreased from 14 to 6.7 per 1000 patients.[5]

Two fundamental consequences of neuropathy are encountered in clinical practice: Charcot fractures, correctly termed *neuroarthropathy,* and ulceration.

Care of the Insensitive Foot

Skin breakdown in the patient with neuropathy is a common problem. It is remarkable how noncompliant patients with diabetes tend to be. Although theoretically it might be expected that patients with deformity, ulceration, and even infection would take care of themselves and their feet, this is quite incorrect. On the contrary, it is common to find a patient walking on a foot that is markedly swollen, infected, and ulcerated. Even after prolonged treatment and rehabilitation, when appropriate shoes have been provided these patients still wear potentially harmful stylish shoes. This problem has been identified frequently in patients with a neuropathy. Once patients lose feeling in a part of the body, such as the feet, they tend to think of these regions as no longer part of themselves, often regarding their feet as dead. These patients require a tremendous amount of care, time, and education. It is only by repeatedly reinforcing this educational program that patients will make a conscious effort to take care of themselves. This education and support should be given with an appropriate amount of caring and understanding on the part of the therapist, because these patients frequently have a poor self-image and a negative view of their disease process.

In addition to the sensory neuropathy, the skin of the foot is invariably dry as a result of autonomic neuropathy that leads to a lack of sweating.[6] This is associated with increased keratinization, particularly on the plantar weight-bearing surfaces. Normally, feet and superficial layers of skin are constantly kept moist by sweat, and in this state the keratin is soft. With the absence of moisture, the keratin cracks, and although this condition is limited to the outer epidermal layers, it is often associated with a chronic dermatitis. On the plantar aspect of the foot, these keratin cracks in the skin become inflamed and thickened. Callus forms and stimulates further cyclic build-up of callus along the edges of the cracked skin until the cracks are torn open, leading to inflammation, ulceration, and infection. The skin should therefore be kept moist, preventing these cyclic changes. However, the patient should be told that moisturizing creams are harmful because they accumulate and are associated with allergic reactions if used for a prolonged period. Perhaps the best moisturizer is water; the feet should be soaked in cool water for 20 minutes a day followed by drying and rubbing the skin with petroleum jelly. Patients are instructed to decrease the repetitive build-up of keratin by using pumice stones and to avoid paring the calluses themselves.

The foot should be protected from excessive mechanical pressure, because damage to the insensitive foot by external forces can occur in a number of ways. The only source of constant pressure on the foot is circumferential tension, such as occurs from the shoe or a strap. The pressure occurs at right angles to the edge of the foot, and the patient can be shown an example of what happens by tying a piece of string around the hand, noting the points at which pressure areas occur. Although the tension from the string (and the tight shoe) is equal all around the foot, the pressure resulting from this tension is least on the dorsum of the foot and greatest on its medial and lateral borders. In the presence of any forefoot deformity, particularly hallux valgus, greater pressure is exerted over the medial border of the foot. Patients often purchase loose-fitting shoes in an attempt to avoid this extra pressure, but this only produces increased friction on other parts of the foot, further potentiating ulceration.

Tight shoes, therefore, are a source of constant pressure, particularly if worn for a number of hours, and will cause a pressure ulceration. This is particularly a problem with new shoes. A second form of damage occurs as a result of much higher pressure, which can break the surface of the skin — for example, stepping on a sharp stone or a thumbtack. The third and most common form of skin breakdown occurs through constant, repetitive, but moderate pressures resulting from prolonged standing or walking.[7] Patients should be instructed to look for areas of pressure or redness and feel for warmth over the foot, particularly after wearing new shoes. These shoes should be stretched and worn only for short periods of time until they are softened and broken in. Only leather shoes should be used by patients with neuropathy because shoe surfaces made of artificial materials do not stretch and do not adapt well to local increasing pressure. Shoes should be changed frequently during the course of the day and different shoes rotated so that localized pressure necrosis is unlikely to occur. The insides of the shoes should be checked regularly for cracks in the soles and wrinkles in the lining of the shoe. Patients are instructed to check inside the shoe to ensure that no foreign objects have fallen inside. Shoes with buckles and straps that may cause ridging should be avoided.

The most significant source of abnormal pressures in the foot is from repetitive overuse stresses resulting from excessive standing or walking. The tissues are structurally abnormal as a result of prior scarring from previous ulcerations. These patients are unable to alter their gait, and they do not limp as a result of these abnormal stresses; therefore, if these repetitive minor overuse injuries continue, blisters form which are followed by ulceration. Although they lack protective sensation, patients should understand that ulcers do not just develop, and that there are warning signs they can watch for to prevent ulceration. They should also understand that they can reduce the pressure and stresses on the foot by shoe modifications. This can be accomplished either by using a rigid-soled rocker-bottom shoe or by using molded inlays to accommodate the foot.[8]

Body weight is transmitted throughout the foot, generating forces and pressures directly; therefore, the pressure is greatest on the plantar aspect of the foot. When standing, both feet share the load, and the pressure is approximately 20 pounds per square inch, but this changes when one foot is off the ground. During the stance phase of gait, however, particularly during toe-off, the forefoot bears significantly increased loads of up to 60 pounds per square inch. These kind of pressures clearly can be responsible for inflammation and ulceration if the overuse continues. These forces can be dissipated by the use of soft inner soles, provided that shoes with extra depth are worn. These molded inlays will have no effect whatever unless more room is provided for the foot by an extra-depth shoe.

Molded insoles, particularly those made with Plastizote and firmer grades of Plastizote such as Aliplast and Pelite, are extremely durable. These are closed-cell foams that are heat moldable but are poor conductors of heat, and they can therefore be molded directly to the foot without causing burns. These molded inlays can therefore be made into a perfect fit for the foot. Various composite inlays can also be fashioned with varying densities of support to give increased durability to the inlay. These are far preferable to soft, commercially available prefabricated arch supports, which I believe are contraindicated in patients who lack protective sensation. These molded insoles should be used in extra-depth shoes, which are now easily obtainable.

The foot is particularly vulnerable when in single stance phase and during roll-off or toe-off when the weight-bearing part of the foot is bending and undergoing shear stress. These local increases in pressure and shear stress can be minimized by preventing the bending of the foot through creation of a rigid sole, and by keeping the ground contact point further back, near the center of the shoe.[9] This can be done by wearing a custom-made rocker-bottom shoe. When obtaining the mold for the foot, the toes should be extended so that the toe of the shoe is slightly turned up and allows the heel to lift while walking without the toes touching the ground.

Neuropathic Ulceration: The Total Contact Cast

Although there are numerous methods available to treat the neuropathic ulcer, I have found the total contact cast to be reliable, cost effective, and associated with little morbidity. The cast functions by reducing the pressure over the wound and by redistributing the weight-bearing load of the entire plantar surface of the foot and leg, which is further reduced with foam padding directly over the ulcer.[10-13] Immobilization of the foot decreases the spread of local inflammation, limiting the stress on granulation tissue and the skin edges.[14] The swelling begins to reduce after about 24 hours in the cast, and the interstitial fluid pressure diminishes, improving the microcirculation and facilitating healing of the ulcer.

Decision-making regarding treatment of neuropathic ulceration is a team effort and depends on successful communication among the physician, cast technician, physical therapist, and footwear specialist. The cast is only one method for healing the ulcer; if it is utilized without careful team planning, it is likely to fail, and ulceration will recur. Particular attention should be directed toward providing safe and effective footwear once healing has occurred.

Furthermore, the therapist should identify any factors that have precipitated ulceration. Patient education is therefore critical and is an integral part of the treatment process. This is accomplished by modifying the patient's environment, shoewear, patterns of walking, and particularly the daily care of the feet. Generally, all ulcerations on the plantar weight-bearing surface of the foot are amenable to initial treatment with the total contact cast. Ulcers that are actively draining should be débrided first, and osteomyelitis should be ruled out prior to treatment with the cast. Débridement of necrotic tissue and appropriate wound care with whirlpool and antibiotic therapy is required before casting is initiated. With more active drainage, the cast changes are performed more frequently during the initial weeks until the wound is stable.[15,16] Patients should be able to comply with restricted weight-bearing during the initial 24 hours after casting. Once the cast is dry, full

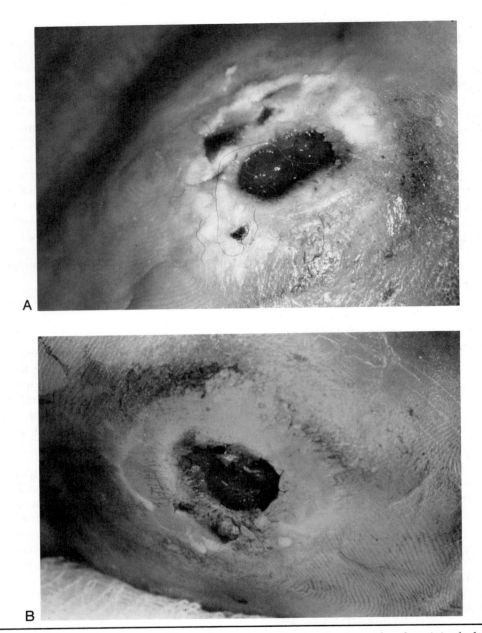

Fig. 58-1. **(A)** Prior to the application of the total contact cast, the ulcer has heaped-up keratinized edges. **(B)** The edges of the ulcer are shaved down so that a smooth border is present between the bed of the ulcer and the surrounding skin.

weight-bearing may commence, because this is an ambulatory treatment program. If there is significant swelling of the foot and ankle, casting may still be used, but the swelling should be brought under control prior to initiating the cast treatment. This may take a number of days or even weeks, particularly if the edema is chronic. Nevertheless, if the therapist is prepared to change the cast at frequent intervals during the first 2 weeks, the cast treatment works well to decrease this edema. Serious complications of casting

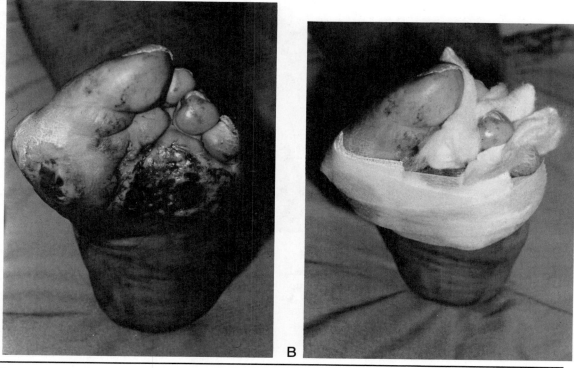

Fig. 58-2. (A) Ulcer on the plantar surface of the foot. **(B)** A gauze bandage is applied to the ulcer, and cotton inserted between the toes.

may occur when attention is not given to problems with swelling. Although patients lack protective sensation, they are usually able to cope with simple instructions regarding a loose-fitting cast, and they are told to avoid bearing weight until a new, snug-fitting cast is applied.

Fabrication of the cast commences with preparation of the wound by débridement of all necrotic tissue, particularly in the depths of the ulcer. The wound edges are trimmed and shaved, removing all callus and excess keratin so that a smooth transition from the wound to the adjacent surrounding skin bed is present (Fig. 58-1). The wound is cleansed with an appropriate antibacterial solution such as povidone-iodine, and a sterile dressing is applied (Fig. 58-2). Only one layer of a 2 × 2-inch gauze pad is used to prevent excessive bulk and therefore pressure over the affected area. Strategic areas of the foot and ankle are protected with padding to guard against addi-

tional skin breakdown and maceration. The rest of the casting is done as follows:

1. Cotton padding is applied between the toes to avoid pressure from rubbing.
2. Four-inch stockinette is applied from the knee to the toes. The end of the stockinette is folded back over the top of the toes and taped securely with paper tape (Fig. 58-3). Wrinkling of the stockinette should be avoided, and it is cut transversely across the anterior ankle to avoid creasing in this area. It is therefore preferable to overlap the stockinette wherever possible to avoid friction directly beneath these areas of wrinkling. In these areas, the stockinette is also taped into position.
3. Low-density ½-inch thickness closed-cell foam is then applied over the toes and extended to cover any bony prominence, such as the first and fifth metatarsal heads and the malleoli. The proximal edge of the foam must be beveled to provide a smooth transition to the adjacent skin. This foam padding is also applied directly over the wound using ⅛-inch cut-out pads, which are also beveled. The malleoli are protected with

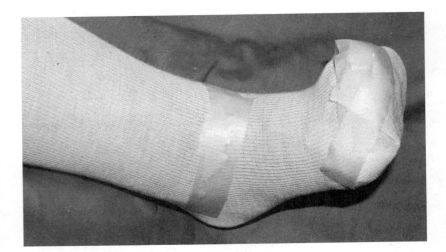

Fig. 58-3. A single layer of stockinette is applied from the knee to cover the toes. The crease at the ankle and forefoot is cut, and the edge is folded over and secured with tape.

this foam, and adhesive-backed felt is also applied over the dorsum of the foot, extending proximally up the leg to pad the anterior tibial crest (Figs. 58-3 through 58-5).

4. The cast is applied with the patient in the prone position, maintaining the knee in 90° of flexion and the ankle in 5° of dorsiflexion (Figs. 58-6 and 58-7).
5. The padding and stockinette are rechecked for shifts in position or wrinkles and any final corrections made.
6. The inner layers of the cast shell are important because

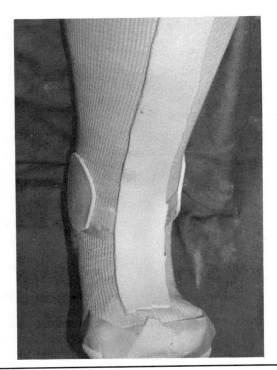

Fig. 58-4. Adhesive-backed ⅛-inch felt is applied to the malleoli and along the tibial crest.

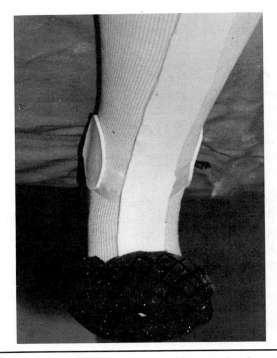

Fig. 58-5. Closed-cell foam is applied to the forefoot, and the edges are bevelled. This foam can be applied to bony prominences to pad the area directly under the ulcer.

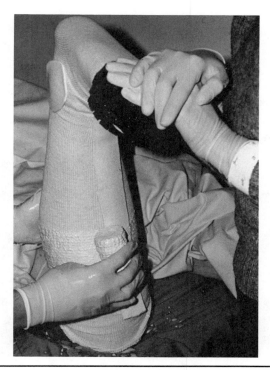

Fig. 58-6. The cast is applied with the patient in the prone position. Elasticized plaster is rolled without tension from 2 inches below the knee to cover the foot.

improves gait and also provides a broader area of weight-bearing during ambulation, thereby improving balance.

10. The cast is reinforced with Fiberglas covering the toes. The patient is instructed to avoid bearing weight for 12 to 24 hours and may commence with full weight-bearing activities thereafter.

Healing of the ulcer usually occurs between 3 and 6 weeks later. As discussed earlier, management of the wound is only one aspect of treatment. It is important to anticipate healing by providing the patient with appropriate shoewear with protective molded Plastizote inserts for ambulation. These shoes should be available once the ulcer has healed, and I typically take the molds of the feet once swelling has been reduced to anticipate final healing. Recurrent ulceration is common and depends on the site of the ulcer and the presence of deformity. However, recurrences can be treated with another short period of total contact casting. Nevertheless, the global problem should be addressed, including patient education, and pro-

they most closely approximate the skin, and care must be taken to avoid wrinkling of the plaster or tenting over bony prominences. The first layer is applied loosely with elasticized plaster because it adheres to the folds and contours of the ankle and foot quite precisely. The elasticized plaster should not be over-stretched, particularly over the bony prominences.

7. The plaster is applied from 1 inch distal to the fibular neck to the toes, and covers the distal foam by approximately 1 inch. Two rolls of 4-inch width plaster are generally adequate. The plaster should be molded carefully to conform to the leg, foot, and ankle until it begins to harden.

8. Two additional rolls of 4-inch plaster are applied from the distal third of the leg to cover the foot to reinforce the inner shell. This plaster should be smoothed and contoured until firm.

9. A rocker bottom on the cast is ideal and can be built into the cast itself by layering plaster onto the bottom of the cast from the heel to an area just proximal to the metatarsal heads. This should be tapered toward the toes so that on weight-bearing, the toes are approximately 1½ inches off the floor (Fig. 58-8). This rocker

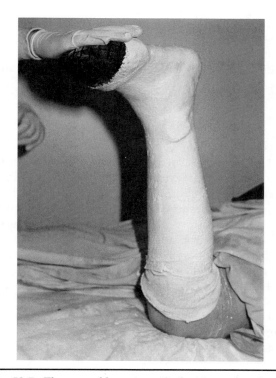

Fig. 58-7. The second layer is applied with regular plaster; two rolls of 4-inch plaster is sufficient.

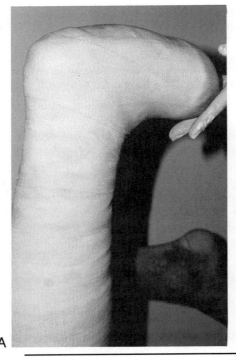
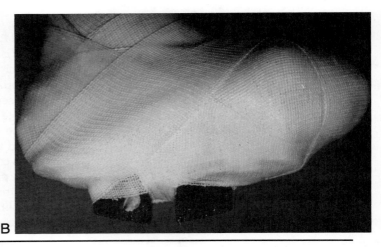

Fig. 58-8. **(A)** The cast is reinforced with Fiberglass, and a rocker bottom sole created by layering the plaster. **(B)** An alternative to the rocker bottom sole is a cast heel, which also facilitates walking, particularly in inclement weather.

tective footwear, including molded orthoses, should be employed.

Management of Neuroarthropathy

During the initial stages of this disease process, the foot is typically warm and swollen (Fig. 58-9). It is not uncommon for patients with neuroarthropathy to be treated for cellulitis or even to undergo surgical drainage for presumed deeper infection during this acute inflammatory phase. Although diagnosis of acute neuroarthropathy can be difficult, it is made on the basis of painless swelling associated with warmth of the affected area and various radiographic changes.[17-29] It is important to recognize that the patient may not have diabetes, because patients with preclinical diabetes may also develop a neuroarthropathy. No correlation exists between the severity or control of the diabetes and the extent of neuropathy and neuroarthropathy. Therefore, in the absence of an obvious source of infection, all patients with or without diabetes who have a warm, swollen, painless foot should be treated presumptively for a neuroarthropathic process.

Radiographs are often helpful, but the typical changes of neuroarthropathy, such as fragmentation and new bone formation, often are not present during the acute stage. Radiographs can therefore be misleading, because little other than soft tissue swelling or subtle subluxation may be seen during this acute stage. It is particularly important to obtain weight-bearing radiographs of the foot and ankle. Non–weight-bearing views do not reveal the true pathologic process, and, when subluxation or impending dislocation is present, it can only be adequately shown if the radiographs are obtained in the weight-bearing position.

The pathologic process of neuroarthropathy is not well understood. Clearly, the fracture is not always associated with significant trauma, and often a history of even minor trauma is lacking. Most likely a combination of events is associated with the onset of

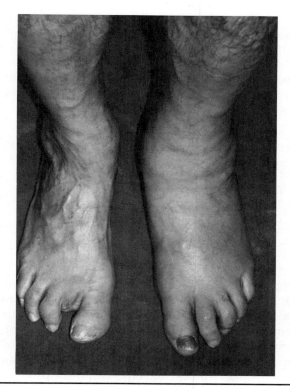

Fig. 58-9. This patient had a 3-week history of painless swelling of the foot. He has all the stigmata of an acute neuroarthropathic or Charcot fracture of the foot.

acute neuroarthropathy. It is my contention that the basic process may not even be a fracture, but rather a disruption of the ligamentous support to the joints. This is then followed by minor fracture or fragmentation, culminating in the gross fracture process associated with continued weight-bearing. It is the process of ligamentous instability that is probably responsible for most cases of acute neuroarthropathy.

The patient with an acute neuroarthropathy is at significant risk. The foot requires rest, best obtained by an initial period of hospitalization, during which time the patient can be taught about the nature of neuropathy and deformity. Because most diabetic patients are extremely noncompliant, without a careful program of education, they will place weight on the foot and complicate the fracture management further. I recommend that, during this initial acute phase, the foot be immobilized and the patient be required to avoid weight-bearing for approximately 6 to 8 weeks. Restriction of activities and ambulation in these patients is difficult to enforce. Nevertheless, strict avoidance of weight-bearing and elevation of the foot should be encouraged during the acute inflammatory phase.

When the warmth begins to subside, ambulation may commence. I have found the use of a total contact cast to be extremely effective in controlling the swelling and in keeping these patients ambulatory. It is imperative to change the cast frequently during the initial stages of ambulation, because the edema is rapidly dissipated with this ambulatory treatment program. If the foot is swollen, the first cast change is performed between 2 and 5 days after being placed, followed by regular cast changes at 1- to 2-week intervals thereafter. The duration of casting is determined to some extent by the nature and site of the deformity in the foot and ankle, but my preference is to prolong this period for approximately 9 to 12 months after the acute episode. Immobilization is continued until the disease process is quiescent, as determined by the absence of warmth and swelling, which can be demonstrated clinically and radiographically. Thermistor testing is an accurate way to monitor the fluctuations of warmth in the foot. I use thermistors frequently and encourage patients to purchase a cutaneous thermometer to determine daily changes in temperature, which can then be used to assess potential areas of imminent breakdown. A technetium bone scan obtained at 3- to 6-month intervals will also demonstrate gradually decreasing activity.

Once the neuropathic process has entered a subacute phase, which usually occurs between 2 and 4 months, an alternative to the total contact cast that can be employed is a total contact bivalved cast mold. The cast is made in a manner similar to that described above, is split medially and laterally, and then is lined with varying densities of Plastizote and secured with Velcro straps. This enables the patient to bathe and preserves the pliability of the skin. The inner lining shell of the cast is changed every 1 to 2 months, because this has a tendency to soften, flatten, and "bottom out."

Once the disease process has subsided completely, a decision should be made about permanent bracing. Generally, deformity in the hindfoot and ankle should be braced permanently with a double upright brace or, as I prefer, a Plastizote-lined polypropylene ankle-foot orthosis. All deformity of the midfoot requires protection with a total contact molded shoe or, at the least, an extra-depth shoe with molded Plastizote inlays. Approximately 40 percent of patients will develop a neuroarthropathic process in the opposite foot, and because the deformity can be minimized if treated early, patients should understand the nature of the disease and be alert to the onset of warmth and painless swelling of the foot or ankle.[24,26]

POST-TRAUMATIC CONDITIONS OF THE FOOT AND ANKLE

Perhaps one of the most perplexing problems in treating the injured foot is to decide what exactly is causing the pain, because chronic pain is not easily focused or located by the patient and the physician must resort to indirect methods of diagnosis. Frequently, regional nerve and soft tissue blocks are helpful in assessing the traumatized foot.

Unfortunately, many of the clinical conditions occurring in the injured foot and ankle overlap, and it is often difficult to separate one from another. The history of the injury and treatment are of paramount importance. An inconsequential or trivial injury is typically associated with reflex sympathetic dystrophy. The overall appearance of the foot may help determine what the underlying problem is, because chronic swelling, skin changes, intrinsic atrophy, and clawing of the toes are each suggestive of different conditions. The use of differential nerve blocks is extremely helpful. For the foot and ankle, I use a mixture of 1 percent lidocaine and 0.5 percent bupivacaine. Whenever these agents are used, it is important to inject only small volumes to prevent dissipation of the anesthetic to adjacent structures, which may complicate the overall picture. In addition to clinical examination and differential nerve, soft tissue and intra-articular blocks, technetium bone scan imaging is particularly helpful. If performed correctly, a three-phase bone scan should distinguish inflammatory changes in the soft tissues, joints, and osseous structures. Electrophysiologic testing with electromyography and nerve conduction studies is also helpful and should be undertaken in all patients with chronic pain.

The patient with chronic foot pain should be evaluated consistently, with careful attention to the following:

1. History of the injury
2. Physical examination, including skin, subcutaneous tissues, mobility of joint, deformity, and gait
3. Differential nerve, soft tissue, and joint blocks
4. Radiographs and stress radiographs
5. Technetium bone scan
6. Electromyography and nerve conduction studies

Regional Nerve Blockade of the Foot and Ankle

Regional anesthesia is an extremely effective method for use in chronic pain syndromes of the foot and ankle. Often these patients are unable to localize the source of the pain, and the description of their symptoms is also at times confusing. In many patients chronic pain is diffuse, and it is difficult to differentiate neuritic, arthritic, and other soft tissue pain syndromes. Differential blocks of the ankle and subtalar joints and the surrounding soft tissue structures will often clarify the problem, facilitating treatment. A thorough knowledge of the anatomy of the foot is of course helpful in planning these blocks.

Before instituting the nerve or soft tissue block, the patient's anxiety should be allayed. Patients will tolerate the block if the physician takes the time to explain the expected effect of the anesthetic and, at the same time, administers the block very slowly. It is best to wait at least 30 to 60 minutes before performing any extensive manipulation or surgical procedure, so that the efficacy of the anesthesia can be adequately assessed. If the patient becomes extremely anxious during any procedure while local or regional anesthesia is being used, the effect of the block may be masked, and it may be better to re-examine the patient at another time with adequate sedation (oral diazepam) taken 1 hour prior to the administration of the regional anesthetic agent.

For an effective block, I use an equal mixture of 1 percent lidocaine (Xylocaine) and 0.5 percent bupivacaine (Marcaine). Unless the intent is to prolong the effect of the block, the anesthetic agents should not contain epinephrine. I have not experienced any problems when using epinephrine, provided that the block is administered proximally in the foot or ankle and never used for digital blockade.

The posterior tibial nerve is blocked two finger-breadths posterior to the medial malleolus at approximately a 45° inclination from the perpendicular to the anteroposterior surface of the ankle (Fig. 58-10). If the posterior tibial artery is palpable, this may be used as a landmark with the injection site just posterior to it. The needle should be aspirated as it is advanced to preclude intravascular injection. The patient must be warned about the possibility of paresthesias, which are described well to them before giving the block. This is far preferable to a violent withdrawal of the foot if the nerve is inadvertently punctured with the needle. Although paresthesia in the foot is a reliable indicator of the position of the needle, intraneural injection causes exquisite pain and should be avoided. While injecting in the region of the posterior tibial nerve, it is useful to place the index finger of the opposite hand over the flexor retinaculum and palpate the injectable material as it distends the tissues. This appears to be the most reliable method of ascertaining an accurate block of the posterior tibial nerve. Usually, a total of 10 ml of the anesthetic agent is infiltrated to block the posterior tibial nerve.

The superficial peroneal nerve is blocked by subcutaneous infiltration across the dorsum of the midfoot, or more proximally at the medial edge of the fibula at the level of the ankle. Depending on the region of the foot that is being assessed, the sural and saphenous nerve may be blocked as well with subcutaneous infiltration. The sural nerve innervates the lateral border of the foot and can be blocked either distally in the foot or more proximally posterior to the fibula. The saphenous nerve innervates the medial aspect of the ankle and the medial non–weight-bearing surface of the foot and is blocked subcutaneously at the level of the medial malleolus.

The terminal sensory innervation of the deep peroneal nerve supplies the dorsum of the first webspace of the foot, but the nerve also has a significant motor branch to the extensor digitorum brevis muscle. Both the motor and sensory branches are blocked by deeper insertion of the needle, because the nerve is not subcutaneous as is the superficial peroneal nerve but lies deep to the extensor retinaculum. The nerve lies in a constant position between the extensor hallucis longus and the extensor digitorum longus tendons at the level of the ankle joint.

It is not usually necessary to block all the nerves of the foot, and under most circumstances, each nerve may be blocked selectively to determine its role in causing the patient's symptoms. I typically block one nerve with small volumes (1 to 2 ml) of anesthetic and wait 20 minutes before blocking the next nerve. This is time consuming, but it is extremely effective in determining what area of the foot is uncomfortable in patients with chronic pain.

Chronic Compartment Syndromes of the Foot

Compartment syndromes of the extremities have been well documented as a complication of trauma and, over the past decade, understanding of the pathophysiology of this condition and its treatment have increased significantly. If diagnosis and treatment are carried out expeditiously, many of the potential complications of myoneural ischemia can be avoided. Although compartment syndromes of the foot have received much attention recently, the signs and symptoms of increased intracompartmental pressures within the foot are often overlooked, which may lead to the development of profound myoneural ischemia.[30,31] The consequences of untreated compartment syndromes of the foot are significant, because these patients have profound sensorimotor disturbances and marked clinical dysfunction.

Patients complain of chronic pain with stiffness, particularly in the midfoot and forefoot, associated with a deep sense of aching and cramping. Sensory changes may also be present, depending on the site of the injury, and some patients have burning, tingling, and a sense of numbness in the midfoot and forefoot, which is difficult to differentiate from a tarsal tunnel syndrome. The delicate balance between the intrinsic and extrinsic flexors of the metatarsophalangeal joints is lost, because the intrinsic muscles atrophy. The toes are typically hyperextended at the metatarsophalangeal and flexed at the interphalangeal joints

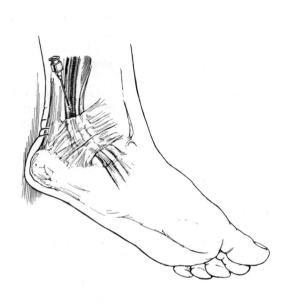

A

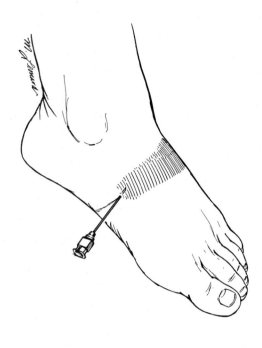

B

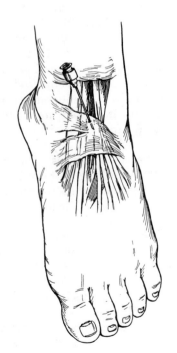

C

Fig. 58-10. Techniques of the posterior tibial **(A)**, superficial peroneal **(B)**, and deep peroneal **(C)** nerve blocks. Note that the deep peroneal nerve lies beneath the extensor retinaculum, whereas the superficial peroneal, sural, and saphenous nerves are subcutaneous.

as a result of this intrinsic muscle atrophy. The extrinsic extensors hyperextend the metatarsophalangeal joints while the long flexor tendons flex both the proximal and distal interphalangeal joints. These deformities become fixed, and because the intrinsic tendons now lie dorsal to the axis of the metatarsal head, their function is further impaired and progressively worsening atrophy occurs. Other intrinsic muscles, including the abductor hallucis, abductor digiti quintae, and extensor brevis, also undergo partial atrophy, and the foot loses its contour and bulk. With this generalized atrophy, discomfort occurs from pressure over the bony prominences of the foot. The foot is invariably stiff from joint and muscle contractures, frequently the result of inadequate treatment at the time of the original injury.[31]

The goal of treatment in these patients should be to re-establish a plantigrade weight-bearing surface of the forefoot. This is often difficult owing to intrinsic muscle atrophy and distal subluxation of the metatarsal fat pad, but a combined physical therapy and surgical program is often successful. Soft tissue releases of both the metatarsophalangeal and proximal interphalangeal joints should be performed to realign the toes. In the presence of fixed contracture, a proximal interphalangeal joint resection arthroplasty or arthrodesis is preferred. This is followed by vigorous manipulations of the forefoot in an effort to relocate the metatarsal fat pad more proximally. At this stage, treatment should be directed toward improving soft tissue mobility. Combinations of paraffin wax, massage, light ultrasound, and hydrotherapy are utilized, and patients are encouraged to exercise and massage their feet.

Unfortunately, often other associated injuries requiring treatment are also present. Not infrequently, traumatic arthritis occurs in the tarsometatarsal, midtarsal, or subtalar joints, and chronic pain from nerve entrapment, tarsal tunnel syndrome, and reflex sympathetic dystrophy may be present, requiring investigation. These conditions are discussed in subsequent sections.

Post-traumatic Arthritis of the Foot

Although traumatic arthritis may occur in the forefoot, midfoot, and hindfoot, the tarsometatarsal, midtarsal, and subtalar joints are involved most fre-quently. Traumatic arthritis of the tarsometatarsal joint after injury is common, often regardless of the initial treatment. Unfortunately, there are multiple small articulations that are often difficult to reduce, and fracture fragments are small and frequently associated with chondral injury.

The morbidity after fracture and dislocation of the tarsometatarsal complex has been described previously. It is an interesting observation that the medial joints, and particularly the second metatarsocuneiform joint, are most likely to develop symptoms after injury. The medial joints of the tarsometatarsal joint have a minimal excursion of movement. The normal range of motion in the sagittal plane of the fifth metatarsal is approximately 14°, the fourth metatarsal 11°, the third metatarsal 2°, the second metatarsal 1°, and the first metatarsal 7°.[32] Despite these minimal arcs of motion, it is precisely these joints that are associated with painful degenerative arthrosis after injury. The metatarsocuboid joint rarely develops symptoms after injury despite a range of motion that is 10 times that of the medial joints. Exactly why the more mobile lateral articulations seldom become symptomatic and the second metatarsal–middle cuneiform joint invariably becomes so is unclear. This may have something to do with the relative frequency with which these joints of the tarsometatarsal complex are injured. Nevertheless, even in the presence of significant radiographic arthrosis, the lateral joints rarely develop.

Management of the degenerative arthritis consists of immobilizing the foot with a rigid orthotic device to prevent pronation of the articulation during the midstance phase of gait. Unfortunately, a rigid orthosis is seldom tolerated by the patient, because the edge of the device is too hard and rubs against prominent osteophytes along the medial tarsometatarsal joint. Although the more flexible accommodative orthoses are well tolerated, they are less likely to control motion at the joint. Nevertheless, the more rigid variety of accommodative orthoses are optimal, and I use a combination of leather, Pelite and firmer densities of Plastizote. If this orthosis is insufficient, a firmer device using polyethylene or Fiberglas materials, such as Rheodur, would be appropriate. If these accommodative orthoses do not alleviate discomfort, further structural immobilization with a polypropylene molded ankle-foot orthosis (MAFO) is often helpful. This can be lined with low-density Plastizote to avoid medial impingement.

If a combination of nonsteroidal anti-inflammatory medication, physical therapy modalities, and orthotic and brace support fails, arthrodesis of the tarsometatarsal joints is indicated.[33,34] Unfortunately, the results after arthrodesis have not been consistently good, and not infrequently patients continue to experience discomfort and mild pain. This may be due to a combination of dystrophic soft tissue changes, neuritis, or areas of traumatic arthrosis not incorporated into the arthrodesis. Although the degenerative changes involve predominantly the metatarsocuneiform articulation, the intercuneiform joints may also be disrupted and should be incorporated into the arthrodesis. Nerve injury, particularly involving the deep peroneal nerve, is common, either as a result of the injury or as a consequence of subsequent surgery. These dystrophic changes are extremely difficult to manage, and patients are often better off in more sedentary occupations and activities.

Painful Sequelae After Calcaneus Fractures

The painful sequelae of calcaneus fractures serve to illustrate many of the problems in managing chronic injury to the foot and ankle. Successful rehabilitation involves a team effort, including rehabilitation nurses, physiotherapists, orthotists, vocational guidance counselors, and physicians. The tremendous disability caused by this injury, and its devastating effect upon what most frequently are young men in the most productive years of their lives, has been recognized. The adverse effects occurring after calcaneus fractures are diverse and demonstrate a need for critical evaluation of the physical, social, and psychiatric problems incurred by these patients. Many patients have chronic pain stemming from arthritis, neuritis, tendinitis, and dystrophic changes in the soft tissues.[35-42] To some extent many of these problems may result from inadequate or inappropriate primary treatment, and although significantly comminuted fractures may have a poor outcome regardless of initial treatment, many of these can by and large be avoided. The specific problems are numerous, and include focal bone and soft tissue impingement, nerve-related pain, subtalar arthritis, calcaneal fibu-

lar abutment, and the smashed heel pad syndrome. Diffuse, poorly localized pain occurs after unrecognized compartment syndromes and chronic pain syndromes, reflex sympathetic dystrophy, and entrapment neuropathies.

Many approaches have been used to treat these problems, ranging from shoe modifications to physiotherapy, surgical reconstruction, and judicious neglect. Controversy as to the appropriate late treatment of calcaneus fractures stems from the relatively unsatisfactory results frequently reported, as well as the devastating physical and psychosocial disability that patients with this injury commonly incur. Many of these patients have sustained their injuries during their prime productive years. Most patients are between the ages of 20 and 40 years, and they are faced with a series of physical and social setbacks, because many of them are unable to return to work in their previous occupations.

Most patients experience lateral foot pain, but it is often difficult to differentiate and isolate the source from which the pain is arising. Lateral foot and ankle pain may arise from calcaneal fibular abutment, discrete peroneal tendinitis, irritation of the sural nerve, or subtalar arthritis. With most varieties of calcaneus fracture, a depression of the posterior tuberosity occurs, and loss of height is accompanied by widening of the heel, which often tilts into varus position. This increased width is easy to demonstrate radiographically with a standing axial tangential view of the calcaneus or a mortise view of the ankle. By far the most specific imaging method for visualizing calcaneal fibular abutment and the overall congruency of the subtalar joint is a computed tomogram.

In addition to the lateral foot and ankle symptoms, medial pain often occurs, typically caused by tibial nerve entrapment or osseous impingement from fracture fragments with medial protrusion. Diffuse discomfort is frequently the result of either a chronic pain syndrome, tibial nerve entrapment and a traumatic tarsal tunnel syndrome, reflex sympathetic dystrophy, or the manifestations of chronic myoneural ischemia from an undiagnosed compartment syndrome. Central heel pad pain results from irreversible disruption of the architecturally septated compartments of the heel pad. The heel pad is uniquely structured so as to encapsulate fat globules in separate compartments, providing cushioning but also resiliency with weight-bearing. With crushing of the heel pad, the interdigitating fibrous septa are disrupted and unfortunately can never be restored. Painful atrophy occurs because this intimate lattice arrangement is lost and cannot be replaced. Although it is not possible to eliminate this discomfort completely, most patients gain some improvement with appropriate heel cups and soft cushioned orthoses, particularly those made of Sorbithane.

Management of these conditions can be extremely frustrating. In many instances the patients are themselves despondent, often clinically depressed, with little to look forward to. The social impact of the injury on their marriage and family may be significant, and it is important to identify evidence of alcohol or drug abuse. Potential sources of secondary gain involving litigation and any outstanding compensation should also be identified and the effect on the patient's treatment program analyzed. It is useful to identify the patient's activities of daily living, ambulation, and work requirements as well as expectations and goals regarding treatment. Since most of these injuries are sustained in the work environment, a rehabilitation nurse who can function as employer liaison should be consulted throughout the course of therapy.

In establishing the source of pain, differential lidocaine blocks are extremely useful. An attempt is made to isolate parts of the foot and assess the impact of the local anesthetic on the patient's symptoms. Because branches of the tibial nerve may also innervate parts of the subtalar joint through the tarsal canal, this block is performed at a second visit. Very small volumes of lidocaine are used. Initially, the peroneal tendon sheath is infiltrated proximal to the fibula with 2 ml. This is followed with a block of the sural nerve, 1 inch proximal to the fibula using 1 ml of lidocaine. The subtalar joint is blocked last, through the sinus tarsi. Significant fibrosis is invariably present around the joint and it is difficult to enter the joint with the needle. For this reason, entering the sinus tarsi is generally sufficient because the nerve to the joint capsule enters through the sinus tarsi and tarsal canal. After each block, the patient is asked to walk about for approximately 10 minutes, and the

foot is re-examined to assess the efficacy of the block. The last block to be administered is given medially and the tibial nerve is blocked with 5 ml of 1 percent plain lidocaine, 1½ inches proximal to the medial malleolus. In this way, all the branches, including the calcaneal, lateral plantar, and medial plantar nerves, are anesthetized and the overall contribution of the tibial nerve to the pain can be assessed.

Occasionally, following all these blocks, the patient continues to complain of pain in the region of the ankle as well as the midfoot and forefoot. If pain is localized at the ankle, a tibiotalar impingement should be suspected. With the crushing of the heel and loss of the heel height, the talus is forced into the calcaneus, and as it assumes a more horizontal position, the talar declination angle decreases. As the talus tilts upward, dorsiflexion of the foot is limited, and anterior tibiotalar abutment occurs. If undiagnosed, this may be the source of chronic ankle pain and may eventually lead to formation of large anterior osteophytes. This is easily demonstrated both clinically and radiographically with decreased excursion of the foot in dorsiflexion and osteophytes visible on a weight-bearing lateral radiograph of the foot. Any vague diffuse pain still present may be attributable to reflex sympathetic dystrophy or another variety of chronic pain syndrome.

All patients should undergo an initial course of rehabilitation with physical therapy. I emphasize daily exercise in a swimming pool, massage, and manipulation of the ankle and hindfoot to improve motion, particularly in the sagittal plane. It is generally fruitless to attempt mobilization of the subtalar joint, which often needlessly increases the patient's discomfort. The soft tissue should be treated with techniques aimed at decreasing swelling and inflammation. I use lateral cortisone injections quite liberally.

Common among therapists and physicians is an attitude of nihilism in treating these patients, who are frequently treated for years without ever returning to work or reasonable activities of daily living. However, it is important to recognize that only a small percentage of these patients actually improve with a conservative rehabilitation program. In our series of 54 patients with 57 fractures who were evaluated at an average of 23 months after injury, only three patients were improved sufficiently from aggressive rehabilitation to the point that surgery was not necessary.[42] For this reason, physicians probably should be more aggressive with earlier surgical reconstruction, because in this same group 72 percent of all patients returned to work and to their preinjury activity level, and 62 percent were able to return to construction and heavy labor.

Reflex Sympathetic Dystrophy

Reflex sympathetic dystrophy (RSD) is a pernicious complication that may follow any injury whether major or insignificant. Generally, the patient's symptoms are vastly out of proportion to the magnitude of the injury. Many terms have appeared in the literature to describe this condition, including major causalgia, Sudek's atrophy, and minor causalgia. However, these are all recognizably distinct entities that differ according to the nature of the injury, the clinical presentation, and the treatment. This disorder is discussed more fully in Chapter 47.

Management of Chronic Swelling of the Foot

Feet swell in association with acute inflammatory or traumatic conditions, and if these go untreated the swelling becomes chronic. Resolution of edema can be difficult and frustrating, and it is probably helpful to commence with an overview of the physiology of venous return from the foot, the concepts of which have changed dramatically over the past few years. Venous emptying from the lower limb depends on an effective muscle pump to provide the impetus for flow as well as venous valves to prevent reversal of blood back toward the foot.[43,44] One postulate has been that venous emptying of the foot occurs through weight-bearing as a result of blood being forced into the deep veins from the sole of the foot, assisted by a negative pressure. However, Gardner and Fox have demonstrated that a discrete pump is present in the foot by which venous return is facilitated.[43] It is of extreme importance to understand that muscular action is not necessary for the foot pump to work. Gardner and Fox have shown, for example, that applying weight to a paralyzed leg with the knee flexed will stimulate venous return.[43] The plantar veins empty predominantly through flattening of the plantar arch during weight-bearing and contraction

of the intrinsic muscles. During weight-bearing, the arch of the foot flattens, and the blood in the veins is literally forced out. The deep veins of the foot do not empty into the superficial venous system of the foot, and retrograde emptying of the plantar veins is prevented not by a system of valves, but merely by tension in the plantar aponeurosis. This system of venous emptying provides a good explanation of symptoms of venous disease, because if either is incompetent, a condition of venous hypertension and swelling of the foot results.[45]

The calf muscle pump is considered to be the mechanism that provides the forward flow of venous blood. There are, however, other muscle pumps in the thigh and leg; video phlebography has even shown the existence of a muscle pump in the foot.[45-47] The most important of these muscle pumps is in the foot and is activated by weight-bearing. Interestingly enough, the pump is unaffected by muscular actions such as ankle movement. Duplex ultrasound and video phlebography have demonstrated that, with weight-bearing, the pump is activated and the large venous plexus on the plantar lateral aspect of the foot empties. Furthermore, this pumping action during weight-bearing can be simulated with an inflatable bladder around the foot, which delivers a compressive force to the foot.

An understanding of the physiology of venous return from the foot is of practical importance in managing acute or chronic venous stasis. To enhance reduction of swelling, many different varieties of pneumatic devices have been used to enhance venous emptying. However, most of the commercially available pneumatic compression devices have varying cycles with long inflation times and are suitable only for intermittent use in the setting of a physical therapy center. Furthermore, these devices are generally applied around the entire lower leg and the entire envelope is inflated synchronously, thereby compromising venous return, because the proximal veins collapse and trap blood in the peripheral system.

However, a pneumatic impulse device has been developed that more accurately mimics the action of the muscle pump of the foot by an intermittent and sudden compression (AV Impulse System, Novamedix, UK). A small plastic inflation bladder is placed under the arch of the foot and attached to the compression device. The compressed air cycles every 20 seconds, and is delivered with an inflation time of 0.4 second and an inflation pressure of approximately 100 mm Hg with a 3-second duration of inflation.[48] This AV Impulse pump differs from the pneumatic devices in that the rapid rise in compression pressure (less than 0.4 second) imitates the physiologic action of ambulation.

Provided that the air vents intermittently into a small pneumatic pad around the foot, imitating the action of walking, edema decreases rapidly. The intermittent compression device has been used successfully for management of acute and chronic edema. This is particularly useful in the patient with swelling from chronic neuroarthropathy and in the setting of trauma and chronic postsurgical swelling. I have used this pump device either at different periods of the day or even continuously, with due care for patients with neuropathy, who may not be able to tolerate prolonged or sustained periods of pumping without developing pressure ischemia.

I also have evaluated edema in the foot in patients after a wide variety of conditions — acute trauma, major surgery to the foot and ankle, chronic postsurgical swelling, and chronic neuropathic arthropathy. The subtle reductions in swelling were monitored utilizing volumetric analysis with water displacement, and dramatic reduction of swelling was found in all these groups. This has proved to be an extremely effective method for mobilizing swelling in the foot, one that is superior to other currently available systems.

Perhaps of even greater significance is the prevention of swelling in the first place. This would be consistent with current principles of fracture care, utilizing rigid internal fixation and earlier mobilization. This early fostering of range of motion prevents or decreases joint contracture, swelling, stiffness, and ultimately the chronic form of swelling and fibrosis, which are so difficult to treat. To a large extent, this "fracture disease" can be prevented by early mobilization of the foot and ankle. The trauma from the fracture produces tearing of the soft tissues with associated hemorrhage into small compartments of the foot. The resulting interstitial edema and a lymphatic stasis heralds the onset of chronic fibrosis, scarring, and swelling.[49] The resorption of the posttraumatic hematoma occurs by small lymphatic vessels and veins. However, the arteriolar-venular gradient is insufficient within itself to provide the sufficient venous return necessary for drainage of swollen tissue. Both the lymphatic and capillary circulations depend primarily on the milking action of muscular contraction, particularly during ambulation, for decreasing swelling. This lymphatic and capillary stasis edema can be prevented through early range-of-motion exercises, especially important because immobilization of a severe fracture for the appropriate length of time invariably produces fibrous ankylosis. Atrophy occurs, and when associated with tenosynovitis and scarring of the tendon sheaths, range of motion in the foot and ankle is further decreased.

These concepts were recognized many years ago by Lapidus, who used utilized immediate mobilization and swimming pool exercises for many fractures of the foot. In many patients, this is not easy because of pain from the injury and the prerequisites of fracture treatment. Although this may not be practical for certain injuries, the concept is apt and is consistent with a more rapid recovery.

Management of Chronic Infection of the Foot and Ankle

One of the more useful techniques of managing acute or chronic infections of the foot is through the induction of active hyperemia using warm compresses. This has been particularly applicable to the neuropathic foot, and I use this technique regularly with chronic ulceration and draining wounds of the foot and ankle. The use of warm compresses in the treatment of superficial skin and wound infections has been described in the literature for centuries.[50,51] Clare, in a treatise on management of abscesses and other wound infections, wrote in 1779, "the ingredients of a poultice should be boiled together and stirred; it should have an unctuous surface and be applied warm . . . cataplasms are exceedingly useful where there is tension and pain; for where the discharge is acrid they adsorb the offending matter, and by their warmth and consistance give ease, and aiding Nature in her healing intentions."[50] These methods were still being utilized in the early part of the 20th century: ". . . put soothing or exciting bandages on the sick portions of the body, the wet linen folded up in six to twelve layers and moistened with water of 72–100 degrees Fahrenheit according to the nature of the boil . . . when the compress begins to get dry it is to be renewed every 6–8 hours."[51]

Since the introduction of antibiotics in the 1940s these time-honored methods of treatment have been utilized less frequently, and the application of compresses is rarely mentioned in current surgery texts. It has been my experience that patients are generally treated with a variety of antibiotics with or without appropriate bed rest or elevation of the extremity. Although these modalities are of paramount importance in managing the local infection, the use of warm compresses has significantly enhanced the recovery process. I employ warm compresses now as an adjunct to immobilization, parenteral antibiotic therapy, and, when indicated, surgical débridement. The compress also is the initial treatment of postoperative wound infections, cellulitis, diabetic infections, and other primary and chronic infections of the foot. It is similarly utilized in conjunction with incision and drainage for deeper abscesses and infections of the plantar fascial spaces.

After initial cultures, combined blood count, determination of sedimentation rate, and appropriate radiographic imaging studies, patients are placed on bed rest with elevation of the extremity, parenteral antibiotics, and immediate application of compresses. A povidone-iodine–soaked gauze sponge is applied to the open wound and covered with a warm (95° to 105°F) moist towel wrapped around the foot (Fig. 58-11). Three layers of thin, commercial impermeable plastic (Saran Wrap) are applied, followed by two layers of plastic-lined disposable absorbent pads (Chucks). The compress is completely changed every 12 hours and generally discontinued by 48 hours, although I have used them for up to 4 days when continued benefit is apparent. Maceration of the skin after each dressing change is common but is not a serious problem and should not be a contraindication to treatment.

The induction of active hyperemia by use of heat has been described in various texts as part of the treatment of the inflammatory process for centuries. My treatment differs from that described historically, because the compress is changed every 12 hours, and not more frequently. This procedure relies on retention of body heat and moisture in the dressing to provide the increased superficial blood flow to the skin and subcutaneous tissues. It is important to recognize that this technique does not replace incision and drainage of an abscess or adequate surgical débridement of the wound where indicated. The use of warm compresses is not the definitive treatment but rather an adjunct to patient care. This contrasts with earlier reports, in which the warm compress may have been relied on for definitive treatment: "the fears of the patient have often prevented incisions, particularly in abscesses of the breast, the female being disposed to try every method rather than endure the knife . . . cases have happily succeeded by the repetition of emollient poultices."[50]

USE OF ORTHOSES IN REHABILITATION OF THE FOOT

Pads, molds, orthoses, and braces for the foot and ankle form an integral part of rehabilitation and are discussed briefly here. First, a word about semantics and terminology: There is no such thing as an "orthotic," a word that is an adjective. The correct terms are an orthotic device or an orthosis. An orthotic device attempts to adjust and interface the anatomic relationships of the forefoot and hindfoot with the walking surfaces. This is achieved by the contour of the orthosis, which causes it to move into specific positions at various times during the gait cycle. There is a big difference between an orthosis that is molded according to the contours of the foot and an accommodative orthosis. The former is referred to as either a biomechanical or a functional orthosis and is capable of controlling the position of the foot during gait. The functional orthosis is made by first taking a plaster imprint or mold of the foot. From this mold, or negative, a positive impression is made by pouring or filling the negative with plaster of Paris in liquid form. The final functional orthotic device is cast by pressing or creating a press fit against the positive mold with varying densities of materials according to prescription.

Three different types of foot orthoses are commonly used, each with their own specific indications. It is quite clear that as the orthosis becomes stiffer, the

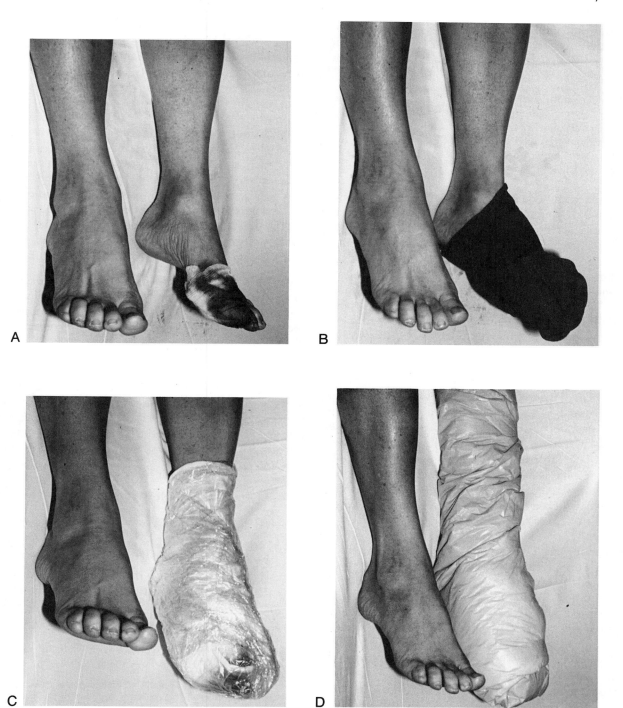

Fig. 58-11. This patient has a chronic infection of the hallux. The wound is covered with a povidone-iodine–soaked gauze sponge **(A)**, and wrapped with a warm, moist towel. **(B)**. This is then wrapped in approximately three layers of impermeable plastic sheeting **(C)**, and finally covered with a large towel or blanket **(D)**.

potential for controlling pathologic aspects of gait and deformity is greater. Generally three different varieties of orthotic devices are used commonly in practice:

1. Rigid orthotic devices, which are made from harder Fiberglas-type materials, such as Rheodur.
2. Softer accommodative inserts made of rubber, felt, or combinations, such as Spenco.
3. Flexible semirigid orthotic devices, which are made of harder rubber or softer plastics.

Many accommodative orthoses are available commercially. Typically, these are used in elderly patients with metatarsalgia and in patients with neuropathy, intrinsic atrophy, neuromuscular deformities, and particularly an insensitive foot. These orthoses are not in any way rigid or mechanically controlled and cannot alter foot function. They offer no protection from abnormal hindfoot mechanics, such as abnormal pronation, and have little applicability in runners because pronation and resupination of the foot cannot be controlled. These in-shoe pads, however, are extremely effective in minimizing external friction and pressure and in redistributing the weight-bearing forces of the midfoot and forefoot. Either the pads can be applied to the shoe, or temporary adhesive pads can be used directly on the foot. Adhesive moleskin is particularly useful in this regard because it can be adapted to the various needs of the foot. Adhesive felt is also useful and can be purchased in thicknesses ranging from $\frac{1}{8}$ inch to 1 inch. I use these adhesive-backed felts liberally and apply them either to the shoe or to the patient's foot.

It is important for rehabilitation personnel to familiarize themselves with various materials used for accommodative orthoses. Spenco (Spenco Medical Corporation, Waco, TX) is a nitrogen-impregnated rubber and is available commercially. It is typically used as full-length inner soles and is now available for purchase in most athletic shoe stores. These inner soles really do very little for the foot, and although I do not use them frequently, they sometimes are adapted by adding adhesive-backed felt pads to support the forefoot in the presence of painful metatarsalgia. Plastizote is a softer material, which comes in three different grades of density. The softest, Plastizote #1, tends to compress easily and to "bottom out" after a few months of wear, when it should be re-placed, particularly when employed for the insensate foot. Plastizote is the mainstay of treatment for patients with insensitivity. The material is soft, fairly durable, and, most importantly, heat moldable without generating enough heat during this process to burn the patient. Cork can be used quite advantageously, because it also meets some of the prerequisites for soft materials. I have used cork and rubber together or commercially available cork-rubber mixtures such as Corex (Mayflower Podiatry Supplies, Los Alamitos, CA), which are quite useful because they can be easily shaped with a grinder. The cork-rubber combination preserves its shape and does not bottom out as readily as Plastizote. Nevertheless, it is not moldable and for this reason is used as an adjunct to combination inserts, such as Plastizote and rubber.

Rigid orthotic devices are fabricated after a plaster mold impression is taken from the foot. The type of orthotic device fabricated does not simply support the arch, but attempts to control elements of movement of the foot. These orthoses have no long-term "curative" properties and only work while being worn in the shoe. An analogous situation is with eyeglasses, which improve vision only while they are being worn; once they are removed, the eyes return to their previous myopic state. The goal of these rigid orthotic devices is to alter the biomechanical properties of the foot during gait so that the foot and leg can function more normally.

REFERENCES

1. Bell ET: Incidence of gangrene of the extremities in nondiabetic and in diabetic persons. Arch Pathol 49:469, 1950
2. Cameron CC, Lennard-Jones JE, Robinson DM: Amputations in the diabetic: outcome and survival. Lancet 2:605, 1964
3. Most R, Sinnock P: The epidemiology of lower extremity amputations in diabetic individuals. Diabetes Care 6:87, 1983
4. Wagner FW: The diabetic foot. Orthopaedics 10:163, 1987
5. Davidson JK, Alogna M, Goldsmith M et al: Assessment of program effectiveness at Grady Memorial Hospital. p. 329. In Steiner S, Lawrence PA (eds): Educating Diabetic Patients. Springer Verlag, New York, 1981
6. Goodman J, Bessman AM, Teget B, Wagner FW Jr: Risk factors in local surgical procedures for diabetic gangrene. Surg Gynecol Obstet 143:587, 1976
7. Bauman JH, Girling JP, Brand PW: Plantar pressures and trophic ulceration: evaluation of footwear. J Bone Joint Surg [Br] 45:652, 1963
8. Holstein P, Larsen K, Sager P: Decompression with aid of insoles in treatment of diabetic neuropathic ulcers. Acta Orthop Scand 47:463, 1976
9. Birke JA, Sims S, Buford WL: Walking casts: effect on plantar foot pressures. J Rehabil Res Dev 22:18, 1985

10. Coleman WC, Brand PW, Birke JA: The total contact cast: a therapy for plantar ulceration on insensitive feet. J Am Podiatr Med Assoc 74:548, 1984

11. Helm PA, Walker SC, Pullium G: Total contact casting in diabetic patients with neuropathic foot ulcerations. Arch Phys Med Rehabil 65:691, 1984

12. Pring DJ, Casiebanca N: Simple plantar ulcers treated by below-knee plaster and molded double-rocker plaster shoe: a comparative study. Lepr Rev 53:261, 1982

13. Sinacore DR: Total contact casting in the treatment of diabetic neuropathic ulcers. In Levin ME, O'Neal LW (eds): The Diabetic Foot. 4th Ed. CV Mosby, St. Louis, in press

14. Stokes IAF, Faris IB, Hutton WC: The neuropathic ulcer and loads on the foot in diabetic patients. Acta Orthop Scand 46:839, 1975

15. Livingston R, Jacobs RL, Karmody A: Plantar abscess in the diabetic patient. Foot Ankle 5:205, 1985

16. Kelly PJ, Coventry MB: Neurotrophic ulcers of the feet: review of 47 cases. JAMA, 168:388, 1958

17. Boehm HJ: Diabetic Charcot joint: report of case and review of literature. N Eng J Med 267:185, 1962

18. Clohisy DR, Thompson RC: Fractures associated with neuropathic arthropathy in adults who have juvenile-onset diabetes. J Bone Joint Surg [Am] 70:1192, 1988

19. Cohn BT, Brahms MA: Diabetic arthropathy of the first metatarsal cuneiform joint. Orthop Rev 16:465, 1987

20. Harris JR, Brand PW: Patterns of disintegration of the tarsus in the anaesthetic foot. J Bone Joint Surg [Br] 48:4, 1966

21. Frykberg RG, Kozak GP: Neuropathic arthropathy in the diabetic foot. Am Fam Physician 17:105, 1978

22. Heiple KG, Cammarn MR: Diabetic neuroarthropathy with spontaneous peritalar fracture-dislocation. J Bone Joint Surg [Am] 48:1177, 1966

23. Jacob JE: Observations of neuropathic (Charcot) joints occurring in diabetes mellitus. J Bone Joint Surg [Am] 40:1043, 1958

24. Johnson JTH: Neuropathic fractures and joint injuries. Pathogenesis and rationale of prevention and treatment. J Bone Joint Surg [Am] 49:1, 1967

25. Lesko P, Maurer RC: Talonavicular dislocations and midfoot arthropathy in neuropathic diabetic feet: natural course and principles of treatment. Clin Orthop 240:226, 1989

26. Miller DS, Lichtman WF: Diabetic neuropathic arthropathy of feet. Arch Surg 70:513, 1955

27. Newman JH: Non-infective disease of the diabetic foot. J Bone Joint Surg [Br] 63:593, 1981

28. Robillard R, Gagnon P-A, Alareie R: Diabetic neuroarthropathy: report of four cases. Can Med Assoc J 91:795, 1964

29. Sinah S, Munichoodappa CS, Kozak GP: Neuroarthropathy (Charcot joints) in diabetes mellitus. Medicine 51:191, 1972

30. Myerson MS: Acute compartment syndromes of the foot. Bull Hosp Joint Dis 47:2, 1987

31. Myerson MS: The diagnosis and treatment of compartment syndromes of the foot. Orthopedics 13:711, 1990

32. Ouzounian T, Shereff M: In vitro determination of midfoot motion. Foot Ankle 10:140, 1989

33. Johnson JE, Johnson KA: Dowel arthrodesis for degenerative arthritis of the tarsometatarsal (Lisfranc) joints. Foot Ankle 6:243, 1986

34. Cotton FJ: Old Fractures of the os calcis. Ann Surg 74:294, 1921

35. Deyerle WM: Long-term follow-up of fractures of the os calcis. Diagnostic peroneal synoviagram. Orthop Clin North Am 4:213, 1973

36. James ETR, Hunter GA: The dilemma of painful old os calcis fractures. Clin Orthop 177:112, 1983

37. Johansson JE, Harrison J, Greenwood FAH: Subtalar arthrodesis for adult traumatic arthritis. Foot Ankle 2:294, 1982

38. Mann RA: The tarsal tunnel syndrome. Orthop Clin North Am 5:109, 1974

39. Meyer JM, Lagier R: Posttraumatic sinus tarsi syndrome: an anatomical and radiological study. Acta Orthop Scand 48:121, 1977

40. Miller WE, Lichtblau PO: The smashed heel. South Med J 58:1229, 1985

41. McLaughlin HL: Treatment of late complications after os calcis fractures. Clin Orthop 30:111, 1963

42. Quill GE, Myerson MS: Late reconstruction following calcaneus fractures. Presented at Annual AOFAS Meeting, Banff Springs, Alberta, Canada, 1990

43. Gardner AMN, Fox RH: The venous pump of the human foot. Bristol Med-Chir J 98:109, 1983

44. Gardner AMN, Fox RH: The return of blood to the heart against the force of gravity. p. 56. In Negus D, Jantet G (eds): Phlebology '85. John Libbey, London, 1986

45. Lundstrom B, Osterman G: Assessment of deep venous insufficiency by ascending phlebography. Acta Radiol [Diagn] (Stockh) 24:375, 1983

46. Watkins PJ: Foot blood flow in diabetic neuropathy. J R Soc Med 76:996, 1983

47. Bishara RA, Sigel B, Rocco K et al: Deterioration of venous function in normal lower extremities during daily activity. J Vasc Surg 3:700, 1986

48. Brown JG, Ward PE, Wilkinson AJ, Mollan RAB: Impedance plethysmography: a screening procedure to detect deep-vein thrombosis. J Bone Joint Surg [Br] 69:264, 1987

49. Fox RH, Gardner AMN: Video-phlebography in the investigation of venous physiology and disease. p. 68. In Negus D, Jante G (eds): Phlebology '85. John Libbey, London, 1986

50. Clare P: An essay on the cure of abscesses by caustic, and on the treatment of the wounds and ulcers. London, 28, 1779

51. Lewis D: The Practice of Surgery. Vol. I. p. 124. WF Prior Co., Philadelphia, 1933

Section VI
APPENDICES

APPENDIX I

Skeletal Anatomy*

* All figures except AI-18, AI-19, AI-24, and AI-25 are from Crafts RC: A Textbook of Human Anatomy. 3rd Ed., Churchill Livingstone, New York, 1985, with Figures AI-18, AI-19, AI-24, and AI-25 are from Quain: Elements of Anatomy, 1900, courtesy of Longman Group Ltd.

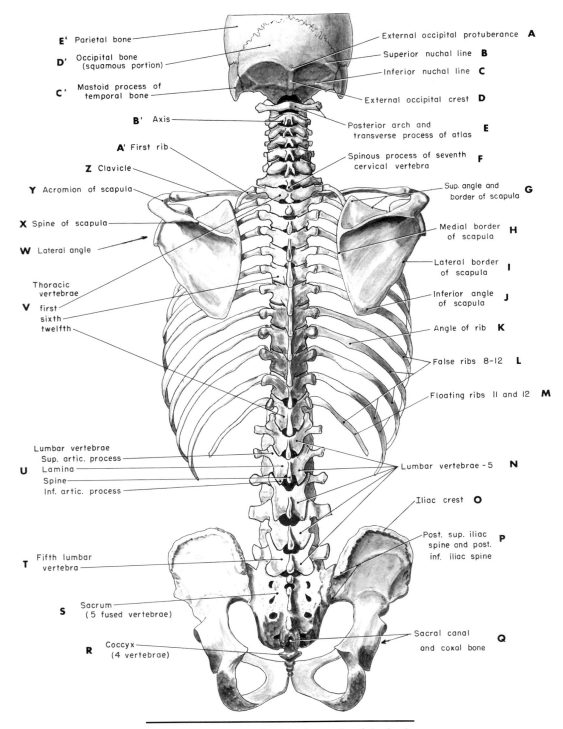

Fig. AI-1. Bones involved in the study of the back.

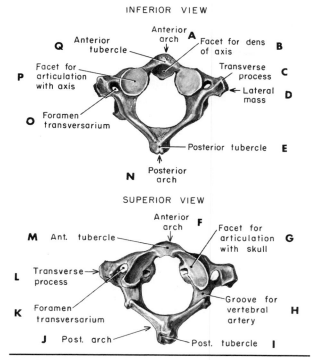

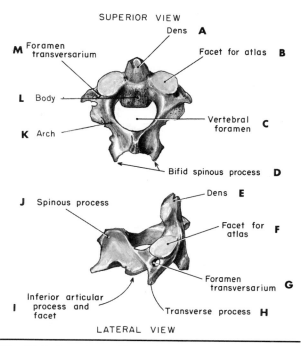

Fig. AI-2. Inferior and superior views of the first cervical vertebra, the atlas.

Fig. AI-3. Superior and lateral views of the second cervical vertebra, the axis.

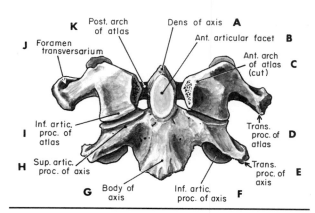

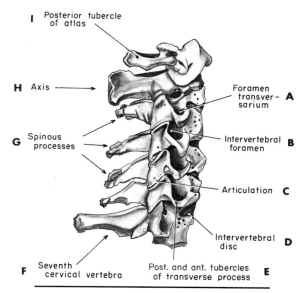

Fig. AI-4. Anterior view of atlas and axis. The anterior tubercle of the atlas has been removed to show the relationship of the anterior arch to the dens of the axis.

Fig. AI-5. Lateral view of cervical vertebrae.

SUPERIOR VIEW

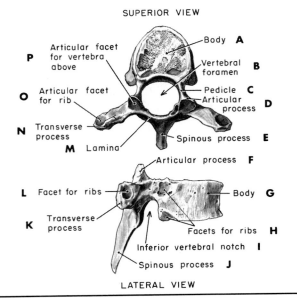

Fig. AI-6. Superior and lateral views of a typical thoracic vertebra.

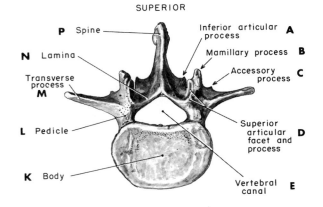

Fig. AI-7. Superior and lateral views of a lumbar vertebra.

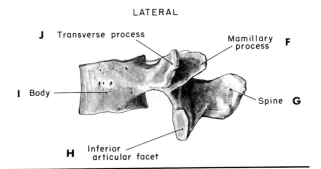

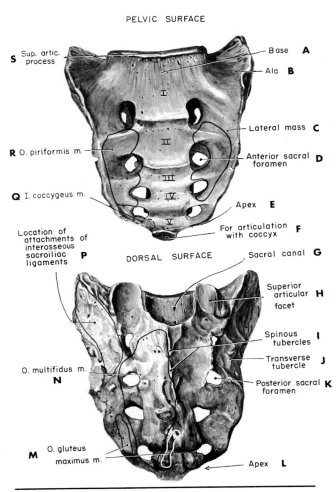

Fig. AI-8. Pelvic and dorsal surfaces of sacrum with muscle attachments outlined.

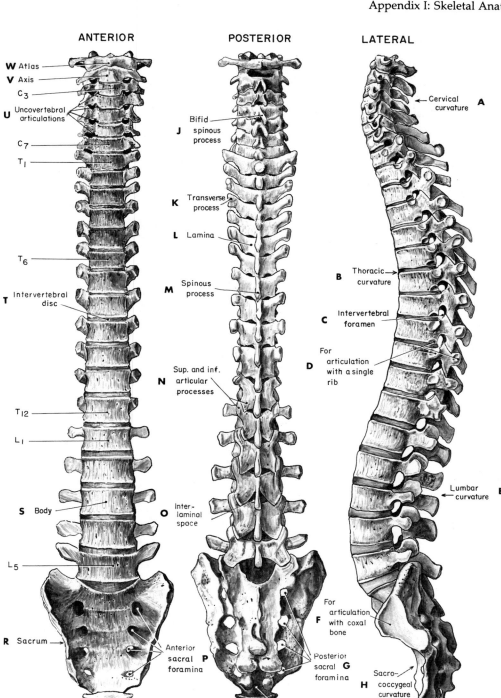

ANTERIOR

W Atlas
V Axis
C$_3$
U Uncovertebral articulations
C$_7$
T$_1$
T$_6$
T Intervertebral disc
T$_{12}$
L$_1$
S Body
L$_5$
R Sacrum
Anterior sacral foramina
Q Coccyx

POSTERIOR

J Bifid spinous process
K Transverse process
L Lamina
M Spinous process
N Sup. and inf. articular processes
O Inter-laminal space
P Posterior sacral foramina
G
Sacral canal **I**

LATERAL

Cervical curvature **A**
B Thoracic curvature
C Intervertebral foramen
D For articulation with a single rib
Lumbar curvature **E**
F For articulation with coxal bone
H Sacro-coccygeal curvature

Fig. AI-9. Anterior, posterior, and lateral views of the vertebral column.

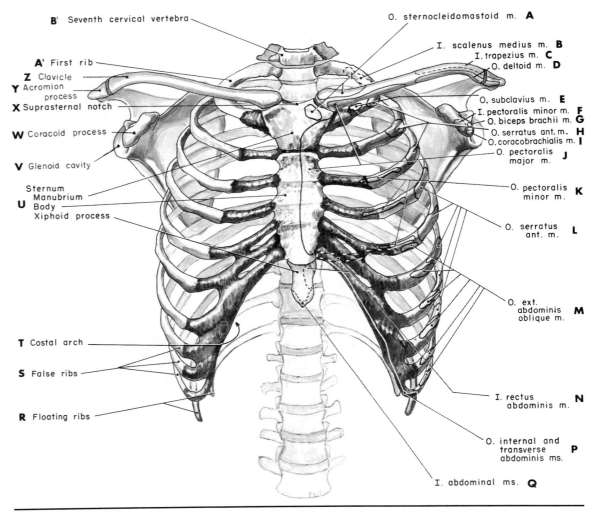

B' Seventh cervical vertebra

A' First rib
Z Clavicle
Y Acromion process
X Suprasternal notch
W Coracoid process
V Glenoid cavity
Sternum
Manubrium
U Body
Xiphoid process

T Costal arch
S False ribs
R Floating ribs

O. sternocleidomastoid m. **A**
I. scalenus medius m. **B**
I. trapezius m. **C**
O. deltoid m. **D**
O. subclavius m. **E**
I. pectoralis minor m. **F**
O. biceps brachii m. **G**
O. serratus ant. m. **H**
O. coracobrachialis m. **I**
O. pectoralis major m. **J**
O. pectoralis minor m. **K**
O. serratus ant. m. **L**
O. ext. abdominis oblique m. **M**
I. rectus abdominis m. **N**
O. internal and transverse abdominis ms. **P**
I. abdominal ms. **Q**

Fig. AI-10. The thoracic cage, showing manner of attachment of ribs to sternum. The darker shaded areas are the cartilaginous portions of the ribs. Origins and insertions of muscles are outlined.

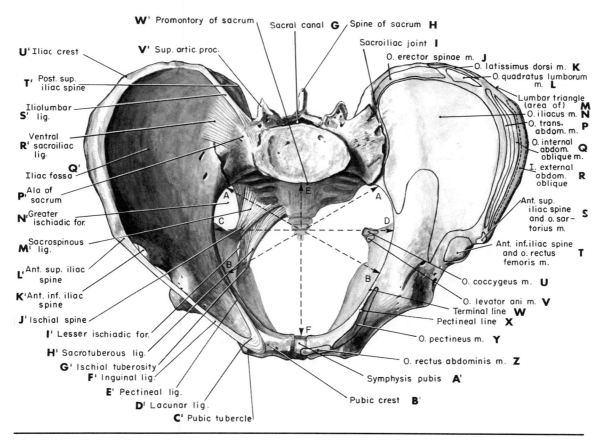

Fig. AI-11. The male bony pelvis, showing attachments of muscles on the left and ligaments on the right. Note the location of the pubic symphysis (A') and crest (B'), pectineal line (X), anterior superior iliac spine (S), and the iliac crest (U'). Note also the attachments of the inguinal ligament (F') and its continuation as the lacunar (D') and pectineal (E') ligaments.

Labels in the figure:

W' Promontory of sacrum
Sacral canal **G**
Spine of sacrum **H**
Sacroiliac joint **I**
O. erector spinae m. **J**
O. latissimus dorsi m. **K**
O. quadratus lumborum m. **L**
Lumbar triangle (area of) **M**
O. iliacus m. **N**
O. trans. abdom. m. **P**
O. internal abdom. oblique m. **Q**
I. external abdom. oblique **R**
Ant. sup. iliac spine and o. sartorius m. **S**
Ant. inf. iliac spine and o. rectus femoris m. **T**
O. coccygeus m. **U**
O. levator ani m. **V**
Terminal line **W**
Pectineal line **X**
O. pectineus m. **Y**
O. rectus abdominis m. **Z**
Symphysis pubis **A'**
Pubic crest **B'**
C' Pubic tubercle
D' Lacunar lig.
E' Pectineal lig.
F' Inguinal lig.
G' Ischial tuberosity
H' Sacrotuberous lig.
I' Lesser ischiadic for.
J' Ischial spine
K' Ant. inf. iliac spine
L' Ant. sup. iliac spine
M' Sacrospinous lig.
N' Greater ischiadic for.
P' Ala of sacrum
Q' Iliac fossa
R' Ventral sacroiliac lig.
S' Iliolumbar lig.
T' Post. sup. iliac spine
U' Iliac crest
V' Sup. artic. proc.

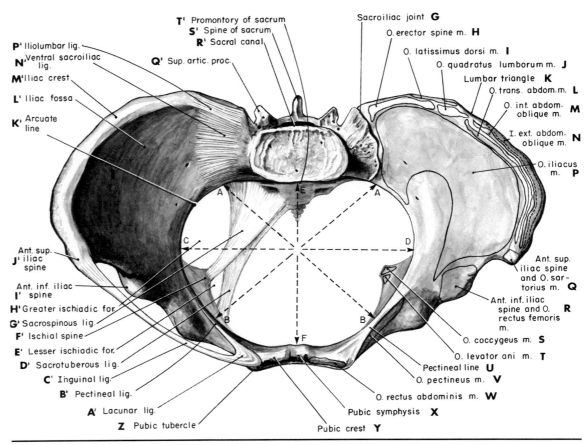

Fig. AI-12. The female bony pelvis, with origins and insertions of muscles indicated on the left and the ligaments shown on the right. A—sacroiliac joint; B—iliopubic eminence; C and D—middle of pelvic brim; E—sacral promontory; F—pubic symphysis.

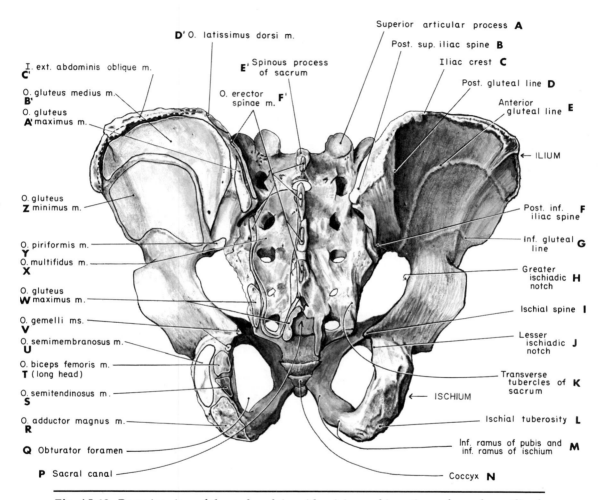

Fig. AI-13. Posterior view of the male pelvis, with origins and insertions of muscles outlined.

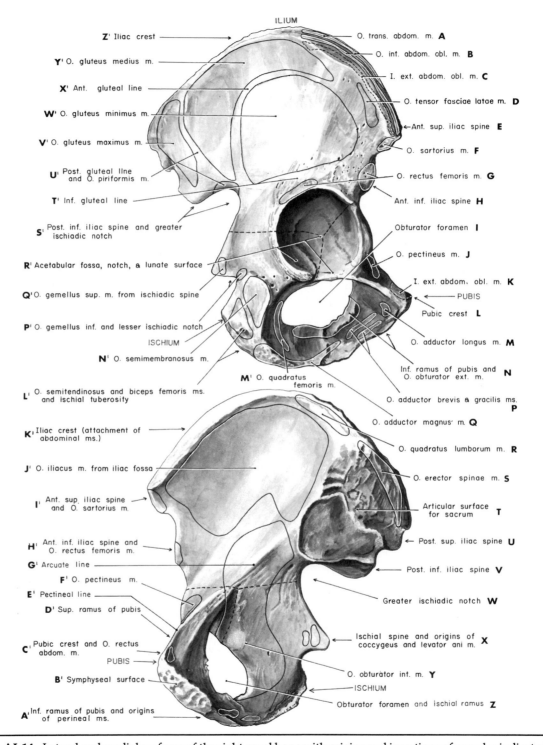

Fig. AI-14. Lateral and medial surfaces of the right coxal bone with origins and insertions of muscles indicated.

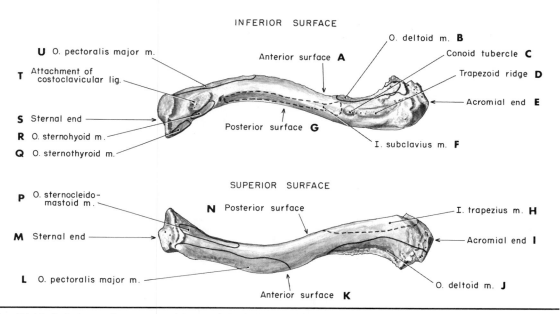

INFERIOR SURFACE

U O. pectoralis major m.

T Attachment of
   costoclavicular lig.

O. deltoid m. **B**

Anterior surface **A**

Conoid tubercle **C**

Trapezoid ridge **D**

Acromial end **E**

S Sternal end

R O. sternohyoid m.

Q O. sternothyroid m.

Posterior surface **G**

I. subclavius m. **F**

SUPERIOR SURFACE

P O. sternocleido-
   mastoid m.

N Posterior surface

M Sternal end

I. trapezius m. **H**

Acromial end **I**

L O. pectoralis major m.

O. deltoid m. **J**

Anterior surface **K**

Fig. AI-15. Inferior and superior surfaces of the left clavicle with origins and insertions of muscles outlined.

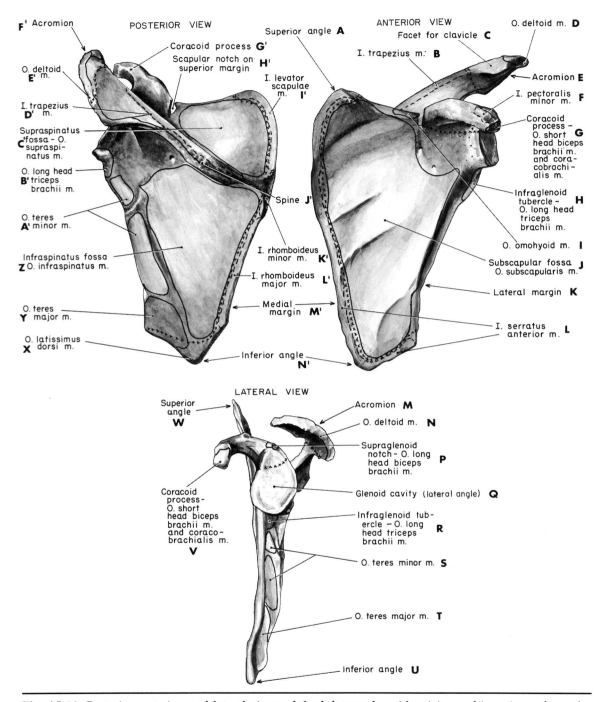

Fig. AI-16. Posterior, anterior, and lateral views of the left scapula, with origins and insertions of muscles outlined. (Crosses indicate location of epiphyseal lines.)

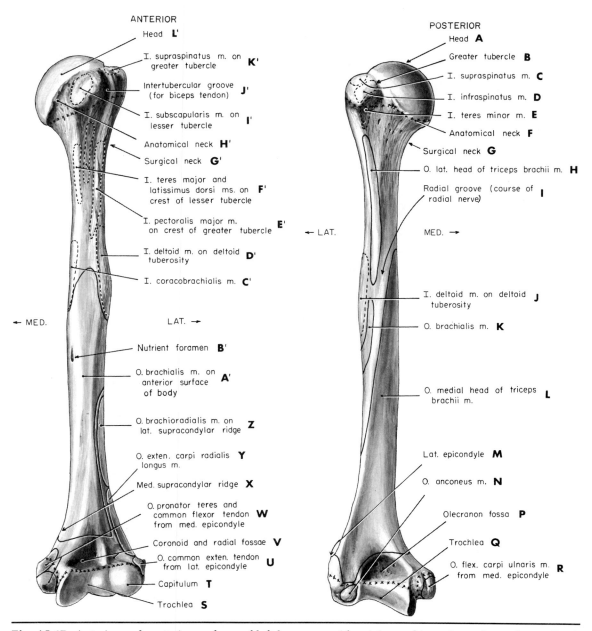

ANTERIOR

Head **L'**

I. supraspinatus m. on greater tubercle **K'**

Intertubercular groove (for biceps tendon) **J'**

I. subscapularis m. on lesser tubercle **I'**

Anatomical neck **H'**

Surgical neck **G'**

I. teres major and latissimus dorsi ms. on crest of lesser tubercle **F'**

I. pectoralis major m. on crest of greater tubercle **E'**

← LAT.

I. deltoid m. on deltoid tuberosity **D'**

I. coracobrachialis m. **C'**

← MED.

LAT. →

Nutrient foramen **B'**

O. brachialis m. on anterior surface of body **A'**

O. brachioradialis m. on lat. supracondylar ridge **Z**

O. exten. carpi radialis longus m. **Y**

Med. supracondylar ridge **X**

O. pronator teres and common flexor tendon from med. epicondyle **W**

Coronoid and radial fossae **V**

O. common exten. tendon from lat. epicondyle **U**

Capitulum **T**

Trochlea **S**

POSTERIOR

Head **A**

Greater tubercle **B**

I. supraspinatus m. **C**

I. infraspinatus m. **D**

I. teres minor m. **E**

Anatomical neck **F**

Surgical neck **G**

O. lat. head of triceps brachii m. **H**

Radial groove (course of radial nerve) **I**

MED. →

I. deltoid m. on deltoid tuberosity **J**

O. brachialis m. **K**

O. medial head of triceps brachii m. **L**

Lat. epicondyle **M**

O. anconeus m. **N**

Olecranon fossa **P**

Trochlea **Q**

O. flex. carpi ulnaris m. from med. epicondyle **R**

Fig. AI-17. Anterior and posterior surfaces of left humerus, with origins and insertions of muscles outlined. (Crosses indicate location of epiphyseal lines.)

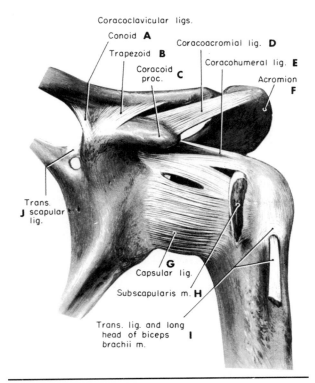

Coracoclavicular ligs.

Conoid **A**

Trapezoid **B**

Coracoid proc. **C**

Coracoacromial lig. **D**

Coracohumeral lig. **E**

Acromion **F**

Trans. scapular lig. **J**

Capsular lig. **G**

Subscapularis m. **H**

Trans. lig. and long head of biceps brachii m. **I**

Fig. AI-18. Anterior view of left shoulder. Apertures in capsule are for connections between the joint cavity and surrounding bursae.

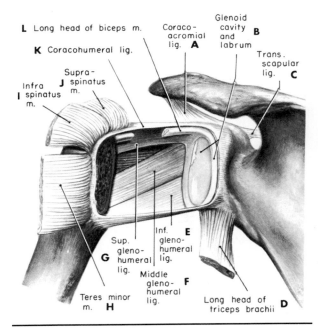

L Long head of biceps m.

K Coracohumeral lig.

Coraco-acromial lig. **A**

Glenoid cavity and labrum **B**

Trans. scapular lig. **C**

Infra spinatus m. **I**

Supra-spinatus m. **J**

Inf. gleno-humeral lig. **E**

Sup. gleno-humeral lig. **G**

Middle gleno-humeral lig. **F**

Teres minor m. **H**

Long head of triceps brachii **D**

Fig. AI-19. A posterior view of the anterior capsule of the left shoulder joint, made possible by removal of the head of the humerus.

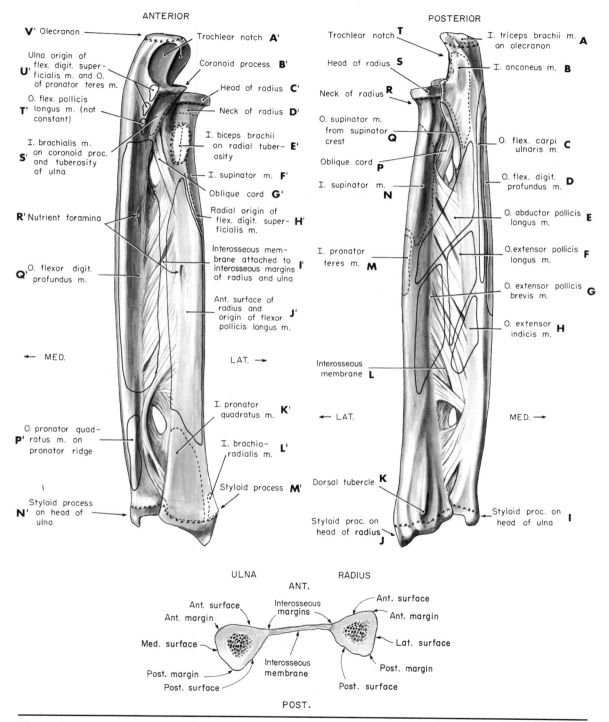

Fig. AI-20. Anterior and posterior surfaces of left ulna and radius and the interosseous membrane. Origins and insertions of muscles have been outlined. (Crosses indicate location of epiphyseal lines.) Cross section below shows margins and surfaces.

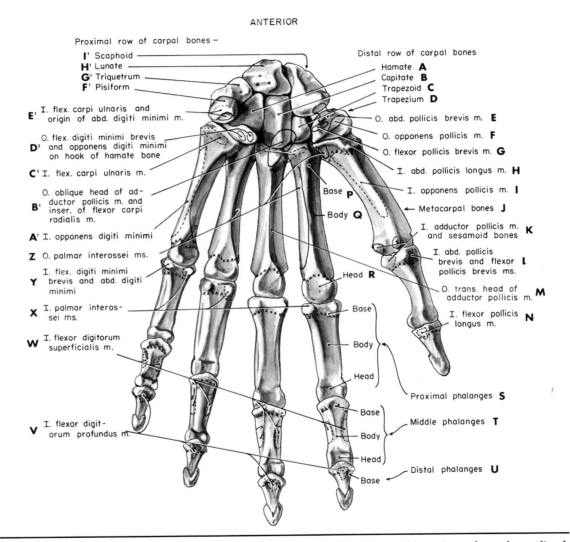

ANTERIOR

Proximal row of carpal bones —

I' Scaphoid
H' Lunate
G' Triquetrum
F' Pisiform

Distal row of carpal bones

Hamate **A**
Capitate **B**
Trapezoid **C**
Trapezium **D**

E' I. flex. carpi ulnaris and origin of abd. digiti minimi m.

O. abd. pollicis brevis m. **E**

O. flex. digiti minimi brevis
D' and opponens digiti minimi
on hook of hamate bone

O. opponens pollicis m. **F**

O. flexor pollicis brevis m. **G**

C' I. flex. carpi ulnaris m.

I. abd. pollicis longus m. **H**

O. oblique head of ad-
B' ductor pollicis m. and
inser. of flexor carpi
radialis m.

I. opponens pollicis m. **I**

Base **P**

Metacarpal bones **J**

Body **Q**

A' I. opponens digiti minimi

I. adductor pollicis m. **K**
and sesamoid bones

Z O. palmar interossei ms.

Head **R**

I. abd. pollicis
brevis and flexor **L**
pollicis brevis ms.

I. flex. digiti minimi
Y brevis and abd. digiti
minimi

Base

O. trans. head of **M**
adductor pollicis m.

X I. palmar interos-
sei ms.

Body

I. flexor pollicis
longus m. **N**

W I. flexor digitorum
superficialis m.

Head

Proximal phalanges **S**

Base

Middle phalanges **T**

V I. flexor digit-
orum profundus m.

Body

Head

Distal phalanges **U**

Base

Fig. AI-21. Anterior surface of the bones of left wrist and hand with origins and insertions of muscles outlined. (Crosses indicate location of epiphyseal lines.)

POSTERIOR

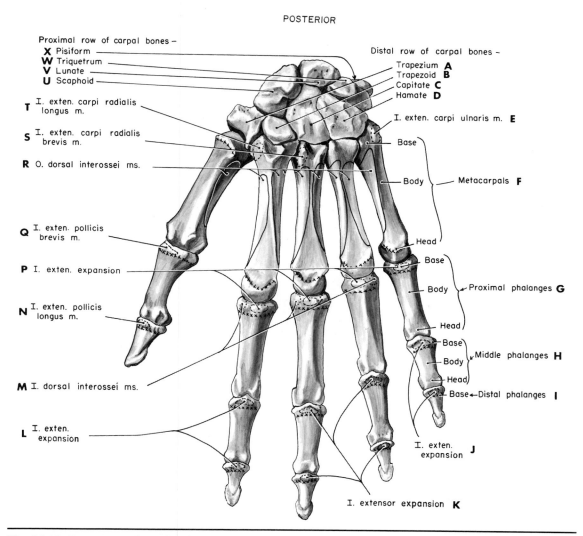

Proximal row of carpal bones —
X Pisiform
W Triquetrum
V Lunate
U Scaphoid

Distal row of carpal bones —
Trapezium **A**
Trapezoid **B**
Capitate **C**
Hamate **D**

T I. exten. carpi radialis longus m.

S I. exten. carpi radialis brevis m.

R O. dorsal interossei ms.

I. exten. carpi ulnaris m. **E**

Base

Body — Metacarpals **F**

Q I. exten. pollicis brevis m.

P I. exten. expansion

N I. exten. pollicis longus m.

Head

Base

Body — Proximal phalanges **G**

M I. dorsal interossei ms.

Head
Base
Body — Middle phalanges **H**
Head
Base ←Distal phalanges **I**

L I. exten. expansion

I. exten. expansion **J**

I. extensor expansion **K**

Fig. AI-22. Posterior surface of the bones of left wrist and hand with origins and insertions of muscles outlined. (Crosses indicate location of epiphyseal lines.)

ANTERIOR

POSTERIOR

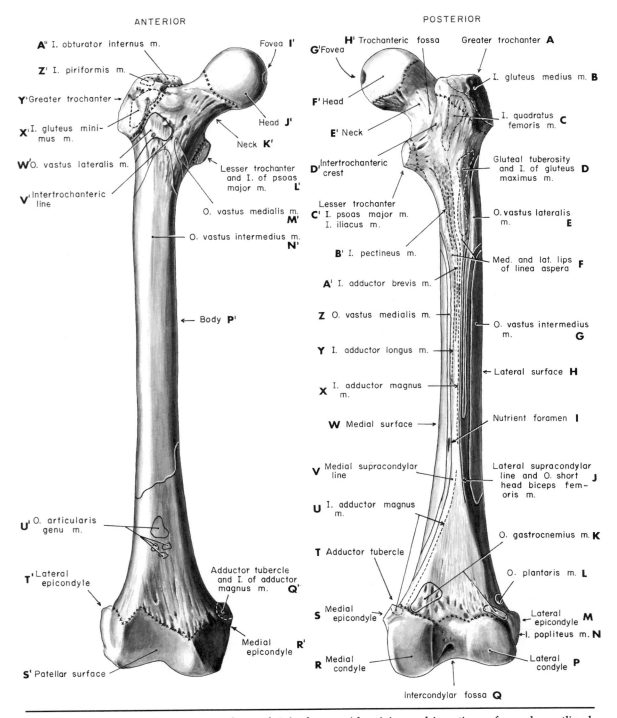

A″ I. obturator internus m.

Z′ I. piriformis m.

Y′ Greater trochanter →

X′ I. gluteus minimus m.

W′ O. vastus lateralis m.

V′ Intertrochanteric line

Fovea **I′**

Head **J′**

Neck **K′**

Lesser trochanter and I. of psoas major m. **L′**

O. vastus medialis m. **M′**

O. vastus intermedius m. **N′**

← Body **P′**

U′ O. articularis genu m.

T′ Lateral epicondyle

Adductor tubercle and I. of adductor magnus m. **Q′**

Medial epicondyle **R′**

S′ Patellar surface

H′ Trochanteric fossa

G′ Fovea

F′ Head

E′ Neck

D′ Intertrochanteric crest

Lesser trochanter
C′ I. psoas major m.
I. iliacus m.

B′ I. pectineus m.

A′ I. adductor brevis m.

Z O. vastus medialis m.

Y I. adductor longus m.

X I. adductor magnus m.

W Medial surface →

V Medial supracondylar line

U I. adductor magnus m.

T Adductor tubercle

S Medial epicondyle

R Medial condyle

Greater trochanter **A**

I. gluteus medius m. **B**

I. quadratus femoris m. **C**

Gluteal tuberosity and I. of gluteus maximus m. **D**

O. vastus lateralis m. **E**

Med. and lat. lips of linea aspera **F**

O. vastus intermedius m. **G**

← Lateral surface **H**

Nutrient foramen **I**

Lateral supracondylar line and O. short head biceps femoris m. **J**

O. gastrocnemius m. **K**

O. plantaris m. **L**

Lateral epicondyle **M**

I. popliteus m. **N**

Lateral condyle **P**

Intercondylar fossa **Q**

Fig. AI-23. Anterior and posterior surfaces of right femur with origins and insertions of muscles outlined. (Crosses indicate location of epiphyseal lines.) The insertion of the obturator externus muscle into the trochanteric fossa is hidden from view by the overhanging greater trochanter.

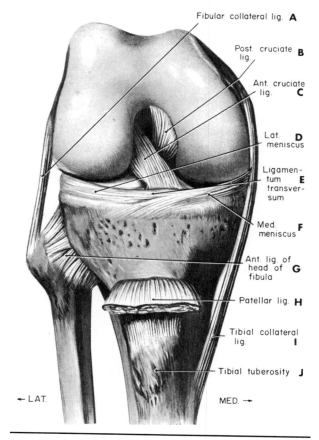

Fibular collateral lig. **A**

Post. cruciate lig. **B**

Ant. cruciate lig. **C**

Lat. meniscus **D**

Ligamentum transversum **E**

Med. meniscus **F**

Ant. lig. of head of fibula **G**

Patellar lig. **H**

Tibial collateral lig. **I**

Tibial tuberosity **J**

← LAT.   MED. →

Fig. AI-24. Right knee joint—anterior view of cruciate ligaments.

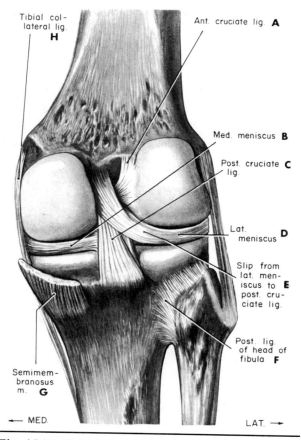

Tibial collateral lig. **H**

Ant. cruciate lig. **A**

Med. meniscus **B**

Post. cruciate lig. **C**

Lat. meniscus **D**

Slip from lat. meniscus to post. cruciate lig. **E**

Post. lig. of head of fibula **F**

Semimembranosus m. **G**

← MED.   LAT. →

Fig. AI-25. Right knee joint—posterior view of cruciate ligaments.

Fig. AI-26. Anterior and posterior surfaces of the right patella.

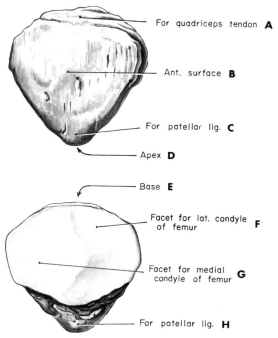

For quadriceps tendon **A**

Ant. surface **B**

For patellar lig. **C**

Apex **D**

Base **E**

Facet for lat. condyle of femur **F**

Facet for medial condyle of femur **G**

For patellar lig. **H**

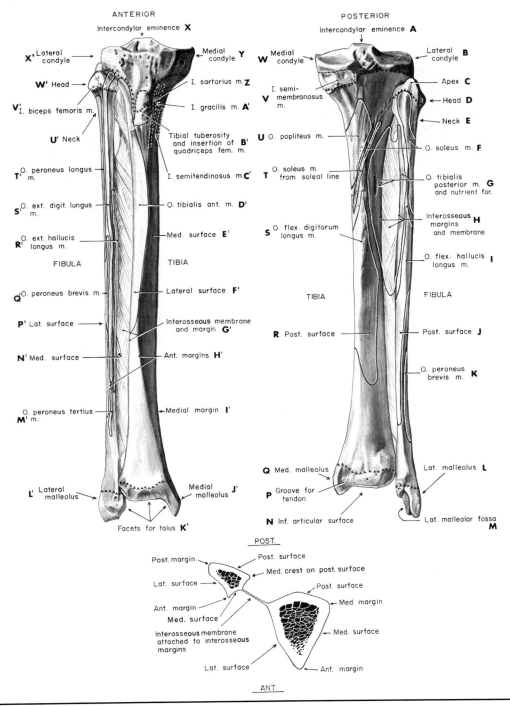

Fig. AI-27. Anterior and posterior surfaces of the right tibia and fibula with origins and insertions of muscles outlined. The interosseous membrane has been included. (Crosses indicate position of epiphyseal lines.) Cross section below clarifies the margins and surfaces.

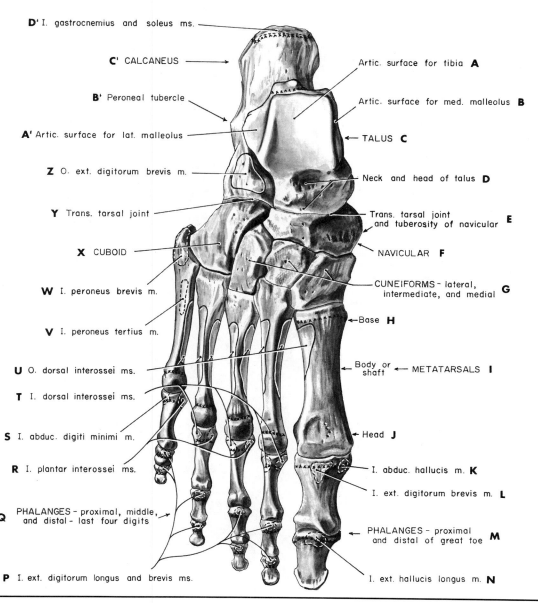

D' I. gastrocnemius and soleus ms.

C' CALCANEUS

B' Peroneal tubercle

A' Artic. surface for lat. malleolus

Z O. ext. digitorum brevis m.

Y Trans. tarsal joint

X CUBOID

W I. peroneus brevis m.

V I. peroneus tertius m.

U O. dorsal interossei ms.

T I. dorsal interossei ms.

S I. abduc. digiti minimi m.

R I. plantar interossei ms.

Q PHALANGES – proximal, middle, and distal – last four digits

P I. ext. digitorum longus and brevis ms.

Artic. surface for tibia **A**

Artic. surface for med. malleolus **B**

TALUS **C**

Neck and head of talus **D**

Trans. tarsal joint and tuberosity of navicular **E**

NAVICULAR **F**

CUNEIFORMS – lateral, intermediate, and medial **G**

Base **H**

Body or shaft ← METATARSALS **I**

Head **J**

I. abduc. hallucis m. **K**

I. ext. digitorum brevis m. **L**

PHALANGES – proximal and distal of great toe **M**

I. ext. hallucis longus m. **N**

Fig. AI-28. Bones of the right foot (dorsal surface) with origins and insertions of muscles outlined. (Crosses indicate location of epiphyseal lines.) Note how the epiphyseal lines indicate that the bone missing in the great toe is the metatarsal and not a phalanx.

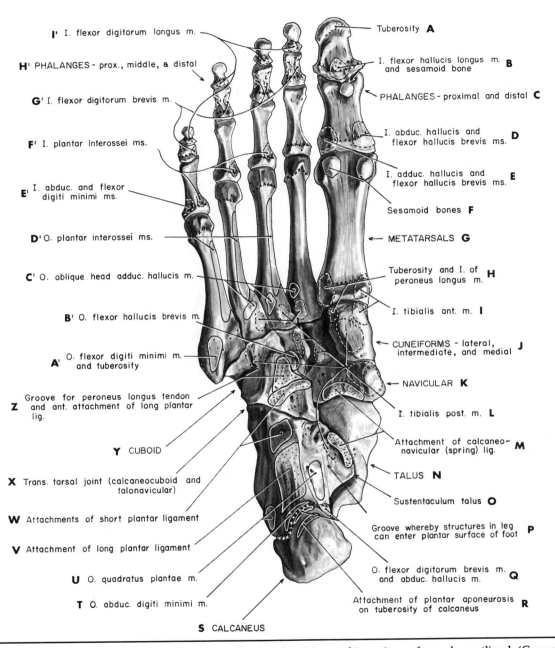

I' I. flexor digitorum longus m.

H' PHALANGES - prox., middle, a distal

G' I. flexor digitorum brevis m.

F' I. plantar interossei ms.

E' I. abduc. and flexor digiti minimi ms.

D' O. plantar interossei ms.

C' O. oblique head adduc. hallucis m.

B' O. flexor hallucis brevis m.

A' O. flexor digiti minimi m. and tuberosity

Z Groove for peroneus longus tendon and ant. attachment of long plantar lig.

Y CUBOID

X Trans. tarsal joint (calcaneocuboid and talonavicular)

W Attachments of short plantar ligament

V Attachment of long plantar ligament

U O. quadratus plantae m.

T O. abduc. digiti minimi m.

S CALCANEUS

Tuberosity A

I. flexor hallucis longus m. and sesamoid bone B

PHALANGES - proximal and distal C

I. abduc. hallucis and flexor hallucis brevis ms. D

I. adduc. hallucis and flexor hallucis brevis ms. E

Sesamoid bones F

METATARSALS G

Tuberosity and I. of peroneus longus m. H

I. tibialis ant. m. I

CUNEIFORMS - lateral, intermediate, and medial J

NAVICULAR K

I. tibialis post. m. L

Attachment of calcaneo-navicular (spring) lig. M

TALUS N

Sustentaculum talus O

Groove whereby structures in leg can enter plantar surface of foot P

O. flexor digitorum brevis m. and abduc. hallucis m. Q

Attachment of plantar aponeurosis on tuberosity of calcaneus R

Fig. AI-29. Bones of the right foot (plantar surface) with origins and insertions of muscles outlined. (Crosses indicate location of epiphyseal lines.)

APPENDIX II

Common Abbreviations used in Orthopaedic Surgery and Rehabilitation

MICHAEL J. BOTTE   MATTHEW BERCHUCK
REID ABRAMS   MARY ANN E. KEENAN

The following list contains some of the common abbreviations used in orthopaedic and rehabilitation textbooks, scientific manuscripts, medical records, and verbal communication. These are listed in this appendix because of their frequent use and concomitant cause of confusion. These are not necessarily "official" abbreviations, but rather have been compiled from observations made by the authors and as noted by their frequent verbal and written use. The authors neither recommend nor discourage the use of these abbreviations, and the list is not meant to be all-inclusive. The list has been provided to clarify abbreviations that are commonly used but not always explained or understood.

aa.	artery
AAHKS	Association for Arthritic Hip and Knee Surgery
AAOS	American Academy of Orthopaedic Surgeons
ABD	abduction
AbDM	abductor digiti minimi
ABJS	Association of Bone and Joint Surgeons
AbPB	abductor pollicis brevis
AbPl	abductor pollicis longus
AC	acromioclavicular (e.g., AC joint)
ACL	anterior cruciate ligament
ACORE	Advisory Council for Orthopaedic Resident Education
ACPOC	Association of Children's Prosthetic and Orthotic Clinics
ADD	adduction
ADL	activities of daily living
AdP	adductor pollicis
ADQ	adductor digiti quinti
AE	above elbow (e.g., AE amputation)
AEA	above-elbow amputation
AFO	ankle-foot orthosis
AG	antigravity
AGF	angle of greatest flexion
AK	above knee (e.g., AK amputation)
AKA	above-knee amputation; also known as
ALL	anterior longitudinal ligament
ALS	amyotrophic lateral sclerosis; anterolateral sclerosis
Anes.	anesthesia
ANS	autonomic nervous system
ant.	anterior
AO	Arbeitsgemeinschaft fuer Osteosynthesfragen (Swiss-based group involved in research and development of methods of internal fixation of fractures)
AOA	American Orthopaedic Association
AOFAS	American Orthopaedic Foot and Ankle Society
AOS	Academic Orthopaedic Society
AP	anteroposterior (e.g., AP roentgenogram); adductor pollicis
APB	abductor pollicis brevis
APL	abductor pollicis longus
AROM	active range of motion
ASAP	as soon as possible
ASES	American Shoulder and Elbow Surgeons
ASIA	American Spinal Injury Association
ASIF	Association for the Study of Internal Fixation (American-based group involved in research and development of methods of internal fixation of fractures)
ASIS	anterior superior iliac spine
ASSH	American Society for Surgery of the Hand
AV	arteriovenous
AVF	arteriovenous fistula
AVM	arteriovenous malformation
BE	below elbow (e.g., BE amputation)
BEA	below-elbow amputation
bilat.	bilateral

BK	below knee (e.g., BK amputation)
BKA	below-knee amputation
BME	brief maximal effort
BP	blood pressure
Bx	biopsy
C1 to C7	cervical vertebrae 1 to 7
CB	contrast bath
CBC	complete blood count
CC	chief complaint
CDH	congenital dislocation of the hip; congenital dysplasia of the hip
CMC	carpometacarpal (e.g., CMC joint)
CMT	Charcot-Marie-Tooth disease
CNS	central nervous system
c/o	complaint of
CO	cervical orthosis
collat.	collateral
COMSS	Council of Musculoskeletal Specialty Societies
CORR	*Clinical Orthopaedics and Related Research*
CP	cerebral palsy
CPM	continuous passive motion
CR	closed reduction; capillary refill
CREST	*c*alcinosis cutis, *R*aynaud's phenomenon, *e*sophogeal dysmotility, *s*clerodactyly, *te*langiectasia
CRIF	closed reduction, internal fixation (of fracture)
CSF	cerebrospinal fluid
C-spine	cervical spine
CSRS	Cervical Spine Research Society
CT	computed tomography; carpal tunnel
CTLO	cervicothorocolumbar orthosis
CTLS	cervicothoracolumbosacral (e.g., CTLS orthosis)
CTO	cervicothoracic orthosis
CTR	carpal tunnel release
CTS	carpal tunnel syndrome
CV	cerebrovascular
CVA	cerebrovascular accident
cva	costovertebral angle
CVP	central venous pressure
CXR	chest x-ray
DBS	Denis Browne splint
DCP	dynamic compression plate
decub.	decubitus position
DHS	dynamic hip screw
DI	dorsal interosseous
DIP	distal interphalangeal (e.g., DIP joint)
DIPJ	distal interphalangeal joint
DISH	diffuse idiopathic skeletal hyperostosis

DISI	dorsiflexion intercalary segmental instability
Disl.	dislocation
DJD	degenerative joint disease
DKB	deep knee bends
DOA	date of admission; dead on arrival
DOE	date of examination
DP	distal phalanx; dorsalis pedis (artery)
DPC	distal palmar crease; delayed primary closure (of wound)
DTRs	deep tendon reflexes
DVT	deep vein thrombosis
Dx	diagnosis
ECG	electrocardiogram (graph)
ECRB	extensor carpi radialis brevis
ECRL	extensor carpi radialis longus
ECU	extensor carpi ulnaris
EDB	extensor digitorum brevis
EDC	extensor digitorum comminis
EDL	extensor digitorum longus
EDM	extensor digiti minimi
EDQ	extensor digiti quinti
EEG	electroencephalogram (graph)
EHB	extensor hallucis brevis
EHL	extensor hallucis longus
EIP	extensor indicis proprius
EKG	electrocardiogram
EMG	electromyography, electromyogram
EOM	extraocular movement
EPB	extensor pollicis brevis
EPL	extensor pollicis longus
ERE	external rotation in extension
ERF	external rotation in flexion
ESR	erythrocyte sedimentation rate
EUA	exam under anesthesia
EWHO	elbow-wrist-hand orthosis
Ex Fix	external fixator
FA	false aneurysm
FABER	flexion in abduction and external rotation
FADIR	flexion in adduction and internal rotation
FB	foreign body
FCR	flexor carpi radialis
FCU	flexor carpi ulnaris
FDB	flexor digitorum brevis
FDL	flexor digitorum longus
FDP	flexor digitorum profundus
FDS	flexor digitorum superficialis
FES	function electrical stimulation
FFC	fixed flexion contracture
FFP	fresh frozen plasma
FH	family history

FHB	flexor hallucis brevis
FHL	flexor hallucis longus
FOB	foot of bed (e.g., elevate FOB)
FOSA	Federation of Spine Associations
FPB	flexor pollicis brevis
FPL	flexor pollicis longus
Fract.	fracture
FROM	full range of motion
FTSG	full-thickness skin graft
FUO	fever of unknown (or undetermined) origin
FWB	full weight bearing
Fx	fracture
GAD	gadolinium
GI	gastrointestinal
gr. troch.	greater trochanter
GU	genitourinary
Hb	hemoglobin
Hc	hematocrit
Hct	hematocrit
HCTU	home cervical traction unit
HD	heloma durum (hard corn)
HEENT	head, eyes, ears, nose, throat
Hgb	hemoglobin
H&H	hematocrit and hemoglobin
HKAFO	hip-knee-ankle-foot orthosis
HM	heloma molle (soft corn)
HNP	herniated nucleus pulposus
HO	heterotopic ossification
HOB	head of bed (e.g., elevate HOB)
HP	hot pack
H&P	history and physical
HT	hand therapy; hammer toe; Hubbard tank
HTO	high tibial osteotomy
HV	hallux valgus
Hx	history
IAA	International Arthroscopy Association
ICS	intercostal space
ICT	intermittent cervical traction
I&D	incision and drainage; irrigation and débridement
IDK	internal derangement of the knee
IHW	inner heel wedge
IM	intramedullary (e.g., IM rod)
inf.	inferior
INFH	ischemic necrosis of the femoral head
IP	interphalangeal (e.g., IP joint)
IPJ	interphalangeal joint
IRE	internal rotation in extension
IRF	internal rotation in flexion
IS	interspace

ISK	International Society of the Knee
ITB	iliotibial band
ITT	internal tibial torsion
IV	intravenus
JBJS	*Journal of Bone and Joint Surgery*
JHS	*Journal of Hand Surgery*
JOR	*Journal of Orthopaedic Research*
JPO	*Journal of Pediatric Orthopaedics*
KAFO	knee-ankle-foot orthosis
KS	Knee Society
KSHR	Kiros Society for Hand Research
L1 to L5	lumbar vertebrae 1 to 5
LAC	long arm cast
lam.	laminectomy
LAS	long arm splint
lat.	lateral
LATS	long arm thumb spica
LCL	lateral collateral ligament
LCP	Legg-Calvé-Perthes disease
LE	lower extremity; lupus erythematosus
lig.	ligament
LLC	long leg cast
LLD	leg length discrepancy
LLE	left lower extremity
LLL	left lower limb
LLQ	left lower quadrant
LLWC	long leg walking cast
LOM	limitation of motion
LP	lumbar puncture
LROM	limited range of motion
LS	lumbosacral
L/S	lumbosacral
LSO	lumbosacral orthosis
L-spine	lumbar spine
LUE	left upper extremity
LUL	left upper limb
LUQ	left upper quadrant
MAL	midaxillary line
MCL	medial collateral ligament; midclavicular line
MCP	metacarpophalangeal (e.g., MCP joint)
MCPJ	metacarpophalangeal joint
MD	muscle disease; muscular dystrophy
med.	medial
MHW	medial heel wedge
MI	myocardial infarction
mm.	millimeter; muscle; mucous membrane
MM	mucous membrane
MMT	manual muscle testing

MPV	metatarsus primus varus
MRI	magnetic resonance imaging
MS	multiple sclerosis
MSL	midsternal line
MTA	metatarsus adductus
MT bar	metatarsal bar
MTJ	midtarsal joint
MTP	metatarsophalangeal (e.g., MTP joint)
MTPJ	metatarsophalangeal joint
MTV	metatarsus varus
n.	nerve
NASS	North American Spine Society
NCN	National Council of Nurses
NCV	nerve conduction velocity
NHP	nursing home placement
NP	nucleus pulposis
NV	neurovascular
N/V	neurovascular
NWB	non–weight bearing
OCD	osteochondritis dissecans
OD	osteochondritis dissecans; oculus dexter (right eye)
ODM	opponens digiti minimi
OOB	out of bed
OOP	out of plaster
OP	opponens pollicis
OPD	outpatient department
OPLL	ossification of the posterior longitudinal liagment
OR	operating room
ORA	Orthopaedic Rehabilitation Association
ORIF	open reduction, internal fixation (of fractures)
ORS	Orthopaedic Research Society
OS	oculus sinister (left eye)
OT	occupational therapy
OTA	Orthopaedic Trauma Association
OU	both eyes
OW	opening wedge (osteotomy)
PA	posteroanterior (e.g., PA roentgenogram)
PAL	posterior axillary line
PB	peroneus brevis; paraffin bath
PCE	physical capacities evaluation
PCL	posterior cruciate ligament
PE	pulmonary embolism; physical examination
pect.	pectoralis
PEMF	pulsating electromagnetic fields
PERRLA	pupils equal, round, reactive to light, accommodation
PFC	pelvic flexion contraction

PFFD	proximal femoral focal deficiency
phal.	phalanx, phalanges
PI	palmar interossei; primary investigator
PIP	proximal interphalangeal (e.g., PIP joint)
PIPJ	proximal interphalangeal joint
PL	palmaris longus
PLL	posterior longitudinal ligament
Plt	platelet
PMD	progressive muscular dystrophy
PNF	proprioceptive neuromuscular facilitation
PNS	peripheral nervous system
PO	postoperatively
POSNA	Pediatric Orthopaedic Society of North America
post.	posterior
PQ	pronator quadratus
PR	pelvic rock
preop	preoperatively
PREs	progressive resistive exercises
PROM	passive range of motion
PT	physical therapy; pronator teres; prothrombin time
PTB	patellar tendon–bearing (cast)
PTT	patellar tendon transfer; partial thromboplastin time
PVA	Paralyzed Veteran's of America
PVD	peripheral vascular disease
PVS	pigmented villonodular synovitis
PW	plantar wart
PWB	partial weight bearing
px	pneumothorax
quad	quadriceps; quadrilateral; quadriplegic
RA	rheumatoid arthritis
RBC	red blood cell count
rbc	red blood cell count
RJOS	Ruth Jackson Orthopaedic Society
RLE	right lower extremity
RLL	right lower limb
ROM	range of motion
RR	recovery room
RUE	right upper extremity
RUL	right upper limb
RUQ	right upper quadrant
S1 to S5	sacral vertebrae 1 to 5
SAC	short arm cast
SAS	short arm splint
SC	sternoclavicular (e.g., SC joint)
SCFE	slipped capital femoral epiphysis
SCI	spinal cord injury
SDD	sterile dry dressing

SI	sacroiliac (e.g., SI joint)
SICOT	International Society of Orthopaedic Surgery and Traumatology
SLC	short leg cast
SLE	systemic lupus erythematosus
SLR	straight leg raising
SLS	short leg splint
SPLATT	split anterior tibial tendon transfer
SQ	subcutaneous
SRS	Scoliosis Research Society
staph	*Staphylococcus*
STJ	subtalar joint
S-T-P	superficialis-to-profundus (tendon transfer)
strep	*Streptococcus*
STS	soft tissue swelling
STSG	split-thickness skin graft
sup.	superior
sx	symptoms
sympt	symptoms
T1 to T12	thoracic vertebrae 1 to 12
TA	tibialis anterior
TAL	tendo-Achilles lengthening
TAM	total active motion
TB	tuberculosis
TBC	tuberculosis
TBI	traumatic brain injury
T&C	type and crossmatch
TDWB	touchdown (or toe down) weight bearing
TENS	transcutaneous electrical nerve stimulation
TEV	talipes equinovarus
TFR	toe flexor release
TG	tendon graft
THA	total hip arthroplasty
THR	total hip replacement
TIA	transient ischemic attack
TJA	total joint arthroplasty
TJR	total joint replacement
TKA	total knee arthroplasty
TKR	total knee replacement
T-L	thoracolumbar
TLS	thoracolumbosacral (e.g., TLS orthosis)
TLSO	thoracolumbosacral orthosis
TMT	tarsometatarsal
tomo	tomogram
TPM	total passive motion
troch	trochanter
TS	thumb spica (cast)
T-spine	thoracic spine
T&S	type and screen

TT	tendon transfer; tilt table; tourniquet time
TTT	total tourniquet time
tx	traction
UE	upper extremity
UN	ulnar nerve
URI	upper respiratory tract infection
US	ultrasound
UTI	urinary tract infection
VATER	*v*ertebral anomalies, *a*nal atresia, *t*racheo-*e*sophageal fistula, *r*adial and *r*enal anomalies
VDDR	vitamin D–dependent rickets
VDRO	varus derotation osteotomy
VDRR	vitamin D–resistant rickets
VISI	volar flexion intercalary segmental instability
VS	vital signs
VSS	vital signs stable
WBAT	weight bearing as tolerated
WBC	white blood cell count
WC	wheel chair
WEST	work evaluation systems technology
WFE	Williams flexion exercises
WHO	wrist-hand orthosis
WNL	within normal limits
WPB	whirlpool bath
X Fix	external fixator
XIP	x-ray in plaster
XOP	x-ray out of plaster

SUGGESTED READINGS

Blauvelt CT, Nelson R: A Manual of Orthopaedic Terminology. 4th Ed. CV Mosby Co, St. Louis, 1990

Friel JP: Dorland's Illustrated Medical Dictionary. 25th Ed. WB Saunders, Philadelphia, 1974

Hoppenfeld S: Physical Examination of the Spine and Extremities. Appleton-Century-Crofts, Norwalk, CT, 1976

Lovell WW, Winter RB: Pediatric Orthopaedics. 2nd Ed. JB Lippincott, Philadelphia, 1986

Mallon WJ, McNamara MJ, Urbaniak JR: Orthopaedics for the House Officer. Williams & Wilkins, Baltimore, 1990

Rockwood CA Jr, Green DP: Fractures in Adults. Vol. 1–2. JB Lippincott, Philadelphia, 1984

Rockwood CA Jr, Green DP: Fractures in Children. Vol. 3. JB Lippincott, Philadelphia, 1984

Wilson JD, Braunwald E, Isselbacher KJ et al: Harrison's Principles of Internal Medicine. 12th Ed. McGraw-Hill, Inc, New York, 1991

APPENDIX III

Definitions of Common Anatomic Terms Used in Orthopaedic Surgery and Rehabilitation

MICHAEL J. BOTTE
REID ABRAMS
MARY ANN E. KEENAN

Allogenous: material (usually refers to tissue, such as a graft) taken from another host of the same species

Allograft: graft taken from different host of same species

Antebrachium: forearm

Anulus: ring-shaped opening

Aponeurosis: flattened, expanded tendon or end of a tendon that attaches to a muscle (usually a flat muscle)

Apophysis: portion of bone that contributes to growth, but is the point of strong tendinous insertion rather than a part of the joint

Articulation: connection between bones; a joint

Autogenous: material (usually refers to tissue, such as a graft) taken from the same host

Autograft: graft taken from same host

Autonomic nervous system: provides innervation of smooth muscle, heart muscle, and glands; consists of craniosacral (parasympathetic) and thoracolumbar (sympathetic) portions

Belly: midportion or fleshy part of a muscle

Body: broadest or longest mass of a bone

Central nervous system: the brain and spinal cord

Condyle: the expanded, rounded portion of bone, usually at the end of a long bone, that encompasses or is next to the articular portion of a bone

Crest: ridge or border of a bone

Cribriform: resembling a sieve

Deltoid: shaped like the Greek letter delta

Diaphysis: the shaft of a long bone

Diarthrosis: movable joint

Eminence: low convexity of a bone, sometimes barely perceptible

Endosteum: condensed layer of fibrous tissue containing osteogenic cells, lining the medullary canal of a long bone

Epiphyseal plate (line): growth center for elongation of bone, located between epiphysis and metaphysis

Facet: small articular area

Falciform: sickle shaped

Foramen: hole, perforation

Fornix: vaultlike space

Fossa: shallow depression

Fundus: base

Genu: knee

Glenoid: resembling a shallow cavity

Insertion: relatively movable part of a muscle attachment

Isthmus: narrow portion of the canal in the shaft of a long bone

Lamella: small plate or thin layer

Lamina: plate or layer

Linea: line

Macula: spot

Mastoid: shaped like a breast

Metaphysis: portion of a long bone between the diaphysis (shaft) and epiphysis

Origin: relatively fixed part of a muscle attachment

Process: projection

Protuberance: swelling (usually smaller than process)

Ramus: platelike branch of a bone

Raphe: a seam; the union of two parts in a line

Sesamoid: a small round bone found within a tendon or a muscle; functions to increase movement in a joint by improving the angle of approach of tendon into its insertion

Sheath: protective covering

Spine: pointed projection of bone

Suture: interlocking of jagged edges

Teres: round

Thenar: relating to the palm or plantar aspect of foot

Trochlea: spool shaped

Tubercle: small bump

Tuberosity: large projection or bump on bone

Uncinate: hooked; process shaped like a hook

SUGGESTED READINGS

Blauvelt CT, Nelson R: A Manual of Orthopaedic Terminology. 4th Ed. CV Mosby Co, St. Louis, 1990

Friel JP: Dorland's Illustrated Medical Dictionary. 25 th Ed. WB Saunders, Philadelphia, 1974

Hoppenfeld S: Physical Examination of the Spine and Extremities. Appleton-Century-Crofts, Norwalk, CT, 1976

Mallon WJ, McNamara MJ, Urbaniak JR: Orthopaedics for the House Officer. Williams & Wilkins, B altimore, 1990

Pansky B: Review of Gross Anatomy. 5th Ed. Macmillan Publishing Co, New York, 1984

Williams PL, Warwick R., Dyson M, Bannister LH: Gray's Anatomy. 27th British Ed. Churchill Livingstone, Edinburgh, 1989

APPENDIX IV   Common Terms of Position, Direction, and Movement

REID ABRAMS
MARY ANN E. KEENAN

Abduction: drawing away from the midline

Adduction: drawing toward the midline

Anatomic position: standing erect, arms at the sides, palms of the hands turned forward

Anterior: in front of

Anteversion: in reference to the neck of the humerus or femur, relates to an anterior rotation

Apposition: contact of two adjacent parts

Caudad: refers to an orientation toward the feet from a specific reference point

Cephalad: refers to an orientation toward the head from a specific reference point

Circumduction: movement of a ball-and-socket joint in a circular motion

Coronal: longitudinal plane passing through the body from side to side (i.e., from left to the right, or vice versa)

Distal: farther from the root, midline, or cranium

Dorsal: toward the rear, back; also back of the hand, top of the foot

Dorsiflexion: refers to pulling the wrist, foot, or toes up (toward the dorsal surface) evert: to turn outward

External rotation: in the frontal plane, rotation away from the midline

Frontal: (see coronal)

Inferior: lower, farther from crown of head

Internal rotation: in the frontal plane, rotation toward the midline

Inversion: to turn inward

Lateral: farther from midline (or center plane)

Longitudinal: refers to long axis

Medial: nearer to midline (or center plane)

Median: midway, in the middle

Midline: a line between two equal halves of the body, dividing the body into a right and left side

Midsagittal: vertical plane at midline dividing body in right and left halves

Oblique: slanting, diagonal

Opposition: applied mostly to the thumb but also to the little finger; denotes the motion required to bring the thumb against the little finger (pulp surfaces). For the thumb, opposition is the combined action of abduction, pronation, rotation, and flexion

Palmar: palm side of hand

Plantar: bottom or sole side of foot

Plantar flexion: refers to pulling the toes or foot downward (toward the plantar surface)

Posterior: rear or back

Pronation: rotational movement of the forearm or ankle to place the palm downward or the plantar surface of the foot outward

Prone: body lying face down

Proximal: near to the limb root, or near to the midline or cranium

Radial deviation: angulation of the wrist toward the radius (or lateral deviation)

Retroversion: in reference to the neck of the humerus or femur, relates to posterior rotation

Sagittal: vertical plane or section dividing body into right and left portions

Superficial: nearer to surface

Superior: upper, nearer to crown of head

Supination: rotational movement of the forearm or ankle to place the palm upward or plantar surface of the foot inward

Supine: body lying face up

Transverse: at right angles to long axis, plane or section dividing body into upper and lower parts

Ulnar deviation: angulation of the wrist toward the ulna (or medial deviation)

Valgus: refers to distal part that is angled away from or laterally from midline

Varus: refers to distal part that is angled medially relative to the proximal part

Ventral: situated before or in front of

Vertical: refers to long axis in erect position

Volar: palm side of hand (palmar is now usually preferred term)

SUGGESTED READINGS

Blauvelt CT, Nelson R: A Manual of Orthopaedic Terminology. 4th Ed. CV Mosby Co, St. Louis, 1990

Friel JP: Dorland's Illustrated Medical Dictionary. 25th Ed. WB Saunders, Philadelphia, 1974

Hoppenfeld S: Physical Examination of the Spine and Extremities. Appleton-Century-Crofts, Norwalk, CT, 1976

Mallon WJ, McNamara MJ, Urbaniak JR: Orthopaedics for the House Officer. Williams & Wilkins, Baltimore, 1990

Pansky B: Review of Gross Anatomy. 5th Ed. Macmillan Publishing Co, New York, 1984

Williams PL, Warwick R., Dyson M, Bannister LH: Gray's Anatomy. 27th British Ed. Churchill Livingstone, Edinburgh, 1989

APPENDIX V

Muscles of the Limbs: Origin, Insertion, Action, Innervation

MICHAEL J. BOTTE
REID ABRAMS

MATTHEW BERCHUCK
MARY ANN E. KEENAN

Table AV-1. Muscles of the Shoulder Girdle

Muscle	Origin	Insertion	Action	Innervation (Nerve Roots)
Trapezius	External occipital protuberance, sup. nuchal line of occipital bone, ligamentum nuchae, spinous proc. C7 and T1–T12 vertebrae, supraspinous lig.	Post. border of lat. clavicle, med. margin of acromion, post. border of scapular spine	Rotation of scapula to raise point of shoulder; adduction of scapula; tilting of chin	Spinal accessory n. (cranial I) (C3, 4)
Latissimus dorsi	Spine of lower 6 thoracic vertebrae, lumbar aponeurosis, supraspinous lig., post. iliac crest, lower four ribs	Intertuburcular groove of humerus	Adduction, extension, internal rotation of arm	Thoracodorsal n. (C6–8)
Levator scapulae	Post. tubercles, transverse process C1–C4	Medial border of scapula sup. to spine	Elevation, rotation of scapula	Dorsal scapular n. (C5)
Rhomboid minor	Lig. nuchae, spines C7–T1	Medial border of scapula at level of scapular spine	Adduction, elevation rotation of scapula; stabilization of scapula against thorax	Dorsal scapular n. (C5)
Rhomboid major	Spines T2–T5, supraspinous lig.	Medial border of scapula inf. to spine	Adduction, elevation of scapula	Dorsal scapular n. (C5)
Platysma	Fascia over pect. mj. and deltoid	Mandible, skin of lower face	Elevation of skin from clavicle; drawing of lower lip down and back; assistance of jaw opening	Facial n. (cranial VII)
Pectoralis major	Med. clavicle, lat. sternum to 7th costal cartilage, costal carts. 2–6; aponeurosis of ext. abd. oblique.	Crest of gr. tubercle of humerus	Forward flexion, adduction, medial rotation of arm	Medial (C8, T1) and lat. (C5–7) pectoral nerves
Pectoralis minor	Ribs 3–5	Coracoid process of scapula	Depression and forward displacement of scapula	Medial pectoral n. (C8, T1)
Subclavius	Upper border and costal cart. of 1st rib	Inf. surface of clavicle	Depression and ant. displacement of clavicle	N. to subclavius (C5, 6)
Serratus anterior	Outer surface of ribs 1–9	Costal surface of vertebral border of scapula	Abduction of scapula	Long thoracic n. (C5–7)
Deltoid	Lat. 1/3 of clavicle, acromion, spine of scapula	Deltoid tuberosity of humerus	Abduction, forward flexion or extension of humerus	Axillary n. (C5, 6)

(Continued)

875

Table AV-1. Muscles of the Shoulder Girdle *(continued)*

Muscle	Origin	Insertion	Action	Innervation (Nerve Roots)
Subscapularis	Costal surface of scapula (subscapular fossa)	Lesser tuberosity of humerus	Internal rotation, adduction of humerus	Upper and lower subscapular nerves (C5, 6)
Supraspinatus	Supraspinatus fossa of scapula	Sup. aspect of gr. tuberosity of humerus	Abduction of humerus; stabilizes humeral head in glenoid fossa to assist deltoid in shoulder abduction	Suprascapular n. (C5, 6)
Infraspinatus	Infraspinatus fossa of scapula	Gr. tuberosity of humerus (inferior to supraspinatus insertion)	External rotation of humerus	Suprascapular n. (C5, 6)
Teres major	Dorsal surface of inf. angle of scapula	Medial lip of bicipital groove of humerus	Internal rotation, adduction of humerus	Lower subscapular n. (C5, 6)
Teres minor	Dorsal surface of lat. border of scapula	Gr. tuberosity of humerus (inf. to infraspinatus insertion)	Adduction, external rotation of humerus	Axillary n. (C5, 6)

Table AV-2. Muscles of the Arm

Muscle	Origin	Insertion	Action	Innervation
Coracobrachialis	Coracoid process of scapula	Medial humeral diaphysis	Forward flexion, adduction of humerus	Musculocutaneous n. (C5, 6)
Biceps brachii	Short head from coracoid process, long head from supraglenoid tuberosity	Radial tuberosity, lacertus fibrosus	Flexion, supination of forearm	Musculocutaneous n. (C5, 6)
Brachialis	Distal 2/3 of humerus	Coronoid process of ulna	Flexion of forearm	Musculocutaneous (and occasionally radial) n. (C5–7)
Triceps brachii	Long head from infraglenoid tuberosity of scapula, lat. head from posterolateral humerus, medial head from distal post. humerus	Olecranon, deep fascia of forearm	Extension of forearm, adduction of arm (long head)	Radial n. (C6, 7)

Table AV-3. Muscles of the Forearm

Muscle	Origin	Insertion	Action	Innervation
Anconeus	Lat. epicondyle of humerus, post. capsule of elbow	Lat. side of olecranon and post. surface of ulna	Extension of forearm	Radial n. (C7, 8)
Brachioradialis	Lat. supracondylar ridge of humerus, lat. intermuscular septum	Lat., distal radius, styloid process	Flexion of forearm; assistance of pronation of forearm (when forearm is supinated); assistance of forearm supination (when forearm is pronated)	Radial n. (C5, 6)
Pronator teres	Humeral head from medial epicondylar ridge of humerus, ulnar head from medial side of coronoid process of ulna	Lat. radial diaphysis	Pronation of forearm; assistance of forearm flexion	Median n. (C6, 7)
Flexor carpi radialis	Medial epicondyle of humerus (common flexor origin)	Base of index and long metacarpals	Flexion, radial deviation of wrist; assistance of flexion and pronation of forearm	Median n. (C6, 7)
Palmaris longus	Medial epicondyle of humerus (common flexor origin)	Palmar fascia	Flexion of wrist; assistance of flexion, pronation of forearm	Median n. (C6, 7)
Flexor carpi ulnaris	Humeral head: medial epicondyle of humerus (common flexor origin); ulnar head: proximal ulna	Pisiform, hamate, and base of 5th metacarpal	Flexion, ulnar deviation of wrist; assistance of flexion of forearm	Ulnar n. (C8, T1)
Flexor digitorum superficialis	Humeral head: medial epicondyle of humerus (common flexor origin); ulnar head: coronoid process of ulna; radial head: oblique line of radial diaphysis	Palmar middle phalanges of digits	Flexion of proximal interphalangeal joints; assistance of flexion of metacarpophalangeal joints, forearm, and wrist	Median n. (C7, C8)
Flexor digitorum profundus	Medial ant. surface of ulna, interosseous membrane, deep fascia of forearm	Palmar distal phalanges	Flexion of distal interphalangeal joints; assistance of flexion of proximal interphalangeal joints, metacarpophalangeal joints, and wrist	Median n. to radial 2 digits, ulnar n. to ulnar 2 digits (C7, C8)
Flexor pollicis longus	Palmar surface of radius, interosseus membrane, medial border of coronoid process	Base, palmar distal phalanx of thumb	Flexion of thumb interphalangeal joint	Median n. (C8, T1)
Pronator quadratus	Distal palmar ulna	Distal palmar radius	Pronation of forearm	Median n. (C8, T1)
Extensor carpi radialis longus	Lat. supracondylar ridge of humerus, lat. intermuscular septum	Dorsal base of index metacarpal	Extension, radial deviation of wrist	Radial n. (C6, 7)
Extensor carpi radialis brevis	Common extensor origin from lat. epicondyle of humerus, radial collateral ligament of elbow joint, intermuscular septum	Dorsal base of long finger metacarpal	Extension, radial deivation of wrist	Post. interosseous of radial (C6, 7)

(Continued)

Table AV-3. Muscles of the Forearm *(continued)*

Muscle	Origin	Insertion	Action	Innervation
Extensor digitorum communis	Common extensor origin from lat. epicondyle of humerus, intermuscular septum	Dorsal bases of middle and distal phalanges	Extension of digits, assistance of wrist extension	Post. interosseous n. (C6, 7)
Extensor digiti minimi	Common extensor origin from lat. epicondyle of humerus, intermuscular septum	Dorsal base of distal phalanx of little finger	Extension of little finger	Posterior interosseous n. (C7, 8)
Extensor carpi ulnaris	Common extensor origin from lat. epicondyle of humerus, post. border of ulna	Dorsomedial base of little finger metacarpal	Extension, ulnar deviation of wrist	Post. interosseous n. (C6, 7)
Supinator	Lat. epicondyle of humerus, lat. capsule of elbow, supinator crest and fossa of ulna	Radiopalmar surface of proximal radius	Supination of forearm	Radial n. (C6, 7)
Abductor pollicis longus	Dorsal surface of mid-diaphysis of radius and ulna, interosseous membrane	Radial base of thumb metacarpal	Abduction of thumb; assistance of wrist abduction	Post. interosseous n. (C6, 7)
Extensor pollicis brevis	Dorsal surface of radial diaphysis, interosseous membrane	Base of proximal phalanx or thumb	Extension of proximal phalanx (and metacarpal) of thumb	Post. interosseous n. (C6, 7)
Extensor pollicis longus	Dorsal surface of ulnar diaphysis, interosseous membrane	Dorsal base, distal phalanx of thumb	Extension of distal phalanx of thumb; assistance of extension of proximal phalanx and metacarpal of thumb	Post. interosseous n. (C6, 7)
Extensor indicis proprius	Dorsal distal ulnar diaphysis, interosseous membrane	Dorsal proximal phalanx of index finger	Extension of proximal phalanx of index finger	Post. interosseous n. (C6, 7)

Table AV-4. Intrinsic Muscles of the Hand

Muscle	Origin	Insertion	Action	Innervation
Abductor pollicis brevis	Transverse carpal lig., scaphoid tubercle, palmar trapezium	Radial base proximal phalanx of thumb	Palmar abduction of proximal phalanx of thumb	Recurrent br. of median n. (C8, T1)
Opponens pollicis	Transverse carpal lig., palmar trapezium	Radiopalmar surface of thumb metacarpal	Opposition of thumb to digits (palmar abduction, pronation of thumb)	Recurrent br. of median n. (C8, T1)
Flexor pollicis brevis	Transverse carpal lig., palmar trapezium	Base of proximal phalanx of thumb	Flexion of proximal phalanx of thumb	Recurrent br. of median n. (C8, T1), occasionally deep br. of ulnar n. to deep head

(Continued)

Table AV-4. Intrinsic Muscles of the Hand *(continued)*

Muscle	Origin	Insertion	Action	Innervation
Adductor pollicis	Oblique head from palmar trapezium, trapezoid, and capitate; transverse head from palmar surface of long finger metacarpal	Ulnar side of base of proximal phalanx of thumb	Adduction of thumb; assistance of opposition	Deep br. of ulnar n. (C8, T1)
Palmaris brevis	Ulnar side of transverse carpal lig., palmar aponeurosis	Skin on ulnar border of palm	Corrugation of skin on ulnar palm (deepening of palm)	Superficial br. of ulnar n. (C8, T1)
Abductor digiti minimi	Pisiform, tendon of flexor carpi ulnaris	Ulnar aspect of proximal phalanx of little finger, aponeurosis of extensor digiti minimi	Abduction of little finger from palm	Deep br. of ulnar n. (C8, T1)
Flexor digiti minimi	Transverse carpal lig., hook of hamate	Ulnar side, base of proximal phalanx of little finger	Flexion of proximal phalanx of little finger	Deep br. of ulnar n. (C8, T1)
Opponens digiti minimi	Transverse carpal lig., hook of hamate	Ulnar side of metacarpal of little finger	Opposition of little finger to thumb; flexion of metacarpal of little finger anteriorly out of palm	Deep br. of ulnar n. (C8, T1)
Lumbricales	Four lumbricales arise from tendons of flexor digitorum profundus	Join with interossei to form lateral bands that become dorsal hood with the extensor digitorum communis tendons; ultimate insertions include base of the middle phalanx (central slip) and base of distal phalanx	Extension of the proximal interphalageal joints, flexion of metacarpophalangeal joints	Median n. to radial 2 lumbricales, ulnar n. to ulnar 2 lumbricales (C8, T1)
Dorsal interossei	Four dorsal interossei each from sides of adjacent two metacarpals	1st into radial side of proximal phalanx of index finger, 2nd into radial side of proximal phalanx of long finger, 3rd into ulnar side of proximal phalanx of long finger, 4th into ulnar side of proximal phalanx of ring finger; all interossei also with variable contributions to lat. bands to form part of the dorsal hood	Abduction of index, long, ring fingers from midline of hand; flexion of proximal phalanges; extension of middle phalanges	Deep br. of ulnar n. (C8, T1)
Palmar interossei	Three palmar interossei: 1st from ulnar side of index metacarpal, 2nd from radial side of ring metacarpal, 3rd from radial side of little finger metacarpal	1st into ulnar side of proximal phalanx of index, 2nd into radial side of proximal phalanx of ring finger, 3rd into radial side or proximal phalanx of little finger	Adduction of digits	Deep br. of ulnar n. (C8, T1)

Table AV-5. Muscles of the Hip, Thigh, and Iliac Region

Muscle	Origin	Insertion	Action	Innervation
Psoas major	Ant. surface of transverse processes and bodies of lumbar vertebrae, corresponding disks	Lesser trochanter of femur	Flexion of hip; flexion of vertebral column on pelvis when femur is fixed	Second, third lumbar n. (L3, 4)
Psoas minor	Vertebral margins of 12th thoracic and 1st lumbar vertebrae, corresponding disks	Pectineal line, iliopectineal eminence of pelvis	Flexion of vertebral column	First or second lumbar n. (L1, 2)
Iliacus	Sup. 2/3 of iliac fossa, iliac crest, ant. sacroiliac, lumbosacral, iliolumbar lig., ala of sacrum	Tendon of psoas major, lesser trochanter, capsule of hip joint	Flexion of hip; flexion of pelvis on hip when femur is fixed	Femoral n. (L2, 3)
Sartorius	Ant. sup. iliac spine	Proximal medial tibia (joins with insertions of gracilis and semitendinosus to form "pes anserinus")	Flexion of hip, flexion of knee, external rotation of tibia	Femoral n. (L2, 3)
Rectus femoris	Straight head from ant. inf. iliac spine, reflected head from upper margin of acetabulum	Sup. border of patella (and into tibial tuberosity through patellar ligament)	Extension of knee; flexion of hip	Femoral n. (L3, 4)
Vastus lateralis	Intertrochanteric line, gr. trochanter, gluteal tuberosity, linea aspera, lateral intermuscular septum	Lat. border of patella (and into tibial tuberosity through patellar ligament)	Extension of knee	Femoral n. (L3, 4)
Vastus intermedius	Upper 2/3 of ant. and lat. femur, distal 1/2 of linea aspera, upper part of lat. supracondylar line, lat. intermuscular septum, vastus tubercle	Deep surface of tendon of rectus femoris and vasti muscles (and into tibial tuberosity through patellar ligament	Extension of knee	Femoral n. (L3, 4)
Vastus medialis	Distal 1/2 intertrochlear line, linea aspera, medial supracondylar line, medial intermuscular septum, tendon of adductor magnus	Medial aspect of patella, tendon of rectus femoris (and into tibial tuberosity through patellar ligament)	Extension of knee	Femoral n. (L3, 4)
Pectineus	Pectineal line, pubis between iliopectineal eminence and pubic tubercle	Line extending from lesser trochanter to linea aspera	Adduction, flexion, internal rotation of femur	Femoral n. (L3, 4)
Gracilis	Inf. 1/2 pubic symphysis, sup. 1/2 pubic arch	Proximal medial tibia (joins with insertions of sartorius and semitendinosus to form the "pes anserinus")	Adduction of femur; flexion and internal rotation of tibia	Ant. br. of obturator n. (L2, 3)
Adductor longus	Pubis between crest and symphysis	Central 1/2 of medial lip of linea aspera	Adduction of femur; assistance of flexion of femur	Ant. br. of obturator n. (L2, 3)

(Continued)

Table AV-5. Muscles of the Hip, Thigh, and Iliac Region *(continued)*

Muscle	Origin	Insertion	Action	Innervation
Adductor brevis	Inf. pubic ramus	Proximal femur along line between lesser trochanter to linea aspera	Adduction of femur; assistance of flexion of femur	Ant. br. of obturator n. (L2, 3)
Adductor magnus	Ischial tuberosity, pubic ramus, ischial ramus	Medial femur along line between gr. trochanter to linea aspera, linea aspera, medial supracondylar line, adductor tubercle	Adduction, of flexion, extension of femur	Post. br. of obturator n. (L3–S1)
Gluteus maximus	Post. gluteal line, sacrospinalis tendon, sacrum (dorsal surface), coccyx (dorsal surface), sacrotuberous ligament	Gluteal tuberosity of femur, iliotibial tract	Extension of hip; assistance of adduction and external rotation; extension of truck when femur is fixed	Inf. gluteal n. (L5–S2)
Gluteus medius	Ilium (outer surface from iliac crest and post. gluteal line to ant. gluteal line), gluteal aponeurosis	Gr. trochanter (lat. surface)	Abduction of hip; internal rotation of femur when hip is extended	Sup. gluteal n. (L4–S1)
Gluteus minimus	Ilium (outer surface between ant. and inf. gluteal lines), margin of greater sciatic notch	Gr. trochanter (an. border)	Abduction of hip; internal rotation of femur when hip is extended	Sup. gluteal n. (L4–S1)
Tensor fasciae latae	Ant. portion of outer iliac crest, ant. border of ilium	Iliotibial tract	Flexion, abduction, internal rotation of femur	Sup. gluteal n. (L4–S1)
Piriformis	Pelvic surface of sacrum between ant. sacral foramina, margin of gr. sciatic foramen, sacrotuberous ligament	Gr. trochanter (superior portion)	External rotation of hip; abduction of femur when hip is flexed	1st and 2nd sacral n. (S1, 2)
Obturator internus	Margins of obturator foramen, obturator membrane and fascia	Gr. trochanter (medial surface)	External rotation of hip; abduction of femur when hip is flexed	N. to obturator internus and gemellus sup. (L5–S2)
Gemellus superior	Ischial spine (outer surface)	Gr. trochanter (medial surface)	External rotation of hip	N. to obturator internus and gemellus sup. (L5–S2)
Gemellus inferior	Ischial tuberosity (superior portion)	Gr. trochanter (medial surface)	External rotation of hip	N. to quadratus femoris and gemellus inf. (L4–LS1)
Quadratus femoris	Ischial tuberosity (lateral margin)	Quadrate tubercle of femur, linea quadrata	External rotation, adduction of hip	N. to quadratus femoris and gemellus inf. (L4–S1)
Obturator externus	Outer margin of obturator foramen, outer surface of obturator membrane	Fossa of gr. trochanter	Adduction, external rotation of hip	Posterior br. of obturator n. (L3, 4)
Biceps femoris	Long head: ischial tuberosity and sacrotuberous ligament; short head: lat. lip of linea aspera, lat. supracondylar line of femur, lat. intermuscular septum	Fibular head, lat. condyle of tibia, deep fascia of lat. leg	Flexion of knee; extension of hip; external rotation of tibia when knee is flexed	Sciatic n. (L4–S2)

(Continued)

Table AV-5. Muscles of the Hip, Thigh, and Iliac Region *(continued)*

Muscle	Origin	Insertion	Action	Innervation
Semitendinosus	Superiomedial portion of ischial tuberosity	Proximal medial tibia, deep fascia of leg	Flexion of knee; extension of hip; internal rotation of tibia when knee is flexed	Sciatic n. (L4–S2)
Semimembranosus	Superolateral portion ischial tuberosity	Proximal posteromedial surface of tibia, medial condyle of tibia	Flexion of knee; extension of hip; internal rotation of tibia when knee is flexed	Sciatic n. (L4–S2)

Table AV-6. Muscles of the Calf and Ankle Region

Muscle	Origin	Insertion	Action	Innervation (Nerve Roots)
Tibialis anterior	Lat. condyle of tibia, proximal 2/3 of lat. surface of tibia, interosseus membrane, deep fascia, lat. intermuscular septum	Medial plantar surface of 1st cuneiform, base of 1st metacarpal	Dorsiflexion of ankle; inversion of foot	Deep peroneal n. (L4, 5)
Extensor hallucis longus	Central 1/2 of ant. surface of fibula, adjacent interosseous membrane	Dorsal surface of base of distal phalanx of hallux	Extension of great toe; assistance of dorsiflexion of foot	Deep peroneal n. (L5–S1)
Extensor digitorum longus	Lat. tibial condyle, proximal 3/4 of ant. surface of fibula, interosseous membrane, deep fascia, intermuscular septa	Dorsal surface of bases of middle and distal phalanges of toes 2–5	Extension of toes; assistance of dorsiflexion of foot	Deep peroneal n. (L5–S1)
Peroneus tertius	Inf. ant. surface of fibula, intermuscular septum	Dorsal surface of base and proximal diaphysis of 5th metatarsal	Dorsiflexion of ankle; eversion of foot	Deep peroneal n. (L5–S1)
Gastrocnemius	Medial head: medial femoral condyle and adjacent part of femur, capsule of knee joint, lat. head: lat. femoral condyle and adjacent femur, capsule of knee joint	Calcaneus (through Achilles tendon)	Plantar flexion of ankle; flexion of knee	Tibial n. (S1, 2)
Soleus	Post. surface of head and proximal 1/3 of fibula, central 1/3 of medial tibia, tendinous arch between tibia and fibula	Calcaneus (Achilles tendon)	Plantar flexion of ankle	Tibial n. (L5–S2)
Plantaris	Lat. supracondylar line of femur, oblique popliteal lig. of knee	Calcaneus, medial to Achilles tendon	Plantar flexion of ankle, assistance flexion of knee	Tibial n. (L4–S1)
Popliteus	Lat. femoral condyle, oblique popliteal lig. of knee	Proximal posterior tibia, superior to soleal origin	Flexion of knee; assistance of internal rotation of tibia	Tibial n. (L4–S1)

(Continued)

Table AV-6. Muscles of the Calf and Ankle Region *(continued)*

Muscle	Origin	Insertion	Action	Innervation (Nerve Roots)
Flexor hallucis longus	Distal 2/3 of post. fibula, interosseus membrane, adjacent intermuscular septa and fascia	Plantar base of distal phalanx of hallux	Flexion of distal phalanx of hallux; assistance of flexion of proximal phalanx and plantar flexion of ankle	Tibial n. (S1, 2)
Flexor digitorum longus	Post. surface of central 3/5 of tibia, fascia covering tibialis post.	Plantar base of distal phalanges of toes 2–5	Flexion of distal phalanges of toes 2–5; assistance of flexion of middle and proximal phalanges of toes 2–5; assistance of plantar flexion of ankle	Tibial n. (S1, 2)
Tibialis posterior	Posterolateral proximal tibia, proximal 2/3 of medial surface of fibula, interosseus membrane, deep fascia, intermuscular septum	Medial navicular (tuberosity), plantar surface of cuneiforms, plantar surface of base of metatarsals 1–4, cuboid, and sustentaculum tali	Plantar flexion of ankle; inversion of foot	Tibial n. (L5–S1)
Peroneus longus	Lat. tibial condyle, head and proximal 2/3 of fibula, adjacent fascia, intermuscular septa	Lat. side of 1st cuneiform, base of 1st metatarsal	Eversion of foot; asssitance of plantar flexion of ankle	Superficial peroneal n. (L5–S1)
Peroneus brevis	Distal 2/3 of lat. surface of fibula, adjacent intermuscular septa	Lat. side of base of 5th metatarsal	Eversion of foot; assistance of plantar flexion of foot	Superficial peroneal n. (L5–S1)

Table AV-7. Intrinsic Muscles of the Foot

Muscle	Origin	Insertion	Action	Innervation (Nerve Roots)
Extensor digitorum brevis	Proximal lat. calcaneus, lat. talocalcaneal lig., cruciate crural lig.	Dorsal surface of base of hallux, into lateral sides of tendons of extensor digitorum longus of toes 1–4	Extension of phalanges of toes 1–4	Deep peroneal n. (S1, 2)
Abductor hallucis	Medial calcaneus, laciniate lig., plantar aponeurosis, intermuscular septum	Medial base of proximal phalanx of hallux	Abduction of hallux	Medial plantar n. (S1, 2)
Flexor digitorum brevis	Medial calcaneus, plantar aponeurosis adjacent intermuscular septum	Plantar base of middle phalanx of toes 2–5	Flexion of middle phalanx of toes 2–5; assistance of flexion of proximal phalanges of toes 2–5	Medial plantar n. (S1, 2)
Abductor digiti minimi	Lat. and medial calcaneus, adjacent intermuscular septae	Lat. base of proximal phalanx of 5th toe	Abduction of 5th toe; assistance flexion of 5th toe	Lat. plantar n. (S1, 2)
Quadratus plantae	Medial head: medial calcaneus and medial border of long plantar ligament; lat. head: lateroplantar calcaneus and lat. border of long plantar ligament	Tendons of flexor digitorum longus	Flexion of distal phalanges of toes 2–5	Lat. plantar n. (S1, 2)

(Continued)

Table AV-7. Intrinsic Muscles of the Foot *(continued)*

Muscle	Origin	Insertion	Action	Innervation (Nerve Roots)
Lumbricales	Tendons of the flexor digitorum longus: 1st from medial side of tendon to 2nd toe, 2nd from adjacent side of tendons to 2nd and 3rd toes, 3rd from adjacent sides of tendons to 3rd and 4th toes, 4th from adjacent sides of tendons to 4th and 5th toes	Join tendons of extensor digitorum longus and interossei into bases of terminal phalanges of toes 2–5	Flexion of toes 2–5 at metacarpophalangeal joint; extension of toes 2–5 at interphalangeal joints	Medial, lat. plantar n. (S1, 2)
Flexor hallucis brevis	Medial cuboid, adjacent lat. 3rd cuneiform, prolongation of tendon of tibialis post.	Medial and lateral plantar base of proximal phalanx of hallux through sesmoid bones	Flexion of proximal phalanx of hallux	Medial plantar n. (1st plantar digital) (S1, 2)
Adductor hallucis	Oblique head; bases of metatarsals 2–4; transverse head: capsules of metatarsophalangeal joints and distal plantar metatarsal neck region	Lateral base of proximal phalanx of hallux	Adduction of hallux; assistance of flexion of metatarsophalangeal joint of hallux	Deep br. of lat. plantar n. (S1, 2)
Flexor digiti minimi brevis	Base of 5th metatarsal	Lateral base of proximal phalanx of 5th toe	Flexion of 5th toe	Superificial br. of lat. plantar n. (S1,2)
Dorsal interossei	Each with two heads that arise from adjacent sides of metacarpals	1st into medial side of proximal phalanx of 2nd toe; 2nd into lateral side of proximal phalanx of 2nd toe; 3rd into lateral side of proximal phalanx of 3rd toe; 4th into lateral side of proximal phalanx of 4th toe	Abduction of 2nd, 3rd, and 4th from axis of 2nd toe; assistance of flexion of proximal phalanges and extension of middle phalanges	Superficial and deep br. of lat. plantar n. (S1, 2)
Plantar interossei	Bases and medial sides of 3rd, 4th, and 5th metatarsals	Medial bases of proximal phalanges of toes 3–5	Adduction of toes 3–5 toward axis of 2nd toe; assistance of flexion of proximal phalanges; assistance of extension of middle and distal phalanges	Superficial and deep br. of lat. plantar n. (S1, 2)

SUGGESTED READINGS

Clemente CD: Anatomy: A Regional Atlas of the Human Body. Lea & Febiger, Philadelphia, 1975

Goss CM, Ed. Gray's Anatomy. 29th American ed. Lea & Febiger, Philadelphia, 1973

Netter FH: Atlas of Human Anatomy. Ciba-Geigy Corp, Summit, NJ, 1989

Pansky R: Review of Gross Anatomy. 5th Ed. Macmillan Publishing Co, New York, 1984

Warfel JH: The Extremities. 4th Ed. Lea & Febiger, Philadelphia, 1974

Williams PL, Warwick R, Dyson M, Bannister LH: Gray's Anatomy. 27th British Ed. Churchill Livingstone, Edinburgh, 1989

APPENDIX VI   Normal Joint Range of Motion

The normal range of motion of many joints of the extremities are listed below. It should be kept in mind that variability exists in true "normal" ranges of motion, and while some individuals have inherent laxity in their joints and thus have greater ranges of motion, other individuals may have inherently "stiffer" joints and will exhibit less range of motion. Thus disagreement exists as to the true "normal" ranges of motion, which should be kept in mind in examining this list. In addition, in measuring range of motion of joints, consideration for comparison with the joint on the contralateral side should be made. For accuracy and consistency of measurement, a goniometer should be used for all measurements, and measurements in one patient should be made by the same examiner. Both active and passive range of motion should be recorded.

Joint and Motion	Range (Degrees)
Thumb	
Interphalangeal joint flexion	0–80
Metacarpophalangeal joint flexion	0–50
Carpometacarpal joint flexion	0–15
Digits	
Distal interphalangeal joint flexion	0–90
Proximal interphalangeal joint flexion	0–100
Metacarpophalangeal joint flexion	0–90
Wrist	
Palmar flexion	0–80
Dorsiflexion	0–70
Radial deviation	0–20
Ulnar deviation	0–30
Forearm	
Supination	0–80
Pronation	0–80
Elbow	
Flexion	0–150

Joint and Motion	Range (Degrees)
Shoulder	
Abduction	0–160
Adduction	0–30
Forward flexion	0–160
Extension	0–40
Internal rotation	0–70
External rotation	0–80
Neck	
Forward flexion	0–30
Extension	0–30
Lateral bending (to each side)	0–40
Rotation (to each side)	0–30
Trunk	
Forward flexion	0–90
Lateral bending	0–30
Hip	
Flexion	0–115
Internal rotation	0–30
External rotation	0–50
Abduction	0–50
Adduction	0–30
Knee	
Flexion	0–135
Ankle	
Plantar flexion	0–50
Dorsiflexion	0–20
Hallux	
Metatarsophalangeal joint flexion	0–30
Metatarsophalangeal joint extension	0–50

SUGGESTED READINGS

Friel JP: Dorland's Illustrated Medical Dictionary. 25th Ed. WB Saunders, Philadelphia, 1974

Hoppenfeld S: Physical Examination of the Spine and Extremities. Appleton-Century-Crofts, Norwalk, CT, 1976

Mallon WJ, McNamara MJ, Urbaniak JR: Orthopaedics for the House Officer. Williams & Wilkins, Baltimore, 1990

APPENDIX VII

Manual Muscle Testing and Grading

Table AVII-1. Manual Muscle Testing and Grading

Strength	Muscle Grade
Normal	5
Muscle contraction with full range of motion against gravity with additional resistance	4
Muscle contraction with full range of motion against gravity, but unable to overcome additional resistance	3
Muscle contraction with full range of motion when gravity is eliminated	2
Flicker of muscle contraction	1
No activity	0

SUGGESTED READINGS

Hoppenfeld S: Orthopaedic Neurology. Appleton-Century-Crofts, New York, 1979

Mallon WJ, McNamara MJ, Urbaniak JR: Orthopaedics for the House Officer. Williams & Wilkins, Baltimore, 1990

APPENDIX VIII

Deep Tendon and Superficial Reflexes: Muscles, Peripheral Nerves, and Nerve Roots

Table AVIII-1. Deep Tendon Reflexes

Reflex	Muscle	Peripheral Nerve	Nerve Root
Biceps tendon	Biceps	Musculocutaneous	C5
Brachioradialis	Brachioradialis	Radial	C6
Triceps tendon	Triceps	Radial	C7
Patellar tendon (knee reflex)	Quadriceps	Femoral	L4
Tibialis posterior	Tibialis posterior	Tibial	L5–S1
Ankle reflex (Achilles reflex)	Gastrocnemius-soleus	Tibial	S1

Table AVIII-2. Superficial Reflexes

Reflex	Peripheral Nerve	Nerve Root
Bulbocavernosus	Pudendal	S2–S4
Cremasteric	Genitofemoral	L1
Babinski	Sciatic	S1

SUGGESTED READINGS

Hoppenfeld S: Orthopaedic Neurology. JB Lippincott Co, Philadelphia, 1977

Mallon WJ, McNamara MJ, Urbaniak JR: Orthopaedics for the House Officer. Williams & Wilkins, Baltimore, 1990

The Sacral Lumbar Plexus*

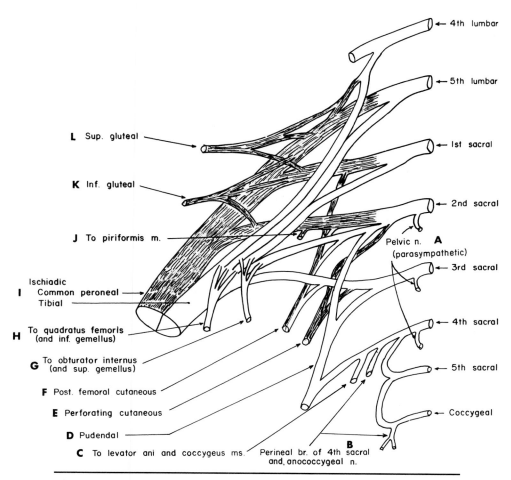

Fig. AIX-1. The sacral plexus. Preaxial nerves are clear, postaxial are shaded.

* Figure AIX-1 is from Crafts RC: A Textbook of Human Anatomy.
3rd Ed. Churchill Livingstone, New York, 1985.

APPENDIX X

The Brachial Plexus*

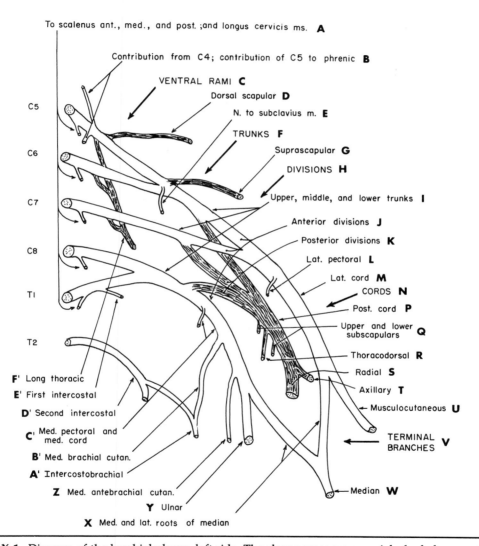

Fig. AX-1. Diagram of the brachial plexus, left side. The clear nerves are preaxial; shaded are postaxial.

* Figure AX-1 is from Crafts RC: A Textbook of Human Anatomy.
3rd Ed. Churchill Livingstone, New York, 1985.

APPENDIX XI Coma Scales

MICHAEL J. BOTTE
MARK S. COHEN

Glasgow Coma Scale for Traumatic Brain Injury

The Glasgow Coma Scale, originally popularized by Jennett et al.,[1] has become a standard for the evaluation of the acute and chronic brain-injured patient.[2]

The coma score equals the sum of eye opening and best motor and verbal response scores (E + M + V)

Table AXI-1. Glasgow Coma Scale

Eye opening (E)	
Spontaneous	4
To loud voice	3
To pain	2
Nil	1
Best motor response (M)	
Obeys	6
Localizes	5
Withdraws (flexion)	4
Abnormal flexion posturing	3
Extension posturing	2
Nil	1
Verbal response (V)	
Oriented	5
Confused, disoriented	4
Inappropriate words	3
Incomprehensible sounds	2
Nil	1

(Table AXI-1). Patients scoring 3 or 4 have an 85% chance of dying or remaining vegetative, whereas scores above 11 indicate 5 to 10% likelihood of death of chronic vegetative state and 85% chance of moderate disability or good recovery. Intermediate scores correlate with proportional chances of patients recovering.

REFERENCES

1. Jennett B et al: Predicting outcome in individual patients after head injury. Lancet 1:1081, 1976
2. Ropper AH: Trauma of the head and spinal cord. pp. 2002–2010. In Wilson JD, Braunwald E, Isselbacher KJ et al (ed): 12th Ed. Harrison's Principles of Internal Medicine. McGraw-Hill, Inc, New York, 1991

Rancho Los Amigos Hospital Adult Head Trauma Service Levels of Cognitive Functioning

The following scale for levels of cognitive functioning was popularized at Rancho Los Amigos Medical Center by Hagen, Malkmus, Durham, and Bowman. A different type of scale than the Glasgow scale, it places more emphasis on cognitive function and behavior, rather than physical or motor functioning.

Table AXI-2. Rancho Los Amigos Levels of Cognitive Functioning

I: No Response	Patient appears to be in a deep sleep and is completely unresponsive to any stimuli presented to him.
II: Generalized Response	Patient reacts inconsistently and nonpurposefully to stimuli in a nonspecific manner. Responses are limited in nature and are often the same regardless of stimulus presented. Responses may be physiologic changes, gross body movements, and/or vocalization. Often the earliest response is to deep pain. Responses are likely to be delayed.
III: Localized Response	Patient reacts specifically but inconsistently to stimuli. Responses are directly related to the type of stimulus presented, as in turning head toward a sound or focusing on an object presented. The patient may withdraw an extremity and/or vocalize when presented with a painful stimulus. He may follow simple commands in an inconsistent, delayed manner, such as closing his eyes, or squeezing or extending an extremity. Once external stimuli are removed, he may lie quietly. He may also show a vague awareness of self and body by responding to discomfort by pulling at nasogastric tube or catheter or resisting restraints. He may show a bias toward responding to some persons (especially family, friends) but not to others.
IV: Confused-Agitated	Patient is in a heightened state of activity with severely decreased ability to process information. He is detached from the present and responds primarily to his own internal confusion. Behavior is frequently bizarre and nonpurposeful relative to his immediate environment. He may cry out or scream out of proportion to stimuli even after removal, may show aggressive behavior, attempt to remove restrains or tubes or crawl out of bed in a purposeful manner. He does not, however, discriminate among persons or objects and is unable to cooperate directly with treatment efforts. Verbalization is frequently incoherent and/or inappropriate to the environment. Confabulation may be present; he may be euphoric or hostile. Thus gross attention to environment is very short and selective attention is often nonexistent. Being unaware of present events, patient lacks short-term recall and may be reacting to past events. He is unable to perform self-care (feeding, dressing) without maximum assistance. If not disabled physically, he may perform such motor activities as sitting, reaching, and ambulating, but as part of his agitated state and not necessarily as a purposeful act or on request.
V: Confused, Inappropriate Nonagitated	Patient appears alert and is able to respond to simple commands fairly consistently. However, with increased complexity of commands or lack of any external structure, responses are nonpurposeful, random, or at best fragmented toward any desired goal. He may show agitated behavior not on an internal basis (as in Level IV), but rather as a result of external stimuli and usually out of proportion to the stimulus. He has gross attention to the environment, but is highly distractible and lacks ability to focus attention to a specific task without frequent redirection back to it. With structure, he may be able to converse on a social-automatic level for short periods of time. Verbalization is often inappropriate; confabulation may be triggered by present events. His memory is severely impaired, with confusion of past and present in his reaction to ongoing activity. Patient lacks initiation of functional tasks and often shows inappropriate use of objects without external direction. He may be able to perform previously learned tasks when structured for him, but is unable to learn new information. He responds best to self, body, comfort, and often family members. The patient can usually perform self-care activities with assistance and may accomplish feeding with maximum supervision. Management on the ward is often a problem if the patient is physically mobile, as he may wander off either randomly or with vague intention of "going home."
VI: Confused-Appropriate	Patient shows goal-directed behavior, but is dependent on external input for direction. Response to discomfort is appropriate and he is able to tolerate unpleasant stimuli (such as nasogastric tube) when need is explained. He follows simple directions consistently and shows carryover for tasks he has relearned (such as self-care). He is at least supervised with old learning; unable to maximally be assisted for new learning with little or no carryover. Responses may be incorrect due to memory problems, but they are appropriate to the situation. They may be delayed to immediate, and he shows decreased ability to process information with little or no anticipation or prediction of events. Past memories show more depth and detail than recent memory. The patient may show beginning

(Continued)

Table AXI-2. Rancho Los Amigos Levels of Cognitive Functioning *(continued)*

	immediate awareness of situation by realizing he does not know an answer. He no longer wanders and is inconsistently oriented to time and place. Selective attention to tasks may be impaired, especially with difficult tasks and in unstructured settings, but is now functional for common daily activities (30 min. with structure). He may show a vague recognition of some staff, has increased awareness of self, family and basic needs (such as food), again in an appropriate manner as in contrast to Level V.
VII. Automatic-Appropriate	Patient appears appropriate and oriented within hospital and home settings, goes through daily routine automatically, but frequently robot-like, with minimal to absent confusion, but has shallow recall of what he has been doing. He shows increased awareness of self, body, family, foods, people, and interaction in the environment. He has superficial awareness of, but lacks insight into, his condition, has decreased judgment and problem-solving ability, and lacks realistic planning for his future. He shows carryover for new learning, but at a decreased rate. He requires at least minimal supervision for learning and for safety purposes. He is independent in self-care activities and supervised in home and community skills for safety. With structure he is able to initiate tasks as social or recreational activities in which he now has interest. His judgment remains impaired, such that he is unable to drive a car. Prevocational or avocational evaluation and counseling may be indicated.
VIII. Purposeful and Appropriate	Patient is alert and oriented, is able to recall and integrate past and recent events, and is aware of and responsive to his culture. He shows carryover for new learning if acceptable to him and his life role, and needs no supervision once activities are learned. Within his physical capabilities, he is independent in home and community skills, including driving. Vocational rehabilitation, to determine ability to return as a contributor to society (perhaps in a new capacity), is indicated. He may continue to show a decreased ability, relative to premorbid abilities, in abstract reasoning, tolerance for stress, and judgment in emergencies or unusual circumstances. His social, emotional, and intellectual capacities may continue to be at a decreased level for him, but functional in society.

APPENDIX XII

Application and Maintenance of the Halo Skeletal Fixator

MICHAEL J. BOTTE   MATTHEW BERCHUCK
THOMAS P. BYRNE   STEVEN R. GARFIN

The halo skeletal fixator, originally developed by Nickel and Perry for the use in cervical spine fusion in patients with poliomyelitis, is now widely used for many types of cervical spine instabilities. Despite its proven effectiveness, certain problems such as pin loosening and infection have been identified. These problems have inspired detailed studies of skull osteology, biomechanics of pin fixation, and techniques of application. Based on these studies, specific recommendations concerning the application and maintenance of the halo have evolved. These are described below along with a step-by-step description of the method of application.

PIN SITE SELECTION

The optimal sites for halo pin insertion have been evaluated in cadaver specimens, radiographic studies, and clinical reviews of pin-related complications. The optimal position for anterior halo pin placement, based on anatomic structures at risk and skull thickness, is in the anterolateral aspect of the skull approximately 1 cm above the orbital rim (eyebrow), cephalad to the lateral two-thirds of the orbit, and below the greatest circumference (equator) of the skull. This area can be considered a safe zone. Placing the pin above the supraorbital ridge will prevent displacement or penetration into the orbit. Placement of the pin below the level of the greatest skull diameter will help prevent cephalad migration of the pin. The safe zone is bordered by the temporalis muscle and fossa laterally and by the supraorbital and supratrochlear nerves and frontal sinus medially. Avoidance of the temporalis muscle and fossa is desirable for two reasons: (1) the cortex in this area is very thin, making skull penetration and/or pin loosening more likely, and (2) penetration of the temporalis muscle by the halo pin can be painful and may impede mandibular motion during mastication. Although placement of pins in the temporalis region has the advantage of hiding the pin scar behind the hairline, the anatomic and mechanical disadvantages of this site do not seem to warrant pin placement there.

Posterior pin placement is less critical, since vulnerable neuromuscular structures are lacking and the skull thickness and contour are more uniform. The posteriolateral aspects of the skull appear optimal at approximately the 4 o'clock and 8 o'clock positions (occiput = 6 o'clock).

ANGLE OF PIN INSERTION

The angle of pin insertion can influence fixation. Cyclic loading comparisons of pins inserted perpendicular to the skull with pins inserted at 15° or 30° angles demonstrated improved pin fixation with perpendicularly inserted pins. This is probably due to the broader pin-bone interface attained with perpendicular pins. With any angulation, the shoulder of the pin may intercept the skull's outer cortex before the tip is fully seated. Although the pin angle is fixed by the ring in current halo equipment, placement of the ring over a relatively flat portion of the skull (i.e., below the equator) may help obtain a perpendicular insertion at the pin-bone interface.

PIN INSERTION TORQUE

The pin insertion torque originally recommended was 5 to 6 inch-pounds (0.57 to 0.68 Newton-meter). This was based primarily on empirical observations. Subsequent laboratory studies on cadavers demonstrated that halo pins inserted at up to 10 inch-pounds (1.13 Newton-meters) barely penetrated the outer table of the skull. Mechanical testing of the

Table AXII-1. Materials for Halo Application

Halo ring (in preselected size)
Sterile halo pins (5, including one spare)
Halo torque screwdrivers (2, nonsterile)
Halo vest (in preselected size)
Halo upright posts and connecting rods
Head board
Spanners (3)
Razors (2)
Povidone-iodine solution
Sterile gloves (2 pairs)
Sterile gauze (4 packs of 2, 4" × 4" size)
Syringes (2, 10-cc)
Needles (4, 25-gauge)
Lidocaine hydrochloride (10 cc of 1% solution)
Crash cart (including manual resuscitator, endotracheal tube)

(From Botte MJ, Garfin SR, Byrne TP et al: The halo skeletal fixator. Clin Orthop Rel Res 239:12, 1989, with permission.)

pin-bone interface with cyclic loading and load-to-failure revealed that a torque of 8 inch-pounds (0.90 Newton-meter) significantly improved the mechanical qualities over those achieved with 6 inch-pounds (0.68 Newton-meter). Clinically, the use of 8 inch-pounds (0.90 Newton-meter) is safe and effective in lowering the incidence of pin loosening and infection when compared with applications at 6 inch-pounds (0.68 Newton-meter).

METHOD OF HALO APPLICATION

Preparation and Selection of Equipment

Application of the halo is easiest when one person positions the head and ring, while two others insert the pins. If available, the use of positioning pins and head holders may decrease personnel needs.

Proper ring and vest size should be determined, followed by a check for all necessary materials and equipment before starting. Suggested materials for halo application are listed in Table AXII-1. Ring size is determined by selecting a ring that provides 1 to 2 cm of clearance around every aspect of the head perimeter. Vest size is determined by measurement of chest circumference using a tape measure. A crash cart with resuscitation equipment should be available throughout the procedure.

Preparation of the Patient

If medical and neurologic status permit, the patient is lightly sedated but kept alert to report any changes in neurologic status during head and neck manipulation. General anesthesia is not recommended, unless it is required for an associated procedure.

The patient is placed supine on the bed or gurney with the head supported beyond the edge. One person is assigned to position and support the head throughout the application procedure. A canvas gurney with snap attachments allows the canvas portion under the head to be released, permitting greater access to the posterior aspect of the head (as the head is hand supported). A head ring support aids control and application.

Four pin sites are selected, two anterior and two posterior. The anterior pin sites are selected in the anterolateral aspect of the skull as described above. Although the specific location of the posterior pins is less crucial, the pins should be placed opposite the corresponding contralateral anterior pin (e.g., right posterolateral diagonal to left anterior lateral). The sites should be inferior to the equator of the skull yet superior enough to prevent ring impingement on the upper helix of the ear. Optimally, the ring will pass approximately 1 cm cephalad to the upper helix of the ear. The hair is shaved at the posterior pin sites, and the skin at all pin sites is prepared with povidone-iodine solution.

Application of the Halo Ring

The preselected ring is positioned below the equator of the skull, approximately 1 cm above the helix of the ear. The middle hole in front can be used to center the ring over the bridge of the nose.

Appropriate holes in the ring are selected for pin placement, and the underlying skin is infiltrated with 1% lidocaine hydrochloride solution. The pins are applied in a sterile fashion. All four pins are advanced to the skin edge prior to penetration. Skin incisions are not necessary. The pins are then advanced using a torque screwdriver, inserting the pins perpendicular to the skull surface. During anterior pin insertion, the patient is asked to close the eyes and relax the forehead to prevent tenting of the skin and allow unencumbered blinking and eye closure. While the ring is held in position, opposite pins are advanced simultaneously through the skin to penetrate the outer cortex of the skull. The remaining pins are advanced in a similar fashion. The pins are tightened sequentially in 2-inch-pound increments until an 8-inch-pound (0.90 Newton-meter) torque is reached. Once the halo is secured, manual traction on the ring can be used to control the cervical spine. Areas of tented skin surrounding the pins should be released with a scalpel to avoid skin tension at the pin site.

Application of the Vest

With continued attention to head position and manual cervical traction, the patient's trunk is elevated 30° and the posterior half of the vest is placed. The anterior half of the vest is then applied and the upright posts and connecting rods are secured to the vest. The head and neck are positioned and all remaining bolts and joints are fastened. The application spanner, wrenches, and torque screwdriver are maintained at the bedside or taped to the front of the vest in case emergency removal of the vest is required. Radiographs of the cervical spine are taken to confirm satisfactory position. Table AXII-2 summarizes the steps in halo fixator application.

CARE AND MAINTENANCE OF THE HALO

Following initial application, the pins are again tightened to 8 inch-pounds (0.90 Newton-meter) at 48 hours after application. Dressings are not used around the pin sites. The sites are kept clean with hydrogen peroxide, cleansing them every other day or as needed. If a pin becomes loose during the course of treatment, the loose pin and remaining pins are retightened to 8 inch-pounds once, if resistance is met within the first two complete rotations of the pin. If no resistance is met, the pin is removed after placement of a new pin in a different location. Placement of a new pin prior to removal of the loose one will help maintain ring fixation to the skull during pin change.

If drainage around a pin develops, cultures should be obtained, appropriate antibiotic therapy initiated, and aggressive local pin care applied. If the drainage

Table AXII-2. Procedure Summary for Application of the Halo Skeletal Fixator

1. Determine ring size (hold ring over head, visualize proper fit)
2. Determine vest size (from chest circumference measurement)
3. Identify pin-site locations (while holding ring in place)
4. Shave hair at posterior pin sites
5. Prepare pin sites with providone-iodine solution
6. Anesthetize skin at pin sites with 1% lidocaine hydrochloride
7. Advance sterile pins to level of skin
8. Have patient close eyes
9. Tighten pins at 2 inch/pound increments in diagonal fashion
10. Seat and tighten pins to 8 inch/pounds torque
11. Apply lock nuts to pins
12. Maintain cervical traction and raise patient trunk to 30°
13. Apply posterior portion of vest
14. Apply anterior portion of vest
15. Connect anterior and posterior portions of vest
16. Apply upright posts and attach ring to vest
17. Recheck fittings, screws, and nuts
18. Tape vest-removing tools to vest
19. Obtain vervical spine roentgenograms

(From Botte MJ, Garfin SR, Byrne TP et al: The halo skeletal fixator. Clin Orthop Rel Res 239:12, 1989, with permission.)

does not respond to treatment or if cellulitis or an abscess develops, the pin should be removed after insertion of a new pin at a different site. Parenteral antibiotic therapy should be instituted and incision, drainage, and irrigation performed as needed.

Slow, continuous bleeding at the pin sites has been shown to occur in patients taking anticoagulants. Tapering the anticoagulant may be required. Pin site packing has not been shown to be effective in patients in whom anticoagulation medication is continued.

Difficulty in swallowing may occur if the head and neck are placed in a position of hyperextension. Readjustment of the halo to provide less cervical extension usually relieves this problem.

Dural puncture may occur if the patient falls on the halo. The patient may complain of headache, malaise, visual disturbances, or other local or systemic symptoms. Clear cerebrospinal fluid leakage around a loose or deeply seated pin may be present. The patient should be hospitalized and parenteral prophylactic antibiotics initiated. The pin should be removed after placement of a new pin at a different site.

An upright position will decrease cranial cerebrospinal fluid pressure and help alleviate leakage. The dural tear should heal in 4 to 5 days. If the leak does not respond, dural repair may be required. Abscesses should be drained.

Decubitus ulcers may develop under the halo vest if it is not adequately padded or if the patient is not appropriately turned or positioned. Patients with neurologic compromise or sensory deprivation are particularly at risk for this complication. Surgical stabilization can be performed to avoid use of the halo in spinal cord injury or in patients with sensory dysfunction. This will minimize skin problems and aid in rapid rehabilitation.

SUGGESTED READINGS

Ballock RT, Botte MJ, Garfin SR: Complications of halo immobilization. p. 376. In Garfin SR (ed): Complications of Spine Surgery. Williams & Wilkins, Baltimore, 1989

Botte MJ, Byrne TP, Garfin SR: Application of the halo fixation device using an increased torque pressure. J Bone Joint Surg [Am] 69:750, 1987

Botte MJ, Byrne TP, and Garfin SR: Use of skin incisions in the application of halo skeletal fixator pins. Clin Orthop (in press)

Botte MJ, Byrne TP, and Garfin SR: The halo skeletal fixator: principals of application and maintenance. Clin Orthop 239:12, 1989

Cooper PR, Maravilla KR, Sklar FH et al: Halo immobilization of cervical spine fractures. Indications and results. J Neurosurg 50:603, 1979

Garfin SR, Botte MJ, Byrne TP, Woo SL-Y: Application and maintenance of the halo skeletal fixator. Update on Spinal Disorders 2:33, 1987

Garfin SR, Botte MJ, Centeno RS, Nickel VL: Osteology of the skull as it affects halo pin placement. Spine 10:696, 1985

Garfin SR, Botte MJ, Nickel VL, Waters RL: Complications in the use of the halo fixation device. J Bone Joint Surg [Am] 68:320, 1986

Garfin SR, Botte MJ, Triggs KJ, Nickel VL: Complications associated with halo pin skull penetration. J Bone Joint Surg 70A:1338, 1988

Garfin SR, Lee TO, Roux RD et al: Structural behavior of the halo orthosis pin-bone interface: Biomechanical evaluation of standard and newly designed stainless steel halo fixation pins. Spine 11:977, 1986

Garfin SR, Roux R, Botte MJ et al: Skull osteology as it affects halo pin placement in children. J Pediatr Orthop 6:434, 1986

Garrett AL, Perry J, Nickel VL: Stabilization of the collapsing spine. J Bone Joint Surg [Am] 43:474, 1961

Kostuik JP: Indications for the use of the halo immobilization. Clin Orthop 154:46, 1981

Nickel VL, Perry J, Garrett AL, Heppenstall M: The halo. A spinal skeletal traction fixation device. J Bone Joint Surg [Am] 50:1400, 1968

Nickel VL, Perry J, Garrett AL, Snelson R: Application of the halo. Orthop Prosthet Appliance J 14:31, 1960

Perry J: The halo in spinal abnormalities. Practical factors and avoidance of complications. Orthop Clin North Am 3:69, 1972

Perry J, Nickel VL: Total cervical spine fusion for neck paralysis. J Bone Joint Surg [Am] 41:37, 1959

Prolo DJ, Runnels JB, Jameson RM: The injured cervical spine. Immediate and long-term immobilization with the halo. JAMA 224:591, 1973

White R: Halo traction apparatus. J Bone Joint Surg [Br] 48:592, 1966

Zwerling MT, Riggins RS: Use of the halo apparatus in acute injuries of the cervical spine. Surg Gynecol Obstet 138:189, 1974

Index

Page numbers followed by f *indicate figures; those followed by* t *indicate tables.*

Position, common terms of, 873–874
Positional tolerance, in spine
    rehabilitation, 775
Positioning, in brain injury, 364
Posterior cord syndrome, in spinal
    cord injury, 414, 415t
Postpolio muscular dystrophy. *See*
    Poliomyelitis, late effects
    of.
Postpoliomyelitis syndrome, 314. *See
    also* Poliomyelitis, late
    effects of.
    anesthesia for, 107
Posttraumatic amnesia, 102
Posttraumatic confusion, duration of,
    in brain injury, 362
Posttraumatic epilepsy, 102
Posttraumatic stress syndrome, 102
Postural drainage, of lung, 35
Pronator quadratus, 877
Pronator teres, 877
Propranolol, in reflex sympathetic
    dystrophy, 652
Proprioception, 806
Prostheses, 127–137. *See also
    anatomical part.*
    for adolescents, 133
    in below-knee amputation,
        129–132
    biomechanics and, 134, 134f
    for children, 133
    definition of, 127
    education for, 127
    future of, 136
    gait and, 134
    historical, 86f, 127
    for infants, 133
    for lower extremity
        rehabilitation, 129f–131f,
        129–132
    recreational, 135f, 135–136
    for skiing, 135
    for sports, 135, 135f
    for upper extremity
        rehabilitation, 132–133
Prosthetics
    rehabilitation engineering center
        for, 156
    in rehabilitation team care, 13
Proteoglycan, in musculoskeletal
    tissue, 210f
Psoas major, 880
Psoas minor, 880

Psychological aspects, 73–81
    disability and, 73–74
        implications of, 76
    of frontal lobe injury, 102
    function and, implications of
        improvement of, 76
    in head injury, 102
    needs determination in, 74–75
        patient and, 75
        staff and, 74–75
    in orthopaedic rehabilitation, 9
    rehabilitation process and, 75–78
        behavioral contracts in,
            77–78
        behavior modification in, 77
        biofeedback in, 77
        emotional aspects in, 75–76
        factors influencing, 75–76
        techniques in, 76–78
    in rehabilitation team care, 14
    in stroke, 340
    team care and, 76
    of temporal lobe injury, 102
    trauma patient and, 101–102
Psychologist
    in spinal cord injury center, 200
    in spine rehabilitation, 774
Psychosocial assessment
    chronic illness in
        family adjustment in, 57
        phases of adjustment in, 57
    definition of, 56–57
    factors involved in, 57
    in rheumatoid arthritis, 562
    social worker and, 56–58
        areas of function of, 56–58
Psychosocial development, in
    myelomeningocele,
    548–549
Psychosocial diagnosis
    social worker and, 58
    in team care, 58
Psychosocial rehabilitation, in spinal
    cord injury, 423
Psychosocial treatment
    advocacy therapy in, 59
    environmental therapy in, 58–59
    family therapy in, 59
    group therapy in, 59
    play therapy in, 59
    psychotherapy in, 58
    sexual counseling in, 59
    social worker and, 58–59

Psychotherapy
    in psychosocial treatment, 58
    in reflex sympathetic dystrophy,
        656
Pulmonary dysfunction, treatment
    goals of, 35
Pulmonary embolism, in trauma
    patient, 99
Purdue Pegboard Test, 174
Putty, therapeutic, in hand
    rehabilitation, 706, 706f

Q

Q (quadriceps)-angle, of
    patellofemoral joint, 792
Quadratus femoris, 881
Quadratus plantae, 883
Quadriceps, and hamstring, co-
    contractions of, in knee
    rehabilitation, 793
Quadriceps fatigue, in postpolio
    syndrome, 504
Quadriceps loading, eccentric, in
    knee rehabilitation, 793
Quadriceps paralysis,
    in postpolio syndrome,
    515–516
Quadriceps weakness, in postpolio
    syndrome, 502
Quadriplegia, high, in spinal cord
    injury,424

R

Radial fracture
    distal
        in brain injury, 404, 405f
        classification of, 711, 712t
        comminuted
            Baltimore Therapeutic
                Exercise Machine for,
                715, 718f
            dynamic wrist flexion-
                extension splints for, 713,
                717f
        cutaneous neuralgia in,
            720–721
        displaced
            external fixation for, 712,
                715f

Social work (*Continued*)
    educational requirements and,
        55–56
    licensing and, 56
    in rehabilitation, 56–60
        community relations and, 61
        discharge planning and, 60
        future directions and, 61
        psychosocial assessment and,
          56–58, 57f
        psychosocial diagnosis and, 58
        psychosocial treatment and,
          58–59
        team care and, 60–61
Social worker, in spinal cord injury
    center, 200
Socioeconomic assessment, in
    rheumatoid arthritis, 562
Soft tissue
    collagen in, 212, 212f
    fixed contracture of, in stroke
      patient, 342
    immobilization of, response to,
      212, 213f
    treatment of, 212–214
      cold in, 213
      electrical stimulation in, 213
      heat in, 213
      joint mobilization in, 213
      motion in, 212–213
      stretching in, 213
Soleus, origin, insertion, and
    innervation of, 882
Soleus muscle flap, in chronic
    osteomyelitis, 662f–663f,
    665, 667–668
Soleus weakness, in postpolio
    syndrome, 504–505, 505f
    ankle dorsiflexion stop orthosis
      for, 505, 505f–506f
    reconstructive surgery for, 513
    signs of, 504, 505f
    test for, 504
Spasticity, 295–307
    in anoxic encephalopathy,
      394–399. *See also*
      Encephalopathy, anoxic
      pediatric, spasticity in.
    in brain injury, 102, 365–374. *See*
      also Brain injury,
      spasticity in.
    in cerebral palsy
      hip pain in, 333

spinal deformity in, 333
    surgery for, 333
characteristics of, 305–306, 306f
clasp-knife response in, 305–306,
    306f
control of, 9
definition of, 295, 342
hyperreflexia in, 306–307
hypertonia in, 306–307
prevention of
    motor nerve block injection in,
      43, 43f
    splinting and casting in, 42,
      42f
in spinal cord injury, 430–435. *See*
    also Spinal cord injury,
    spasticity in.
spinal mechanisms underlying,
    306–307
tendon jerk and clonus in, 306
in upper motoneuron syndrome,
    304
Speech disorders, 52–53
    apraxia, 53
    dysarthria, 52–53
Speech-language pathologist, in
    spinal cord injury center,
    200
Speech-language pathology, 51–54.
    See also Communication
    disorders.
    clinical management of, 53
    communication disorders in,
      52–53
    future directions in, 53–54
    history and emergence of, 51
    qualifications and professional
      standards in, 51–52
    team care in, 53–54
Spenco, for foot orthoses, 838
Spina bifida occulta, 547
Spinal cord
    anatomy of, 296, 296f
    blood supply to, 413, 414f
    gray matter in, 296, 296f–297f
    nerve supply of, 413, 414f
    Rexed's laminae in, 296, 297f
    structure of, 418
    white matter in, 296, 296f
Spinal cord injury, 411–426
    acute care in, future directions in,
      425
    acute management of, 416–418

    abdominal injuries in, 417
    bowel function in, 417–418
    deep venous thrombosis in,
      417
    extremity fractures in, 417
    general care in, 416–417
    positioning in, 416
    pulmonary dysfunction in, 416
    reflex ileus and, 417
    rehabilitation in, 417
    skin care in, 418
    spine alignment in, 416–417
    thoracic injuries in, 417
    thromboembolic disease in,
      417
    urinary function in, 417
anatomy of, 413
anesthesia for, 111
    recovery from, 112
    special problems in, 111–112
autonomic dysreflexia in, 102,
    111–112
case history in, 201–202
categories of, 111, 411
cervical spine in, stabilization of,
    419
complications of, 449–451
    decubitus ulcers as, 424,
      449–451, 450f
    early vs. late admission and,
      205t
    gravitational edema as, 449
    high quadriplegia as, 424
    reflex sympathetic dystrophy
      as, 449
    venous thrombosis as, 449
contractural deformity in,
    435–439. *See also*
    Contractural deformity,
    in spinal cord injury.
definition of, 411
epidemiology of, 411–412
evaluation in, 413–416
extremity fractures in, 427–430.
    See also Fracture, in
    spinal cord injury.
functional goals for, 422, 422t
future directions in, 425–426
general care in, 413
    for acute management, 416–417
halo-brace in, 419
healing of
    ligaments and, 418

Swan-neck deformity
    in motion analysis, 252, 253f
    orthosis for, 564
    in rheumatoid arthritis, 564
Swan-neck orthosis, in rheumatoid
        arthritis, 564
Swiss AO technique, in fracture and
        soft tissue rehabilitation,
        602
Symes' amputation, 616
Symes' prothesis, 616
Sympathectomy, in reflex
        sympathetic dystrophy,
        654–655
Syndesmosis injury, 685–686
Synostosis, in forearm fracture, in
        brain injury, 403
Synovectomy, for rheumatoid
        arthritis, 568–569
Synovial joint space, fluid clearance
        of, during continuous
        passive motion, 284
Synovial tissue, stress deprivation in,
        278

T

Talar process fracture, lateral, 685,
        686f
Talofibular ligament
    anterior, 683
    posterior, 684
Talus, congenital vertical, in
        myelomeningocele, 557
Team care, 11–14
    clinical psychology in, 14
    in hip rehabilitation, 779–780
    intradisciplinary approach in,
        202–203
    kinesiology in, 12–13
    nursing in, 12
    occupational therapy in, 13
    orthotics in, 13
    physical therapy in, 13
    prosthetics in, 13
    rehabilitation engineering in, 12,
        148–149
    social work in, 13–14, 60–61
    in speech-language pathology,
        53–54
    in spinal cord injury, 420
    vocational counseling in, 14

Telephone receiver clip, as function
        enhancer, 120f
Tendon
    immobilization of, response to,
        212, 213f
    rehabilitation of, in fracture care,
        604
Tendon healing, intermittent passive
        motion in, 286
Tendon jerk, in spasticity, 306
Tendon transfers, orthoses after, 124,
        125f
Tensor fasciae latae, 881
Teres major, 876
Teres minor, 876
Tetanic contraction, 260–261, 261f
Thermotherapy, 213, 804–805
Thigh muscles, 880–882
Thomas, Hugh Owen, 87, 92f
Thomas splint, 601–602
Thoracic cage
    muscle attachments of, 848
    skeletal anatomy of, 848
Thoracic-lumbar-sacral orthosis body
        jacket, after spinal fusion
        surgery, 124, 124f
Thoracic spine. See under Spine.
Thoracolumbar spine. See under
        Spine.
Thromboembolic disease, in spinal
        cord injury, 417
Thrombophlebitis
    prophylaxis against, continuous
        passive motion in, 288
    in trauma patient, 99
Thrombosis, deep venous
    in spinal cord injury, 417, 449
    in trauma patient, 99
Thumb-in-palm deformity
    anatomy of, 354–355
    clinical examination in, 253
    diagnostic nerve block for, 253,
        355
    dynamic electromyography in,
        253–255, 254f
    initial management of, 355
    lateral pinch evaluation in,
        253–255, 254f
    in motion analysis, 253–255, 254f
    phenol block for, 355, 371–373,
        372f–373f
    in stroke patient, 354–355
    surgical procedure for, 355

in brain injury, 377–378, 378f
    in Volkmann's ischemic
        contracture, 638–639
Thumb spica splint, for scaphoid
        fracture, 725, 726f
Tibia, anatomy and muscle
        attachments of, 862
Tibia epiphysiodesis, in acute
        poliomyelitis, for
        equalization of leg
        length, 496
Tibial fracture, in brain injury,
        407–408
    casting techniques for, 407
    compartment syndrome in, 408
    external fixation of, 407
    Ilizarov method for, 407, 407f
    intramedullary rod technique for,
        407
    muscle flap coverage in, 407
    peroneal nerve palsy in, 407–408
Tibialis anterior, origin, insertion,
        and innervation of, 882
Tibialis anterior paralysis, in
        postpolio syndrome,
        505–506
Tibialis posterior, origin, insertion,
        and innervation of, 883
Tibialis posterior tendinitis,
        rehabilitation for, 814,
        815f
Tibial nerve block, posterior, for
        chronic foot pain, 829,
        830f
Tinel's sign test
    in peripheral nerve injury, 476t
    in radial neuralgia, 721
Toe clawing
    in brain injury, 380–381, 381f
    in postpolio syndrome, 515
    in spinal cord injury, 438
Toe flexion deformity, in spinal cord
        injury, 438–439
Toileting, in neuromuscular
        disorders, 322–323, 323f
Toilet seat, raised, for hip weakness,
        323, 323f
Tracheostomies, in brain injury, 364
Transcutaneous nerve stimulation, in
        reflex sympathetic
        dystrophy, 655
Trapezius, origin, insertion, and
        innervation of, 875